# SKELETAL TRAUMA
# IN CHILDREN

*Third Edition*

# SKELETAL TRAUMA IN CHILDREN

VOLUME THREE

**NEIL E. GREEN, M.D.**

Professor and Vice Chairman
Department of Orthopaedic Surgery
Head of Pediatric Orthopaedics
Vanderbilt University School of Medicine and Medical Center
Nashville, Tennessee

**MARC F. SWIONTKOWSKI, M.D.**

Professor and Chairman
Department of Orthopaedic Surgery
University of Minnesota Medical School
Minneapolis, Minnesota

**SAUNDERS**
An Imprint of Elsevier Science

**SAUNDERS**
*An Imprint of Elsevier Science*

The Curtis Center
Independence Square West
Philadelphia, Pennsylvania 19106

SKELETAL TRAUMA IN CHILDREN                                    ISBN 0–7216–9294–X

---

### Notice

Orthopaedic medicine is an ever-changing field. Standard safety precautions must be followed, but as new research and clinical experience broaden our knowledge, changes in treatment and drug therapy may become necessary or appropriate. Readers are advised to check the most current product information provided by the manufacturer of each drug to be administered to verify the recommended dose, the method and duration of administration, and contraindications. It is the responsibility of the treating physician, relying on experience and knowledge of the patient, to determine dosages and the best treatment for each individual patient. Neither the Publisher nor the editor assumes any liability for any injury and/or damage to persons or property arising from this publication.

THE PUBLISHER

---

First Edition 1994. Second Edition 1998.

**Library of Congress Cataloging-in-Publication Data**

Skeletal trauma in children / [edited by] Neil E. Green, Marc F. Swiontkowski.—3rd ed.
    p. ; cm.
    "Volume three."
    Includes bibliographical references and index.
    ISBN 0–7216–9294–X
    1. Fractures in children.   2. Dislocations in children.   I. Green, Neil E.   II. Swiontkowski,
Marc F.
    [DNLM: 1. Fractures—Child.   2. Dislocations—Child.   WE 175 S6273 2003]
    RD101 .S55 2003
    617.1'5'083—dc21                                                      2001049611

*Acquisitions Editor:* Richard Lampert
*Developmental Editor:* Faith Voit
*Senior Project Manager:* Natalie Ware

GW/EBA

Printed in the United States of America.

Last digit is the print number:   9   8   7   6   5   4   3   2   1

# CONTRIBUTORS

**Mohammed J. Al-Sayyad, M.D., F.R.C.S.(C.), Dipl. Sports Medicine**

Clinical Fellow, University of Minnesota and Riverside University Hospital, Minneapolis, Minnesota

*Fractures and Dislocations of the Foot and Ankle*


**Peter F. Armstrong, M.D., F.R.C.S.(C.)**

Director of Medical Affairs, Shriners Hospitals for Children, Tampa, Florida

*Fractures of the Forearm, Wrist, and Hand*


**Fred F. Behrens, M.D.**

Professor and Chair, Department of Orthopaedics, New Jersey Medical School; Attending, University Hospital, Newark, New Jersey

*Fractures with Soft Tissue Injuries; Fractures of the Tibia and Fibula*


**S. Terry Canale, M.D.**

Professor and Chairman, University of Tennessee—Campbell Clinic Department of Orthopaedic Surgery, The University of Tennessee; Chief of Orthopaedics, LeBonheur Children's Medical Center, Memphis, Tennessee

*Physeal Injuries*


**Howard M. Clarke, M.D., Ph.D., F.R.C.S.(C.), F.A.A.P., F.A.C.S.**

Associate Professor, Surgery, University of Toronto; Staff Surgeon, Surgery Department, Division of Plastic Surgery Hospital for Sick Children, Toronto, Ontario, Canada

*Fractures of the Forearm, Wrist, and Hand*


**Kathryn E. Cramer, M.D.**

Associate Professor, Wayne State University School of Medicine; Attending, Children's Hospital of Michigan and Detroit Receiving Hospital, Detroit, Michigan

*Child Abuse*


**Alvin H. Crawford, M.D., F.R.C.S.**

Professor of Pediatric Orthopaedic Surgery, University of Cincinnati College of Medicine; Director of the Department of Orthopaedic Surgery, Children's Hospital Medical Center, Cincinnati, Ohio

*Fractures and Dislocations of the Foot and Ankle*


**Neil E. Green, M.D.**

Professor and Vice Chairman, Department of Orthopaedic Surgery; Head of Pediatric Orthopaedics, Vanderbilt University School of Medicine and Medical Center, Nashville, Tennessee

*Fractures and Dislocations about the Elbow; Child Abuse*


**Robert N. Hensinger, M.D.**

Professor, University of Michigan Medical School; Chairman, University of Michigan Health System, Department of Orthopaedic Surgery, Ann Arbor, Michigan

*Complications of Fractures in Children*


**Ginger E. Holt, M.D.**

Assistant Professor of Orthopaedic Surgery, Department of Orthopaedics and Rehabilitation, Vanderbilt University School of Medicine and Medical Center, Nashville, Tennessee

*Pathologic Fractures in Children*


**Eric T. Jones, M.D., Ph.D.**

Clinical Professor of Orthopedic Surgery, West Virginia University, Morgantown, West Virginia

*Skeletal Growth and Development as Related to Trauma*


**V. Elaine Joughin, M.D., F.R.C.S.(C.)**

Alberta Children's Hospital, Calgary, Alberta, Canada

*Fractures of the Forearm, Wrist, and Hand*


**Eric C. McCarty, M.D.**

Assistant Professor, Department of Orthopaedics and Rehabilitation, Vanderbilt University Medical Center, McGogin Sports Medicine Center, Nashville, Tennessee

*Anesthesia and Analgesia for the Ambulatory Management of Children's Fractures*


**Gregory A. Mencio, M.D.**

Associate Professor, Department of Orthopaedics and Rehabilitation, Vanderbilt University Medical Center, Nashville, Tennessee

*Anesthesia and Analgesia for the Ambulatory Management of Children's Fractures*


**Linda J. Michaud, M.D.**

Associate Professor of Clinical Physical Medicine and Rehabilitation and Clinical Pediatrics, University of Cincinnati College of Medicine; Director, Division of Pediatric Physical Medicine and Rehabilitation, Cincinnati Children's Hospital Medical Center, Cincinnati, Ohio

*Rehabilitation of the Child with Multiple Injuries*


**James F. Mooney, III, M.D.**

Chief, Department of Pediatric Orthopaedics, Children's Hospital of Michigan, Detroit, Michigan

*Fractures and Dislocations about the Shoulder*

**M.L. Chip Routt, Jr., M.D.**

Professor, Department of Orthopedic Surgery, University of Washington—Harborview Medical Center, Seattle, Washington

*Fractures of the Femoral Shaft*


**Sanjeev Sabharwal, M.D.**

Assistant Professor of Orthopaedics, New Jersey Medical School; Attending, University Hospital, Newark, New Jersey

*Fractures with Soft Tissue Injuries*


**Thomas A. Schildhauer, M.D.**

Oberarzt, Chirurgische Klinik und Poliklinik, BG-Kliniken Bergmannsheil, Ruhr-Universität Bochum, Bochum, Germany

*Fractures of the Femoral Shaft*


**Herbert S. Schwartz, M.D.**

Professor, Orthopaedic Surgery and Pathology, Vanderbilt University School of Medicine, Nashville, Tennessee

*Pathologic Fractures in Children*


**Louise Z. Spierre, M.D.**

Pediatric Physiatrist and Medical Director, Pediatric Rehabilitation Services, Saint Mary's Duluth Clinic, Duluth, Minnesota

*Rehabilitation of the Child with Multiple Injuries*


**J. Andy Sullivan, M.D.**

Professor and Chair, Department of Orthopedic Surgery, University of Oklahoma College of Medicine and Medical Center; Attending, Children's Hospital of Oklahoma, Oklahoma City, Oklahoma

*Fractures of the Spine in Children*


**Marc F. Swiontkowski, M.D.**

Professor and Chairman, University of Minnesota Department of Orthopaedic Surgery, Minneapolis; Chief of Orthopaedic Surgery, Regions Hospital, St. Paul; Staff Orthopaedist, Henepin County Medical Center, Minneapolis, Minnesota

*Fractures and Dislocations about the Hips and Pelvis*


**George H. Thompson, M.D.**

Professor, Orthopaedic Surgery and Pediatrics, Case Western Reserve University; Director, Pediatric Orthopaedics, Rainbow Babies and Children's Hospital, Cleveland, Ohio

*The Multiply Injured Child; Fractures of the Tibia and Fibula*


**Lawrence X. Webb, M.D.**

Professor, Department of Orthopaedics, Wake Forest University School of Medicine, Winston-Salem, North Carolina

*Fractures and Dislocations about the Shoulder*


**John H. Wilber, M.D.**

Professor of Orthopaedic Surgery, Case Western Reserve University; Director of Orthopaedic Trauma, University Hospital of Cleveland and Metro Health Medical Center, Cleveland, Ohio

*The Multiply Injured Child*


**R. Baxter Willis, M.D., F.R.C.S.(C.)**

G. Dean MacEwen Professor of Orthopaedics, Louisiana State University Health Sciences Center; Chairman, Department of Orthopaedics, Children's Hospital, New Orleans, Louisiana

*Fractures of the Forearm, Wrist, and Hand*


**James G. Wright, M.D., M.P.H., F.R.C.S.C.**

Professor, Departments of Surgery, Public Health Science, and Health Policy, Management and Evaluations, University of Toronto; Robert B. Salter Chair in Surgical Research; Program Head, Population Health Sciences, Research Institute; Investigator, Canadian Institutes for Health Research, The Hospital for Sick Children, Toronto, Ontario, Canada

*Outcomes Assessment in Children with Fractures*


**Nancy L. Young, Ph.D.**

Assistant Professor, Department of Paediatrics, Health Policy, Management and Evaluations, and Graduate Department, Rehabilitative Sciences, University of Toronto; Scientist, Community Health Systems Resource Group, The Hospital for Sick Children, Toronto, Ontario, Canada

*Outcomes Assessment in Children with Fractures*


**Lewis E. Zionts, M.D.**

Professor, Departments of Orthopaedics and Pediatrics, Keck School of Medicine, University of Southern California; Director of Pediatric Orthopaedics, Women's and Children's Hospital and Los Angeles County/University of Southern California Medical Center, Los Angeles, California

*Fractures and Dislocations about the Knee*

# PREFACE TO THE THIRD EDITION

The Second Edition of Skeletal Trauma in Children provided the reader with advanced analysis and recommendation for the full spectrum of musculoskeletal injuries in children. We added more advanced forms of fracture care than were available in the First Edition and provided expanded reference lists and treatment recommendations based on greater analysis of outcome.

The recognition that children's diaphyseal fractures are not always best treated by nonoperative means was clearly explained in the chapters of the Second Edition. Additional treatment options for diaphyseal fractures involving minimal surgical incisions were spelled out in detail. For example, the morbidity coming from traditional traction and cast treatment of femur fractures was clearly described. The risk of complications of operative management of long bone fractures, such as overgrowth, infection, and non-union were clearly described. The Second Edition added new chapters on the assessment of outcome of musculoskeletal injury, which has proved to be a widely used reference in the pediatric musculoskeletal injury community. In fact, evidence obtained by this relatively new field has provided much of the rationale for a more invasive treatment of skeletal injuries in children.

In the Third Edition, we add two new chapters. The chapter on Anesthesia and Analgesia for the Ambulatory Management of Children's Fractures stems from our long-standing academic interest in the best ways to manage pain in children, while achieving safe and accurate reduction. As is the tradition of this book with management of individual injuries, we have provided descriptors for the full spectrum of options with recommended treatment. Secondly, we have added a chapter on Rehabilitation of the Child with Multiple Injuries. This chapter will prove to be a useful reference in defining the role of rehabilitation services in obtaining optimum outcome for children with multiple injuries, especially those with a concomitant head injury.

As in the first two Editions, we do not spend much time reviewing treatment of historical interest only. We have updated the treatment of all musculoskeletal injuries in this Volume to continue to enable the reader to find quickly and review the details about what is considered to be the current, best method of treatment for individual pediatric musculoskeletal injuries. Our contributors again have labored many hundreds of hours individually and in teams to provide you, the reader, with this current compendium. Most importantly, organizing the material in a way useful to working surgeons should provide the orthopaedic surgeon with more confidence and result in better outcomes for children with musculoskeletal injuries.

*Neil E. Green, M.D.*
*Marc F. Swiontkowski, M.D.*

# PREFACE TO THE FIRST EDITION

Orthopaedic surgery is becoming highly subspecialized, with increasing numbers of graduating residents seeking subspecialty training in the form of postresidency fellowships. In spite of this trend toward a focused practice within orthopaedic surgery, most orthopaedic surgeons continue to care for the traumatized patient. This volume is therefore designed with the practitioner in mind. Our goal was to produce a practical yet comprehensive text that covered the field of pediatric musculoskeletal trauma. The design of the chapters allows the reader to quickly find the pertinent information about a specific injury without the distraction of too much historical perspective. Extensive bibliographies have been provided so that in-depth research may be undertaken if desired. We have sought to provide the reader with up-to-date concepts concerning the treatment of fractures in children. The chapter authors have been selected because of their expertise in specific areas of pediatric orthopaedic trauma. Half of the contributors are orthopaedic trauma surgeons with an interest in pediatric orthopaedic trauma, and the other half are pediatric orthopaedic surgeons who are involved in the care of musculoskeletal trauma in the pediatric patient.

Some forms of treatment may still be controversial, and alternative means of therapy are described. Nevertheless, treatment that today is considered on the cutting edge may well become the standard tomorrow. Until recently, operative treatment of children's fractures was rarely considered appropriate except in the case of open fractures. We have come to realize, however, that some fractures in children may be best managed operatively. We have reflected this trend in the writing of this text.

This text has been written to accompany the first two adult volumes entitled *Skeletal Trauma. Skeletal Trauma in Children,* however, is able to stand alone because it deals entirely with pediatric orthopaedic trauma.

*Neil E. Green, M.D.*
*Marc F. Swiontkowski, M.D.*

# ACKNOWLEDGMENTS

Throughout the years involved in preparing the Third Edition, many individuals at Elsevier Science provided an important role in the development, writing, and editing of this text. We would like to thank, particularly, Richard Lampert, who has continued to oversee the process at Elsevier Science. Faith Voit also assisted us. Artists Philip Ashley and Ted Huff provided the great majority of expert illustrations for the text.

I, Neil Green, warmly thank several people who helped throughout the production of the book. Joan Lorber was instrumental in communicating with the publisher and the contributors in coordinating the final revisions of the chapters. Debbie Chessor's photography reproduced beautifully. I wish to express how much my father, Dr. H. Howard Green, meant to me and how much he influenced the direction of my academic career. As a practicing orthopaedic surgeon, he showed enormous compassion for his patients, as well as the intellect and medical ability that he passed on to three sons. Other thanks must be extended to the many orthopaedic educators with whom I have worked, including Drs. J. Leonard Goldner, James Urbaniak, and Ben Allen. I express sincere thanks to Dr. Paul P. Griffin, who is the ultimate Pediatric Orthopaedic Surgeon, and with whom I worked after first arriving at Vanderbilt. Finally, thanks are given to Dr. Gregory Mencio, with whom I have worked for more than ten years. His view of the care of pediatric orthopaedic trauma mirrors mine.

I, Marc Swiontkowski, acknowledge that the material presented in this text has been edited based on the extensive experience provided by my practice at Vanderbilt University Medical Center with Dr. Neil Green from 1985 to 1988. The experience was expanded upon at Harborview Medical Center in Seattle from 1988 to 1997. Work there with Drs. Catherine Kramer and M. L. Chip Routt, Jr., was especially beneficial. I especially recognize the mentoring provided by my teachers, Drs. Frederick N. Elliott, J. Paul Harvey, Jr., and Sigvard T. Hansen, Jr., whose examples at critical points in my career have had deep and long-lasting effects. Since moving to the University of Minnesota in 1997, additional experience in managing children's fractures has been provided by collaborative work with Drs. Thomas Varecka, Richard Kyle, Andrew Schmidt, Ed Rutledge, and David Templeman at Hennepin County Medical Center, and Drs. Peter Cole, Joel Smith, Greg Brown, John Stark, and Tom Lange at the Regions Medical Center in St. Paul. Collaboration with the Gillette Pediatric Orthopaedic Group, ably led by Dr. Steven Koop, has been an additional inspiration. Without the continued assistance of Catherine Girard, this volume would not have been completed in such a satisfactory fashion.

# CONTENTS

CHAPTER 1

*Skeletal Growth and Development as Related to Trauma* 1

Eric T. Jones, M.D., Ph.D.


CHAPTER 2

*Physeal Injuries* 17

S. Terry Canale, M.D.


CHAPTER 3

*Pathologic Fractures in Children* 57

Herbert S. Schwartz, M.D.
Ginger E. Holt, M.D.


CHAPTER 4

*The Multiply Injured Child* 73

John H. Wilber, M.D.
George H. Thompson, M.D.


CHAPTER 5

*Fractures with Soft Tissue Injuries* 104

Fred F. Behrens, M.D.
Sanjeev Sabharwal, M.D.


CHAPTER 6

*Complications of Fractures in Children* 124

Robert N. Hensinger, M.D.


CHAPTER 7

*Outcomes Assessment in Children with Fractures* 153

James G. Wright, M.D., M.P.H., F.R.C.S.C.
Nancy L. Young, Ph.D.


CHAPTER 8

*Fractures of the Forearm, Wrist, and Hand* 166

Peter F. Armstrong, M.D., F.R.C.S.(C.)
V. Elaine Joughin, M.D., F.R.C.S.(C.)
Howard M. Clarke, M.D., Ph.D., F.R.C.S.(C.), F.A.A.P.,
F.A.C.S.
R. Baxter Willis, M.D., F.R.C.S.(C.)


CHAPTER 9

*Fractures and Dislocations about the Elbow* 257

Neil E. Green, M.D.


CHAPTER 10

*Fractures and Dislocations about the Shoulder* 322

Lawrence X. Webb, M.D.
James F. Mooney, III, M.D.


CHAPTER 11

*Fractures of the Spine in Children* 344

J. Andy Sullivan, M.D.


CHAPTER 12

*Fractures and Dislocations about the Hips and Pelvis* 371

Marc F. Swiontkowski, M.D.


CHAPTER 13

*Fractures of the Femoral Shaft* 407

M.L. Chip Routt, Jr., M.D.
Thomas A. Schildhauer, M.D.


CHAPTER 14

*Fractures and Dislocations about the Knee* 439

Lewis E. Zionts, M.D.


CHAPTER 15

*Fractures of the Tibia and Fibula* 472

George H. Thompson, M.D.
Fred F. Behrens, M.D.


CHAPTER 16

*Fractures and Dislocations of the Foot and Ankle* 516

Alvin H. Crawford, M.D., F.R.C.S.
Mohammed J. Al-Sayyad, M.D., F.R.C.S.(C.)

CHAPTER 17

*Child Abuse* 587
    Kathryn E. Cramer, M.D.
    Neil E. Green, M.D.

CHAPTER 18

*Anesthesia and Analgesia for the Ambulatory Management of Children's Fractures* 606
    Eric C. McCarty, M.D.
    Gregory A. Mencio, M.D.

CHAPTER 19

*Rehabilitation of the Child with Multiple Injuries* 619
    Louise Z. Spierre, M.D.
    Linda J. Michaud, M.D.

*Index* 627

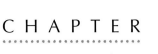

# C H A P T E R 1

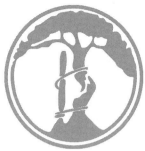

# Skeletal Growth and Development as Related to Trauma

Eric T. Jones, M.D., Ph.D.

The effect of growth on trauma to the musculoskeletal system may be positive or negative. Adult bone is dynamic; it is constantly involved in bone turnover and remodeling in response to aging and changes in stress on the skeleton. Bone in children undergoes a rapid, steady state of change. The pediatric skeleton not only remodels in response to alterations in stress but also grows in length and width in addition to changing shape, alignment, and rotation as it matures. An understanding of these changing forces and their effect on skeletal trauma in children is important in determining the treatment of injured bones and joints.

Factors affecting the growth of bone and particularly the physis are variable and incompletely understood. The physis responds to various growth-regulating hormones (thyroxine, estrogen, testosterone), parathyroid hormone, and corticosteroids, as well as the peptide signaling proteins transforming growth factor β (TGF-β), platelet-derived growth factor (PDGF), and bone morphogenetic protein (BMP), in addition to immunoregulatory cytokines (interleukin-1 [IL-1] and IL-6).[1, 4, 5] Diurnal variation in the growth of bone has been shown to reflect the levels of the different hormones.[4] Mechanical factors also have control over growth rates. This control is particularly evident in femoral overgrowth, in which disruption of the periosteal sleeve and increasing vascularity of the bone by fracture increase longitudinal growth.[4, 18] It has been postulated that mechanical factors, such as tension within the surrounding periosteum, may have some control over the growth rate.[18, 21]

The principles of fracture treatment are the same for all ages, anatomic alignment being the primary concern. The fracture should not be malaligned or malrotated. Although some angulation is acceptable when treating fractures in children, it is best to keep the amount of angulation as small as possible by routine fracture treatment methods, whatever the patient's age. Multiple attempts at anatomic reduction in a child may actually cause harm and should be avoided. The small amount of angulation associated with torus or so-called buckle fractures in children can virtually always be accepted.

Marked bowing, which can be seen in greenstick fractures in the forearm, should usually be corrected by completing the fracture and restoring alignment.[16]

Bone healing in children is generally rapid, primarily because of the thickened, extremely osteogenic periosteum. The age of the patient directly affects the rate of healing of any fracture: the younger the child, the more rapidly the fracture heals. At birth, femoral shaft fractures heal in 3 or 4 weeks, but as the child ages, the healing rate approaches that of an adult. A femoral shaft fracture in an adolescent heals in 12 to 16 weeks (Fig. 1–1).

Injuries to the growth plate heal more rapidly than shaft fractures do. Physeal injuries, in almost all parts of the body, heal in approximately 3 weeks.[22] The age-related rate of healing is due to the osteogenic activity of the periosteum. The periosteum thins as the child grows older, thereby lessening osteogenic activity.

Treatment of trauma to the pediatric skeleton is generally routine. Dislocations and ligamentous injuries are uncommon in children in comparison with adults, but ligamentous injuries may occur in older children, in whom the epiphysis and metaphysis are more securely attached. Most injuries, though, are simple fracture patterns caused by low-velocity trauma such as falls. In most cases, closed reduction followed by a short time in a cast restores normal function to a pediatric extremity. However, a number of pitfalls can make treatment of pediatric fractures difficult and demanding, particularly fractures of the growth plate.

## HISTORY AND DIAGNOSIS

In infants, a history is not usually available, and the child does not always cooperate with either the physical examination or the treatment. Radiographs of an infant can be difficult to obtain and interpret (Fig. 1–2), especially those of bones in the elbow and hip region, which may require comparison views. Anteroposterior

1

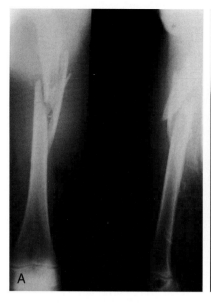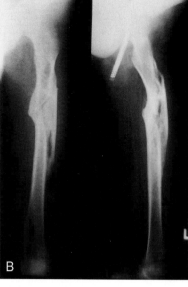

FIGURE 1–1. *A,* Radiograph of a comminuted subtrochanteric fracture of the femur in an 11-year-old boy. *B,* Ten weeks after fracture, the bone is healed. In an adult, this fracture would be difficult to treat nonoperatively and could require 3 to 6 months to heal.

and lateral views, including the joints above and below the injured area, constitute a minimal radiographic evaluation. Usually, routine radiographs coupled with a good physical examination can establish the diagnosis. Often, however, two views of the side opposite the injury are helpful in an infant, particularly in injuries to the elbow. Arthrograms of the elbow or hip or ultrasonography can be useful as a diagnostic aid when radiographs are confusing.[9]

Children with multiple trauma, head injuries, or both can have occult axial fractures and epiphyseal injuries, which are difficult to diagnose or suspect even with a good physical examination. In these children, a bone scan may be useful to assist in diagnosing fractures unidentified by routine screening radiographs.[13]

Fractures through the growth plate in children can be difficult to interpret if the fracture is not displaced (Fig. 1–3). A thorough physical examination can usually identify this type of injury, which occurs most commonly at the distal end of the radius or fibula. Palpation at the

tip of the lateral malleolus usually identifies a ligament injury; swelling and tenderness at the growth plate region can identify a fracture undetected by radiographs. Often, a small metaphyseal fragment on the radiograph suggests physeal injury.

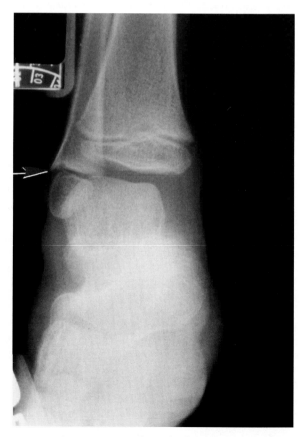

FIGURE 1–3. Anteroposterior radiograph of the ankle of a 6-year-old boy who injured his ankle and had obvious swelling and tenderness over the distal fibular growth plate but not over the tip of the fibula. Radiographically, subtle widening is apparent, but otherwise, the radiograph looks entirely normal. The diagnosis is made by physical examination.

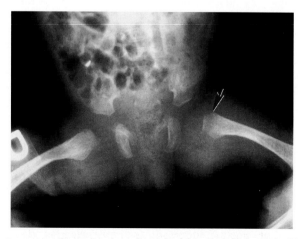

FIGURE 1–2. Anteroposterior radiograph of the pelvis of a 1-month-old infant who sustained an intertrochanteric fracture *(arrow)* of the left hip. Initially, a septic hip was diagnosed. Infection may be confused with fracture in a child, especially in the inflammatory phase of healing.

The dependence of healing capacity on age is significant. Every age group has its typical injury. Most infants and newborns (up to 2 years of age) sustain their fractures by having someone else injure them. Above 2 years of age, the child is walking and running and beginning to pursue various activities. Children most commonly fracture the forearm and usually the distal end of the radius.[17, 20] Clavicular fractures are common in infancy and the preschool age group, but their incidence decreases with increasing age. Forearm fractures, though common in young children, show a progressive increase into the teenage years.

Most injuries occur when the child is playing with relatively simple toys. More severe injuries are caused by automobiles, lawn mowers, all-terrain vehicles, and the like. As a child approaches the midteens, injuries are much like those of an adult. The age at which the growth plates close varies greatly and depends on hereditary factors and hormonal variation. Skeletal age is an important factor in the consideration of injuries in children in that the closer the child to the end of growth, the less prominent the role of the growth plate in treatment of the injury.

The effect of growth on fracture healing usually aids the orthopaedist in fracture treatment. A certain amount of angulation and deformity will remodel with growth. The amount is dependent on the age of the child, location of the injury in the bone, degree of deformity, and whether the deformity is in the plane of motion of the adjacent joint.[3] Increased blood flow to the injured area can result in accelerated growth of the injured bone (as well as surrounding bones), which can lead to overgrowth (usually associated with the femur or humerus). Growth, however, can produce deformity if the growth plate is injured or if trauma has altered muscle forces on an extremity, as it does in a head-injured child.

Finally, child abuse must be considered in all children's injuries and should always be suspected when treating this age group for fracture.[14] Care must be taken to ensure that the child is checked for abuse on initial assessment and for possible subsequent injuries during follow-up. Parents or guardians of children who are not brought back for follow-up appointments for fractures should be contacted and asked to schedule a return visit.

## FORMATION OF BONE

Embryonic bone forms through either membranous or endochondral ossification. In the former, mesenchymal cells proliferate to form membranes primarily in the region in which flat bones will be fabricated.[21] Endochondral ossification is bony replacement of a cartilage model and is the mode of formation of long bones.

### Membranous Bone Formation

Membranous bone formation increases the diameter of long bones and is responsible for the creation of flat bones such as the scapula, skull, and in part, the clavicle and pelvis. Flat bones are formed as mesenchymal cells condense into sheets that eventually differentiate into osteoblasts. Surface cells become the periosteum. Primary bone is remodeled and transformed into cancellous bone, to which the periosteum adds a compact cortical bone cover. This type of growth is independent of a cartilage model.

Membranous bone growth also enlarges the diameter of the diaphyseal portion of long bones. As endochondral ossification lengthens bones, proliferation of bone occurs beneath the periosteum through membranous bone formation. This type of bone formation is also apparent in subperiosteal infection and after bone injury when periosteal bone forms around fracture hematoma (Fig. 1–4).

### Endochondral Ossification

Endochondral ossification requires the presence of a cartilage anlage. Early in gestation, mesenchymal cells aggregate to form models of the future long bones. A cartilage model develops, and the peripheral cells organize into a perichondrium.[18, 21] The cartilage cells enlarge and degenerate, and the matrix surrounding them calcifies. This ossification begins in the center of the diaphysis and is called the primary ossification center. Vascular buds enter the ossification center and transport new mesenchymal cells capable of differentiating into osteoblasts, chondroclasts, and osteoclasts. These cells align themselves on the calcified cartilage and deposit bone. Primary cancellous bone is thus formed. Ossification expands toward the metaphyseal regions.

Long bone growth continues as the terminal ends of the cartilage model keep growing in length by cartilage cell proliferation. This growth continues in this manner until after birth, when secondary ossification centers (epiphyses) develop.

The mass of cartilage found between the epiphyseal and diaphyseal bone in later postnatal development thins to become the epiphyseal plate, which continues as the principal contributor to the growth (in length) of long bones until maturation is reached. The girth of the long bone is provided by the cambium layer of the periosteum.[17] Successive surfaces of compact bone are added to the exterior while remodeling by resorption of the interior (endosteal) surface takes place.

Once the physis is established between the epiphysis and metaphysis, the periosteal ring becomes relatively firmly attached at the level of the zone of hypertrophied cells. This periphyseal periosteal collar is referred to as the fibrous ring of Lacroix.[17] The zone of Ranvier, the cellular segment responsible for growth in diameter of the physis,[17] is located in the same area. The periosteum is firmly attached at this level. Even when the periosteum is torn over the diaphysis, it usually remains attached at the physis.

Injury to bones results in acceleration of both endochondral and membranous bone formation, particularly in the area of injury, but normal growth in surrounding bones may likewise be increased by the greater blood flow to the injured extremity.[10]

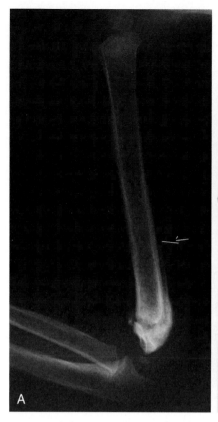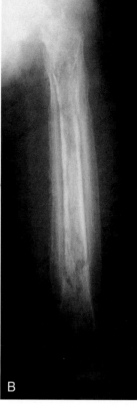

FIGURE 1–4. *A,* Radiograph of a healing supracondylar fracture illustrating the periosteum stripped *(arrow)* to nearly the midshaft of the humerus. The bridging periosteal bone stabilizes this fracture in about 3 weeks. *B,* The large periosteal involucrum that surrounds the former bone (sequestrum) in a femur with osteomyelitis. The periosteum can be stimulated to remanufacture an entire cortex around this area such that when the sequestered bone is removed, the periosteal bone will form a new (larger-diameter) femoral diaphysis.

## BIOLOGY OF FRACTURE HEALING

Fracture healing is usually divided into three stages: (1) inflammatory, (2) reparative, and (3) remodeling.

Fracture healing involves both membranous and endochondral ossification. Injuries to the pediatric skeleton always involve a variable amount of surrounding soft tissue injury. Unlike the soft tissues, which heal by replacement of the injured tissue with collagen scar tissue, bone heals by replacing the area that is injured with normal bony tissue.

The blood supply to the bone is an important part of fracture healing, and significant soft tissue injury delays healing. The normal process of fracture healing in any part of the bone follows a set chronologic order. Any of these phases may be disrupted or delayed by excessive adjacent soft tissue injury.

### Inflammatory Phase

The inflammatory phase of fracture healing "sets the stage" for cartilage and bone formation by supplying the building blocks necessary for repair and remodeling. When bone is injured, the bone, periosteum, and soft tissue (mostly muscle) around the fracture begin to bleed. Hematoma collects at the fracture site, both inside and outside the bone. This hematoma may dissect along the periosteum, which is easily elevated or was elevated

at the time that the fracture was maximally displaced. The more severe the soft tissue injury, the more displaced the fracture, and the more the periosteum is torn, the larger the area that fills with hematoma. The role of hematoma is to serve as a source of signaling agents capable of initiating cellular events critical to fracture healing.

Current research suggests that these agents are divided into two groups: peptide signaling proteins (TGF-β, fibroblast growth factor [FGF], PDGF, and BMPs) and immunoregulatory cytokines (IL-1 and IL-6).[5] The peptide signaling proteins are derived from platelets and extracellular bone matrix and are critical for regulation of cell proliferation and mesenchymal stem cell differentiation. TGF-β is a multifunctional growth factor that controls tissue differentiation in fracture repair. FGFs increase the proliferation of osteoblasts and chondrocytes and may stimulate the formation of new blood vessels. PDGF acts on mesenchymal cell precursors to stimulate osteoblast differentiation. BMPs are a class of proteins produced in the early stages of fracture repair and strongly stimulate endochondral ossification. The immunoregulatory cytokines are released from inflammatory cells present in the hematoma and serve to regulate the early events in fracture healing.

In open fractures, part of the hematoma is lost through the skin, thereby taking some of the osteo-inductive components of the hematoma away. When open fractures are irrigated and débrided and the fracture is washed out, much of the hematoma is lost. A smaller hematoma reaccumulates after surgery. This loss of osteoinductive potential probably slows the onset of the inflammatory response and delays healing of the fracture.

The bone, for at least a millimeter or two directly adjacent to the fracture site, loses its blood supply. After initial reabsorption of the dead bone along the fracture line, the fracture line in children usually becomes more visible radiographically 2 or 3 weeks after injury.

Pediatric bone is more vascular than that of an adult and is able to generate a greater hyperemic and inflammatory response. The more mature (less porous) the cortex, the slower the vascular response to injury. Vasodilatation and the cellular inflammatory response begin shortly after fracture, and the injured area is filled with inflammatory cells such as polymorphonuclear leukocytes and macrophages. The hematoma and inflammatory response also incite the release of molecules such as growth factors and cytokines from the platelets.[11] In the initial phase of fracture healing, after the hematoma has formed, a scaffolding of fibrovascular tissue replaces the clot with collagen fibers. These fibers eventually become the collagen of the woven bone of the primary callus that forms around the fracture.

The vascular response aids in initiating the cellular response to fracture. A number of TGF-β subtypes help mediate cellular and tissue responses to inflammation and tissue repair.[11] During the inflammatory phase of fracture healing, TGF-β from the extracellular matrix of bone and also from platelets controls the mesenchymal precursor cells that may form osteoblasts and osteoclasts. The maximal cellular response is ongoing within 24 hours of injury and occurs first in the subperiosteal region of the fracture.[24]

Osteogenic induction is stimulation by growth factors to convert the multipotential cells into osteoprogenitor cells. The osteoprogenitor cells on the undersurface of the periosteum help form periosteal bone.

The osteogenic cells that originate from the periosteum help manufacture the external callus. Endochondral bone formation from the endosteal areas combines with subperiosteal bone formation to bridge the fracture.

The more motion, the lower the oxygen tension and the more cartilage that is formed. Cartilage is later ossified as microvascular supply returns to the area. The dead bone at the fracture surface is revascularized in a process that occurs faster in more vascular areas such as the metaphysis (as compared with the diaphysis).

The subperiosteal callus in children initially stabilizes the area so that the fracture may be clinically healed by the external callus by the end of the reparative phase. During remodeling, this callus decreases and is replaced with the endochondral ossified bone that has formed at the fracture surface.

## Reparative Phase

The reparative phase of fracture healing is highlighted by the development of new blood vessels and the onset of cartilage formation. The surrounding soft tissue provides vascular ingrowth initially to the periosteal area and subsequently to the endosteal area. Before fracture, the cortical blood supply is primarily from endosteal bone and branches out radially from inside the medullary canal. During the reparative phase, most of the blood supply to the cortex arises from outside the bone rather than inside.

Rat models of fracture healing reveal that intramembranous and endochondral bone formation is initiated during the first 10 days. Inflammatory mediators in the fracture hematoma recruit chondrocytes capable of producing fracture callus. The hematoma initiates and is eventually replaced by the ingrowth of fibrovascular tissue. This developing construct provides structural support to stabilize the bone ends. This primitive tissue is eventually replaced through endochondral and intramembranous bone formation.

Endochondral bone formation results from calcification of the cartilage anlagen that forms adjacent to the fracture site. Intramembranous bone formation occurs at the periphery as undifferentiated mesenchymal cells in the periosteum differentiate into osteoblasts capable of forming bone without a preceding cartilage model.

Tissue differentiation during the reparative phase is strongly influenced by local mechanical factors. Fracture healing is classically divided into primary and secondary healing. Primary healing results from rigid stabilization (i.e., plate immobilization) and involves a direct attempt by the cortex to bridge the fracture gap. Bridging occurs through direct haversian remodeling by intramembranous bone formation.

Secondary healing results from treatment of fractures with less rigid methods (i.e., fracture bracing). Motion at the fracture site, the presence of a fracture gap, and an intact tissue envelope encourage the formation of abundant callus. The callus formed subsequently undergoes endochondral ossification. Ideal fracture treatment most likely involves early rigidity to ensure adequate vessel ingrowth, followed by progressive loading and motion to stimulate ample callus formation.

As the periosteum produces bone beneath it, the periosteum is pushed away from the bone and makes a collar of bone around the area of injury. Initially, this tissue is more cartilaginous and fibrous and is not very well ossified. It may not show up well on a radiograph until the blood supply is adequate enough to allow mineralization and conversion to bone.

An important process that occurs between the reparative and remodeling phases is clinical union of the fracture, which takes place when the bony callus surrounds the fracture fragments and joins the callus coming from the other side. At this point the bone may be stable clinically, and although some plastic deformation is still possible with appropriate force, the bone is usually strong enough that the patient can begin to use the extremity in a more normal way.

Clinical union has occurred when the fracture site does not move during gross examination, when attempts to move the fracture do not cause pain, and when radiographs demonstrate bone across the fracture. This point demarcates the end of the reparative phase and the beginning of the remodeling phase.

## Remodeling Phase

Remodeling is the final phase of bone healing. It may last for a short time in a young child or continue throughout growth or even beyond the end of growth in an older child. Once the bone is clinically stabilized, the ongoing stresses and strains on the bone that normally help cause modeling are responsible for remodeling this early soft woven bone. The bone usually returns to normal both radiographically and clinically.

One complete skeletal turnover occurs during a child's first year of life. This turnover declines to about 10% per year in late childhood and continues at about this rate or a little slower for life.[6] Remodeling does not result from the activity of a single type of cell such as osteoclasts or osteoblasts, but rather results from coordinated absorption and formation of bone over large regions around the fracture. The bioelectric forces exert control over a large part of the bone, not just from cell to cell.

The control mechanisms for the remodeling phase of bone are essentially the electrical behavior that is responsible for modeling bone according to Wolff's law. As bone is subjected to the stresses of use during normal activities, the bone remodels appropriately for those stresses. Because a child's bone is normally modeling anyway and is actively changing and continuing to remodel in response to growth and stress, a child's bone remodels significantly faster than an adult's.

Systemic factors can affect the rate of bone healing. In addition to the age of the patient, hormonal factors that help promote bone healing are growth hormone, thyroid hormone, calcitonin, insulin, antibiotic steroids, and vitamins A and B.[18] Certain types of electrical currents, magnetic fields, hyperbaric oxygen, and exercise can also positively influence bone healing.

Factors that discourage bone healing are diabetes, corticosteroids, and certain endocrinopathies. Denervation, irradiation, and high doses of hyperbaric oxygen also slow the healing of fractures.

Cartilage does not heal in the same phases as bone. When the physis is injured, it does not heal by the formation of callus. Inflammatory and reparative phases occur in cartilage healing, but no remodeling phase.[4, 18]

## DIFFERENCES BETWEEN PEDIATRIC AND ADULT FRACTURE HEALING

One of the primary differences between pediatric and adult bone is the very thick periosteum in children. The periosteum around the fracture site walls off the hematoma and is stripped from the bone as bleeding occurs—a primary factor in the amount of new bone formed around a fracture. The area of bone necrosis on either side of the fracture surface must be replaced by viable bone through the process of bone resorption and deposition. This process leads to an initial radiographic appearance of sclerosis at the fracture site because new bone is being formed on the existing necrotic bone. The area around the necrotic bone elicits an inflammatory response. Because pediatric bone is more vascular than adult bone, the inflammatory (hyperemic) response is more rapid and significant. Temperatures as high as 40°C may be noted immediately after major long bone fractures. This hyperemic inflammatory reaction is also responsible for growth stimulation, which may result in overgrowth of the bone. Because of this response, the early stage of fracture healing is much shorter in a child than in an adult.[18, 20, 22]

The initial cellular repair process, which consists of organization of hematoma and fibrovascular tissue growth, is of much greater importance in adult bone than in pediatric bone. Periosteal callus bridges this area long before the underlying hematoma forms a cartilage anlagen that goes on to ossify.

Once cellular organization from the hematoma has passed through the inflammatory process, repair of the bone begins in the area of the fracture. In children, the periosteum is the primary producer of new bone through membranous ossification. This process considerably supplements endochondral (organizing hematoma) bone formation. In most children, by 10 days to 2 weeks after fracture, a rubber-like bone forms around the fracture and makes it difficult to manipulate. The fracture site is still tender, however, and not yet ready for mobilization of the adjacent joints. Fracture stabilization occurs earlier in children than in adults.

As part of the reparative phase, cartilage formed as the hematoma organizes is eventually replaced by bone through the process of endochondral bone formation, much the same as endochondral bone is formed in utero.

The remodeling phase of fracture healing may continue for some time, particularly in more displaced fractures. Remodeling is accelerated by motion of the adjacent joints and use of the extremity. The stresses and strains of regular use of the bone directly promote remodeling of the fractured bone into a bone that closely resembles the original structure. Because the mechanisms involved in fracture healing are the same as those in the growth process, particularly in the remodeling phase, bone heals much more rapidly in children than in adults.

The hematoma, which forms in the inner portion of the bone, is invaded by inflammatory cells and subsequently by type II collagen. Endochondral bone may be formed deep in a fracture, whereas membranous (periosteal) bone is rapidly and abundantly bridging the fracture peripherally.

The major reason for the increased speed of healing of children's fractures is the periosteum, which contributes the largest part of new bone formation around a fracture. Children have significantly greater osteoblastic activity in this area because bone is already being formed beneath the periosteum as part of normal growth. This already active process is readily accelerated.

In radiographs of bones that were fractured several months previously, transverse lines may be seen in the metaphyseal region. These lines are usually referred to as Harris growth arrest lines[12] or the transverse lines of Park.[19] These transversely oriented trabeculae occur in bones that are normally growing rapidly (e.g., femur, tibia) and in those in which the trabeculae are predominantly longitudinally oriented (Fig. 1–5). When growth

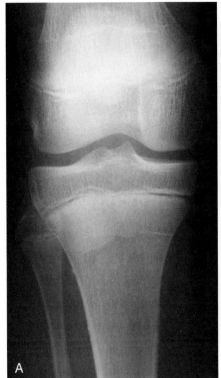
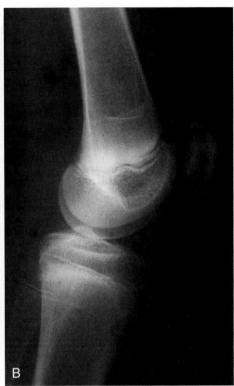

FIGURE 1–5. Anteroposterior (A) and lateral (B) radiographs of the knee of a 12-year-old child 6 months after a femoral shaft fracture. Arrest lines parallel to the physis can be seen in the metaphyseal area of the distal ends of the femur and tibia and the fibula. The temporary depression of growth at the time of injury results in more horizontal trabeculae being laid down, thereby increasing the density of bone at that level.

deceleration occurs, as happens immediately after fracture of an extremity, the bone is, in effect, standing still and making transversely oriented trabeculae, formations that increase local bone density and are evident radiographically after further growth. Arrest lines should parallel the physeal contour. Lines that do not may indicate an area of physeal damage or an osseous bridge.[19]

Usually, these transverse trabeculae are transmitted symmetrically throughout the skeleton because the growth slowdown is systemic. The physes that grow more rapidly (e.g., distal end of the femur, proximal end of the tibia) have arrest lines farthest from the physis. In the metaphyseal areas of bones, where the slowest growth occurs, transverse trabeculae may be difficult to see radiographically or may not form at all.

Physes that do not grow rapidly under normal circumstances form primarily transversely oriented trabeculae, so arrest lines are not often seen in these slower-growing bones. Transversely oriented Harris lines may result from any type of stress on bone that causes a temporary slowdown in the formation of longitudinally oriented bone. Such stresses include systemic illness, fever, and starvation.[17]

## Anatomy of Pediatric Bones

As the skeleton of a child grows, it develops from a relatively elastic and rubbery type of biomechanical material to the more rigid structure of an adult skeleton. Because of the amount of radiolucent cartilage material in pediatric bone, comparison films are often necessary to determine whether a radiograph is abnormal. The types of injuries may also be different in children; for example, ligamentous injuries and dislocations are rare. Valgus stress injuries around the knee frequently lead to ligamentous and intra-articular ligamentous and meniscal injuries in adults. In children, the distal femoral or proximal tibial physis is more likely to be injured because it is the weak link (Fig. 1–6). Ligament injuries in skeletally immature children are uncommon, but they do occur.

Pediatric bony injuries are more often treated by closed reduction than by open reduction because of the short time to union and the ease of obtaining and maintaining anatomic reduction, especially in extra-articular fractures (Fig. 1–7). The quality of anesthesia/analgesia provided to the child is strongly correlated with the quality of the reduction.[1]

## Remodeling

The remodeling ability of bone in children may make reduction accuracy somewhat less important than it is in adults. Remodeling may occur readily in the plane of a joint (Fig. 1–8), but it occurs far less readily, if at all, in children with rotational deformity and angular deformity not in the plane of the joint.[3, 21]

Angulation in the midportion of long bones is not usually acceptable and does not remodel very well. In children younger than 8 to 10 years, residual angulation is more acceptable. If the angulation is less than 30° and is within the plane of the joint, remodeling toward

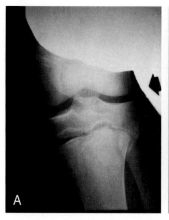
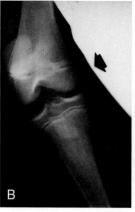
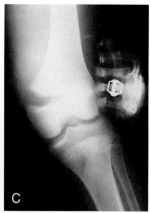

FIGURE 1–6. Stress films illustrating injuries to the proximal tibial physis (A), the medial collateral ligament (B), and the distal femoral physis (C) in skeletally immature children.

FIGURE 1–7. A, Anteroposterior and lateral radiographs of a 15-year-old boy who sustained a displaced transverse fracture of the diaphysis of his tibia. B, Follow-up at 4 months shows abundant periosteal healing, although a portion of the fracture line is still evident. It is characteristic for pediatric long bone fractures to heal early with periosteal callus; secondarily, the diaphysis heals and remodels.

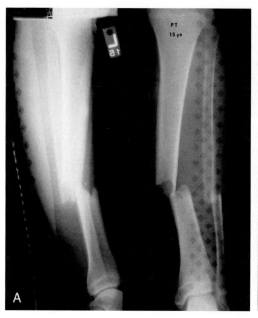
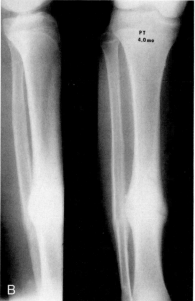

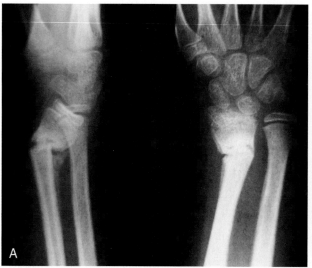
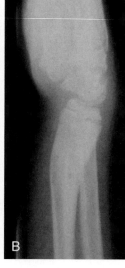

FIGURE 1–8. A, Radiograph of the distal portion of the radius in an 11-year-old girl at the time of cast removal 6 weeks after injury. B, A lateral radiograph taken 3 months later shows considerable remodeling of the fracture in the plane of the joint.

normal alignment can be expected.[18] Side-to-side (bayonet) apposition of bone is acceptable as long as alignment is accurate (Fig. 1–9). This position leads to prompt, strong union with solid periosteal bone bridging.

The younger the child, the greater the amount of remodeling that can be expected. The capacity for remodeling is not, however, reason to treat injuries less than completely. The age of the child, the distance from the physis, and the amount of angulation are the primary considerations. Remodeling does not occur in displaced intra-articular fractures. In children, remodeling is often relied on in the treatment of proximal humeral and distal radial injuries. Although operative treatment is required for the best initial radiographic alignment, remodeling usually results in excellent restoration of the anatomy.

Delayed union and nonunion rarely, if ever, occur in children. In a series of over 2000 fractures in children, not a single case of nonunion was seen.[2] Probably, the only exceptions occur in older children with open injuries that have severe soft tissue injury or become infected. Refracture is uncommon, although in malaligned forearm fractures, refracture may occur after mobilization. Myositis ossificans and stiffness in joints secondary to fractures are exceedingly rare. Physical therapy to regain motion is seldom necessary except in head-injured children.

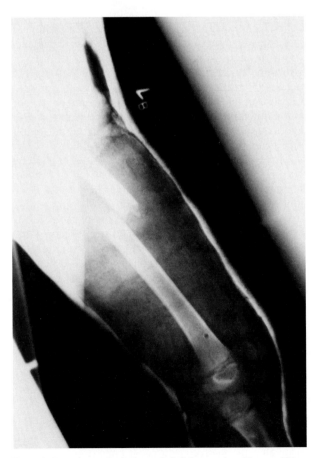

**FIGURE 1–9.** Radiograph of a femoral shaft fracture in a 10-year-old boy in a cast. The fracture was placed in about 1 cm of overlap (bayonet apposition) to allow for expected overgrowth of the extremity after fracture.

## Anatomic Differences

The most obvious anatomic difference in the pediatric skeleton is the presence of growth plates and the thick periosteum. Growth plate injuries and epiphyseal injuries can lead to growth disturbance that may be significant (Fig. 1–10). Often, injury to the growth plate and epiphysis parallels adult intra-articular injuries. Just as adult intra-articular injuries require anatomic reduction, so do pediatric articular injuries. As noted earlier, the periosteum in children is much thicker, more active, less readily torn, and more easily stripped from the bone than in adults. The periosteum helps both in reduction (where it serves as a hinge) and in maintenance of reduction and contributes immensely to rapid fracture healing.

The periosteum in children is much less frequently disrupted around the entire circumference of the bone and exhibits a much greater osteogenic potential than in adults. The intact periosteum helps reduce the amount of displacement and is, in general, the primary reason for more stable fractures in children. Callus forms much more quickly in children, and bones heal faster because of the osteogenic periosteum and the greater vascularity of growing bone.

Occasionally, plain x-ray studies are not sufficient to demonstrate the anatomy of a pediatric joint injury, and it may be necessary to perform arthrography, computed tomography, or magnetic resonance imaging to adequately visualize the fracture, particularly around the elbow or in the newborn hip. Each part of the developing bone has its own characteristic injuries, growth, and remodeling patterns.

### EPIPHYSIS

At birth, most epiphyses are completely cartilaginous structures. The length of time for formation of the secondary ossification center within the epiphysis varies, with the distal portion of the femur being formed first.[3] A global type of growth plate is present in the epiphysis. When the epiphysis is entirely cartilaginous, the physis is almost completely protected from injury. Once bone has formed within the epiphysis, it is more likely to be broken. When the epiphysis is nearly all bone, it is subject to injury, much like the remainder of the bones.

### PHYSIS

The growth plate remains cartilaginous throughout development. As the child grows older, the physis becomes thinner and it is easier to disrupt the growth plate by injury. The most common location of injury in Salter-Harris type I injuries is through the lower hypertrophic zone of the physis. Infants and newborns have fewer mammillary processes that stabilize the epiphysis on the metaphysis. However, with further growth, particularly in the distal femoral region, prominent mammillary processes help the physis secure the epiphysis to the metaphysis. The proximal femoral physis

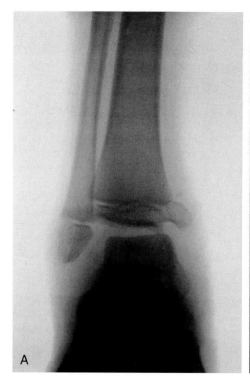 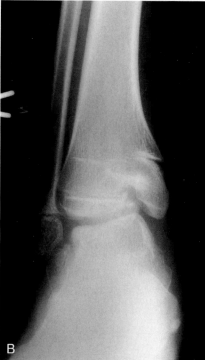

FIGURE **1–10.** *A,* Radiograph of a 7-year-old boy who sustained a fracture of the medial malleolus, as shown in this mortise view. The fracture was treated with closed reduction and application of a long leg cast. *B,* Mortise view of the ankle of the same patient 4 years after his injury. The medial malleolar portion of the epiphysis has healed to the metaphyseal area of this Salter type IV injury. He has not only an incongruous growth plate but also an incongruous ankle joint. Intra-articular fractures such as this one should be treated with open reduction and internal fixation to anatomically restore both the joint surface and the growth plate.

changes considerably and forms into what are essentially two separate physeal areas: the capital femoral epiphysis and, below it, the trochanteric apophysis.

## METAPHYSIS

The metaphysis is the trumpet-shaped end of long bones. It has a thinner cortical area and increased trabecular bone and is wider than the corresponding diaphyseal part of the bone. Porosity in the metaphyseal area is greater than in the diaphyseal area, and the periosteum is more firmly attached in the metaphyseal area as it gets closer to the physis.

Most bone remodeling occurs in the metaphyseal region of a bone after fracture. Periosteal bone forms in the area joining the diaphysis to the epiphysis. This area progressively transforms back into a trumpet-shaped metaphyseal cortex with longitudinal growth.

## DIAPHYSIS

The diaphysis is the principal portion of the long bone and is extremely vascular in the newborn. With further growth it becomes less vascular, and the cortical bone thickens. The diaphysis grows in diameter by periosteum-mediated membranous bone formation.

## Biomechanical Differences

Pediatric bone is less dense and more porous and is penetrated by more vascular channels than adult bone.[15, 21] It has a comparatively lower modulus of elasticity, lower bending strength, and lower mineral content.[7] Immature bone has greater porosity on cross section, and immature cortical bone has a greater number of osteon systems traversing the cortex than mature bone. The periosteum is strong and can serve as a hinge for reduction and maintenance of fracture reduction. The increased porosity of pediatric bone helps prevent propagation of fracture lines. It is uncommon to see comminuted fractures in children. A comparison of load deformation curves of fractures in pediatric and adult bone shows a long plastic phase in children.[7] The porosity and rough mechanical fracture surface prolong the time and energy absorption before bone is broken. Adult bone almost always fails in tension, whereas bone in children can fail either in tension or in compression.

When bones are bent, stress on the tension side is about the same as on the compression side. Because bone has a lower yield stress in tension than in compression, bone yields first on the tension side. As the bending continues, a crack travels across the bone from the tension side toward the compression side.

Depending on the amount of energy to be absorbed, the large pores in growing bone may stop propagation of the fracture line, which may leave a portion of the cortex intact on the compression side and result in a greenstick fracture.[16] If enough plastic deformity is present in the remaining cortex, it may be necessary to complete the fracture as part of treatment. Completing the fracture is usually done by reversing the deformity so that the remaining cortex is placed on the tension side.

Bone is said to be elastic if it returns to its original shape after the load is removed. If bone does not return to its original shape and residual deformity remains after the load is released, bone has undergone plastic deformation. Such deformation results from failure in com-

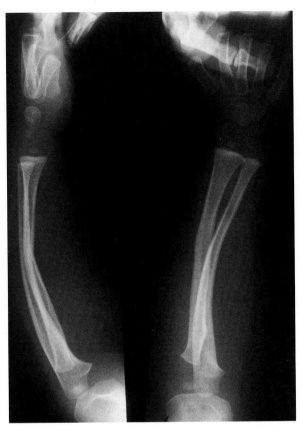

FIGURE **1–11.** Plastic deformation in the radius and ulna of a 2-year-old after a fall. The bones are plastically deformed at the midshaft, with volar compression and dorsal tension failure, but without fracture propagation.

pression on one side of the bone and failure in tension on the opposite side. Incomplete failure in tension in which the fracture line does not propagate through bone results in plastic deformity of bone (Fig. 1–11).

## CLASSIFICATION OF CHILDREN'S FRACTURES

Pediatric fractures can be classified into five types: (1) plastic deformation, (2) buckle fracture (near the metaphysis), (3) greenstick fracture, (4) complete fracture, and (5) epiphyseal fracture.

### Plastic Deformation

Plastic deformation of bone is essentially unique to children. It is most commonly seen in the ulna and, occasionally, the fibula. If bending of bone occurs to such a degree that there is microscopic failure in compression on the concavity of the bone and microscopic failure in tension on the convexity but a fracture on the tension side does not propagate, permanent deformation of the bone ensues when the force is removed. If no hematoma is formed, periosteal elevation and significant callus

formation may not occur, but the bone may be permanently deformed in a plastic fashion. If the deformity occurs in a child younger than 4 years or if the deformation is less than 20°, the angulation usually corrects with growth.[16]

### Buckle Fractures

Buckle fracture, also an injury primarily of childhood, is a compression failure of bone that usually occurs at the junction of the metaphysis and diaphysis. In the metaphysis, where porosity is greatest, bone in compression may be buckled by the denser bone of the diaphysis (Fig. 1–12). This injury is similar to a diaphyseal greenstick fracture. Failure on the tension side propagates the fracture, and failure on the compression side buckles the more cortical diaphyseal bone into the more membranous metaphyseal bone. This injury is commonly referred to as a torus fracture because of its similarity to the raised band around the base of a classical Greek column.

### Greenstick Fractures

Greenstick fractures occur when a bone is bent and the tension side of the bone is adversely affected. The bone begins to fracture, but the fracture line does not propagate entirely through the bone. Failure on the

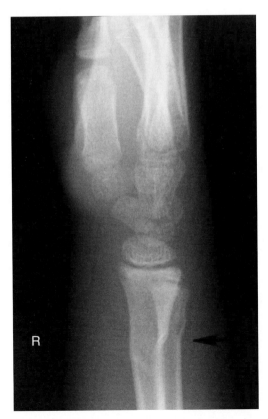

FIGURE **1–12.** Torus fractures usually occur at the junction (*arrow*) of metaphyseal and diaphyseal bone. The more porous metaphyseal bone fails in compression.

compression side of the bone allows plastic deformity to occur. In an adult without porous bone and deformity on the compression side, the fracture line virtually always propagates through the bone. Because compressive bone undergoes plastic deformation, it does not recoil to an anatomic position and must be completely broken to restore normal alignment.

## Complete Fractures

Fractures that propagate completely through a bone may be described in several ways, as follows.

### SPIRAL FRACTURES

Spiral fractures are usually created by a rotational force on the bone. They are low-velocity injuries commonly associated with child abuse. An intact periosteal hinge enables an orthopaedic surgeon to reduce the fracture by reversing the rotational injury.

### OBLIQUE FRACTURES

Oblique fractures occur diagonally across diaphyseal bone, usually at about 30° to the axis of the bone.[22] Analogous to complete fractures in an adult, these injuries usually cause significant disruption of the periosteum. Because these fractures are unstable and may be difficult to hold in anatomic reduction, alignment is important. Fracture reduction is attempted by immobilizing the extremity while applying traction.

### TRANSVERSE FRACTURES

Transverse fractures through pediatric bone usually occur from three-point bending and are readily reduced by using the periosteum on the concave side of the fracture force. The periosteum on the side opposite the apex of the force is torn. The three-point bending type of immobilization usually maintains this diaphyseal fracture in a reduced position (Fig. 1–13).

Butterfly fragments are not common in pediatric injuries but result from a mechanism similar to that causing a transverse fracture, with the butterfly fragment remaining on the side of the apical force of the three-point bend. This injury occurs in the highly cortical area of the diaphysis—usually in the midshaft of the femur, tibia, or ulna (Fig. 1–14).

## Epiphyseal Fractures

Injuries to the epiphysis of a bone usually involve the growth plate. Problems after injury to the growth plate are not common, but any time the physis is injured, the potential for deformity exists. The distal radial physis is the most frequently injured physis.[17] Usually, the growth plate repairs well and rapidly, and most physeal injuries heal in 3 to 6 weeks. Damage to the plate can occur by crushing, vascular compromise of the physis, or bone growth bridging from the metaphysis to the bony portion

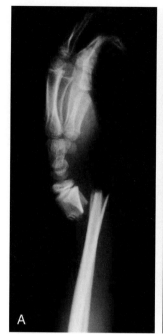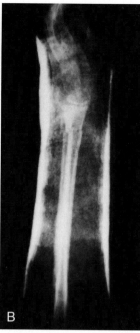

**FIGURE 1–13.** *A* and *B,* Lateral radiographs of a dorsally displaced distal radial and ulnar fracture, which is easily reduced by using the intact dorsal periosteum to aid in locking the distal fragments in place.

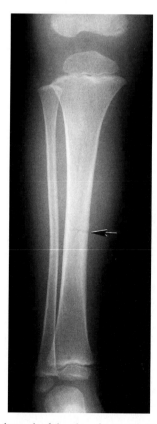

**FIGURE 1–14.** Radiograph of the tibia of a 2-year-old with incomplete fracture of the tibia *(arrow)* and plastic deformity of the fibula. The lateral apical three-point stress on the tibia resulted in a tension-generated fracture whose propagation was halted before it reached the lateral cortex. The injury lacked sufficient energy to generate a butterfly fragment on the lateral side.

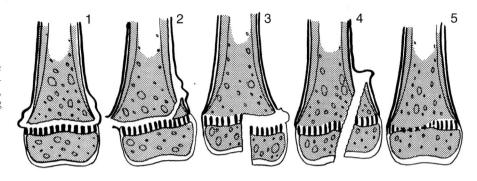

**FIGURE 1–15.** Illustration of the Salter-Harris classification of epiphyseal injuries (see text). (From Salter, R.B.; Harris, W.R. J Bone Joint Surg Am 45:587, 1963.)

of the epiphysis. The damage can result in progressive angular deformity, limb length discrepancy, or joint incongruity.

Injury to the physis has been studied by many researchers over the years.[8, 20, 22] Their studies show an age-dependent change in the stability of the epiphysis on the metaphysis. The physis and epiphyses are firmly connected externally by periosteum and internally by the mammillary processes. The physis is a hard, rubbery material that is more susceptible to injury by rotation than by angulation or traction.

Injuries involving the growth plate usually occur at the junction of calcifying cartilage cells and those that are uncalcified.[23] With epiphyseal injury, the growth plate is generally attached to the epiphyseal side of the fracture, and anatomic reduction of the joint surface usually results in anatomic reduction of the growth plate. In distal femoral epiphyseal injuries, the germinal part of the plate is often "scraped off" the epiphyseal portion either during fracture or during fracture reduction. These injuries are likely to result in growth plate damage.

Epiphyseal injuries are usually classified by the Salter-Harris classification system,[23] which is based on the radiographic appearance of the fracture (Fig. 1–15). Injury may occur to the epiphysis and growth plate or to the perichondrial ring. In a type I fracture, the epiphysis separates completely from the metaphysis without any radiographically evident fracture through bone.

The plane of cleavage in physeal injuries is usually through the zone of hypertrophic cells and degenerating cartilage cell columns. The remaining growth plate remains attached to the epiphysis. The fracture plane does not always propagate directly through the hypertrophic zone but may at some places undulate into the germinal zone of the physis or into segments of the metaphysis. Changes in contour are caused by the mammillary processes extending into the metaphysis. The distal femoral growth plate is shaped such that fragments of the metaphysis are often broken off when the growth plate is injured.

In type I injuries, the periosteum usually remains attached to the growth plate, thereby preventing significant displacement of the epiphysis. In patients with very little periosteal disruption, slight widening of the physis may be the only radiographic sign of an injury through the physis (Fig. 1–16). Although type I injuries are not

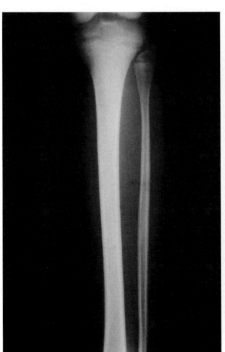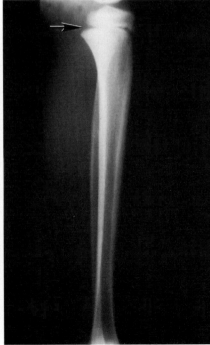

**FIGURE 1–16.** Anteroposterior and lateral radiographs of the tibia of a 10-year-old child who had proximal tibial pain and swelling. This proximal tibial epiphyseal injury (*arrow*) was missed in the emergency room. Salter type I injuries are often subtle and require close correlation between the physical examination and the radiograph.

usually associated with vascular change, complete separation of the capital femoral epiphysis can result in avascular necrosis and growth arrest of the proximal end of the femur. The larger the ossification center, the greater the tendency of the injury to produce a metaphyseal fragment on the compression side of the injury.

In a type II fracture, the most common Salter-Harris fracture pattern, the injury passes through the growth plate and out through a portion of the metaphysis. The periosteum is usually damaged on the tension side, but the fracture leaves the periosteum intact in the region of the metaphyseal fragment.

As in a type I injury, the line of fracture separation occurs along the hypertrophic and calcified zones of the physis. However, propagation along this junction is more variable in a type II injury. As the fracture line courses toward the compression side of the injury, it propagates through the metaphyseal area. The periosteal attachment along the metaphyseal fragment can be used to aid in reduction of the injury.

Growth disruption secondary to type I and type II injuries is infrequent, although it can occur, particularly if the circulation to the epiphysis is disrupted. Anatomic reduction is not generally required with type I and type II injuries. These injuries are adjacent to the joint, and the entire growth plate is intact. Remodeling usually occurs rapidly if the bone is angulated.

A type III fracture is intra-articular and passes through the epiphysis until it reaches the growth plate. The fracture line then courses through the growth plate to the periosteal surface. This type of fracture usually occurs when the growth plate is beginning to undergo closure. Problems pertaining to growth arrest may not be major, particularly in distal fibular injuries, but such may not be the case for injuries around the elbow. With anatomic reduction of the articular surface, the physis is usually anatomically reduced as well. In that situation, growth arrest is not generally a problem, even in skeletally immature children.

A type IV injury is also intra-articular and involves the epiphysis as well as the metaphysis. The fracture line crosses through the growth plate. The injury is similar to a type III fracture in that the articular surface must be anatomically reduced. A vertical split of all zones of the physis occurs, and the physis must be anatomically reduced to restore the architecture of the growth plate and minimize the risk of osseous bridge formation.

Considerable debate exists concerning type V injuries. The original type V injury as described by Salter was a crush injury to the growth plate.[19] A type V fracture may be difficult to recognize on initial radiographs because it may appear to be type I. These injuries are very uncommon, but any injury accompanied by clinical swelling and tenderness around the growth plate and associated with considerable axial load should be suspected to be type V.

The Salter-Harris classification is useful as a rapid means of describing an epiphyseal injury based on radiographic interpretation. A more complex and inclusive classification scheme was proposed by Ogden.[20] It includes nine types of fractures that are further divided into subtypes A through D. The Ogden classification has not been used to any extent because of its complexity.

Other injuries to the epiphysis are avulsion injuries of the tibial spines and injuries to the muscle attachments to the pelvis. Osteochondral fractures of the articular surface of the femur, patella, and talus are among other epiphyseal injuries that do not involve the growth plate.

## SUMMARY

Injury to the growing skeleton is common both as an isolated event and in a multiply injured child. Skeletal injuries in children should be treated as early as possible because they heal more rapidly than adult injuries do. Growth usually aids in the care of a traumatized extremity in that it speeds fracture healing because the repair processes are ongoing and no time is lost in calling up the repair troops. The thick osteogenic periosteum aids in reduction of the fracture and rapidly provides a bridge over the broken bone.

Porous growing bone affords fracture patterns that are biomechanically different from those of adult bone but that are, in general, easier to treat. Nearly all fractures in children can be treated with a cast without worry about stiff joints or the need for physical therapy to mobilize injured joints.

Although growing bone is well equipped to deal with trauma, some injuries may damage the growth mechanisms so severely that they cannot recover. Others have that potential if the orthopaedist is not wary and ready to act rapidly to restore normal growth as well as function.

### REFERENCES

1. Beaty, J.H., ed. Orthopaedic Knowledge Update 6. American Academy of Orthopaedic Surgeons, Rosemont, IL, 1999, pp. 129–138.
2. Beckman, F.; Sullivan, J. Some observations of fractures of long bones in children. Am J Surg 51:722–741, 1941.
3. Bount, W. Fractures in Children. Baltimore, Williams & Wilkins, 1955.
4. Brighton, C.T. The growth plate and its dysfunctions. Instr Course Lect 36:3–25, 1987.
5. Buckwalter, J.A.; Einhorn, T.A.; Simon, S.R., eds. Orthopaedic Basic Science, 2nd ed. Rosemont, IL, American Academy of Orthopaedic Surgeons, 2000, pp. 377–381.
6. Buckwalter, J.A.; Glimcher, M.J.; Cooper, R.R.; Recker, R. Bone biology. J Bone Joint Surg Am 77:1276–1284, 1995.
7. Currey, J.D.; Butler, G. The mechanical properties of bone tissue in children. J Bone Joint Surg Am 57:810–814, 1975.
8. Dale, G.G.; Harris, W.R. Prognosis of epiphyseal separation: An experimental study. J Bone Joint Surg Br 40:122, 1958.
9. Davidson, R.S.; Markowitz, R.I.; Dormans, J.; Drumond, D.S. Ultrasonographic evaluation of the elbow in infants and young children after suspected trauma. J Bone Joint Surg Am 76:1804–1813, 1994.
10. Edvardson, P.; Syversen, S.M. Overgrowth of the femur after fractures of the shaft in childhood. J Bone Joint Surg Br 58:339–346, 1976.
11. Einhorn, T.A. Enhancement of fracture-healing. J Bone Joint Surg Am 77:940–953, 1995.
12. Harris, H.A. The growth of long bones in childhood. Arch Intern Med 38:785–793, 1926.

13. Heinrich, S.D.; Gallagher, D.; Harris, M.; Nadell, J.M. Undiagnosed fractures in severely injured children and young adults: Identification with technetium imaging. J Bone Joint Surg Am 76:561–572, 1994.

14. King, J.; Diefendorf, D.; Apthorp, J. Analysis of 429 fractures in 189 battered children. J Pediatr Orthop 51:722–741, 1941.

15. Light, T.R.; Ogden, D.A.; Ogden, J.A. The anatomy of metaphyseal torus fractures. Clin Orthop 188:103–111, 1984.

16. Mabrey, J.D.; Fitch, R.D. Plastic deformation in pediatric fractures: Mechanism and treatment. J Pediatr Orthop 9:310–314, 1989.

17. Neer, C.S., II; Horwitz, B.Z. Fractures of the epiphyseal plate. Clin Orthop 41:24–32, 1965.

18. Ogden, J.A. Anatomy and physiology of skeletal development. In: Ogden, J.A., ed. Skeletal Injury in the Child. Philadelphia, Lea & Febiger, 1982, pp. 16–40.

19. Ogden, J.A. Growth slowdown and arrest lines. J Pediatr Orthop 4:409–415, 1984.

20. Ogden, J.A. Injury to growth mechanisms of the immature skeleton. Skeletal Radiol 6:237–253, 1963.

21. Ogden, J.A. The uniqueness of growing bones. In: Rockwood, C.A., Jr.; Wilkins, K.E.; King, R.E., eds. Fractures in Children, Vol. 3. Philadelphia, J.B. Lippincott, 1984, pp. 1–86.

22. Rang, M. Injuries of the epiphysis, growth plate and perichondrial ring. In: Rang, M., ed. Children's Fractures. Philadelphia, J.B. Lippincott, 1983, pp. 10–25.

23. Salter, R.B.; Harris, W.R. Injuries involving the epiphyseal plate. J Bone Joint Surg Am 45:587–622, 1963.

24. Tonna, E.A.; Cronkite, E.P. Cellular response to fracture studied with tritiated thymidine. J Bone Joint Surg Am 43:352–362, 1961.

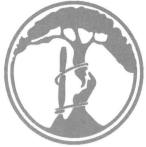

# CHAPTER 2

# Physeal Injuries

S. Terry Canale, M.D.

The physes appear to be the weakest area in children's bones, and they are also the structures that must be preserved if normal growth is to occur. It is mandatory to treat all physes as gently as possible and to delay prognosis until the time for growth disturbance has passed. Just as all children are different, injuries to different physes respond differently. Each physeal injury must be approached as a distinct entity, with the patient's age, the location of the injury, the type of injury, the growth potential of the affected area, the degree of displacement, and the time from injury to treatment kept in mind. It should also be remembered that management of the complications of physeal injuries is difficult and complex.

## PATHOLOGY

### Relevant Anatomy

The physis is the primary center for growth of the skeleton. Initially, primary physes are relatively discoid areas of rapidly maturing cartilage, but with increasing biomechanical stress, especially shear stress, the physes undergo changes in contour, or undulations.[64, 73] Planar physes contribute primarily to longitudinal growth, and spherical physes contribute almost exclusively to circumferential expansion of the bone. The physes also differ in morphology according to their location in the skeleton. The rapidly growing distal femoral physis, for example, has elongated cell columns, in contrast to the shortened cell column formation in the slowly growing phalangeal physis.

Cartilage cells grow continually on the side of the physis facing the epiphysis of a long bone, whereas on the metaphyseal side, cartilage continually breaks down and is replaced by bone. When the skeleton has achieved its adult size, the physes are resorbed and replaced by bone that joins the epiphysis permanently to the metaphysis. In males, most fusions are complete at about

20 years of age; in females, growth in length of the bones ceases about 2 years earlier. The annual rate of bone renewal during the first 2 years of life is 50%, as opposed to 5% in adults.

The physis can be divided into zones according to function (Fig. 2–1). The zone of growth is concerned with both longitudinal and circumferential growth of the bone. The zone of matrix formation undergoes several biochemical changes necessary for eventual ossification. In the zone of cartilage transformation, tissue is mineralized to create bone matrix (the primary spongiosa), and the original bone surrounding the cartilaginous septum is gradually removed and replaced with more mature secondary spongiosa that no longer contains remnants of the cartilaginous precursor. Ranvier described a circumferential notch containing cells, fibers, and a bony lamina located at the periphery of the physis; this area of active peripheral cellular addition to the physis contributes to latitudinal growth (appositional growth). The periosteal sleeve is firmly attached to each end of a bone at the zone of Ranvier and the perichondrium of the epiphysis and appears to be an anatomic restraint to rapid, uncontrolled longitudinal growth.[100, 174, 178]

Physes have been described as either pressure (compressive) or traction (tensile) responsive; the latter have been referred to as apophyses. Studies have demonstrated significant histologic differences in the two types of physes in the tibial tuberosity, and similar structural changes are believed to exist in other apophyses.

The metaphysis is the area of most rapid change in bone structure. As the physis is replaced by primary spongiosa, this bone is apposed to the surfaces of the longitudinal matrix between the cell columns, where it is rapidly remodeled and replaced by more mature bone. The metaphysis represents the transition zone from the wider physis to the narrow diaphysis.

The blood supply of the physis is from three sources: the epiphyseal circulation, the metaphyseal circulation, and the perichondrial circulation.[136] The epiphyseal circulation varies with the location and growth of the secondary ossification center. Vessels enter and disperse

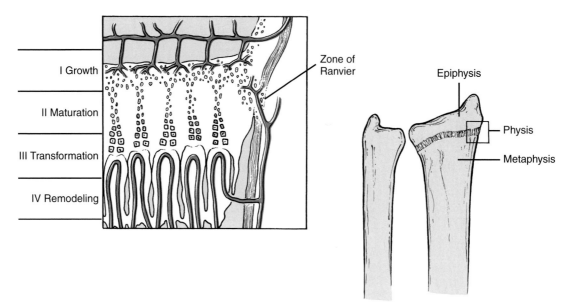

FIGURE 2–1. Zones of the physis according to function. I, growth; II, maturation; III, transformation; IV, remodeling. (Redrawn from Ogden, J.A. Skeletal Injury in the Child, 2nd ed. Philadelphia, Lea & Febiger, 1990.)

throughout the chondroepiphysis within cartilage canals. These canals course throughout the epiphysis, except for the avascular articular cartilage region, and branch out into the germinal cell regions of the physis. The vessels may occasionally communicate with the metaphyseal circulation. Each canal contains a central artery, veins, and a complex capillary network surrounding the central vessels. As ossification progresses, these vessels are incorporated into the osseous vasculature; one or two vessels usually develop as the predominant blood supply.

## Incidence

Physeal injuries have been reported to occur in approximately 30% of long bone fractures in children.[111, 112, 134] The distal end of the radius,[125] distal end of the tibia,[35] and phalanges of the fingers[54] have each been reported to be a frequent site of physeal injury. Regardless of the particular site of injury, it appears that distal physes are injured more frequently than proximal physes.[107, 125] Physeal injuries occur approximately twice as often in boys as in girls, probably because the physes remain open longer in boys and are exposed to more trauma through athletic activities. Most physeal fractures occur in boys between the ages of 12 and 15 years and in girls between the ages of 9 and 12 years.[153]

Athletics play an important role in physeal injuries. Watkins and Peabody[192] found that of 394 sports injuries in children and adolescents, most of the 195 chronic injuries affected cartilage, physes, and apophyses. Some specific physeal injuries are associated with specific sports, such as "Little League elbow" and "gymnast's wrist." Several studies have described stress injuries to the distal portions of the radius and ulna in competitive adolescent gymnasts and found radiographic evidence of premature closure of the physis and, later, shortening of the radius.[2, 4, 5, 27, 33, 60, 176, 185, 203] DiFiori and col-

leagues[49] found evidence of stress injuries of the distal radial physis in 25% of 44 nonelite gymnasts, all of whom had more than normal positive ulnar variance. They suggested that these injuries might be caused by growth inhibition of the distal end of the radius, growth stimulation of the ulna, or a combination of the two. Chang and associates[36] also found that chronic, repetitive stress in the wrists of adolescent gymnasts led to a disturbance in distal radial growth with resultant ulnar-plus variance. Kolt and Kirkby[90] detected physeal injuries in 12% of a group of 65 elite and subelite female gymnasts. Apple and McDonald[6] reported that chronic, repetitive cyclic loading in the lower extremity produced no harmful effect on the physes and that young runners experienced no more injuries than adult runners did. Micheli[118] also found no deleterious effects from weight training in immature athletes. Turz and Crost,[187] however, reported that 12% of the children in their study who required hospitalization for a sports injury experienced angulation or shortening of a limb or limited joint motion.

The strength of the physis is related to its morphology and to the intercellular matrix. In the first two zones of the physis, the cartilage matrix is abundant and the physis is strong. In the third zone, the enlarged chondrocytes decrease the capacity to withstand shearing, bending, and tension stress. This zone appears to be the weakest part of the physis. Harris[67] demonstrated that when the proximal tibial epiphysis is separated from the metaphysis, the plane of cleavage consistently passes through this third zone. The fourth zone is reinforced by calcification but is still weaker than the first and second zones. Fractures generally involve the third and fourth zones. Trabecular formation in the metaphysis also contributes to the strength of the physis, but the metaphysis is susceptible to compression or torus forces. As long as the epiphysis is cartilaginous, it serves as a sort of shock absorber and transmits forces directly into the metaphysis, which as a result may sustain a torus fracture. As the epiphysis ossifies, this shock-absorbing ability lessens, and forces are transmitted more directly into the physis, where shearing may occur through the third and fourth zones.

The dense periosteal attachments around the periphery of the physis also appear to increase the resistance to shear and tensile forces, especially as they blend into the epiphyseal perichondrium and joint capsule–ligament complex. The periosteum is attached relatively loosely to the metaphysis; the diaphyseal periosteum is even more loosely attached and does not appear to offer any mechanical protection for the diaphysis. Bright and co-workers[22] showed that the load-to-failure value of epiphyseal cartilage with intact periosteum is almost twice that of epiphyseal cartilage with the periosteum removed. As a checkrein on the epiphysis once the physis has failed, the periosteum may prevent marked displacement if its fibers are not ruptured. This function may explain why epiphyseal injury often occurs without radiographic evidence of significant displacement.

## MECHANISM OF INJURY

The mechanism of injury to the physeal structures depends to some extent on the age of the child. Bright and associates[22] showed experimentally that the tensile strength of the physis increases with age. Chung and co-workers[39] found that the perichondrial complex provides significant strength to the physis in childhood but less so in adolescence. In infancy and early childhood, when the physis is relatively thick, shearing or avulsion forces are most commonly involved. In older children and adolescents, physeal fracture-separation is most often caused by a combination of shearing and angular forces. Near the end of skeletal growth, when part of the physis has closed, intra-articular shearing forces, with or without angular forces, may lead to an intra-articular fracture. Momentary, transient dislocation or near-dislocation of a joint secondary to an avulsion or shearing force may also cause an intra-articular fracture. A severe abduction or adduction angular force applied to a joint that normally only flexes or extends exerts a severe compression force on the physis.

Though long a matter of controversy, the role of compression in physeal injuries is now generally accepted. Aminian and Schoenecker[5] and Abram and Thompson[2] described premature physeal closure after nonphyseal fractures of the distal third of the radius. These authors suggested that the growth arrest was most likely caused by a compression injury to the physis at the time of the wrist fracture rather than by ischemia, as proposed by Peterson and Burkhart.[152]

Keret and co-workers[85] described asymmetric premature closure of the proximal tibial physis in a patient with fractures of the contralateral tibia and ankle; the physeal damage was not diagnosed at the time of injury. Hresko and Kasser[72] reported seven cases of physeal arrest about the knee in patients who had nonphyseal injuries of the lower extremities. Their patients were between the ages of 10 and 12 years, and all physeal arrests involved the posterolateral part of the distal end of the femur or the anterior part of the proximal end of the tibia. No patient had evidence of iatrogenic trauma to the physis, such as that caused by pin placement or other surgical procedures.

The harmful effect of chronic, repetitive stress on the physes has long been recognized, from the Little League elbow and shoulder syndromes to growth disturbances of the wrist in gymnasts. Physeal growth arrest of the distal phalanx of the thumb has also been reported in adolescent piano players.[7, 84]

In addition to macrotrauma or microtrauma, the growth mechanisms may be damaged by surgical procedures such as the insertion of pins or screws,[79, 103] by irradiation,[44, 162, 184] by chemotherapy,[162, 188] by disease such as infection or neoplasm,[41, 66] or by congenital conditions such as metabolic or hematologic disorders.[88, 161, 170] Intraosseous fluid infusion, an effective technique used in emergency departments to aid in the resuscitation of pediatric patients, has raised concern about the possibility of physeal injury. Bielski and colleagues[11] constructed an experimental rabbit model to simulate intraosseous infusion in human infants in order to determine the effects on the physis and growth rate of the infused bone. No growth disturbance occurred in any of the infused tibias. Gross and microscopic changes were confined to metaphyseal bone and completely resolved after 3 weeks. They noted no evidence of physeal injury or change in growth rate in any of the rabbit models.

Radiotherapy for musculoskeletal neoplasms can cause physeal damage and growth arrest when the physis is included in the radiation field.[162] Pateder and associates[145] investigated the molecular mechanisms involved in radiation-induced arrest of bone growth in an avian model and found that exposure of physeal chondrocytes to radiation resulted in a specific pattern of biochemical and morphologic alterations that were dependent on dose and progressed over time. When administered before radiotherapy, the radioprotectant compound amifostine ($S$-2[3-aminopropylamino]-ethylphosphorothioic acid) has been demonstrated to provide differential protection of normal cells from the damaging effects of ionizing radiation. Tamurian and co-workers[184] found in a laboratory study involving a rat model that amifostine reduced the anticipated growth loss normally resulting from a single 12.5-Gy radiation dose by 48.9% in the femur, 13.1% in the tibia, and 27.6% overall in the total limb. Also using a rat model, Damron and colleagues[44] found that growth loss and limb discrepancy were significantly reduced in proportion to increasing amifostine doses. In a later study, the growth loss resulting from the combination of amifostine and five-fraction irradiation was statistically significantly lower than that from five-fraction irradiation alone.

### Consequences of Injury

The most obvious and catastrophic consequence of physeal injury is disruption of longitudinal growth of the bone. Complete growth arrest may result in significant

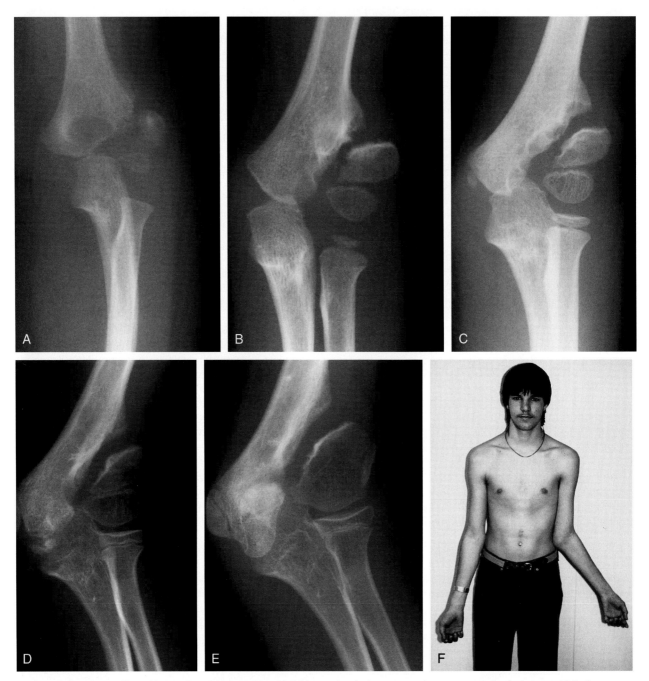

**FIGURE 2–2.** *A,* Fracture of lateral humeral condyle in a 5-year-old child treated with observation only. *B,* One year after fracture, established nonunion is evident. *C,* Three years after fracture, the capitellum and condyle appear to be migrating proximally. *D,* Five years after fracture, established cubitus valgus is apparent in addition to the nonunion. *E,* Ten years after fracture, a severe cubitus valgus deformity is present; the patient suffered mild ulnar nerve symptoms. *F,* Eleven years after fracture, the patient has an unsightly cubitus valgus deformity. (*A–F,* From Canale, S.T.; Beaty, J.H., eds. Operative Pediatric Orthopaedics. St. Louis, Mosby–Year Book, 1991.)

limb length inequality with functional impairment. Partial growth arrest may lead to angular deformity or progressive shortening. Nonunion (e.g., after fracture of the lateral humeral condyle [Fig. 2–2]), malunion, and avascular necrosis (e.g., after injury to the capital femoral epiphysis) may also occur. Infrequently, arteriovenous malformation may cause accelerated growth.

Several reports have demonstrated that the prognosis for future growth is dependent on the location of the lesion in the physis. If the fracture is limited to the layer

of hypertrophic cells, healing is usually uneventful. If the fracture reaches the layer of germinal cells or crosses the entire physis, growth disturbance is more likely[167] (Fig. 2–3). Gomes and co-workers,[62] in an experimental study in rats, correlated growth disturbance with the Salter-Harris types of fractures. They reported transitory growth arrest and increased thickening of the zone of hypertrophic cells after type I and type II fractures, but a nearly normal physis was seen within 25 days. After type III injuries, an angular deformity occurred that increased with time. After type IV injuries, a step-off developed on the articular surface and became more severe with time. According to these investigators, no compressive force was applied to produce the bony bridges, so these alterations are probably secondary and may be triggered by the presence of the osseous callus itself, which fills the gap and maintains the interruption of the growth cartilage, thus establishing a bony bridge between the epiphyseal and metaphyseal bone.

Circulation plays an important role in the genesis of these deformities because the bony bridge is preceded by early anastomosis between the epiphyseal and metaphyseal vessels through the gap in the growth cartilage. These findings support the impression of other investigators that permanent damage to the physis and the consequent bone deformity in these two types of injuries (Salter-Harris types III and IV) are caused by the establishment of early anastomotic connections between the epiphyseal and metaphyseal vessels. In a study in rabbits, Gomes and Volpon[61] noted that compression of the fragments of Salter-Harris types III and IV fractures prevented the formation of vascular anastomoses between the epiphyseal and metaphyseal vessels and resulted in osseous union without callus or bony bar formation. They recommend rigid internal fixation of types III and IV fractures.

## COMPLETE GROWTH ARREST

Complete cessation of growth after physeal injury is infrequent, and its significance depends on the age of the patient. An adolescent near the end of skeletal growth may not have any functional sequelae; however, in younger children, a substantial limb length discrepancy may develop.

## PARTIAL GROWTH ARREST

Partial growth arrest produces angular and longitudinal growth abnormalities. The arrest occurs when a bridge of bone forms across the physis from the metaphysis to the epiphysis and tethers growth. Growth of the remaining physis causes angular deformity. The size and location of the bony bar determine the clinical deformity. For example, laterally situated bony bars about the knee produce genu valgum deformities, whereas anterior bars produce genu recurvatum. If the bar is in the center of the physis, growth of the periphery may cause cupping, tenting, or a dip deformity of the metaphysis and relative shortening of the bone with little angular deformity.

Bright[20] classified partial growth arrest as peripheral, central, and combined and reported that 60% of cases of partial growth arrest in his series of 225 patients were caused by peripheral lesions. Partial arrest occurs almost twice as often in boys as in girls. The physes of the distal end of the femur, distal and proximal ends of the tibia, and distal portion of the radius are most frequently affected.

All bony bars result from damage to the physeal cells, most commonly from fracture. They may also occur after other kinds of physeal damage, such as infection, tumor, radiation, thermal burns, and the insertion of metal across the physis. Neural and vascular abnormalities have also been shown to alter physeal growth, and, for some

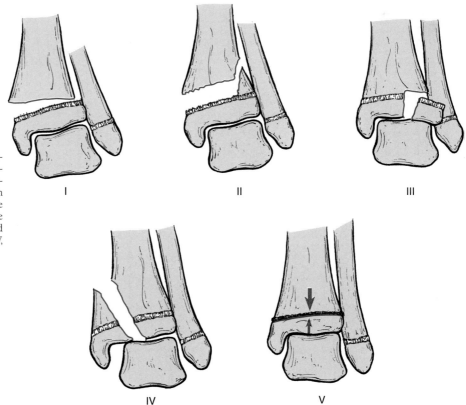

FIGURE 2–3. Salter-Harris classification of physeal injury. I, pure separation through the physis; II, metaphyseal spike; III, separation through the physis and vertically through the epiphysis; IV, fracture through the metaphysis, through the physis, and vertically through the epiphysis; V, pure compression injury.

I

II

III

IV

V

bony bars, no cause was apparent. Of all the causes of bony bars, perhaps the only preventable one is iatrogenic damage from metal pins or screws placed across the physis. A small, smooth pin placed perpendicularly across the center of the physis for a short time (2 to 3 weeks) rarely causes growth arrest; however, a threaded wire placed obliquely across a physis and left in place for a few weeks usually results in a bony bar.

## Commonly Associated Injuries

Injuries most commonly associated with physeal fractures are those to the neurovascular and ligamentous structures near the physis. Avulsion of the physis as a result of ligamentous injury occurs most often at the tibial spine, at the ulnar styloid, and in the phalanges. Neurovascular injuries are most common with supracondylar humeral and proximal tibial fractures. Dislocation of the joint or an ipsilateral shaft fracture is seen most frequently with medial epicondylar fractures, about half of which are associated with partial or complete elbow dislocation; however, ipsilateral fractures of the shafts of other long bones are often seen with the physeal injury.

Combinations of physeal injury and ligamentous disruption are most common about the knee.[10, 50, 51] Avulsion of the tibial spine is often associated with injury to the cruciate ligaments. Posterior displacement of a fracture fragment may cause impingement, occlusion, intraluminal damage, or transection of the popliteal artery (Fig. 2–4).

Recurvatum deformity of the tibia after femoral fractures in children is believed to be iatrogenically induced; however, Bowler and associates[18] believe that it is the result of physeal injury incurred at the time of trauma rather than injury caused by a tibial traction pin. They reported premature closure of the anterior portion of the proximal tibial physis, along with associated genu recurvatum deformity, in two adolescent boys who sustained closed femoral fractures. Neither was treated with proximal tibial traction. One patient was managed by skin traction and spica casting, and the other was treated with distal femoral pin traction. Etchebehere and co-workers[52] used three-phase bone scintigraphy to document the metabolic activity of the distal femoral and proximal tibial physes after femoral fractures in 18 children (average age of 6 years) and suggested that this activity may explain overgrowth after femoral fracture.

The increased tibial valgus that often occurs after tibial metaphyseal and diaphyseal fractures in children has been attributed to both physeal overgrowth and eccentric growth.[71, 75, 78, 82, 123] Ogden and colleagues,[133] however, reported that their data suggested that the progressive valgus angulation is an accelerated physiologic response. In the 17 children in their study, they found not only generalized overgrowth of the injured tibia, both proximally and distally, but also asymmetric proximal medial overgrowth in every patient. In five of six patients with Harris lines, distal as well as proximal tibial

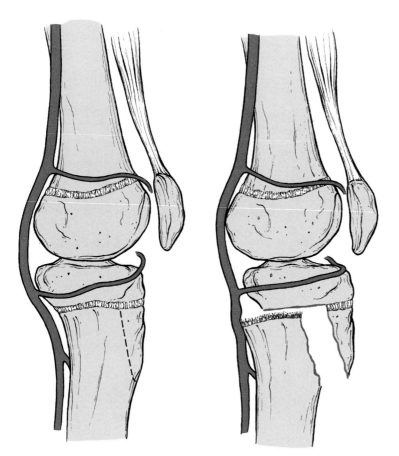

FIGURE 2–4. Displacement of a fracture fragment may cause impingement, occlusion, intraluminal damage, or transection of the popliteal artery after posterior displacement of the tibia in a Salter-Harris type I physeal injury.

metaphyseal overgrowth was present, but the distal line was always parallel to the physis and did not contribute to the valgus angulation.

## Classification

The first classification scheme for physeal fractures was proposed by Foucher in 1863.[57] In 1898, Poland[156] advanced his four-part classification (Fig. 2–5), and Aitken[3] in 1965 divided these fractures into three types. The Salter-Harris[167] classification, presented in 1963, has been the most widely used. It is based on the mechanism of injury, the relationship of the fracture line to various cellular layers of the physis, and the prognosis concerning subsequent growth disturbance.

This radiographic classification includes five types of fractures: type I, complete separation of the epiphysis and physis from the metaphysis, with fracture through the zone of hypertrophic cells (Fig. 2–6); type II, similar to type I, except that a metaphyseal fragment is present on the compression side of the fracture (Thurston-Holland sign) (Fig. 2–7); type III, physeal separation with fracture through the epiphysis into the joint (Fig. 2–8); type IV, fracture through the metaphysis, physis, and epiphysis and into the joint (Fig. 2–9); and type V, compression or crushing injury to the physis.

Rang[158] added type VI to the Salter-Harris classification: avulsion injury to the peripheral portion of the physis, after which bony bridge formation may result in considerable angular deformity because of its peripheral location (Fig. 2–10). Weber[194] added intra-articular and extra-articular designations to the Salter-Harris classification.

Ogden[134] included injuries to other growth mechanisms, such as the metaphysis, diaphysis, periosteum, zone of Ranvier, and perichondrium, in his extensive nine-part classification scheme, which follows (see Fig. 2–5).

**Type I.** The epiphysis and some of the contiguous physis separate from the metaphysis with osseous fragments (type IA), the fracture line undulates through a zone of hypertrophic cartilage cells, and little or no displacement of the epiphyseal fragment occurs. Type IB fractures occur in children with systemic disorders affecting ossification of the metaphysis. Type IC fractures have an associated injury to the germinal portion of the physis.

**Type II.** In type II, the most common physeal injury, the line of fracture passes through hypertrophic and provisionally calcified zones, but propagation across the physeal-metaphyseal junction is variable. A small triangular metaphyseal fragment (Thurston-Holland sign) is diagnostic, with displacement being variable. Type IIB involves further propagation of the fracture forces on the tensile side to create a free metaphyseal fragment. Type IIC includes a thin layer of metaphysis along with or instead of the triangular fragment, with the fracture traversing most of the metaphysis. Type IID includes compression of the metaphysis into the physis.

**Type III.** This lesion is an intra-articular fracture involving the epiphysis, with the plane of fracture occurring from the articular surface through the epiphysis, epiphyseal ossification center, and physis. In type IIIA, the fracture line extends along the hypertrophic zone of the physis toward the periphery. In type IIIB, a transverse fracture propagates through the primary spongiosa, with a thin layer of metaphyseal bone left with the epiphyseal fragment. Type IIIC includes injuries to epiphyses that have undergone major contour changes, such as the ischial tuberosity, and propagation of the epiphyseal fracture may not involve a joint (Fig. 2–11). These mostly nonarticular injuries occur primarily in the pelvis, where epiphyses are attached to contiguous structures through radiolucent cartilage and fibrocartilage, such as the symphysis pubis. When the epiphysis is avulsed from the metaphysis, the cartilaginous-fibrocartilaginous attachment is attenuated or fractured, which may cause growth disturbance.

**Type IV.** The fracture line involves the articular surface; extends through the epiphysis, across the full thickness of the physis, and through a segment of the metaphysis (type IVA); and causes a complete longitudinal split of all zones of the physis. In type IVB, further propagation of the fracture through the remaining portion of the physis creates an additional free fragment. In type IVC, the epiphyseal fracture propagates through radiolucent cartilage. Type IVD fractures are usually caused by severe trauma, such as lawn mower injuries, and result in multiple metaphyseal-physeal-epiphyseal fragments (Fig. 2–12).

**Type V.** A compression force is transmitted through segments of the epiphysis and physis, where it disrupts germinal regions of the chondrocytes and adjacent hypertrophic regions and damages the vascular supply; this pattern is difficult, if not impossible, to appreciate on plain radiographs. Type V injuries include those caused by electric shock, irradiation, and frostbite.

**Type VI.** This fracture involves the peripheral region of the physis, especially the zone of Ranvier, and may result from a glancing type of trauma involving primarily avulsion of the overlying skin or subcutaneous tissue, such as might occur from a bicycle or lawn mower accident, deep extension of infection, or a severe burn. Rang described this fracture as occurring in sports injuries secondary to avulsion of the ligamentous attachments adjacent to the physis.[158]

**Type VII.** These fractures are completely intraepiphyseal, with propagation from the articular surface through the epiphyseal cartilage and into the secondary ossification center. Type VIIA involves propagation of the fracture through both the epiphyseal and articular cartilage and the bone of the secondary ossification center (Fig. 2–13). Type VIIB involves propagation of the fracture primarily through the cartilaginous portions, with involvement of some of the preossifying regions.

**Type VIII.** These injuries affect metaphyseal growth and remodeling mechanisms and cause transient vascular compromise.

**Type IX.** This type comprises selective injuries to the diaphyseal growth mechanism of appositional, membranous bone formation from the periosteum. These injuries may be associated with severe fragmentation of portions of the diaphysis.

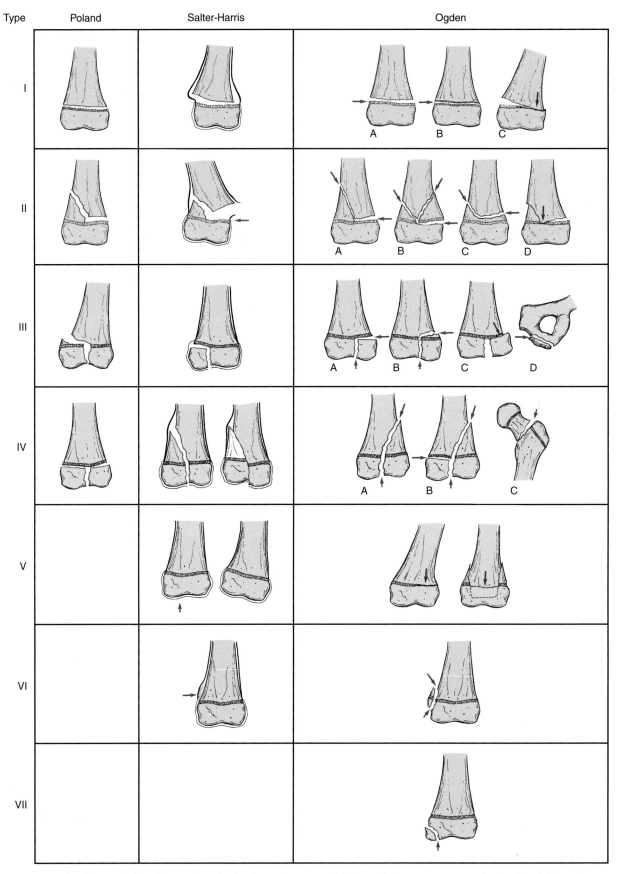

**Figure 2–5.** Classification of physeal injuries by Poland, Salter and Harris, and Ogden. All three systems are similar but, from left to right, are increasingly complex. The Salter-Harris classification is a refinement of Poland's system; Ogden's classification, which is all-inclusive, adds more subclasses. (From Canale, S.T. Fractures in children. In: Crenshaw, A.H., ed. Campbell's Operative Orthopaedics, 7th ed. St. Louis, C.V. Mosby, 1987.)

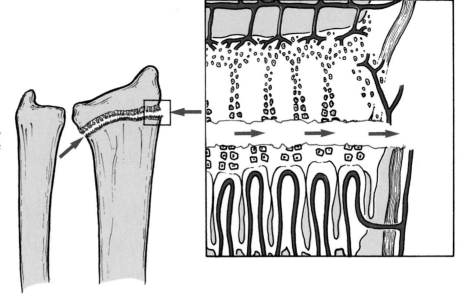

FIGURE 2–6. Salter-Harris type I injury with physeal separation through the zone of hypertrophic cells.

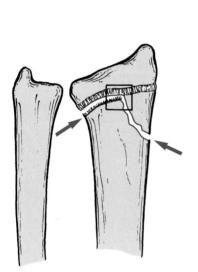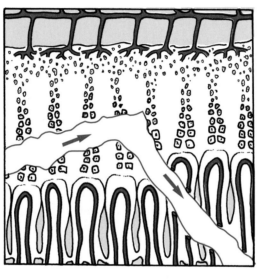

FIGURE 2–7. A Salter-Harris type II injury is similar to type I but has a metaphyseal spike.

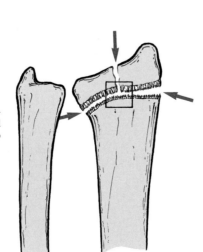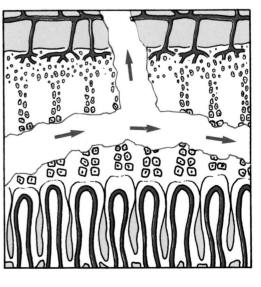

FIGURE 2–8. Salter-Harris type III injury with physeal separation and extension across the epiphysis into the joint.

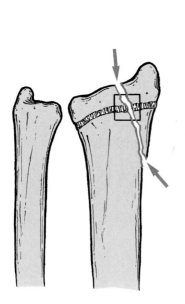

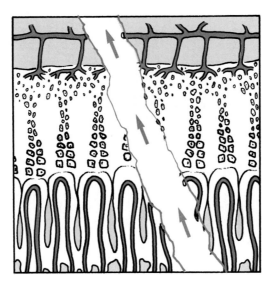

FIGURE 2–9. Salter-Harris type IV injury with a metaphyseal spike; the physis and epiphysis are both involved.

Types VIII and IX fractures are nonphyseal injuries that may affect metaphyseal and diaphyseal remodeling and growth.

Peterson[150, 151] described two physeal fractures that had not been previously classified: a fracture completely across the metaphysis with extension to the physis, usually with no extension of the fracture along the physis (Fig. 2–14), and a fracture in which a portion of the physis is missing (Fig. 2–15). This type is always an open

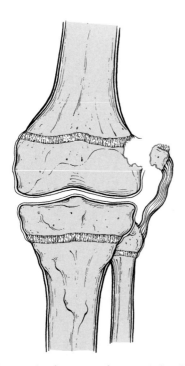

FIGURE 2–10. Example of a type VI fracture, as described by Rang: avulsion of the attachment of the fibular collateral ligament at the physis, which can cause peripheral growth arrest and severe angular deformity. (Redrawn from Weber, B.G.; Brunner, C.; Freuler, F. Treatment of Fractures in Children and Adolescents. New York, Springer-Verlag, 1980.)

fracture that requires initial surgery; premature physeal closure usually develops and necessitates later reconstructive surgery.[184]

Several authors have devised classification schemes for specific anatomic locations: distal tibial injuries—Chadwick and Bentley[35]; tibial tuberosity fractures—Watson-Jones[193]; proximal humeral fractures—Neer and Horowitz[125]; lateral condylar fractures—Milch[121]; medial condylar fractures—Kilfoyle[86]; distal humeral epiphyseal separations—DeLee and colleagues[47]; olecranon epiphyseal fractures—Grantham and Kiernan[63] and Wilkins[196]; radial neck fractures—Vostal,[189] Newman,[127] O'Brien,[130] Jeffrey,[81] and Wilkins[196]; Monteggia fractures—Bado,[8] Wiley and Galey,[195] and Letts and co-workers[106]; thumb metacarpal fractures—O'Brien[129]; and phalangeal physeal fractures—Wood[199] and O'Brien.[129] Scuderi and Bronson[171] described a classification of triradiate cartilage fractures (Fig. 2–16). These specific classification schemes are discussed in the chapters that deal with specific injuries.

For most physeal injuries, the Salter-Harris classification with the addition of Rang's type VI fracture is adequate and most easily applied. More complicated injuries may benefit from more specific classification according to one of the more detailed systems.

## DIAGNOSIS

Most patients with physeal injury can attribute it to a specific traumatic incident. Pain and localized tenderness are the most common symptoms. Swelling and effusion are variable signs that depend on the severity and anatomic location of the injury. Children, however, are not good historians, and physeal injuries can occur in a variety of ways. Musharafieh and Macari[124] reported that, of 38 children with diagnoses of wrist sprains, 33 had Salter-Harris type I fractures of the distal end of the radius. In addition to specific trauma, the physes may

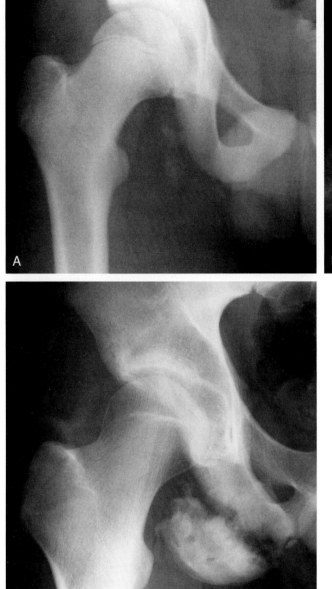

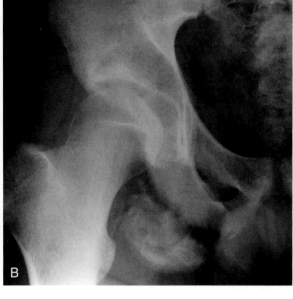

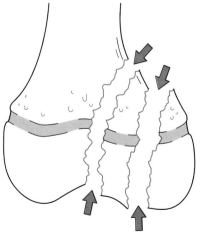

FIGURE **2–11.** Ischial tuberosity fracture. *A*, Large avulsion of the ischial tuberosity in a 13-year-old girl. *B*, Six months after injury, a large area of ossification can be seen. *C*, Three years after injury, an ununited ischial tuberosity is evident.

be damaged by infection (Brodie's abscess), pathologic processes (tumor, pathologic fracture, chondromalacia, bone cyst), metabolic disease, congenital abnormalities such as neurofibromatosis or syphilis, endocrine disorders, radiation or chemotherapy, or child abuse (Fig. 2–17).

## Radiographic Evaluation

Because of the chondro-osseous nature and irregular contours of the physes, some acute physeal injuries are not clearly seen on plain radiographs.[163] Slight widening of the physis may be the only sign of minimal displacement of an epiphyseal fragment. The small metaphyseal fragment (Thurston-Holland sign) may be difficult to appreciate. Two views taken at 90° planes to

FIGURE **2–12.** Ogden type IVD injuries are caused by severe trauma that produces multiple metaphyseal-physeal-epiphyseal fragments.

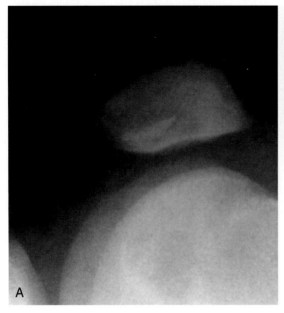

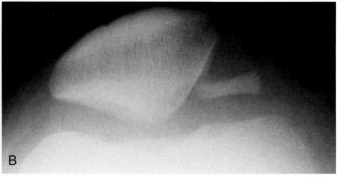

Figure 2–13. *A* and *B,* Osteochondral fracture of the patella in a child (Ogden type VIIA).

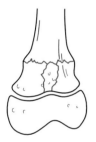
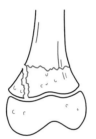
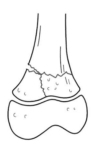
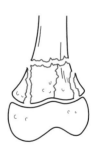

Figure 2–14. Fracture of the metaphysis, with extension to the physis. (From Peterson, H.A. J Pediatr Orthop 14:431, 1994.)

each other may help delineate the fracture, and comparison films of the opposite extremity are invaluable for determining whether physeal injury has occurred. Oblique views may be helpful in injuries to the forearm or lower part of the leg. Varus and valgus stress views are useful for injuries about the knee and elbow to demonstrate gapping between the epiphysis and metaphysis. Identical views of the contralateral extremity can help establish whether occult separation of the physis (Salter-Harris type I injury) has occurred. Kleinman and Marks[89] described the radiographic characteristics of a "corner fracture" caused by child abuse (see Fig. 2–17). A metaphyseal fragment (the corner) is displaced, with the

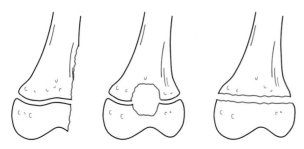

Figure 2–15. Fractures of the physis, with a portion of the physis missing. (From Peterson, H.A. J Pediatr Orthop 14:431, 1994.)

now-ossified epiphysis giving the characteristic appearance (Fig. 2–18).

## Special Studies

Tomograms may be necessary in acute injuries to delineate fragmentation and the orientation of fragments. Tomogram cuts should be made at 0.5-cm intervals rather than at the standard 1 cm. Computed tomography (CT), especially with sagittal and coronal reconstruction, may be necessary to determine the exact nature of severely comminuted epiphyseal and metaphyseal fractures that are not clearly seen on plain radiographic views.[202] Loder and associates[108] reported that helical CT scanning accurately predicted the location and size of bony bars in five children in whom bar excision was planned. As advantages of helical CT scanning, they cite excellent bony detail, radiation dose of a half to a fourth that of conventional tomography, and rapidity of scanning (approximately 20 seconds) without the necessity of sedation. Nuclear bone scanning may not be especially helpful in physeal fractures because the physes are normally relatively active on nuclear scans of children; increased uptake may occur at several physes in an extremity secondary to trauma, infection, or neoplasm. Magnetic resonance imaging (MRI) has proved reliable

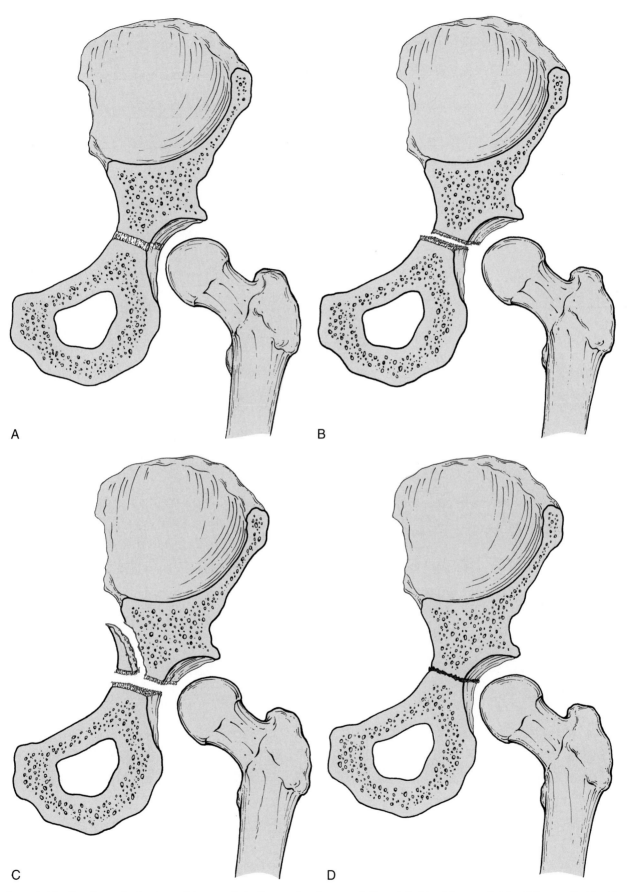

**FIGURE 2–16.** Classification by Scuderi and Bronson of triradiate cartilage fractures. *A,* Normal. *B,* Salter I fracture. *C,* Salter II fracture. *D,* Salter V fracture. (*A–D,* From Scuderi, G.; Bronson, M.J. Triradiate cartilage injury; report of two cases and review of the literature. Clin Orthop 217:179, 1987.)

**FIGURE 2–17.** Physeal fractures caused by child abuse in an infant. *A,* Bilateral transepiphyseal hip fractures. *B,* Distal (corner) and proximal femoral physeal fractures. *C* and *D,* Distal tibial physeal fractures (corner). *E,* Six months after the injuries, proliferative callus formation is evident in the femur.

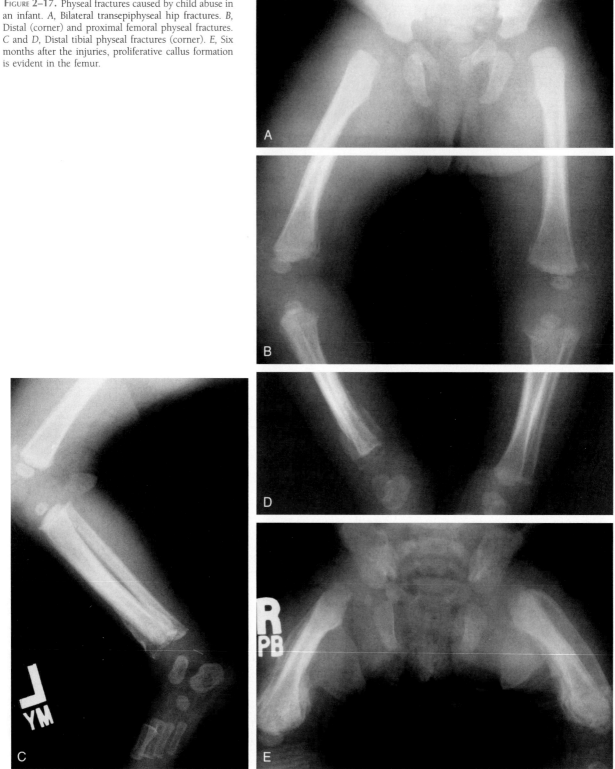

for evaluation of physeal injuries[14, 42, 69, 87, 173] (Fig. 2–19). Smith and colleagues[177] noted that MRI performed in the acute period (within 10 days of fracture) provides the most accurate evaluation of physeal fracture anatomy and can demonstrate transphyseal bridging or altered arrest lines in physeal fractures before they become apparent on radiographs. Petit and co-

workers[154] compared radiographic and MRI evaluation of 19 acute distal tibial fractures and found that only one was misclassified from the radiographs. MRI did not cause the treatment plan to be changed in any patient. Although fracture lines and fragments were more easily seen on MRI, especially Salter-Harris type IV and triplane fractures, the authors recommended that gradient-echo

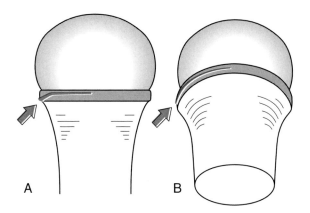

FIGURE 2–18. *A,* When the fracture line *(arrow)* is incomplete (it extends across only a portion of the metaphysis), the appearance suggests a focal, triangularly shaped peripheral fragment encompassing the subperiosteal bone collar. *B,* When the fracture line *(arrow)* is tipped obliquely, the peripheral margin of the fragment is projected as a curvilinear density. (*A, B,* From Kleinman, P.K.; Marks, S.C. J Bone Joint Surg Am 77:1471, 1995.)

MRI be limited to complex fractures. Carey and associates,[31] however, in their comparison of radiographic and MRI evaluation of 14 patients with known or suspected physeal injuries, found that MRI changed the Salter-Harris classification in 2 of 9 with fractures visible on radiographs, detected occult fractures in 5 of 14, and resulted in a change in management in 5 of 14.

Ultrasonography has been reported to be able to document soft tissue injury without fracture; Boker and Burbach[13] described the use of ultrasonography for the diagnosis of separation of the proximal humeral epiphysis in newborns, and Brown and Eustace reported the ultrasound diagnosis of a neonatal transphyseal supracondylar humeral fracture.[24] Arthrography may be necessary to confirm suspected physeal injuries, especially in the hip and elbow. An arteriogram may be indicated if vascular injury is suspected.

## Differential Diagnosis

Physeal fractures may be simulated by variations in normal growth patterns (Fig. 2–20), infection, congenital conditions, metabolic disorders, or neoplasms.

## MANAGEMENT

Treatment of physeal injuries is based on the severity of the injury, its anatomic location, and the age of the patient. Many concepts of remodeling after angulation of a fracture have been described. Ryoppy and Karaharju[166] listed several factors contributing to the remodeling process in a long bone, including asymmetric epiphyseal growth, changes in the process of resorption, and apposition in the metaphysis. Longitudinal growth is generally accepted as a major means of remodeling, as is stimulation of growth by a diaphyseal fracture. Abraham[1] demonstrated that after osteotomy, the radius and tibia of an immature monkey remodeled 5° each year until maturity and that the periosteum and physis contributed equally to the correction. Valgus, varus, and flexion deformities corrected to the same degree. Epiphysiodesis of the adjacent physes did not prevent correction of the shaft of the bone. Remodeling of the osteotomy site was radiographically characterized by bone deposition on the concave side, with no significant resorption on the convex side. Pauwels[146] demonstrated that the physis responds eccentrically to change and pressure and that, through selective growth in different regions, it attempts to remodel itself perpendicular to the major traction forces moving across the physis. This characteristic may explain the gradual correction of some deformities, in accordance with the Heuter-Volkmann principle.

An injury that may cause disabling sequelae in a young child may result in little or no impairment in an

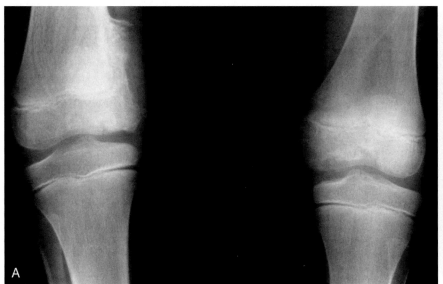
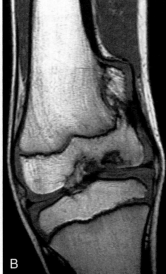

FIGURE 2–19. *A,* Bony formation in right knee after Salter-Harris type II fracture of the distal femur. *B,* MRI defines extent of bony bar and identifies a traumatic osteochondral defect.

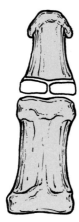

FIGURE 2–20. Fissuring of the epiphysis of the proximal phalanx of the great toe is not a fracture. (Redrawn from Lyritis, G. Skeletal Radiol 10:250, 1983.)

adolescent nearing the end of skeletal growth. If a child has several years of growth remaining before closure of the physes and if the epiphyses are still capable of growth, most deformities in the plane of motion of the joint will remodel.

Different physes have different growth potentials. Pritchett[157] used teleradiographs of the upper extremities of 244 healthy, well-nourished children, taken at 6-month intervals from the age of 7 years until skeletal maturity, to determine the growth remaining at both physes of the humerus, radius, and ulna. He found that in this time span the humerus grows approximately 1.2 cm each year in girls and 1.3 cm in boys, the ulna grows approximately 1 cm each year in girls and 1.1 cm in boys, and the radius grows approximately 0.9 cm each year in girls and 1 cm in boys. These data allow accurate prediction of growth and growth discrepancy in the upper extremity and help to more precisely determine the appropriate time for equalization procedures.

The greatest discrepancy between the physes of the same bone probably exists in the humerus. In this bone, the distal physis provides only 20% of the longitudinal growth and is therefore less capable of correcting angular deformity, except in the sagittal plane. Conversely, the proximal physis provides 80% of the growth of the diaphysis and can often completely remodel the entire proximal end of the humerus within a year. In the femur, the reverse is true. The distal physis contributes 70% of the growth of the femur, and the capital femoral physis contributes only 30% of the entire length of the femur. For this reason, proximal femoral physeal arrest in an older child rarely causes significant leg length inequality and only minimal coxa vara deformity. Injury to the distal femoral physis may result in significant limb shortening and angulation. In the tibia, the proximal physis contributes considerably more growth than the distal physis does; conversely, the distal radial physis contributes more growth than the proximal physis does.

Most children's fractures heal twice as fast as adults' fractures, and most purely epiphyseal separations heal in half the time of a long bone fracture in a child. Thus, whereas an adult tibial fracture may require 12 to 18 weeks for healing, the same fracture in a child may require only 6 to 9 weeks and a purely epiphyseal separation, only 3 to 5 weeks. Supracondylar femoral fractures in adults may require 20 weeks for healing, whereas in children, 8 to 10 weeks is sufficient. Usually, only 5 to 6 weeks of immobilization is required for Salter-Harris type I or II fractures of the distal femoral physis.

The time between injury and initial treatment is also an important factor. For closed reduction, ideally, the injury should be only several hours old. When the injury is several days old, a decision must be made whether the deformity is sufficient to warrant initial reduction or, if the original reduction has been lost, whether a second closed reduction is indicated. The age of the patient, the severity of the deformity, and the plane of the deformity should all be considered. The younger the patient, the more correction that can be anticipated, especially if the angulation is in the plane of flexion or extension.

Establishing the time of the last oral intake of the child is also important in deciding whether general anesthesia is feasible. Serious complications from aspiration can occur when a child with a full stomach is anesthetized for reduction of a closed fracture, which may have been unnecessary. Although regional anesthesia, such as axillary blocks or Bier blocks, is difficult in children, it may be supplemented with a "pediatric cocktail." Often, for simple epiphyseal separations, no anesthesia is preferable to multiple anesthetic injections into the fracture site. In any case, gentle reduction is mandatory. Traction rather than forceful manipulation should be used to avoid physeal damage. Multiple attempts at closed reduction should be avoided. If the fracture cannot be reduced in one or two gentle attempts with the child under local or regional anesthesia, closed reduction with general anesthesia should be considered. If significant deformity persists after closed reduction, especially in Salter-Harris types III and IV injuries, open reduction and internal fixation may be indicated.

If open reduction and internal fixation are indicated, the periosteum around the epiphysis may be resected for better exposure and more accurate reduction; however, the fragment should not be completely denuded of soft tissue attachments, through which it receives its blood supply. If the periosteum is elevated near the epiphysis, Bright[20] recommended careful resection for about 1 cm on either side of the physis to prevent the formation of a bony bridge between the epiphysis and metaphysis.

Periosteum interposed in the fracture site has been implicated in the formation of bony bars.[104, 160, 198] Although no studies have shown that entrapped periosteum has an adverse effect on healing of physeal fractures, several studies have reported that periosteum folded into a physeal defect results in the creation of a bony bar and physeal growth arrest.[20, 80, 197] In a proximal tibial physeal fracture model in animals, Phieffer and associates[155] found that fracture alone resulted in physeal injury with the formation of a small histologic bar but no clinically evident growth arrest. Interposition of periosteum in the fracture site resulted in the formation of a small histologic bar and a small, but statistically significant increase in leg length discrepancies when compared with fracture alone.

Treatment of specific physeal injuries is described in later chapters; the general guidelines given here are based on the Salter-Harris classification of physeal fractures.

Type I injuries (separation of the epiphysis from the metaphysis) can usually be treated by closed reduction and casting because the periosteal sleeve is generally intact. At sites where the periosteum is thin (such as the femur or radius), internal fixation may be required after open or closed reduction. Occasionally, closed reduction cannot be achieved because of interposed periosteum (medial malleolus) or muscle or tendon (deltoid or biceps in the proximal part of the humerus).

Type II fractures (fracture-separation of the epiphysis, fracture of the metaphysis) can usually be managed by closed reduction by using the intact hinge of periosteum.

Types III and IV fractures (intra-articular fracture involving the physis, epiphysis, and metaphysis) require anatomic reduction, usually involving open reduction and internal fixation with smooth pins that avoid the physis. Foster and colleagues[56] described the use of a free fat interpositional graft (Langenskiöld procedure) in the treatment of three acute severe physeal injuries (two distal tibial, one distal femoral). At follow-up periods of 5.5, 2.5, and 2 years, all physes were open with normal growth. Although none of the three children was skeletally mature at the time of follow-up and the continuance of physeal growth was not known, Foster and co-workers recommended the "anticipatory Langenskiöld" procedure for acute physeal injuries in which growth arrest is expected. They suggested that this measure might avoid the standard surgical procedures, such as osteotomies, that are used to treat the results of growth arrest.

Type V (compression) fractures are rarely diagnosed acutely, and treatment is delayed until the development of a bony bridge across the physis is apparent.[115]

Some important points to remember in the treatment of physeal injuries include the following:

1. Displacement is often minimal or absent; however, if at all in doubt, the extremity should be splinted and the injury reexamined in 1 or 2 weeks for periosteal reaction indicating a Salter-Harris type I physeal injury.
2. When attempting closed reduction through manipulation and traction, great care must be taken to achieve gentle reduction with the musculature as relaxed as possible to avoid "grating" the physis on metaphyseal or epiphyseal fragments. To circumvent physeal damage, the reduction should be 75% traction and 25% manipulation.
3. Restoration of the congruency of both the articular surface and the physis is essential if it has been disrupted, especially in young children. After a Salter-Harris type I or II injury without intra-articular disruption and in the plane of motion of the joint, a considerable amount of remodeling can be expected; less than satisfactory reduction can and should be accepted in preference to repeated attempts at reduc-

tion that may damage the germinal cells of the physis. No definite degree of angulation can be called acceptable in children's fractures. In general, greater angular deformity can be tolerated in the upper extremity than in the lower extremity, more valgus deformity can be tolerated than varus deformity, and more flexion deformity can be tolerated than extension deformity. In the lower extremity, more deformity can be tolerated proximally than distally (the same varus angle in the hip can be better compensated than in the knee and is least compensated in the ankle). Spontaneous correction of angular deformities is greatest when the angulation is in the plane of motion of a nearby hinged joint; for example, in fractures just proximal to the knee, elbow, or wrist, angulation with its apex toward the flexor aspect of the joint usually results in surprisingly little deformity. Function usually returns to normal unless the fracture occurs near the end of growth. Angulation in any other direction will probably persist to some extent. Rotational deformities are permanent.
4. The undulating contour of the physes must be borne in mind. Before open reduction and internal fixation are undertaken, the surgical approaches to and anatomy of the physes should be known. Birch and colleagues[12] published an excellent description of the major physes and the most appropriate approach to each.
5. Internal fixation should be adequate for rigid fixation, but not more than necessary, and should be easily removable.
6. Smooth rather than threaded pins should be used, and the physis should be avoided if possible (Fig. 2–21A); pins should parallel the physis in the epiphysis and metaphysis. Smooth oblique pins should be inserted across the physis only if satisfactory internal fixation cannot be achieved with transverse fixation (Fig. 2–21B). Böstman and colleagues[15, 16] reported the experimental use of biodegradable pins (cylindrical rods made of polylactide-glycolide copolymer) for transepiphyseal fracture fixation, thus avoiding the need to remove implants. They described the use of this device in three supracondylar fractures of the elbow and three fractures of the physes of the first metatarsal, distal end of the tibia, and medial humeral epicondyle. Preliminary results at 1 year showed no evidence of growth impairment or failure of fixation. The authors believe that because the cross-sectional area of the pin is only 1.8 mm, which falls within the experimentally observed safe limit of 3% of the physis, these pins will not damage the physis; conclusive evidence requires larger numbers of patients and longer follow-up, however.
7. Neurovascular status must be carefully evaluated before treatment, after treatment, and during convalescence. Unfortunately, uncertainty about the neurovascular status of an extremity before treatment and resultant neurovascular compromise after treatment are common and can cause medicolegal problems.[191]
8. Parents should be warned of the possibility of complications such as bony bridge formation, angular deformity, and avascular necrosis.

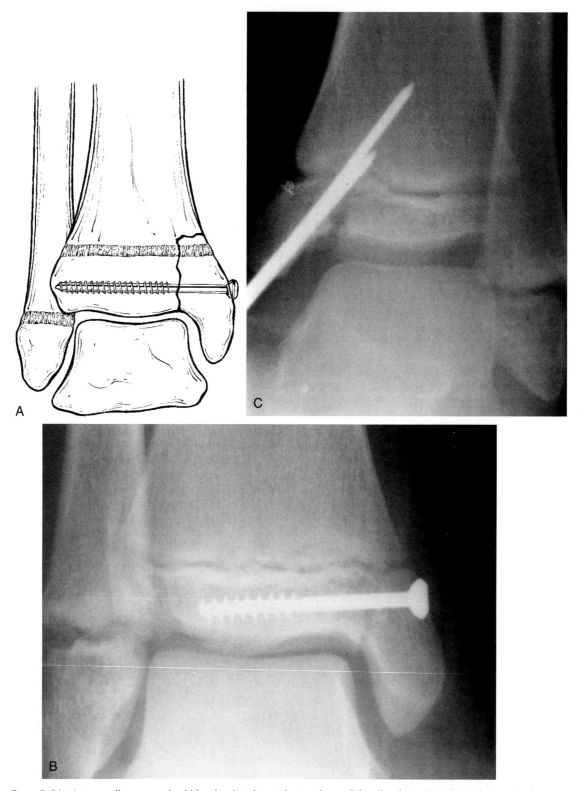

FIGURE 2–21. *A,* A cancellous screw should be placed in the epiphysis only, parallel to the physis. *B,* Radiograph showing the screw in place. *C,* Smooth pins may cross the physis, as in this Salter-Harris type III fracture, even though parallel transverse pins are preferred, when possible.

9. Long-term follow-up is essential to determine whether complications will occur. All physeal separations, regardless of type, should be checked within the first week after reduction to ensure that reduction has not been lost or to allow a second reduction, if necessary, before healing has occurred. After 7 to 14 days, Salter-Harris types I and II fractures can generally be expected to heal without loss of reduction. Salter-Harris types III and IV fractures treated by closed reduction should be carefully examined every

5 to 7 days for the first 3 weeks to be sure that the fracture fragments are not displaced. If adequate radiographs cannot be taken through the plaster cast, the cast should be removed. Depending on the type and location of the fracture, long-term follow-up is essential. Parents should be informed of the possibility of growth arrest and angulation deformity, and the importance of returning for follow-up examination at 6 to 12 months should be emphasized. At long-term follow-up, Harris growth lines should be examined to make sure that they are parallel to the physis (see further on).

## CHARACTERISTICS OF SOME COMMONLY INJURED PHYSES

Although growth disturbance can occur after injury to any physis, it is more likely with injury to some physes than to others. Growth disturbance has been reported after injuries to the triradiate cartilage,[25, 70] the physes of the spine[101, 200] and the clavicle,[68] and those of the hands and feet,[105, 128] but such disturbances are relatively infrequent.

**Proximal Femur.** In epiphyseal separations of the hip joint, with or without displacement of the fragment from the acetabulum, avascular necrosis occurs in a large percentage of patients regardless of treatment (Fig. 2–22). In older children (10 years and above), closed reduction and pinning can be performed; premature physeal closure causes little limb length discrepancy.

**Distal Femur.** Salter-Harris types III and IV fractures of the distal femoral physis often cause significant shortening and angular deformity.[43] Type II lesions, which are usually benign lesions in other physes, are especially prone to complications such as premature physeal closure. The portion of the physis attached to the metaphyseal fragment does not fuse prematurely or form bony bridges, whereas the unattached portion may.

**Proximal Tibia.** Unrecognized Salter-Harris type III fractures cause premature physeal closure, with subsequent varus or valgus deformity.[140, 144, 159, 175] Anterior closure results in hyperextension deformity. Salter-Harris types I or II fractures with posterior displacement may cause catastrophic vascular compromise of the popliteal vessels. Chow and co-workers[37] reported 16 patients with avulsion fractures of the proximal tubercle, two thirds of which were Salter-Harris types I and II injuries and were treated conservatively; type III fractures involving the knee joint were internally fixed. Final results were good in all patients, except for minor complications such as a prominent, uncomfortable tibial tubercle (Fig. 2–23).

**Distal Tibia.** Salter-Harris types III and IV fractures almost always occur at the medial plafond. Fixation should be obtained with transverse pins through the epiphysis or metaphyseal spike; oblique pins may cause premature physeal closure and formation of a bony bridge. Fixation should be with smooth K-wires or screws that do not cross the physis but traverse only the metaphysis and epiphysis (Fig. 2–24). Types I and II fractures can usually be treated by closed means.[33] However, if a large fragment of periosteum is caught in the fracture site and is

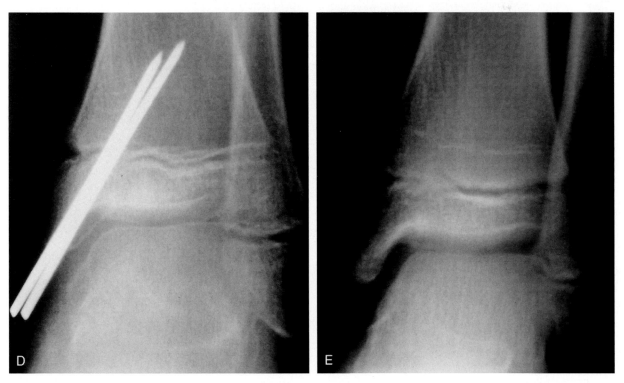

FIGURE 2–21 *Continued. D,* At the time of union and pin removal. *E,* At 2 years, symmetric growth (note the parallel "injury line" proximally) and no bony bridge formation. (*B–E,* From Canale, S.T.; Beaty, J.H., eds. Operative Pediatric Orthopaedics. St. Louis, Mosby–Year Book, 1991.)

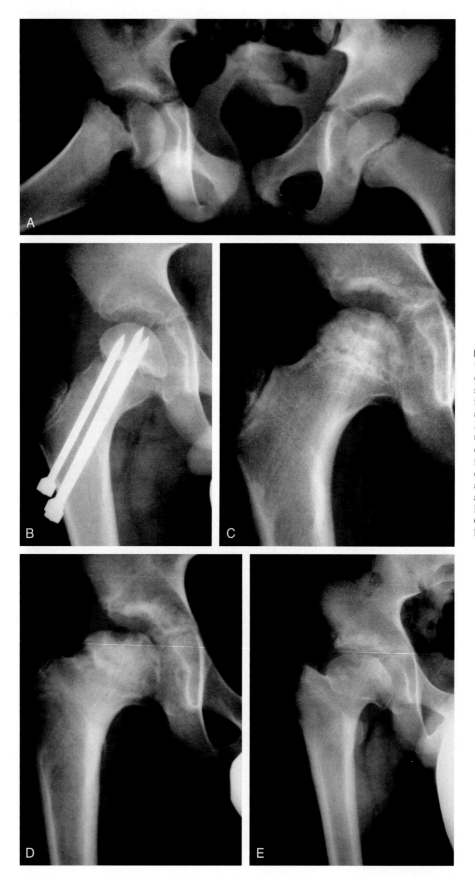

**FIGURE 2–22.** *A,* Type I transepiphyseal fracture in a 6-year-old child. *B,* After closed reduction and fixation with smooth pins. *C,* One year after the fracture, the pins have been removed, and avascular necrosis has developed. *D,* During the course of abduction treatment. *E,* Four years after treatment of avascular necrosis, the femoral neck is short because of premature physeal closure; however, the head is reasonably well shaped, and the result is acceptable. (*A–E,* From Canale, S.T.; Beaty, J.H., eds. Operative Pediatric Orthopaedics. St. Louis, Mosby–Year Book, 1991.)

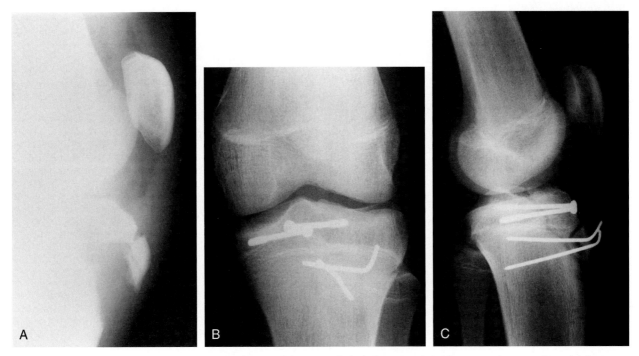

FIGURE 2–23. *A,* Severe Salter-Harris type III or IV fracture of the proximal tibial physis. *B and C,* After open reduction and internal fixation.

preventing adequate reduction and resulting in an unacceptable varus or valgus deformity, open reduction and internal fixation may be necessary[198] (Fig. 2–25). DeSanctis and associates[48] reported that of 113 children with fractures of the distal ends of the tibia and fibula, 10 had growth disturbances. They suggested that the mechanism most likely to damage the physis is adduction-supination with compression, which can produce Salter-Harris type III, IV, or V fractures. These authors recommended open reduction and internal fixation, but noted that poor results occurred even after surgical treatment.

**Calcaneal Physis (Apophysis).** Walling and colleagues[190] described 12 open and closed fractures of the calcaneal apophysis. Open injuries occurred in young children and were associated with subsequent maldevelopment of the posterior portion of the calcaneus from

damage to the growth mechanism. Two adolescent patients had slipped calcaneal apophyses (type I injury), similar to slipped capital femoral epiphyses, and three patients had splitting fractures through the apophysis and physis into the main part of the calcaneus (type IV injury). The authors concluded that injuries to the calcaneal apophysis are comparable to growth mechanism injuries in the long bones (Fig. 2–26). Long-term effects that disrupt the normal developmental process may lead to a deformed calcaneus and hinder weight bearing, especially when concomitant soft tissue injuries are present.

**Proximal Humerus.** Fractures at this location are most commonly Salter-Harris type II injuries; they occur in younger children and remodel satisfactorily (Fig. 2–27A). Open or percutaneous pin fixation is rarely necessary, except when soft tissue (such as the deltoid,

FIGURE 2–24. *A,* Salter-Harris type IV fracture of the distal tibial physis. *B,* After open reduction and internal fixation with cancellous screws.

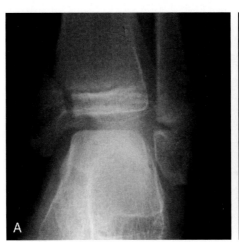
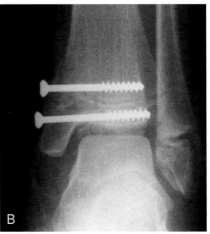

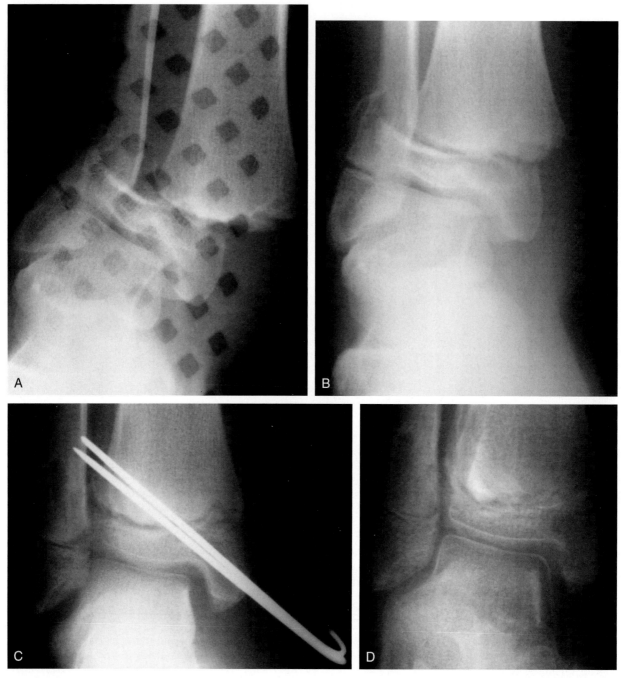

FIGURE 2–25. *A,* Salter-Harris type I fracture of the distal tibial physis in an older child. *B,* After closed reduction, residual angulation is 17°. *C,* After open reduction and internal fixation with smooth pins, a flap of periosteum was found to be caught in the fracture. *D,* At early follow-up, no evidence of a bony bridge can be seen. (*A–D,* From Canale, S.T.; Beaty, J.H., eds. Operative Pediatric Orthopaedics. St. Louis, Mosby–Year Book, 1991.)

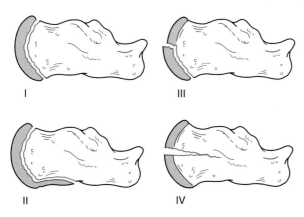

FIGURE 2–26. Schematic depiction of the patterns of growth mechanism fractures affecting the calcaneal apophyseal and physeal regions. The numbers I to IV correspond to the same types of fracture patterns involving the typical long bone physeal-epiphyseal regions. (From Walling, A.K.; Grogan, D.P.; Carty, C.T.; Ogden, J.A. J Orthop Trauma 4:349, 1990.)

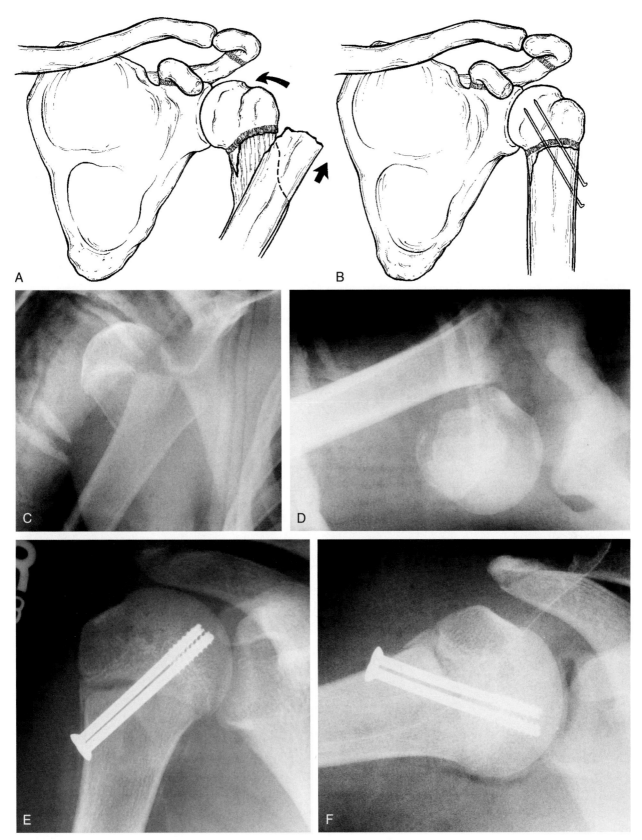

FIGURE 2–27. *A,* Remodeling potential of a proximal humeral epiphyseal fracture because of a periosteal sleeve. *B,* Closed reduction and percutaneous pinning of the proximal humeral epiphyseal separation with two wires cross the physis. *C* and *D,* Anteroposterior and lateral views of the displaced proximal humeral fracture in an unacceptable position. *E* and *F,* After limited open reduction and internal fixation. (*A,* Redrawn from Ogden, J.A. Skeletal Injury in the Child. Philadelphia, Lea & Febiger, 1982. *B,* Redrawn from Magerl, F. Fractures of the proximal humerus. In: Weber, B.G.; Brunner, C.; Freuler, F., eds. Treatment of Fractures in Children and Adolescents. Berlin, Springer-Verlag, 1980.)

biceps tendon, or periosteum) is interposed in the fracture site (Fig. 2–27B).

**Distal Humerus.** Fracture-separation of the entire distal end of the humerus should not be confused with elbow dislocation or fracture of the lateral condyle (Fig. 2–28). Lateral condylar fractures almost always require open reduction and internal fixation (Fig. 2–29). Rutherford[165] reported 39 lateral humeral condylar fractures treated with open reduction and internal fixation. He found that physeal arrest was rare despite malreduction and that the fishtail deformity commonly associated with malreduction did not necessarily predict avascular necrosis.

Medial epicondylar fractures are relatively uncommon. Fracture fragments may be caught in the joint after elbow dislocation, but the fracture can generally be reduced with closed maneuvers (Fig. 2–30). Salter-Harris types I and II fractures of the radial neck can usually be treated in closed fashion with manual reduction or manipulation with a percutaneous pin to achieve an acceptable position of less than 45° of angulation. If open reduction and internal fixation are indicated, adequate fixation should be used to maintain the reduction.

Normal secondary ossification centers of the olecranon should not be confused with physeal fractures (Fig. 2–31). Significant olecranon physeal fractures should be treated as in adults. Closed treatment by lengthy immobilization with the arm in extension to allow apposition and healing may permanently impair flexion of the elbow.

**Distal Radius.** Most Salter-Harris types I and II fractures in this area can be reduced by closed manipulation; the periosteal hinge that is usually present allows easy closed reduction. Rarely, a periosteal flap may prevent reduction, and open reduction and internal fixation may be necessary. Conversely, both-bone fractures of the distal portion of the forearm may be completely displaced and difficult to "hook on" with closed methods.

**Distal Ulna.** Diagnosing this physeal injury may be difficult because of the late ossification of the distal ulnar physis, and concomitant ulnar physeal injuries should be suspected in any injury to the distal end of the radius, especially when an ulnar metaphyseal or styloid fracture is not readily evident. Golz and co-workers[60] reviewed 18 patients with injuries involving the distal ulnar physis.

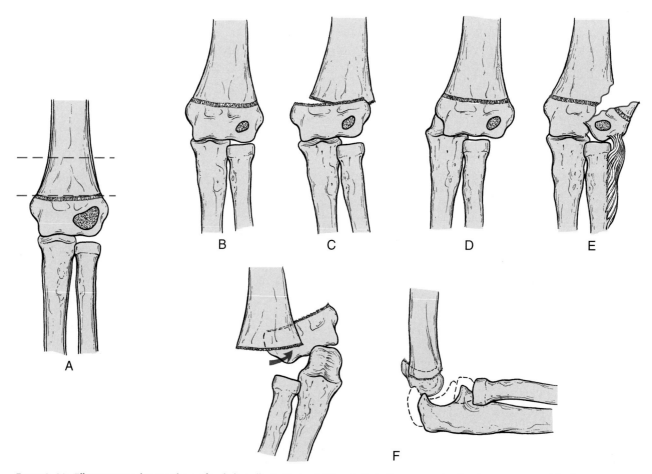

**FIGURE 2–28.** Elbow injuries that may be confused clinically. *A,* Horizontal lines indicate the area proximally where a supracondylar fracture occurs and distally where an epiphyseal fracture-separation occurs in the wide part of the distal end of the humerus in young children. *B,* Normal elbow before three centers of ossification appear. *C,* Separation of the entire distal humeral epiphysis. *D,* Dislocation of the elbow. *E,* Fracture of the lateral condyle. *F,* Fracture-separation of the entire distal humeral epiphysis with posteromedial displacement; note the radial head and proximal part of the ulna being displaced as a unit in relation to the distal end of the humerus. (*A–E,* Redrawn from Mizuno, K.; Hirohata, K.; Kashiwagi, D. J Bone Joint Surg Am 61:570, 1979. *F,* Redrawn from Barrett, W.P.; Almquist, E.A.; Staheli, L.T. J Pediatr Orthop 4:618, 1984.)

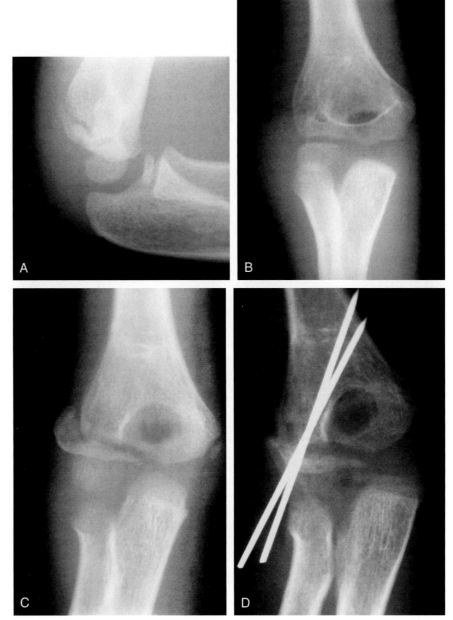

FIGURE 2–29. *A* and *B*, An undisplaced lateral condylar fracture was treated in a long arm cast. *C*, A "Jones view" at 3 weeks shows displacement. *D* and *E*, After open reduction and fixation with smooth wires.

*Illustration continued on following page*

Type I injuries were the most common fracture, with premature physeal closure and ulnar shortening occurring in 55% of the patients. Other effects included radial bowing, ulnar angulation of the distal end of the radius, and ulnar translocation of the carpus. Galeazzi fracture-dislocations in children are rare. An equivalent injury in children is a fracture of the radius with separation of the distal ulnar physis (Salter-Harris type II epiphyseal fracture). The ulnar physis avulses before failure of the triangular fibrocartilage complex (Fig. 2–32). Soft tissue interposition may block reduction and necessitate open reduction (Fig. 2–33). Landfried and colleagues[96] reported three cases, all treated by open reduction and internal fixation. They emphasized the potential for growth disturbance.

## TREATMENT OF COMPLICATIONS

### Growth Acceleration

Fracture of the physis with displacement of the epiphysis may rarely result in accelerated growth of the affected bone. Because of rapid healing of the physis, the increased vascular response to injury is usually briefer than after other fractures, and increased growth is rarely significant. Growth acceleration after physeal injury may be associated with the use of implants or fixation devices, which may stimulate longitudinal growth. For the rare limb length discrepancy caused by accelerated growth that requires treatment, epiphysiodesis may be performed in young patients, or a

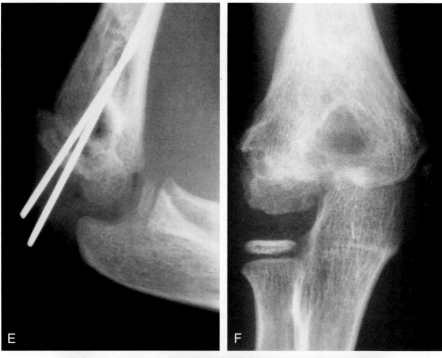

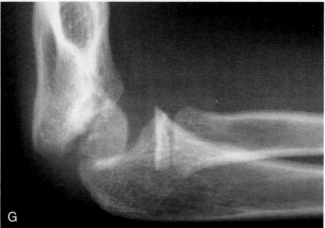

FIGURE **2–29** *Continued. F* and *G,* At 6 months, the wires have been removed and union is complete. (*A–G,* From Canale, S.T.; Beaty, J.H., eds. Operative Pediatric Orthopaedics. St. Louis, Mosby–Year Book, 1991.)

shortening procedure may be done in skeletally mature patients.[28, 30, 141]

## Growth Arrest

### COMPLETE GROWTH ARREST

Complete cessation of growth after physeal injury is uncommon. If it occurs near the end of skeletal growth, it causes no significant impairment. In younger patients, however, complete physeal arrest may lead to a substantial limb length discrepancy. The younger the child, the greater the problem. In adolescents, epiphysiodesis of the contralateral physis may be indicated if it can be done without producing disproportionate extremities (Fig. 2–34). If more than 6 cm of correction is required, epiphysiodesis probably is not indicated. If epiphysiodesis is not feasible, a lengthen-

ing procedure may be considered. Ilizarov[76] and De Bastiani and colleagues,[45, 46] as well as others,[64] have described a technique of limb lengthening by slow distraction with a dynamic axial fixator (callotasis). Callus is formed in response to proximal submetaphyseal corticotomy when distraction is begun 2 weeks later. Once the desired length is obtained, the fixator is worn without distraction until callus formation is evident on radiographs. De Bastiani and coauthors[45] reported mean lengthening of 22% in 100 bony segments in 50 patients with limb length inequality and in 23 with achondroplasia.

These investigators also reported lengthening by chondrodiastasis or controlled symmetric distraction of the physis with the dynamic axial fixator.[46] Fjeld and Steen,[55] however, noted growth retardation after experimental lengthening by physeal distraction. In 7 of their 22 animal models, the physes of the lengthened bones appeared to close earlier than did those

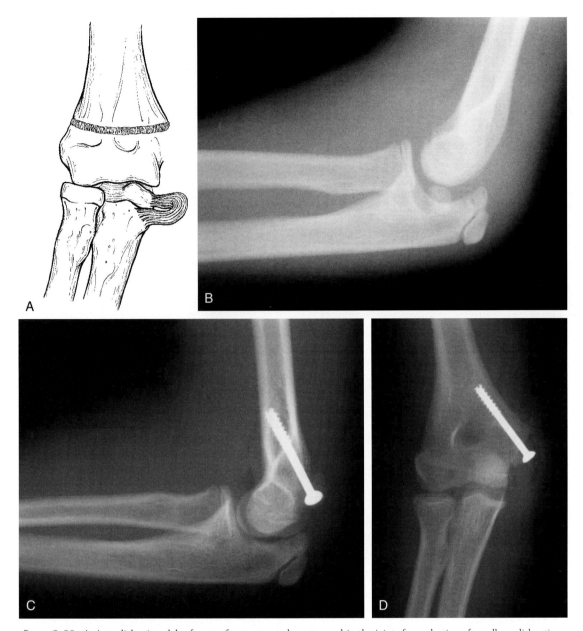

FIGURE **2–30.** *A,* A medial epicondylar fracture fragment may be entrapped in the joint after reduction of an elbow dislocation. *B,* Lateral radiograph revealing a subluxed elbow and medial epicondylar fragment in the joint. *C* and *D,* Anteroposterior radiograph after open reduction and internal fixation with a screw.

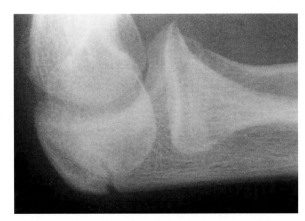

FIGURE **2–31.** Delayed fusion of a secondary ossification center may be confused with an olecranon fracture. (From Canale, S.T.; Beaty, J.H., eds. Operative Pediatric Orthopaedics. St. Louis, Mosby–Year Book, 1991.)

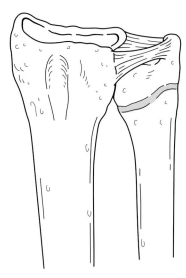

FIGURE 2–32. Attachment of the triangular fibrocartilage complex. The ulnar attachment is at the base of the styloid, and the radial side is on the edge of the articular surface and the radius. (From Landfried, M.J.; Stenclik, M.; Susi, J.G. J Pediatr Orthop 11:332, 1991.)

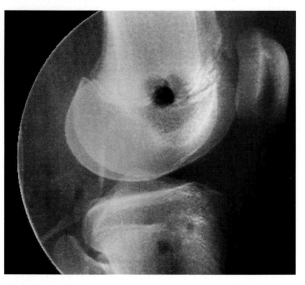

FIGURE 2–34. Lateral radiograph after percutaneous epiphysiodesis of the distal end of the femur; note the "bull's-eye" effect.

of the controls, and growth retardation ranging from 40% to 70% occurred in all animals. They concluded that physeal distraction is a valid method of limb lengthening but appears to have a consistently harmful effect on the physis and should be used only in patients near skeletal maturity. Transplantation of a physis on a vascular pedicle has been reported, but this procedure is not a well-established option.

## PARTIAL GROWTH ARREST

Premature partial arrest of growth of a physis produces angular and longitudinal abnormalities of the involved

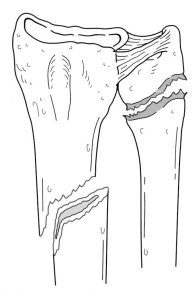

FIGURE 2–33. Fracture pattern. Periosteum was interposed and was blocking fracture reduction. An intact triangular fibrocartilage complex with an epiphyseal fracture is also apparent. (From Landfried, M.J.; Stenclik, M.; Susi, J.G. J Pediatr Orthop 11:332, 1991.)

bone and is much more common than complete growth arrest. Partial arrest occurs when a bridge of bone forms across the physis from the metaphysis to the epiphysis. This bar tethers growth in one area, and as the remaining physis grows, angular deformity occurs. The size and location of the bar determine the clinical deformity.

Any injury to physeal cells may cause formation of a bony bar. The most common cause is fracture, although infection, tumors, irradiation, thermal burns, and metal implants across the physis may also result in the formation of a bony bar. Some authors have suggested factors such as neural and vascular abnormalities, reduced vascular supply from any cause, and metabolic abnormalities. The most common sites of bony bars are the proximal tibial and distal femoral physes, which account for 60% and 70% of the growth of their respective bones.

Clinical signs of bony bar formation are usually angular deformity and shortening of the involved extremity. Growth disturbance lines (Harris lines) associated with episodes of illness or injury in children and adolescents appear in the long bones after shaft fractures. Fractures of the femur, tibia, or fibula cause growth disturbance lines at all the fast-growing physes in both the fractured and the contralateral extremities.[58, 59, 83, 131, 137] Closure of the periphery of the physis or partial arrest after trauma results in a tilt deformity of the extremity; analysis of the character and displacement of Harris lines aids in the diagnosis of physeal arrest. The sclerotic line first appears 6 to 12 weeks after fracture. If the line extends across the width of the metaphysis parallel to the physis in both planes, growth of the entire physis is likely (Fig. 2–35). Focal defects in the line may indicate areas of growth impairment. If the line remains parallel to the physis, angular deformity is unlikely. An oblique line not parallel to the physis is an early warning that growth arrest may occur, especially at the periphery. If the entire physis is involved, comparison of the location of the Harris lines in

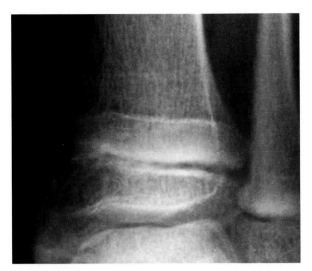

**FIGURE 2–35.** A growth disturbance line parallel to the physis indicates no partial or total growth arrest.

helpful to determine the configuration and area involved by the bony bar and to delineate the configuration and area of the remaining normal physis.

Carlson and Wenger[32] described a method for producing a schematic cross-sectional map on graph paper from data obtained by biplane polytomography (Fig. 2–36). They reported that this map helps identify the lesions that should be treated surgically and aids in planning the surgical approach and resection. They advise that the best results are obtained when 2 years of longitudinal growth remains and the physeal bar involves less than half the physis. Broughton and co-workers[23] reported the results of epiphysiolysis (bony bar resection) in 13 children with partial growth arrest, 8 of whom were monitored to skeletal maturity and the other 5 for at least 4 years. They found epiphysiolysis to be most effective for small bars and those affecting only the central area of the physis. Ogden[135] noted that if more than 40% to 50% of the area of the physis is involved with a bony bridge, an acceptable result is unlikely. Surgery must be performed meticulously and requires familiarity with physeal anatomy in general and the specific anatomy of the bony bridge to be treated.

Treatment of bony bars depends on the age of the patient, the specific physis, and the area of the physis involved. In adolescents with little remaining growth, observation may be the best treatment. In younger patients with significant growth remaining, surgical options include (1) arrest of the remaining growth of the injured physis, which should be considered in older children with mild angular deformity and expected minor limb length discrepancy; (2) arrest of the remaining physis and the physis of the adjacent bone; (3) arrest of the remaining growth of the injured physis, the physis

the injured extremity with those in the contralateral extremity and adjacent physis is also helpful.

In addition to routine radiographs, scanograms should be obtained to document lengths of the extremities. Bone age must be determined to assess the potential for remaining growth. Huurman and colleagues[74] described a simple, rapid, and accurate method for measuring limb length discrepancies with CT. In their technique, the patient receives less radiation, some of the computation errors are eliminated, the cost is comparable to that of scanograms, and joint contractures do not prohibit accurate measurement. Polytomograms are

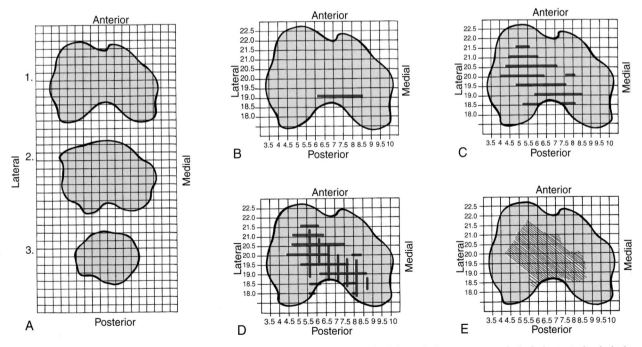

**FIGURE 2–36.** Carlson and Wenger method of mapping physeal bars. *A,* Outlines: *1,* distal femoral physis; *2,* proximal tibial physis; *3,* distal tibial physis. *B,* Anteroposterior projection level indicated by a *thick straight line. C,* All anteroposterior levels plotted from tomograms. *D,* Lateral projection levels plotted. *E,* Final cross-sectional map of the physeal bar. (*A–E,* Redrawn from Carlson, W.O.; Wenger, D.R. J Pediatr Orthop 4:232, 1984.)

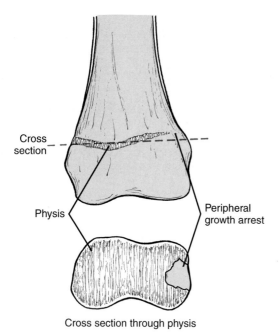

Cross section

Physis

Peripheral growth arrest

Cross section through physis

**FIGURE 2–37.** Type I peripheral growth arrest may cause rapid angular deformity. (Redrawn from Bright, R.W. In: Rockwood, C.A., Jr.; Wilkins, K.E.; King, R.E., eds. Fractures in Children. Philadelphia, J.B. Lippincott, 1984.)

of the adjacent bone, and the corresponding physes of the contralateral bones; (4) combinations of physeal arrest with opening or closing wedge osteotomies to correct the angular deformity; (5) opening or closing wedge osteotomy without physeal arrest, which may require several osteotomies because of recurrence of the deformity; (6) lengthening or shortening of the involved bone (shortening should be considered only for the femur); (7) resection of the bony bar and insertion of interposition material; (8) resection of the bony bar and osteotomy for correction of the angular deformity; and (9) various combinations of these techniques.

Bright[20] classified partial growth arrest into three types according to location and treatment: type I, peripheral; type II, central; and type III, combined. Type I lesions can be approached through a peripheral incision; the periosteum is elevated and the bony bridge is resected through a small window (Fig. 2–37). Type II lesions require a more extensive and difficult approach. The skin incision is the same, but the periosteal flap is kept entirely on the metaphyseal side of the physis. A metaphyseal window is made close to the bony bridge, through which it is removed with a curette and dental bur (Fig. 2–38). Type III lesions cause extensive angular deformities and require removal of the bony bridge and osteotomy for correction (Fig. 2–39). According to Bright,[20] varus or valgus angulation of 15° or less does not require corrective osteotomy in young children if adequate bony bridge resection is accomplished. Both Bright[20] and Langenskiöld and associates[97, 98] recommend osteotomy for angulation only if it is more than 25° to 30° for deformities in the plane of motion of the adjacent joint (Fig. 2–40). Bright[20, 21] reported that angular deformities correct within a year of restoration of longitudinal growth and more quickly if the deformity is in the plane of joint motion.

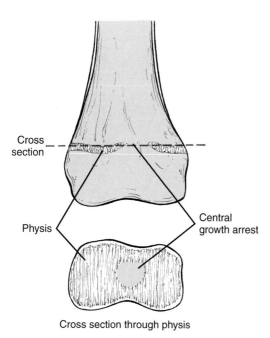

Cross section

Physis

Central growth arrest

Cross section through physis

**FIGURE 2–38.** Type II central growth arrest with physeal tenting into the metaphysis; the entire perichondral ring is open and intact to provide longitudinal growth. (Redrawn from Bright, R.W. In: Rockwood, C.A., Jr.; Wilkins, K.E.; King, R.E., eds. Fractures in Children. Philadelphia, J.B. Lippincott, 1984.)

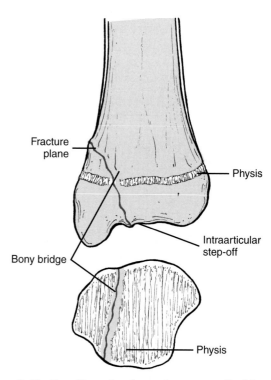

Fracture plane

Physis

Intraarticular step-off

Bony bridge

Physis

**FIGURE 2–39.** Type III combined growth arrest usually follows a Salter-Harris type III or IV fracture that was incompletely reduced. (Redrawn from Bright, R.W. In: Rockwood, C.A., Jr.; Wilkins, K.E.; King, R.E., eds. Fractures in Children. Philadelphia, J.B. Lippincott, 1984.)

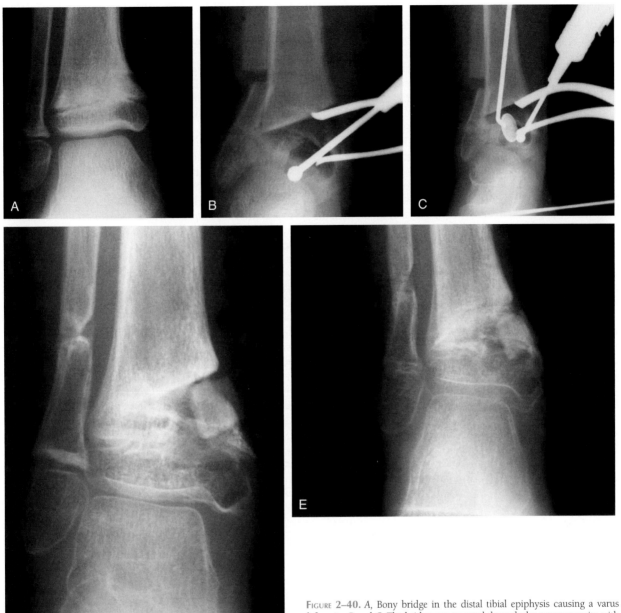

FIGURE 2–40. *A,* Bony bridge in the distal tibial epiphysis causing a varus deformity. *B* and *C,* The bridge was resected through the osteotomy site with the aid of a laminar spreader; a dental mirror and bur ensure removal of all of the bridge. *D* and *E,* At early follow-up.

Resection with interposition material to prevent formation of a bony bar was evaluated experimentally by Peterson.[148, 149] Among interposition materials tested were gold leaf, rubber film, Gelfoam, bone wax, methyl methacrylate, muscle, fat, and cartilage. The results of his study and those of other authors, including Langenskiöld and Bright, are varied, but evidence suggests that formation of a bony bar can be prevented or inhibited by the use of fat or other interposition materials; conversely, when no interposition material is used, bar formation recurs consistently.[26, 180] Peterson[149] reported the successful use of methyl methacrylate with barium (cranioplast) as an interposition material in 68 patients. Olin and colleagues[142] developed a procedure for transplanting free autogenous iliac crest physeal grafts into defects in the lateral aspect of the distal femoral physes of

rabbits. The transplant was composed of a fibrocartilaginous layer, cartilage similar to physeal cartilage, and a physis. Their results showed that such a transplant can prevent bony bridge formation, growth arrest, or development of a valgus deformity when placed in the lateral femoral condyle after excision of a focal bony bridge. Mayr and associates[113] described reconstruction of the distal tibial physis with an autologous graft from the iliac crest consisting of apophyseal cartilage and perichondrium. Three years after surgery, the stability of the ankle was excellent, with adequate growth of the reconstructed physis.

Langenskiöld and co-workers[98, 99] reported that in skeletally immature pigs, osseous cavities filled with autogenous fat elongated with growth and, as the cavity elongated, the fat expanded to fill the defect.[126, 127]

Histologic analysis demonstrated living adipose tissue, which has been shown to have an inhibitory effect on osteogenesis. These investigators also preferred fat for interposition in the belief that the chemical and physical properties of fat contribute more than simple interposition to prevent recurrence of the bony bridge. Ogden[134] reported the use of fat interposition in open reduction and internal fixation of acute Salter-Harris type IV fractures. He recommended, in addition to fat interposition, removal of the metaphyseal side of the small type IV fracture fragment (Thurston-Holland sign), especially at the malleoli, to convert the fracture to a type III injury and help prevent the formation of bony bridges. Enough fat can usually be taken at the edge of the operative site, but when the bridge resection is large, fat may be taken from the gluteal area.

Physeal transfer may offer a method of replacing the damaged physis.[132, 201] Lalanandham and associates[95] monitored the viability and metabolism of cartilage transplanted to the physeal regions of rabbits. In addition to measuring growth, they performed histochemical and autoradiographic studies. Their results indicated that avascular cartilage transplants could remain viable, could synthesize proteoglycan, and were associated with growth, though less than normal growth. Nettelblad and co-workers[126] in 1984 showed that free microvascular physeal transfers were superior to nonmicrovascular transfers in rabbits. They found that a vascularized physeal graft could be transplanted from its normal site to the contralateral site with maintenance of normal growth capacity. However, they believe that clinical applications are minimal until further investigations determine how the transplanted physis reacts when transferred to a heterotopic anatomic site with altered stress. Bowen and colleagues[17] developed a method for transferring the metaphysis and epiphysis of the distal end of the ulna in dogs and microsurgically revascularizing them from the pedicle of the anterior interosseous vessels. When both circulations were revascularized, the grafts retained their structural integrity, and growth continued at rates only slightly lower than normal (mean of 85%). If either or both circulations were not revascularized, growth rates were lower, and skeletal collapse of the ischemic bone was frequent. These investigators also developed a method of skeletal fixation but found the long-term clinical results to be unsatisfactory because of fracture of the graft after a mean of 8.2 weeks. Boyer and co-workers[19] compared the growth in vascularized physeal allograft transplants, autografts, and nonoperated physes in rabbits, with and without immunosuppression with cyclosporine. They found that the proximal tibial physeal autografts, with or without cyclosporine, and allografts with cyclosporine grew at rates similar to that of the nonoperated physes. These authors suggested that development of specific immunosuppressive techniques could allow successful transplantation of physeal allografts in children.

Whatever surgical technique is chosen, a knowledge of the underlying physeal anatomy and the relationship of overlying structures to the physis is essential. Birch and colleagues[12] examined by anatomic dissection the most commonly affected physes—the distal radial, distal femoral, proximal tibial, and distal tibial and fibular physes—and described their surgical anatomy. Their observations and recommendations are summarized in the following paragraphs.

**Distal Radial Physis.** The physis of the distal end of the radius is completely extracapsular and is easily exposed by any direct approach on its volar, dorsal, or radial aspect; it is obscured by the ulna medially. The volar metaphysis is cloaked by the pronator quadratus and is best exposed through the volar approach of Henry, but with the radial artery retracted radially rather than ulnarly.

**Distal Femoral Physis.** The synovial reflection of the suprapatellar pouch obscures portions of the anterior, medial, and lateral aspects of the distal end of the femur and must be bluntly dissected anteriorly. The capsular attachment extends to the level of the physis anteriorly and posteriorly. The insertion of the adductor magnus tendon medially and the intermuscular septum laterally serve as landmarks to the level of the physis. This physis is best exposed through a posteromedial approach as described by Trickey[186] and a direct posterior exposure, with mobilization and protection of the neurovascular bundle.

**Proximal Tibial Physis.** The physis of the proximal end of the tibia is completely extracapsular. The medial aspect of the physis is covered by the medial collateral ligament and tendons of the pes anserinus; in direct exposure, these structures can be mobilized and retracted without difficulty. The anterolateral and anteromedial aspects of the metaphysis are easily accessible, but care must be taken to avoid injury to the apophysis of the tibial tubercle. The posterior aspects of the physis and the metaphysis are obscured in the midline by the popliteus muscle, and this posterolateral region is the least surgically accessible. The posteromedial aspect of the metaphysis can be approached through a modification of the Banks-Laufman[9] exposure of the posteromedial portion of the tibia. After developing the interval between the semitendinosus and the medial aspect of the gastrocnemius, the popliteus muscle is mobilized and reflected distally and laterally.

**Distal Tibial and Fibular Physes.** The distal tibial physis is entirely extracapsular. The anterior and posterior tibiofibular ligaments insert across the anterolateral and posterolateral aspects of the physis of the distal end of the fibula. Direct exposure is difficult only on the lateral aspect of the tibia, where the physis is obscured by the overlying fibula.

## Apophyseal Injuries

An apophysis is defined as a bony prominence onto which muscles or tendons are attached. In children, each apophysis is connected to bone through a histologically recognizable physis. The shape and size of an apophysis are influenced by the forces placed on it by its muscle or tendon attachments. Because of the forces affecting them, these structures are called traction apophyses. Some apophyses have only a single muscle or tendon attachment, whereas others are attached to whole muscle groups.

Initially, the apophyses appear as cartilaginous prominences at the ends of or along the sides of bones; later, centers of ossification develop similar to those of other physes. The ossification centers then either fuse with an associated epiphysis, such as the tibial tubercle fusing with the proximal tibial epiphysis, or remain as isolated centers of ossification. Eventually, the physeal plate between the ossification center and the shaft of the bone disappears as bony fusion is achieved. Because the attachments to the apophysis are very strong, excessive force usually causes avulsion or fracture through the apophysis rather than pulling of the tendon from its insertion (Fig. 2–41).

Most commonly, problems with the apophyses are inflammation or partial avulsion caused by repetitive microtrauma (traction apophysitis). These injuries typically occur in active adolescents between the ages of 8 and 15 years and are usually manifested as periarticular pain. Common sites of apophyseal injury are the knee (Osgood-Schlatter disease and Sinding-Larsen-Johansson syndrome), heel (Sever's disease), medial epicondyle of the humerus (so-called Little League elbow), ischial tuberosity,[53, 116] and spine.[29]

Osgood-Schlatter disease is a traction apophysitis of the tibial tubercle that commonly occurs in boys 13 to 14 years of age and girls 10 to 11 years of age. Inflammation and new bone formation at the tendon insertion are characteristic.[92, 139] Differential diagnoses include patellar peritendinitis, Sinding-Larsen-Johansson syndrome, avulsion fracture of the tibial tuberosity, tumor, and infection. The diagnosis of Osgood-Schlatter disease is based on clinical signs and symptoms such as pain, heat, tenderness, and usually local swelling and prominence in the area of the tibial tuberosity. Pain typically occurs when the knee is extended against resistance. The most important radiographic sign is soft tissue swelling anterior to the tibial tuberosity. Lazovic and colleagues[102] recommended ultrasonography for diagnosis of apophyseal injuries because it requires no radiation exposure

and allows early detection of injury even when an ossification center is not present in the apophysis. The condition usually resolves within 1 to 2 years, but, in about 10% of patients, the formation of a discrete ossicle and bursa causes pain and tenderness.

Reduction of stress on the apophysis is the objective of management and can usually be obtained with some restriction of activity and the use of knee pads for sports in which direct knee contact occurs. If the pain is severe, the extremity may be immobilized in a commercial knee immobilizer for 6 weeks. In chronic conditions, the ossicle may become so painful that it requires excision.[122] Avulsion fracture of the proximal tibial apophysis is relatively uncommon but does occur.[38] Zimbler and Merkow[204] described a genu recurvatum deformity caused by Osgood-Schlatter disease; this abnormality was originally described in 1952 by Stirling[181] as a complication of Osgood-Schlatter disease. It rarely requires treatment.

Sinding-Larsen-Johansson syndrome is a traction apophysitis of the distal pole of the patella and is the juvenile equivalent of the "jumper's knee" seen in mature patients. It also occurs in patients with cerebral palsy who walk in a crouched position. According to Medlar and Lyne,[114] the condition occurs most commonly in boys between the ages of 10 and 13 years, is usually unilateral, and requires 3 to 12 months for resolution. Inflammation is localized to the tendon attachment of the distal patellar pole and is followed by calcification in distinct radiographic stages. Treatment is the same as for Osgood-Schlatter disease.

Accessory ossicles of the malleoli in skeletally immature individuals, as described by Ogden and Lee,[138] may develop in either malleolus. Although they appear to be separate entities on radiographs, these foci are not anatomically separate. Ossicles are usually asymptomatic, but they can be injured acutely or chronically. The diagnosis of such injury by conventional radiographs is limited. A bone scan may be positive if a stress fracture is present. An ossicle may also be avulsed as a ligament failure analogue, similar to a sleeve fracture of the patella.

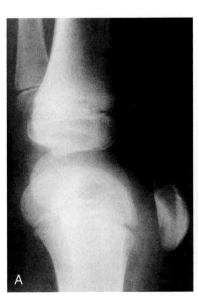
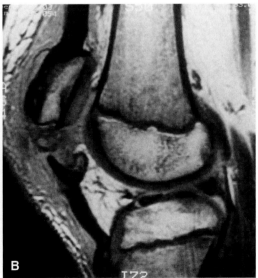

FIGURE 2–41. *A*, Lateral radiograph of the right knee showing a small avulsion fracture of the inferior pole of the patella and patella alta. *B*, Magnetic resonance image of the right knee in the sagittal plane showing an avulsion fracture of the inferior pole of the patella with an attached sleeve of cartilage. (*A, B*, From Shands, P.A.; McQueen, D.A. J Bone Joint Surg Am 77:1721, 1995.)

Traction (avulsion) apophysitis of the medial malleolus can occur after sports activity in children. Ishii and co-workers[77] reported three children with chronic injuries of the medial tibial malleolus caused by traction injuries during sports. All three had swelling of the medial malleolus, tenderness over its anterior part, and pain on forced valgus movement of the foot. Radiographs revealed bilateral accessory ossification centers, and MRI demonstrated partial avulsion or an avulsion fracture of the apophyseal cartilage and fragmentation of the accessory centers.

Sever's disease[172] (calcaneal apophysitis) is a frequent overuse syndrome in growing children. It is most often seen in those who are in a growth spurt and involved in vigorous physical activity. The calcaneal apophysis appears in boys at an average age of 7.9 years and in girls at an average age of 5.6 years. It is initially an area of irregular ossification of less density than the surrounding bone and is located in the lower portion of the posterior surface of the calcaneus. The most frequent differential diagnosis is retrocalcaneal bursitis. In calcaneal apophysitis, the heel is tender when the apophysis is compressed on its medial and lateral sides, and dorsiflexion of the ankle is limited. In retrocalcaneal bursitis, the point of maximal tenderness is immediately anterior to the Achilles tendon at the superior border of the calcaneus when compression is applied from the medial and lateral sides. Radiographic findings in Sever's disease are controversial. Some believe that the appearance of the calcaneal apophysis is changed in symptomatic patients, whereas others believe that the radiographs reflect normal variations attributable to skeletal age, weight, activity, and flexibility. In patients with unilateral heel pain, radiographs may help rule out other pathologic conditions such as tumor, infection, or fracture. Treatment consists of activity restriction and the use of heel cups and Plastizole inserts.[120] Immobilization in a short leg cast for 4 to 6 weeks may be indicated for patients with acute symptoms. Lokiec and Wientroub[109] described osteochondritis of the medial plantar apophysis of the calcaneus that caused medial plantar heel pain in a 15-year-old basketball player. The lesion was detected radiographically and by increased focal uptake on bone scan. Conservative treatment resulted in complete pain relief and a normal calcaneal appearance with union of the osteochondral fragment; no recurrence was noted during a 3-year follow-up.

Iliac apophysitis was reported in 18 adolescent runners by Clancy and Foltz[40] in 1976. They postulated that the mechanism of injury was an inflammatory reaction of the unfused iliac apophysis caused either by repetitive muscular contraction or by subclinical stress fractures of the apophysis. All their patients were able to return to running after 4 to 6 weeks of rest. Kujala and colleagues[93] reviewed 14 patients with ischial apophysitis and 21 with avulsion of the ischial tuberosity and found that patients with apophysitis (14.1 years) were younger than those with avulsion (18.9 years); apophysitis usually healed with no complications, while avulsion often caused prolonged pain that required surgery. Lombardo and co-workers[110] reported a bilateral radiographic abnormality, "discontinuity" of the anterior part of the iliac apophysis, in 9 of 13 adolescent athletes with

a diagnosis of "hip-pointer" injuries. They believed this discontinuity to be an anatomic anomaly that was vulnerable to injury by either repetitive or acute trauma. The discontinuity disappeared at skeletal maturity in all nine patients; eight of the nine improved with a regimen of reduced activity, with total resolution of symptoms in 1 to 8 months. One cross-country runner continued to have symptoms for 4 years. Takayanagi and colleagues[183] reported a patient who had knee pain 10 years after avulsion of the ischial tuberosity; he had significant bone and muscle atrophy of the thigh, and the knee pain was relieved after strengthening of the hamstrings. In a patient with sciatic nerve palsy, Spinner and associates[179] found a large ossified fragment within the biceps muscle of the thigh abutting the sciatic nerve at the level of the lesser trochanter. The fragment resulted from an unrecognized apophyseal avulsion fracture of the ischial tuberosity that the patient had sustained while sprinting 27 years earlier. Avulsion of the pelvic apophysis is usually caused by sudden contraction of the hamstrings, adductor magnus, iliopsoas, and hip flexors in athletes participating in sports involving a high contraction rate or forceful hamstring stretch, such as sprinting, long jumping, or hurdling (Fig. 2–42). These avulsions have

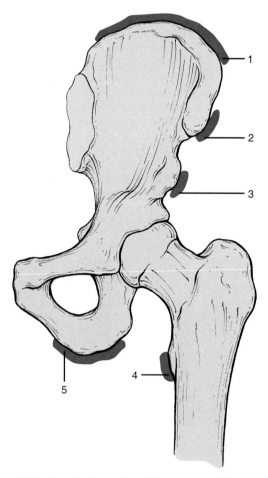

**FIGURE 2–42.** Sites of pelvic avulsion fractures reported by Fernbach and Wilkinson. *1,* Iliac crest; *2,* anterior superior iliac spine; *3,* anterior inferior iliac spine; *4,* lesser trochanter; *5,* ischium/ischial apophysis. (Redrawn from Fernbach, S.K.; Wilkinson, R.J. AJR Am J Roentgenol 137:581, 1981.)

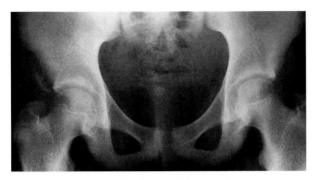

**FIGURE 2–43.** Avulsion of the anterior inferior iliac spine in a soccer player caused by resisted flexion of the hip.

been classified as apophysiolysis (undisplaced), acute avulsion fractures, and old ununited avulsions (Fig. 2–43). Pain in the groin and buttock is the most common symptom. With separation of the ischial apophysis, the gap is palpable and should be sought after any suspected hamstring injury.[169] Radiographs confirm the diagnosis (see Fig. 2–11). Conservative management is generally sufficient if the displacement is minimal; wide separation of the fracture fragments may require surgical intervention if symptoms persist. Wooton and colleagues[200] reported chronic disability in three athletes with nonunion or avulsion of the ischial tuberosity; all resumed their sport after open reduction and internal fixation of the fracture. These workers also successfully treated one acute fracture with wide displacement by open reduction and internal fixation and recommend such management for acute fractures with more than 2 cm of displacement.

Vertebral apophysitis, or "atypical Scheuermann's disease," is frequently associated with repetitive sports activity and may represent compression fractures caused by repetitive microtrauma, most commonly in the thoracolumbar spine[65, 119, 168] (Fig. 2–44). Acute injuries of the vertebral ring apophyses and intervertebral discs have also been reported in adolescent athletes, especially those involved in jumping sports such as gymnastics and in weightlifting.[182] The ring apophysis is separated from the vertebral body by a cartilaginous layer and may be displaced by trauma. Although radiographs may be normal initially, injury to the vertebral ring apophysis may be followed by prolapse of disc material, reduction of disc height, and disc degeneration; thus, long-term follow-up of athletes with back symptoms is essential. Peh and co-workers[147] found that posterior lumbar vertebral apophyseal ring fractures were difficult to identify on MRI and recommended careful review of radiographs, supplemented by targeted CT, for diagnosis.

Olecranon apophysitis may be caused by abnormal stress of the triceps attachment on the olecranon apophysis.[143] Kovach and associates[91] and Micheli[117] have reported persistence of the separated olecranon secondary ossification center into adulthood.

Medial epicondylar apophysitis occurs most frequently in children and adolescents involved in throwing sports, especially baseball, but it has been reported in other sports, including gymnastics, wrestling, and weightlifting (Fig. 2–45). Repetitive microtrauma is caused by tension stress across the medial epicondyle and collateral ligaments. With excessive throwing action, the medial epicondyle may become prominent and painful. Active adolescent baseball pitchers frequently have accelerated growth and widening of the medial epicondylar apophysis; fragmentation of the apophysis is occasionally noted. The pain generally resolves with rest, usually with no significant sequelae.

Avulsion of the medial epicondyle may result from a valgus injury to the elbow or occasionally from forceful pull of the forearm flexor muscles. These avulsions are usually minimally displaced and can be treated with 2 to

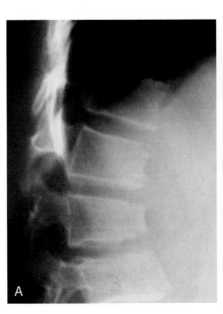
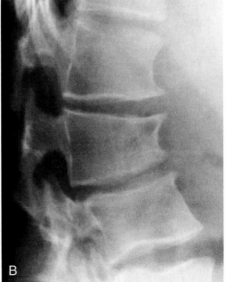

**FIGURE 2–44.** *A,* A radiograph of a 12-year-old gymnast with nagging back pain shows thoracolumbar Scheuermann's disease. *B,* At the age of 19 years, she is pain free, but this radiograph shows permanent wedging.

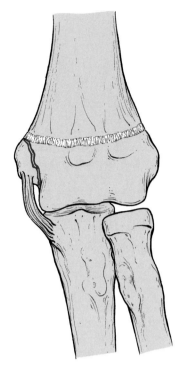

**FIGURE 2–45.** Medial epicondylar apophysitis.

3 weeks of immobilization (Fig. 2–46). If valgus instability is suspected, stress radiographs should be obtained. Surgical treatment may be required for instability, entrapment of the fragment within the joint, or ulnar nerve dysfunction.

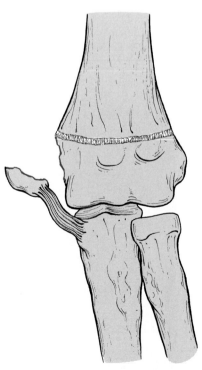

**FIGURE 2–46.** Medial epicondylar avulsion.

## REFERENCES

1. Abraham, E. Remodeling potential of long bones following angular osteotomies. J Pediatr Orthop 9:37, 1989.
2. Abram, L.J.; Thompson, G.H. Deformity after premature closure of the distal radial physis following a torus fracture with a physeal compression injury. J Bone Joint Surg Am 69:1450, 1987.
3. Aitken, A.P. Fractures of the epiphyses. Clin Orthop 41:19, 1965.
4. Albanese, S.A.; Palmer, A.K.; Kerr, D.R.; et al. Wrist pain and distal growth plate closure of the radius in gymnasts. J Pediatr Orthop 9:23, 1989.
5. Aminian, A.; Schoenecker, P.L. Premature closure of the distal radial physis after fracture of the distal radial metaphysis. J Pediatr Orthop 15:495, 1995.
6. Apple, D.F., Jr.; McDonald, A. Long-distance running and the immature skeleton. Orthopedics 3:929, 1981.
7. Attkiss, K.J.; Buncke, H.J. Physeal growth arrest of the distal phalanx of the thumb in an adolescent pianist: A case report. J Hand Surg [Am] 23:956, 1998.
8. Bado, J.L. The Monteggia lesion. Clin Orthop 50:71, 1967.
9. Banks, S.W.; Laufman, H. An Atlas of Surgical Exposures of the Extremities. Philadelphia, W.B. Saunders, 1953.
10. Bertin, K.C.; Goble, E.M. Ligament injuries associated with physeal fractures about the knee. Clin Orthop 177:188, 1983.
11. Bielski, R.J.; Bassett, G.S.; Fideler, B.; Tolo, V.T. Intraosseous infusions: Effects on immature physis—an experimental model in rabbits. J Pediatr Orthop 13:511, 1993.
12. Birch, J.G.; Herring, J.A.; Wenger, D.R. Surgical anatomy of selected physes. J Pediatr Orthop 4:224, 1984.
13. Boker, F.H.L.; Burbach, T. Ultrasonic diagnosis of separation of the proximal humeral epiphysis in the newborn. J Bone Joint Surg Am 72:187, 1990.
14. Borsa, J.J.; Peterson, H.A.; Ehman, R.L. MR imaging of physeal bars. Radiology 199:683, 1996.
15. Böstman, O.; Makela, E.A.; Sodergard, J.; et al. Absorbable polyglycolide pins in internal fixation of fractures in children. J Pediatr Orthop 13:242, 1993.
16. Böstman, O.; Makela, E.A.; Tormala, P.; Rokkanen, P. Transphyseal fracture fixation using biodegradable pins. J Bone Joint Surg Br 71:706, 1989.
17. Bowen, C.V.A.; Ethridge, G.P.; O'Brien, B.M.; et al. Experimental microvascular growth plate transfers. Part 2—Investigation of feasibility. J Bone Joint Surg Br 70:311, 1988.
18. Bowler, J.R.; Mubarak, S.J.; Wenger, D. Tibial physeal closure and genu recurvatum after femoral fracture: Occurrence without a tibial traction pin. J Pediatr Orthop 10:653, 1990.
19. Boyer, M.I.; Danska, J.S.; Nolan, L.; et al. Microvascular transplantation of physeal allografts. J Bone Joint Surg Br 77:806, 1995.
20. Bright, R.W. Partial growth arrest: Identification, classification, and results of treatment [abstract]. Orthop Trans 6:65, 1982.
21. Bright, R.W.; Elmore, S.M. Physical properties of epiphyseal plate cartilage. Surg Forum 19:463, 1968.
22. Bright, R.W.; Burstein, A.H.; Elmore, S.M. Epiphyseal-plate cartilage: A biomechanical and histological analysis of failure modes. J Bone Joint Surg Am 56:688, 1974.
23. Broughton, N.S.; Dickens, D.R.V.; Cole, W.G.; Menelaus, M.B. Epiphysiolysis for partial growth plate arrest: Results after four years or at maturity. J Bone Joint Surg Br 71:13, 1989.
24. Brown, J.; Eustace, S. Neonatal transphyseal supracondylar fracture detected by ultrasound. Pediatr Emerg Care 13:419, 1997.
25. Bucholz, R.W.; Ezaki, M.; Ogden, J.A. Injury to the acetabular triradiate physeal cartilage. J Bone Joint Surg Am 64:600, 1982.
26. Bueche, M.J.; Phillips, W.A.; Gordon, J.; et al. Effect of interposition material on mechanical behaviour in partial physeal resection: A canine model. J Pediatr Orthop 10:459, 1990.
27. Caine, D.; Howe, W.; Ross, W.; Bergman, G. Does repetitive physical loading inhibit radial growth in female gymnasts? Clin J Sports Med 7:302, 1997.
28. Canale, S.T. Special techniques. In: Canale, S.T.; Beaty, J.H., eds. Operative Pediatric Orthopaedics. St. Louis, Mosby–Year Book, 1991.
29. Canale, S.T. Sports medicine. In: Canale, S.T.; Beaty, J.H., eds. Operative Pediatric Orthopaedics. St. Louis, Mosby–Year Book, 1991.

30. Canale, S.T.; Russell, T.; Holcomb, R. Percutaneous epiphysiodesis: Experimental study and preliminary clinical results. J Pediatr Orthop 6:150, 1986.

31. Carey, J.; Spence, L.; Blickman, H.; Eustace, S. MRI of pediatric growth plate injury: Correlation with plain film radiographs and clinical outcome. Skeletal Radiol 27:250, 1998.

32. Carlson, W.O.; Wenger, D.R. A mapping method to prepare for surgical excision of a partial physeal arrest. J Pediatr Orthop 4:232, 1984.

33. Carter, S.R.; Aldridge, M.J. Stress injury of the distal radial growth plate. J Bone Joint Surg Br 70:834, 1988.

34. Chadwick, C.J. Spontaneous resolution of varus deformity of the ankle following adduction injury of the distal tibial epiphysis. J Bone Joint Surg Am 64:774, 1982.

35. Chadwick, C.J.; Bentley, G. The classification and prognosis of epiphyseal injuries. Injury 18:157, 1987.

36. Chang, C.Y.; Shih, C.; Penn, I.W.; et al. Wrist injuries in adolescent gymnasts of a Chinese opera school: Radiographic survey. Radiology 195:861, 1995.

37. Chow, S.P.; Lam, J.J.; Leong, J.C.Y. Fracture of the tibial tubercle in the adolescent. J Bone Joint Surg Br 72:231, 1990.

38. Christie, M.J.; Dvonch, V.M. Tibial tuberosity avulsion fracture in adolescents. J Pediatr Orthop 1:391, 1981.

39. Chung, S.M.K.; Batterman, S.C.; Brighton, C.T. Shear strength of the human femoral capital epiphyseal plate. J Bone Joint Surg Am 58:94, 1976.

40. Clancy, W.G., Jr.; Foltz, A.S. Iliac apophysitis and stress fractures in adolescent runners. Am J Sports Med 4:214, 1976.

41. Clayer, M.; Boatright, C.; Conrad, E. Growth disturbances associated with untreated benign bone cysts. Aust N Z J Surg 67:872, 1997.

42. Craig, J.G.; Cramer, K.E.; Cody, D.D.; et al. Premature partial closure and other deformities of the growth plate: MR imaging and three-dimensional modeling. Radiology 210:835, 1999.

43. Czitrom, A.A.; Salter, R.B.; Willis, R.B. Fractures involving the distal femoral epiphyseal plate of the femur. Int Orthop 4:269, 1981.

44. Damron, T.A.; Spadaro, J.A.; Margulies, B.; Damron, L.A. Dose response of amifostine in protection of growth plate function from irradiation effects. Int J Cancer 90:73, 2000.

45. De Bastiani, G.; Aldegheri, R.; Renzi-Brivio, L.; Trivella, G. Limb lengthening by callus distraction (callotasis). J Pediatr Orthop 7:129, 1987.

46. De Bastiani, G.; Aldegheri, R.; Renzi-Brivio, L.; Trivella, G. Chondrodiastasis-controlled symmetrical distraction of the epiphyseal plate. Limb lengthening in children. J Bone Joint Surg Br 68:550, 1986.

47. DeLee, J.C.; Wilkins, K.E.; Rogers, L.F.; Rockwood, C.A. Fracture-separation of the distal humeral epiphysis. J Bone Joint Surg Am 62:46, 1980.

48. de Sanctis, N.; Della Corte, S.; Pempinello, C. Distal tibial and fibular epiphyseal fractures in children: Prognostic criteria and long-term results in 158 patients. J Pediatr Orthop B 9:40, 2000.

49. DiFiori, J.P.; Puffer, J.C.; Mandelbaum, B.R.; Dorey, F. Distal radial growth plate injury and positive ulnar variance in nonelite gymnasts. Am J Sports Med 25:763, 1997.

50. Eady, J.L.; Cardenas, C.D.; Sopa, D. Avulsion of the femoral attachment of the anterior cruciate ligament in a seven-year-old child. J Bone Joint Surg Am 64:1376, 1982.

51. Edwards, P.H., Jr.; Grana, W.A. Physeal fractures about the knee. J Am Acad Orthop Surg 3:63, 1995.

52. Etchebehere, E.C.; Caron, M.; Pereira, J.A.; et al. Activation of the growth plates on three-phase bone scintigraphy: The explanation for the overgrowth of fractured femurs. Eur J Nucl Med 28:72, 2001.

53. Fernbach, S.K.; Wilkinson, R.J. Avulsion injuries of the pelvis and proximal femur. AJR Am J Roentgenol 137:581, 1981.

54. Fischer, M.D.; McElfresh, E.C. Physeal and periphyseal injuries of the hand. Patterns of injury and results of treatment. Hand Clin 10:287, 1994.

55. Fjeld, T.O.; Steen, H. Growth retardation after experimental limb lengthening by epiphyseal distraction. J Pediatr Orthop 10:463, 1990.

56. Foster, B.K.; John, B.; Hasler, C. Free fat interpositional graft in acute physeal injuries: The anticipatory Langenskiöld procedure. J Pediatr Orthop 20:282, 2000.

57. Foucher, M. De la divulsion des epiphyses. Congr Med France (Paris) 1:63, 1863.

58. Frick, S.L.; Shoemaker, S.; Mubarak, S.J. Altered fibular growth patterns after tibiofibular synostosis in children. J Bone Joint Surg Am 83:247, 2001.

59. Garn, S.M.; Silverman, F.N.; Hertzog, K.P.; Rohmann, C.G. Lines and bands of increased density: Their implication to growth and development. Med Radiogr Photogr 44:58, 1968.

60. Golz, R.J.; Grogan, D.P.; Greene, T.L.; et al. Distal ulnar physeal injury. J Pediatr Orthop 11:318, 1991.

61. Gomes, L.S.; Volpon, J.B. Experimental physeal fracture-separations treated with rigid internal fixation. J Bone Joint Surg Am 75:1756, 1993.

62. Gomes, L.S.; Volpon, J.B.; Gonclaves, R.P. Traumatic separation of epiphyses: An experimental study in rats. Clin Orthop 236:286, 1988.

63. Grantham, S.A.; Kiernan, H.A. Displaced olecranon fractures in children. J Trauma 15:197, 1975.

64. Greco, F.; de Palma, L.; Specchia, N.; Mannarini, M. Growth-plate cartilage metabolic response to mechanical stress. J Pediatr Orthop 9:520, 1989.

65. Greene, T.L.; Hensinger, R.N.; Hunter, L.Y. Back pain and vertebral changes simulating Scheuermann's disease. J Pediatr Orthop 5:1, 1985.

66. Grogan, D.P.; Love, S.M.; Ogden, J.A.; et al. Chondro-osseous growth abnormalities after meningococcemia: A clinical and histopathological study. J Bone Joint Surg Am 71:920, 1989.

67. Harris, H. The vascular supply of bone, with special reference to the epiphyseal cartilage. J Anat 64:3, 1929.

68. Havranek, P. Injuries of the distal clavicular physis in children. J Pediatr Orthop 9:213, 1989.

69. Havranek, P.; Lizler, J. Magnetic resonance imaging in the evaluation of partial growth arrest after physeal injuries in children. J Bone Joint Surg Am 73:1234, 1991.

70. Heeg, M.; Visser, J.D.; Oostvogel, H.J.M. Injuries of the acetabular triradiate cartilage and sacroiliac joint. J Bone Joint Surg Br 70:34, 1988.

71. Herring, J.A.; Moseley, C. Posttraumatic valgus deformity of the tibia. J Pediatr Orthop 4:654, 1984.

72. Hresko, M.T.; Kasser, J.S. Physeal arrest about the knee associated with non-physeal fractures in the lower extremity. J Bone Joint Surg Am 71:698, 1989.

73. Hunziker, E.B.; Schenk, R.K.; Cruz-Orive, L.M. Quantitation of chondrocyte performance in growth-plate cartilage during longitudinal bone growth. J Bone Joint Surg Am 69:162, 1987.

74. Huurman, W.W.; Jacobsen, F.S.; Anderson, J.C.; Chu, W.K. Limb-length discrepancy measured with computerized axial tomographic equipment. J Bone Joint Surg Am 69:699, 1987.

75. Hynes, D.; O'Brien, T. Growth disturbance lines after injury of the distal tibial physis: Their significance in prognosis. J Bone Joint Surg Br 70:231, 1988.

76. Ilizarov, G.A. The tension-stress effect on the genesis and growth of tissues. Part I. The influence of stability of fixation and soft-tissue preservation. Clin Orthop 238:249, 1989.

77. Ishii, T.; Miyagawa, S.; Hayashi, K. Traction apophysitis of the medial malleolus. J Bone Joint Surg Br 76:802, 1994.

78. Jackson, D.W.; Cozen, L. Genu valgum as a complication of proximal tibial metaphyseal fractures in children. J Bone Joint Surg Am 53:1571, 1971.

79. Janarv, P.M.; Wikstrom, B.; Hirsch, G. The influence of transphyseal drilling and tendon grafting on bone growth: An experimental study in the rabbit. J Pediatr Orthop 18:149, 1998.

80. Jarry, L.; Uhthloff, H.K. Pluripotency of periosteum and endosteum in fracture healing. J Bone Joint Surg Br 51:387, 1969.

81. Jeffrey, C.C. Fracture of the head of the radius in children. J Bone Joint Surg Br 32:314, 1950.

82. Jordon, S.E.; Alonso, J.E.; Cook, F.F. The etiology of valgus angulation after metaphyseal fractures of the tibia in children. J Pediatr Orthop 7:450, 1987.

83. Karrholm, J.; Hansson, L.I.; Slevik, G. Roentgen stereophotogrammetric analysis of growth pattern after supination-adduction ankle injuries in children. J Pediatr Orthop 2:271, 1982.

84. Kasdan, M.L. Physeal growth arrest of the distal phalanx of the thumb in an adolescent pianist: A case report. J Hand Surg [Am] 23:532, 1998.

85. Keret, D.; Mendez, A.A.; Harcke, H.T.; MacEwen, G.D. Type V physeal injury: A case report. J Pediatr Orthop 10:545, 1990.

86. Kilfoyle, R.M. Fracture of the medial condyle and epicondyle of the elbow in children. Clin Orthop 41:43, 1965.

87. Kim, I.O.; Kim, H.J.; Cheon, J.E.; et al. MR imaging of changes of the growth plate after partial physeal removal and fat graft interposition in rabbits. Invest Radiol 35:712, 2000.

88. Kim, H.W.; Morcuende, J.A.; Dolan, L.A.; Weinstein, S.L. Acetabular development in developmental dysplasia of the hip complicated by lateral growth disturbance of the capital femoral epiphysis. J Bone Joint Surg Am 82:1692, 2000.

89. Kleinman, P.K.; Marks, S.C. Relationship of the subperiosteal bone collar to metaphyseal lesions in abused infants. J Bone Joint Surg Am 77:1471, 1995.

90. Kolt, G.S.; Kirkby, R.J. Epidemiology of injury in elite and subelite female gymnasts: A comparison of retrospective and prospective findings. Br J Sports Med 33:312, 1999.

91. Kovach, J., II; Baker, B.E.; Mosher, J.F. Fracture separation of the olecranon ossification center in adults. Am J Sports Med 13:105, 1985.

92. Kujala, U.M.; Kvist, M.; Heinonen, O. Osgood-Schlatter's disease in adolescent athletes: Retrospective study of incidence and duration. Am J Sports Med 13:236, 1985.

93. Kujala, U.M.; Orava, S.; Karpakka, J.; et al. Ischial tuberosity apophysitis and avulsion among athletes. Int J Sports Med 18:149, 1997.

94. Labelle, H.; Bunnell, W.P.; Duhaime, M.; Poitras, B. Cubitus varus deformity following supracondylar fractures of the humerus in children. J Pediatr Orthop 2:539, 1982.

95. Lalanandham, T.; Ehrlich, M.G.; Zaleske, D.J.; et al. Viability and metabolism of cartilage transplanted to physeal regions. J Pediatr Orthop 10:450, 1990.

96. Landfried, M.J.; Stenclik, M.; Susi, J.G. Variant of Galeazzi fracture-dislocation in children. J Pediatr Orthop 11:332, 1991.

97. Langenskiöld, A. Surgical treatment of partial closure of the growth plate. J Pediatr Orthop 1:3, 1981.

98. Langenskiöld, A.; Osterman, K.; Valle, M. Growth of fat grafts after operation for partial bone growth arrest: Demonstration by computed tomography scanning. J Pediatr Orthop 7:389, 1987.

99. Langenskiöld, A.; Videman, T.; Nevalainen, T. The fate of fat transplants in operations for partial closure of the growth plate: Clinical examples and an experimental study. J Bone Joint Surg Br 68:234, 1986.

100. Langenskiöld, A. Role of the ossification groove of Ranvier in normal and pathologic bone growth: A review. J Pediatr Orthop 18:173, 1998.

101. Lawson, J.P.; Ogden, J.A.; Bucholz, R.W.; Hughes, S.A. Physeal injuries of the cervical spine. J Pediatr Orthop 7:428, 1987.

102. Lazovic, D.; Wenger, U.; Peters, G.; Gosse, F. Ultrasound for diagnosis of apophyseal injuries. Knee Surg Sports Traumatol Arthrosc 3:234, 1996.

103. Leet, A.I.; Mackenzie, W.G.; Szoke, G.; Harcke, H.T. Injury to the growth plate after Pemberton osteotomy. J Bone Joint Surg Am 81:169, 1999.

104. Lesko, P.D.; Georgis, T.; Slabaugh, P. Case report. Irreducible Salter-Harris type II fracture of the distal radial epiphysis. J Pediatr Orthop 7:719, 1987.

105. Letts, M.; Esser, D. Fractures of the triquetrum in children. J Pediatr Orthop 13:228, 1993.

106. Letts, M.; Locht, R.; Wiens, J. Monteggia fracture-dislocations in children. J Bone Joint Surg Br 67:724, 1985.

107. Leung, A.G.; Peterson, H.A. Fractures of the proximal radial head and neck in children with emphasis on those that involve the articular cartilage. J Pediatr Orthop 20:7, 2000.

108. Loder, R.T.; Swinford, A.E.; Kuhns, L.R. The use of helical computed tomographic scan to assess bony physeal bridges. J Pediatr 17:356, 1997.

109. Lokiec, F.; Wientroub, S. Calcaneal osteochondritis: A new overuse injury. J Pediatr Orthop B 7:243, 1998.

110. Lombardo, S.J.; Ratting, A.C.; Kerlan, R.K. Radiographic abnormalities of the iliac apophysis in adolescent athletes. J Bone Joint Surg Am 65:444, 1983.

111. Mann, D.C.; Rajmaira, S. Distribution of physeal and non-physeal fractures of long bones in children aged 0 to 16 years. J Pediatr Orthop 10:713, 1990.

112. Marcus, R.E.; Mills, M.F.; Thompson, G.H. Multiple injury in children. J Bone Joint Surg Am 65:1290, 1983.

113. Mayr, J.M.; Pierer, G.R.; Linhart, W.E. Reconstruction of part of the distal tibial growth plate with an autologous graft from the iliac crest. J Bone Joint Surg Br 82:558, 2000.

114. Medlar, R.C.; Lyne, E.D. Sinding-Larsen-Johansson disease. J Bone Joint Surg Am 60:1113, 1978.

115. Mendez, A.A.; Bartal, E.; Grillot, M.B.; Lin, J.J. Compression (Salter-Harris type V) physeal fracture: An experimental model in the rat. J Pediatr Orthop 12:29, 1992.

116. Metzmaker, J.N.; Pappas, A.M. Avulsion fractures of the pelvis. Am J Sports Med 13:349, 1985.

117. Micheli, L.J. The traction apophysitis. Clin Sports Med 6:389, 1986.

118. Micheli, L.J. Overuse injuries in children's sport: The growth factor. Orthop Clin North Am 14:337, 1983.

119. Micheli, L.J. Low-back pain in the adolescent: Differential diagnosis. Am J Sports Med 7:361, 1979.

120. Micheli, L.J.; Ireland, M.L. Prevention and management of calcaneal apophysitis in children: An overuse syndrome. J Pediatr Orthop 7:34, 1987.

121. Milch, H. Fractures and fracture-dislocations of humeral condyles. J Trauma 4:592, 1964.

122. Mital, M.A.; Matza, R.A.; Cohen, J. The so-called unresolved Osgood-Schlatter lesion. J Bone Joint Surg Am 62:732, 1980.

123. Murakami, S.; Yamamoto, H.; Furuya, K.; Tomimatsu, T. Irreducible Salter-Harris type II fracture of the distal tibial epiphysis. J Orthop Trauma 8:524, 1994.

124. Musharafieh, R.S.; Macari, G. Salter-Harris I fractures of the distal radius misdiagnosed as wrist sprain. J Emerg Med 19:265, 2000.

125. Neer, C.S.; Horowitz, B. Fractures of the proximal humeral epiphyseal plate. Clin Orthop 41:24, 1965.

126. Nettelblad, H.; Randolph, M.A.; Weiland, A.J. Free microvascular epiphyseal-plate transplantation. J Bone Joint Surg Am 66:1421, 1984.

127. Newman, J.H. Displaced radial neck fractures in children. Injury 9:114, 1977.

128. Noonan, K.J.; Saltzman, C.L.; Dietz, F.R. Open physeal fractures of the distal phalanx of the great toe. J Bone Joint Surg Am 74:122, 1994.

129. O'Brien, E.T. Fractures of the hand and wrist region. In: Rockwood, C.A., Jr.; Wilkins, K.E.; King, R.E., eds. Fractures in Children. Philadelphia, J.B. Lippincott, 1984.

130. O'Brien, P.I. Injuries involving the radial epiphysis. Clin Orthop 41:51, 1965.

131. O'Brien, T.; Millis, M.B.; Griffin, P.P. The early identification and classification of growth disturbances of the proximal end of the femur. J Bone Joint Surg Am 68:970, 1986.

132. O'Driscoll, S.W.; Keeley, F.W.; Salter, R.B. Durability of regenerated articular cartilage produced by free autogenous periosteal grafts in major full-thickness defects in joint surfaces under the influence of continuous passive motion: A follow-up report at one year. J Bone Joint Surg Am 70:595, 1988.

133. Odgen, J.A.; Ogden, D.A.; Pugh, L.; et al. Tibia valga after proximal metaphyseal fractures in childhood: A normal biologic response. J Pediatr Orthop 15:489, 1995.

134. Ogden, J.A. Skeletal Injury in the Child, 2nd ed. Philadelphia, Lea & Febiger, 1990.

135. Ogden, J.A. Current concepts review: The evaluation and treatment of partial physeal arrest. J Bone Joint Surg Am 69:1297, 1987.

136. Ogden, J.A. The uniqueness of growing bones. In: Rockwood, C.A.; Wilkins, K.E.; King, R.E., eds. Fractures in Children. Philadelphia, J.B. Lippincott, 1984.

137. Ogden, J.A. Growth slowdown and arrest lines. J Pediatr Orthop 4:409, 1984.

138. Ogden, J.A.; Lee, J. Accessory ossification patterns and injuries of the malleoli. J Pediatr Orthop 10:306, 1990.

139. Ogden, J.A.; Southwick, W. Osgood-Schlatter's disease and development of the tibial tuberosity. Clin Orthop 116:180, 1976.

140. Ogden, J.A.; Tross, R.B.; Murphy, M.J. Fractures of the tibial tuberosity in adolescents. J Bone Joint Surg Am 62:205, 1980.

141. Ogilvie, J. Epiphysiodesis: Evaluation of a new technique. J Pediatr Orthop 6:174, 1986.

142. Olin, A.; Creasman, C.; Shapiro, F. Free physeal transplantation in the rabbit: An experimental approach to focal lesions. J Bone Joint Surg Am 66:7, 1984.

143. Pappas, A.M. Elbow problems associated with baseball during childhood and adolescence. Clin Orthop 164:30, 1982.

144. Pappas, A.M.; Anas, P.; Toczylowski, H.M., Jr. Asymmetrical arrest of the proximal tibial physis and genu recurvatum deformity. J Bone Joint Surg Am 66:515, 1989.

145. Pateder, D.B.; Eliseev, R.A.; O'Keefe, R.J.; et al. The role of autocrine growth factors in radiation damage to the epiphyseal growth plate. Radiat Res 155:847, 2001.

146. Pauwels, F. Biomechanics of the Locomotor Apparatus. Berlin, Springer-Verlag, 1980.

147. Peh, W.C.; Griffith, J.K.; Yip, D.K.; Leong, J.C. Magnetic resonance imaging of lumbar vertebral apophyseal ring fractures. Australas Radiol 42:34, 1998.

148. Peterson, H.A. Partial growth plate arrest. In: Morrissy, R.T., ed. Lovell and Winter's Pediatric Orthopaedics, 3rd ed. Philadelphia, J.B. Lippincott, 1990.

149. Peterson, H.A. Partial growth plate arrest and its treatment. J Pediatr Orthop 4:246, 1984.

150. Peterson, H.A. Physeal fractures. Part 2. Two previously unclassified types. J Pediatr Orthop 14:431, 1994.

151. Peterson, H.A. Physeal fractures. Part 3. Classification. J Pediatr Orthop 14:439, 1994.

152. Peterson, H.A.; Burkhart, S.S. Compression injury of the epiphyseal growth plate: Fact or fiction? J Pediatr Orthop 1:377, 1981.

153. Peterson, H.A.; Madhok, R.; Benson, J.T.; et al. Physeal fractures. Part 1. Epidemiology in Olmsted County, Minnesota, 1979–1988. J Pediatr Orthop 14:423, 1994.

154. Petit, P.; Panuel, M.; Faure, F.; et al. Acute fracture of the distal tibial physis: Role of gradient-echo MR imaging versus plain film examination. AJR Am J Roentgenol 166:1203, 1996.

155. Phieffer L.S.; Meyer, R.A. Jr.; Gruber, H.E.; et al. Effect of interposed periosteum in an animal physeal fracture model. Clin Orthop 376:15, 2000.

156. Poland, J. Traumatic Separation of the Epiphyses. London, Smith Elder, 1898.

157. Pritchett, J.W. Growth and predictions of growth in the upper extremity. J Bone Joint Surg Am 70:520, 1988.

158. Rang, M. The Growth Plate and Its Disorders. Baltimore, Williams & Wilkins, 1969.

159. Rhemrev, S.J.; Sleeboom, C.; Ekkelkamp, S. Epiphyseal fractures of the proximal tibia. Injury 31:131, 2000.

160. Riseborough, E.J.; Barrett, I.R.; Shapiro, F. Growth disturbances following distal femoral epiphyseal fracture-separations. J Bone Joint Surg Am 65:885, 1983.

161. Rodgers, W.B.; Schwend, R.M.; Haramillo, D.; et al. Chronic physeal fractures in myelodysplasia: Magnetic resonance analysis, histologic description, treatment, and outcome. J Pediatr Orthop 17:615, 1997.

162. Roebuck, D.J. Skeletal complications in pediatric oncology patients. Radiographics 19:873, 1999.

163. Rogers, L.F.; Poznanski, A.K. Imaging of epiphyseal injuries. Radiology 191:297, 1994.

164. Rosenberg, L.C. The physis as an interface between basic research and clinical knowledge [editorial]. J Bone Joint Surg Am 66:815, 1984.

165. Rutherford, A. Fractures of the lateral humeral condyle in children. J Bone Joint Surg Am 67:851, 1985.

166. Ryoppy, S.; Karaharju, E.O. Alteration of epiphyseal growth by an experimentally produced angular deformity. Acta Orthop Scand 45:290, 1974.

167. Salter, R.B.; Harris, W.R. Injuries involving the epiphyseal plate. J Bone Joint Surg Am 45:587, 1963.

168. Savini, R.; Di Silvestre, M.; Gargiulo, G.; Picci, P. Posterior lumbar apophyseal fractures. Spine 16:1118, 1991.

169. Schlonsky, J.; Olix, M.L. Functional disability following avulsion fracture of the ischial epiphysis. J Bone Joint Surg Am 54:641, 1972.

170. Schmidt, T.L.; Kalamchi, A. The fate of the capital femoral physis and acetabular development in developmental coxa vara. J Pediatr Orthop 2:534, 1982.

171. Scuderi, G.; Bronson, M.J. Triradiate cartilage injury: Report of two cases and review of the literature. Clin Orthop 217:179, 1987.

172. Sever, J.I. Apophysitis of the os calcis. N Y Med J, May 1, 1912.

173. Shands, P.A.; McQueen, D.A. Demonstration of avulsion fracture of the inferior pole of the patella by magnetic resonance imaging. J Bone Joint Surg Am 77:1721, 1995.

174. Shapiro, F.; Holtrop, M.E.; Glimcher, M.J. Organization and cellular biology of the perichondrial ossification groove of Ranvier. J Bone Joint Surg Am 59:703, 1977.

175. Shelton, W.R.; Canale, S.T. Fractures of the tibia through the proximal tibial epiphyseal cartilage. J Bone Joint Surg Am 61:167, 1979.

176. Shih, C.; Chang, C.Y.; Penn, I.W.; et al. Chronically stressed wrists in adolescent gymnasts: MR imaging appearance. Radiology 195:855, 1995.

177. Smith, B.C.; Rand, F.; Jaramillo, D.; Shapiro, F. Early MR imaging of lower-extremity physeal fracture-separations: A preliminary report. J Pediatr Orthop 14:526, 1994.

178. Speer, D.P. Collagenous architecture of the growth plate and perichondrial ossification groove. J Bone Joint Surg Am 64:399, 1982.

179. Spinner, R.J.; Atkinson, J.L.; Wenger, D.E.; Stuart, M.J. Tardy sciatic nerve palsy following apophyseal avulsion fracture of the ischial tuberosity. Case report. J Neurosurg 89:819, 1998.

180. Staheli, L.T.; Williamson, V. Partial physeal growth arrest and treatment by bridge resection and fat interposition. J Pediatr Orthop 10:769, 1990.

181. Stirling, R.I. Complications of Osgood-Schlatter's disease [abstract]. J Bone Joint Surg Br 34:149, 1952.

182. Sward, L.; Hellstrom, M.; Jacobsson, B.; et al. Acute injury of the vertebral ring apophysis and intervertebral disc in adolescent gymnasts. Spine 15:144, 1990.

183. Takayanagi, H.; Watanabe, H.; Shinozaki, T.; Takagishi, K. Overgrowth of the ischial tuberosity complicating femoral bone and muscle atrophy: Implications for a delayed complication of malunited apophyseal avulsion fracture. Am J Orthop 27:308, 1998.

184. Tamurian, R.M.; Damron, T.A.; Spadaro, J.A. Sparing radiation-induced damage to the physis by radioprotectant drugs: Laboratory analysis in a rat model. J Orthop Res 17:286, 1999.

185. Tolat, A.R.; Sanderson, P.L.; De Smet, L.; Stanley, J.K. The gymnast's wrist: Acquired positive ulnar variance following chronic epiphyseal injury. J Hand Surg [Br] 17:678, 1992.

186. Trickey, E.L. Rupture of the posterior cruciate ligament of the knee. J Bone Joint Surg Br 50:334, 1968.

187. Turz, A.; Crost, M. Sports-related injuries in children: A study of their characteristics, frequency, and severity, with comparison to other types of accidental injuries. Am J Sports Med 14:294, 1986.

188. van Leeuwen, B.L.; Kamps, W.A.; Jansen, H.W.; Hoekstra, J.H. The effect of chemotherapy on the growing skeleton. Cancer Treat Rev 26:363, 2000.

189. Vostal, O. [Fracture of the neck of the radius in children.] Acta Chir Traumatol Cech 37:294, 1970.

190. Walling, A.K.; Grogan, D.P.; Carty, C.T.; Ogden, J.A. Fractures of the calcaneal apophysis. J Orthop Trauma 4:349, 1990.

191. Waters, P.M.; Kolettis, G.J.; Schwend, R. Acute median neuropathy following physeal fractures of the distal radius. J Pediatr Orthop 14:173, 1994.

192. Watkins, J.; Peabody, P. Sports injuries in children and adolescents treated at a sports injury clinic. J Sports Med Phys Fitness 36:43, 1996.

193. Watson-Jones, R. Fractures and Joint Injuries. Baltimore, Williams & Wilkins, 1946.

194. Weber, B.G. Fibrous interposition causing valgus deformity after fracture of the upper tibial metaphysis in children. J Bone Joint Surg Br 59:290, 1977.

195. Wiley, J.J.; Galey, J.P. Monteggia injuries in children. J Bone Joint Surg Br 67:728, 1985.

196. Wilkins, K.E. Fractures and dislocations of the elbow region. In: Rockwood, C.A., Jr.; Wilkins, K.E.; King, R.E., eds. Fractures in Children. Philadelphia, J.B. Lippincott, 1984.

197. Wirth, T.; Byers, S.; Byrd, R.W.; et al. The implantation of cartilaginous and periosteal tissue into growth plate defects. Int Orthop 18:200, 1994.

198. Wood, K.B.; Bradley, J.P.; Ward, W.T. Pes anserinus interposition in a proximal tibial physeal fracture. Clin Orthop 264:239, 1991.
199. Wood, V.E. Fractures of the hand in children. Orthop Clin North Am 7:527, 1976.
200. Wooton, J.R.; Cross, M.J.; Holt, K.W.G. Avulsion of the ischial apophysis: The case for open reduction and internal fixation. J Bone Joint Surg Br 72:625, 1990.
201. Yamauchi, T.; Yajima, H.; Tamai, S.; Kizaki, K. Flap transfers for the treatment of perichondrial ring injuries with soft tissue defects. Microsurgery 20:262, 2000.
202. Young, J.W.R.; Bright, R.W.; Whitley, N.O. Computed tomography in the evaluation of partial growth plate arrest in children. Skeletal Radiol 15:530, 1986.
203. Zehntner, M.K.; Jakob, R.P.; McGanity, P.L.J. Case report. Growth disturbance of the distal radial epiphysis after trauma: Operative treatment by corrective radial osteotomy. J Pediatr Orthop 10:411, 1990.
204. Zimbler, S.; Merkow, S. Genu recurvatum: A possible complication after Osgood-Schlatter disease: Case report. J Bone Joint Surg Am 66:1129, 1984.

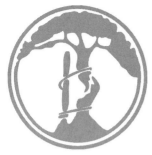

# CHAPTER 3

# Pathologic Fractures in Children

Herbert S. Schwartz, M.D.
Ginger E. Holt, M.D.

Pathologic fractures are fractures through diseased bone, and in children, such fractures are caused by a spectrum of conditions different from those in adults. Children's diseases frequently associated with pathologic fractures include noncancerous benign bone tumors and congenital or genetic abnormalities affecting the skeleton. Polyostotic disease with fracture affecting the immature skeleton is often caused by osteomyelitis, histiocytosis, vascular neoplasms, and metastasis (neuroblastoma and Wilms's tumor). Rarely, sarcomas may initially be manifested as fractures, but fractures more typically occur during neoadjuvant chemotherapy for osteosarcoma. In contrast, causes of pathologic fractures in the adult skeleton, especially in individuals older than 40 years, include the malignancies myeloma, metastatic carcinoma, lymphoma, and rarely, sarcomas of bone. Occasionally, giant cell tumors and enchondromas are identified. Elderly individuals frequently present with pathologic fractures from osteoporosis or Paget's disease, in addition to metastasis (Table 3–1).

The axial skeleton is a frequent repository for metastatic foci because of its rich vascular supply when compared with the appendicular skeleton. The site, age, and plain radiographic appearance create a differential diagnosis for pathologic fractures that remains broad. As a result, each case must be approached from a perspective that encompasses age, symptoms, image appearance, and an understanding of bone biology. Algorithms rarely suffice in pediatric orthopaedics or orthopaedic oncology.

The goal of this chapter is to introduce the reader to the multitude of variables involved in the successful treatment of pediatric pathologic fractures. A diagnosis *must* be made before embarking on any treatment strategy. Tissue documentation by biopsy is highly recommended to confirm the diagnosis of a pathologic fracture as the initial symptom. Depending on the confidence of the treating surgeon, a radiographic diagnosis may substitute for a tissue one, for example, in unicameral bone cysts (UBCs). After carefully weighing and balancing these variables, an optimal treatment strategy can be formulated for a particular child. A different child with the same fracture may benefit from a different treatment. It is not our intent to provide a cookbook algorithmic treatment approach, for that is to the detriment of patient care. It can be said that pediatric orthopaedics and orthopaedic oncology are two orthopaedic surgical subspecialties that require a high degree of cognitive decision making. Treatment of children's pathologic fractures is even more complex.

## BONE PHYSIOLOGY

Bone is a specialized connective tissue with matrix consisting predominantly of type I collagen. It is a dynamic organ that receives one fifth of the cardiac output and is one of the only organs capable of true regeneration. Shaping of the skeleton and the build-up of bone mass during childhood and adolescence are a result of the constant interplay between bone formation and bone resorption. Bone remodeling continues throughout life. The average individual reaches peak bone mass in the third decade of life, with the adult skeleton containing approximately 2 million bone-remodeling units. Each unit comprises a spatial and temporal group of organized cells responsible for osteoclastic bone resorption and osteoblastic bone formation in response to local and environmental stimuli. Various pathologic states interfere with this remodeling process.

Bone resorption is mediated by the osteoclast, a multinucleated giant cell derived from granulocyte-macrophage precursors. Bone formation requires the presence and function of the osteoblast, which is derived from mesenchymal fibroblast-like cells. Net bone formation occurs by the process of coupling (contiguous and concurrent bone formation and resorption). Under normal circumstances, 88% to 95% of the bone surface area is quiescent while the remainder is involved in active remodeling. The total length of time required to complete

TABLE 3–1 • • • • • • • • • • • • • • • • • • • • • • • • • • • • • • • • • • • •

## Age Distribution of Common Orthopaedic Bone Tumors

| Age (yr) | Tumor | |
| --- | --- | --- |
| | **Benign** | **Malignant** |
| 0–5 | Chondroma | Neuroblastoma |
| | Unicameral bone cyst | (metastatic) |
| | Osteoid osteoma | Rhabdomyosarcoma |
| | Nonossifying fibroma | (metastatic) |
| | Fibrous dysplasia | Ewing's sarcoma |
| | | Osteosarcoma |
| | | Lymphoma |
| 10–40 | Chondroma | Osteosarcoma |
| | Osteoid osteoma | Ewing's sarcoma |
| | Aneurysmal bone cyst | Lymphoma |
| | Unicameral bone cyst | |
| | Nonossifying fibroma | |
| | Fibrous dysplasia | |
| | Eosinophilic granuloma | |
| | Chondroblastoma | |
| | (skeletally immature) | |
| | Giant cell tumor | |
| | (skeletally mature) | |
| 40+ | Chondroma | Carcinoma |
| | Giant cell tumor | Multiple myeloma |
| | Hemangioma | Lymphoma |
| | | Chondrosarcoma |
| | | Osteosarcoma |
| | | Chordoma |

• • • • • • • • • • • • • • • • • • • • • • • • • • • • • • • • • • • • • • • • • •

a remodeling cycle for a typical bone-remodeling unit in a young adult is estimated to be 200 days. One bone-remodeling unit takes approximately 3 weeks to complete bone resorption, whereas it takes 3 months to form bone. Bone formation is quicker in children.

What is a pathologic fracture? Is it a radiologic, clinical, or combination diagnosis? Must the bone be completely or incompletely broken or displaced (or both) in one or more planes? Must the patient have symptoms or pain with activity? Can the bone be microscopically, but not macroscopically fractured? These issues are pertinent because it is important to understand and develop proper treatment strategies based on answers to these questions. For the purposes of discussion in this chapter, a pathologic fracture will be defined as a clinically symptomatic interruption in the cortex of a diseased bone. Although fractures are typically macroscopic, it does not necessarily have to be so. A child's bone is much more plastic than that of an adult. Bending without complete fiber separation occurs in a child and may be clinically relevant.

Bone strength is related to a combination of material and structural properties. The mineral component of bone is responsible for most of its compressive strength, whereas both mineral and protein components are important for strength in tension.[5] Normal activity results in forces of compression, tension, and torsion. However, bone is weakest in torsion, and even a small cortical defect can significantly reduce torsional strength. For example, a 6-mm drill hole in the tibial shaft cortex, such as that generated to obtain a bone biopsy specimen, reduces torsional strength by 50%.[4]

Tumor present at a fracture delays, alters, or prevents bone healing. In certain instances, the rapid growth of the tumor cells overwhelms the reparative process of bone. In metastatic bone disease, damage to the skeleton is usually much more extensive than can be expected simply from the amount of malignant cells present. Much evidence has now shown that most of the tumor-induced skeletal destruction is mediated by osteoclasts. Malignant cells secrete factors that both directly and indirectly stimulate osteoclastic activity.[22] These factors include a variety of cytokines: interleukin-1 (IL-1), IL-6, tumor necrosis factor, IL-11, IL-13, and IL-17. IL-1 is the most powerful stimulator of bone resorption in vitro. Growth factors identified in tumorous bone include transforming growth factor $\alpha$, transforming growth factor $\beta$, and epidermal growth factor. Paracrine factors that also stimulate osteoclastic activity include prostaglandin E and parathyroid hormone–related protein (PTH-rP), and these factors are typically produced by malignant cells. PTH-rP is immunologically distinct from parathyroid hormone, but the two hormones have significant homology at the amino terminal of the molecule, which is necessary for osteoclast stimulation.[32] This peptide has recently been found to be important in the osteolysis induced by metastatic breast cancer and in the hypercalcemia of lung cancer.

Healing of pathologic fractures has been found to correlate most closely with tumor type and patient survival.[11] Resection of the tumor deposit is an important part of the management of pathologic fractures. Thus, the biology of the bone and its biomechanics in conjunction with tumor pathology are important contributing variables to understand when planning the overall treatment of pathologic fractures.

The most important task to be performed when a pathologic fracture is first detected is to establish the diagnosis with certainty. A radiographic diagnosis can be accurate, especially for UBCs; however, it is not a substitute for a tissue-confirmed diagnosis. Consequently, it is recommended that a biopsy be strongly considered for all initial manifestations of pathologic and other neoplasms of bone. Biopsy is a complex cognitive skill that is dependent on a careful physical examination, history, and interpretation of radiographic staging studies, including proper assessment of local, regional, and distant disease. It is crucial to determine whether polyostotic bone involvement is present. The surgeon is best able to interpret the diagnostic, anatomic, and pathologic significance of musculoskeletal disease and should thus review the images personally.

Biopsies are best performed by individuals who perform them on a daily basis. Complications from an improperly selected biopsy site are frequent and can be devastating.[18] Nondiagnostic or nonrepresentative harvesting of lesional tissue delays the diagnosis, and biopsy performed before complete imaging can hamper treatment planning. Only after a tissue diagnosis is made can proper treatment ensue. Treatment must be based on an accurate diagnosis and understanding of bone biology (component 1) in conjunction with the pathology (component 2). Function is the third key element (compo-

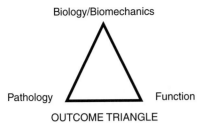

Biology/Biomechanics

Pathology         Function

OUTCOME TRIANGLE

FIGURE 3–1. Outcome triangle for pathologic fractures (see text).

nent 3) that is weighed in the balance when developing an overall treatment strategy.

# OUTCOME TRIANGLE

It is an error to treat a pathologic fracture as though it were a fracture through normal bone. Unfortunately, it is far too common for an orthopaedic surgeon to emphasize the type and choice of internal fixation implant rather than the timing and planning of surgery for a pathologic fracture. To achieve satisfactory treatment and outcomes in individuals with pathologic fractures requires that this dangerous reflex be harnessed. Proper treatment planning depends on weighing and taking into account all variables about a particular pathologic fracture and the individual before developing a treatment strategy. A multitude of treatment variables can be schematically represented in the three points of the outcome triangle (Fig. 3–1). A thorough and properly weighted evaluation of the triad of variables in the outcome triangle will more likely result in a favorable outcome for a patient with a pathologic fracture than will the more traditional orthopaedic surgical approach. The three variables are bone biology (component 1), including biomechanics; pathology (component 2); and function (component 3).

## Outcome, Part I—Bone Biology

Bone biology, the first part of the triad, includes the cellular makeup of the fractured bone and its biomechanical environment. Each bone is different, and each site within a bone is different, depending on age. The healing potential of a bone is a function of certain variables, including remodeling potential, age, vascularity, position relative to the physis, and the density of bone-remodeling units. Of course, these variables can be affected by the pathologic process. Osteopetrosis, or marble bone disease, is a congenital disease manifested by deficient or absent osteoclasts. It frequently results in pediatric pathologic fractures (Fig. 3–2). The lineage and the sequence of growth and differentiation factors necessary to convert primitive monocyte precursors to functioning osteoclasts have recently been elaborated in an elegant series of experiments.[6, 17, 29] The first regulating factor converts the primitive monocyte-macrophage stem cell into a macrophage precursor. This transcription factor is labeled PU.1. Experimental knockout mice deficient in PU.1 lack macrophages and osteoclasts, and the condition is lethal.[34] Mouse mutants deficient in macrophage colony-stimulating factor lack osteoclasts but contain immature macrophages; osteopetrosis develops in these mice but is cured by bone marrow transplantation.

Osteoprotegerin (OPG), a novel glycoprotein that regulates bone resorption, is a member of the tumor necrosis factor receptor superfamily. It is a decoy receptor

FIGURE 3–2. Initial films of a pathologic fracture of the femur of a child with osteopetrosis (A). The healed fracture shows little remodeling (B).

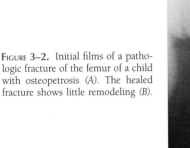
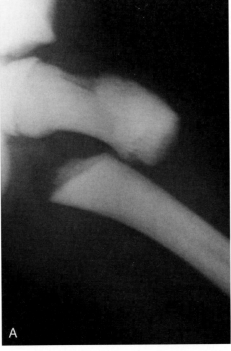
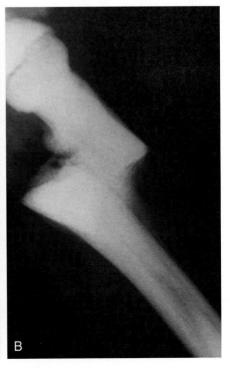

that competes with RANK (receptor for activation of nuclear factor κB [NF-κB]) for RANK ligand, which is responsible along with c-*fos* for differentiating the macrophage into an early osteoclast. OPG itself is a macrophage receptor similar to RANK, and it impedes osteoclastogenesis. Mice lacking αvβ3 integrin or c-*src* have substantial osteoclast numbers, but the cells fail to polarize. It allows conversion of an immature osteoclast into a functioning osteoclast with a ruffled border. SRC knockout experiments yield nonfunctional osteoclasts lacking cathepsin K, carbonic anhydrase II, or the proton-transporting adenosine triphosphate synthase pump. These nonfunctional osteoclasts are incapable of creating an acidic microenvironment and thus cannot resorb bone. Therefore, overproduction of OPG results in limited osteoclast formation and the clinical syndrome of osteopetrosis. Decreased OPG production results in too many osteoclasts being produced and the clinical syndrome of osteoporosis. Administration of recombinant OPG to normal adult mice causes a profound, yet nonlethal form of osteopetrosis. Thus, age and cellular makeup can help in understanding and determining the extent and healing potential of the bone and can serve as a guide for treatment.

Figure 3–2 depicts a subtrochanteric fracture in an osteopetrotic pediatric femur with no evidence of osteoclast function. Marrow formation is absent. A transverse fracture has occurred as a result of the pathologic process and brittleness of the bone. The fracture can heal, but without significant remodeling potential. This outcome can be anticipated by the lack of bone resorption units, or osteoclasts. Understanding the disease process and the healing potential of the bone will help guide the treatment strategy. For instance, intramedullary implants will probably be difficult or impossible to insert, and extramedullary implants will create significant stress risers and subject the bone to additional delayed fractures. Therefore, biologic manipulation (bone marrow transplantation) of the fracture and secondary bone healing may offer the most advantageous treatment strategy.

Neurofibromatosis provides another example of how understanding bone biology and its relationship to disease affects the healing potential when dealing with a pathologic fracture. Union is compromised and fracture healing adversely affected because of the nonanatomic biomechanics and poor vascularity at the site. An anterolateral tibial bow is associated with neurofibromatosis type 1 approximately half the time. The pseudarthrosis is not usually present at birth and therefore not truly congenital, but it occurs during the first decade of life. The dysplastic, hamartomatous bone is poorly vascularized and unable to withstand the continual stresses applied, with resultant fracture and angulation (Fig. 3–3). Manifestations of the disease alter with time, thereby limiting the usefulness of many of the morphologic classification systems currently in use. Union is best achieved by correcting the biomechanical and biologic environment because the pathology is of limited consequence in neurofibromatosis. Excision of the pseudarthrosis in conjunction with bone grafting and intramed-

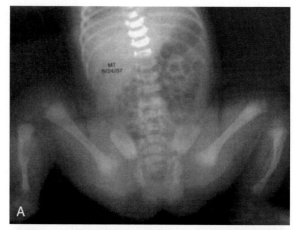

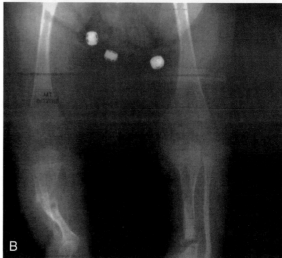

**FIGURE 3–3.** Pseudarthrosis of the tibia from neurofibromatosis. *A,* Radiograph of a newborn demonstrating a pathologic fracture of the right tibia and an impending fracture of the left tibia. *B,* Radiograph of a 1-year-old demonstrating bilateral pathologic fractures resulting in tibial pseudarthroses.

ullary fixation is a common procedure after failure of early treatment, including total contact bracing. Autogenous bone grafting is of assistance. A vascularized fibular graft or distraction osteogenesis can also be considered, depending on the circumstances.[33] Realignment of the limb to create compressive rather than tension forces at the pseudarthrosis site is beneficial. A Syme amputation can result in spontaneous union.[14]

Pathologic fractures of certain bones can help dictate their management. High stress is concentrated on the tension areas of weight-bearing bones, including the femoral neck and diaphysis of the tibia. Far more load is applied to weight-bearing bones than to non–weight-bearing bones. Fractures of vertebral bodies create the potential for spinal cord injuries. Vertebrae plana is caused by localized histiocytosis (eosinophilic granuloma) of the vertebral body. The natural history is one of spontaneous resolution without operative intervention, but a tissue diagnosis is often necessary, especially if monostotic disease is present, to rule out a malignant etiology. Infrequently, vertebrae plana can result in a neurologic deficit.[13] Figure 3–4 portrays the natural history of vertebrae plana without surgical intervention.

The biology of pathologic fracture healing is affected by the administration of chemotherapy or by irradiation of the injured site, an issue especially important in malignant pathologic fractures. The administration of chemotherapy or radiation therapy to pathologic fractures secondary to sarcoma typically facilitates fracture healing. Although it is generally recognized that chemotherapy and radiation therapy delay the normal bone's cellular response to heal a fracture, in the presence of rapidly dividing malignant cells, cytotoxic therapy provides a net positive result. Chemotherapy or external-beam radiation therapy, by destroying more cancerous than normal cells, creates a more favorable milieu for fracture healing. This effect of therapy on bone is another example demonstrating the need to understand bone biology to facilitate fracture healing.

## Outcome, Part II—Pathology

The pathology component of the outcome triangle is based on an understanding of the disease and its biologic behavior and natural history. A thorough understanding of the disease entity and its pathologic behavior is paramount in determining how best to treat it. Treatment of a pathologic fracture is therefore dependent on knowing the diagnosis, which can only be established with certainty from a properly obtained and representative biopsy sample. Although a plethora of pathologic entities may affect bone and thus make it susceptible to fracture, the modes of treatment are far less in number.

Groups of pathologic entities that can result in pathologic fracture include (1) genetic or metabolic bone disease abnormalities (e.g., osteogenesis imperfecta [OI] or osteopetrosis), (2) nutritional or environmental disturbances (e.g., rickets), (3) benign bone tumors (e.g., cysts, cartilage, fibrous tumors), (4) skeletal sarcomas (e.g., osteosarcoma, Ewing's sarcoma), and (5) skeletal metastases (e.g., neuroblastoma, rhabdomyosarcoma). These five disease categories represent a multitude of diagnoses, both neoplastic and non-neoplastic. Rather than elaborating on each pathologic entity, it is convenient to group them by pathobiologic activity (Table 3–2).

Management of pathologic fractures is predicated on an understanding of the biologic relationship between the pathology and the bone. Both active and inactive UBCs, or growing and static cartilage neoplasms of bone, may be encountered. Fibrous dysplasia in a femoral neck is not the same as fibrous dysplasia in the diaphysis of a long bone. Despite histologic similarities, a nonossifying fibroma occupying three quarters of the diameter of a long bone has consequences different from those of a fibrous cortical defect. Hence, the key to understanding neoplastic and non-neoplastic pathologic fractures is to understand the effect that the lesion has on a bone and how to best correct the problems caused by it. Treatment is not based on memorizing the textbook definition of a particular tumor. Instead, proper treatment depends on developing an understanding of the relationship of the pathology to the specific bone and subsequently formulating a method to augment fracture healing for the particular individual.

Pathology alone does not dictate management. Consequently, the plan of this section is to group treatment

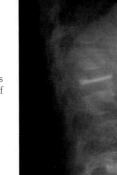

FIGURE 3–4. Localized histiocytosis demonstrated as L1 vertebrae plana. *A* and *B,* Reconstitution of vertebral body height over a 6-year time interval.

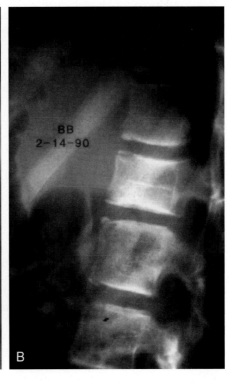

● ● ● ● ● ● ● ● ● ● ● ● ● ● ● ● ● ● ● ● ● ● ● ● ● ● ● ● ● ● ● ● ● ● ● ● ● ● ● ● ● ● ● ● ● ● ● ● ● ● ● ● ● ● ●

Musculoskeletal-Related Disorders

| Disease | Inheritance | Genetics | Defect |
|---|---|---|---|
| Ewing's sarcoma | — | t(11,22) | Loss of tumor suppressor gene(s) and creation of a fusion product |
| Osteosarcoma | — | 17p13, p53 | Loss of tumor suppressor gene(s) |
| | | 13q14 | Retinoblastoma gene type 1 |
| Achondroplasia | AD | 4p16 | *FGFR-3* gene |
| | | | Abnormal enchondral bone formation |
| Neurofibromatosis | | | |
| NF1 | AD | 17q11 | Neurofibromin |
| NF2 | AD | 22q11 | Schwannomin |
| Osteogenesis imperfecta | | | |
| Clinical group I mild | AD | α1, #17 | 50% decreased type I collagen |
| | | α2, #7 | |
| Clinical group II lethal | AR | | Unstable triple helix |
| Clinical group III deforming | AR | | Abnormal type I |
| Clinical group IV moderate | AD | | Shortened pro-α chains |
| Osteopetrosis | | | |
| Mild, tarda | | SRC, OPG, RANK | Osteoclasts lack complete differentiation |
| Malignant, infantile | | M-CSF; PU.1 | Defective osteoclastogenesis |
| Rickets | | | |
| Vit D–deficient diet | | | Decreased Vit D intake |
| | | | Leads to secondary hyperparathyroidism |
| Vit D dependent | AR | 12q14 | Lack renal 25 (OH)-Vit D$_1$ α-hydroxylase |
| Vit D resistant | X-linked dominant | | Impaired renal tubular phosphate resorption (PEX, cellular endopeptidase) |
| Fibrous dysplasia | — | | G$_s$ α (receptor-coupled signaling protein for cAMP) |
| Osteochondromatosis | — | 8q24.1/11p11 | *EXT1, EXT2* genes |

*Abbreviations:* AD, autosomal dominant; AR, autosomal recessive; cAMP, cyclic adenosine monophosphate; M-CSF, macrophage colony-stimulating factor; OPG, osteoprotegerin; RANK, receptor for activation of nuclear factor κB; #, chromosome number.

options into three categories and give appropriate pathologic examples for each. The treatment categories are (1) nonoperative management, (2) intralesional surgery with or without bone grafting or implants, and (3) wide tumor resection with reconstruction of the skeletal defect. Irrespective of the treatment option, strong consideration and respect must be given to the viability and preservation of the physis and epiphysis to avoid the consequences of limb length inequality or deformity. Pathology is but one of the triad of components that make up the outcome triangle and must be weighed in the overall equation for optimal management of a particular pathologic fracture.

*Nonoperative management* requires a surgeon confident in the diagnosis and outcome. Patience and experience result from an understanding of the natural history of the disease and the morbidity of surgical intervention. Inherited genetic diseases such as OI or osteopetrosis frequently result in pathologic fractures that are often managed nonoperatively. Figure 3–2 presents the natural history of pathologic fracture healing managed nonoperatively. Osteopetrotic bone lacks ruffled bordered osteoclasts, and thus the ability to resorb bone is compromised. Medullary canals are atrophic or absent, but bone formation is not impaired. As a result, fracture healing occurs but remodeling is slower. The bone is often more brittle than normal bone. Thus, intramedullary or extramedullary implants can create more problems than secondary bone healing alone. Excellent clinical outcomes may result in osteopetrotic pathologic

fractures when a conservative management approach is undertaken.

OI is a syndrome resulting from a mutation in one of the two genes controlling type I collagen synthesis, and most fit into four clinical types. Type II OI results from the replacement of a helical glycine with a larger amino acid. The mutant chain wrecks helix formation, and normal collagen falls to 20%. Type I OI mutations prematurely terminate the message for 50% of collagen synthesis. Types III and IV are disruptions in mineralization.[23, 30] Hydroxyapatite matrix formation is imperfect and therefore results in a structurally weakened bone lattice. The bone fragility in OI has a variable clinical spectrum in terms of the degree of fracture and age at initial evaluation. Weight-bearing bones are treated differently from non–weight-bearing bones. The age of the patient and the proximity of the fracture line to the physis are important considerations in management. Remodeling bone formation and bone resorption both behave and occur in a nearly normal fashion. In Figure 3–5, nonoperative management and pathologic fracture healing are shown in a patient with OI. Nonoperative management is indicated for upper extremity fractures that can be successfully treated without angular deformity. Lower extremity fractures, especially after deformity has occurred, are best treated with internal fixation and frequently require multiple osteotomies. The Sheffield telescopic intramedullary rod appears to be associated with fewer complications than the Bailey-Dubow rod or the nonelongating rod of Sofield and Millar.[24] The

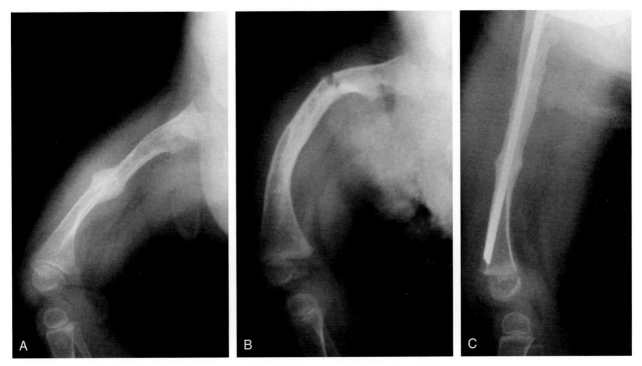

**FIGURE 3–5.** Sequential lateral views of the femur of a child with osteogenesis imperfecta show deformity from sequential fractures and healing (A), refracture (B), and healing after shish-kebab realignment osteotomies of the femur (C).

ultimate goal in treatment is to maintain mobility, which is often accomplished by maintaining length and preventing deformity. Figure 3–5 depicts a fracture that has healed initially by nonoperative treatment, but the deformity of the femur was so great that intramedullary fixation and multiple osteotomies were required. Fracture immobilization in children with OI can also be a

problem because it induces disuse osteoporosis. Therefore, casting of these fractures must emphasize stability.

Nutritional rickets is a condition in which polyostotic pathologic fractures may occur. Figure 3–6 shows an adolescent with primary hyperparathyroidism and multiple brown tumors, identified on staging radiographic studies. A symptomatic distal radial pathologic fracture

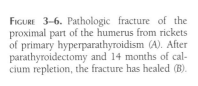

**FIGURE 3–6.** Pathologic fracture of the proximal part of the humerus from rickets of primary hyperparathyroidism (A). After parathyroidectomy and 14 months of calcium repletion, the fracture has healed (B).

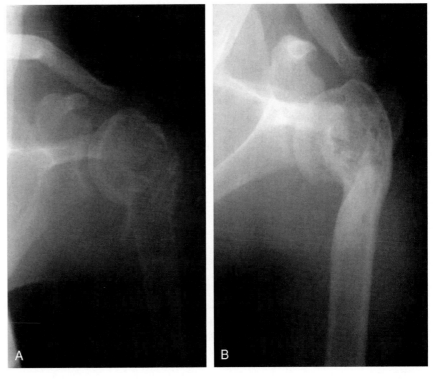

brought the child to medical attention, but detection of hypercalcemia and analysis of a bone biopsy specimen were required to establish the diagnosis. Once the diagnosis was determined with certainty, skeletal treatment was clearly best approached in a conservative manner. After removal of the parathyroid adenoma, commencement of skeletal calcium repletion allowed fracture healing to begin. Therefore, the fracture management goals were to maintain alignment while calcium homeostasis normalized. Parathyroidectomy and parenteral calcium repletion over a period of 3 to 4 months were necessary before initiation of fracture healing. Any surgical implant would serve little purpose in this case.

UBCs are frequently manifested as pathologic fractures in children and are typically treated nonoperatively. These fractures occur on the metaphyseal side of a long bone with the cyst abutting the physis. Often, it is not the tumor itself but rather a pathologic fracture that causes pain and prompts the child to complain. The typical radiographic finding is that of a "fallen leaf" sign. One must ask where the "leaf" falls from. In fact, the "leaf" represents a piece of cortical bone that has fractured, become displaced, and fallen into the fluid-filled cavity inside the bone. The fractures may be displaced or nondisplaced or shatter like an eggshell. Frequently, UBCs require only nonoperative treatment (Fig. 3–7). Uneventful fracture healing is likely. A repeat fracture in the future may occur as a result of the biomechanical inferiority of the hollow cystic bone structure.

The pathogenesis of UBCs remains an enigma. Etiologies range from the synovial cysts postulated by Mirra and colleagues[19] to dysplastic bone formed in response to trauma.[15] Vascular phenomena have also been attributed to the etiology of UBCs and vary from venous occlusion of the intramedullary space to the presence of inflammatory cytokine mediators in the cyst fluid that incite osteolysis.[16] It is not known whether the inflammatory mediators are the cause or a result of the bone resorption. Another etiology is the theory that vascular occlusion induces increased venous pressure, which results in bone resorption. These theories all suggest a non-neoplastic origin of UBCs and explain their conservative management strategy.

Nonoperative management should be the first treatment option. Should this option fail in that the bone does not reconstitute early and repeated fractures occur, measures that wash out the inflammatory mediators or lower the interstitial cavity pressure are frequently performed. Trephination procedures involve the insertion of at least two needles into the cavity and injecting methylprednisolone into the cyst as proposed by Scaglietti and associates or irrigation with normal saline under fluoroscopic guidance.[25] Additionally, the trocar can be injected with a variety of substances, including autogenous bone marrow, allograft, demineralized bone matrix, or other bone graft substitutes. Overall, a review of the literature reveals that local recurrence rates after triple injection range from 15% to 88%.[37] This outcome does not differ greatly from the published recurrence rates after open surgical procedures that expose the cavity in an attempt to fill it with an autogenous bone graft, allograft, or in some cases, calcium sulfate. Because

recurrence rates are high, physicians are reminded to manage these problems conservatively. Nonoperative management or injection techniques should be offered preferentially. Metal implants are rarely, if ever, used to treat these fractures, which have excellent remodeling potential because no true cellular (neoplastic) damage is involved in these lesions. Such considerations are especially pertinent for proximal humeral UBCs. A proximal femoral UBC warrants caution because intraarticular pathologic neck fractures and their sequelae are orthopaedic problems.

Fibrous cortical defects are benign bone tumors that are typically detected on incidentally performed radiographs. Their natural history is one of slow ossification. They are often polyostotic (20%) and are typically located in the long bones of the lower extremities. Until the lesion ossifies, the cortical lesions may represent stress risers. As a result, they can be the nidus for a fracture line. Figure 3–8 presents an oblique, low-energy spiral fracture through the distal tibial metaphysis in association with a fibrous cortical defect. The figure demonstrates noneventful healing in a cast in this skeletally immature child. Remodeling has occurred, with subsequent partial obliteration of the benign bone tumor. A fibrous cortical defect appears to be histologically identical to its larger counterpart, nonossifying fibroma. Nonossifying fibromas involve the medullary canal and are typically surgically treatable lesions. They will be discussed later.

Osteochondromas are benign bone tumors with cartilaginous caps. They seldom, if ever, are associated with pathologic fractures because the bone is often stronger in these areas than the contralateral uninvolved side. They can result in angular deformities that may require corrective surgery later in childhood.[7]

*Benign bone tumors with true growth potential are frequently treated operatively with intralesional curettage.* Such benign bone tumors include nonossifying fibroma, aneurysmal bone cyst, eosinophilic granuloma (histiocytosis), and chondroblastoma. These lesions have radiographic and clinical features that overlap with those of malignant bone tumors. In addition, osteomyelitis has clinical and radiographic findings in common with malignant bone tumors. Therefore, the reader is reminded that a pathologic diagnosis by biopsy is warranted. Continued neoplastic growth potential is likely for some of these benign bone tumors. Treatment options depend on establishing a diagnosis and involve eradication of the tumor by intralesional resection, followed by skeletal reconstruction. Skeletal reconstruction usually entails bone grafting (autogenous graft or allograft) with or without internal fixation with a metallic implant. Figure 3–9 depicts a pathologic fracture through a diaphyseal eosinophilic granuloma (localized histiocytosis). The differential diagnosis for this lesion with poor radiographic margins includes Ewing's sarcoma and osteomyelitis. The pathologic fracture resulted in displacement and is best managed by biopsy confirmation followed by vigorous (intralesional resection) curettage, bone grafting, and internal fixation with a plate and screws. Occasionally, the trauma of fracture may be sufficient to disturb the local blood supply and eradicate

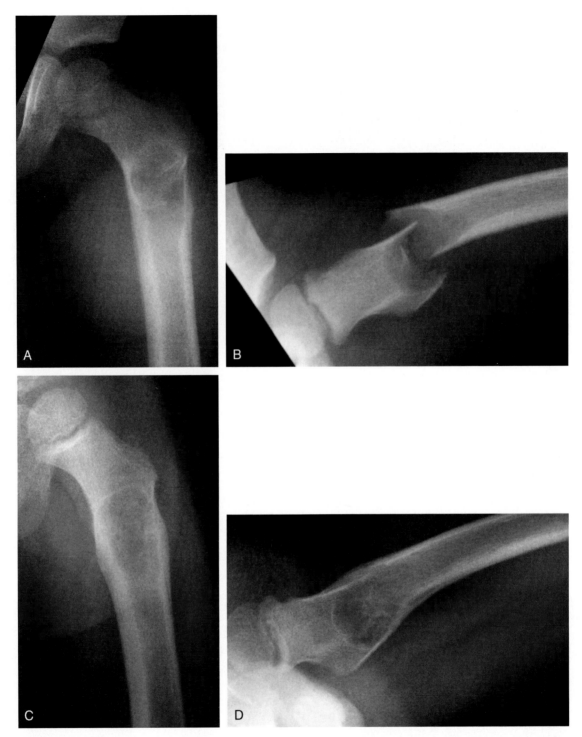

**FIGURE 3–7.** Anteroposterior *(A)* and lateral *(B)* views of the femur of a 2-year-old boy who presented with pain and inability to bear weight following a fall. After 6 weeks' treatment in a spica cast, the anteroposterior *(C)* and lateral *(D)* radiographs show healing of the fracture and early filling of the cyst with bony matrix.

the neoplasm. However, after a thorough biopsy, it is wise to proceed with complete intralesional resection.

Skeletal reconstruction with a bone graft or bone graft substitute appears to be indicated. Many surgeons now prefer to avoid the morbidity of iliac bone graft harvesting by using the variety of bone graft substitutes now available on the market. However, no reliable, controlled documented published series have compared

bone graft substitutes with autogenous bone grafts in humans at this time, especially in children, who have the greater potential for bone regrowth. Part of the reason for the paucity of controlled trials is that it is hard to noninvasively measure bone regrowth at the pathologic fracture site. The size of the eradicated tumor cavity and the pathology differ so greatly from patient to patient that uniformity in treatment is hard to achieve. Nonetheless,

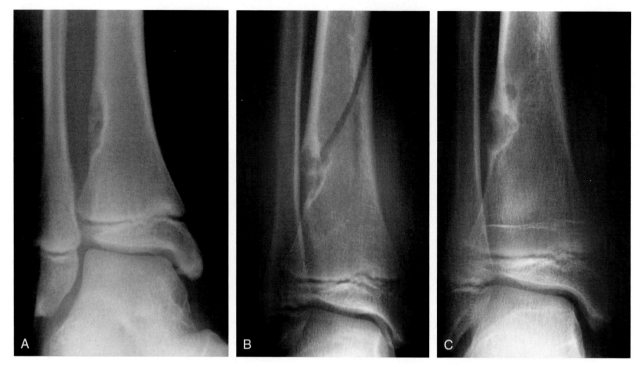

**FIGURE 3–8.** A fibrous cortical defect (*A*), which was identified as an incidental finding, becomes a stress riser when torsional force is applied (*B*). Healing of the fracture and remodeling have partially obliterated the lesion (*C*).

it appears that calcium sulfate, allografts with or without demineralized bone matrix, or autogenous bone grafts or bone marrow result in successful bone healing at pathologic fracture sites after curettage in the range of 50%.[20] This success rate encourages surgeons to try these measures before proceeding with the separate incision necessary for iliac crest bone graft harvesting.

The use of metallic implants remains controversial. Intramedullary devices offer biomechanical advantages in comparison to extramedullary devices. Intramedullary fixation of skeletally immature long bones is gaining popularity, although the risk of avascular necrosis and alteration of the physis remains real.[21] Fifty adolescents from 10 to 16 years of age were treated by inserting antegrade intramedullary devices through the greater trochanteric apophysis for traumatic femoral fractures. In no patient did deformity or avascular necrosis develop at an average follow-up of 16.2 months (range, 6 to 60). This issue is better discussed in other chapters in this textbook, but intramedullary devices appear to be safe.[3]

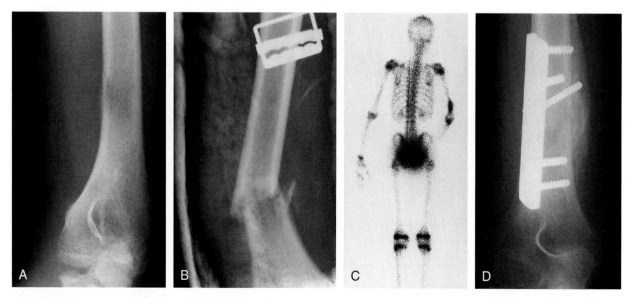

**FIGURE 3–9.** The same young man as in Figure 3–4 developed an unrelated lesion of the distal humerus (*A*). This lesion is purely lytic, with no obvious fracture but with periosteal new bone. Following a fracture through this lesion (*B*), an early bone scan (*C*) shows increased activity. Bone graft and internal fixation (*D*) led to good fracture and lesional healing of this eosinophilic granuloma.

Because of the greater reparative capacity of children's fractures than fractures in adults, the strength of the implant frequently does not need to be as great. After a pathologic fracture treated by curettage and bone grafting, it is common to insert internal fixation devices, such as a plate and screws, to prevent a torsional fracture through stress risers created by the bone defect. The typical six to eight cortices required for screw purchase on each side of the fracture site are not indicated, as is dogma for adult fracture osteosynthesis. Children's bones typically withstand earlier loading and are more pliable than those of adults. Early healing and weight bearing are thus possible.

Fibrous dysplasia and enchondromas are special instances of benign bone tumors that can be associated with pathologic fractures. Their respective polyostotic forms (polyostotic fibrous dysplasia, with or without Albright's disease, or Ollier's disease, Fig. 3–10) require complex treatment strategies because of the increased tumor burden in the fractured bone or in neighboring bones. Oftentimes, these fibrous and cartilaginous lesions may in fact overlap histologically. Malunions, angular deformities, and limb length inequalities present long-term challenges for the orthopaedic surgeon. Such reconstruction strategies are best deferred to other chapters.

Surgical indications for acute pathologic fractures should include fractures causing persistent pain or progressive deformity, in addition to correcting the obvious radiographic skeletal fracture. Chronic symptoms are usually the result of multiple and repeated microfractures, which often precede frank fractures. Treatment is best geared to correcting the biomechanical deformity rather than resecting all of the tumor. Frequently, tumor resection is not advised.[9] The shepherd's crook deformity in fibrous dysplasia of the femoral neck is best treated with mechanical implantation (see Fig.

3–10). Enneking and Geran used fibulas or grafts of cortical bone inserted into the intramedullary portion of the head, neck, and shaft, similar to a second-generation intramedullary nail.[9] Twelve of their 15 patients initially presented with a fatigue fracture. No attempt was made to resect the tumor. Osteotomies may be required to restore normal anatomic alignment to the proximal end of the femur. In these situations, intramedullary devices have proved superior to extramedullary devices.[10]

The weight-bearing status of the bone can also affect treatment strategies. Skeletally immature weight-bearing long bones of the lower extremity affected with symptomatic fibrous dysplasia are best treated by open reduction and internal fixation with an intramedullary device.[31] In contrast, upper extremity non–weight-bearing long bones were satisfactorily treated by closed methods. The data imply that continued weight bearing on a biomechanically deficient pathologic bone results in pain and progressive deformity from repeated microfracture. Eventually, a stress fracture or obvious displaced fracture is radiographically identified. Therefore, internal stabilization with an implant is preferred to minimize pain, deformity, and suffering. The growth potential of these neoplasms remains but is often of a nonthreatening magnitude. Clinical and radiographic follow-up through at least skeletal maturity is recommended. Malignant transformations of enchondromas in Ollier's disease, although termed chondrosarcomas, are not life threatening, especially when occurring in the appendicular skeleton.[26] Therefore, an emphasis on early biomechanical treatment of pathologically weakened bone appears to be a priority.[28]

Nonossifying fibromas, typically when they exceed 50% of the bone's diameter, result in pathologic fracture in weight-bearing long bones. For these reasons, prophylactic fixation after biopsy confirmation and intralesional curettage is indicated for symptomatic lesions.[2] The

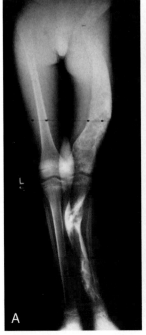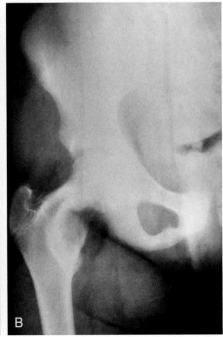

**FIGURE 3–10.** *A,* Fibrous dysplasia. A standing anteroposterior view shows the legs of an individual with severe, unilateral fibrous dysplasia. These untreated femoral and tibial deformities result in painful limitation of any weight-bearing activities. *B,* Fibrous dysplasia in this proximal femur caused a painful limp and early varus deformity.

superiority of autogenous bone grafts over bone graft substitutes in pediatric patients has not been proved.

*Wide, margin-free surgical resection of bone tumors is typically reserved for skeletal sarcomas.* Pathologic fractures occurring through skeletal sarcomas are complicated orthopaedic and oncologic conditions that are best treated by an experienced multidisciplinary management team. This team is large and encompasses medical and nonmedical professionals who care for children with a pathologic fracture through a malignant bone tumor.

Clearly, the method of diagnosis remains of paramount importance, for even the placement of a needle puncture or biopsy tract can jeopardize limb survival. Pathologic fractures through skeletal sarcomas such as osteosarcoma come in varied patterns. They can be the initial manifestation of the disease, or they can occur after diagnosis and neoadjuvant chemotherapy. Osteosarcomas that are initially manifested as a pathologic fracture frequently do so with displacement and local hemorrhage (Fig. 3–11). This complication presents the management

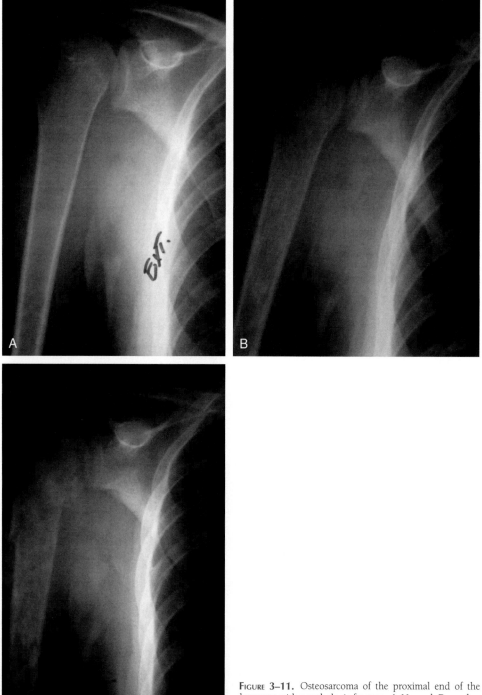

**FIGURE 3–11.** Osteosarcoma of the proximal end of the humerus with a pathologic fracture. *A,* Normal, December 1999. *B,* Tumor destruction, August 2001. *C,* Pathologic fracture, September 2001.

team with the problem of malignant cell contamination of the fracture hematoma. Pathologic fractures that occur after neoadjuvant therapy are typically those of mechanical insufficiency and result in angular deformity. The risk of tumor seeding is less than after acute manifestations. The recent literature suggests that with aggressive combination treatment, event-free survival rates for patients treated with limb salvage versus amputation after pathologic fractures associated with osteosarcoma are similar.[1, 27] However, these articles also suggest that the local recurrence rate is less in individuals treated with amputation than with limb salvage, thus supporting the hypothesis that malignant cells seed the fracture hematoma. The studies are not randomized. Patients treated by amputation are probably self-selected and therefore have the largest fracture hematoma associated with them. Local recurrence rates in limbs salvaged after acute pathologic fracture are two to four times those seen in nonpathologic fractures. Consequently, the local recurrence rate after limb salvage appears to be higher than after amputation. Because almost all patients in whom a local recurrence develops die, it appears that pathologic fractures are a serious consequence of osteosarcoma that may preclude limb salvage. Limb-preserving radical resection combined with aggressive chemotherapy appears to bring the overall survival rate of limb salvage close to that of ablative procedures.

Wide surgical resection may also be indicated for metastatic lesions that are infrequently associated with pathologic fractures in the immature skeleton, including patients with metastatic rhabdomyosarcoma or younger children with metastatic neuroblastoma. Depending on the stage, disease-free interval, and functional condition of the child, variables may dictate whether a wide surgical resection may be indicated. The longer the event-free survival period before diagnosis of an isolated metastasis, the more likely that a wider resection margin is needed.

After wide resection, the reconstruction alternatives are more complex than after intralesional or nonoperative management. Large skeletal defects need to be managed with structural allografts or megaprosthesis arthroplasties. Often, composites of the two are indicated. Expandable prostheses offer limb-lengthening options for young children with a large skeletal defect adjacent to a joint. Further discussion of reconstructive options is beyond the scope of this chapter. Limb salvage options are available but need to be carefully weighed against those of amputation or the intermediary procedure of Van Ness rotationplasty.

## Outcome, Part III—Function

To maximize the return of skeletal function after a pathologic fracture, one must be able to answer the question of how the pathologic fracture has altered the patient's or child's activity level and lifestyle. It is not sufficient to treat a radiograph, nor is it sufficient to use an algorithm to determine the next step. All pathologic fractures are not the same. Rather, each pathologic fracture, especially in a child, is as different as the tumor

pathology, stage, age at diagnosis, and the child's needs. The orthopaedic surgeon must individualize treatment plans.

The functional condition of the child immediately after a pathologic fracture can help guide the treatment strategy. Pain is frequently the acute problem and should therefore be the first consideration, providing that neurovascular compromise is not an issue. Whether traction or hospitalization is required needs to be evaluated. Basic orthopaedic tenets apply. Oftentimes, a sling is all that is necessary, such as after a minimally displaced pathologic fracture in the proximal end of the humerus from a UBC. Perhaps, further imaging of the fracture site is indicated if the trauma sustained by the child does not typically result in a fracture or a particular fracture pattern. A high index of suspicion is often necessary to search for an underlying pathology.

After comfort and safety from neurovascular injury are ensured, mobility should be considered next. Pathologic fractures seldom result in open fractures. Will casting allow a child to be mobile? Will the child's mobility alter fracture union rates? Will immobilization produce a decrease in bone mineral density and worsen the child's functional outcome, as is frequently seen in OI? Will surgical intervention diminish the need for a postoperative cast? Will open reduction and internal fixation allow earlier weight bearing? If return to weight bearing will not occur sooner with a more aggressive treatment strategy, what are its indications? Is more than one skeletal lesion present? Will the repair of a distal long bone lesion create a secondary lesion more proximally located in the same bone? It is not reasonable to fix one part of the bone if the remaining bone remains structurally compromised.

What is the natural history of a pathologic fracture? Will the fracture spontaneously resolve, as is seen in vertebrae plana? See Figure 3–4. Oftentimes, an eosinophilic granuloma of a non–weight-bearing bone, such as the clavicle, will heal spontaneously after a pathologic fracture. If surgical intervention will not offer significant advantages in terms of functional improvement in the long or short term, it should not be an option when considering only musculoskeletal rehabilitation. Restoration of anatomic alignment and prevention of deformity are important considerations, as are maintenance of the viability of the physis and elimination of future limb length inequality. The morbidity associated with surgery may weigh more as a detriment than as an advantage.

Financial considerations need to be evaluated in the treatment and functional outcome. The cost savings of internal fixation are having an increased socioeconomic impact on the physician. Hospital traction for a sustained period may not offer any functional improvement when compared with immediate skeletal stabilization. The cost savings may push the equation toward internal fixation.

The psychosocial adaptation of the child or patient reacting to a pathologic fracture and its treatment is another variable to be considered in the functional portion of the outcome triangle. This variable especially comes into play in the management of skeletal sarcomas, when limb salvage versus amputation options frequently present a dilemma to the family and surgeon. Multiple studies have not demonstrated any adverse psychologic outcome from childhood amputation, but clearly, the stigma and fear of amputation are concerns in our society.[35, 36] Additionally, long-term financial analyses have demonstrated that the cost of amputation to society is far greater than limb salvage. This difference increases exponentially the younger the children and the longer their survival.[12] The Van Ness rotationplasty offers an alternative to amputation by providing a more efficient gait. The rotationplasty converts an above-knee amputee into a below-knee amputee by using the rotated ankle as a knee joint. Plantar flexion of the ankle is converted to knee extension by transposing the ankle joint and rotating it 180°. The psychosocial adaptation of a child seen in public with the foot pointing backward can have serious consequences. However, studies have not demonstrated any deleterious long-term psychologic sequelae of such procedures.[35] Recent advances in limb salvage techniques and implants have diminished the need for this procedure. Distraction osteogenesis with ring fixators placed on an extremity for the greater part of a year may also have an adverse impact on the psychologic makeup of the child. How the child is able to cope with the fixator, adapt in school, and maintain mobility are important considerations to be evaluated.

Functional outcome rating scores for extremities, especially after a large skeletal reconstruction, are not commonly used in practice. The Toronto Extremity Salvage Score (TESS) is a well-studied and validated outcome instrument.[8] It is currently being evaluated and applied to extremities after limb salvage reconstruction in adults. Although this instrument does not directly apply to most pathologic fractures in children, knowledge of the rating system by the treating surgeon provides a "conscience" that may help direct management strategies toward a more optimal functional result. Another existing rating system includes the extremity-specific American Academy of Orthopaedic Surgeons Functional Rating System. The components of any validated functional outcome instrument combine objective measures with the subjective perception of the patient. Though possibly difficult in a child, it is important to consider these variables when planning a treatment strategy. It may often be necessary for the parent's wishes and desires to give way to the priorities of oncologic and orthopaedic management. Functional restoration therefore remains a critical component in the overall treatment plan.

## CONCLUSION

Pathologic fractures in children occur from a variety of causes. No single approach is best, nor is an algorithm appropriate for every use. One must develop a cognitive treatment strategy that weighs the pros and cons and considers the variables as described by the outcome triangle. The clinician-scientist must consider bone biology and biomechanics at the fracture site. Determining lesional pathology is of paramount importance, whether it be from a neoplastic or non-neoplastic entity, so that bone healing can be maximized. Time-efficient,

child-protective skeletal restoration is the measured impact of the surgeon's intervention. This strategy must be individualized for every situation.

Combinations of diseases, fracture sites, and children are many, whereas treatment options are fewer. Options include nonoperative management with observation and intralesional resection with or without bone grafting and with or without internal fixation. Third, wide resection with megaprosthetic or biologic reconstruction of skeletal defects may be required. A thoughtful, disciplined, and patterned approach will most often be successful.

The goals for treatment of a child's pathologic fracture are all based on the establishment of a diagnosis. Only after establishing the diagnosis with certainty can a proper treatment strategy be formulated. Fracture management is then based on answering the questions posed by the outcome triangle. The goals of treatment are five: (1) pain relief and comfort for the child; (2) achievement of local control or containment of the pathologic entity; (3) skeletal stabilization, preservation of growth, and return to anatomic alignment; (4) fracture union; and (5) restoration of function. Maintaining perspective by "keeping your eye on the ball" will facilitate optimal patient care and minimize the confounding variables that seem to plague the treatment of pathologic fractures.

### REFERENCES

1. Abudu, A.; Sferopoulos, N.K.; Tillman, M.R.; et al. The surgical treatment and outcome of pathologic fractures in localized osteosarcoma. J Bone Joint Surg Br 78:694–698, 1996.
2. Arata, M.A.; Peterson, H.A.; Dahlin, D.C. Pathologic fractures through non-ossifying fibromas: Review of the Mayo Clinic experience. J Bone Joint Surg Am 63:980–988, 1981.
3. Beaty, J.H.; Austin, S.M.; Warner, W.H.; et al. Interlocking intramedullary nailing of femoral shaft fractures in adolescents: Preliminary results and complications. J Pediatr Orthop 14:178–183, 1994.
4. Brooks, D.B.; Burstein, A.H.; Frankel, V.H. The biomechanics of torsional fractures: The stress concentration effect of a drill hole. J Bone Joint Surg Am 52:507–514, 1970.
5. Burstein, A.H.; Zika, J.M.; Heipole, K.G.; Klein, L. Contribution of collagen and mineral to the elastic-plastic properties of bone. J Bone Joint Surg Am 57:956–961, 1975.
6. Bucay, N.; Sarosi, I.; Dostan, C.R.; et al. Osteoprotegerin-deficient mice developed early onset osteoporosis and arterial calcification. Genes Dev 12:1260–1268, 1998.
7. Chin, K.R.; Kharrazi, F.D.; Miller, B.S.; et al. Osteochondromas of the distal aspect of the tibia or fibula. Natural history and treatment. J Bone Joint Surg Am 82:1269–1278, 2000.
8. Davis, A.M.; Bell, R.S.; Badley, E.M.; et al. Evaluating functional outcome in patients with lower extremity sarcoma. Clin Orthop 358:90–100, 1999.
9. Enneking, W.F.; Geran, P.F. Fibrous dysplasia of the femoral neck. J Bone Joint Surg Am 68:1415–1422, 1986.
10. Freeman, B.; Bray, E.W.; Meier, L.C. Multiple osteotomies with Zickel nail fixation for polyostotic fibrous dysplasia involving the proximal part of femur. J Bone Joint Surg Am 69:691–698, 1987.
11. Gainor, B.J.; Buckart, P. Fracture healing in metastatic bone disease. Clin Orthop 178:297–302, 1983.
12. Grimer, R.J.; Carter, S.R.; Pynsent, P.R. The cost effectiveness of limb salvage for bone tumors. J Bone Joint Surg Br 79:558–561, 1997.
13. Green, N.; Robertson, W.W.; Kilroy, A.W. Eosinophilic granuloma of the spine with associated neural deficient. J Bone Joint Surg Am 62:1198–1202, 1980.
14. Guille, J.T.; Kumar, S.J.; Shah, A. Spontaneous union of a congenital pseudoarthrosis of the tibia after Syme amputation. Clin Orthop 351:180–185, 1998.

15. Jaffe, H.L.; Lichtein, L. Solitary unicameral bone cyst with emphasis on the roentgen picture. The pathologic picture and the pathogenesis. Arch Surg 44:1004–1025, 1942.
16. Komiya, S.; Minamitani, K.; Sasaguri, Y.; et al. Simple bone cyst: Treatment by trepanation and studies on bone resorptive factors in cyst fluid with a theory of its pathogenesis. Clin Orthop 287:204–211, 1993.
17. Lacey, D.L.; Timms, E.; Tan, H.L.; et al. Osteoprotegerin ligand is a cytokine that regulates osteoclast differentiation and activation. Cell 93:165–176, 1998.
18. Mankin, H.J.; Mankin, C.J.; Simon, M.A. The hazards of the biopsy, revisited. J Bone Joint Surg Am 78:656–663, 1996.
19. Mirra, J.M.; Bernard, G.W.; Bullough, P.G.; et al. Cementum-like bone production in solitary bone cyst: Reported of three cases. Clin Orthop 135:295–307, 1978.
20. Mirzayan, R.; Panossian, V.; Avedian, R.; et al. The use of calcium sulfate in the treatment of benign bone lesions. J Bone Joint Surg Am 83:355–358, 2001.
21. Momberger, N.; Stevens, P.; Smith, J.; et al. Intramedullary nailing of femoral fractures in adolescence. J Pediatr Orthop 20:482–484, 2000.
22. Mundy, G.R. Mechanisms of bone metastasis. Cancer 80(Suppl 8): 1546–1556, 1997.
23. Sillence, D.O. Osteogenesis imperfecta; an expanding panorama of variance. Clin Orthop 159:11–25, 1981.
24. Wilkinson, J.M.; Scott, B.W.; Clarke, A.M.; Bell, M.J. Surgical stabilisation of the lower limb in osteogenesis imperfecta using the Sheffield telescopic intramedullary rod system. J Bone Joint Surg Br 80:999–1004, 1998.
25. Scaglietti, O.; Marchetti, P.G.M.; Bartolozzi, P. Final results obtained in the treatment of bone cysts with methylprednisolone acetate (Depo-Medrol) and a discussion of results achieved in other bone lesions. Clin Orthop 165:33–42, 1982.
26. Schwartz, H.S.; Zimmerman, N.B.; Simon, M.A.; et al. The malignant potential of enchondromatosis. J Bone Joint Surg Am 69:269–274, 1987.
27. Scully, S.P.; Temple, H.T.; O'Keefe, R.J.; et al. The surgical treatment of patients with osteosarcoma who have sustained a pathologic fracture. Clin Orthop 324:227–232, 1996.
28. Shapiro, F. Ollier's disease. An assessment of angular deformity, shortening, and pathologic fracture in twenty-one patients. J Bone Joint Surg Am 64:95–103, 1982.
29. Simonet, W.S.; Lacey, D.L.; Dunstan, C.R.; et al. Osteoprotegerin: Novel secreted protein involved in the regulation of bone density. Cell 89:309–319, 1997.
30. Smith, R. Osteogenesis imperfecta—where next? J Bone Joint Surg Br 79:177–178, 1997.
31. Stephenson, B.; London, M.D.; Hankin, F.M.; Kaufer, H. Fibrous dysplasia and analysis of options for treatment. J Bone Joint Surg Am 69:400–409, 1987.
32. Suva, L.J.; Winslow, G.A.; Wettenhall, R.E.; et al. A parathyroid hormone–related protein implicated in malignant hypercalcemia: Cloning and expression. Science 237:893–896, 1987.
33. Traub, J.A.; O'Connor, W.; Musso, P.D. Congenital pseudoarthrosis of the tibia: A retrospective review. J Pediatr Orthop 19:735–740, 1999.
34. Trondavi, M.M.; McKercher, S.R.; Anderson, K.; et al. Osteopetrosis in mice lacking haematopoietic transcription factor PU.1. Nature 386:81–84, 1997.
35. Weddington, W.W.; Segraves, K.B.; Simon, M.A. Psychological outcome of extremity sarcoma survivors undergoing amputation or limb salvage. J Clin Oncol 3:1393–1399, 1985.
36. Weddington, W.W.; Segraves, K.B.; Simon, M.A. Current and lifetime incidence of psychiatric disorders among a group of extremity sarcoma survivors. J Psychosom Res 30:121–125, 1986.
37. Wilkins, R.M. Unicameral bone cysts. J Am Acad Orthop Surg 8:217–224, 2000.

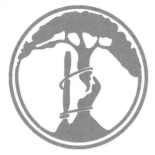

# CHAPTER 4

# The Multiply Injured Child

John H. Wilber, M.D.
George H. Thompson, M.D.

Children who are victims of severe trauma often sustain musculoskeletal injuries. However, they may also suffer injuries to other body areas that can be severe and life threatening. Although severe trauma is a major cause of morbidity and death in this age group, children and young adolescents are better able to survive it and often respond to treatment better than adults do. Long-term morbidity or disability is caused predominantly by injuries to the central nervous system (CNS) and musculoskeletal system.[164] Therefore, careful, coordinated, and integrated management of all injuries is mandatory to minimize morbidity and mortality.[57, 181] This chapter deals with the assessment of children who have sustained injuries to the musculoskeletal system and other body areas or organ systems. It is not our intent to discuss in detail specific isolated musculoskeletal injuries or their treatment; this information is presented in other chapters. The focus is on evaluating and prioritizing treatment of a multiply injured child with musculoskeletal injuries, with special consideration of aspects of care that may differ when dealing with multiple rather than isolated injuries.

## PATHOLOGY

It has been well documented in both the adult and the pediatric literature that an individual with multiple injuries must be managed differently from someone in whom similar injuries have occurred in isolation.* Concomitantly, it must be appreciated that assessment and management of a multiply injured patient may differ for adults and children. The anatomic, biomechanical, and physiologic differences in the musculoskeletal systems of adults and children have an important influence on orthopaedic treatment, as well as the incidence,

distribution, and management of injuries to other body areas and organ systems.[61, 193, 221, 222, 237]

## ANATOMIC DIFFERENCES

Anatomic differences in the pediatric skeleton are multiple and vary with age and maturity. These differences include the presence of preosseous cartilage, physes, and thicker, stronger periosteum that produces callus more rapidly and in greater amounts than in adults. Because of the effects of age and growth, children vary in body size and proportions.

The size of the child is important not only in the response to trauma but also in the severity and constellation of injuries. Being variably smaller, children sustain a different complex of injuries than adults do in a similar traumatic situation. An example is a pedestrian struck by a motor vehicle. In adults, injury to the tibia or knee is common because these structures are at the level of the automobile's bumper. In children, depending on their height, the bumper usually causes a fracture of the femur or pelvis or, in toddlers, a chest or head injury. Because the mass of a child's body is proportionately less, a child is much more likely to become a projectile when struck, with further injuries caused by secondary contact with the ground or another object. A classic example is Waddell's triad, which consists of an ipsilateral femoral shaft fracture, chest contusion, and contralateral head injury[221] (Fig. 4–1). Because of their smaller size, children are also more likely to be trapped beneath a moving object such as a motor vehicle and sustain crush injuries, fractures, and soft tissue damage. Crush injuries are relatively common in children; they often result in severe soft tissue loss, which has a worse prognosis.[148]

A child's body proportions, being quite different from those of an adult, can produce a different spectrum of injuries. A child's head is larger in proportion to the body, and the younger the child, the more extreme this

---

*See References 5, 57, 71, 76, 80, 99, 157, 181, 218, 230, 270.

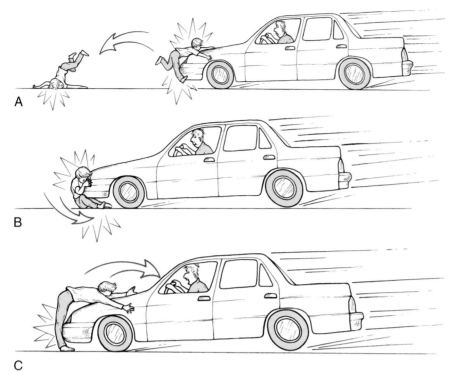

A

B

C

FIGURE **4–1.** Different injury patterns resulting from a similar car-versus-pedestrian mechanism. *A,* A typical Waddell triad in which the child sustains an ipsilateral femoral and chest injury from the initial impact of the car and is then thrown forward and strikes the contralateral side of the head on the ground. *B,* A smaller child being struck by the car and sustaining chest and head injuries from a direct blow on the bumper and then sustaining lower extremity crush injuries from being dragged underneath the car. *C,* An adolescent being struck, sustaining tibia or knee injuries from the bumper, and then being thrown forward and sustaining chest, head, and neck injuries from impact on the windshield.

disproportion.[121] This comparatively larger head size makes the head and neck much more vulnerable to injury, especially with falls from a height, because the weight of the head often causes it to strike the ground first. In contrast, adults are more likely to protect themselves with their extremities or try to land on their feet. The relative shortness of children's extremities, especially the arms, and a lack of strength often prevent them from adequately protecting themselves during a fall. This theory is supported by the high incidence of head injuries suffered by young children as a result of falls[22, 170, 202, 238] (Fig. 4–2).

## BIOMECHANICAL DIFFERENCES

The material properties, or composition, of bone in children is quite different from those of adult bone. Children, including those who are victims of multiple trauma, demonstrate unique fracture patterns. These patterns include compression (torus), incomplete tension-compression (greenstick), plastic or bend deformation,[160] complete, and epiphyseal fractures. These fracture patterns result from the presence of the physes, the thicker periosteum, and the material properties of the bone itself. Complete fractures occur more commonly in children with multiple trauma because they are associated with high-velocity injuries. Biomechanically, the pediatric skeletal system responds differently to an applied force than the adult skeleton does. Pediatric bone has a lower ash content and increased porosity, properties indicative of less mineralization.[61] Such bone composition results in increased plasticity and less energy needed for bone failure. This difference decreases with skeletal maturity.

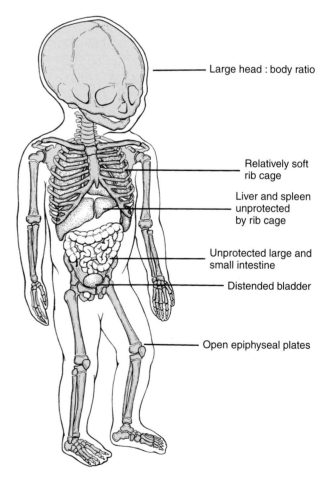

Large head : body ratio

Relatively soft rib cage

Liver and spleen unprotected by rib cage

Unprotected large and small intestine

Distended bladder

Open epiphyseal plates

FIGURE **4–2.** Anatomic differences predispose a child to injuries different from those of an adult. These differences include a disproportionately large head, pliable rib cage with exposed liver and spleen below its margin, unprotected large and small bowel, distended bladder above the pelvic brim, and open physes.

Bending is the most common mode for failure in long bones. Stress on the tension side of a bone with a low-yield stress initiates a fracture that is followed by compression on the opposite side. As bending continues, the fracture line eventually travels the entire width of the bone. Currey and Butler[61] demonstrated that although pediatric bone is weaker, it has a greater capacity to undergo plastic deformation than adult bone does. Because pediatric bone yields at a lower force, the stress in the bone is less and the energy to propagate the fracture is less. These factors account for the compression, greenstick, and plastic deformation fracture patterns. The increased porosity of pediatric bone, which was previously thought to play a major role in the different fracture patterns, is no longer accepted as a theory. Currey[60] studied impact energy absorption in 39 human femurs ranging from 3 to 95 years old and found no relationship between porosity and the impact energy absorbed.

Ligaments frequently insert into the epiphyses. As a consequence, traumatic forces applied to an extremity may be transmitted to the physis. The strength of the physis is enhanced by the perichondrial ring and, in some cases, by interdigitating mammillary bodies. In spite of this enhanced strength, however, the physis is not as strong biomechanically as the ligaments or metaphyseal or diaphyseal bone. Consequently, physeal fractures are relatively common in multiply injured children, and ligamentous injuries are less common than in adults. Ligamentous injuries do occur, however, and are probably more frequent than previously reported.

Because pediatric bone is more deformable and fractures with less force, it also affords less protection to the internal organs and other structures. The plasticity of bones can allow internal injuries without obvious external trauma, as reflected in the increased incidence of cardiac and pulmonary injury without apparent damage to the thoracic cage and a high incidence of abdominal injuries without significant injury to the pelvis, abdomen, or lower ribs.[34, 77, 251] Injuries to the liver and spleen are more common in children because of less rib coverage of these structures, as well as the greater pliability of the ribs. Children also have less soft tissue coverage, including muscle mass and strength, to protect the skeletal system from trauma. The lower mass of soft tissue may contribute to injury to the internal organs.

## PHYSIOLOGIC DIFFERENCES

Children respond differently from adults to the metabolic and physiologic stress of trauma. The total blood volume is smaller, depending on the size of the child, so less blood loss can be tolerated and hypovolemia develops more rapidly because the smaller volumes lost represent a larger percentage of the total.[161] The higher ratio of surface area to volume also makes children more vulnerable to hypothermia.[232] Klein and Marcus[141] showed that the metabolic response is significantly different in adults and children. Whereas adults have a significant increase in their metabolic rate from the stress of trauma, children have minimal or no change. This minimal response to stress is believed to be caused by the

significantly higher baseline metabolic rate of children, which needs to be increased only a small amount to accommodate the increased metabolic demands. The accelerated metabolic rate, together with the ability to metabolize lipid stores, provides a possible explanation for the increased survival rates in children after severe trauma.

Physiologically, pediatric fractures have the capacity to heal rapidly, remodel, overgrow, and become progressively deformed or shortened if the physis is injured. For these reasons, pediatric fractures secondary to severe trauma require careful management. Musculoskeletal morbidity is a common sequela of multiple trauma.[126, 164] The ultimate consequences of injury are often not known for many years, and long-term follow-up is therefore necessary.

## INCIDENCE

Trauma is the leading cause of death in children 14 years of age and younger. It accounts for approximately 50% of all deaths in children[99] as compared with 10% in the overall population of the United States. Fifteen thousand children 14 years old or younger die of accidental injuries each year in the United States, and an additional 19 million are injured severely enough to seek medical care or to have their activities restricted.[1, 5, 189] Haller[111] reported that more than 100,000 children are permanently crippled each year as a result of accidents. Marcus and coworkers,[164] in a study of multiple injuries in children, found that long-term morbidity was directly related to the severity of the head and musculoskeletal injuries. Fortunately, most injuries in children are minor; the most common are caused by falls resulting in injury to a single extremity, usually the upper extremity. Chan and associates[48] in 1989 showed that approximately 13% of the children being evaluated in the emergency department of an urban teaching hospital had serious injuries. Gallagher and colleagues[89] in 1984 and Tsai[278] in 1987 showed a bimodal age distribution of traumatic injuries in children, the first being in the first year of life and the second being an increase through the adolescent years. Chan and associates[48] showed a steady increase in the number of age-associated injuries with respect to both total number and severity. Although the exact incidence and rate of severe traumatic injuries are not truly known, it has been shown in multiple studies that the incidence increases as the child begins to interact with the adult world, especially with motor vehicles.[48, 99, 125, 129] The majority of injuries in the earlier years occur where younger children spend the most time, usually in or about the home. This pattern changes as children get older, spend more time away from home, and begin to enter the adult world.

## MECHANISM OF INJURY

As in adults, the severity of the injuries sustained by children is directly related to the ultimate force applied.

The two most common mechanisms of severe injury in children are falls and motor vehicle–related accidents.

## Falls

Gratz[99] reported that most pediatric injuries are caused by simple falls, which account for 46% of injuries overall. According to Hall and coworkers,[110] falls account for 46% of all childhood deaths from trauma. Nonetheless, falls are only the seventh leading cause of death in children from all causes. Falls have an increasing importance in younger children in that they are the third leading cause of mortality in children aged 1 to 4 years. Even simple falls in an infant or young child can be significant. According to these investigators, falls contributed to 41% of deaths in this age group.[110] Musemeche and associates[185] showed that falls occur predominantly in the younger population, with a mean age of 5 years and a 68% male preponderance. Seventy-eight percent of the falls occurred from a height of two stories or less and occurred at or near the home. Most patients sustained a single major injury that usually involved the head or skeletal system, although the incidence and spectrum of injury have been shown to vary with age.[238] Long bone fractures predominate in children, whereas the incidence of spine and the total number of fractures are increased in adolescents. Fortunately, children can survive falls from significant heights, although serious injuries do occur.[22, 45, 238, 291] As would be expected, morbidity and mortality rates increase with the height of the fall, the latter usually being related to falls of a distance exceeding 10 feet. Falls from windows are a particular urban problem, especially for children 4 years and younger.[22]

## Motor Vehicle Accidents

By far, the most common cause of multiple injury to children is motor vehicle accidents—as both occupants and pedestrians. This fact is well documented in publications on multiply injured children[137, 157, 164, 252] (Table 4–1). In the 1989 series by Kaufmann and colleagues[137] of 376 multiply injured children, motor vehicle–related accidents accounted for 58% of the overall injuries and 76% of the severely injured children. Marcus and coworkers[164] and Loder[157] reported a 91% and 96% incidence of motor vehicle–related mechanisms of injury in their respective series. Although the mechanism of injury was not analyzed by age, the incidence of motor vehicle–related injuries increases with age. According to the *Injury Mortality Atlas of the United States, 1979–1987,* deaths from motor vehicle accidents are lowest from birth to 14 years (5.9 to 10 per 100,000 population), with the peak occurring in the 15- to 24-year-old age group (26 to 45 per 100,000).[127] Males in this age group have twice the mortality rate of females. Scheidler and colleagues demonstrated that being an unrestrained child or adolescent and being ejected from the vehicle tripled the risk for mortality and significantly increased injury severity scores.[239]

## ASSOCIATED INJURIES

By definition, a multiply injured child has injuries involving more than one organ system. It is critical to recognize, evaluate, and treat all injuries sustained. Although many injuries occur in isolation or in random combination, numerous others have been shown to occur in an associated pattern. One of the more common groups of associated injuries is that described as Waddell's triad.[221] A history of a child being struck by a car and a diagnosis of any one of the triad of injuries should alert the physician to evaluate the other associated areas. This admonition holds true for all known injury patterns.

## Spinal Injuries

The presence of facial injuries, including lacerations, contusions, and fractures, has been shown to be associated with an increased incidence of cervical spine injury in both children and adults.[150, 154] The presence of a spinal fracture at any level in a multiple-trauma patient is associated with a greater incidence (5% to 10%) of noncontiguous fractures at other levels of the spine.[104, 109, 187, 210] Because children are more elastic than adults, the force of injury can be transmitted over multiple segments and result in multiple fractures. In addition, certain anatomic differences have an effect on the type of injury, such as the increased cartilage-to-bone ratio, the presence of secondary ossification centers, variations in the normal planes of the articular facet, and increased laxity. Thus, any child presenting with head, facial, or spinal injury at any level should have a careful evaluation of the entire spinal column, especially a head-injured child who is either comatose or unable to cooperate in the examination. chest.[241, 258, 259] In a multiply injured child, a spinal injury must be assumed to be present until proved

| TABLE 4–1 | | | |
|---|---|---|---|
| **Mechanism of Injury** | | | |
| **Mechanism** | **Marcus et al. (1983) (N = 74) (%)** | **Loder (1987) (N = 74) (%)** | **Kaufmann et al. (1990) (N = 376) (%)** |
| Motor vehicle accidents | | | |
| Occupant | 9 | 35 | 18 |
| Pedestrian | 76 | 33 | 23 |
| Bicycle | 3 | 18 | 17 |
| Motorcycle | 3 | 5 | 0 |
| Train | 6 | 1 | 0 |
| Falls | 3 | 4 | 24 |
| Other | 0 | 4 | 19 |

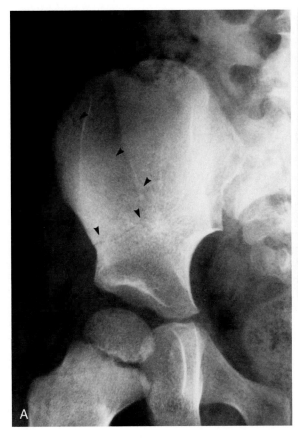

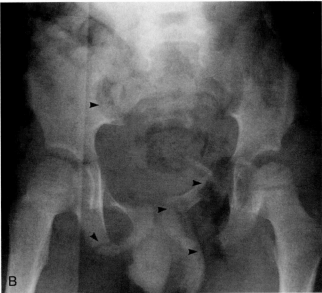

FIGURE 4–3. *A,* Anteroposterior radiograph of a 4-year-old child demonstrating a nondisplaced stable fracture of the iliac wing with no associated intrapelvic or infra-abdominal injuries. *B,* Anteroposterior pelvic radiograph of a 5-year-old who was run over by a truck and sustained multiple pelvic injuries and multiple associated injuries, including proximal femoral fractures, degloving soft tissue injuries, rectal perforation, and bladder rupture.

otherwise by physical examination and radiographic evaluation.

## Rib Fractures

The validity of fracture of the first rib as a marker for severe trauma is well documented in the adult literature.[3] Harris and Soper[115] in 1990 demonstrated the same association in pediatric multiple-trauma patients. Fractures of the first rib are associated with a high incidence of other injuries, including clavicle fractures, additional rib fractures, head injuries, great vessel injuries, pneumothoraces, and lung and cardiac contusions.

Multiple rib fractures are also a marker of severe trauma in pediatric patients. Garcia and associates[92] reported a 42% mortality rate in pediatric patients with multiple rib fractures; the risk of mortality increases with the number of ribs fractured. They found that a head injury with multiple rib fractures signified an even worse prognosis with a 71% mortality rate. Because head injuries are associated with a higher incidence of mortality and long-term disability, it is critical to recognize this relationship. Multiple rib fractures in a child younger than 3 years should also alert the physician to the possibility of child abuse; 63% of the patients in this age group in the series of Garcia and colleagues were victims of child abuse.[92] Multiple fractures in different stages of healing are also a sign of child abuse and should

raise the physician's suspicion accordingly (see Chapter 17).

## Pelvic Fractures

Pelvic fractures in children are uncommon and, as in adults, are usually the result of high-velocity trauma.* Simple or isolated, nondisplaced pelvic fractures have low morbidity and mortality rates and tend to not be associated with other injuries (Fig. 4–3). Fortunately, most pelvic injuries in children are simple nondisplaced fractures. Conversely, severe, displaced pelvic fractures have a 63% to 87% incidence of associated injuries.[103, 229, 269] Associated injuries include head injuries; other fractures, including open fractures; hemorrhage; genitourinary injuries; and abdominal injuries. A sacral fracture, which is common in pelvic fractures, may have associated neurologic deficits. The presence of severe pelvic fractures should alert the physician to possible injuries to the abdominal and pelvic contents, particularly genitourinary injuries such as urethral lacerations (especially in males) and bladder rupture. Abdominal injuries may include rectal lacerations, tears of the small or large intestine, and visceral rupture of the liver, spleen, and kidneys. Blood at the urethral meatus, a high-riding or nonpalpable prostate gland on rectal examination, and

---

*See references 24, 29, 38, 42, 93, 103, 139, 172, 173, 184, 186, 215, 223, 226, 229.

blood in the scrotum are indications of serious damage to the genitourinary system. Such genitourinary complications must be investigated further, usually with a retrograde urethrogram, before attempting to insert a Foley catheter.[83] Rectal or vaginal lacerations indicate that the pelvic fracture may be open. A diverting colostomy may be necessary for these individuals to decrease the risk of infection. If a pelvic fracture is diagnosed and if it is necessary to perform peritoneal lavage, a supraumbilical approach is recommended instead of the routine infraumbilical approach because the former approach may avoid false-positive findings secondary to pelvic bleeding. Unstable fractures, such as vertical shear or wide pelvic diastasis, are often associated with significant hemorrhage and hypovolemic shock secondary to retroperitoneal bleeding[223] (see Chapter 12). Significant hemorrhage requiring transfusion occurs in 27% to 46% of pediatric pelvic fractures.[269] Control of hemorrhage is important because persistent bleeding may lead to coagulopathy and hypothermia.

## Lap Belt Injuries

In an automobile accident, the use of a lap belt without shoulder restraint may produce a constellation of injuries referred to as the seat belt syndrome.[2, 8, 96, 236, 248, 260] These injuries in children include flexion-distraction injury to the lumbar spine (Chance's fracture), small bowel rupture, and traumatic pancreatitis. Ecchymosis in a lap belt distribution should alert the physician to search for a lumbar fracture.[248] Head and extremity injuries are unusual, but can occur, in sharp contrast to an unrestrained passenger, who usually sustains severe head and solid organ injuries.[122, 227]

## Other Injury Patterns

Understanding injury patterns and the types of associated injury can be helpful in evaluating a multiply injured patient. However, almost any combination can occur in a child, and the injury patterns are most closely related to the mechanism, the total force applied, and the age of the patient. According to Peclet and colleagues,[202] head injuries are most common in child abuse victims, occupants in vehicular accidents, and children sustaining falls; nearly 40% of abused children suffer injuries to the head and face. In their study, thoracic and abdominal injuries were most common in children with penetrating injuries (gunshot and stab wounds), whereas extremity injuries predominated in bicyclists and pedestrians. These investigators also showed that the types of injuries change with age: burns and foreign bodies accounted for most injuries to children aged 1 to 2 years, as compared with a median age of 7 years for pedestrian bicycle injuries and 12 years for gunshot and stab wounds. Falls and traffic-related injuries predominated in children 5 to 10 years of age. Children who sustained injuries from falls were significantly younger than those with traffic-related injuries. The pattern of injuries from falls also changes

with age. Sawyer and associates found that adolescents sustain a greater number of vertebral fractures and total fractures per fall whereas children have a greater number of long bone fractures.[238] Because the mechanisms of injury change with age, injury patterns and associated injuries also vary accordingly.

## TRAUMA SCORING SYSTEMS

It is obvious that a multiply injured child has a spectrum of injuries of varying degrees of severity. The need for a measure of the severity of trauma is well recognized, both to assist in management and as a predictor of outcome. This need has been documented in adult trauma patients, and several systems have been developed, including the Injury Severity Score[12, 13, 54]; Shock Index[41]; Trauma Score[47]; Revised Trauma Score[46]; Glasgow Coma Scale[264]; Abbreviated Injury Scale[51, 52, 101]; TRISS-Scan, a combination of the Trauma Score, Injury Severity Score, and patient age[32, 135]; Acute Trauma Index[177]; and Hannover Polytrauma Score.[192] Similar systems have been recommended for pediatric patients, the most widely used being the Modified Injury Severity Scale (MISS)[169, 171] and, the Pediatric Trauma Score (PTS).[266, 267]

Significant controversy exists regarding which is the best trauma scoring system to use and whether specific pediatric scores are needed. Two studies both showed that the Trauma Score and the TRISS-Scan showed the greatest accuracy as regards survival prediction.[199, 294] The need for pediatric-specific scores was therefore questioned. Nevertheless, the MISS and PTS can be useful in assessing and monitoring the outcomes of multiply injured children.

## Modified Injury Severity Scale

The MISS represents an adaptation of the Abbreviated Injury Scale—1980,[52] combined with the Glasgow Coma Scale for neurologic injuries.[264] The pediatric MISS categorizes injuries into five body areas: (1) neurologic system, (2) face and neck, (3) chest, (4) abdomen and pelvic contents, and (5) extremities and pelvic girdle[169, 171] (Table 4–2). The severity of each injury is rated on a scale of 1 to 5, with 1 point for minor injury, 2 points for moderate injury, 3 points for severe but not life-threatening injury, 4 points for severe injury but with probable survival, and 5 points for critical injury with uncertain survival. The Glasgow Coma Scale is used for grading neurologic injuries[264] (Table 4–3). The usefulness of the Glasgow Coma Scale has been well established in head injuries in both adult and pediatric populations.

The MISS score is determined by the sum of the squares of the three most severely injured body areas. The MISS has been shown to be an accurate predictor of morbidity and mortality in pediatric trauma. Mayer and associates[171] found that scores of 25 points or more were associated with an increased risk of permanent disability.

TABLE 4–2 ....................................................................................

The Modified Injury Severity Scale (MISS) for Multiply Injured Children

| Body Area | 1—Minor | 2—Minor | 3—Severe, Not Life Threatening | 4—Severe, Life Threatening | 5—Critical, Survival Uncertain |
|---|---|---|---|---|---|
| Neural | GCS score of 13–14 | GCS score of 9–12 | GCS score of 9–12 | GCS score of 5–8 | GCS score of 4 |
| Face and neck | Abrasion or contusions of the ocular apparatus or lid Vitreous or conjunctival hemorrhage Fractured teeth | Undisplaced facial bone fracture Laceration of the eye, disfiguring laceration Retinal detachment | Loss of an eye, avulsion of the optic nerve Displaced facial fracture "Blow-out" fracture of the orbit | Bone or soft tissue injury with minor destruction | Injuries with airway obstruction |
| Chest | Muscle ache or chest wall stiffness | Simple rib or sternal fracture | Multiple rib fractures Hemothorax or pneumothorax Diaphragmatic rupture Pulmonary contusion | Open chest wounds Pneumomediastinum Myocardial contusion | Lacerations, tracheal hemomediastinum Aortic laceration Myocardial laceration or rupture |
| Abdomen | Muscle ache, seat belt abrasion | Major abdominal wall contusion | Contusion of abdominal organs Retroperitoneal hematoma Extraperitoneal bladder rupture | Minor laceration of abdominal organs Intraperitoneal bladder rupture Spine fractures with paraplegia | Rupture or severe laceration of abdominal vessels or organs |
| Extremities and pelvic girdle | Minor sprains Simple fractures and dislocations | Open fractures of digits Nondisplaced long bone or pelvic fractures | Thoracic or lumbar spine fractures Displaced long bone or multiple hand or foot fractures Single open long bone fracture Pelvic fractures with displacement Laceration of major nerves or vessels | Multiple closed long bone fractures Amputation of limbs | Multiple open long bone fractures |

GCS, Glasgow Coma Scale.
Adapted from Mayer, T., et al. J Pediatr Surg 15:719–726, 1980.

A score of more than 40 points was usually predictive of death. In their initial study, a score of 25 points or more was associated with 40% mortality and 30% disability, whereas a score of 24 points or less was associated with no deaths and only a 1% disability rate. Their mean MISS score for death was 33.4 points; for permanent disability, it was 30.2 points.

Marcus and coworkers[164] in 1983 used the MISS in their series of 34 multiply injured children and showed a progressive increase in disability and mortality with increasing scores. The mean score was 22 points, with a range of 10 to 34 points. Children with scores of 25 points or less had a 30% incidence of impairment, children with scores of 26 to 40 points had a 33% incidence of impairment, and children with scores of more than 40 points had a 100% incidence of impairment. Contrary to the findings of Mayer and associ-

ates,[171] children with scores over 40 were able to survive, but not without significant disability.

Loder[157] in 1987 also confirmed the relationship of increasing MISS scores with increasing mortality and morbidity in his series of 78 multiply injured children. He reported a mean MISS score of 28 points (range, 10 to 57 points). No deaths occurred in children with MISS scores of less than 40 points. The mortality rate for those with MISS scores above 40 points was 50%, and above 50 points it increased to 75%. Thus, the effectiveness of the MISS score in predicting both morbidity and mortality is well documented in several studies, although the absolute percentages vary.

Garvin and colleagues[93] in 1990 demonstrated the accuracy of the MISS in predicting morbidity and mortality after pediatric pelvic fractures. Disrupted pelvic fractures had a higher MISS score than did nondisrupted

---

**TABLE 4–3** ..............................................

Glasgow Coma Scale

---

**EYE OPENING**

4. Spontaneous
3. To speech
2. To pain
1. None

**BEST VERBAL RESPONSE**

5. Oriented
4. Confused
3. Inappropriate
2. Incomprehensible
1. None

**BEST MOTOR RESPONSE**

6. Obeys commands
5. Localizes pain
4. Withdraws
3. Flexes to pain
2. Extends to pain
1. None

..................................................

From Teasdale, G.; Bennett, B. Lancet 2:81–84, 1974.

---

fractures, and the former were associated with an increased incidence of morbidity and mortality.

Yue and associates[296] used the MISS in comparing the extent of injuries and the results of nonoperative versus operative or rigid stabilization in the management of ipsilateral pediatric femur and tibia fractures, the "floating" knee. The scores were useful in comparing the severity of injuries in both groups of patients.

## Pediatric Trauma Score

The index used to predict injury severity and mortality in children is the PTS.[136, 266, 267] This score is based on six components: (1) size, (2) airway, (3) systolic blood pressure, (4) CNS injury, (5) skeletal injury, and (6) cutaneous injury. Each category is scored +2 (minimal or no injury), +1 (minor or potentially major injury), or −1 (major or immediately life-threatening injury), depending on severity, and these points are added (Table 4–4). One major advantage of this system is that it is based on

criteria that can be easily obtained either at the scene of the accident or in the emergency room, and it can thus be used for triage purposes. Tepas and coworkers[266] in 1988 demonstrated a direct linear relationship between the PTS and the Injury Severity Scale and found that the PTS was an effective predictor of both morbidity and mortality. No deaths occurred in children with a PTS greater than 8 points; those with a PTS below zero had 100% mortality. The PTS allows for rapid assessment of trauma severity in a multiply injured child, which assists in appropriate field triage, transport, and early emergency treatment of these patients. It is recommended that children with a PTS of 8 points or less be transported to a pediatric trauma center for management.

## CONSEQUENCES OF INJURY
..................................................

### Mortality

Mortality rates in children vary greatly as a result of differences in the mechanism of injury, severity of injury, and age of the patient. Unlike adults, who have a trimodal distribution of mortality from trauma, children follow a bimodal curve. Peclet and colleagues[202] in 1990 demonstrated that the majority of deaths in children occurred within the first hour after injury, with another peak occurring at approximately 48 hours. In their series, 74% of deaths occurred within the first 48 hours. Overall, the mortality rate was 2.2% for all patients admitted to the trauma service. Not all the patients in this series were multiply injured, thus explaining the low mortality rate. In series dealing only with multiply injured children, van der Sluis and coauthors,[280] Mayer and associates,[171] Wesson and coworkers,[289] and Loder[157] reported mortality rates of 20%, 15%, 13%, and 9%, respectively. These series did not include children who were dead on arrival in the emergency department.

The fact that mortality rates are closely associated with the severity of injury is not surprising. The higher the MISS score or the lower the PTS, the greater the rate of mortality. In spite of obvious differences from adults, children tend to have similar outcomes from trauma when equivalent injuries are compared. This finding was supported by the work of Eichelberger and colleagues,[73]

---

**TABLE 4–4** ..............................................

Pediatric Trauma Score

|  | Severity Points | | |
|---|---|---|---|
| **Component** | **+2** | **+1** | **−1** |
| Size | >20 kg | 10–20 kg | <10 kg |
| Airway | Normal | Maintainable | Unmaintainable |
| Central nervous system | Normal | Obtunded | Comatose |
| Systolic blood pressure | >90 mm Hg | 90–50 mm Hg | <50 mm Hg |
| Open wounds | None | Minor | Major or penetrating |
| Skeletal | None | Closed fracture | Open or multiple fractures |

..................................................

Adapted from Tepas, J.J., III, et al. J Trauma 28:425–429, 1988.

who used a statistical method based on the Trauma Score, MISS, and age. These investigators were unable to show statistically significant differences between the various pediatric age groups and the adult population. Other studies have documented higher survival rates in severely injured children than in adults with a similar degree of injury.[157, 164] This concept is accepted by many but may not be true, as shown by Eichelberger and colleagues[73, 74] and Nakayama and associates.[188] Head injuries are consistently associated with higher mortality rates than are other types of injuries.

## Morbidity

Unlike a child with an isolated injury, which is usually associated with rapid healing, good function, and minimal residual disability, a multiply injured child has a significantly higher risk of residual disability. Morbidity in children is usually related to injuries to the CNS and musculoskeletal system.[81, 164, 280, 289] At a 6-month follow-up in a study by Wesson and coworkers[289] of severely injured children, 54% still had one or more functional limitations, with 4% in a vegetative state, 11% severely disabled, 32% moderately disabled, and 53% healthy. The cause of the disability at 6 months was head injury in 44% and musculoskeletal injury in 32%. These findings are consistent with other reported series. In the series by Marcus and coworkers,[164] 10 of the 32 survivors had residual disabilities. Five were related to head injury with residual seizures and spasticity. The remainder were from musculoskeletal injuries and included nonunion, malunion, and growth disturbances. Feickert and coauthors, in a series of severely head-injured children, reported that 39% still had severe neurologic impairment at the time of discharge.[81] The incidence and severity of the residual disability increased with the severity of the overall injury, as reflected in a higher MISS score. In children, disability often occurs late and is progressive because of the fact that children are still growing and normal growth patterns have been disrupted.

## TRAUMA EVALUATION AND MANAGEMENT

### Field Management before Transport

Successful management of a multiply injured child requires rapid, systematic assessment, with early emphasis on the treatment of life-threatening conditions. Treatment is initiated in the field with advanced life support techniques. The importance of treatment in the field, or during the prehospital phase, is well documented.[6, 123, 219, 240] Because mortality follows a bimodal distribution in pediatric multiple-trauma patients, with most deaths occurring shortly after the accident, an efficient and effective system of prehospital care is mandatory.[89, 278] Delays in treatment have been shown

by Seelig and associates[242] and by Holmes and Reyes[123] to significantly increase mortality. If surgery for life-threatening conditions was delayed more than 4 hours after injury, mortality was approximately 90%, whereas if surgery was performed within 4 hours, mortality was reduced to 30%. Functional recovery was also improved with more rapid surgical care. Delay in diagnosis and treatment has been shown to be particularly detrimental to those with head injury. A severely injured child is at greatest risk for delays in diagnosis and treatment.[87] The goal of field treatment is to evaluate the patient rapidly, stabilize life-threatening conditions, prepare the patient for transport by immobilizing injured areas, and deliver the patient to a center equipped for resuscitation and definitive treatment.

Early resuscitation plus stabilization of a pediatric trauma patient requires specialized equipment, including small-diameter airway tubes, small-bore intravenous needles, modified backboards, small cervical collars, and splints of appropriate size. As in adults, it is critical to immobilize the patient properly before transport to avoid further damage to injured parts, especially when dealing with spinal injuries and extremity fractures. Preventable deaths in multiply injured children have been placed into three major categories by Dykes and associates[71]: (1) respiratory failure, (2) intracranial hematoma, and (3) inadequately treated hemorrhage. Treatment of respiratory failure and hemorrhage can be initiated in the field. Optimal treatment of an intracranial hematoma, however, requires rapid field triage and transport for immediate surgical decompression. Ramenofsky and colleagues[218] showed a 53% incidence of preventable deaths, with field treatment errors occurring in 36% of cases and transport errors in 23%. The importance of appropriate field treatment cannot be overemphasized.

The use of pediatric air ambulance programs has been shown to be safe and effective and to allow earlier specialized medical care for severely injured children.[147]

## Pediatric Trauma Centers

Because most children sustaining multiple injuries require specialized care, they should be rapidly transported to a center that is able to institute the necessary treatment. The American College of Surgeons (ACS) has set standards categorizing the level of trauma care that an institution can provide to both adult and pediatric trauma victims.[5] These levels of care are categorized into pediatric trauma centers, adult trauma centers (level I, II, or III), and adult trauma centers with added qualifications to treat children. The ACS has also set guidelines regarding when a patient should be transferred to a pediatric trauma center (Table 4–5). Transport of an injured child to a facility lacking the capability of adequately handling these injuries significantly delays appropriate treatment and may allow inappropriate treatment to be initiated by a well-intentioned but inexperienced physician or staff member. Improved outcomes for trauma victims treated at trauma centers are well documented in both the pediatric and adult literature.[36, 71, 132, 137, 209, 218, 290] Osler and colleagues

**TABLE 4–5**

Guidelines for Pediatric Trauma Center Referral

More than one body system injury
Injuries that require pediatric intensive care
Shock that requires more than one blood transfusion
Fractures with neurovascular injuries
Fractures of the axial skeleton
Two or more major long bone fractures
Potential replantation of an amputated extremity
Suspected or actual spinal cord injury
Head injuries with any of the following:
    Orbital or facial bone fractures
    Altered state of consciousness
    Cerebrospinal fluid leak
    Changing neurologic status
    Open head injury
    Depressed skull fracture
    Requirements of intracranial pressure monitoring
Ventilatory support required

From American College of Surgeons Committee on Trauma. Advanced Trauma Life Support Course. Instructor's Manual. Chicago, American College of Surgeons, 1993.

reported that although pediatric trauma centers have overall higher survival rates for multiply injured children than adult trauma centers do, the difference decreases when controlled for Injury Severity Score, PTS, age, mechanism, and ACS verification status.[198]

## Trauma Team

In a multiply injured child, the complexity and number of injuries mandate a team approach. A multidisciplinary approach with members of specialties working as equal partners usually allows optimal care.[132] In most cases, the team leader should be a pediatric surgeon who specializes in the care of multiply injured children. This person should take primary responsibility for supervising the resuscitation effort, coordinating team members, and making critical decisions regarding treatment priorities. The members of the team are drawn from the pediatric surgical subspecialties and include a thoracic surgeon, cardiovascular surgeon, orthopaedic surgeon, neurosurgeon, urologist, pediatric anesthesiologist, and plastic surgeon. Additional members include emergency department physicians and nurses, pediatric intensive care physicians and nurses, respiratory therapists, and physicians and nurses from rehabilitation services. Social workers, psychologists, and counselors also have an important role in the treatment of these patients.

## Primary Survey and Resuscitation

The principles of evaluation and stabilization of a pediatric trauma patient have been established as guidelines and protocols by the ACS for advanced trauma life support.[5] Although these guidelines are similar to those for adults, pediatric patients require special consideration because of unique anatomic, physiologic, and patho-

physiologic differences.[75] The initial treatment consists of basic resuscitative measures, with the major focus on diagnosis and treatment of life-threatening injuries. These measures are considered the primary survey, with attention directed toward the treatment of problems with the airway, breathing, and circulation (the ABCs of initial resuscitation). The primary survey concludes with a brief neurologic examination and complete exposure of the patient for further assessment.

## AIRWAY AND BREATHING

Assessment of the airway is a primary consideration in all trauma patients. Patency of the airway must be assessed from the oral pharynx to the trachea. Evaluation, treatment, and maintenance of the airway must be performed with control and stabilization of the neck because of an increased incidence of cervical spine injuries in these children. Children have considerable variation in the anatomy of the upper airway that depends on their size and age. In spite of age, the jaw thrust maneuver is best for restoring airway patency; debris can be cleared from the mouth manually or with suction, if available. The neck is stabilized with in-line cervical traction. It is important to realize that infants are obligatory nasal breathers and that any injury that occludes the nasal passages also occludes the upper airway. These injuries include nasal fractures, foreign material in the nostrils, and bleeding within the nasal passages. Iatrogenically inserted tubes, such as nasogastric tubes, can also contribute to nasal occlusion. Thus, in an infant, both the oral pharynx and the nasal passage need to be cleared to restore the airway.

If a patent airway cannot be guaranteed with these maneuvers, an airway must be established with the use of an endotracheal tube. An oral airway is not recommended in children. Because the trachea varies in length and diameter according to the child's size and age, the diameter of the endotracheal tube chosen also varies. Two helpful rules may be used when choosing an endotracheal tube. The first is to base the size of the tube on the size of the external nares or the size of the child's little finger.[195] The other is the following formula[6, 72, 146]:

$$\text{Endotracheal tube (internal diameter in millimeters)} = 16 + \text{patient's age} \div 4$$

A full complement of endotracheal tube sizes must be available for dealing with multiply injured children. These tubes should be uncuffed, which allows for a loose fit in the trachea to prevent subglottic edema, ulceration, and eventual stenosis.

Passage of an endotracheal tube in a child is complicated by several factors, including the child's inability to cooperate, the flexed position of the head because of the large occiput, and the cephalic position of the larynx and glottis. The shortness of the trachea in young children also increases the potential for bronchial intubation; consequently, the presence of such intubation needs to be evaluated clinically by auscultation of breath sounds and by a postintubation anteroposterior (AP) radiograph of the chest.[50] Because the child's trachea is not calcified and is soft, the tip of the endotracheal tube can often be palpated to confirm its position. A pulse oximeter (oxygen saturation monitor) may be helpful in documenting tracheal versus esophageal intubation.

If the upper airway of a child is acutely obstructed and an adequate nasotracheal or endotracheal airway cannot be established, a surgical airway must be urgently created. A needle cricothyrotomy can be performed quickly and safely to establish a temporary airway and is the treatment of choice.[35, 191, 255] Surgical cricothyrotomy is rarely indicated because of its association with subglottic tracheal stenosis. A large-bore needle (14 or 16 gauge) can be directly inserted percutaneously into the trachea through the cricothyroid membrane to temporarily achieve an airway.[255]

Considerations for emergency needle cricothyrotomy include laryngeal fracture, major foreign bodies that cannot be removed manually, severe oropharyngeal bleeding prohibiting intubation, edema of the glottis, and facial or mandibular fractures. Because needle cricothyrotomy with the use of jet insufflation is only a temporary airway, if it is deemed that an oral or nasal airway cannot be achieved rapidly, provision must be made to convert the needle cricothyrotomy into a surgical cricothyrotomy. The cricothyrotomy should be performed in the operating room under controlled conditions to decrease the risk of subglottic tracheal stenosis. Surgical cricothyrotomy is not recommended in children younger than 12 years because of this potential complication.

As previously mentioned, while the airway is being established, care must be taken to stabilize the neck. All patients should be considered to have a cervical spine injury until proved otherwise. Temporary stabilization of the neck with sandbags and a backboard can be used, although these restraints should be replaced by a rigid cervical collar as soon as possible. A modified backboard should be used for young children and infants because of the large size of the head in relation to the trunk. Herzenberg and coworkers[121] demonstrated that the neck is flexed when the child is placed on a standard backboard, thus potentially displacing an unstable cervical spine injury (Fig. 4-4). A backboard with an occipital cutout or a pad under the trunk to elevate it is used to prevent flexion of the cervical spine. In-line traction is used in all patients when trying to establish the airway. A lateral radiograph of the cervical spine is always obtained after the primary survey. Major head and facial injuries should increase the physician's suspicion of potential cervical spine injuries.[150] In a comatose or uncooperative patient, a normal lateral radiograph of the cervical spine is inadequate evidence to rule out spinal injuries. The neck is protected until a full radiographic series (AP, oblique, and odontoid views) and clinical evaluation can be performed. Computed tomography (CT) is necessary if a fracture or the suggestion of a fracture is noted on these radiographs.

Once an airway has been established, adequate ventilation needs to be maintained. The adequacy of ventilation is evaluated both clinically and with arterial blood gas values. A pulse oximeter is also a rapid, noninvasive, and effective means of monitoring ventilation. Symmetric movement of the chest, auscultation for symmetric breath sounds, and palpation for equal chest expansion are necessary to ensure adequate ventilation. A posteroanterior (PA) or AP radiograph of the chest needs to be obtained to evaluate the position of the endotracheal tube, as well as assess for injuries to the thorax (rib fractures), heart, lungs, and great vessels. Because the thoracic cage in children is very compliant, pediatric patients can have significant lung and cardiac injuries without obvious external damage to the chest and without rib fractures.[34, 77, 251] The presence of a fracture

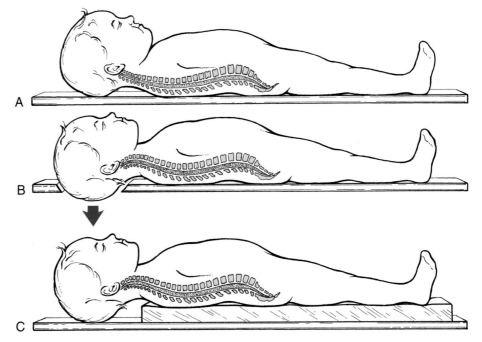

FIGURE 4-4. Standard adult backboard. *A,* The enlarged occiput causes a child to flex the head forward. *B* and *C,* Appropriate positioning on a modified board with either the occipital area cut out or a pad under the thorax to prevent flexion of the cervical spine.

of the first rib or multiple ribs indicates severe trauma and an increased risk for associated injuries.[92, 115]

**Life-Threatening Ventilation Abnormalities.** Injuries that may have a life-threatening effect on ventilation include tension pneumothorax, open pneumothorax, massive hemothorax, and flail chest. Because infants and small children ventilate primarily with the diaphragm, any injury or condition that compromises diaphragmatic excursion restricts ventilation. Potential injuries that affect diaphragmatic excursion include diaphragmatic rupture and intra-abdominal injuries.

*Gastric Distention.* Severe gastric distention can decrease diaphragmatic excursion considerably. Gastric decompression should be performed in all children with signs of ventilatory compromise. Decompression can be achieved easily with the passage of a small nasogastric or orogastric tube. Because of particulate matter, a tube smaller than a No. 10 French tube will not adequately aspirate the gastric fluid and stomach contents and should not be used.

*Tension Pneumothorax.* A pneumothorax under pressure may initially be managed by the insertion of a large-caliber intravenous catheter, such as a 14- or 16-gauge Angiocath, into an intercostal space. Such treatment relieves the pressure and converts it into a simple pneumothorax, which can be managed with the use of a chest tube. Large penetrating chest wounds are initially treated with an occlusive dressing and positive-pressure ventilation. A flail chest is diagnosed by the observation of paradoxical motion with respirations.[69] If the child also has signs of inadequate ventilation, it should be treated with endotracheal intubation and mechanical ventilation.

## CIRCULATION AND RESUSCITATION

**Shock.** It is critical to recognize and treat shock in the immediate phases of the primary survey. A child's response to shock is different from that of an adult. A child is often able to maintain normal blood pressure by increasing the heart rate along with significant peripheral constriction while in the supine position. Signs of shock in children include tachycardia, tachypnea, poor peripheral perfusion (cool extremities), diminished responsiveness, decreased urine output, and a systolic blood pressure less than 70 mm Hg.[5]

A decrease in blood pressure is not usually seen or is a very late finding; absence of hypotension, however, does not rule out shock. A child can often compensate for a 15% to 20% blood volume loss without a decline in blood pressure. The absolute blood pressure is not critical, and ACS guidelines state that it is unwise and time consuming to obtain blood pressure readings during the acute resuscitative phase.[5] Blood pressure measurement can be performed once the child has been stabilized. A guide for normal blood pressure in children is a systolic pressure of 80 mm Hg plus twice the child's age in years, with diastolic pressure being two thirds of systolic pressure. Because infants are relatively incapable of increasing their cardiac stroke volume, their only way to increase cardiac output is by increasing the heart rate. Thus, the heart rate must be monitored closely. Normal vital signs by age are presented in Table 4–6.

**Cardiac Tamponade.** Tamponade occurs when the pericardial space surrounding the heart fills with fluid (usually blood) and prevents the normal distention and contractility of the heart. This cardiac compression results in a progressive decrease in cardiac output and, ultimately, heart failure. The clinical findings of cardiac tamponade include Beck's triad: muffled heart sounds, distended neck veins, and pulsus paradoxus. Initial emergency management consists of pericardiocentesis with the use of a long, plastic-sheathed needle that is attached to an electrocardiogram monitor and inserted through a subxiphoid route. The need for emergency surgical drainage of the pericardium can be temporarily delayed by leaving the plastic sheath in place for continued drainage.

**Hemorrhage.** Severe exsanguinating hemorrhage requires prompt identification and treatment, usually by direct pressure. It is not wise to probe wounds and use clamps, which can cause further damage. If direct pressure does not stop the bleeding, the use of a temporary tourniquet is recommended. It is important to note the time of tourniquet application and to plan definitive treatment so that the tourniquet can be removed before permanent ischemic damage occurs. Treatment of shock should proceed concomitantly with an evaluation to determine its cause. If an obvious external source of blood loss is not found, one must assume that the patient is bleeding into a major body cavity. The presence of a head injury or multiple extremity fractures does not usually account for blood loss causing signs of shock, and thus other causes should

| TABLE 4–6 |
|---|

Approximate Weight, Blood Volume, Vital Signs, and Maintenance Fluids by Age

| Age | Approximate Weight (kg) | Blood Volume (mL/kg) | Pulse | Systolic Blood Pressure (mm Hg) | Respiration | Maintenance Fluid/24 hr (DR ¼ NS) |
|---|---|---|---|---|---|---|
| Birth | 3.5 | 90 | 140–160 | 80 | 40 | 100 mL/kg |
| 6 mo | 6.0 | 90 | 140–160 | 80 | 40 | 100 mL/kg |
| 1 yr | 12.0 | 85 | 120–160 | 90 | 30 | 1000 mL + 50 mL/kg over 10 kg |
| 4 yr | 16.0 | 80 | 120–140 | 90 | 30 | 1000 mL + 50 mL/kg over 10 kg |
| 10 yr | 35.0 | 75 | 100–120 | 100 | 20 | 1500 mL + 20 mL/kg over 20 kg |
| 15 yr | 55.0 | 70 | 80–100 | 110 | 20 | 1500 mL + 20 mL/kg over 20 kg |

be investigated.[14] An unstable pelvic fracture can result in significant blood loss and requires urgent reduction and stabilization,[235] which can be done with the temporary use of a pneumatic antishock garment, a spica cast, an anterior external fixator, or open fixation with a plate. Cotler and colleagues[55] treated patients with displaced pelvic fractures and ongoing hemorrhage with an immediate spica cast and reported less blood transfused after cast application. This technique may be definitive management in certain pediatric pelvic fractures. A simple anterior external fixation frame can be safely and rapidly applied with a single pin (4 or 5 mm, depending on the size of the child) into each anterior iliac crest at the level of the gluteal ridge. These pins are then connected with a single anterior bar that adequately holds the pelvis closed. Sufficient space should be allowed for access to the abdomen. Satisfactory results have been reported with external fixation in pediatric pelvic fractures.[4, 21, 216, 225, 276] If emergency laparotomy is needed, a pubic diastasis can be plated through this incision by using a two-hole plate. A pelvic clamp for the posterior pelvic ring has been developed and used,[91] but experience with this clamp in the pediatric population is limited. A steep learning curve and multiple potential complications have been reported in the adult population.[94] Reduction of a displaced pelvic fracture decreases pelvic volume and hemorrhage, relieves pain, and provides immobilization.

**Resuscitation.** As in adults, two peripheral percutaneous intravenous lines should be inserted during the initial survey. These lines should be placed in the upper extremity, although the lower extremities can be used if venous access is inadequate or cannot be achieved. If percutaneous intravenous lines cannot be inserted, cutdowns must be performed. The most common sites for cutdowns are the greater saphenous vein on the medial aspect of the ankle, the cephalic vein at the elbow, and the external jugular vein of the neck. The use of percutaneous subclavian vein central lines is not routinely recommended in children, especially those younger than 2 years, because of the difficulty of insertion and the potential for complications. They can be used in older children, although such lines are not generally necessary except for monitoring purposes. After adequate venous access has been achieved, other resuscitative measures can be instituted.

The primary objective of the initial resuscitation of a pediatric patient is to determine the degree of blood loss and the subsequent amount of blood replacement. Fluid or blood replacement must be rapid enough to maintain stable vital signs and adequate urinary output. In a child with signs of shock, a bolus of lactated Ringer's solution with 5% dextrose should be given at approximately 20 mL/kg body weight. A positive response includes a decrease in heart rate, an increase in blood pressure, improved peripheral circulation, increased urine output, and improved sensorium. If no signs of improvement are apparent, a second bolus of the same volume should be given.[5, 76, 161, 244] If still no obvious improvement is seen after the second bolus, type-specific blood at 20 mL/kg body weight or type O Rh-negative packed red blood cells at 10 mL/kg should be administered. Blood less than

5 days old is recommended for transfusion because it has higher levels of 2,3-diphosphoglycerate, which improves delivery of oxygen to tissues.[203] When large volumes are required, the blood should be passed through a warming device to avoid hypothermia. Blood loss replacement in a child is based on the 3 for 1 rule: 3 mL of lactated Ringer's solution with 5% dextrose for 1 mL of blood loss. In a child with severe head injury, fluid administration should be adequate but judicious to avoid overhydration and increased intracranial pressure; monitoring of intracranial pressure is required.

**Acid-Base Balance.** During resuscitation, pediatric patients may have acid-base complications. Most will resolve with adequate ventilation and perfusion. If the pH falls below 7.2, sodium bicarbonate ($NaHCO_3$) should be administered according to the following formula[5]:

$$\text{Body weight (kg)} \times 0.3 \times \text{base deficit} = \text{total } NaHCO_3$$

Half may be given as a bolus, with the remainder given at a rate of 3 to 5 mEq/min after adequate ventilation has been established. If carbon dioxide cannot be excreted, $NaHCO_3$ will not correct the acidosis.

After resuscitation, maintenance fluids must be administered (see Table 4–6).

**Hypothermia.** Hypothermia can be a significant problem in a child because of the volume of fluids needed for resuscitation and the high ratio of body surface area to body mass. Every attempt should be made to use warmed fluids. Other means of maintaining body temperature include keeping the child covered, increasing the room temperature, and using overhead heaters and heating blankets. Hypothermia in a small child or infant can significantly complicate resuscitation because it may render the patient refractory to the usual therapy for shock.[232] Hypothermia stimulates catecholamine secretion and muscle shivering and hence results in metabolic acidosis with the potential for negative effects on pharmacokinetics. Coagulation disorders may also develop and aggravate the condition. The child's temperature should be maintained at 36°C or 37°C.

## Secondary Survey

In the secondary survey, the history is completed and a comprehensive physical examination is performed. A trauma radiographic series is obtained concomitantly. The examination proceeds systematically, with evaluation of the head, spine, chest, abdomen, and extremities to determine the extent of the injuries and prioritize subsequent treatment. The secondary survey is followed by definitive management of the injuries.

### TRAUMA RADIOGRAPHIC SERIES

During the primary survey, plans should be made for obtaining a radiographic trauma series: a lateral view of the cervical spine, a supine AP view of the chest, and an AP view of the pelvis. These radiographs do not take precedence over the treatment of immediate life-threatening injuries. Depending on the size of the child, the chest and pelvic radiographs may be obtained on a single cassette, thus saving time and reducing the need to move the child. These radiographs are obtained during the secondary survey.

**Lateral Cervical Spine Radiograph.** As mentioned previously, a lateral radiograph of the neck is used to screen for cervical spine injuries.[65, 130, 156, 217] Dietrich and coworkers[65] in 1991 found that lateral radiographs of the cervical spine were 98% accurate in recognizing the presence of pediatric cervical spine fractures. Though useful as a screen, lateral radiographs cannot be used as the sole measure for determining cervical spine injury in an uncooperative or unresponsive child. AP, open-mouth odontoid, and oblique views are necessary to complete the radiographic assessment of any child in which the lateral screening view is suggestive of a fracture. Lateral neck radiographs in a young child can be difficult to interpret. An atlantodens interval of up to 5 mm is normal in a child. Displacement of more than 5 mm is considered abnormal and indicative of a tear of the transverse atlantal ligament.[155, 204] This injury is best assessed on controlled flexion-extension lateral radiographs in a conscious, cooperative child. In extension, overriding of the anterior arch of the atlas on top of the odontoid can be seen in up to 20% of children.[204] It is not unusual to find slight subluxation in the upper cervical spine, especially at the C2-3 level and, to a lesser extent, the C3-4 level. Such subluxation is normal and is called pseudosubluxation of childhood.[44] It can be distinguished from abnormal by the posterior cervical line of Swischuk.[262] Variations in the curvature and growth of the cervical spine can resemble an injury.[156] Marked angulation at a single interspace suggestive of an injury to the interspinous or posterior longitudinal ligament can occur in up to 16% of normal children.[44] Wedging of the C3 vertebral body is also a normal finding in 7% of infants and young children.[261] CT is necessary in those with a fracture or suspicion of a fracture. Magnetic resonance imaging (MRI) is performed if neurologic signs or deficits are noted. The child should be treated with external support by in-line traction or sandbags or be placed in a rigid collar and assumed to have a cervical spine injury until proved otherwise. It must also be remembered that children, because of their elasticity, can sustain a spinal cord injury without a radiographic abnormality (SCIWORA).[200, 295]

**Anteroposterior Chest Radiograph.** The supine AP chest radiograph is extremely useful in evaluating for the presence of suspected injuries noted during the primary survey, to check on the response to any treatment rendered for these conditions, and to assess for more subtle injuries not suspected. Injuries that can be diagnosed on a chest radiograph include pneumothorax, hemopneumothorax, pulmonary contusion, aortic arch injury (mediastinal widening), disruption of the trachea or a bronchus, diaphragmatic rupture, rib fracture or fractures, and thoracic spine injury. As stated previously, because of the compliance of the ribs, a child can sustain significant internal injury without obvious damage to the chest.[34, 77, 251] The diagnosis of a fracture of the first rib or multiple ribs is a marker of severe trauma and warrants further evaluation.[92, 115]

**Anteroposterior Pelvic Radiograph.** This radiograph is useful for evaluating injuries to the pelvis. Although minor nondisplaced pelvic fractures may not be associated with significant complications, severe displaced pelvic fractures have an increased risk for associated injuries and therefore a much worse prognosis.* Associated injuries occur in 63% to 87% of children with pelvic fractures.[103, 229, 269]

Fractures and dislocations of the hip and proximal ends of the femurs can also be assessed on a routine AP pelvic radiograph. A pelvic CT scan is indicated if an injury to the sacrum, sacroiliac joint, or acetabulum is suspected clinically or by standard radiographs (see Chapter 12). Posterior pelvic injuries may not be well visualized on standard radiographs; CT has been shown to be the best radiographic procedure for evaluating these types of injuries.[247]

**Other Radiographs.** Findings on clinical evaluation of the extremities, including palpation, should be used as the basis for obtaining radiographs of the extremities. These radiographs are of lower priority and should not take precedence over the assessment and treatment of any life-threatening conditions. When radiographs are obtained, they should be orthogonal, with two views 90 degrees apart (AP or PA and lateral). They should include the joints above and below if a fracture is present. Comparison views are only occasionally necessary in a child. Appropriate placement of the child or infant on a large plate often gives a single AP view of the entire body (babygram), which can be an extremely helpful screening technique. The use of a technetium bone scan has been recommended by Heinrich and associates for a multiply injured pediatric patient with head injuries to assist in the diagnosis of musculoskeletal injuries.[118]

## HEAD INJURIES

Head injuries in a child may have a poor prognosis and a high incidence of morbidity and mortality.[20, 31, 81, 126, 265] Rapid evaluation and treatment are therefore indicated. Signs of external injury, including scalp lacerations, hematomas, and facial lacerations or fractures, should increase suspicion of potential severe intracranial injury. The eyes should be evaluated both with regard to pupil size and reactivity and for evidence of increased intracranial pressure by funduscopic examination. A neurologic evaluation, including assessment of cranial nerves, motor function, strength, sensation, deep tendon reflexes, and rectal sphincter tone, should be performed and carefully documented. The Glasgow Coma Scale score should be determined and recorded[264] (see Table 4–3). CT is indicated in any child sustaining a head injury, especially if unconscious or semiconscious. If surgery and thus anesthesia are necessary, CT is required to clear the child for surgery. In a hemodynamically unstable child who warrants emergency surgery to

---

*See references 24, 29, 38, 42, 93, 103, 139, 172, 173, 184, 186, 215, 223, 229.

control hemorrhage, CT may have to be delayed until the patient is stabilized and then performed before surgical treatment is continued. Herniation syndromes and expanding mass lesions must be decompressed urgently. Children with signs of increased intracranial pressure should have direct intracranial pressure measurements monitored routinely.[43] Such measurement can be done safely and greatly aids in the treatment of this condition.

It is important to remember that uncorrected hypovolemic shock may further compromise a severe brain injury. Hypoxemia caused by shock may result in a secondary brain injury. Hypoxemia must be corrected by intubation, adequate ventilation with supplemental oxygen, and fluid or blood replacement. Restriction of fluids to minimize cerebral edema is not appropriate until after hemodynamic stabilization.

## SPINE AND SPINAL CORD INJURIES

Vertebral injuries may be present with or without spinal cord injury. In a child who is a victim of multiple trauma, a spinal column injury should be presumed until ruled out by physical and radiographic evaluation. Information regarding the mechanism of injury, the use of restraints or seat belts (in motor vehicle accidents), the child's neurologic status at the scene of the accident, and any change in neurologic status is important to obtain during the initial evaluation. Any child sustaining an injury above the clavicle or a head injury resulting in loss or alteration of consciousness should be suspected of having a cervical spine injury. Injuries produced by high-velocity accidents should also arouse suspicion of vertebral column injuries. As stated previously, a SCIWORA is also possible.[200, 295]

Examination of a child with a suspected spinal injury is carried out with the patient supine, in a neutral position, and with stabilization of the head and neck. In small children, it is appropriate to place a pad beneath the trunk to avoid hyperflexion of the neck because of the disproportion in head size.[121] The child should be protected in this manner until definitive radiographs have been obtained. A careful physical examination is performed, with particular attention directed to the presence of prominent spinous processes, local tenderness, pain with attempted motion, edema, ecchymoses, visible deformities, and muscle spasms. In suspected cervical spine injuries, it is also important to assess for tracheal tenderness or deviation and the presence of retropharyngeal hematoma. A careful neurologic examination, including muscle strength, sensory changes, alterations in deep tendon reflex, and autonomic dysfunction, must be performed and accurately recorded. Autonomic dysfunction is identified by the lack of bladder and rectal control.

In spinal cord injuries, it is important to determine whether the lesion is complete or incomplete. The presence of superficial (pinprick) and deep pain discrimination indicates an incomplete lesion and intact lateral column function. Posterior column function is assessed by position and vibratory sensation. Because of the phenomenon of sacral sparing, it is important that sensation to the anal, perianal, and scrotal areas be tested.

Evaluation for sacral sparing should include sensory perception and voluntary contraction of the rectum. The presence of sacral spearing indicates that the paralysis is not complete and is a good prognostic sign with respect to neurologic recovery. Detailed sensory examination can be extremely difficult, if possible at all, in younger children.

The evaluation of muscle function and sensation determines the level of spinal cord injury. Sledge and colleagues[249] demonstrated the value of MRI in assessing thoracolumbar fractures, spinal stability, and the spinal cord injury pattern. The latter could be used in predicting clinical outcome.

Spinal shock may occur after spinal cord injury. The pulse rate is not usually increased with this type of shock, and blood pressure typically falls to approximately 80 mm Hg systolic as blood pools from the dilated visceral vessels. Flaccid muscle paralysis, flaccid sphincters, and absent deep tendon reflexes are associated with spinal shock. The presence of a bulbocavernosus reflex may be important in distinguishing spinal shock from true spinal cord injury. After completion of a careful neurologic evaluation, spinal radiographs must be obtained.

Lateral cervical spine and AP chest radiographs are obtained on every patient sustaining multiple trauma. In the lateral radiograph of the cervical spine, it is important that all seven vertebrae be identified. Occasionally, the patient's shoulders must be pulled down to visualize C6 and C7. Other cervical radiographs include AP, oblique, and odontoid views. Occasionally, CT or MRI may be necessary to confirm a cervical spine injury and to determine its stability. Lateral flexion and extension radiographs are dangerous and must be performed under appropriate supervision. When injuries to the thoracic and lumbar spine are suspected, AP and lateral radiographs are obtained. Occasionally, oblique radiographs of the lumbar spine may be useful.

Treatment of any vertebral column and associated spinal cord injury is under the direction of the orthopaedic surgeon and neurosurgeon (see Chapter 11), preferably at a pediatric trauma center. In unstable cervical spine fractures or fracture-dislocations, stabilization by the application of tongs and traction may be appropriate. However, traction should be used cautiously to avoid distraction. Traction weights should be applied sequentially and stabilization assessed by repeat lateral radiographs. The use of steroids in acute spinal cord injuries has been shown to be effective in improving neurologic recovery when these agents are given in the first 8 hours after injury.[33] Steroid use is controversial and has not been selectively studied in children or adolescents.

## CHEST INJURIES

The child's chest is very compliant, and significant intrathoracic injury may occur without obvious external trauma.[34, 77, 251] The chest should be evaluated by palpation, percussion, and auscultation in addition to an AP chest radiograph. The presence of a first-rib fracture or multiple rib fractures is an indicator of severe injury, and other associated injuries must be sought.[92, 115] Conditions previously stabilized in the primary survey should undergo definitive treatment during the secondary survey. Definitive treatment may include the insertion of a chest tube for a pneumothorax or drainage of a hemopneumothorax. The diagnosis of blunt cardiac contusion requires a high index of suspicion. It is usually associated with severe trauma to multiple systems, and serial electrocardiograms and cardiac enzyme determinations are indicated.[67]

Although rupture of the aorta is rare in children, a widened mediastinum warrants an aortogram. Bronchial injuries and diaphragmatic rupture occur more frequently. Pulmonary contusions are quite common with blunt chest trauma in children and are often complicated by aspiration of gastric contents.[251]

Diaphragmatic injuries are fortunately rare but are life threatening when they occur. According to Brandt and colleagues,[34] they are always associated with either penetrating or high-velocity blunt trauma. Diaphragmatic injuries are usually diagnosed with the trauma chest radiograph, although they can be missed. The incidence of associated injuries is high, and emergency surgical repair is essential.

## ABDOMINAL INJURIES

The majority of serious abdominal injuries in children are the result of blunt trauma, although penetrating trauma has an increasing incidence in the inner-city population, especially in adolescent males.[127] Serious injuries to the abdominal contents can be inflicted with less force than in an adult because of the anatomic differences in children. The costal margin is higher than in an adult, thus affording less protection to the upper abdominal viscera. In addition, children have less abdominal musculature and a more compliant pelvis.

Routine examination of an injured child's abdomen may be difficult because of the patient's fear, inability to cooperate, and generalized response to pain. In addition, a child's typical response of aerophagia, which results in gastric distention, increases the difficulty of an examination. In an attempt to reduce this problem, all children sustaining blunt abdominal trauma should have a nasogastric tube inserted and the gastric contents aspirated. In the distended state, the bladder in infants and small children can extend up to the umbilicus, and it is helpful to insert a Foley catheter to decompress the bladder, provided that the child has no evidence of pelvic fracture or genitourinary injury. The presence of gross hematuria after catheterization is more suggestive of urologic injury than is microscopic hematuria, and further investigation of the urinary tract is necessary.[269] Serial abdominal examinations in an injured child in the absence of pelvic or genitourinary injuries are critical.

A child who presents with signs of peritoneal irritation, a distended abdomen, or signs of hypovolemia without obvious external blood loss needs further urgent diagnostic studies. A child with peritoneal irritation and unstable vital signs requires emergency laparotomy. Those with stable vital signs may undergo further evaluation by peritoneal lavage, CT, or ultrasonography in combination with serial clinical examinations and assessment of vital signs.

Peritoneal lavage is a sensitive study for demonstrating intra-abdominal bleeding.[68, 70, 211] Peritoneal lavage in a child may be difficult because of a lack of cooperation, distention of the stomach or bladder (or both), and thinness of the abdominal wall, which allows sudden penetrations and iatrogenic visceral injury. The recommended technique is similar to that for an adult. After passage of a nasogastric tube and Foley catheter, the catheter is inserted with an open technique, and 10 mL/kg body weight (up to 1 L) of lactated Ringer's solution is infused into the abdominal cavity over a 10-minute period. The solution is then reaccumulated by gravity drainage into an empty intravenous bag lowered to the floor and analyzed.[5] Criteria for positive lavage findings are similar to those for adults and are presented in Table 4–7.

An abdominal CT scan is frequently necessary to evaluate abdominal injury in children,[53, 134] especially for assessing possible splenic, hepatic, and renal injuries. CT has the advantages of being noninvasive and enabling more specific evaluation of solid visceral injuries. Its disadvantages include added time needed for scanning, radiation exposure, expense, and less specificity in evaluating perforations and injuries to the small or large bowel. The issue of when to use peritoneal lavage, CT, or both is controversial.[97, 165] In general, CT has replaced peritoneal lavage in evaluating a traumatized patient who has stable vital signs and does not require immediate surgery for other associated injuries. Peritoneal lavage remains the test of choice in patients with multiple injuries requiring immediate surgical intervention. The relative indications for peritoneal lavage versus CT are listed in Table 4–8. Initial screening with peritoneal lavage followed by serial CT scans in a stable child has been recommended by Rothenberg and associates.[234]

Ultrasonography has been recommended as a triage procedure to replace initial CT and peritoneal lavage.[159, 201] It has the benefits of being rapid, versatile, and cost-effective. Luks and coworkers[159] reported a sensitivity of 89% and specificity of 96%. Patrick and colleagues[201] also showed that ultrasound was a reliable procedure for triaging blunt abdominal trauma and that it had significant cost savings in that it decreased the

| TABLE 4–7 | | | |
|---|---|---|---|
| *Criteria for Positive Peritoneal Lavage in Children* | | | |
| **Test** | **Positive** | **Intermediate** | **Negative** |
| RBC count (per mm³) | >100,000 | 50,000–100,000 | <540,000 |
| WBC count (per mm³) | >500 | 100–500 | <100 |
| Bile | + | | |
| Bacteria | + | | |

Aspiration of 10 mL of gross blood is considered positive, and lavage is not necessary.
RBC, red blood cell; WBC, white blood cell.
Modified from Joyce, M. In: Marcus, R.E., ed. Trauma in Children. Rockville, MD, Aspen, 1986, pp. 13–38; Eichelberger, M.R.; Randolph, J.G. In: Moore, E.E.; Eisenman, B.; Van Way, C.E., eds. Critical Decisions in Trauma. St Louis, C.V. Mosby, 1984, p. 344.

**TABLE 4–8** ...............................................................

Indications for Peritoneal Lavage versus Abdominal Computed Tomography

| Peritoneal Lavage | Abdominal CT |
|---|---|
| Central nervous system injury/an unresponsive child | Stable vital signs |
| Unexplained shock | Suspected intra-abdominal injury |
| Penetrating chest injury below the nipple | Slowly declining hematocrit |
| Major thoracic injury | Neurologic injuries |
| Major orthopaedic injury above and below the diaphragm | Multiple injuries requiring general anesthesia |
| Patient going to the operating room for other system injury | Blood in urine |
| Abdominal signs or symptoms | |

Data from Drew, R., et al. Surg Gynecol Obstet 145:885, 1977; Meissner, M., et al. Am J Surg 161:552–555, 1991.

need for more expensive CT scans. This diagnostic procedure is operator dependent, and considerable experience is required.

The spleen is the most commonly injured intra-abdominal organ in children, but treatment is quite different from that for adults. Unlike the situation in adults, treatment of splenic injuries in children is initially nonoperative in an attempt to salvage the organ.[66, 78, 125] Several considerations influence this nonoperative approach. First, the incidence of late malignant sepsis after splenectomy in children is well documented.[85] Second, the capsule of the pediatric spleen is thicker than that in an adult, which allows for surgical repair. Third, a child's spleen often stops bleeding spontaneously. The spleen is best evaluated with the use of serial CT scans or radioisotope imaging. Children who present with evidence of massive bleeding require emergency operative treatment, with every attempt made to repair and salvage the spleen. Patients with stable vital signs and hematocrit levels can be observed in the pediatric or surgical intensive care unit and monitored with a repeat CT scan in 5 to 7 days. Surgical intervention is indicated during that time if the patient has signs of continued bleeding, such as a progressive decline in hematocrit, or shows signs of increasing peritoneal irritation.

Hepatic injuries (the liver is the second most commonly injured abdominal organ in children) are also managed nonoperatively, if possible. Close serial clinical examinations and monitoring are indicated, in addition to initial and follow-up CT scans.[16, 133]

Penetrating abdominal injuries such as gunshot or stab wounds should not be treated conservatively and require mandatory laparotomy.[180] CT scans and peritoneal lavage are not considered necessary in penetrating trauma.

## EXTREMITY INJURIES

In general, definitive evaluation and management of extremity injuries have a low priority during both the primary and the secondary surveys. Extremity injuries are rarely life threatening and should never take precedence over the evaluation and treatment of serious injuries. Initial treatment of extremity injuries should include covering all wounds with sterile dressing, realigning deformed extremities, and splinting all potentially injured extremities. A neurovascular examination

both before and after splinting is essential. Open wounds of the extremity require antibiotics and possibly tetanus prophylaxis (Tables 4–9 and 4–10). Wounds should never be left uncovered, and multiple inspections of the wounds should be avoided. Inappropriate handling of wounds has been shown to significantly increase the rate of infection.[279] The resulting infections are usually with nosocomial organisms, with the added problem of multiple-drug resistance. All wounds in proximity to a fracture should be considered communicating and the fracture treated as an open fracture.

Assessment of extremity injuries includes visual inspection of the entire extremity, which mandates the removal of all clothing. All extremities are palpated for evidence of tenderness, swelling, crepitus, and instability, and all joints are inspected both visually and manually for signs of swelling, effusion, and deformity. Range of motion and ligamentous stability are assessed. All major joints are examined, with special attention to the knees. Ligamentous injury to the knee is commonly associated with other injuries, such as femoral shaft fractures and posterior hip dislocation, and the knee injury is often

**TABLE 4–9** ....................................

Schedule of Active Immunization against Tetanus

| Dose | Age/Interval | Vaccine |
|---|---|---|
| **AGE YOUNGER THAN 7 YEARS** | | |
| Primary 1 | Age 6 wk or older | DPT |
| Primary 2 | 4–8 wk after the first dose | DPT |
| Primary 3 | 4–8 wk after the second dose | DPT |
| Primary 4 | About 1 yr after the third dose | DPT |
| Booster | 4–6 yr of age | DPT |
| Additional boosters | Every 10 yr after the last dose | Td |
| **AGE 7 YEARS AND OLDER** | | |
| Primary 1 | First visit | Td |
| Primary 2 | 4–6 wk after the first dose | Td |
| Primary 3 | 6 mo–1 yr after the last dose | Td |
| Boosters | Every 10 yr after the last dose | Td |

.............................................................

DPT, diphtheria and tetanus toxoids and pertussis vaccine absorbed; Td, tetanus and reduced-dose diphtheria toxoids absorbed (for adults only).

From Cates, T.R. In Mandell, G.L.; Douglas, R.G., Jr.; Bennett, J.E., eds. Principles and Practice of Infectious Diseases. New York, Churchill Livingstone, 1990, pp. 1946–1982.

**TABLE 4–10** ............................................

Guide to Tetanus Prophylaxis

| History of Tetanus Immunization (Doses) | Clean, Minor Wounds | | All Other Wounds | |
|---|---|---|---|---|
| | *Td* | *TIG* | *Td* | *TIG* |
| Uncertain or less than 2 | Yes | No | Yes | Yes |
| 2 | Yes | No | Yes | No* |
| 3 or more | No† | No | No‡ | No |

............................................

*Yes if older than 24 hours.
†Yes if more than 10 years since the last dose.
‡Yes if more than 5 years since the last dose (more frequent boosters are not needed and can accentuate side effects).
Td, tetanus toxoid; TIG, tetanus immune globulin.
From Cates, T.R. In: Mandell, G.L.; Douglas, R.G., Jr.; Bennett, J.E., eds. Principles and Practice of Infectious Diseases. New York, Churchill Livingstone, 1990, pp. 1946–1982.

missed[140]; instability on examination may represent a physeal injury.

**Vascular Injuries.** Injuries to major arteries in association with extremity fractures are uncommon in children.[86, 190, 243, 250, 284] Shaker and colleagues[243] reported that only 8 of 118 children (7%) younger than 15 years with upper and lower extremity fractures had vascular injuries; most were the result of supracondylar fractures of the distal end of the humerus. Between zero and 18% of open tibial fractures (usually type IIIC by definition; see Table 5–1) have associated vascular injuries.* These injuries frequently lead to amputation. Vascular injuries can also occur after closed proximal tibial metaphyseal fractures and knee dislocations.[86, 190, 221] Displaced pelvic fractures can result in injuries to the paravaginal, superior gluteal, and internal iliac arteries.[226] These vascular injuries can give rise to large retroperitoneal hematomas. Fortunately, most hemorrhage from pelvic fractures comes from small arterial injuries rather than major vessels. Prompt clinical recognition, radiographic evaluation, and repair or reconstruction are necessary for limb salvage. The cardinal signs of arterial injury include pulselessness, pain, pallor, paresthesias, and paralysis.[183, 284] However, the presence of palpable pulses or Doppler-documented flow does not rule out an arterial injury. Compartment syndromes can have many of the same features as an arterial injury, especially in the forearm and lower part of the leg. Thus, careful evaluation is necessary.

Knee dislocation, displaced proximal tibial fractures, and multiple ligamentous injuries are highly associated with injuries to the popliteal artery and warrant further evaluation.[86, 190, 221] Such evaluation can include arteriography, duplex sonography, and use of the Doppler systolic arterial pressure index.[131, 174] In this last method, described by Johansen and associates[131] in 1991, the Doppler arterial pressure in the injured extremity is divided by the pressure in an uninjured extremity. A value of less than 0.90 was found to have a

sensitivity and specificity of 95% and 97%, respectively, for a major arterial injury. The negative predictive value for an index greater than 0.90 was 99%. This finding was confirmed in a clinical trial, and these authors now recommend using this noninvasive test for exclusion arteriography in patients at risk for silent arterial injuries of an extremity. This test is rapid as well as cost-effective and can save valuable time during the secondary survey. However, it does not disclose injuries to the profunda femoris, profunda brachii, and peroneal arteries. It may also not recognize lesions that do not reduce blood flow to the extremity, such as intimal flaps and small pseudoaneurysms.

When an arterial injury is suspected or diagnosed clinically, an arteriogram should be considered. Common indications for arteriographic evaluation of the extremities include dislocation of the knee, absent or asymmetric distal pulses, displaced pelvic fractures with hypotension, signs of peripheral ischemia, and severe open fractures. A formal arteriogram can be performed in injured extremities without significant ischemia. A single-plane, single-bolus arteriogram should be performed in the operating room when the extremity is ischemic and prompt revascularization is essential. In an older child or adolescent, the technique is the same as that used in adults.[195] In an infant or small child, a cutdown is usually necessary for vascular access to avoid iatrogenic injury to the vessels. Angiography and embolization with clotted blood, Gelfoam, or other material can be effective in controlling hemorrhage after pelvic fractures.[15, 269] Compartment syndromes can occur after vascular repair, so fasciotomies are recommended at the time of repair.[233]

Radiographs should be obtained for all extremities with a suspected injury. Initial radiographs in a single plane can be used for screening assessment, although orthogonal views are recommended before definitive treatment is planned. In an infant or small child, a single cassette can be used to obtain a radiograph of the whole body, including the extremities. This technique is used purely for screening purposes, and the need for additional specific views must be based on the results of evaluation. In an unresponsive or multiply injured patient, a technetium bone scan can be helpful to identify undiagnosed skeletal injuries.[118]

**Compartment Syndromes.** Compartment syndromes do occur in children and are related to the severity of the trauma[166, 167, 182, 233] (see Chapter 5). The lower part of the leg and the forearm are the most common sites for compartment syndromes and are usually the result of tibial shaft (see Chapter 5) and supracondylar fractures of the distal portion of the humerus. The presence of a displaced supracondylar fracture and a displaced ipsilateral forearm fracture increases the risk for compartment syndrome.[23] Compartment syndromes can also occur in other areas, such as the foot. The presence of open fractures does not preclude a compartment syndrome.[40, 58, 59, 124, 128, 142, 231] Assuming that an open fracture has decompressed the adjacent compartments is a mistake inasmuch as compartment syndrome develops in approximately 3% of open tibial fractures. Careful evaluation of injured extremities should therefore include

_____

*See references 39, 40, 58, 59, 102, 124, 128, 142, 231, 253.

assessment for signs of compartment syndrome. The most important findings include swelling and tenseness of the compartment and exaggerated pain with passive stretch of the distal joints. Paresthesias, pulselessness, and paralysis are late findings, and the absence of these signs does not rule out this diagnosis. Compartment pressures should be measured in all children with signs consistent with compartment syndrome. Uncooperative children or those with head injuries need to be evaluated very carefully because they will lack the usual symptoms. Rapid surgical treatment with the release of all involved compartments is critical to reduce potential complications.[95, 166, 167, 182, 183, 233] In the forearm, separate incisions are used to decompress the volar or extensor compartment[233] (Fig. 4–5). The Henry approach, which entails division of the lacertus fibrosus, allows excellent exposure and decompression. In the lower part of the leg, the double-incision technique is recommended to decompress the four compartments[233] (Fig. 4–6).

## FRACTURE MANAGEMENT OF A MULTIPLY INJURED CHILD

Once the extremity injuries have been defined during the secondary survey, definitive treatment needs to be prioritized and planned.[57, 181, 273] Extremity injuries that have a high priority include major joint dislocations, open joint injuries, open fractures, fractures associated with vascular injury, and unstable pelvic injuries in children who are hemodynamically unstable. The need for stabilization of long bone fractures, especially the femoral shaft, is well documented in adult victims of multiple trauma and is probably equally important in adolescents.[30, 140, 230] Its importance is not as clear in children and infants, although stabilization of these fractures can certainly aid in nursing care, mobility of the child, and control of pain and blood loss. Loder[157]

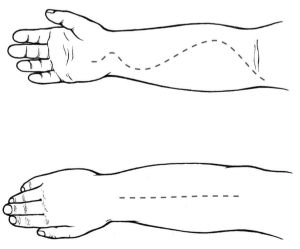

**FIGURE 4–5.** Standard fasciotomy sites for the forearm. Henry's approach is used for the volar surface with a straight dorsal incision.

showed that early stabilization of fractures in a multiply injured child reduces the number of days in both the intensive care unit and the hospital. It also decreases the duration of ventilatory support and the overall complication rate in comparison to children with delayed skeletal stabilization. A study by Hedequist and associates[116] has questioned the beneficial effect of early femoral stabilization with regard to pulmonary complications. It is important to re-emphasize that extremity injuries are not life-threatening injuries and should not supersede the latter. They can, however, be limb threatening and should not be neglected. Long-term morbidity is most frequently associated with inadequate treatment of extremity injuries.[157, 164] Because children's fractures tend to heal more rapidly than do similar fractures in adults, plans for surgical intervention need to be completed earlier in the hospital course; otherwise, the option for fracture reduction surgery may be lost, and osteotomies may be required.

## Indications for Surgical Management

Most pediatric fractures and dislocations can be managed satisfactorily by closed reduction techniques and cast immobilization or traction with the use of skin or skeletal techniques.[27, 112, 193, 207, 208, 221, 222, 263, 287] However, in specific situations, surgical management may be more advantageous and result in decreased morbidity and better functional results.[270, 271] A multiply injured child and skeletally immature adolescent are major examples. Indications for operative treatment of pediatric fractures have been outlined by Thompson and associates.[271] These indications include displaced epiphyseal fractures, displaced intra-articular fractures, unstable fractures, multiple injuries, and open fractures. The last indication is frequently present in a multiply injured child. Common fractures in each of the five categories are presented in Table 4–11.

In deciding on early and definitive management, several important factors must be considered: the prognosis for survival and residual disability, whether standard closed methods of treatment will adversely affect the management of other body area injuries, and whether other body area injuries have a potentially deleterious effect on the musculoskeletal injuries if the latter are managed in closed fashion. If the prognosis is favorable and either of the last two factors is positive, the surgical option may be advantageous in the overall management of the child.[270] Possible examples include a child with a flail chest and a closed femoral shaft fracture. The femoral fracture should not be treated by skeletal traction because of possible compromise in care of the chest. Likewise, a child with a head injury who is combative or spastic may not be a candidate for conservative fracture management, especially a femoral shaft fracture, because of the difficulty in maintaining satisfactory alignment. In both situations, it would be more appropriate to surgically stabilize the fractures. It must be remembered that children tend to survive more serious injuries than adults do; thus, in all but the most extreme cases, survival should be expected.

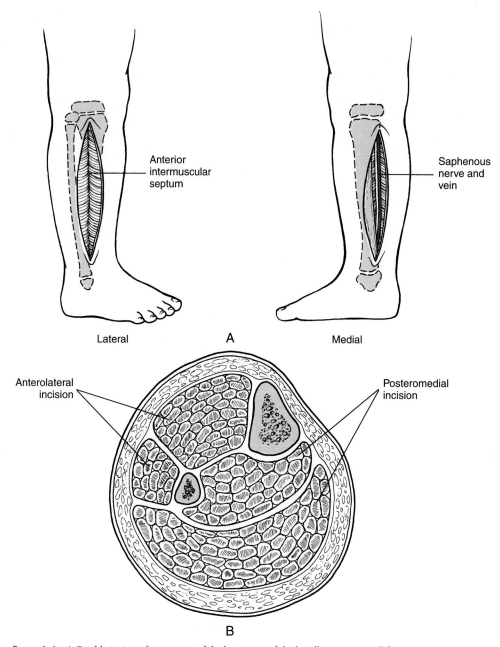

**Figure 4–6.** *A,* Double-incision fasciotomies of the lower part of the leg allow access to all four compartments. Care must be taken on the medial side to avoid injury to the saphenous nerve and vein. *B,* Cross section of the lower portion of the leg demonstrating access to the four compartments through the double incisions.

## Timing of Fracture Management

Severely injured children, as well as adults, are in their best physiologic state immediately after resuscitation. Delaying definitive treatment frequently allows secondary complications to occur, such as pulmonary atelectasis, fat emboli, contamination of abrasions and wounds, fluid and electrolyte imbalance, and deep venous thrombosis, which may preclude surgical management for several weeks. This delay may result in subsequent musculoskeletal complications such as nonunion and malunion.[149, 164] If the musculoskeletal injuries are closed, the other body area injuries do not require

surgery, and the child's condition is critical, closed management may be the most appropriate initial method, even if less than optimal alignment is achieved. Definitive management may be delayed several days, pending survival of the child. If surgery for other body areas must be performed on the day of injury, operative fracture management should be performed concomitantly, if possible. Loder[157] showed that children undergoing immediate surgical stabilization of fractures had fewer complications than did those whose stabilization was delayed. Because fractures heal rapidly in children, delays in treatment may significantly increase the difficulty of operative repair, if needed.

Serious burns are another possible indication for early operative stabilization of associated fractures.[25] Open fractures and periarticular fractures associated with serious burns should be treated as soon as possible. If treatment is initiated within 48 hours, the risk of secondary infection is decreased. After 48 hours, the risk for deep infection about the implant will be high. These fractures are then better managed by external fixation or limited internal fixation.

## Epiphyseal Fractures

Fractures involving the epiphysis and physeal growth plate are common injuries in children who are victims of multiple trauma. Peterson and Peterson[206] found that upper extremity physeal injuries occur more frequently than those of the lower extremities (1.6:1). The physis of the distal end of the radius was the most frequently injured physis, followed by the distal tibial and finger phalangeal physes. Distal physes of long bones were found to be injured more often than proximal physes, except for the humerus. The peak age of the incidence of physeal injuries is 12 to 13 years, with males predominating.

The most widely used classification of epiphyseal plate fractures is that of Salter and Harris[237] (see Fig. 2–5), and it has been demonstrated to be simple, accurate, and prognostically significant. A more complex classification was proposed by Ogden.[194] The Salter-Harris classification differentiates five types of epiphyseal fracture: in type I, the epiphysis is completely separated from the metaphysis without any bone fracture; in type II, the fracture extends partially along the physis and then exits through a

portion of the metaphysis and produces the Thurston-Holland sign; in type III, the fracture extends partially through the physis and then extends through the epiphysis into the joint; in type IV, the fracture extends obliquely across the metaphysis, the physis, and the epiphysis and enters the joint; and in type V, a nondisplaced crush injury to the physis, no definite fracture line is visible radiographically.

Type I and type II fractures do not disturb the germinal layer of the physis and therefore usually have an excellent prognosis after closed reduction and cast immobilization. Displaced type III and type IV fractures require anatomic reduction, usually by open reduction plus internal fixation (ORIF), to restore alignment of the physis, as well as the articular surface of the joint. The prognosis is usually good, provided that vascularity to the fracture fragment remains intact and the reduction is anatomic. If anatomic alignment of these fractures is not achieved, an osseous bridge may form across the physeal plate and result in premature physeal closure or asymmetric growth; central bridges result in shortening, and peripheral bridges tend to produce angular deformities. These bony bridges can occasionally be resected and fat or Silastic interposed to prevent re-formation. These techniques can be effective in restoring longitudinal growth.[37, 144, 205] A type V fracture has a poor prognosis because of the inherent damage to the physis, which leads to a growth disturbance. This injury is typically recognizable only in retrospect and is not usually amenable to resection.

## Principles of Surgical Management

The principles of surgical management of fractures in a multiply injured child and skeletally immature adolescent are distinctly different from those in a mature adolescent and adult. Spiegel and Mast[254] listed five general principles applicable to the operative management of pediatric fractures; these principles apply to multiple injuries, as well as isolated fractures requiring surgical intervention:

1. Multiple closed reductions of an epiphyseal fracture are contraindicated because they may cause repetitive damage to the germinal cells of the physis, thereby predisposing to premature closure and late deformity.

2. At surgery, anatomic alignment is mandatory, especially for displaced intra-articular and epiphyseal fractures.

3. Internal fixation devices, if used, should be simple when possible, such as K-wires, and should be removed as soon as the fracture has healed.

4. Rigid fixation to allow immediate mobilization of the extremity is not usually the goal; rather, the goal is stability sufficient to hold the fragments in anatomic alignment with a supplemental cast.

5. External fixators, when used, are removed as soon as possible, and cast immobilization is substituted when the soft tissue problems have been corrected or when the fracture is stable. However, in a multiply

---

**TABLE 4–11** ....................................

Common Indications for Operative Management and Internal Fixation of Fractures in Children

| Indication | Common Location |
|---|---|
| Displaced epiphyseal fractures (especially types III and IV) | Lateral condyle<br>Radial head<br>Phalanx<br>Distal femur<br>Proximal tibia<br>Distal tibia |
| Displaced intra-articular fractures | Olecranon<br>Radial neck<br>Femoral neck<br>Patella |
| Unstable fractures | Distal humerus (supracondylar)<br>Radial/ulnar diaphysis<br>Phalanx<br>Spine |
| Multiply injured children (especially with head injury) | Femoral diaphysis<br>Tibial diaphysis<br>Pelvis<br>Spine |
| Open fractures | Severe soft tissue loss |

From Thompson, G.H.; Wilber, J.H. In: Marcus, R.E., ed. Trauma in Children. Rockville, MD, Aspen, 1986, pp. 99–146.

injured patient, the internal or external fixation must be of sufficient strength to allow for mobilization of the child.

Thus, planning for appropriate surgical procedures is based on the age and size of the child, the bone fractured, and the extent and severity of other injuries.

## Surgical Techniques

Three basic surgical techniques are used in the management of pediatric fractures, including multiple trauma: ORIF, closed reduction and internal fixation, and external fixation.[270]

### ORIF

Displaced epiphyseal fractures, especially Salter-Harris type III and IV intra-articular fractures,[237] and unstable fractures, such as those involving the forearm diaphysis and the spine, as well as ipsilateral fractures of the femur and tibia ("floating" knee),[28, 296] may require ORIF. Indications in a multiply injured child include closed fractures, especially of the femoral shaft, and other fractures with neurovascular injuries requiring repair. Fractures are usually stabilized before vascular repair, provided that the ischemia time is not significantly prolonged, but stabilization should not take precedence over vascular repair if the warm ischemia time is approaching 6 hours.[243, 293] Occasionally, open fractures, especially those of the femur or tibia, may be candidates for ORIF.[113, 151] Closed femoral shaft fractures can also be treated by ORIF.[88, 143, 286]

**Internal Fixation Devices.** The type of internal fixation used during open reduction depends on the goals of management and the age of the patient. As stated by Spiegel and Mast[254] and by others, the goal of fracture surgery in children is not usually rigid internal fixation but rather attainment and maintenance of anatomic alignment. Thus, most fractures can be managed by simple internal fixation devices such as K-wires, Steinmann pins, cortical screws, and cannulated screws.[254, 270, 271] The fractured extremity is protected postoperatively with external immobilization, typically a plaster cast, until satisfactory union is obtained. This type of management usually allows the child sufficient mobilization to enhance overall care.

Compression plates and screws can be used for unstable diaphyseal fractures, especially those of the femoral shaft, in children and skeletally immature adolescents to achieve satisfactory mobilization. Publications have reported excellent results with the use of compression plates and screws in young children with closed femoral shaft fractures, especially those who are victims of multiple trauma.[88, 143, 286] In children, internal fixation devices are removed soon after fracture union to minimize the risk of physeal injury and prevent incorporation of the device into the growing bone. They should also be used with caution in type I and II open fractures because of an increased risk of infection after their use in children.

## CLOSED REDUCTION AND INTERNAL FIXATION

Closed reduction plus internal fixation is indicated for certain displaced epiphyseal, intra-articular, and unstable metaphyseal or diaphyseal fractures. In children, this technique generally refers to percutaneous fixation with K-wires or Steinmann pins. Pediatric fractures amenable to closed reduction and percutaneous internal fixation include humeral supracondylar, phalangeal, and femoral neck fractures. Anatomic alignment must be attainable by closed reduction before this method can be used. Failure to obtain anatomic alignment is an indication for open reduction.

The literature suggests that certain pediatric fractures, especially those involving the forearm and femoral shaft, be managed by closed intramedullary nailing. Unstable and open forearm fractures are also becoming a common indication.[7, 49, 145, 158, 212, 228, 245, 282]

The most common indication for intramedullary nailing in children is a femoral shaft fracture, especially in victims of multiple trauma.* The tibia is a much less common indication, although successful results have been reported.[213]

These implants are inserted under fluoroscopic control, and prophylactic antibiotics are used in all cases. The results are superior to those of closed management. Two basic techniques may be used—reamed and unreamed nails. Reamed nails, including those that can be locked proximally, distally, or both, are used predominantly in older adolescent femoral fractures with the same technique as in adults.[19, 291] Numerous publications have reported avascular necrosis of the capital femoral epiphysis (femoral head) after reamed intramedullary nailing of the pediatric femur.[10, 19, 176, 196, 268] This complication appears to be caused by damage to the anastomotic arterial ring at the base of the femoral neck, by direct damage to the lateral ascending cervical arteries to the femoral head, or by intracapsular tamponade. Avascular necrosis has also been reported after closed intramedullary shortening in an adolescent.[175] Premature closure of the greater trochanteric apophysis has also been described after intramedullary femoral rodding.[98, 220] This problem can produce an increase in femoral neck valgus. Gonzalez-Herranz and coworkers[98] found that 30% of 34 children who underwent femoral rod placement had abnormalities in growth of the proximal end of the femur. This abnormal proximal femoral growth was most likely to occur in children younger than 13 years, in whom they recommended other methods of management. Because of anatomic considerations and the risk of distal femoral physeal and greater trochanteric apophyseal injuries, reamed nails are recommended primarily for older adolescents. However, it has been reported that reamed nails can be inserted through the tip of the greater trochanter, thereby avoiding injuries to the retinacular vessels.[179, 277] Multiple flexible nails are used for intramedullary stabilization in children and adolescents, particularly for

---

*See references 19, 56, 82, 84, 90, 113, 117, 119, 120, 140, 151, 152, 153, 162, 179, 214, 224, 272, 281, 283, 285, 292, 297, 298.

length-stable fracture patterns.[56, 87, 214] The complication rate is low.

**Internal Fixation Devices.** Steinmann pins, K-wires, and cannulated screws are the most commonly used devices in closed reduction with internal fixation.[271] They are inserted percutaneously after closed reduction and can either traverse the fracture or be placed above and below the fracture and secured with an external fixation clamp or incorporated into a plaster cast. Smooth pins or wires may be placed across a physis if necessary for fracture fixation. These devices are usually removed as soon as the fracture has healed.

Unreamed and reamed intramedullary nails may be used in selected cases. As stated previously, reamed nails are used almost exclusively for the femoral shaft in adolescents. The unreamed rods used for younger children include Rush pins, Ender nails, and small-diameter (2.5 to 4 mm) flexible rods of titanium or stainless steel. Rush pins do not usually provide rigid fixation, and the extremity must be supported by a cast. Ender and flexible rods, however, can provide both alignment and length, as well as rotational stability.* These nails are prebent to conform to the anatomic curves of the involved bone, inserted to provide three-point fixation, and then anchored in the proximal and distal metaphyses. This technique allows end-to-end contact and maintenance of normal bone curvature. The secondary muscles provide additional support. Slight movement occurs at the fracture site and stimulates callus formation. These devices have a high success rate and low incidence of complications.

## EXTERNAL FIXATION

Common indications for external fixation of pediatric fractures include type II and III open fractures; fractures associated with severe burns; fractures with bone or extensive soft tissue loss that may require reconstructive procedures such as free vascularized grafts or skin grafts; fractures requiring distraction, such as those with significant bone loss; unstable pelvic femoral and tibial fractures; fractures in children with associated head injuries and spasticity; and fractures associated with vascular or nerve repairs or reconstruction.† Fractures, especially open fractures of the femur[9, 26, 62, 64, 178, 231] and tibia,‡ are the most common long bones treated by external fixation.

Advantages of external fixation include rigid immobilization of fractures; direct surveillance of the limb and associated wounds; facilitation of wound management, such as repeated débridement, flap procedures, and dressings; patient mobilization for treatment of other injuries and transportation for diagnostic and therapeutic procedures; and possible insertion with local anesthesia in severely injured patients. The major complications of external fixation are pin tract infections and refracture after removal.[178, 253]

---

*See references 56, 82, 84, 117, 152, 153, 162, 213, 214, 281, 285.
†See references 4, 9, 21, 26, 64, 79, 100, 138, 148, 211, 225, 273–275.
‡See references 39, 40, 58, 59, 102, 124, 128, 142, 231, 253.

**External Fixation Devices.** A multitude of external fixators are commercially available, and newer multiplane devices are continually being developed. Transcutaneous pins incorporated into casts[17, 59] or connected by a tube of methylmethacrylate[63] can be substituted if necessary. The use of half-pins is preferred to minimize additional muscle and soft tissue damage and possible neurovascular injury.[113] Ring fixators are not commonly used as an external fixation device in pediatric fractures but can be considered. During the insertion of any external fixation device, care must be taken to avoid the epiphysis and physis. Meticulous daily pin care is mandatory to minimize the risk of infection. It is recommended that the fixator be removed once satisfactory skin coverage has been obtained or when sufficient callus formation to provide fracture stability is demonstrated radiographically. Protection in a plaster cast after removal of the external fixator is suggested. Tolo reported refracture of 3 of 14 tibial fractures (21%) 5 to 10 months after removal of a Hoffman device.[275] Whether the refracture was secondary to stress shielding or to relative ischemia from the severe local trauma at the site of injury is not known. As experience has been gained with the use of external fixators in children in the past decade, the incidence of refracture has decreased.[64, 79, 100, 230, 274] However, Miner and Carroll reported refracture in 8 of 37 (22%) femoral fractures treated by external fixation between 1992 and 1998.[178]

## Open Fractures

Open fractures are one of the most serious injuries to the pediatric musculoskeletal system. They are usually caused by high-velocity trauma and are increasing in frequency, especially in multiply injured children. In a series of multiply injured children reported by Marcus and coworkers,[164] 10% of the fractures were open. Approximately 25% to 50% of children with open fractures have other body area injuries. The objectives of treatment of open fractures in children are the same as for adults: preventing wound sepsis, healing soft tissue injuries, achieving bony union, and returning the patient to optimal function.[105–107]

All open fractures are graded according to the size of the wound, the extent of the soft tissue injury, and the degree of contamination because these factors affect the prognosis. The most widely used classification was developed by Gustilo and associates[105–107] (see Table 5–1). In a type I open fracture, the wound is less than 1 cm long. It is usually a clean puncture wound from a spike of bone that has pierced the skin. The fracture is generally simple, transverse, or short oblique, with minimal comminution and soft tissue damage. In a type II open fracture, the wound is more than 1 cm in length, but the soft tissue damage is not extensive. A slight or moderate crushing injury, moderate comminution of the fracture site, and moderate contamination may be present. Type III injuries are characterized by extensive damage to the skin and soft tissue, including muscle and possibly neurovascular structures. A significant degree of contamination is present. This type of injury is usually caused by high-velocity trauma and results in considerable fracture comminution and instability.

Type III open fractures are subdivided into three additional categories.[106] In type IIIA, soft tissue coverage of the fractured bone is adequate despite the extensive soft tissue injury. This group includes segmental or severely comminuted fractures from high-energy trauma, regardless of the size of the wound. Type IIIB open fractures have extensive injury or loss of soft tissue, with periosteal stripping and exposure of bone. Massive contamination and comminution of these fractures are common. After débridement and irrigation is completed, a segment of bone is exposed, and a local or free flap is needed for coverage. A type IIIC injury includes any open fractures associated with arterial injury that must be repaired, regardless of the degree of soft tissue injury. The incidence of wound infection, delayed union, nonunion, amputation, and residual disability is directly related to the classification of the open fracture.

Methods of achieving the goals of management as described by Gustilo and associates[105–108] include emergency initial care; thorough initial evaluation to diagnose other life-threatening injuries; appropriate antibiotic therapy; extensive and possible repeat wound débridement; fracture stabilization; local wound care; rarely, autogenous cancellous bone grafts; and rehabilitation. Each of these measures is discussed in detail in Chapter 5. Open fractures are frequently managed by external fixation. These devices stabilize the fracture and allow restabilization and access to the associated wounds for repeated débridement and bone grafting procedures. External fixation also allows the child to be more mobile for the evaluation and treatment of other body area injuries. Open fractures of the tibia and fibular shaft are the most common, as well as the most difficult.* Open fractures of the pelvis are uncommon but are associated with an approximately 50% mortality.[269] The cause of death is either hemorrhage early or sepsis later.

# REHABILITATION

Once the soft tissue and body cavity injuries have healed and bone union has occurred, rehabilitation of the child is important. Rehabilitation typically consists of range-of-motion exercises followed by strengthening of the musculature. It is important that these children undergo long-term follow-up to determine ultimate outcome with respect to function and growth of the injured extremities. Follow-up should continue until skeletal maturity to monitor growth of the injured extremities.

Formal physical therapy and rehabilitation are not generally necessary for the majority of injured children. Most of these injuries are simple, low-velocity injuries that heal rapidly because of resiliency of the child. In a multiply injured child, however, such is not usually the case. Because of the severity and complexity of the injuries, long hospitalization and multiple surgeries are often required. Although it has been shown that a child

can tolerate prolonged immobilization without the usual complications seen in an adult, such as joint stiffness, severe muscular atrophy, and disuse osteoporosis, complications can and do occur, and a good result cannot always be assumed. Significant long-term disability, most often related to injuries to the CNS and musculoskeletal system, can occur in children. Aggressive treatment has been shown to decrease these complications and improve the overall result.[157] Further detail is provided in Chapter 5.

## Physical Therapy

Physical therapy should be initiated as soon as the child's medical condition permits. Early physical therapy consists of gentle range-of-motion exercises of the noninjured or stabilized extremities to avoid soft tissue contractures and joint stiffness. Such therapy is especially important in a head- or spine-injured patient. More physical therapy can be instituted as the child's condition allows, including transfer training, resistive strengthening, and eventually ambulation. Each case must be dealt with individually because the spectrum and severity of injuries dictate the type and level of therapy. Close communication and cooperation between the physician and therapist are extremely important. Most physical therapy can be initiated while the child is still in the trauma center. Once the child's condition no longer requires that level of specialization, transfer to a different facility can be considered, possibly another acute care facility that is not a trauma center but is more accessible to the family or a long-term rehabilitation facility if acute care is no longer necessary. Children are often transferred long distances to be treated at trauma centers, and these distances can become a burden for families. Therefore, when the child's condition improves, every effort should be made to transfer the child to a facility closer to home. Some trauma centers are equipped with facilities for both acute care and long-term rehabilitation services. This type of center enables transfer from acute care to long-term care status while maintaining continuity of treatment by many of the same physicians and therapists. Such continuity is desirable because children develop important relationships with and dependencies on the treating physicians and therapists and severing these relationships can be extremely traumatic to the patient.

Children with severe head, spinal, and musculoskeletal injuries are most often in need of prolonged rehabilitation and are more likely to have permanent disabilities.[157, 164, 168, 171] Severe head injuries account for the majority of long-term rehabilitation, as well as most long-term disabilities. Children with head injuries require specialized facilities equipped for long-term rehabilitation—both physical rehabilitation and rehabilitation of cognitive capacities, including speech and learning. Multiple fractures in the absence of CNS injury can also result in long-term disability requiring prolonged rehabilitation. In addition to the usual procedures, specialized treatment with orthoses, prostheses, and appliances is often necessary for rehabilitation to optimal function. Fitting and the use of orthoses and

---

*See references 39, 40, 58, 59, 102, 124, 128, 142, 231, 253.

prostheses in children are specialized because the child continues to grow, and close monitoring and frequent modifications are necessary. The appropriate use of physical therapy can significantly improve the outcome in these children.

## Psychologic Rehabilitation

Psychologic rehabilitation of an injured child is as important as physical rehabilitation.[163, 256, 257] The physical trauma often creates severe psychologic trauma that in many cases is overlooked. After the initial traumatic event, the patient is faced with continued pain from the injury and often multiple, painful surgical procedures; disfigurement and loss of body image; and prolonged separation from parents, siblings, family, friends, and home. This psychologic trauma is not limited to the child but also affects the parents and family and often the person who feels responsible for the injury.[288] Dysfunctional behavior is frequently seen in children after trauma and includes phobias, scholastic difficulties, depression, and rage attacks.[18] This behavior is manifested not only by children with head injuries but also by those with severe injuries without CNS involvement. Delays in the normal developmental processes are common, and in many cases, the child is noted to regress. Such reactions can be considered normal, although they can become extreme. They are usually most pronounced 1 month after injury. In children without neurologic injury, it can take up to 12 months before the child approaches the preinjury level of function.[256, 257] The use of rigid fracture stabilization that permits the child to be mobile appears to lessen child and family stress and allow more rapid psychosocial recovery.[257]

These psychologic problems cannot be avoided completely, but they can certainly be lessened by appropriate early intervention with the patient and family. The physicians and staff must be aware of these problems and try to be as supportive as possible. It is important to spend time with the patient and family and inform them of the injuries sustained, what is to be expected, the types of procedures to be performed, and the prognosis. Painful procedures should be explained in detail and their importance stressed. Children should be allowed to express their fears and concerns and be made to feel a part of the process. They must be given assurances that they have not lost total control over their environment. The family should be allowed to be with the child as much as physically possible. It is often desirable to allow one family member to remain in the patient's room. Many rooms are equipped with extra beds so that parents can sleep in the room with their child. Social and psychologic counseling is often necessary, especially when the child or family appears to have problems coping with the situation. Marcus[163] has generalized a child's normal and abnormal psychologic responses to trauma (Table 4–12).

The effect of the trauma and all the circumstances and associated consequences on the entire family cannot be ignored. Harris and associates showed that two thirds of the uninjured siblings showed aggressive behavior and

**TABLE 4–12** ....................................

Normal and Abnormal Psychologic Responses of Children to Trauma

1. Impact phase—crying, screaming, panic
2. Rebound phase—defensive response
   Avoidance of feelings and thoughts regarding the situation
   Behavioral withdrawal and regression
   Increased dependency
   Nightmares, increased startle responses
3. Reintegration and recovery phase
   Preoccupation with the traumatic experience (thoughts, feelings, play activities)
   Possible continued sleep problems and disturbing dreams
4. Post-traumatic phase
   Intensity of experiences diminished (thoughts, feelings)
   Normal sleep
   Return to pretrauma personality function
   Return to self-confidence and self-esteem
5. Pathologic responses
   Prolongation of phases 1–3 beyond expected
   Phase 4 impaired (chronic anxiety, depression, behavioral problems, sleep disturbances, nightmares, guilt, withdrawal, excessive hostility)
   Low self-confidence and self-esteem
   Obsession with trauma
   Neurotic symptoms (tics, neuroses, encopresis, or other regressive patterns)

....................................................

From Marcus, I.M. In: Marcus, R.E., ed. Trauma in Children. Rockville, MD, Aspen, 1986, pp. 245–257.

one third of the parents involved had marriage problems traceable to the event. Though probably not preventable, these problems need to be recognized and addressed.[114]

## Education

Children who require prolonged hospitalization and rehabilitation will have their schooling interrupted, in many cases for an extended period. This interruption in schooling may put them significantly behind the level of their peers, which will give them an added problem when they are ready to return to school. It is important to initiate schooling and tutoring in the hospital as soon as the patient's condition allows while recognizing that the duration of tutoring may be lengthy. Harris and colleagues showed that 80% of all polytraumatized children required special schooling for years after the event.[114] Thirty-two percent of the polytraumatized pediatric patients in the series by van der Sluis and coworkers required transfer to a school offering education of a lower standard.[280] Children with a severe head injury face another spectrum of problems because they may require a specialized educational program as part of the rehabilitation process.

### REFERENCES

1. Accidental Death and Disability. The Neglected Disease of Modern Society. Washington, DC, National Academy of Sciences–National Research Council, 1966.
2. Agram, P.F.; Donkle, D.E.; Winn, D.G. Injuries to a sample of seatbelted children evaluated and treated in a hospital emergency room. J Trauma 27:58–64, 1987.

3. Albers, J.E.; Rath, R.K.; Glaser, R.S.; et al. Severity of intrathoracic injuries associated with first rib fractures. Ann Thorac Surg 33:614–618, 1982.

4. Alonso, J.E.; Horowitz, M. Use of the AO/ASIF external fixator in children. J Pediatr Orthop 7:594–600, 1987.

5. American College of Surgeons Committee on Trauma. Advanced Trauma Life Support Course. Instructor's Manual. Chicago, American College of Surgeons, 1993.

6. American National Standards Institute. Tracheal Tubes and Cuffs. New York, American National Standards Institute, 1974.

7. Amit, Y.; Salai, M.; Chechik, A.; et al. Closing intramedullary nailing for the treatment of diaphyseal forearm fractures in adolescence: A preliminary report. J Pediatr Orthop 5:143–146, 1985.

8. Anderson, P.A.; Henley, M.B.; Rivara, F.P.; et al. Flexion distraction and Chance injuries to the thoracolumbar spine. J Orthop Trauma 5:153–160, 1991.

9. Aronson, J.; Tursky, E.A. External fixation of femur fractures. J Pediatr Orthop 12:157–163, 1992.

10. Astion, D.J.; Wilber, J.H.; Scoles, P.V. Avascular necrosis of the capital femoral epiphysis after intramedullary nailing for a fracture of the femoral shaft. A case report. J Bone Joint Surg Am 77:1092–1094, 1995.

11. Baker, C.C.; Oppenheimer, L.; Stephens, B.; et al. Epidemiology of traumatic deaths. Am J Surg 140:144, 1980.

12. Baker, S.P.; O'Neill, B. The injury severity score: An update. J Trauma 16:882–885, 1976.

13. Baker, S.P.; O'Neill, B.; Hadden, W., Jr.; et al. The injury severity score: A method of describing patients with multiple injuries and evaluating emergency care. J Trauma 14:187–196, 1974.

14. Barlow, B.; Niemirska, M.; Gandhi, R.; Shelton, M. Response to injury in children with closed femur fractures. J Trauma 27:429–430, 1987.

15. Barlow, B.; Rottenberg, R.W.; Santalli, T.V. Angiopathic diagnosis and treatment of bleeding by selective embolization following pelvic fractures in children. J Pediatr Surg 10:939–942, 1975.

16. Bass, B.; Eichelberger, M.R.; Schisgall, R.; et al. Hazards of nonoperative therapy of hepatic injury in children. J Trauma 24:978–982, 1984.

17. Bassey, L.O. The use of P.O.P. integrated pins as an improvisation on the Hoffmann's apparatus: Contribution to open fracture management in the tropics. J Trauma 29:59–64, 1989.

18. Basson, M.D.; Guinn, J.E.; McElligott, J.; et al. Behavior disturbances in children after trauma. J Trauma 31:1363–1368, 1991.

19. Beaty, J.H.; Austin, S.M.; Warner, W.C.; et al. Interlocking intra-medullary nailing of femoral-shaft fractures in adolescents: Preliminary results and complications. J Pediatr Orthop 14:178–183, 1984.

20. Becker, D.P.; Miller, J.D.; Ward, J.D.; et al. The outcome from severe head injury with early diagnosis and intensive management. J Neurosurg 47:491–502, 1977.

21. Behrens, F. External fixation in children: Lower extremity. Instr Course Lect 39:205–208, 1990.

22. Benoit, R.; Watts, D.D.; Dwyer, K.; et al. Windows 99: A source of suburban pediatric trauma. J Trauma 49:477–481, 2000.

23. Blakemore, L.C.; Cooperman, D.R.; Thompson, G.H.; et al. Compartment syndrome in ipsilateral humerus and forearm fractures in children. Clin Orthop 376:32–38, 2000.

24. Blasier, R.D.; McAfee, J.; White, R.; Mitchell, D.T. Disruption of the pelvic ring in pediatric patients. Clin Orthop 376:87–95, 2000.

25. Blasier, R.D. Treatment of fractures complicated by burn or head injuries in children. J Bone Joint Surg Am 81:1038–1043, 1999.

26. Blasier, R.D.; Aronson, J.; Tursky, E.A. External fixation of pediatric femur fractures. J Pediatr Orthop 17:342–346, 1997.

27. Blount, W.P. Fractures in Children. Baltimore, Williams & Wilkins, 1954.

28. Bohn, W.W.; Durbin, R.A. Ipsilateral fractures of the femur and tibia in children and adolescents. J Bone Joint Surg Am 73:429–439, 1991.

29. Bond, S.J.; Gotschall, C.S.; Eichelberger, M.R. Predictors of abdominal injury in children with pelvic fractures. J Trauma 31:1169–1173, 1991.

30. Bone, L.B.; Johnson, K.D.; Weigelt, S.; et al. Early vs. delayed stabilization of femoral fracture. A preoperative randomized study. J Bone Joint Surg Am 71:336–340, 1989.

31. Bowers, S.A.; Marshall, L.F. Outcome in 200 consecutive cases of severe head injury in San Diego County: A prospective analysis. Neurosurgery 6:237–242, 1980.

32. Boyd, C.R.; Tolson, M.A.; Copes, W.S. Evaluating trauma care: The TRISS method. J Trauma 27:370–378, 1987.

33. Bracken, M.B.; Shephard, M.J.; Collins, W.F.; et al. A randomized, controlled trial of methyl prednisolone or naloxone in the treatment of acute spinal-cord injury. N Engl J Med 322:1405–1411, 1990.

34. Brandt, M.L.; Luks, F.I.; Spigland, N.A.; et al. Diaphragmatic injury in children. J Trauma 32:298–301, 1992.

35. Brantigan, C.O.; Grow, J.B. Cricothyroidotomy: Elective use in respiratory problems requiring tracheotomy. J Thorac Cardiovasc Surg 71:72–81, 1976.

36. Breaux, C.W.; Smith, G.; Georgeson, K.E. The first two years' experience with major trauma at a pediatric trauma center. J Trauma 30:37–43, 1990.

37. Bright, R.W. Operative correction of partial epiphyseal plate closure by osseous-bridge resection. J Bone Joint Surg Am 56:655–664, 1974.

38. Bryan, W.J.; Tullos, H.S. Pediatric pelvic fractures: A review of 52 patients. J Trauma 19:799–805, 1979.

39. Buckley, S.L.; Smith, G.R.; Sponseller, P.D.; et al. Severe (type III) open fractures of the tibia in children. J Pediatr Orthop 16:627–634, 1996.

40. Buckley, S.L.; Smith, G.; Sponseller, P.D.; et al. Open fractures of the tibia in children. J Bone Joint Surg Am 72:1462–1469, 1990.

41. Burri, C.; Allgöwer, M. Central venous pressure and shock index in the severely injured. Helv Chir Acta 39:107–111, 1972.

42. Canale, S.T.; King, R.E. Pelvic and hip fractures. Part I: Fractures of the pelvis. In: Rockwood, C.A., Jr.; Wilkins, K.E.; King, R.E., eds. Fractures in Children, 3rd ed. Philadelphia, J.B. Lippincott, 1991, pp. 991–1046.

43. Caniano, D.A.; Nugent, S.K.; Rogers, M.C.; et al. Intracranial pressure monitoring in the management of the pediatric trauma patient. J Pediatr Surg 15:537–542, 1980.

44. Cattell, H.S.; Filtzer, D.L. Pseudosubluxation and other normal variation in the cervical spine in children: A study of one hundred and sixty children. J Bone Joint Surg Am 47:1295–1298, 1985.

45. Chadwick, D.L.; Chin, S.; Salerno, C.; et al. Death from falls in children: How far is fatal? J Trauma 31:1353–1355, 1991.

46. Champion, H.R.; Sacco, W.J.; Copes, W.S.; et al. A revision of the Trauma Score. J Trauma 29:623–629, 1989.

47. Champion, H.R.; Sacco, W.J.; Carnazzo, A.J.; Fouty, W.J. Trauma Score. Crit Care Med 9:672–676, 1981.

48. Chan, B.S.H.; Walker, P.J.; Cass, D.T. Urban trauma: An analysis of 1,116 pediatric cases. J Trauma 29:1540–1547, 1989.

49. Cheng, J.C.Y.; Ng, B.K.W.; Ying, S.Y.; Lam, P.K.W. A 10-year study of the changes in the pattern and treatment of 6,493 fractures. J Pediatr Orthop 19:344–350, 1999.

50. Coldiron, J.S. Estimation of nasotracheal tube length in neonates. Pediatrics 41:823–828, 1968.

51. Committee on Injury Scaling. The Abbreviated Injury Scale. 1990 Revision. Morton Grove, IL, American Association for Automotive Medicine, 1990, pp. 1–66.

52. Committee on Injury Scaling. The Abbreviated Injury Scale— 1980 Revision. Morton Grove, IL, American Association for Automotive Medicine, 1980.

53. Cooney, D.R. Splenic and hepatic trauma in children. Surg Clin North Am 61:1165–1180, 1981.

54. Copes, W.S.; Champion, H.R.; Sacco, W.J.; et al. The Injury Severity Score revisited. J Trauma 28:69–77, 1988.

55. Cotler, H.B.; LaMont, J.G.; Hansen, S.T., Jr. Immediate spica casting for pelvic fractures. J Orthop Trauma 2:222–228, 1988.

56. Cramer, K.E.; Tornetta, P., III; Spero, C.R.; et al. Ender rod fixation of femoral shaft fractures in children. Clin Orthop 376:119–123, 2000.

57. Cramer, K.E. The pediatric polytrauma patient. Clin Orthop 318:125–135, 1995.

58. Cramer, K.E., Limbird, T.J.; Green, N.E. Open fractures of the diaphysis of the lower extremity in children. Treatment, results and complications. J Bone Joint Surg Am 74:218–232, 1992.

59. Cullen, M.C.; Roy, D.R.; Crawford, A.H.; et al. Open fractures of the tibia in children. J Bone Joint Surg Am 78:1039–1047, 1996.

60. Currey, J.D. Changes in the impact energy absorption of bone with age. J Biomech 12:459–469, 1979.

61. Currey, J.D.; Butler, G. The mechanical properties of bone tissue in children. J Bone Joint Surg Am 57:810–814, 1975.

62. Davis, T.J.; Topping, R.E.; Blanco, J.S. External fixation of pediatric femoral fractures. Clin Orthop 318:191–198, 1995.

63. Demetriades, D.; Nikolaides, N.; Filiopoulos, K.; Hager, J. The use of methylmethacrylate as an external fixator in children and adolescents. J Pediatr Orthop 15:499–503, 1995.

64. de Sanctis, N.; Gambardella, A.; Pempinello, C.; et al. The use of external fixators in femur fractures in children. J Pediatr Orthop 16:613–620, 1996.

65. Dietrich, A.M.; Ginn-Pease, M.E.; Bartkowski, H.M.; et al. Pediatric cervical spine features: Predominantly subtle presentation. J Pediatr Surg 26:995–1000, 1991.

66. Douglas, G.L.; Simpson, J.S. The conservative management of splenic trauma. J Pediatr Surg 6:565, 1971.

67. Dowd, M.D.; Krug, S. Pediatric blunt cardiac injury: Epidemiology, clinical features, and diagnosis. J Trauma 40:61–67, 1996.

68. Drew, R.; Perry, J.F., Jr.; Fischer, R.P. The expediency of peritoneal lavage for blunt trauma in children. Surg Gynecol Obstet 145:885, 1977.

69. Duff, J.H.; Goldstein, M.; McLean, A.P.H.; et al. Flail chest: A clinical review and physiological study. J Trauma 8:63–74, 1968.

70. DuPriest, R.W., Jr.; Rodriguez, A.; Shatney, C.H. Peritoneal lavage in children and adolescents with blunt abdominal trauma. Am Surg 48:460–462, 1982.

71. Dykes, E.H.; Spence, L.J.; Bohn, D.J.; Wesson, D.E. Evaluation of pediatric trauma care in Ontario. J Trauma 29:724–729, 1989.

72. Eckenhoff, J. Some anatomic considerations of infant larynx influencing endotracheal anesthesia. Anesthesiology 12:401, 1951.

73. Eichelberger, M.R.; Mangubat, E.A.; Sacco, W.S.; et al. Comparative outcomes of children and adults suffering blunt trauma. J Trauma 28:430–434, 1988.

74. Eichelberger, M.R.; Mangubat, E.A.; Sacco, W.J.; et al. Outcome analysis of blunt injury in children. J Trauma 28:1109–1117, 1988.

75. Eichelberger, M.R.; Randolph, J.G. Pediatric trauma: Initial resuscitation. In: Moore, E.E.; Eiseman, B.; Van Way, C.E., eds. Critical Decisions in Trauma. St. Louis, C.V. Mosby, 1984, p. 344.

76. Eichelberger, M.R.; Randolph, J.G. Pediatric trauma. An algorithm for diagnosis and therapy. J Trauma 23:91–97, 1983.

77. Eichelberger, M.R.; Randolph, J.G. Thoracic trauma in children. Surg Clin North Am 61:1181–1197, 1981.

78. Ein, S.H.; Shandling, B.; Simpson, J.S.; Stephens, C.A. Nonoperative management of traumatized spleen in children. How and why. J Pediatr Surg 12:117–119, 1978.

79. Evanoff, M.; Strong, M.L.; MacIntosh, R. External fixation maintained until fracture consolidation in the skeletally immature. J Pediatr Orthop 13:98–101, 1993.

80. Faist, E.; Baue, A.E.; Dittmer, H.; et al. Multiple organ failure in polytrauma patients. J Trauma 23:775–785, 1983.

81. Feickert, H.-J.; Drommer, S.; Heyer, R. Severe head injury in children: Impact of risk factors on outcome. J Trauma 47:33–38, 1999.

82. Fein, L.H.; Pankovich, A.M.; Spero, C.M.; Baruch, H.M. Closed flexible intramedullary nailing of adolescent femoral shaft fractures. J Orthop Trauma 3:133–141, 1989.

83. Flaherty, J.J.; Kelley, R.; Burnett, B.; et al. Relationship of pelvic bone fracture patterns to injuries of urethra and bladder. J Urol 99:297–300, 1968.

84. Flynn, J.M.; Hresko, T.; Reynolds, R.A.K.; et al. Titanium elastic nails for pediatric femur fractures: A multicenter study of early results with analysis of complications. J Pediatr Orthop 21:4–8, 2001.

85. Francke, E.L.; Neu, H.C. Postsplenectomy infection. Surg Clin North Am 61:135–155, 1981.

86. Friedman, R.J.; Jupiter, J.B. Vascular injuries and closed extremity fractures in children. Clin Orthop 188:112–119, 1984.

87. Furnival, R.A.; Woodward, G.A.; Schunk, J.E. Delayed diagnosis of injury in pediatric trauma. Pediatrics 98:56–63. 1996.

88. Fyodorov, I.; Sturm, P.F.; Robertson, W.W., Jr. Compression plate fixation of femoral shaft fractures in children aged 8 to 12 years. J Pediatr Orthop 19:578–581, 1999.

89. Gallagher, S.S.; Finison, K.; Guyer, B.; et al. The incidence of injuries among 87,000 Massachusetts children and adolescents: Results of the 1980–81 state-wide children injury prevention surveillance system. Am J Public Health 74:1340–1347, 1984.

90. Galpin, R.D.; Willis, R.B.; Sabano, N. Intramedullary nailing of pediatric femoral fractures. J Pediatr Orthop 14:184–189, 1994.

91. Ganz, R.; Krushell, R.J.; Jakob, R.P.; Kuffer, J. The antishock pelvic clamp. Clin Orthop 267:71–78, 1991.

92. Garcia, V.F.; Gotschall, C.S.; Eichelberger, M.R.; Bowman, L.M. Rib fractures in children: A marker of severe trauma. J Trauma 30:695–700, 1990.

93. Garvin, K.L.; McCarthy, R.E.; Barnes, C.L.; Dodge, B.M. Pediatric pelvic ring fractures. J Pediatr Orthop 10:577–582, 1990.

94. Ghanayem, A.J.; Stover, M.D.; Goldstein, J.A.; et al. Emergent treatment of pelvic fractures: Comparison of methods for stabilization. Clin Orthop 318:75–80, 1995.

95. Gilberman, R.H.; Zakaib, G.S.; Murbarak, S.J.; et al. Decompression of forearm compartment syndromes. Clin Orthop 134:225–229, 1978.

96. Glassman, S.D.; Johnson, J.R.; Holt, R.T. Seatbelt injuries in children. J Trauma 33:882–886, 1992.

97. Goldstein, A.S.; Sclafani, S.J.; Kupferstein, N.H.; et al. The diagnostic superiority of computerized tomography. J Trauma 25:938–946, 1985.

98. Gonzalez-Herranz, P.; Burgos-Flores, J.; Rapariz, J.M.; et al. Intramedullary nailing of the femur in children. Effects on its proximal end. J Bone Joint Surg Br 77:262–266, 1995.

99. Gratz, R.R. Accidental injury in childhood: A literature review on pediatric trauma. J Trauma 19:551–555, 1979.

100. Gregory, R.J.H.; Cubison, T.C.S.; Pinder, I.M.; Smith, S.R. External fixation of lower limb fractures of children. J Trauma 33:691–693, 1992.

101. Greenspan, L.; McLellan, B.A.; Greig, H. Abbreviated Injury Scale and Injury Severity Score: A scoring chart. J Trauma 25:60–64, 1985.

102. Grimard, G.; Naudie, D.; Laberge, L.C.; Hamby, R.C. Open fractures of the tibia in children. Clin Orthop 332:62–70, 1996.

103. Grisoni, N.; Connor, S.; Marsh, E.; et al. Pelvic fractures in a pediatric Level I trauma center. J Orthop Trauma (in press).

104. Gupta, A.; El Masri, W.S. Multilevel spinal injuries: Incidence, distribution, and neurologic patterns. J Bone Joint Surg Br 71:692–695, 1989.

105. Gustilo, R.B.; Merkow, R.L.; Templeman, D. Current concepts review. The management of open fractures. J Bone Joint Surg Am 72:299–304, 1990.

106. Gustilo, R.B.; Mendoza, R.M.; Williams, D.N. Problems in the management of type II (severe) open fractures: A new classification of type III open fractures. J Trauma 24:742–746, 1984.

107. Gustilo, R.B. Principles of the management of open fractures. In: Gustilo, R.B., ed. Management of Open Fractures and Their Complications. Philadelphia, W.B. Saunders, 1982.

108. Gustilo, R.B.; Anderson, J.T. Prevention of infection in treatment of 1025 open fractures of long bones: Retrospective and prospective analysis. J Bone Joint Surg Am 58:453–458, 1976.

109. Hadden, W.A.; Gillespie, W.J. Multiple level injuries of the cervical spine. Injury 16:628–633, 1985.

110. Hall, J.R.; Reyes, H.M.; Horvat, M.; et al. The mortality of childhood falls. J Trauma 29:1273–1275, 1989.

111. Haller, J.A., Jr. Pediatric trauma. The No. 1 killer of children. JAMA 249:47, 1983.

112. Handelsman, J.R. Management of fractures in children. Surg Clin North Am 63:629–670, 1983.

113. Hansen, S.T. Internal fixation of children's fractures of the lower extremities. Orthop Clin North Am 21:353–363, 1990.

114. Harris, B.H.; Schwaitzberg, S.D.; Seman, T.M.; Herrman, C. The hidden morbidity of pediatric trauma. J Pediatr Surg 24:103–106, 1989.

115. Harris, G.J.; Soper, R.T. Pediatric first rib fractures. J Trauma 30:343–345, 1990.

116. Hedequist, D.; Starr, A.J.; Wilson, P.; Walker, J. Early versus delayed stabilization of pediatric femur fractures: Analysis of 387 patients. J Orthop Trauma 13:490–493, 1999.

117. Heinrich, S.D.; Drvaric, D.M.; Darr, K.; MacEwen, G.D. The operative stabilization of pediatric diaphyseal femur fractures with flexible intramedullary nails: A prospective analysis. J Pediatr Orthop 14:501–507, 1994.

118. Heinrich, S.D.; Gallagher, D.; Harris, M.; Nadell, J.M. Undiagnosed fractures in severely injured children and young adults: Identification with technetium imaging. J Bone Joint Surg Am 76:561–572, 1994.

119. Heinrich, S.D.; Drvaric, D.; Darr, K.; MacEwen, G.D. Stabilization of pediatric diaphyseal femur fractures with flexible intramedullary nails (a technique paper). J Orthop Trauma 6:452–459, 1992.

120. Herndon, W.A.; Mahnken, R.F.; Ynrgve, D.A.; Sullivan, J.A. Management of femoral shaft fractures in the adolescent. J Pediatr Orthop 9:29–32, 1989.

121. Herzenberg, J.E.; Hensinger, R.N.; Dedrick, B.K.; Phillips, W.A. Emergency transport and positioning of young children who have an injury to the cervical spine. J Bone Joint Surg Am 71:15–22, 1989.

122. Hoffman, M.A.; Spence, L.J.; Wesson, D.E.; et al. The pediatric passenger: Trends in seatbelt use and injury patterns. J Trauma 27:974–976, 1987.

123. Holmes, M.J.; Reyes, H.M. A critical review of urban pediatric trauma. J Trauma 24:253–255, 1984.

124. Hope, P.G.; Cole, W.G. Open fractures of the tibia in children. J Bone Joint Surg Br 74:546–553, 1992.

125. Howman-Giles, R.; Gilday, D.W.; Venagopal, S.; et al. Splenic trauma: A nonoperative management and long term follow up by scintiscan. J Pediatr Surg 12:121, 1978.

126. Hu, X.; Wesson, D.E.; Logsetty, S.; Spence, L.J. Functional limitations and recovery in children with severe trauma: A one-year follow-up. J Trauma 37:209–213, 1994.

127. Injury Mortality Atlas of the United States, 1979–1987. Washington, DC, U.S. Department of Health and Human Services, 1987.

128. Irwin, A.; Gibson, P.; Ashcroft, P. Open fractures of the tibia in children. Injury 26:21–24, 1995.

129. Izant, R.J.; Hubay, C.A. The annual injury of 15,000,000 children. A limited study of childhood accidental injury and death. J Trauma 6:65–74, 1966.

130. Jaffe, D.M.; Binns, H.; Radkowski, M.A.; et al. Developing a clinical algorithm for early management of cervical spine injury in child trauma victims. Am J Emerg Med 16:270–276, 1987.

131. Johansen, K.; Lynch, K.; Paun, M.; Copass, M. Non-invasive vascular tests reliably exclude occult arterial trauma in injured extremities. J Trauma 31:515–522, 1991.

132. Joyce, M. Initial management of pediatric trauma. In: Marcus, R.E., ed. Trauma in Children. Rockville, MD, Aspen, 1986 pp. 13–38.

133. Karp, M.P.; Cooney, D.R.; Pros, G.A.; et al. The non-operative management of pediatric hepatic trauma. J Pediatr Surg 18:512–518, 1983.

134. Karp, M.P.; Cooney, D.R.; Berger, P.E.; et al. The role of computed tomography in the evaluation of blunt abdominal trauma in children. J Pediatr Surg 16:316, 1981.

135. Kaufmann, C.R.; Maier, R.V.; Kaufmann, E.J.; et al. Validity of applying TRISS analysis to injured children. J Trauma 31:691–697, 1991.

136. Kaufmann, C.R.; Maier, R.V.; Rivara, F.P.; Carrico, J. Evaluation of the Pediatric Trauma Score. JAMA 263:69–72, 1990.

137. Kaufmann, C.R.; Rivara, F.P.; Maier, R.V. Pediatric trauma: Need for surgical management. J Trauma 29:1120–1126, 1989.

138. Kendra, J.C.; Price, C.T.; Songer, J.E.; Scott, D.S. Pediatric applications of dynamic axial external fixation. Contemp Orthop 19:477–486, 1989.

139. Keshishyan, R.A.; Rozinov, V.M.; Malakhov, O.A.; et al. Pelvic polyfractures in children: Radiographic diagnosis and treatment. Clin Orthop 320:28–33, 1995.

140. Kirby, R.M.; Winquist, R.A.; Hansen, S.T., Jr. Femoral shaft fractures in adolescents: A comparison between traction plus cast treatment and closed intramedullary nailing. J Pediatr Orthop 1:193–197, 1981.

141. Klein, L.; Marcus, R.E. Trauma in children: Management, prognosis and metabolism. In: Marcus, R.E., ed. Trauma in Children. Rockville, MD, Aspen, 1986, pp. 1–12.

142. Kreder, H.J.; Armstrong, P. A review of open tibia fractures in children. J Pediatr Orthop 15:482–488, 1995.

143. Kregor, P.J.; Song, K.M.; Routt, M.L., Jr.; et al. Plate fixation of femoral shaft fractures in multiply injured children. J Bone Joint Surg Am 75:1774–1780, 1993.

144. Langenskiold, A.; Osterman, K. Surgical elimination ofd post-traumatic partial fusion of the growth plate. In: Houghton, G.R.; Thompson, G.H., eds. Problematic Musculoskeletal Injuries in Children. London, Buttersworth, 1983, pp. 14–31.

145. Lascombes, P.; Prevot, J.; Ligier, J.N.; et al. Elastic stable intramedullary nailing in forearm shaft fractures in children: 85 cases. J Pediatr Orthop 10:167–171, 1990.

146. Lee, K.W.; Dougal, R.M.; Templeton, J.J.; et al. Selection of endotracheal tubes in infants and children [abstract]. American Academy of Pediatrics annual meeting, Section of Anesthesiology, Las Vegas, NV, 1980, p. 15.

147. Letts, M.; McCaffrey, M.; Pang, E.; Lalonde, F. An analysis of an air-ambulance program for children. J Pediatr Orthop 19:240–246, 1999.

148. Letts, R.M.: Degloving injuries in children. J Pediatr Orthop 6:193–197, 1987.

149. LeWallen, R.P.; Peterson, H.A. Non-union of long bone fractures in children: A review of 30 cases. J Pediatr Orthop 5:135–142, 1985.

150. Lewis, V.L.; Manson, P.N.; Morgan, R.F.; et al. Facial injuries associated with cervical fractures: Recognition patterns and management. J Trauma 25:90–93, 1985.

151. Lhowe, D.W.; Hansen, S.T. Immediate nailing of open fractures of the femoral shaft. J Bone Joint Surg Am 70:812–820, 1988.

152. Ligier, J.N.; Metaizeau, J.P.; Prevot, J.; Lascombes, P. Elastic intramedullary nailing of femoral shaft fractures in children. J Bone Joint Surg Br 70:74–77, 1988.

153. Ligier, J.N.; Metaizeau, J.P.; Prevot, J.; Lascombes, P. Elastic stable intramedullary pinning of long bone shaft fractures in children. Z Kinderchir 40:209–212, 1985.

154. Lim, L.H.; Lam, L.K.; Moore, M.H.; et al. Associated injuries in facial fractures: Review of 839 patients. Br J Plast Surg 46:635–638, 1993.

155. Locke, G.R.; Gardner, J.I.; Van Epps, E.F. Atlas-dens interval (ADI) in children: A survey based on 200 normal cervical spines. AJR Am J Roentgenol 97:135–140, 1966.

156. Loder, R.T. Imaging of the pediatric spine. In: Betz, R.R., Mulcahey, M.J., eds. The Child with a Spinal Cord Injury. Rosemont, IL, American Academy of Orthopaedic Surgeons, 1996, pp. 47–60.

157. Loder, R.T. Pediatric polytrauma: Orthopaedic care in hospital course. J Orthop Trauma 1:48–54, 1987.

158. Luhmann, S.J.; Gordon, J.E.; Schoenecker, P.L. Intramedullary fixation of unstable both-bone forearm fractures in children. J Pediatr Orthop 18:451–456, 1998.

159. Luks, F.I.; Lemire, A.; St.-Vil, D.; et al. Blunt abdominal trauma in children: The practical value of ultrasonography. J Trauma 34:607–611, 1993.

160. Mabrey, J.D.; Fitch, R.D. Plastic deformation in pediatric fractures: Mechanism and treatment. J Pediatr Orthop 9:310–314, 1989.

161. Mangubat, E.; Eichelberger, M. Hypovolemia shock in pediatric patients: A physiologic approach to diagnosis and treatment. Trauma Clin Update Surg 2:1–8, 1985.

162. Mann, D.C.; Weddington, J.; Davenport, K. Closed Ender nailing of femoral shaft fractures in adolescents. J Pediatr Orthop 6:651–655, 1986.

163. Marcus, I.M. Emotional and psychological implications of trauma. In: Marcus, R.E., ed. Trauma in Children. Rockville, MD, Aspen, 1986, pp. 245–257.

164. Marcus, R.E.; Mills, M.; Thompson, G.H. Multiple injury in children. J Bone Joint Surg Am 65:1290–1294, 1983.

165. Marx, J.A.; Moore, E.E.; Jordan, R.C.; et al. Limitations of computed tomography in the evaluation of acute abdominal trauma: A prospective comparison with diagnostic peritoneal lavage. J Trauma 25:933–937, 1985.

166. Matsen, F.A.; Veith, R.G. Compartmental syndromes in children. J Pediatr Orthop 1:33–41, 1981.

167. Matsen, F.A.; Winquist, R.A.; Krugmire, R.B. Diagnosis and management of compartmental syndromes. J Bone Joint Surg Am 62:286–291, 1980.

168. Mayer, B.W. Pediatric Anesthesia. A Guide to Its Administration. Philadelphia, J.B. Lippincott, 1981, pp. 51–64, 251.

169. Mayer, T.; Walker, M.L.; Clark, P. Further experience with the modified abbreviated injury severity scale. J Trauma 24:31–34, 1984.

170. Mayer, T.; Walker, M.L.; Johnson, D.G.; Matlak, M.E. Causes of morbidity and mortality in severe pediatric trauma. JAMA 245:719–721, 1981.

171. Mayer, T.; Matlak, M.E.; Johnson, D.G.; Walker, M.L. The modified injury severity scale in pediatric multiple trauma patients. J Pediatr Surg 15:719–726, 1980.

172. McDonald, G.A.: Pelvic disruptions in children. Clin Orthop 151:130–134, 1980.

173. McIntyre, R.C.; Bensard, D.D.; Moore, E.E.; et al. Pelvic fracture geometry predicts risk of life-threatening hemorrhage in children. J Trauma 35:423–429, 1993.

174. Meissner, M.; Paun, M.; Johansen, K. Duplex scanning for arterial trauma. Am J Surg 161:552–555, 1991.

175. Mileski, R.A.; Garvin, K.L.; Huurman, W.W. Avascular necrosis of the femoral head after closed intramedullary femoral shortening in an adolescent. J Pediatr Orthop 15:24–26, 1995.

176. Mileski, R.A.; Garvin, K.L.; Crosby, L.A. Avascular necrosis of the femoral head in an adolescent following intramedullary nailing of the femur. A case report. J Bone Joint Surg Am 76:1706–1708, 1994.

177. Milholland, A.V.; Cowley, R.A.; Sacco, W.J. Development and prospective study of an anatomical index and an acute trauma index. Ann Surg 45:246–254, 1979.

178. Miner, T.; Carroll, K.L. Outcomes of external fixation of pediatric femoral shaft fractures. J Pediatr Orthop 20:405–410, 2000.

179. Momberger, N.; Stevens, P.; Smith, J.; et al. Intramedullary nailing of femoral fractures in adolescents. J Pediatr Orthop 20:482–484, 2000.

180. Moore, E.E.; Moore, J.B.; VanDuzer-Moore, S.; et al. Mandatory laparotomy for gunshot wounds penetrating the abdomen. Am J Surg 140:847, 1980.

181. Moulton, S.L. Early management of the child with multiple injuries. Clin Orthop 376:6–14, 2000.

182. Mubarak, S.J.; Carroll, N.C. Volkmann's contracture in children: Aetiology and prevention. J Bone Joint Surg Br 61:285–293, 1979.

183. Mubarak, S.J.; Owens, C.A.; Hargens, A.R.; et al. Acute compartment syndromes: Diagnosis and treatment with the aid of the Wick catheter. J Bone Joint Surg Am 60:1091–1095, 1978.

184. Murr, P.C.; Moore, E.E.; Lipscomb, R.; et al. Abdominal trauma associated with pelvic fracture. J Trauma 20:919–923, 1980.

185. Musemeche, C.A.; Barthel, M.; Cosentino, C.; Reynolds, M. Pediatric falls from height. J Trauma 31:1347–1349, 1991.

186. Musemeche, C.A.; Fischer, R.P.; Cotler, H.B.; Andrassy, R.J. Selective management of pediatric pelvic fractures. A conservative approach. J Pediatr Surg 22:538–540, 1987.

187. Myer, P.R., Jr. Surgery of Spine Trauma. New York, Churchill Livingstone, 1989, pp. 197–198.

188. Nakayama, D.K.; Copes, W.S.; Sacco, W.J. The effect of patient age upon survival in pediatric trauma. J Trauma 31:1521–1526, 1991.

189. National Safety Council. Accident Facts. Chicago, National Safety Council, 1982.

190. Navarre, J.R.; Cardillo, P.J.; Gorman, J.F.; et al. Vascular trauma in children and adolescents. Am J Surg 143:229–231, 1982.

191. Neff, C.C.; Pfister, R.C.; VanSonnenberg, E. Percutaneous transtracheal ventilation: Experimental and practical aspects. J Trauma 23:84–90, 1983.

192. Oestern, H.J.; Tscherne, H.; Sturm, J.; Nerlich, M. Classification of the severity of injury. Unfallchirurg 88:465–472, 1985.

193. Ogden, J.A. Skeletal Injury in the Child, 2nd ed. Philadelphia, W.B. Saunders, 1990.

194. Ogden, J.A. Skeletal growth mechanism injury patterns. J Pediatr Orthop 2:371–377, 1982.

195. O'Gorman, R.B.; Feliciano, D.V. Arteriography performed in the emergency center. Am J Surg 152:323, 1986.

196. O'Malley, D.E.; Mazur, J.M.; Cummings, R.J. Femoral head avascular necrosis associated with intramedullary nailing in an adolescent. J Pediatr Orthop 15:21–23, 1995.

197. O'Neill, J.A. Special pediatric emergencies. In: Boswick, J.A., ed. Emergency Care. Philadelphia, W.B. Saunders, 1981, p. 13.

198. Osler, T.M.; Vane, D.W.; Tepas, J.J.; et al. Do pediatric trauma centers have better survival rates than adult trauma centers? An examination of the National Pediatric Trauma Registry. J Trauma 50:96–99, 2001.

199. Ott, R.; Krämer, R.; Martas, P.; et al. Prognostic value of trauma scores in pediatric patients with multiple injuries. J Trauma 49:729–736, 2000.

200. Pang, D. Spinal cord injury without radiographic abnormality (SCIWORA) in children. In: Betz, R.R.; Mulcahey, M.J., eds. The Child With a Spinal Cord Injury. Rosemont, IL, American Academy of Orthopaedic Surgeons, 1996, pp. 139–160.

201. Patrick, D.A.; Bensard, D.B.; Moore, E.E.; et al. Ultrasound is an effective triage tool to evaluate blunt abdominal trauma in the pediatric population. J Trauma 45:57–63, 1998.

202. Peclet, M.H.; Newman, K.D.; Eichelberger, M.R.; et al. Patterns of injury in children, J Pediatr Surg 25:85–90, 1990.

203. Pediatric transfusions practice. In: Snyder, E.L., ed. Blood Transfusion Therapy. Arlington, VA, American Association of Blood Banks, 1983, p. 49.

204. Pennecot, G.F.; Gouraud, D.; Hardy, J.R.; et al. Roentgenographical study of the stability of the cervical spine in children. J Pediatr Orthop 4:346–352, 1984.

205. Peterson, H.A. Partial growth plate arrest and its treatment. J Pediatr Orthop 4:246–258, 1984.

206. Peterson, C.A.; Peterson, H.A. Analysis of the incidence of injuries to the epiphyseal growth plate. J Trauma 12:275–281, 1972.

207. Pollak, A.N.; Cooperman, D.R.; Thompson, G.H. Spica cast treatment of femoral shaft fractures in children. The prognostic value of the mechanism of injury. J Trauma 37:223–229, 1994.

208. Pollen, A.G. Fractures and Dislocations in Children. Baltimore, Williams & Wilkins, 1973.

209. Potoka, D.A.; Schall, L.C.; Gardner, M.J.; et al. Impact of pediatric trauma centers on mortality in a statewide system. J Trauma 49:237–245, 2000.

210. Powell, J.N.; Waddell, J.P.; Tucker, W.S.; Tranfeldt, E.E. Multiple-level noncontiguous spinal fractures. J Trauma 29:1146–1151, 1989.

211. Powell, R.W.; Smith, D.E.; Zarins, C.K.; et al. Peritoneal lavage in children with blunt abdominal trauma. J Pediatr Surg 11:973–977, 1976.

212. Pugh, D.M.W.; Galpin, R.D.; Carey, T.P. Intramedullary Steinmann pin fixation of forearm fractures in children: Long-term results. Clin Orthop 376:39–48, 2000.

213. Qidwai, S.A. Intramedullary Kirschner wiring for tibia fractures in children. J Pediatr Orthop 21:294–297, 2001.

214. Qidwai, S.A.; Khatlak, Z.K. Treatment of femoral shaft fractures by intramedullary Kirschner wires. J Trauma 48:256–259, 2000.

215. Quinby, W.C., Jr. Fractures of the pelvis and associated injuries in children. J Pediatr Surg 11:353–364, 1966.

216. Quinten, J. External fixation in child traumatology. Orthopaedics 7:463–470, 1984.

217. Rachesky, I.; Boyce, W.T.; Duncan, B.; et al. Clinical prediction of cervical spine injuries in children: Radiographic abnormalities. Am J Dis Child 141:199–201, 1987.

218. Ramenofsky, M.L.; Luterman, A.; Quindlen, E.; et al. Maximum survival in pediatric trauma: The ideal system. J Trauma 24:818–823, 1984.

219. Ramenofsky, M.L.; Luterman, A.; Currer, P.W.; et al. EMS for pediatrics: Optimal treatment or unnecessary delay? J Pediatr Surg 18:498–504, 1983.

220. Raney, E.M.; Ogden, J.A.; Grogan, D.P. Premature greater trochanteric epiphysiodesis secondary to intramedullary femoral rodding. J Pediatr Orthop 13:516–520, 1993.

221. Rang, M. Children's Fractures, 2nd ed. Philadelphia, J.B. Lippincott, 1983.

222. Rang, M.; Thompson, G.H. Children's fractures: Principles and management. Reconstr Surg Traumatol 17:2–15, 1979.

223. Reed, M.H. Pelvic fractures in children. J Can Assoc Radiol 27:255–261, 1976.
224. Reeves, R.B.; Ballard, R.I.; Hughes, J.L. Internal fixation versus traction and casting of adolescent femoral shaft fractures. J Pediatr Orthop 10:592–595, 1990.
225. Reff, R.B. The use of external fixation devices in the management of severe lower extremity and pelvic injuries in children. Clin Orthop 188:21–33, 1984.
226. Reichard, S.A.; Helikson, M.A.; Shorter, N.; et al. Pelvic fractures in children—review of 120 patients with a new look at general management. Pediatr Surg 15:727–734, 1980.
227. Reid, A.B.; Letts, R.M.; Black, G.B. Pediatric Chance fractures: Association with intra-abdominal injuries and seatbelt use. J Trauma 30:384–391, 1990.
228. Richter, D.; Ostermann, P.A.W.; Ekkernkamp, A.; et al. Elastic intramedullary nailing: A minimally invasive concept in the treatment of unstable forearm fractures in children. J Pediatr Orthop 18:457–461, 1998.
229. Rieger, H.; Brug, E. Fractures of the pelvis in children. Clin Orthop 336:226–239, 1997.
230. Riska, E.B.; von Bonsdorff, H.; Hakkinen, S.; et al. Prevention of fat embolism by early internal fixation of fractures in patients with multiple injuries. Injury 8:110–116, 1976.
231. Robertson, P.; Karol, L.A.; Rab, G.T. Open fractures of the tibia and femur in children. J Pediatr Orthop 16:621–626, 1996.
232. Roe, C.F.; Santulli, T.V.; Blair, C.S. Heat loss in infants during general anesthesia and operations. J Pediatr Surg 1:266, 1966.
233. Rorabeck, C.H. A practical approach to compartment syndromes. Part III. Treatment. Instr Course Lect 32:102–113, 1983.
234. Rothenberg, S.; Moore, E.E.; Maxx, J.A.; et al. Selective management of blunt abdominal trauma in children. The triage role of peritoneal lavage. J Trauma 27:1101–1106, 1987.
235. Rothenberger, D.A.; Fischer, R.P.; Perry, J.F., Jr. Major vascular injuries secondary to pelvic fractures: An unsolved clinical problem. Am J Surg 136:660–662, 1978.
236. Rumball, K.; Jarvis, J. Seat-belt injuries of the spine in young children. J Bone Joint Surg Br 74:571–574, 1992.
237. Salter, R.B.; Harris, W.R. Injuries involving the epiphyseal growth plate. J Bone Joint Surg Am 45:587–622, 1963.
238. Sawyer, J.R.; Flynn, J.M.; Dormans, J.P.; et al. Fracture patterns in children and young adults who fall from significant heights. J Pediatr Orthop 20:197–202, 2000.
239. Scheidler, M.G.; Shultz, B.L.; Schall, L.; Ford, H.R. Risk factors and predictors of mortality in children after ejection from motor vehicle crashes. J Trauma 49:864–868, 2000.
240. Schwab, C.W.; Peelet, M.; Zachnowski, S.W.; et al. The impact of an air ambulance system on an established trauma center. J Trauma 25:580–586, 1985.
241. Sclafani, S.J.; Florence, L.O.; Phillips, T.F.; et al. Lumbar arterial injury: Radiologic diagnosis and management. Radiology 165:709–714, 1987.
242. Seelig, J.M.; Becker, D.P.; Miller, J.D.; et al. Traumatic acute subdural hematoma: Major mortality reduction in comatose patients treated within four hours. N Engl J Med 304:1511–1518, 1981.
243. Shaker, I.J.; White, J.J.; Signer, R.D.; et al. Special problems of vascular injuries in children. J Trauma 16:863–867, 1976.
244. Shires, G.T.; Canizaro, P.C. Fluid resuscitation in the severely injured. Surg Clin North Am 53:1341–1365, 1973.
245. Shoemaker, S.D.; Comstock, C.P.; Mubarak, S.J.; et al. Intramedullary Kirschner wire fixation of open or unstable forearm fractures in children. J Pediatr Orthop 19:329–337, 1999.
246. Siemens, R.A.; Fulton, R.L. Gastric ruptures as a result of blunt trauma. Am Surg 43:229, 1977.
247. Silber, J.S.; Flynn, J.M.; Katz, M.A.; et al. Role of computed tomography in the classification and management of pediatric pelvic fractures. J Pediatr Orthop 21:148–151, 2001.
248. Sivit, C.J.; Taylor, G.A.; Newman, K.D.; et al. Safety-belt injuries in children with lap-belt ecchymosis: CT findings in 61 patients. AJR Am J Roentgenol 157:111–114, 1991.
249. Sledge, J.B.; Allred, D.; Hyman, J. Use of magnetic resonance imaging in evaluating injuries to the pediatric thoracolumbar spine. J Pediatr Orthop 21:288–293, 2001.
250. Smith, C.; Green, R. Pediatric vascular injuries. Surgery 90:20–31, 1981.

251. Smyth, B.T. Chest trauma in children. J Pediatr Surg 14:41, 1979.
252. Snyder, C.L.; Jain, V.N.; Saltzman, D.A.; et al. Blunt trauma in adults and children. J Trauma 30:1239–1245, 1990.
253. Song, K.M.; Sangeorzan, B.; Benirschke, S.; Browne, R. Open fractures of the tibia in children. J Pediatr Orthop 16:635–639, 1996.
254. Spiegel, P.G.; Mast, J.W. Internal and external fixation of fractures in children. Orthop Clin North Am 11:405–421, 1980.
255. Spoerel, W.E.; Narayanan, P.S.; Singh, N.P. Transtracheal ventilation. Br J Anaesth 43:932, 1971.
256. Stancin, T.; Kaugars, A.S.; Thompson, G.H.; et al. Child and family functioning 6 and 12 months after a serious pediatric fracture. J Trauma 51:69–76, 2001.
257. Stancin, T.; Taylor, H.G.; Thompson, G.H.; et al. Acute psychological impact of pediatric orthopaedic trauma with and without accompanying brain injuries. J Trauma 45:1031–1038, 1998.
258. Sturm, J.T.; Hynes, J.T.; Perry, J.F., Jr.; et al. Thoracic spinal fractures and aortic rupture: A significant and fatal association. Ann Thorac Surg 50:931–933, 1990.
259. Sturm, J.T.; Perry, J.F., Jr. Injuries associated with fractures of the transverse processes of the thoracic and lumbar vertebrae. J Trauma 24:597–599, 1984.
260. Sturm, P.F.; Glass, R.B.J.; Sivit, C.J.; Eichelberger, M.R. Lumbar compression fractures secondary to lap-belt use in children. J Pediatr Orthop 15:521–523, 1995.
261. Swischuk, L.E.; Swischuk, P.N.; John, S.D. Wedging of C-3 in infants and children: Usually a normal finding and not a fracture. Radiology 188:523–526, 1993.
262. Swischuk, L.E. Anterior displacement of C2 in children: Physiologic or pathologic? Radiology 122:759–763, 1977.
263. Tachdjian, M.O. Pediatric Orthopedics, 2nd ed., Vol. 4. Philadelphia, W.B. Saunders, 1990.
264. Teasdale, G.; Bennett, B. Assessment of coma and impaired consciousness: A practical scale. Lancet 2:81–84, 1974.
265. Tepas, J.J., III; DiScala, C.; Ramenofsky, M.L.; et al. Mortality and head injury: The pediatric perspective. J Pediatr Surg 25:92, 1990.
266. Tepas, J.J.; Ramenofsky, M.L.; Mollitt, D.L.; et al. The pediatric trauma score as a predictor of injury severity: An objective assessment. J Trauma 28:425–429, 1988.
267. Tepas, J.J., III; Mollitt, D.L.; Talbert, J.L.; Bryant, M. The pediatric trauma score as a predictor of injury severity in the injured child. J Pediatr Surg 22:14–18, 1987.
268. Thometz, J.G.; Lamdan, R. Osteonecrosis of the femoral head after intramedullary nailing of a fracture of the femoral shaft in an adolescent. A case report. J Bone Joint Surg Am 77:1423–1426, 1995.
269. Thompson, G.H.; Tynan, M. Complications of pelvic fractures in children. In: Epps, C., ed. Complications of Surgery. Philadelphia, J.B. Lippincott, 1995, pp. 125–154.
270. Thompson, G.H.; Wilber, J.H. Fracture management in the multiply injured child. In: Marcus, R.E., ed. Trauma in Children. Rockville, MD, Aspen, 1986, pp. 99–146.
271. Thompson, G.H.; Wilber, J.H.; Marcus, R.E. Internal fixation of fractures in children and adolescents. A comparative analysis. Clin Orthop 188:10–20, 1984.
272. Timmerman, L.A.; Rab, G.T. Intramedullary nailing of femoral shaft fractures in adolescents. J Orthop Trauma 7:331–337, 1993.
273. Tolo, V.T. Orthopaedic treatment of fractures of the long bones and pelvis in children who have multiple injuries. Inst Course Lect 49:415–423, 2000.
274. Tolo, V.T. External fixation in multiply injured children. Orthop Clin North Am 21:393–400, 1990.
275. Tolo, V.T. External skeletal fixation in children's fractures. J Pediatr Orthop 3:435–442, 1983.
276. Torode, I.; Zieg, D. Pelvic fractures in children. J Pediatr Orthop 5:76–84, 1985.
277. Townsend, D.R.; Hoffinger, S. Intramedullary nailing of femoral shaft fractures in children via the trochanter tip. Clin Orthop 376:113–118, 2000.
278. Tsai, A. Epidemiology of pediatric prehospital case. Ann Emerg Med 16:284–292, 1987.
279. Tscherne, H.; Gotzen, L. Fractures with Soft Tissue Injuries. Berlin, Springer-Verlag, 1984.

280. van der Sluis, C.K.; Kingma, J.; Eisma, W.H.; tenDuis, H.J. Pediatric polytrauma: Short-term and long-term outcomes. J Trauma 43:501–505, 1997.

281. Verstreken, L.; Delronge, G.; Lamoureaux, J. Orthopaedic treatment of pediatric multiple trauma patients. A new technique. Int Surg 73:177–179, 1988.

282. Verstreken, L.; Delronge, G.; Lamoureaux, J. Shaft forearm fractures in children. Intramedullary nailing with immediate motion: A preliminary report. J Pediatr Orthop 8:450–453, 1988.

283. Viljanto, J.; Linna, M.I.; Kiviluoto, H.; Paananen, M. Indications and results of operative treatment of femoral shaft fractures in children. Acta Chir Scand 141:366–369, 1975.

284. Voto, S.J.; Pigott, J.; Riley, P.; Donovan, D. Arterial injuries associated with lower extremity fractures. Orthopaedics 11:357–360, 1988.

285. Vransky, P.; Bourdelat, D.; Al Faour, A. Flexible stable intramedullary pinning technique in the treatment of pediatric fractures. J Pediatr Orthop 20:23–27, 2000.

286. Ward, W.W.; Levy, J.; Kaye, A. Compression plating for child and adolescent femur fractures. J Pediatr Orthop 12:626–632, 1992.

287. Weber, B.G.; Brunner, C.; Freuler, F., eds. Treatment of Fractures in Children and Adolescents. Berlin, Springer-Verlag, 1980.

288. Wesson, D.E.; Scorpio, R.J.; Spence, L.J.; et al. The physical, psychological, and socioeconomic costs of pediatric trauma. J Trauma 33:252–257, 1992.

289. Wesson, D.E.; Williams, J.I.; Spence, L.J.; et al. Functional outcome in pediatric trauma. J Trauma 29:589–592, 1989.

290. Wesson, D.E.; Williams, J.I.; Salmi, L.R.; et al. Evaluating a pediatric trauma program: Effectiveness versus preventable death. J Trauma 28:1226–1231, 1988.

291. Williams, R.A. Injuries in infants and small children resulting from witnessed and corroborated free falls. J Trauma 31:1350–1352, 1991.

292. Winquist, R.A.; Hansen, S.T., Jr.; Clawson, D.K. Closed intramedullary nailing of femoral fractures. A report of five hundred and twenty cases. J Bone Joint Surg Am 66:529–539, 1984.

293. Wolma, F.J.; Larrieu, A.J.; Alsop, G.C. Arterial injuries of the legs associated with fractures and dislocations. Am J Surg 140:806–809, 1980.

294. Yian, E.H.; Gullahorn, L.J.; Loder, R.T. Scoring of pediatric orthopaedic polytrauma: Correlation of different injury scoring systems and prognosis for hospital course. J Pediatr Orthop 20:203–209, 2000.

295. Yngve, D.A.; Harris, W.P.; Herndon, W.A.; et al. Spinal cord injury without osseous spine fracture. J Pediatr Orthop 8:153–159, 1988.

296. Yue, J.J.; Churchill, R.S.; Cooperman, D.R.; et al. The floating knee in the pediatric patient. Nonoperative versus operative stabilization. Clin Orthop 376:124–136, 2000.

297. Ziv, I.; Blackburn, N.; Rang, M. Femoral intramedullary nailing in the growing child. J Trauma 24:432–434, 1984.

298. Ziv, I.; Rang, M. Treatment of femoral fractures in the child with head injury. J Bone Joint Surg Br 65:276–278, 1983.

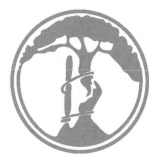

# CHAPTER 5

# Fractures with Soft Tissue Injuries

Fred F. Behrens, M.D.
Sanjeev Sabharwal, M.D.

## CHARACTERISTICS

Although skeletal maturity and preexisting conditions (e.g., osteogenesis imperfecta) influence the injury patterns of open fractures and dislocations, the kinetic energy $E_k = mv^2/2$, more than any other variable, determines the severity and specific features of a particular injury. Thus, closed pediatric fractures are largely caused by low-energy domestic activities and play, whereas violent traffic and other accidents are responsible for over 80% of open fractures in those older than 2 years.[33, 47, 77, 78] Even in adolescents, athletic activities account for less than 5% of open fractures. Although some open fractures occur through the physes, the majority are located in the diaphyses.

Open fractures in children younger than school age are rare because of their small body mass, the large amount of protective subcutaneous fat, and their limited exposure to high-risk activities; in addition, massive violence in this age group leads to loss of life rather than limb injury. The substantial energy involved in the creation of open fractures also causes more associated injuries.

## CLASSIFICATIONS

As many other fracture classifications, those focusing on the severity of the soft tissue injury lack verification or have interobserver concurrence of 60% or less.[16, 44] None have been tested in children. However, they tend to establish a diagnostic framework, increase awareness of injury severity, and provide some treatment guidance.

### Open Fractures

Most classifications of open musculoskeletal injuries account for the size, severity, and extent of the soft tissue lesion but neglect such modifying factors as wound contamination, fracture pattern, and associated injuries. The open fracture classification that is currently most popular for both children and adults was developed by Gustilo and Anderson in 1976 and divides fractures into three types according to soft tissue severity. It was further refined in 1984 to allow for better differentiation of the most severe injuries[31] (Table 5–1).

In type I open fractures, the wound is less than 1 cm long. It is often a clean puncture wound in which a spike of bone has pierced the skin. These fractures are accompanied by little soft tissue damage and no sign of crushing injury. The fracture is usually simple, transverse, or short oblique, with little comminution.

In type II open fractures, the laceration is more than 1 cm in length, but no extensive soft tissue damage is present. These fractures are associated with a slight or moderate crushing injury, moderate comminution at the fracture site, and moderate contamination.

Type III injuries are characterized by extensive damage to skin, muscle, bone, and possibly neurovascular structures. A high degree of contamination may be present. Type III injuries are divided into three subgroups. In type IIIA, soft tissue coverage of the fractured bone is adequate despite the extensive injury. This subtype includes segmental and severely comminuted fractures from high-energy trauma regardless of the size of the wound. Type IIIB injury has extensive soft tissue disruption or loss, with periosteal stripping and exposure of bone. Massive contamination and comminution of the fractures are common. A local or free flap is generally needed to obtain satisfactory wound coverage. Type IIIC includes any open fractures associated with an arterial injury that needs repair regardless of the extent of soft tissue damage. The incidence of wound infection, delayed union, nonunion, amputation, and residual disability is directly related to the type of soft tissue injury. The more severe the injury, the greater the risk of complications.[31, 40, 41]

Open fractures inflicted by lawn mowers and tornados

**TABLE 5–1** . . . . . . . . . . . . . . . . . . . . . . . . . . .

Classification of Open Fractures

| Type | Description |
|------|-------------|
| I | Skin opening of 1 cm or less, quite clean. Most likely from inside to outside. Minimal muscle contusion<br>Simple transverse or short oblique fractures |
| II | Laceration more than 1 cm long, with extensive soft tissue damage, flaps, or avulsion. Minimal to moderate crushing component. Simple transverse or short oblique fractures with minimal comminution |
| III | Extensive soft tissue damage, including muscles, skin, and neurovascular structures<br>Often a high-velocity injury with a severe crushing component |
| IIIA | Extensive soft tissue injury with periosteal stripping and bone exposure. Usually associated with massive contamination |
| IIIC | Vascular injury requiring repair |

. . . . . . . . . . . . . . . . . . . . . . . . . . . . . . . . . . . . . .

From Gustilo, R.B.; Mendoza, R.; Williams, D. Problems in the management of type III (severe) open fractures: A new classification of type III open fractures. J Trauma 24:742–746, 1984, © 1984, The Williams & Wilkins Company, Baltimore.

deserve particular attention because both generate highly contaminated open injuries mainly through the impact of flying debris or through the direct force of the cutting blades, which rotate at 3000 rpm and generate about 2100 foot-pounds of kinetic injury.[65] Lawn mower injuries, which often cause compartment syndromes, most commonly afflict children younger than 14 years.[68] Tornado and lawn mower injuries are often complicated by post-traumatic infections with mixed flora, mostly gram-negative bacilli.[60] They should be treated like farm injuries, with broad-spectrum antibiotics, including penicillin, and extensive and repeated débridement.

## The Mangled Extremity

With advances in prehospital resuscitation and the development of free flaps and microvascular reconstruction,[42, 56] many limbs with extensive open fractures that involve vascular compromise[48, 62] or partial amputation[51] can now be salvaged. However, despite the great potential for healing that is typical in children, some of the more severe open fractures are better managed with amputation than with extensive reconstructive procedures that leave the patient with a dubious cosmetic result and only marginal function.[29] To provide some guidance when deciding between limb salvage and amputation, a number of investigators have developed severity indices.[13, 45] In 1990, Johansen and associates[45] developed the Mangled Extremity Severity Score (MESS), which is a rating scale for lower extremity trauma based on skeletal and soft tissue damage, limb ischemia, shock, and age of the patient (Table 5–2). The reliability of this and other injury severity scores in assessing pediatric lower extremity injuries is not known.

## Closed Fractures with Severe Soft Tissue Injuries

It has become increasingly clear that some closed fractures caused by violent force may result in extensive destruction of the soft tissue sleeve surrounding the leg without resulting in an open lesion.[75, 76] These closed fractures with severe soft tissue injury are characterized by skin contusions, deep abrasions, burns, or frank separation of the cutis from the subcuticular tissue. Even in children, these lesions can result in partial or full tissue loss and secondary infection of the fracture site. To avoid catastrophes, these lesions must be treated as open fractures, which facilitates repeated injury evaluation and decreases complications. Tscherne and Oestern[76] provided a classification that describes four grades of these treacherous injuries and may prove useful in choosing among different treatment options (Table 5–3).

## TREATMENT PLAN
. . . . . . . . . . . . . . . . . . . . . . . . . . . . . . . . . . . . . .

### Overview

Although most bony and soft tissue disruptions in children have a greater healing potential, the treatment goals and principles of open musculoskeletal injuries in children are the same as those for adults; the principal goals are (1) restoration and preservation of vital

**TABLE 5–2** . . . . . . . . . . . . . . . . . . . . . . . . . .

Mangled Extremity Severity Score

| Variable | Points |
|----------|--------|
| **SKELETAL/SOFT TISSUE INJURY** | |
| Low energy (stab, simple fracture, "civilian" gunshot wound) | 1 |
| Medium energy (open or multiple fractures, dislocation) | 2 |
| High energy (close-range shotgun or "military" (gunshot wound, crush injury) | 3 |
| Very high energy (above plus gross contamination, soft tissue avulsion) | 4 |
| **LIMB ISCHEMIA** | |
| Pulse reduced or absent but perfusion normal | 1* |
| Pulseless; paresthesias, diminished capillary refill | 2* |
| Cool, paralyzed, insensate, numb | 3* |
| **SHOCK** | |
| Systolic blood pressure always >90 mm Hg | 0 |
| Hypotensive transiently | 1 |
| Persistent hypotension | 2 |
| **AGE (YEARS)** | |
| <30 | 0 |
| 30–50 | 1 |
| >50 | 2 |

. . . . . . . . . . . . . . . . . . . . . . . . . . . . . . . . . . . . . .

*Score doubled for ischemia duration longer than 6 hours.

From Johansen, K.; Daines, M.; Howey, T.; et al. Objective criteria accurately predict amputation following lower extremity trauma. J Trauma 30:568–572, 1990, © 1984, The Williams & Wilkins Company, Baltimore.

**TABLE 5–3**

Classification of Closed Fractures with Soft Tissue Injuries

| | |
|---|---|
| 0 | Minimal soft tissue damage. Indirect violence. Simple fracture patterns. Example: torsion fracture of the tibia in skiers |
| I | Superficial abrasion or contusion caused by pressure from within. Mild to moderately severe fracture configuration. Example: pronation fracture-dislocation of the ankle joint with a soft tissue lesion over the medial malleolus |
| II | Deep contaminated abrasion associated with localized skin or muscle contusion. Impending compartment syndrome. Severe fracture configuration. Example: segmental "bumper" fracture of the tibia |
| III | Extensive skin contusion or crush. Underlying muscle damage may be severe. Subcutaneous avulsion. Decompensated compartment syndrome. Associated major vascular injury. Severe or comminuted fracture configuration |

From Tscherne, H.; Oestern, H.-J. Unfallheilkunde 85:111–115, 1982.

functions, (2) prevention of wound infection, (3) healing of the soft tissue injuries, (4) restoration of bony anatomy and bone union, and (5) recovery of optimal physical and psychosocial function.[7, 32, 75]

These goals are best attained by (1) prompt initial resuscitation, (2) thorough and complete evaluation of life-threatening injuries followed by a full assessment of the fracture site, (3) appropriate antimicrobial therapy, (4) extensive and possibly repeated wound débridement followed by wound coverage, (5) fracture stabilization, (6) autogenous bone grafting when needed, (7) restoration of major bony defects, and (8) comprehensive functional and psychosocial rehabilitation. These interventions often overlap or occur in a modified temporal sequence, depending on age, injury pattern, and associated lesions. They are also highly interdependent; the type and timing of wound closure, for instance, may affect the choice of fracture fixation.

As in adults, open fractures in children are surgical emergencies.[7] Acute care follows the guidelines that have been established for similar lesions in adults. In addition to vigorous acute intervention, the final outcome of these injuries depends on a comprehensive plan of rehabilitation that includes physical therapy as well as educational and socioeconomic support for the family.[7, 13, 25]

## Initial Care

At the scene of the injury, the open wound is covered with a sterile dressing. Profuse bleeding is controlled by local compression. The fracture fragments are aligned by gentle traction and manipulation and are then splinted for transport.[75]

In the emergency room, the patient's vital functions are assessed and monitored, and all organ systems are systematically evaluated. One or more intravenous lines are established. If wound dressings are removed at all, masks and gloves are required. After the history is taken and the physical examination is completed, pertinent

radiographs are obtained and blood is drawn for a complete blood count, typing and crossmatching, and determination of serum electrolytes. Tetanus prophylaxis[17, 30] and the first intravenous dose of a broad-spectrum antibiotic are then given.[32, 67] Any patient with a suspected dysvascular limb is transferred to the operating room without delay for further assessment and possible vascular exploration and repair.[48] Preoperative angiography is not routinely recommended because it further prolongs the warm ischemia time.

## Wound Contamination and Antibiotics

### WOUND CONTAMINATION

It is prudent to consider that all open fractures, dislocations, and closed lesions covered with devitalized tissue are contaminated.[67] Frank infections, however, will develop only if necrotic tissue remains in the wound.[58, 72] Despite the use of systemic antibiotics, Dellinger and colleagues[22] reported that about 16% of all open fractures in adults will eventually become infected. They also reported that infection rates increased from 7% in type I fractures to 56% in type IIIC fractures.[22] Although infection rates in open pediatric fractures are not firmly established, they are assumed to be somewhat lower. Patzakis and Wilkins[67] in 1989 reported only one infection (1.8%) in 55 open fractures in children. In contrast, they had an overall infection rate of 7.2% in 1049 open adult fractures. Typically, the infecting organisms are *Staphylococcus aureus* and aerobic or facultative gram-negative rods in fractures with less severe soft tissue injury, whereas mixed flora prevails in lesions of type IIIB and IIIC severity.[22, 67] Among all open fractures, Patzakis and Wilkins[67] found the highest infection rate in tibial lesions. Infection rates of 1.9% in adults with open fractures have been reported by the Hannover Group, who used aggressive débridement as the mainstay of treatment.[72]

In two studies of open tibial fractures in children, the overall infection rates were 10% and 11%, similar to those reported in adults.[40, 43] No infections developed in type I injuries, whereas in type II lesions, infection rates were 12%, and in type III lesions, 21% and 33%.[40, 43]

### CLOSTRIDIAL INFECTIONS

**Tetanus.** Tetanus is a rare disease, with only about 200 cases of tetanus per year in the United States and a death rate between 10% and 40%.[11, 17] The causative organism is *Clostridium tetani*, a gram-positive rod that grows best under anaerobic conditions and in necrotic tissue. The clinical manifestations are caused by the effects of a neurotoxin on skeletal muscle, peripheral nerves, and the spinal cord. Generalized tetanus starts with cramps in the muscles surrounding the wound, neck stiffness, hyperreflexia, and changes in facial expression. Later, contractions of whole muscle groups cause opisthotonos and acute respiratory failure.

Local tetanus is rare and usually resolves without sequelae.[17]

Tetanus is preventable through active immunization with a formaldehyde-treated tetanospasmin known as tetanus toxoid. In children younger than 7 years, tetanus toxoid is administered in combination with diphtheria toxoid and pertussis vaccine (DPT). The Immunization Practices Advisory Committee recommends routine active immunization for infants and children with diphtheria and tetanus toxoids and pertussis absorbed at the ages of 2 months, 4 months, 6 months, 15 months, and 4 to 6 years.[1] Completion of a primary dose series confers humoral immunity to tetanus for at least 10 years in the majority of those who receive the vaccine (see Table 4–10). A child or adolescent with an open fracture who has not completed the primary series of immunizations or who has not received a booster dose in 10 years should receive tetanus toxoid, which is administered as a 0.5 mL intramuscular injection for patients of all ages.[41a] As has been shown in a 1995 population-based study, immunity cannot be presumed.[30] If the wound is severe, passive immunization with human tetanus immune globulin (HTIG) is added. According to Howell,[41a] "Tetanus immune globulin confers passive immunity for at least 4 weeks. The dose varies with age, but those older than 10 years of age receive 250 units, those 5 to 10 years of age receive 125 units, and those younger than 5 years of age receive 75 units. Tetanus immune globulin and tetanus toxoid should not be administered at the same site but may be administered on the same day. Immune globulin and toxoid are safe during pregnancy." Wounds that are deemed tetanus prone include wounds contaminated with dirt, saliva, or feces; puncture wounds, including nonsterile injections; missile injuries; burns; frostbite; avulsions; crush injuries; and wounds undergoing delayed débridement.[11] Vigorous débridement of open wounds and resection of all nonviable tissue are an integral part of tetanus prevention.

**Gas Gangrene.** Gas gangrene is most frequently caused by *Clostridium perfringens* or *Clostridium septicum*, anaerobic gram-positive spore-forming bacteria that produce numerous exotoxins. Gas gangrene is most frequently seen after primary wound closure, after open crush injuries, and in wounds contaminated by bowel contents or soil.[14, 64, 67] The exotoxins produced by these organisms create local edema, muscle and fat necrosis, and thrombosis of local vessels. The clostridia also generate several gases that dissect into the surrounding tissue and facilitate rapid spread of the infection. In the terminal stages, clostridial infections cause hemolysis, tubular necrosis, and renal failure.[14, 26, 64]

The earliest symptoms of gas gangrene after an open fracture include excruciating pain in the affected area followed by high fever, chills, tachycardia, contusions, and evidence of toxemia. Initially, the skin about the wound is very edematous and cool, but without crepitation. Later, the skin has a brown or bronze coloration, crepitation, and drainage of a thin brownish fluid with a pungent odor. Radiographs demonstrate gas formation within the muscle and intrafascial planes. Gram stain of the exudate reveals gram-positive rods with spores.[27]

Not all post-traumatic crepitation is caused by gas gangrene. It may also be caused by mechanical introduction of air by trauma, surgery, or chemical irrigation,[27] especially in the first 12 hours after injury. Crepitation from gas gangrene usually occurs between 12 and 60 hours after injury; it is initially minimal but progresses with time.[64]

The crucial steps in the treatment of early gas gangrene are radical débridement to remove all necrotic muscle and fasciotomies of all compartments to relieve pressure from the edema and enhance blood flow. Repeated débridement is usually necessary. In addition, the patient should receive intravenous penicillin (several million units a day in divided doses). In allergic patients, intravenous clindamycin (Cleocin Phosphate) or metronidazole (Flagyl) is an acceptable substitute. Because clostridial wounds often grow a mixed flora, a cephalosporin and an aminoglycoside are usually added. The efficacy of polyvalent gas gangrene serum, which can cause sensitivity reactions, remains unproven. Hyperbaric oxygen ventilation may be beneficial[14, 26, 64] because elevated tissue oxygen tension appears to inhibit clostridial growth and the production of exotoxins. This technology, however, is no substitute for meticulous surgical débridement.

## ANTIMICROBIALS

**Systemic Antibiotics.** Approximately 70% of open fractures are contaminated with bacteria at the time of injury. Gram-negative and aerobic gram-positive bacteria are the major pathogens of infections associated with fractures. The risk for the development of an infection in an open fracture depends directly on the severity of the soft tissue injury, the extent of the contamination, the virulence of the involved flora, and the adequacy of surgical débridement.

The use of antibiotics has been demonstrated to be effective in decreasing the risk of infection in open fractures. Patzakis and Wilkins[67] found the infection rate to be 13.9% in 79 patients who received no antibiotics versus 5.5% in 815 patients who were treated with broad-spectrum antibiotics (cephalothin alone or cefamandole plus tobramycin).

Because more than one organism is often present, it is the current practice to use a combination of antibiotics. A cephalosporin (cefazolin or cefamandole) is currently recommended as baseline therapy for all open fractures.[31] For type I lesions, this therapy is initially continued for 24 to 72 hours. One randomized, prospective study in patients aged 14 to 65 years with open fractures showed no difference in the infection rate when comparing 1 day and 5 days of cephalosporin prophylaxis.[21] Type II or III open fractures are treated with a cephalosporin as well as an aminoglycoside to cover both gram-positive and gram-negative bacteria. This combined antibiotic therapy is also continued for 24 to 72 hours. Penicillin is added if the patient is at risk for a clostridial infection. One prospective study in adults showed that ciprofloxacin as a single agent was effective in type I and II open fractures.[66]

Antibiotic therapy is started in the emergency room.

Antibiotics are restarted when another major operation is performed, such as delayed primary or secondary wound closure, elective open reduction and internal fixation, or bone grafting. Prolonged antibiotic therapy does not reduce the rate of wound infections but may promote the development of resistant organisms.[21, 67]

Vigorous, uncompromising resection of all dead soft tissue and the use of systemic antibiotics remain the principal tools in preventing post-traumatic wound infection.

Infection rates in open wounds appear to be further reduced by repeated irrigation with solutions that contain antibiotics such as neomycin, bacitracin, and polymyxin; by the use of iodine-containing solutions,[12] which have a broad bactericidal and spore-killing spectrum; and by the occasional use of antibiotic-containing polymethyl methacrylate beads.[7, 38, 39, 69] These measures are general guidelines. Selection of the optimal antibiotic therapy depends on the regional prevalence of pathogenic bacteria, the profile of nosocomial infections in a particular institution, the emergence of resistance, and the development of new chemotherapeutic agents.[66, 67]

## Wound Care

### IRRIGATION AND DÉBRIDEMENT

In the operating room, after induction of anesthesia the injured extremity is prepared and draped. To avoid contamination of the fracture site, a separate set of instruments is used for the initial part of the procedure: the débridement. Once débridement is completed, the surgical team changes gloves and gowns along with redraping of the operative site before proceeding with fracture fixation and applying the final wound dressing. A pneumatic tourniquet is applied as a safety measure but is not inflated unless massive bleeding occurs. Then follows the most important process in the management of an open fracture: a search for the true extent of the "real injury," which often exceeds the "apparent injury" by a factor of 2 to 3. Many clues alert the surgeon to the true size of the injury zone, including an estimate of the energy involved in the injury event, the size and location of bruises and secondary skin openings, and such radiographic features as air pockets extending along tissue planes and the relationship of bony fragments to neurovascular structures.

This information is used to guide the initiation of débridement—a carefully planned and systematic process that removes all foreign and dead material from the wound. As the first step, the wound edges are liberally extended to allow unobstructed access to the entire injury zone (Figs. 5–1 through 5–13). These incisions should be extensile, should not create flaps, and should respect vascular and neurologic territories. All dead and necrotic skin is resected to a bleeding edge, and necrotic or contaminated subcutaneous tissue and fat are sharply débrided. Contaminated fascia is resected, and prophylactic fasciotomies and epimysiotomies are performed to allow the injured tissue to swell without causing secondary vascular compromise and tissue necrosis. Ischemic muscle is the principal culture medium for bacteria and is radically resected where compromised. The four Cs—consistency, contractility, color, and capacity to bleed—are classic guides to viability but are, unfortunately, not always reliable. The capacity to contract after a gentle pinch with forceps and the presence of arterial bleeding seem to be the best signs of viability.

The intramedullary canal of the principal fracture fragments is carefully inspected and cleansed of any contaminated material. Cancellous bone, if it can be cleaned sufficiently, may serve as excellent graft material. In adults, large nonviable cortical fragments are often retained, but such fragments can be discarded in children, whose capacity for bony regeneration is much

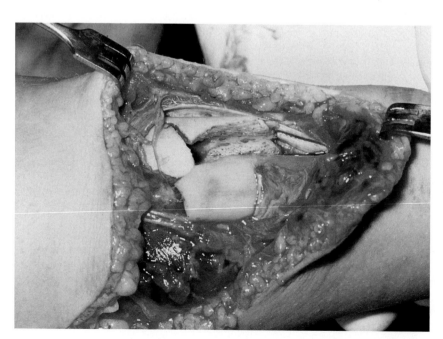

FIGURE 5–1. Type IIIA open tibial fracture in a 7-year-old boy who was hit by a car while crossing a street.

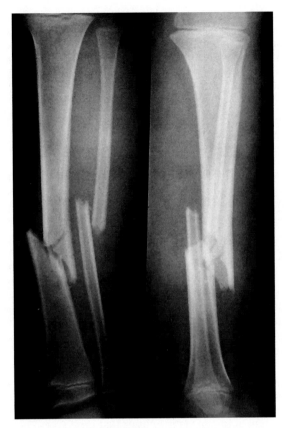

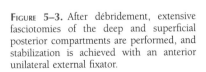
FIGURE 5–2. Tibial radiographs on admission.

greater. Major neurovascular structures must be carefully identified and preserved whenever possible. Débridement is completed when all contaminated, dead, and ischemic tissue is resected and the remaining wound cavity is lined by viable, bleeding tissue.

Throughout the process of débridement, the wound is irrigated with ample amounts of isotonic solution. There appears to be little solid information to document the advantage of adding antibiotics to the irrigant; however, new solutions such as benzalkonium chloride may prove to be superior to normal saline in controlled trials.[18] It aids in the removal of coagulant, fresh blood, foreign material, necrotic tissue, and bacteria. The use of pulsating irrigation with a sprinkler head is optimal,[4] and high pressure should be avoided.[10]

Nerves, vessels, tendons, articular cartilage, and bone, if exposed, are covered with local soft tissue or skin. The surgical extension of the wound, if possible, is usually closed and the remainder of the wound cavity dressed with a bandage soaked in isotonic saline or an antiseptic. Because the extent of soft tissue necrosis is easily underestimated, most open fracture wounds are reevaluated in the operating room within 48 to 72 hours. At that time, it may be necessary to resect more necrotic tissue and do more extensive fasciotomies. The process of débridement is repeated at intervals of 2 to 3 days, or shorter, until the wound can be closed. Perioperative cultures have been abandoned because they are costly and ineffective.[46, 52, 58]

## COMPARTMENT SYNDROMES

Although diagnosis, management, and the long-term effects of compartment syndromes in children have been well delineated, the perception persists that compartment syndromes in open fractures are rare. In fact, increased compartment pressure is most commonly seen in type III open fractures and in children suffering from multiple injuries.[17, 20, 43] Because of their limited ability to communicate, such children are in constant danger that this diagnosis will be missed or delayed, particularly when they are intubated or have a head injury, a peripheral neurologic lesion, or mental impairment. To avoid major disasters, compartment pressures should be promptly determined in any child who is at risk or who

FIGURE 5–3. After débridement, extensive fasciotomies of the deep and superficial posterior compartments are performed, and stabilization is achieved with an anterior unilateral external fixator.

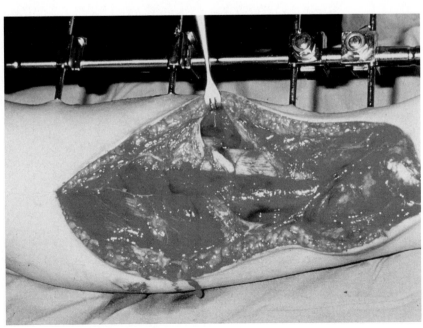

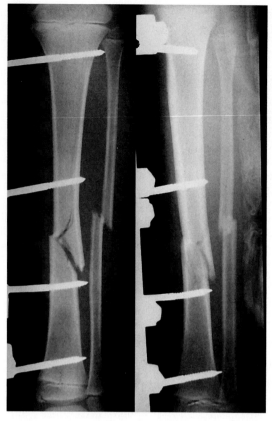

**FIGURE 5–4.** *Left,* external fixation reestablishes proper length and alignment. *Right,* note early osseous union after 6–8 weeks.

has suffered from muscle ischemia for longer than 4 hours.[48] Generally, more than one compartment in a particular extremity segment needs to be decompressed. As a rule, delayed primary closure of all compartment incisions without any need for skin grafting is possible in children.

## AMPUTATION

Trauma is the leading cause of amputations in children.[50] The injuries are most commonly caused by power tools and machinery such as lawn mowers. Other causes include motor vehicle accidents, burns, land mines, gunshots, and blast injuries. In fact, in children younger than 10 years, power lawn mowers accounted for 42% of all amputations. If children younger than 14 years had not been permitted around lawn mowers, approximately 85% of the injuries would have been prevented.[53] In another study of 74 children who sustained traumatic amputations, 53% were unsupervised at the time of the accident.[74] Better public education is needed to lessen the frequency of these devastating injuries.

Although no definite guidelines for amputations in children are available, findings that strongly suggest the need for an amputation include an unrestorable blood supply, warm ischemia time exceeding 6 hours,[49] substantial loss of viable muscle that cannot be replaced with a free flap, the presence of serious secondary bone

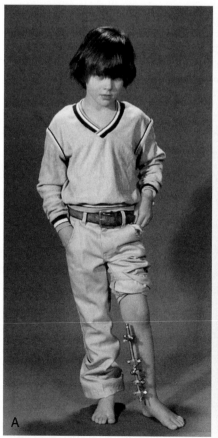

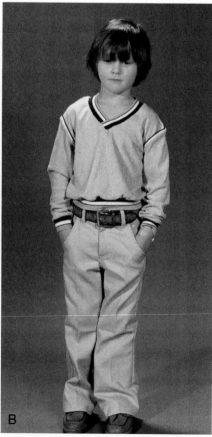

**FIGURE 5–5.** *A,* Four weeks after injury, the patient can bear full weight on the injured leg. *B,* The low-profile external fixator is easily hidden under the pants.

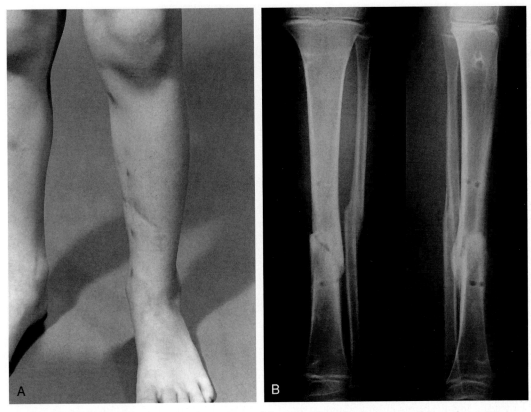

**FIGURE 5–6.** Clinical (*A*) and radiographic (*B*) appearance of the injured limb after fixator removal 3 months postinjury.

or soft tissue injuries involving the same extremity, and possibly a MESS of 7 or higher.[13] In the past, the loss of protective plantar sensation was an additional indication to amputate the foot.[13, 25] However, if the lesion is due to neurapraxia of the posterior tibial nerve, it may recover over time. Data indicate that 70% to 80% of all patients with either direct repair or grafting of a transected

posterior tibial nerve show good end results with successful sensory recovery and no trophic ulceration or any need for ambulatory support.[23, 34, 36, 54, 63] Most of these reports involve adult patients, and most of the grafts were performed on a delayed basis about 6 months after the injury. Whenever possible, the decision to amputate should be made at the initial débridement[7]

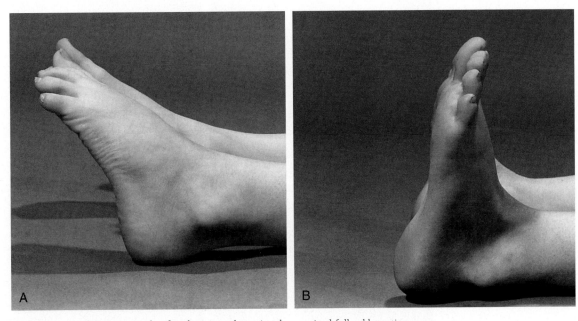

**FIGURE 5–7.** *A* and *B*, Four months after the injury, the patient has regained full ankle motion.

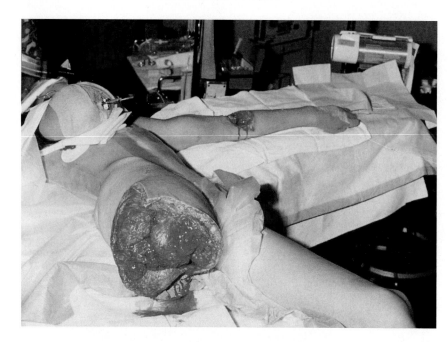

**FIGURE 5–8.** Eleven-year-old boy injured by fast-moving snow removal equipment: traumatic right above-knee amputation and type IIIA open, comminuted, left humeral and closed right forearm fractures.

because at least in adults, primary amputation leads to better long-term results.[12]

A child with a traumatic amputation is managed differently from an adult with a similar injury. The potential for future growth, better healing ability, terminal bony overgrowth, and psychologic and emotional factors all require special consideration.

When possible, preservation of the chondroepiphysis and growth plate should be considered. The distal femoral growth plate, for example, provides 75% of the growth of the femur, and an above-knee amputation done at an early age can lead to an inappropriately short amputation stump that can cause problems with pros-

thetic fitting. An estimate of the growth remaining in the residual limb is required to make a decision on the length of the amputated segment. For instance, an ideal bone length for an adult below-knee amputation is 12.5 to 17.5 cm, depending on body height. In children, a reasonable rule of thumb is to allow for 2.5 cm of bone length for each 30 cm of body height. A partial injury to the open growth plate may cause angular deformities with time, and thus these children need close follow-up until skeletal maturity.

If possible, the articular cartilage at the end of the residual bony segment should be preserved to avoid potential problems with terminal bony overgrowth. This

**FIGURE 5–9.** *A and B,* Plate fixation of a comminuted subtrochanteric femoral fracture to preserve amputation length and gain early soft tissue and bone stability.

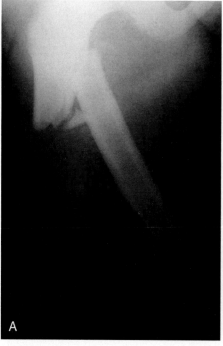
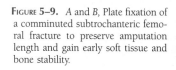
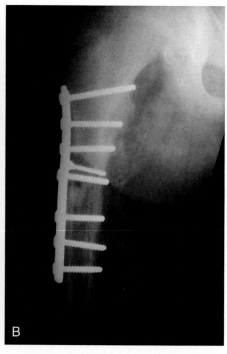

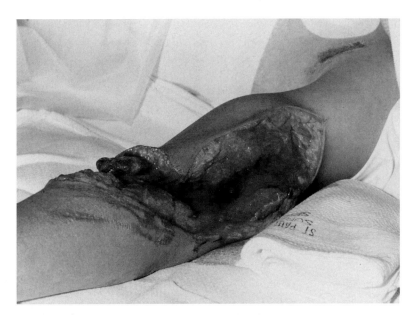

**FIGURE 5–10.** Traumatic wound, lateral aspect of the left arm, overlying comminuted type IIIA humeral fracture. The patient has neurapraxia of the radial nerve.

phenomenon is commonly seen after diaphyseal and metaphyseal amputations and affects the tibia/fibula, humerus, and femur in order of frequency. Occlusion of the medullary canal by a biologic cap consisting of an osteocartilaginous plug can prevent terminal overgrowth. For below-knee amputations, the first metatarsal, talar dome, iliac crest, or ipsilateral fibular head can be used (Figs. 5–14 to 5–17). Biologic capping is recommended at the time of amputation in children younger than 12 years who are undergoing transmetaphyseal or transdiaphyseal amputations of the tibia or humerus.

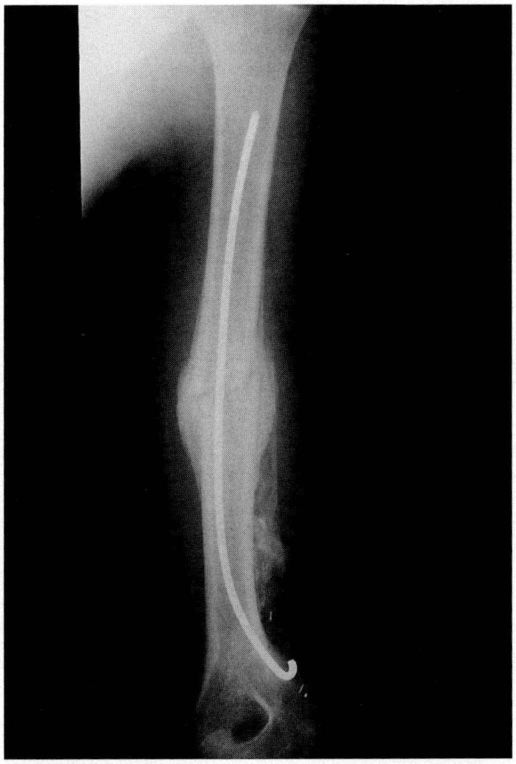

The better healing potential typical in children makes it possible to save more limbs. Skin grafts can be used successfully to conserve limb length without compromising wound healing or prosthetic fitting. Successful lengthening of short residual amputation stumps is feasible.[79]

A child's rapid growth and high demand on the prosthetic device make frequent repair and replacement necessary. Also, the need for appropriate psychologic and emotional support for the child and family needs to be appreciated. Child amputees are often best managed by a multidisciplinary team in a tertiary care center.

## Wound Coverage

As soon as possible, the surgeon must determine the means through which soft tissue coverage will eventually be accomplished. Complex wounds are best assessed early, in conjunction with an expert in soft tissue and microvascular techniques, so that satisfactory wound coverage is completed within 5 to 7 days after the injury and before secondary wound colonization has occurred.[41, 67] Between débridement sessions, the wound is kept moist with dressings soaked in saline or an antiseptic.

Most open fractures of type I to type IIIA severity are covered routinely by delayed primary wound closure or a split-thickness skin graft. For moderate soft tissue defects with exposed bones, nerves, vessels, tendons, or ligaments, local muscle flaps can be ideal. For larger defects and lesions involving the most distal part of the leg, microvascular free flaps are required.[39] Muscle or composite free flaps are indicated for large combined soft tissue and bone defects.[42, 56] In addition to giving excellent coverage, free flaps may diminish low-grade

**FIGURE 5–11.** Humeral fracture healed 8 weeks after intramedullary fixation with a K-wire.

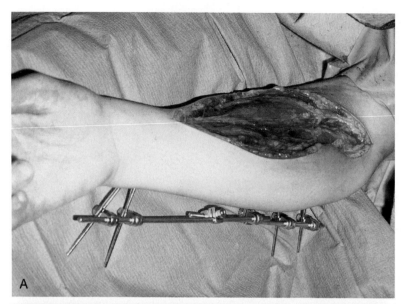

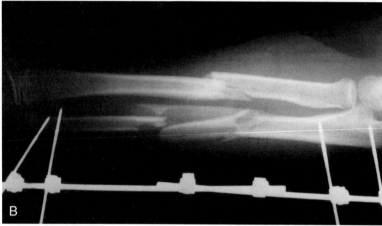

**Figure 5–12.** Clinical (*A*) and radiographic (*B*) status after initial débridement, right forearm fasciotomies, and restoration of ulnar length and alignment with a temporary external fixator.

**Figure 5–13.** Three days after the injury, the patient's forearm wound is reevaluated and found to be clean. The right ulna and radius are plated, and the external fixator is removed.

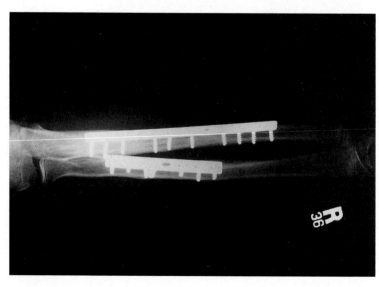

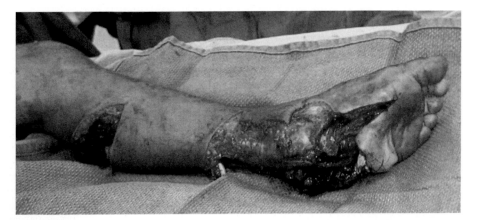

FIGURE 5–14. Six-year-old boy after a severe lawn mower injury to his left leg. This injury was not reconstructible.

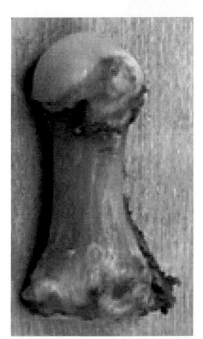

FIGURE 5–15. The first metatarsal salvaged from the amputated leg.

bacterial colonization in the recipient bed and facilitate fracture union.

Although primary wound closure in adults has led to significantly higher rates of infection and nonunion,[70] studies of open tibial fractures in children have reported that primary wound closure was carried out with little ill effect in 55% to 64% of all patients.[19, 29, 39] Recently published reviews have indicated the safety of primary wound closure in selected adult patients.[24] Most open type III fractures require débridement and delayed closure.[5, 15, 71] It must also be remembered that primary wound closure in open fractures is responsible for the majority of cases of gas gangrene.[14, 64]

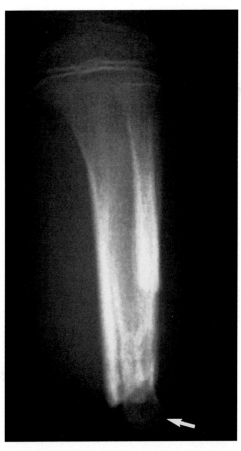

FIGURE 5–17. Radiograph of a tibial stump with an osteochondral graft.

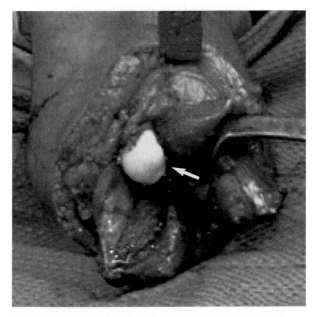

FIGURE 5–16. The first metatarsal was placed into the intramedullary canal of the tibial stump to function as an osteochondral graft.

## ACHIEVING BONE UNION

In children, nonunion of open fractures is uncommon and, as a rule, occurs only after significant bone loss or after major bone resection for the development of post-traumatic osteomyelitis. Fractures with partial bone loss are carefully monitored for 3 to 4 months. The few that have not healed by that time are best managed with a bone graft[6, 73] (Figs. 5–18 to 5–26). Segmental bone loss in younger children, particularly when most of the periosteum has remained intact, is best managed with an autogenous cancellous bone graft. For larger defects in older children, distraction osteogenesis is more reliable.

## FRACTURE FIXATION

### General Concepts

Fixation of the principal fracture fragments reduces pain, prevents additional injuries to surrounding soft tissue, decreases the spread of bacteria, and allows for early soft tissue and bone repair.[6, 59, 67] With few exceptions, indications for the use of particular fixation methods in open fractures are similar to those for closed lesions. However, when compared with closed fractures, those with severe soft tissue injury are generally less stable, demand prolonged observation, require repeated wound

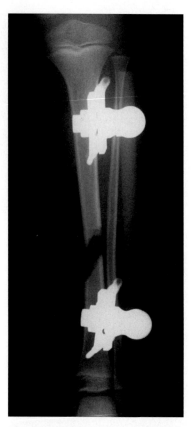

FIGURE 5–19. After repeated débridement, secondary wound closure is performed and the injury stabilized with an anterior external fixator.

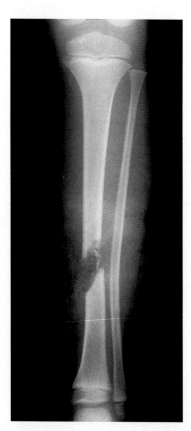

FIGURE 5–18. Two-centimeter bone loss in an 8-year-old boy who sustained a type IIIA open tibial fracture after collision with a car.

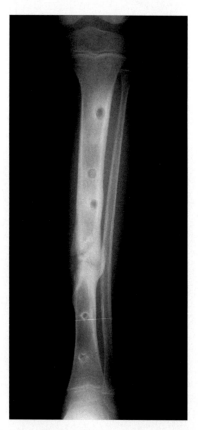

FIGURE 5–20. Eleven months after the initial injury. After failed bone grafting 6 months previously, the fixator was removed and the pinholes curetted. The tibia has been stabilized in a cast for the past month, with no clinical or laboratory indications of a residual infection.

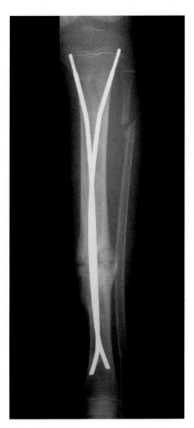

FIGURE 5–21. One month after partial fibulectomy and fracture stabilization with flexible nails.

débridement, and are commonly associated with injuries elsewhere. Operative fixation of open fractures is therefore more often indicated. External and internal fixation techniques allow for easier wound and limb access, facilitate earlier joint mobility and weight bearing, and reduce the length of the hospital stay as well as the frequency of clinic visits and radiographic evaluation when compared with fracture care in casts or traction.

Although the choice of fixation method is largely dependent on the orthopaedic surgeon's preference, consensus is emerging that severely contaminated or type IIIB open injuries are initially best stabilized with a splint or an external fixator.[2, 6] Once a clean wound and a viable soft tissue sleeve have been established, definitive stabilization with a formal cast, a plate, a nail, or an external fixator should follow (see Figs. 5–1 to 5–13; Figs. 5–18 to 5–26).

## Operative Methods

The guidelines and concepts that govern the use of internal and external fixation techniques are similar in children and adults.[9, 61, 73] However, such differences as open growth plates, an increased capability of remodeling, a faster healing rate, and a diminished ability to cooperate, which are typical in children, clearly affect the choice of an optimal implant for a particular injury. In fact, an implant that may be optimal for a particular

fracture in adults can be entirely unsuitable for a similar pediatric lesion.

## PLATES

The large incisions that are often needed for plate application tend to leave unsightly scars and continue to detract from the use of this technique in children. Increased infection rates are also a persistent concern with the use of plates.[71] In addition, substantial overgrowth may occur at the time of both plate application and plate removal.[37, 80]

At this time, plates and screw/plate devices are optimal for the stabilization of displaced open pelvic and hip fractures. Plates may also be preferable to external fixation or a cast for unstable open humeral and forearm fractures, particularly in children older than 10 years (see Figs. 5–8 to 5–13).

## INTRAMEDULLARY NAILS

In children, intramedullary nails are most often used for the stabilization of femur fractures.[28] Flexible stainless steel or titanium rods 2.0 to 4.0 mm in diameter are best suited for stable mid-diaphyseal fractures in younger children.[35] However, rods provide only limited rotational stability, so a temporary hip spica is occasionally indicated. Because injuries to the proximal femoral apophysis appear to be well tolerated

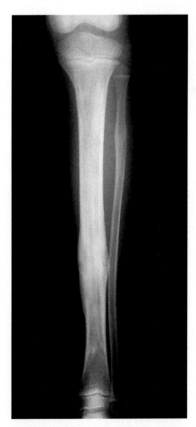

FIGURE 5–22. Six months after elastic nailing and 18 months after the initial injury. The tibia fracture has healed with good alignment and less than 5 mm of shortening.

after the age of 8 years, pediatric locking nails inserted through the greater trochanter are a good option for unstable fractures in older children and adolescents. Standard locking nails that are inserted through the piriformis fossa, however, are contraindicated in those younger than 14 years because of persistent concern about avascular necrosis of the femoral head.[28, 55] In addition, laboratory data indicate that the use of solid intramedullary implants is associated with a lower rate of infection than is the case with slotted implants.[57] Flexible nails may have a place in the treatment of stable tibial fractures or nonunion in older children (see Figs. 5–19 to 5–22).

## EXTERNAL FIXATION

External fixators are ideal for the stabilization of many unstable open shaft fractures in an immature skeleton. The pins can be placed away from the injury site and thus do not interfere with débridement or soft tissue recon-

struction. Even simple fixator constructs are rigid enough to maintain anatomic alignment and allow for almost immediate weight bearing, and the fast healing times typical of children make pin tract complications a rarity. In the early treatment period, the fixator can be removed at any time and be replaced by a plate or an intramedullary nail if so indicated.

In older children and adolescents, devices and components designed for adults are well tolerated. However, for smaller children, fixators used for adult wrist fractures or a combination of smaller pins with adult-sized clamps and connecting rods have proved most appropriate. The pin diameter should not exceed one quarter of the diameter of the bone. Pins with diameters ranging from 2.5 to 4.0 mm are commonly used in children younger than 12 years.[6]

Concern about fixator strength and rigidity often leads to oversized two-plane unilateral and two-plane bilateral frame designs.[6, 8, 9, 73] However, with the exception of athletic or obese teenagers, simple one-plane unilateral

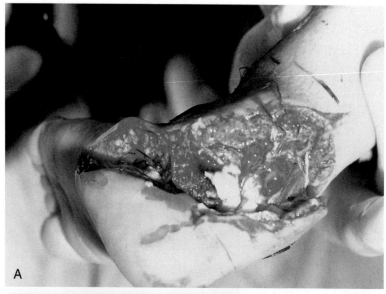

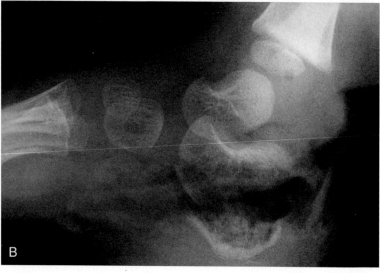

**FIGURE 5–23.** *A* and *B*, Left hindfoot of a 4-year-old boy after a severe lawn mower injury with transection of the Achilles tendon and os calcis. The wound has massive contamination with grass, earth, and machine oil.

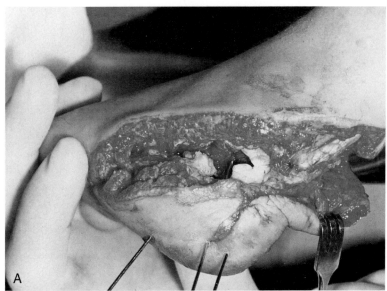

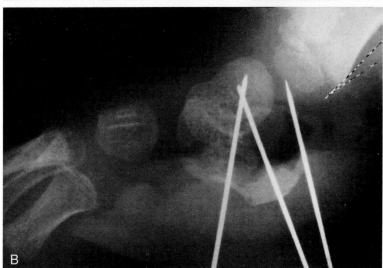

FIGURE **5–24.** *A* and *B,* After repeated débridement, the Achilles tendon is repaired and the os calcis fracture is reduced and stabilized with percutaneous wires.

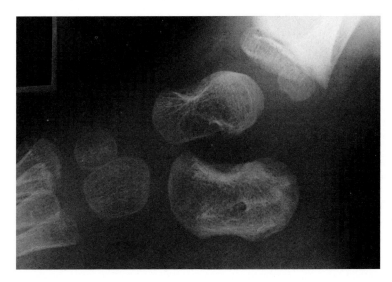

FIGURE **5–25.** One year after the injury, the patient has regained full function in his left foot, and the os calcis has healed.

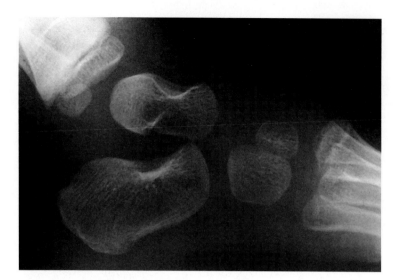

**FIGURE 5–26.** Lateral radiograph comparing the patient's normal right foot 1 year after injury.

frames routinely achieve sufficient rigidity for early unsupported weight bearing. Ring fixators using wires under tension are occasionally indicated for periarticular fractures or comminuted tibial shaft lesions. At times, they are best applied in delayed fashion after the soft tissue wounds have been covered. As in adults, fixators should be kept in place until the fractures have fully healed.[39] Fixator removal—for any reason—halfway through the healing process and placement of the limb in a cast often lead to secondary angulatory deformities.[29]

To provide optimal function and prevent serious side effects, three basic criteria pertain when external fixators are applied: (1) they should not damage vital anatomy, (2) they should provide sufficient wound access for the initial débridement and secondary procedures, and (3) the frame should be appropriate to the mechanical demands of the patient and the injury.[8] Simple means of increasing frame stiffness include using large pins, spreading the pins in each main bony fragment as far apart as possible, placing the longitudinal rods close to the bone, double-stacking the rods, and establishing a second pin plane.[8]

As a limb segment in which the principal long bone lies eccentrically, the tibia is ideally suited for the application of an external frame. The anteromedial third of the tibia represents a safe corridor in which pins can be inserted without the risk of impaling neurovascular structures or myotendinous units. Occasionally, pins and wires may be inserted into the epiphysis. Great care must be taken when pins are placed periarticularly because the undulating shape of the physis creates an unsafe zone that varies in width from 1 to 2 cm.[2] With some care and the use of an image intensifier, epiphyseal pins can be placed safely and may prove highly effective in the management of comminuted metaphyseal injuries. To avoid septic arthritis, pins and wires should not penetrate the joint cavity.

As in adults, external fixators are applied in the operating room under sterile conditions and general anesthesia. The leg is draped so that the knee and ankle joint lie within the operating field because such exposure aids in clinical limb alignment. The most proximal and distal pins are inserted first under image intensification to avoid injuries to the physes. This step is followed by insertion of the remaining screws, including those for a segmental fragment. An image intensifier is used routinely to check pin location and depth of penetration and overall limb alignment.[2, 6] The pins holes are predrilled with a sharp drill bit, and a trocar sleeve is inserted to help protect the soft tissue and facilitate accurate placement. Universal articulations that allow for easy alignment are often used. If a simple fixator device with independent articulations is chosen, care must be taken to avoid malrotation, which is difficult to correct after all the pins have been inserted.[2] Once the frame is applied, final fracture alignment is documented on long films. The pin sites are kept clean by washing the leg once daily with warm soapy water.[2, 73] For younger children, such cleansing is done by the parents, but responsible teenagers can handle this task independently. Unless bone loss has occurred, most patients walk with full weight bearing and little support within 3 weeks.

If healing of a diaphyseal fracture is delayed or a pin gets infected before the fracture is fully consolidated, one might be very tempted to remove the external frame and place the limb in a cast. Unfortunately, this approach frequently leads to secondary deformation of the fracture in the cast and the development of malunion.[39] When faced with delayed union, it is best to keep the fixator in place and support the healing process with an autologous bone graft. Inflamed or infected pins should be managed with improved pin care and a short-term course of oral antibiotics. If this strategy is unsuccessful, the pin should be exchanged and the frame left in place until the fracture has healed. In our hands, the use of titanium pins with a simple regimen of washing the pin sites with soap and water once daily has led to a substantial reduction in pin tract complications.

## Specific Fracture Patterns and Locations

### PERIARTICULAR AND INTRA-ARTICULAR FRACTURES

After adequate débridement, open intra-articular fractures and epiphyseal injuries are anatomically reduced and stabilized with K-wires or screws (see Figs. 5–23 to 5–26). To prevent undue force at the fracture site, the extremity is then protected with a well-padded splint. Once the soft tissue wound has been closed, a plaster cast is applied until the bone has healed and active range-of-motion exercises can be initiated. In the face of a more extensive soft tissue lesion that need prolonged observation and care, a uniplanar transarticular external fixator is preferable to a splint or cast.[33, 80]

### DIAPHYSEAL FRACTURES

**Stable Fractures.** In the upper extremity, stable shaft fractures with mild to moderate soft tissue injuries (type I or type II open fractures) are stabilized with a well-padded splint until the wound has healed. The splint is then replaced and the fracture is managed as a closed fracture with either a formal cast or a sling.

Stable open femoral fractures can be treated in traction until the soft tissue wound has healed. Depending on the age of the child, traction can be replaced by a hip spica cast either immediately or once the fracture fragments have started to consolidate. In older or multiply injured patients, external fixators, flexible intramedullary nails (Ender), or pediatric locking nails inserted through the greater trochanter are generally preferable.

After wound closure, open tibial shaft fractures may be treated in a cast according to the guidelines used for similar closed lesions. If operative fixation is indicated, external fixators are preferable to intramedullary nails or plates (see Figs. 5–1 to 5–7).

**Unstable Fractures.** Diaphyseal fractures that are unstable or complicated by more severe soft tissue injury (all type III open fractures) are best managed with internal or external fixation.

Depending on injury severity and the age of the patient, open unstable humeral fractures are initially stabilized with a coaptation splint or an external fixator. Methods of definitive fracture stabilization include a fracture brace, a small or narrow plate, or an external fixator.

For unstable forearm fractures in younger children, a fixator may be ideal, at least temporarily. In patients older than 10 to 12 years, however, plates are preferable (see Figs. 5–12 and 5–13).

Although unstable open femoral fractures can be managed in traction, this approach is inadequate for polytrauma patients and requires a prolonged hospital stay. In most circumstances, operative fracture fixation is preferable. External fixators that control length, rotation, and angulation can be used reliably in all pediatric age groups.[3] As noted, insertion of rigid locked intramedullary nails through the greater trochanter is an option after the age of 8 years, but standard entry through the piriformis fossa must be avoided in children with open proximal femoral growth plates because of concern about growth abnormalities, in particular, avascular necrosis.

In children with immature skeletons, external fixators remain the method of choice for the fixation of unstable open tibial fractures.

**Traumatic Amputations.** As noted, traumatic amputations in children are managed differently from those in adults because the potential for future growth, better healing ability, terminal bony overgrowth, and psychologic and emotional factors all require special consideration.

## REFERENCES

1. Advisory Committee on Immunization Practices: Adult immunization. MMWR Morb Mortal Wkly Rep 39:37–41, 1990.
2. Alonso, J.; Horowitz, M. Use of the AO/ASIF external fixator in children. J Pediatr Orthop 7:594–600, 1987.
3. Aronson, J.; Tursky, E. External fixation of femur fractures in children. J Pediatr Orthop 12:157–163, 1992.
4. Bach, A.; Hansen, S. Plates versus external fixation in severe open tibial shaft fractures: A randomized trial. Clin Orthop 241:89–94, 1989.
5. Barlett, C.; Weiner, L.; Yang, E. Treatment of type II and type III open tibia fractures in children. J Orthop Trauma 11:357–362, 1997.
6. Behrens, F. External fixation in children: Lower extremity. Instr Course Lect 39:205–208, 1990.
7. Behrens, F. Fractures with soft tissue injuries, In: Browner, B.; Jupiter, J.; Levine, A.; et al., eds. Skeletal Trauma, Philadelphia, W.B. Saunders, 1991, pp. 311–336.
8. Behrens, F.; Johnson, W. Unilateral external fixation: Methods to increase and reduce frame stiffness. Clin Orthop 241:48–56, 1989.
9. Behrens, F.; Searls, K. External fixation of the tibia. J Bone Joint Surg Br 68:246–254, 1986.
10. Bhandari, M.; Schemitsch, E.H.; Adili, A.; et al. High and low pressure pulsatile lavage of contaminated tibial fractures: An in vitro study of bacterial adherence and bone damage. J Orthop Trauma 13:526–533, 1999.
11. Bleck, T. *Clostridium tetani.* In: Mandell, G.; Douglas, R.; Bennet, J., eds. Principles and Practice of Infectious Diseases, 4th ed. New York, Churchill Livingstone, 1995, pp. 2173–2178.
12. Bombelli, R.; Giangrande, A.; Malacrida, V.; Puricelli, G. The control of infection in orthopaedic surgery. Orthop Rev 10:65–72, 1981.
13. Bondurant, F.; Cotler, H.; Buckle, R.; et al. The medical and economic impact of severely injured lower extremities. J Trauma 28:1270–1273, 1988.
14. Brown, P.; Kinman, P. Gas gangrene in a metropolitan community. J Bone Joint Surg Am 56:1445–1451, 1974.
15. Buckley, S.; Smith, G.; Sponseller, P.; et al. Severe (type III) open fractures of the tibia in children. J Pediatr Orthop 16:627–634, 1996.
16. Byrd, H.; Spicer, T.; Cierney, G. Management of open tibial fractures. Plast Reconstr Surg 76:719–728, 1985.
17. Cates, T. *Clostridium tetani* (tetanus). In: Mandell, G.; Douglas, R.; Bennett, J., eds. Principles and Practice of Infectious Disease. New York, Churchill Livingstone, 1990, pp. 1946–1982.

18. Conroy, B.P.; Anglen, J.O.; Simpson, W.A.; et al. Comparison of castile soap, benzalkonium chloride, and bacitracin as irrigation solutions for complex contaminated orthopaedic wounds. J Orthop Trauma 13:332–337, 1999.

19. Cullen, M.; Roy, D.; Crawford, A.; et al. Open fractures of the tibia in children. J Bone Joint Surg Am 78:1039–1046, 1996.

20. DeLee, J.; Stiehl, J. Open tibia fractures with compartment syndrome. Clin Orthop 160:175–184, 1981.

21. Dellinger, E.P.; Caplan, E.S.; Weaver, L.D.; et al. Duration of preventive antibiotic administration for open extremity fractures. Arch Surg 123:333–339, 1988.

22. Dellinger, E.; Miller, S.; Wetz, M.; et al. Risk of infection after open fractures of the arm or leg. Arch Surg 123:1320–1327, 1987.

23. Dellon, A.; McKinnon, S. Results of posterior tibial nerve grafting at the ankle. J Reconstuct Microsurg 7:81–83, 1991.

24. DeLong, W.G.; Born, C.T.; Wei, S.Y.; et al. Aggressive treatment of 119 open fracture wounds. J Trauma 46:1049–1054, 1999.

25. Drennan, J.; Freehafer, A. Fractures of the lower extremities in paraplegic children. Clin Orthop 77:211–217, 1971.

26. Fee, N.; Dobranski, A.; Bisla, R. Gas gangrene complicating open forearm fractures. J Bone Joint Surg Am 59:135–138, 1977.

27. Filler, R.; Griscom, N.; Pappas, A. Post-traumatic crepitation falsely suggesting gas gangrene. N Engl J Med 278:758–761, 1968.

28. Galpin, R.; Willis, R.; Sabano, N. Intramedullary nailing of pediatric femoral fractures. J Pediatr Orthop 14:184–189, 1994.

29. Georgiadis, G.; Behrens, F.; Joyce, M.; et al. Open tibia fractures with severe soft tissue loss: Limb salvage with microvascular tissue transfer versus below knee amputation. Complications, functional results and quality of life. J Bone Joint Surg Am 75:1431–1441, 1993.

30. Gergen, P.J.; McQuillan, G.M.; Kiely, M.; et al. A population-based serologic survey of immunity to tetanus in the United States. N Engl J Med 332:761–766, 1995.

31. Gustilo, R.; Mendoza, R.; Williams, D. Problems in the management of type III (severe) open fractures: A new classification of type III open fractures. J Trauma 24:742–746, 1984.

32. Gustilo, R.; Merkow, R.; Templeman, D. Current concepts review: The management of open fractures. J Bone Joint Surg Am 72:299–304, 1990.

33. Hansen, S. Internal fixation of children's fractures of the lower extremities. Orthop Clin North Am 21:353–363, 1990.

34. Hattrup, S.; Wood, M. Delayed neural reconstruction in the lower extremity: Results of interfascicular nerve grafting. Foot Ankle 7:105–109, 1986.

35. Heinrich, S.; Drvaric, D.; Darr, K.; MacEwen, G. The operative stabilization of pediatric diaphyseal femur fractures with flexible intramedullary nails: A prospective analysis. J Pediatr Orthop 14:501–507, 1994.

36. Higgins, T.; DeLuca, P.; Ariyan, S. Salvage of open tibial fractures with segmental loss of tibial nerve: Case report and review of the literature. J Orthop Trauma 13:380–390, 1999.

37. Highland, T.; Lamont, R. Deep, late infections associated with internal fixation in children. J Pediatr Orthop 5:59–64, 1985.

38. Hitchcock, C. Gas gangrene in the injured extremity. In: Gustilo, R., ed. Mangement of Open Fractures and Their Complications. Philadelphia, W.B. Saunders, 1982, pp. 183–201.

39. Holbrook, J.; Swiontowski, M.; Sanders, R. Treatment of open fractures of the tibial shaft: Ender nailing versus external fixation. J Bone Joint Surg Am 71:1231–1238, 1989.

40. Hope, P.; Cole, W. Open fractures of the tibia in children. J Bone Joint Surg Am 74:546–553, 1992.

41. Horowitz, J.H.; Nichter, L.S.; Kenney, J.G.; Morgan, R.F. Lawn-mower injuries in children: Lower extremity reconstruction. J Trauma 25:1138–1146, 1985.

41a. Howell, J.M., ed. Emergency Medicine, Vol. II. Philadelphia, W.B. Saunders, 1998.

42. Iawya, T.; Kiyonori, H.; Tamada, A. Microvascular free flaps for the treatment of avulsion injuries of the feet in children. J Trauma 22:15–19, 1982.

43. Irwin, A.; Gibson, P.; Ashcroft, P. Open fractures of the tibia in children. Injury 26:21–24, 1995.

44. Jensen, J.E.; Jensen, T.J.; Smith, T.K.; et al. Nutrition in orthopaedic surgery. J Bone Joint Surg Am 64:1263–1272, 1982.

45. Johansen, K.; Daines, M.; Howey, T.; et al. Objective criteria accurately predict amputation following lower extremity trauma. J Trauma 30:568–572, 1990.

46. Kreder, J.; Armstrong, P. The significance of perioperative cultures in open lower extremity fractures. Clin Orthop 302:206–212, 1994.

47. Kurz, W.; Vinz, H. Zur Epidemilogie und Klinik der geschlossenen diaphysaren Unterschenkelfaktur im Kindesalter. Zentralbl Chir 104:1402–1409, 1979.

48. Lange, R.; Bach, A.; Hansen, S.; Johansen, K. Open tibial fractures with associated vascular injuries: Prognosis for limb salvage. J Trauma 25:203–207, 1985.

49. Lawyer, R.; Lubbers, L. Use of the Hoffman apparatus in the treatment of unstable tibial fractures. J Bone Joint Surg Am 62:1264–1273, 1980.

50. Letts, M.; Davidson, D. Epidemiology and prevention of traumatic amputations in children. In: Herring, J.; Birch, J., eds. The Child with Limb Deficiency. Rosemont, IL, American Academy of Orthopaedic Surgeons, 1998.

51. Letts, R. Degloving injuries in children. J Pediatr Orthop 6:193–197, 1987.

52. LLoyd, G. Hippocratic Writings. New York, Pelican Books, 1978.

53. Loder, R.T.; Brown, K.L.; Zelaske, D.J.; Jones, E.T. Extremity lawn mower injuries in children: Report by the Research Committee of the Pediatric Orthopaedic Society of North America. J Pediatr Orthop 17:360–369, 1997.

54. Lusskin, R.; Battista, A.; Lenzo, S.; Price, A. Surgical management of late post-traumatic and ischemic neuropathies involving the lower extremities: Classification and results of therapy. Foot Ankle 7:95–104, 1996.

55. Mazur, J.; O'Malley, D.; Cummings, R. Avascular necrosis of the femoral head following intramedullary nailing in the growing child. Paper presented at The Pediatric Orthopaedic Society of North America, White Sulphur Springs, WV, 1993.

56. Meland, N.; Fisher, J.; Irons, G.; et al. Experience with 80 rectus abdominis free-tissue transfers. Plast Reconstr Surg 83:481–487, 1989.

57. Melcher, G.A.; Claudi, B.; Schlegel, U.; et al. Influence of type of medullary nail on the development of local infection. An experimental study of solid and slotted nails in rabbits. J Bone Joint Surg Br 76:955–959, 1994.

58. Merritt, K. Factors increasing the risk of infection in patients with open fractures. J Trauma 28:823–827, 1988.

59. Merritt, K.; Dowd, J.D. Role of internal fixation in infection of open fractures: Studies with *Staphylococcus aureus* and *Proteus mirabilis*. J Orthop Res 5:23–28, 1987.

60. Millie, M.; Senkowski, C.; Stuart, L.; et al. Tornado disaster in rural Georgia: Triage response, injury pattern and lessons learned. Am Surg 66:223–228, 2000.

61. Mueller, M.; Allgower, M.; Schneider, R.; Willenegger, H. Manual of Internal Fixation, 3rd ed. New York, Springer-Verlag, 1991.

62. Navarre, J.; Cardillo, P.; Gorman, J.; et al. Vascular trauma in children and adolescents. Am J Surg 143:229–231, 1982.

63. Nunley, J.; Gabel, G. Tibial nerve grafting for restoration of plantar sensation. Foot Ankle 14:489–492, 1993.

64. Pappas, A.; Filler, R.; Eraklis, A.; Bernhard, W. Clostridial infections (gas gangrene): Diagnosis and early treatment. Clin Orthop 76:177–184, 1971.

65. Park, W.; DeMuth, W. Wounding capacity of rotary lawn mowers. J Trauma 15:36–38, 1975.

66. Patzakis, M.J.; Bains, R.S.; Lee, J.; et al. Prospective, randomized, double-blind study comparing single-agent antibiotic therapy, ciprofloxacin, to combination antibiotic therapy in open fracture wounds. J Orthop Trauma 14:529–533, 2000.

67. Patzakis, M.; Wilkins, J. Factors influencing infection rate in open fracture wounds. Clin Orthop 243:36–40, 1989.

68. Rosenfield, A.; McQueen, D.; Lucas, G. Orthopedic injuries from the Andover, Kansas, tornado. J Trauma 36:676–679, 1994.

69. Rothenberger, D.; Velasco, R.; Strate, R.; et al. Open pelvic fracture: A lethal injury. J Trauma 18:184–187, 1978.

70. Russel, G.; Henderson, R.; Arnett, G. Primary or delayed closure for open tibial fractures. J Bone Joint Surg Br 72:125–128, 1990.

71. Song, K.; Sangeorzan, B.; Benirschke, S.; Brown, R. Open fractures of the tibia in children. J Pediatr Orthop 16:635–639, 1996.
72. Suedkamp, N.P.; Barbey, N.; Veuskens, A.; et al. The incidence of osteitis in open fractures: An analysis of 948 open fractures (a review of the Hannover experience). J Orthop Trauma 7:473–482, 1993.
73. Tolo, V. External skeletal fixation in children's fractures. J Pediatr Orthop 3:435–442, 1983.
74. Trautwein, L.C.; Smith, D.G.; Rivara, F.P. Pediatric amputation injuries: Etiology, cost and outcome. J Trauma 41:831–838, 1996.
75. Tscherne, H., Gotzen, L. Fractures with Soft Tissue Injuries. Berlin, Springer-Verlag, 1984.
76. Tscherne, H.; Oestern, H. Die Klassifizierung des Weichteilschadens bei offenen und geschlossenen Frakturen. Unfallheilkunde 83:111–115, 1982.
77. Vinz, H. Die Behandlung offener Fracturen bei Kindern. Zentralbl Chir 105:1483–1493, 1980.
78. Vinz, H.; Kurz, W. Die offene diaphysare Unterschenkefractur im Kindesalter. Zentralbl Chir 105:32–38, 1980.
79. Watts, H. Lengthening of short residual limbs in children. In: Herring, J.; Birch, J., eds. The Child with Limb Deficiency. Rosemont, IL, American Academy of Orthopaedic Surgeons, 1998.
80. Weber, B.; Brunner, C.; Freuler, F. Treatment of Fractures in Children and Adolescents. Berlin, Springer-Verlag, 1980.

# CHAPTER 6

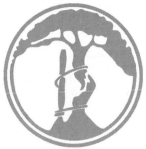
# Complications of Fractures in Children

Robert N. Hensinger, M.D.

## VASCULAR INJURIES

### Arterial Injuries

Penetrating trauma is the most common cause (51%) of arterial injury in children; the remainder are caused by polytrauma from vehicular accidents (30%) and falls (19%).[10] Only 18% of arterial injuries are associated with fractures, usually crush injuries and segmental fractures.[19, 30] Importantly, 45% of patients have injuries to peripheral nerves because of their close association within the neurovascular bundle.[21, 30]

Typically, the artery involved is near the fracture; for example, the common femoral artery is often associated with intertrochanteric fractures of the hip and hip dislocation and the superficial and profunda femoral arteries with subtrochanteric and midshaft fractures.[8, 16] The femoral artery can be injured at the adductor hiatus by a supracondylar femoral fracture.[7] Injury to the popliteal artery or to a combination of the anterior and posterior tibial arteries is usually associated with fracture of the distal femoral (Fig. 6–1) or proximal tibial epiphysis or knee dislocation (32% to 64%).[5, 10, 14, 16, 21, 32]

As in adults, massive bleeding and arterial hemorrhage can occur in children with pelvic fractures. In one study, the mortality rate was 5% in children and 17% in adults.[17] The fracture patterns are usually a combination of anterior and posterior injuries to the pelvic ring, either unilateral or bilateral.[2, 15, 20] O'Neill and colleagues noted that posterior arterial bleeding (internal iliac and posterior branches) was more common in patients with unstable posterior pelvic fractures, whereas anterior arterial bleeding through the pudendal and obturator arteries was more often associated with lateral compression injuries.[24] Injury to the superior gluteal artery was the most common injury associated with posterior pelvic fractures.[24] Eighty percent of children with multiple pelvic fractures had concomitant abdominal or genitourinary injuries; 33% had fractures of the ileum or pelvic rim, and 6% had isolated pelvic fractures.[15] Angiography

to identify the arterial hemorrhage and embolization to control bleeding have been helpful.[20] Similarly, skeletal fixation to reduce the fracture can help control bleeding in pediatric patients at high risk for life-threatening hemorrhage.[20]

The usual signs of vascular compromise are absent distal pulses, lower skin temperature, and poor skin circulation with diminished capillary and venous filling distal to the injury.[19] An angiogram should be considered whenever vascular injury is suspected.[14] Absolute indications for an angiogram are a diminished or absent pulse, large or expanding hematoma, external bleeding, unexplained hypotension, a bruit, and a peripheral nerve injury.[8, 29] If the period of ischemia approaches 6 hours, operative exploration should proceed immediately, and it may be necessary to obtain an angiogram in the operating room.[18] Skeletal injury in the proximity of a major vessel accompanied by a pulse deficit was 100% predictive of a vascular injury in one study.[29] In another report of patients with documented arterial injuries, however, 68% had normal pulses.[21]

Pulses may initially be palpable and then disappear (delayed loss of pulse). Such delayed loss is usually caused by damage to the intima with the subsequent development of thrombosis.[7, 21, 29] Doppler can be very helpful in identifying vascular injuries.[22] However, its reliability is diminished with severe injuries, particularly long bone fractures associated with gunshot wounds. Norman and associates reported a series in which 81% had a normal Doppler examination, yet an occult vascular injury was found on subsequent arteriography in 28%.[22] Most (83%) were minor, but the rest were major, such as a large internal flap, occlusion, pseudoaneurysm, or an arteriovenous fistula. Starr and coworkers found that 32% of their patients with documented arterial injuries had weakly palpable pulses or pulsatile flow that could be detected by Doppler.[31] Damage to the popliteal artery from a knee dislocation is commonly limited to the intima.[8, 11, 12, 16] In children, intimal damage is often more extensive than apparent on simple inspection. Children are particularly prone to

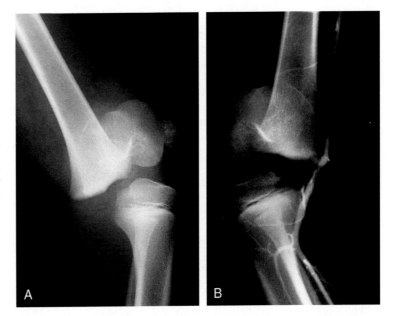

**FIGURE 6–1.** *A,* Supracondylar fracture of the femur in an 8-year-old boy with complete displacement of the distal femoral epiphysis. Decreased pulses and this fracture pattern should make one suspicious of a vascular injury. *B,* An arteriogram demonstrates attenuation of the popliteal artery, but it is still intact. The fracture was reduced and fixed with crossed pins, with subsequent premature growth arrest.

ischemia and gangrene because of arterial spasm, a rare problem in adults.[25, 27] Damron and McBeath recommend that any diminution in pulse, even if the pulse is detectable by Doppler testing, pressure, or palpation, be considered abnormal.[8] The patient should be further evaluated if the pulse does not return after reduction of the fracture or dislocation[7, 23] (Fig. 6–2). Observation of a warm pulseless leg after dislocation of the knee is insufficient. Frequently, these patients have good capillary flow because the amount of flow required to maintain viability of the skin and subcutaneous tissue is much less than that required by muscle.[16] In these circumstances, Green and Allen reported that 90% of the limbs either eventually underwent amputation or had claudication or incapacitating muscle fibrosis and contracture.[16]

Ninety percent of limbs can be salvaged if the circulation is reestablished within 6 hours, whereas revascularization after 8 hours from the time of injury can result in an amputation rate of 72% to 90%.[11, 16] Stanford and colleagues found that the tissues of a child's limb, particularly the nerves and muscles, are at greater risk from prolonged periods of ischemia than adult tissue is.[30] Thus, in children, a delay greater than 6 hours was associated with a poor result in 77%.[30] With massive crush injuries and collateral vessel damage, the 6-hour period of warm ischemia may be too long.[19] Distal compartment syndromes are common after late diagnosis

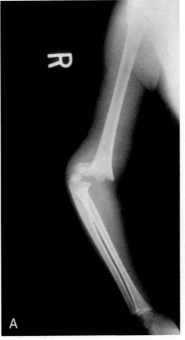
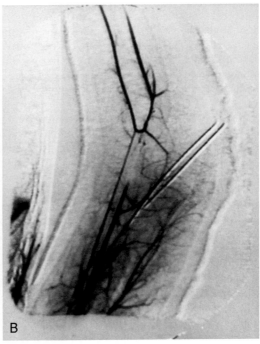

**FIGURE 6–2.** *A,* Supracondylar fracture of the humerus in a 7 year old with absent pulses despite satisfactory reduction and pinning. *B,* Arteriogram demonstrating good collateral circulation, but a complete block of the brachial artery. The artery was explored, an intimal flap was found and resected, and a successful end-to-end anastomosis was performed.

or repair of vascular injuries. Fasciotomies are indicated in children, but not fibulectomy because of the potential for valgus deformity of the ankle.[14, 16, 23]

All major arterial injuries should be repaired; however, repair of venous injuries remains controversial.[10, 19, 28] Ligation of the popliteal artery leads to an alarmingly high rate of amputation—approximately 70% to 86%.[11, 16] In children, autogenous vein grafts are recommended rather than synthetic or bovine material.[32] Spatulation of the ends of the vessels allows for a longer suture line that will accommodate a later increase in vessel size without stricture.[32] Surgical shortening of the bone may facilitate vascular repair, and the leg length discrepancy can be resolved at a later time.

Fracture stabilization can be accomplished by a variety of means. Ideally, if time permits, reduction and fixation of the fracture should precede vascular repair.[14] Initial bony fixation provides maximal skeletal stability and reduces further trauma to the soft tissues, nerves, and collateral blood vessels.[8] Similarly, surgical repair of nerve lacerations is facilitated by bony stabilization. If soft tissue coverage can be achieved, internal fixation is preferred.[6, 31] External fixation, particularly in a severely traumatized limb, has many advantages, including a short operative time.[6] Zehntner and colleagues found that complications were less frequent with initial external fixation of lower extremity fractures than with internal fixation.[34] Indwelling arterial and venous shunts can be helpful in selected cases to reduce the risk of further vessel damage and compartment syndrome.[14, 19] Similarly, temporary shunting can provide a satisfactory solution to the clinical problem of whether an ischemic limb should be revascularized before fracture fixation.[1, 18]

In general, the indications for limb salvage are extended in children because of their greater capacity for healing; however, no data have established the limits of salvage. As an example, successful microvascular intervention for acute vascular injuries in neonates has recently been reported.[13] One must consider the seriousness of associated polytrauma, the degree of damage to the ipsilateral foot, the time required to obtain soft tissue coverage and bone healing, and the potential for rehabilitation.[19] Crush injuries are most often associated with amputation; less often, penetrating injuries lead to amputation.[23] In children, a delay longer than 4 hours was associated with a 50% incidence of long-term severe disability and resulted in late amputation in 30%.[19] Repair of a proximal artery may not result in saving the entire limb but may preserve the knee, which has important functional implications.[21] Navarre and co-workers found that the typical problem was undue optimism with regard to the ability of conservative treatment to achieve limb survival without due consideration of growth demands and potential social and career requirements.[21]

Early complications include wound infection, below-knee amputation, deep vein thrombosis, and motor and sensory deficits.[11] Revascularization does not eliminate the possibility of abnormal growth (overgrowth and undergrowth).[14, 32] All children should be monitored with scanograms until maturity.[32] Loss of normal pulsa-

tile blood flow influences growth; as the child ages, the collateral circulation may not be adequate to meet the increased physiologic demands, and ischemia-like symptoms may be triggered by activity.[14]

## Vascular Injuries Associated with Supracondylar Fractures of the Humerus

Vascular injury is the most serious complication associated with supracondylar fractures; fortunately, it is uncommon.[3, 9] If the child has a pulseless extremity, the fracture should be reduced immediately in an attempt to restore blood supply and avoid compartmental ischemia[4, 7] (see Fig. 6–2). Campbell and colleagues found a brachial artery injury in 38% of the patients who had severe posterior lateral displacement of their supracondylar fracture.[3] Because children are uniquely susceptible to vasospasm, the pulse may not be restored to normal, and a Doppler waveform analysis may be helpful.[32] Many recent technologic improvements such as color-flow duplex scanning and magnetic resonance imaging (MRI) are now available.[26] These techniques are noninvasive and safe for evaluation of the patency of the brachial artery, but they need further study to assess their applicability in clinical practice.[26] Children may have very good secondary capillary perfusion, which can lead to the false assumption that the vascularity is intact. The collateral circulation may be sufficient to maintain a pulse in the distal circulation but not sufficient to maintain perfusion through specific muscle groups.[14] Sabharwal and associates recommended that if the collateral circulation across the elbow is satisfactory, revascularization is not indicated in an otherwise well perfused hand.[26] They concluded that revascularization of a pulseless, but otherwise well perfused limb with a type III supracondylar fracture, though technically feasible and safe, has a high rate of asymptomatic reocclusion and residual stenosis of the brachial artery.[26] With more frequent use of fixation for supracondylar fractures, the incidence of vascular injury seems to have decreased, thus suggesting that some of the previous vascular problems were caused by the flexed position required to maintain the reduction. If the vascular status of the limb is questionable, arteriographic studies should be performed promptly.[4, 7, 14] Similarly, children should have frequent vascular examinations after reduction for signs of vascular insufficiency from intimal tears and brachial artery stenosis.[23]

## COMPARTMENT SYNDROMES

Compartment syndromes can occur in a multiply injured child with the same frequency as in an adult. The condition is caused by swelling and increased pressure in a closed space, such as a fascial compartment, but it can also occur from tight skin or a circumferential cast. If not treated promptly, it results in complete death of the

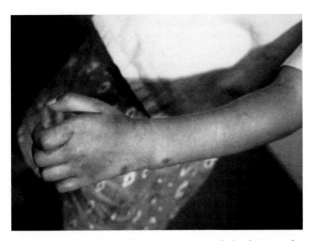

FIGURE 6–3. Volkmann's ischemic contracture of the forearm after treatment of a both-bones fracture and unrecognized compartment syndrome. Note the contracture of the fingers, which are partially insensitive.

structures within the compartment and Volkmann's ischemic contracture (Fig. 6–3). Compartment syndromes occur in the interosseous compartments of the hand and foot, the volar and dorsal compartments of the forearm, the thigh, and all four compartments of the leg.[49, 52, 54, 56] Crush and wringer injuries are the classic causes, but more commonly, compartment syndromes are associated with fractures, severe contusion, drug overdose with limb compression, burns, and vigorous exercise.[50] In children, compartment syndrome can accompany a vascular injury or osteotomy of a bone, especially the proximal end of the tibia.[49] Compartment syndrome may develop after intravenous infiltration or as a complication related to intra-arterial administration of medication through arterial lines.[52] Multiple trauma predisposes a child to compartment syndrome because of additional high-risk factors such as hypotension, vascular injury, and high-energy blunt trauma, which increase tissue necrosis.[55] Compartment syndromes in the thigh have been reported in teenagers after blunt trauma, systemic hypertension, external compression with anti-shock trousers, and vascular injury with or without fracture of the femur.[45, 55] Even children with femoral shaft fractures treated by skin traction may be subject to compartment syndromes.[43] Children who are obtunded and receiving intravenous fluids should be watched carefully for compartment syndrome of the hands.[44]

The injury may be a simple Salter-Harris type I or II fracture of the distal end of the radius or proximal part of the tibia, and compartment syndrome may occur with both open and closed injuries.[35, 42, 51] A common misconception is that an open injury will decompress the compartment. However, not all compartments are successfully relieved by an open injury.[55] Similarly, closed fractures treated with closed intramedullary fixation, such as femoral fractures, are susceptible to compartment ischemia. In restoring femoral length, the muscles are pulled to length, the integrity of the compartments is restored, and a compartment syndrome can occur.[38, 55] Compartment syndromes of the foot in children are usually due to crush injuries and may not be associated

with osseous injury, and neurovascular deficit is infrequent.[56]

As the pressure increases within the space, the first finding or complaint is a decrease in sensation, or paresthesias.[50] Pain, swelling, and tenseness of the compartment are found on physical examination. These symptoms may be difficult to recognize in children who are too young to cooperate with the examination or in those who have a head injury.[36, 47] If the process continues, voluntary use of the muscles is decreased, and eventually complete paralysis ensues. Pain on stretching the involved muscles is a common finding but is subjective and may be the result of trauma. Pulse oximetry was not helpful in the diagnosis of compartment syndrome because a normal reading does not imply adequate tissue perfusion.[46] Conversely, arterial hemoglobin desaturation was not always associated with a rise in compartment pressure.[46] Early ischemia of the nerve may cause anesthesia and obscure this very sensitive finding.[50] An excellent example of this diagnostic dilemma is the loss of toe dorsiflexion after a metaphyseal fracture of the proximal end of the tibia, which may be caused by a direct injury to the peroneal nerve or anterior tibial artery or by an anterior compartment syndrome.[49]

Compartment pressures are seldom high enough to occlude a major artery, so the peripheral pulses are often palpable, and capillary filling is routinely demonstrated in the skin of the hand or foot.[50] With a tissue pressure exceeding 30 mm Hg, capillary pressure is not sufficient to maintain blood flow to the muscles, and necrosis results.[50] With severe intercompartmental edema, the nerves show a gradual decline in action potential amplitude.[40] A complete conduction block can be obtained with a pressure as low as 50 mm Hg and, after 6 to 8 hours of sustained pressure, a pressure of 30 or 40 mm Hg.[40]

Diagnosis or exclusion of compartment syndrome on clinical grounds alone may be impossible.[49] The easiest and quickest method to make the diagnosis is by measuring compartment pressure. It is mandatory that anyone who is managing trauma in children be able to determine these values. Generally, a pressure greater than 30 mm Hg is considered abnormal and demands close observation; a pressure over 40 mm Hg warrants surgical decompression.[49, 50] Children with compartment pressures between 30 and 40 mm Hg can be managed nonoperatively but require excellent observation.[47] Muscle damage is significant when intercompartmental pressures are greater than 30 mm Hg for a period of 6 to 8 hours.[39–41]

Decompression should be performed on anyone who has an interrupted blood supply with an ischemic interval of more than 6 hours.[41] Muscle ischemia exceeding 3 or 4 hours not only endangers muscle function and viability but also causes significant muscle swelling when the circulation is reestablished.[49] Elevated tissue pressure appears to act synergistically with ischemia to produce more severe cellular deterioration than noted with ischemia alone.[38] Children do not differ significantly from adults in that shock, hypoxia, and arterial occlusion may lower tissue pressure tolerance. Elevation of the limb may increase compartment pressure and may be counterproductive if coupled with a decrease in perfusion; this combination may be the mechanism by which ischemic contractures occur after femoral fractures in children.[48] Myoglobinuria may further complicate a compartment syndrome, so adequate hydration and urinary output should be ensured after decompression is accomplished.[48] If a compartment syndrome develops in the hand after the administration of intravenous fluids, it responds well to decompression of the involved compartments and release of the carpal tunnel.[44, 52] Similarly, decompression of the foot requires fasciotomies of all nine compartments.[56] Compartment syndrome does not seem to affect healing of the fracture, and nonunion or delayed union is seldom associated with it.[53] However, the healing time for closed fractures associated with compartment syndrome was noted by Turen and co-workers to be longer, 30.2 versus 17.3 weeks.[57] Interestingly, compartment syndrome lengthens the time for healing of closed fractures, but the healing time was approximately the same as for an open fracture. The method of fixation does not affect the healing time,[53, 57] and external fixation is a satisfactory treatment method.[53]

The duration of the compartment syndrome before definitive surgical decompression is the most important factor in determining the functional outcome.[49] If decompression is accomplished within 12 hours of the first sign or symptom, most patients will have normal function.[49] Late surgical decompression exposes devitalized muscles, which require débridement, and in some instances, infection can ensue and necessitate multiple débridement procedures and antibiotics. Chuang and colleagues recommended exploration and excision of the infarcted muscle within 3 weeks of injury.[37] They found that such a time frame preserves intrinsic hand function and sensation by removing the ischemic environment and preventing the fibrosis that may add to nerve compression and damage.[37]

## FAT EMBOLISM

Fat embolism is a syndrome associated with long bone fractures in which fat emboli to the lungs lead to respiratory problems. It is believed to be caused by dissolution of normal circulating fat; however, the exact mechanism is still unexplained.[61, 65] This condition may be due to actual leaking of fat into the blood stream or a metabolic change that allows normal circulating fat to become free fatty acids. Mudd and associates examined patients who died of fat embolism syndrome after blunt trauma. They found no particular source of the fat, nor was there evidence of bone marrow or myeloid tissue in the lung sections.[67] Many children have fat emboli after injury, but the clinical syndrome develops in very few.[58, 81] Drummond and co-workers reported an incidence of 0.5% in 1800 children with pelvic and femoral fractures as compared with a 5% incidence in adults with similar injuries.[61] However, Fabian and colleagues used more extensive testing and found the minimal incidence in long bone fractures to be 10%.[63] Fat embolism is more often seen in teenagers and late adolescents, and the onset is usually shortly after the injury (within the first 2

to 3 days).[61] Mudd and associates found no correlation with the number or severity of fractures; rather, fat embolism syndrome was more likely to be related to the extensive nature of the soft tissue injuries.[67] The pulmonary changes prevent exchange of oxygen across the alveolar-capillary membrane. In adults, this condition is referred to as adult respiratory distress syndrome. The incidence of fat embolism syndrome is markedly decreased by immediate internal stabilization of long bone fractures as opposed to treatment by traction or late reduction.[64, 66, 68, 71, 72] Fat embolism syndrome has been reported in children with muscular dystrophy and as a complication of closed femoral shortening.[62, 69] Patients who are at risk for the development of fat embolism syndrome should be monitored with pulse oximetry.[62]

With the full-blown syndrome, children have respiratory distress, tachypnea, and a deterioration in blood gas values, particularly $O_2$ saturation.[58] Clinically, the child may appear restless and confused; if untreated, stupor and coma may ensue. Petechiae may develop in the skin and on the chest, axilla, and base of the neck, but they may be transient and are frequently missed.[65] The most significant laboratory finding is a decrease in arterial oxygen tension. Examination for fat in urine and sputum is of little value in comparison to more modern diagnostic measures. Recently, bronchoalveolar lavage for detection of fat-containing cells and retinal examination for cotton-wool spots and retinal hemorrhages have been reported to be helpful in early diagnosis.[59, 60] The chest radiograph classically demonstrates interstitial edema and increased peripheral vascular markings.[65, 70]

If untreated, fat embolism can be lethal; however, early diagnosis and prompt management can usually sustain the patient until the problem clears. Treatment consists of supportive measures for the respiratory problem, including improvement in oxygen saturation (70 mm Hg), and may require endotracheal positive-pressure breathing. Blood volume should be restored and fluid and electrolyte balance maintained. Adequate oxygenation is the most important part of treatment because respiratory failure is the most common cause of death.[61] Treatment with steroids and heparin remains controversial.

## HYPERCALCEMIA OF IMMOBILIZATION

Many children exhibit hypercalcemia after immobilization for a fracture. Cristofaro and Brink reported that 7 of 20 children demonstrated increased serum calcium levels of 10.7 to 13.2 dl (normal, 8.5 to 10.5 dl).[75] Urinary excretion of calcium peaks approximately 4 weeks after immobilization begins and can be expected to return to normal levels with activity.[76, 80] This increased urinary calcium excretion is believed to be part of the normal reparative process. In those who have preexisting metabolic bone disease such as rickets or parathyroid disease, immobilization can further increase serum calcium levels.[80] Similarly, for unexplained reasons, some young patients, usually those 9 to 14 years of age, may have significant blood levels and systemic symptoms.[80]

Symptoms include anorexia, nausea, vomiting, and increased irritability; if severe, generalized seizures, pain with movement, flaccid paralysis, muscle hypertonia, and blurred vision can occur. If the hypercalcemia is not controlled, renal calculi can develop.[75, 76] The serum alkaline phosphatase concentration is usually normal, unlike the case with hyperparathyroidism, in which the serum level is generally high.[76] However, to definitively distinguish the two conditions, a parathyroid hormone assay should be performed.[75]

Intravenous administration of fluids and corticosteroids has been reported to be successful in lowering the serum calcium level until mobilization can be accomplished.[76, 80] Usually, a low calcium diet is recommended. Mithramycin also effectively lowers calcium either by direct antagonism of bone resorption or by interference with the metabolism of parathyroid hormone.[76] In addition, calcitonin has been reported to be effective in acutely lowering serum calcium by inhibiting bone resorption.[73, 77, 79] Appropriate hydration and diuresis can help, as can immediate weight bearing and movement.[76, 78, 80]

Another problem that is similar in nature is acute hypercalcemia after quadriplegia.[73, 74, 77] Particularly in young people, this condition can be troublesome and should be routinely evaluated during the first 6 weeks after the onset of paralysis.

## ECTOPIC BONE FORMATION

Ectopic bone has been reported to appear around all major joints, most often the hip, elbow, and knee[87] (Fig. 6–4). The condition is more common in teenagers, but any age group is at risk. Ectopic bone formation is typically associated with head injury and burns.[87]

Myositis ossificans is associated with burns about the shoulder, distal end of the femur, elbow, and proximal part of the tibia, usually within 4 months after a thermal injury.[86] Mital and colleagues found that heterotopic bone developed in 15% of head-injured children and that coma and spasticity· were the most commonly related factors.[87] Fractures about the pelvis and extensive surgical approaches to repair pelvic fractures increase the risk of myositis ossificans.[90]

The process is usually preceded by an inflammatory response and tenderness near the affected joint in an area of soft tissue and bone trauma. Elevated levels of serum alkaline phosphatase usually precede ossification and remain elevated during active bone formation.[87] Radiographic evidence is apparent within 3 to 4 weeks after the injury.[87] MRI may be helpful in early diagnosis of this condition. A rim with low signal intensity is a common finding, but no unique pattern characterizes myositis ossificans.[82, 85] Initially, the process lacks definable borders and then progresses to a more focal mass with a high central intensity that eventually becomes bone.[82, 83] This pattern is common in the intramuscular type and less so with the periosteal type. Involution is more evident in the intramuscular type.[83] Some resorption may occur after joint movement has begun. Attempts to excise the heterotopic bone should be delayed until the process is completely mature, usually about a year after injury.[89] Some reports have indicated that pharmacologic agents can reduce the incidence of ectopic bone formation. Mital and colleagues found that in head-injured children, salicylates can help minimize or eliminate ectopic bone, particularly after excision.[87] Similarly, indomethacin has been reported to be helpful.[84, 87, 88] Diphosphonates have been used, but because of problems with bone metabolism, they are not currently recommended.[81] Most children can be managed successfully by observation, and the condition can be allowed to run its course because few children have long-term problems.[81]

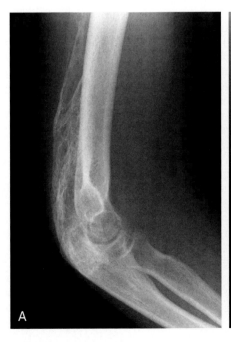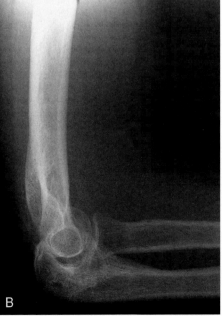

**FIGURE 6–4.** Ectopic bone formation leading to complete elbow ankylosis. Radiographs were obtained before surgery 6 months after a head injury (A) and 6 months after surgical excision (B). (A, B, From Mital, M.A.; et al. J Pediatr Orthop 7:83, 1987.)

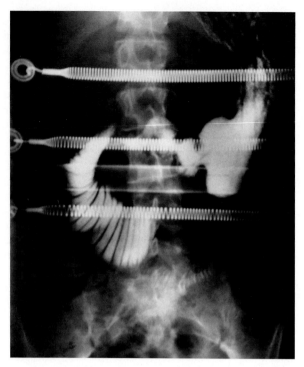

FIGURE 6–5. An upper gastrointestinal series in a patient with superior mesenteric artery syndrome (cast syndrome) demonstrates compression of the fourth portion of the duodenum from the superior mesenteric artery. Complete resolution followed aggressive intravenous hyperalimentation.

## SUPERIOR MESENTERIC ARTERY SYNDROME (CAST SYNDROME)

The superior mesenteric artery syndrome consists of acute gastric dilatation and vomiting. In the past, this syndrome was most often recognized in those treated with a hip spica or body cast, hence the older name *cast syndrome*.[92, 95] However, in more recent times, it has been reported to occur in the absence of a cast, such as after traction for extended periods, spine surgery, and Harrington instrumentation, particularly in the treatment of Scheuermann's kyphosis, and after severe traumatic brain injury.[91, 93, 94] The problem is caused by mechanical obstruction of the third portion of the duodenum by the superior mesenteric artery[91] (Fig. 6–5). It can be caused by hyperlordosis positioning in the cast, but more often it is associated with weight loss and a decrease in the fat protecting the superior mesenteric artery from the duodenum.[91, 92] The angle between the superior mesenteric artery and the aorta becomes more acute and compresses the duodenum.[95] Those with an asthenic body habitus and those who have an alteration in spinal curvature are at greatest risk.[91] If this condition is not treated aggressively, the problem becomes difficult to manage, and patients are subject to progressive weight loss, hypokalemia, and life-threatening dehydration and electrolyte abnormalities.[92, 95]

The syndrome can be reversed by increasing the bulk of retroperitoneal fat. Treatment consists of passing a feeding tube beyond the obstruction or intravenous hyperalimentation plus repositioning (side-lying) to encourage appropriate duodenal drainage.[93, 94] If a cast is

hyperextending the spine, it should be modified. In extreme cases that do not resolve with conservative treatment, complete derotation of the duodenum and colon with stabilization of the mesenteric artery (the Ladd procedure) can resolve the obstruction.[91]

## TRACTION-INDUCED HYPERTENSION

An uncommon event is hypertension associated with traction for a long bone fracture. Hypertension has also been reported to occur during limb lengthening as a result of traction on the bone and its adjacent soft tissue.[96, 100] It may be caused by tension on the sciatic nerve, activation of renin/angiotensin, or prolonged immobilization.[96, 97, 99] Hamdan and co-workers noted elevated blood pressure in 68% of patients undergoing traction, three of whom required treatment.[96] This problem can be controlled by modification of the traction and by hypertension medication until the primary condition has been resolved.[96, 98]

## SPONTANEOUS DEEP VEIN THROMBOSIS

This complication is very uncommon in childhood, with only scattered reports in the literature.[102, 103, 108] Generally, the clinical findings are similar to those found in adults and consist of local discomfort, tenderness and warmth, and often, swelling of the extremity. Deep vein thrombosis should be confirmed by appropriate noninvasive testing and perhaps venograms.[102, 108] A serum lipoprotein(a) (Lp[a]) concentration greater than 30 mg/dl is an important risk factor for thromboembolism in childhood.[107] Children who have venous thromboembolic events should be screened for elevated serum Lp(a).[107] It is likely that many cases are unrecognized.[102, 103] Most children respond to routine treatment, similar to adults.[102, 106] Initial treatment consists of heparin followed by warfarin (Coumadin) over an appropriate period. The problem occurs more often in older teenagers, the obese, and those with local infection in the extremity.[102, 105, 108] Acute pulmonary embolism is extremely rare, but it has been reported and should be managed with the same caution as for an adult.[102]

## MALUNION

The most common malunion experienced by children occurs after a supracondylar fracture of the humerus, usually with a cubitus varus deformity[109] (Fig. 6–6). In the past, the deformity was attributed to a disturbance in elbow growth. However, clinical and experimental evidence indicates that the more common cause is an initial unsatisfactory reduction or early loss of reduction.[109] Unfortunately, the cross section of the proximal humeral

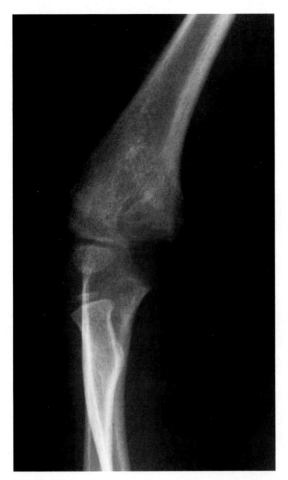

FIGURE 6–6. Supracondylar fracture of the humerus in a 4 year old that healed with a cubitus varus deformity.

fragment is narrow, and unless the distal fragment is reduced anatomically, it is easy for this fragment to rotate and tilt medially with subsequent cubitus varus deformity and limitation of elbow flexion.[118] Growth at the distal end of the humerus contributes only 10% of the

length of the upper extremity, and as a consequence, the potential for subsequent remodeling is limited. The recent popularity of closed reduction with exact anatomic alignment maintained by pin fixation has lessened the frequency of this complication.

Most children do not have a functional deficit but may have a significant cosmetic deformity.[109] If the deformity is present after 1 year and is posing problems, it may be managed by corrective osteotomy. Several authors have described a variety of ways to achieve angular correction.[109, 111, 120] Correction of the rotation, however, is much more difficult but is usually adequately compensated by the shoulder.[120] Fixation of the osteotomy is a problem because of the small size and peculiar shape of the distal end of the humerus, which does not lend itself to standard fixation methods.[109, 111, 120]

A Monteggia lesion consists of a fracture of the ulna and dislocation of the ipsilateral radial head. This lesion can be subtle; in a small child, it is often difficult to assess the relationship of the radial head to the capitellum. As a consequence, an acute lesion is often misdiagnosed, especially in those with associated plastic deformation of the ulna or a greenstick fracture[123] (Fig. 6–7). Similarly, the reduction is often lost (approximately 20%) in the weeks after reduction, especially when the ulnar fracture is oblique.[123] Rodgers and associates published a review of complications and results of reconstruction of Monteggia lesions in children.[123] Attempts at late repair of this lesion were met with considerable problems, including decreased rotation of the forearm, transient motor and sensory ulnar nerve palsies, and residual weakness. However, they believe that the long-term sequelae (pain and weakness) of chronic Monteggia lesions warrant intervention in a skeletally immature patient.[123] If malunion of the ulna prevents reduction, an osteotomy should be performed, preferably one rigidly fixed with a plate and an autogenous bone graft. If the annular ligament needs to be replaced or reconstructed, they recommend a triceps fascia reconstruction as described by Bell Tawse.[123] Complications include malunion of the ulnar shaft, persistent radial head subluxation or

FIGURE 6–7. Monteggia lesion in a 4 year old that was undiscovered for approximately 8 months. The ulnar fracture is healed, yet the radial head remains dislocated. Reduction may require osteotomy of the ulna with rigid plate fixation, reconstruction of the annular ligament, or replacement with the triceps fascia (Bell Tawse procedure).

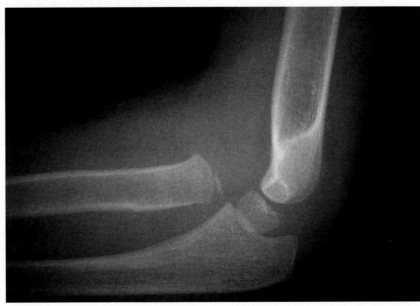

dislocation, and significant loss of pronation[48] and supination.[33]

Another complication related to the elbow is inter-articular entrapment of the medial humeral epicondyle after reduction of an elbow dislocation. Such entrapment may be difficult to visualize radiographically. If not removed from the joint, the epicondyle will severely limit flexion and be painful. This condition should be recognized early and treated appropriately inasmuch as late treatment is difficult and can lead to ulnar neuropathy.[114]

Fractures of the forearm in children are a common cause of malunion because the reduction can easily be lost and difficult to regain[112, 113] (Fig. 6–8). Young children can occasionally remodel the fracture dramatically; as a consequence, physicians have a tendency to depend heavily on remodeling and accept a less than adequate reduction. Price and co-workers recommend acceptance of up to 10° of angulation, 45° of malrotation, and complete displacement before attempting remanipulation or resorting to open reduction and internal fixation.[121] Roberts, in a review of malunion of forearm

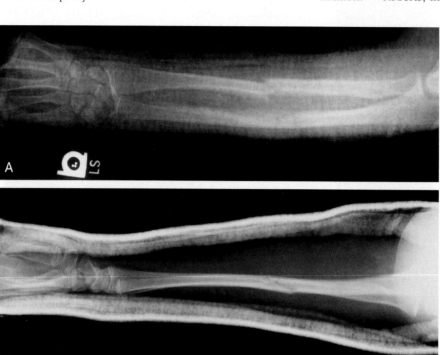

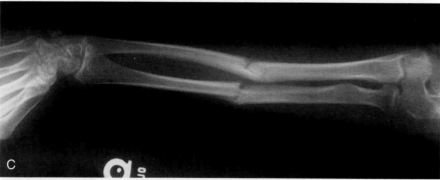

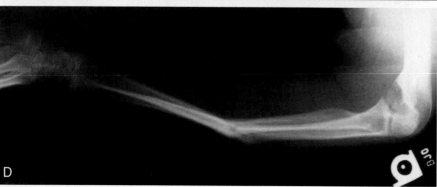

**FIGURE 6–8.** Fracture of the radius and ulna in a 12-year-old girl. Anteroposterior (*A*) and lateral (*B*) views of the injury after satisfactory reduction and cast immobilization. *C* and *D*, Fracture reduction was lost because of early removal of the cast, and open reduction plus plate fixation was required to restore satisfactory alignment. In a girl of this age, spontaneous correction cannot be expected.

fractures, found it important to avoid radial deviation of the radius and to maintain the interosseous gap between the radius and ulna.[122] Although the angulatory deformity has a limited potential for remodeling, rotational deformities do not improve, and they should initially be treated aggressively. Residual rotational deformity can compromise pronation and supination of the forearm, although the clinical significance of this limited rotation has not been clearly established.[121] Remodeling of angulatory deformity is better in the distal third of the radius and ulna than in the midshaft or proximal third and is better in younger children.[112, 113, 115, 125] Diaphyseal fractures of the forearm with radial or ulnar angulation are less likely to remodel completely.[104] In general, midshaft fractures in children younger than 8 years tend to remodel almost completely; however, in children 11 years and older (particularly girls, who mature earlier), spontaneous correction cannot be anticipated and is unpredictable.[104, 115, 128] Late correction is both difficult and embarrassing for the treating surgeon.

Length discrepancy, angulation, and encroachment on the interosseous space are unpredictable indicators of loss of motion. Loss of motion may be caused by soft tissue scarring that produces tension on the interosseous membrane; a few patients with complete remodeling have failed to regain motion.[121] Angulation in the diaphysis is often associated with loss of motion, whereas distal metaphyseal fractures tend to correct and complete range of motion returns.[104] Similarly, anatomic restoration of alignment by open reduction and internal fixation does not always restore full range of motion. Price and co-workers suggest that the shortening resulting from fracture displacement allows for relaxation of the interosseous membrane, which preserves motion.[121] The combination of proximal fracture with angulation, malrotation, and encroachment carries the greatest risk for loss of motion.[121] Price and Tredwell and their co-workers recommend open reduction and internal fixation after a refracture because of the greater likelihood in this circumstance of losing forearm rotation.[121, 126]

In the lower extremity, malunion occurs frequently in a child with a head or spinal cord injury.[110, 116, 117] Ninety percent of head-injured children recover from coma in less than 48 hours. In long-term follow-up, 84% of children who were initially in deep coma (score of 5 to 7 on the Glasgow Coma Scale) were eventually able to walk freely. Thus, one must assume full neurologic recovery.[116] If those with a Glasgow score over 5 do not recover in 3 days, the fracture should be fixed (if the child is older than 5 years).[116, 119, 129] Rigid fixation of long bone fractures aids in nursing care and rehabilitation efforts. Muscle spasticity in the first few days often displaces or angulates fractures immobilized in casts or leads to overriding of fractures in traction[110, 116] (Fig. 6–9). Nonoperative management of fractures in these children results in healing, but with an unacceptable incidence of malunion, angulation, and shortening[116, 119] (Fig. 6–10). Skin insensitivity combined with disorientation may result in skin breakdown with the potential for secondary osteomyelitis.[116] If the child must be moved for special studies such as computed tomog-

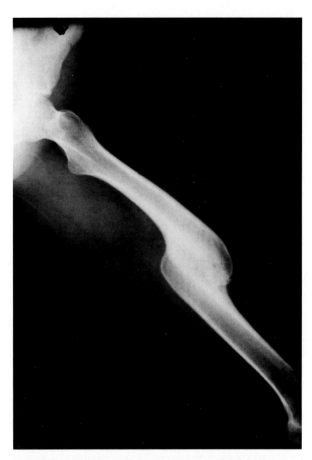

**FIGURE 6–9.** Fifteen-year-old boy with a serious head injury treated with traction for a femoral shaft fracture. Note the shortening and overriding. The patient has recovered and walks with a cane. The leg length discrepancy has caused numerous problems.

raphy (CT) or MRI or requires extensive dressing changes, multiple débridement in the operating room, or whirlpool for burns, the fracture should be stabilized because manipulation of the fracture may increase intracranial pressure. In children with acute quadriplegia or paraplegia, fracture fixation decreases the incidence of skin problems and pressure sores from cast immobilization and the need for external support, which may compromise nursing and rehabilitative efforts.

Bohn and Durbin called attention to the problem of the floating knee, or ipsilateral fracture of the femur and tibia.[110] In general, patients younger than 10 years with this injury respond well to closed treatment, femoral traction (90/90), and a short leg cast followed by a hip spica cast.[110] However, in older children and adolescents whose femoral fractures were treated by traction, these investigators found an increased incidence of complications (40%), including malunion/nonunion, angulation, and refracture.[110] In this group, operative stabilization of the femoral fracture was associated with fewer complications and better results. Importantly, the incidence of tibial complications in this older group was 50%, even in those treated by open reduction or external fixation.[110] The tibial problems may be related to the severity of the injury rather than age.

## SYNOSTOSIS (CROSS UNION)

Cross union is a rare and serious complication of fractures of the forearm. Rotation of the forearm is impossible and may lead to a serious compromise in function. Cross union must be distinguished from myositis ossificans, which is more common and typically less disabling. Most cross unions are confined to the proximal third of the radius and ulna. They are often associated with excision of the radial head after a displaced comminuted fracture, which is a significantly greater risk factor than open reduction alone.[127] Most authors recommend that if open reduction is required, the surgery be performed through two incisions; however, this technique does not necessarily prevent cross union.[127] Similarly, synostosis has been reported after intramedullary fixation of fractures.[101] Other predisposing factors include severe initial displacement, residual displacement, periosteal interposition, delayed surgery, remanipulation, and fracture at the same level of the radius and ulna.[124, 127]

Vince and Miller recommend at least a 1-year interval before excision of a cross union.[127] A bone scan may be useful to establish that the healing reaction is complete and that isotope uptake has returned to the same level as that in the surrounding bone. When excising a synostosis it is important that the bone bridge and its periosteum be removed intact to lessen the chance of recurrence. Several authors suggest interposing fat or Silastic between the radius and ulna to prevent recurrence; however, follow-up data on the success or failure of these proposals are limited.[127] If surgery is delayed too long, soft tissue contractures may preclude recovery of maximal range of pronation and supination (Fig. 6–11).

The same problem can develop between the tibia and the fibula. A similar surgical recommendation could be considered to keep the fibula moving freely at the ankle joint. Another alternative is resection of a portion of the fibula and screw fixation of the distal end of the fibula to the tibial epiphysis.

## LATE ANGULATION

Late angulation is a common problem with fractures of the proximal tibial metaphysis in a young child. Typically, the fracture is a relatively nondisplaced or easily reducible fracture of the proximal tibial metaphysis.[131, 134] It heals uneventfully, but over the ensuing months, progressive valgus angulation develops in the limb and can be alarming in its appearance[131, 134] (Fig. 6–12). Many improve spontaneously, and one should wait at least 18 months to 2 years to be confident that maximal improvement has occurred[130, 136] (Fig. 6–13). Usually, this condition is not associated with fracture of the fibula, but it has been reported with fracture of both bones. Although many theories have been advanced, the most likely mechanism is an increased vascular response leading to stimulation of growth of the medial metaphysis of the proximal end of the tibia.[131–134] In a review of 17 children with this injury, Ogden and colleagues found a generalized increase in growth both proximally and distally and eccentric proximal medial overgrowth in every patient.[133]

Interestingly, proximal metaphyseal osteotomy of the tibia and fibula for correction of the deformity can also initiate a progressive valgus deformity with an unacceptably high rate of recurrence of the angulation.[130, 134] Thus, it is wise to delay surgery until the child is older and less likely to experience this phenomenon.

Varus deformity of the elbow and loss of the carrying angle are common sequelae after lateral humeral condylar fractures.[135] Very few have functional problems, and the cosmetic appearance is usually acceptable. So and associates found that the average angle was 10° in the undisplaced fracture group and 9.6° in the displaced fracture group treated by open reduction, but it was more severe in those whose fractures were not reduced. It is suggested that the increased vascularity on the lateral side of the elbow leads to overgrowth.[135]

## INJURY TO THE TRIRADIATE CARTILAGE

Traumatic disruption of the acetabular triradiate physeal cartilage occurs infrequently. However, children whose

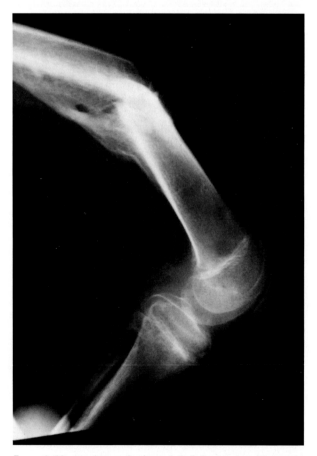

FIGURE **6–10.** Angulation of a femoral shaft fracture in a 13-year-old head-injured patient who was treated with skeletal traction.

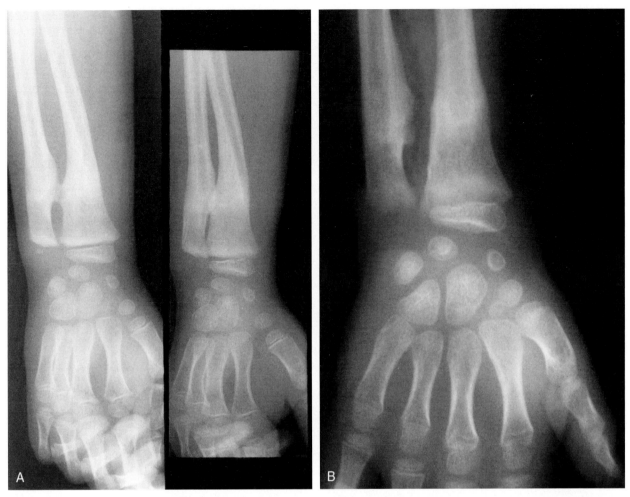

**FIGURE 6–11.** *A,* Anteroposterior and oblique views of the distal end of the forearm and wrist of a 7-year-old boy who sustained a fracture of both bones of the forearm. The fracture healed in a malrotated and angulated position with subsequent synostosis that is easily seen on the oblique view, which separates the radius and ulna. *B,* The traumatic synostosis was resected with interposition of fat. Preoperatively, the patient had no forearm rotation, and postoperatively, he regained 50° of forearm rotation. (*A, B,* Courtesy of Dr. Neil E. Green.)

bone is fractured during the active growth phase have a great potential for early closure and development of a shallow acetabulum.[137, 143] This problem is more common in children younger than 10 years, and in this situation it can lead to incongruity of the hip joint and progressive subluxation requiring acetabular reconstruction.[137, 142–144] Simple displacement of the triradiate cartilage has a more favorable prognosis. In contrast, severe crushing frequently ends in early closure and the worst prognosis.[141] The severe, more crushing type of injury may be difficult to detect on the initial radiographs, and CT scans are helpful.[137] Acetabular injury may be suspected with indirect signs such as concurrent fracture of the neck of the femur, detachment of the proximal femoral epiphysis, traumatic dislocation of the hip, or other pelvic fractures.[144] Frequently, the sacroiliac joint is injured in these severe injuries, thereby leading to further growth disturbance of the ilium.[142] In older children with less growth potential, this pattern is not as troublesome.

Irregularities in growth of the proximal part of the femur may occur as well.[137] As the femoral head

expands, it is displaced laterally and superiorly.[142] It increases pressure against the superior portion of the acetabulum, which can interfere with normal endochondral ossification and increase the acetabular index, similar to the developmental changes accompanying hip subluxation in cerebral palsy.[137] Experimentally induced closure in rabbits further supports this paradigm.[139] If a definite osseous bridge can be identified, resection with fat interposition is recommended.[137] However, the problem is often not discovered until complete closure of the triradiate has occurred.[144]

CT scanning can be helpful in the assessment of pelvic fractures, particularly in patients who may have an osteochondral injury with a retained fragment.[140] If persistent joint widening is noted, one must be very suspicious, even in the absence of a clear history of hip dislocation.[140] An arthrogram may not always be diagnostic.[140] The child may require a bone scan to assess the vascularity of the femoral capital epiphysis.[140] Surgical reduction of pelvic fractures should be considered only in cases of hip instability and severe displacement of the femoral head.[138]

## FRACTURES OF THE FEMORAL SHAFT: THE OVERGROWTH PHENOMENON

It is well known that a fracture of the femur leads to overgrowth averaging 1 cm (range, 0.4 to 2.7 cm).[154, 156] Shapiro found that overgrowth was independent of age, level of the fracture, or position of the fracture at the time of healing (shortened, lengthened, or distracted)[157] and in children younger than 2 years.[155, 157] Stephens and co-workers found that excessive fracture overlap correlated with increased limb growth, which they attributed to more parosteal stripping.[159] Overgrowth occurs in the entire limb, and interestingly, overgrowth of the ipsilateral tibia averaged 0.29 cm (range, 0 to 0.5 cm). The phenomenon occurred in 82% of patients, with 78% of overgrowth occurring in the first 18 months after fracture.[157] In 9%, overgrowth continued throughout the period of remaining growth, though at a slower rate. Staheli noted slightly greater overgrowth in children 4 to 8 years of age.[158] The available evidence suggests that such overgrowth is caused by an increase in vascularity to the bone as a result of the healing reaction.[157] It is an obligatory phenomenon rather than a mechanism to compensate for shortening.[157] This phenomenon has led to the clinical suggestion that the fracture fragments be overlapped approximately 1 to 1.5 cm in a young child, with the expectation that such overlapping will lessen the problem of overgrowth.[153] It may become more troublesome as more

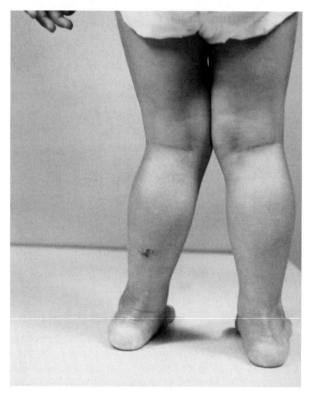

FIGURE 6–12. Clinical appearance of a 2½ year old in whom valgus angulation developed secondary to a fracture of the proximal tibial metaphysis.

femoral shaft fractures are managed by intramedullary fixation or external fixation, which restores the fracture to length.[145, 147, 148]

Hunter and Hensinger reported the problem of complete closure of the epiphyses after fracture of the femur that did not involve the growth plates.[152] In their report, the patient had spontaneous closure of all growth plates of the lower extremity, which led to considerable shortening. Similar cases have been reported sporadically.[146, 149, 153]

Overgrowth is infrequently reported in the upper extremity.[151] In a large study of forearm fractures, overgrowth in the radius or ulna is infrequent and averages 0.44 cm.[150] Davids and co-workers noted that lateral condylar fractures of the humerus can on occasion be complicated by lateral overgrowth and an unsightly appearance.[150]

## GROWTH DISTURBANCES

### Physeal Fractures

Because of the cross-sectional area of the distal femoral physeal plate, the potential for a growth plate injury is great after simple type I and type II Salter-Harris fractures, in contrast to the rare occurrence of a growth plate injury in smaller physes, such as the distal end of the radius. Riseborough and co-workers found an alarmingly high rate of complications: growth arrest and a limb length discrepancy of more than 2.4 cm developed in 56%, and angular deformities greater than 5° requiring osteotomy[175] developed in 26% (see Fig. 6–1A). Growth problems correlate well with the severity of the injury and were seen in all the Salter-Harris types. Fractures in a young child (younger than 11 years) are invariably the result of severe trauma and have the poorest prognosis, with growth problems developing in 83% of these children. Riseborough and co-workers believe that the problem was caused by interruption of the blood supply to this area[175]; however, this conclusion has not been proved. The distal femoral physis has a complex geometric configuration; as a consequence, the damage is not uniform across the physeal cartilage, a circumstance that encourages osseous bridging.

Immobilization in a hip spica cast provides the best result because of more consistent maintenance of reduction than that afforded by a long leg cast. Riseborough and co-workers recommend anatomic reduction and greater use of internal fixation,[175] but it is not guaranteed that this technique will restore normal growth in those who have sustained a severe injury to the growth plate. With a type II fracture-separation, internal fixation of the large metaphyseal fragment provides better results.[175] Because the potential for growth arrest is so high, children should be monitored closely over the period of remaining growth. Tomograms or CT scans with reconstructions are of great value in delineating the presence and extent of a bone bridge. If the resultant bridge is of moderate size, less than 40% of the surface, and

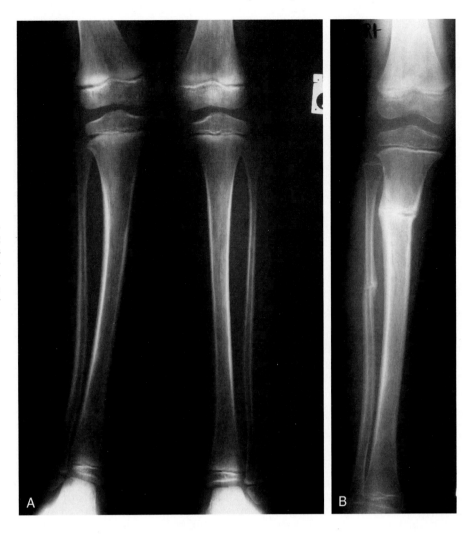

FIGURE **6–13.** *A*, Fracture of the proximal tibial metaphysis in a 7 year old; it was sustained approximately 3½ years before but has not undergone spontaneous remodeling, and the child continues to have a valgus deformity. *B*, Radiograph after a proximal tibial osteotomy to correct the deformity.

surgically accessible, it can be excised. However, if the projected leg length discrepancy is less than 4.8 cm, Riseborough and co-workers advise contralateral distal femoral arrest.[175] Importantly, such arrest does not correct any existing discrepancy but serves only to further limit leg length inequality. With greater differences, limb lengthening will have to be considered. Growth arrest can occur after adjacent fractures in the metaphysis or, less often, the diaphysis,[160, 163] especially with fractures above the femur and near the knee.[163, 165, 166] Such injury often results in delayed recognition of the physeal injury until a gross angular deformity develops. Hresko and Kasser recommend that all adolescents' injuries be monitored expectantly so that they can be detected early.[166]

Changes in the tibiofibular relationship because of growth disturbances after ankle fractures are frequent in children.[168] Fortunately, most occur near the end of growth and, as a consequence, cause only minor problems. Growth arrest of the distal end of the fibula and continued growth of the tibia may initially be compensated by distal sliding of the fibula as a result of traction from the ankle ligaments. If the deformity is of long duration, a valgus deformity will occur (Fig. 6–14). Growth arrest of the distal end of the tibia may cause a varus deformity if the fibula continues to grow (Fig.

6–15). However, the fibula may slide proximally to compensate for tibial overgrowth, with the fibular head becoming more prominent at the knee. Distal fibular growth arrest may be necessary.

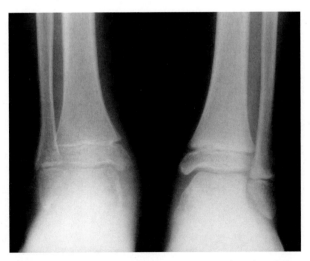

FIGURE **6–14.** Complete closure of the right distal tibial epiphyseal plate occurred in an 11-year-old boy after a direct impact from a fall. Note that the distal fibular growth plate has not closed and that further growth may pose a problem at the ankle.

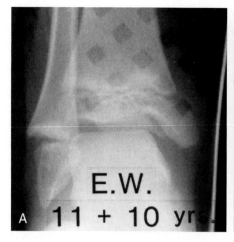
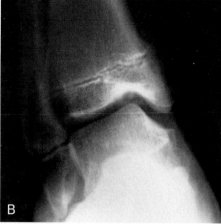

FIGURE **6–15.** *A,* A 12 year old sustained a Salter-Harris type III fracture of the medial malleolus and a type I fracture of the distal end of the fibula. *B,* Development of a bony bar with progressive deformity of the ankle mortise. (*A, B,* From Kling, T.F.; et al. J Bone Joint Surg Am 66:647, 1984.)

## Partial Growth Arrest: Diagnosis, Assessment, and Treatment

One of the unique complications of epiphyseal injuries is the interruption of normal growth of the physis. This disturbance poses a wide range of problems from complete arrest with no further growth to partial arrest and gradual slowing or progressive angulation. Typically, the injury results in a bridge of bone from the metaphysis to the epiphysis, commonly referred to as a bony bar. If the injury is at the periphery, the bar acts as a tether leading to an angular deformity with some decreased growth. If allowed to persist, it will eventually result in complete closure (Fig. 6–16). Central arrest leads to slowing of growth; radiographically, it appears as tenting of the epiphyseal plate with cupping of the epiphysis by the metaphysis. The epiphysis appears to be sucked up into the metaphysis (Fig. 6–17). This situation is more commonly associated with a vascular injury, infection such as meningococcemia, or thermal injury such as frostbite.

Most bony bars occur in fracture patterns that traverse the physis, such as Salter-Harris type IV, but they have been reported after all types of physeal injury. Certain ones are typical; type III injury of the medial malleolus (see Fig. 6–5) and type IV injuries at the distal end of the tibia (see Fig. 6–16) or distal part of the femur have been reported in considerable detail.[169, 173, 177] With the exception of iatrogenic damage from threaded pins or screws across the physis, most cannot be prevented. Evidence indicates that with exact anatomic reduction, some problems can be avoided, or at least minimized, and treatment facilitated. Those who treat these injuries should be cognizant of the potential for bar formation. Children should be closely monitored to detect early bridging. Early diagnosis allows one to deal with the bar much more effectively than if it is discovered late. MRI has been suggested as a method for early detection of growth plate interruption.[167]

The size of the epiphyseal plate, its rate of growth, the age of the patient, and the contour of the physis all play a role in development of the bar.[173, 177] The distal

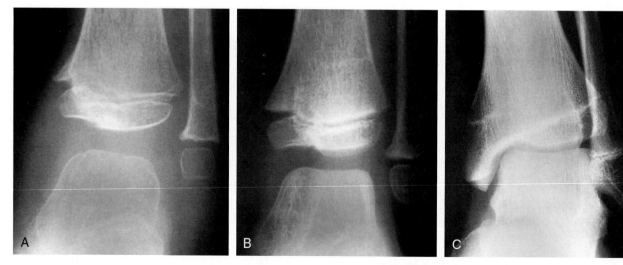

FIGURE **6–16.** A 4 year old sustained a distal tibial fracture, Salter-Harris type IV. *A,* Six months after initial healing. *B,* Two years after injury. *C,* Follow-up at 12 years of age. Note the development of angulation and deformity of the ankle joint with overgrowth of the fibula. (Radiographs courtesy of Dr. Herman D. Hoeksema.)

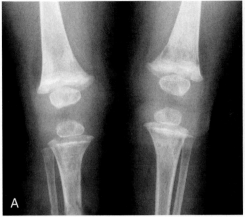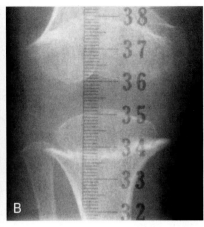

FIGURE 6–17. Central growth arrest after severe meningococcemia at 2 years of age. *A,* Initial normal appearance of the knees. *B,* Two years later, right distal femoral and proximal tibial central growth arrest is apparent. Note that the metaphysis appears to cup the epiphysis and that the epiphyseal plate is tented.

femoral physis is particularly noteworthy because its extreme size and irregularity render it more susceptible to irreversible changes and premature closure.[175] In contrast, the distal end of the radius, though more frequently injured, is less prone to bar formation. Injuries to the distal part of the tibia are particularly subject to bar formation; however, those who sustain such injuries are usually near the end of growth, and as a consequence, the growth disturbance poses fewer problems.[173, 177] The femur is the most common location for growth arrest, followed by the distal end of the tibia and proximal part of the tibia, radius, and humerus.[177] The proximal part of the tibia and distal end of the femur account for only 3% of all physeal injuries but are responsible for most bony bars. This finding is particularly troublesome because they account for 60% to 70% of the growth of the respective bones.[173]

The mechanism of injury and its pathomechanics are important elements of the evaluation inasmuch as many are predictable. MRI can detect early abnormalities in physeal cartilage that often portend subsequent growth disturbances.[167] Later, MRI can provide accurate mapping of physeal bridging and associated growth abnormalities.[167] Polytomography and, more recently, helical CT have been the standard for determining the size and position of the bar.[112] Very thin cuts (anteroposterior and lateral) are used to demonstrate the extent of the formation over the surface of the epiphyseal plate. An excellent paper by Carlson and Wenger provides a detailed description of the technique for mapping partial physeal arrest by using laminagrams before surgical excision[164] (Fig. 6–18).

Recently, helical CT (thin cut) has proved very helpful in preparing physeal maps to determine the extent and location of physeal bony bars. It provides excellent bony detail, and the radiation dose is a half to a quarter of conventional tomography. The rapidity of scanning avoids the need for sedation in a young child.[172, 174] The use of MRI has been helpful in localizing the extent of the lesion (Fig. 6–19), and three-dimensional reconstructions are useful in preoperative planning.[162] Scanograms should be taken to determine the precise length of the extremities and to evaluate the hand and wrist for bone age before planning surgical resection.

A decision to resect the bar or to arrest the remaining growth in the physis must be made. The choice is based on the potential of the bar to cause further length discrepancy or angular deformity and the technical problems involved in removing it.[173] The general recommendation is that if less than 50% of the growth plate is involved and the child has 2 years of growth

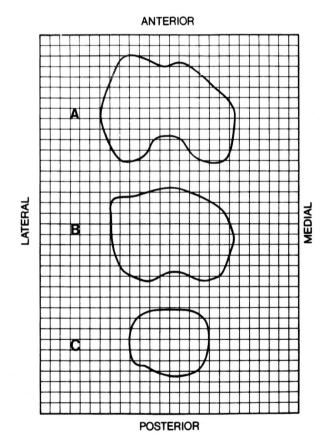

FIGURE 6–18. Outlines that can be used for mapping a physeal bar. *A,* Distal femoral physis. *B,* Proximal tibial physis. *C,* Distal tibial physis. With the use of anteroposterior and lateral tomograms, the extent of the bony bridge is analyzed on each cut by proceeding from the lowest to the highest while making certain to maintain the orientation. The extent of the bony bridge is determined at each level and plotted as a *thick straight line* on the outline. Both anteroposterior and lateral views are plotted on the same graph. This technique determines the exact cross-sectional anatomy of the physeal bar. (*A–C,* From Carlson, W.O.; Wenger, D.R. J Pediatr Orthop 4:232, 1984.)

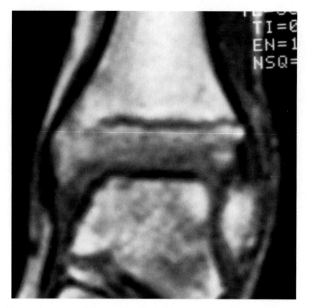

FIGURE **6–19.** Medial growth arrest demonstrated by magnetic resonance imaging of the distal end of the tibia.

remaining, resection should be considered.[173, 177] In general, a leg length discrepancy of 1 inch or less represents little functional impairment, and many discrepancies of up to 2 inches can be adequately compensated by growth arrest of the opposite physis. The decision is further dependent on the percentage of growth contributed by the individual physis to the length of the lower extremity. For example, the distal tibial epiphysis accounts for only 18%, so complete arrest in a teenager is less of a problem; a contralateral epiphysiodesis may be appropriate, which would not be the case in a young child. The decision is much less problematic in the upper extremity because length discrepancy seldom causes functional impairment; many authors recommend

that discrepancies of 4 inches or less are best left untreated. Vocke found that fractures of the radial neck frequently lead to radial head deformity (82%) but to functional problems in only 11%.[176]

If the bar is to be resected, it is important to prevent re-formation. A number of methods that use interposing material to block the healing reaction have been described. Materials include fat, bone wax, Silastic, and Cranioplast. Langenskiold first popularized bar excision in the 1960s, when he resected the bar and filled the space with autogenous fat.[170] He subsequently reported that over the long term, the fat functions as a satisfactory material; it generally prevented bar re-formation and continued to grow with the patient.[171] Silastic was popular but is a controlled substance that cannot be used without investigational permission from the Food and Drug Administration and has recently come under criticism related to its use as a breast implant. Cranioplast has been popularized by Peterson; it is helpful in larger resections, particularly when the bone is structurally weakened, because it is a solid substance that fills the cavity, aids in hemostasis, and decreases the need for postoperative protection.[173] It is important that whatever material is interposed remain in the area of the resection to prevent late bar re-formation.

Peripherally located bars are approached directly, and the periosteum is excised to prevent re-formation (Fig. 6–20). The bar is removed under direct vision with a motorized bur because the bony bar is extraordinarily hard. Magnification may be helpful. Curettes are used as one nears the normal physis. It is important to undermine both the metaphysis and the epiphysis so that the physis is sufficiently exposed to prevent bar formation, but not so much that its vascularity is jeopardized.[173]

Centrally located bars are difficult to resect (Fig. 6–21). They are approached through the metaphysis and generally require a wide metaphyseal window. These bars can be anatomically confusing because they have a volcanic appearance, and resecting the interior can be

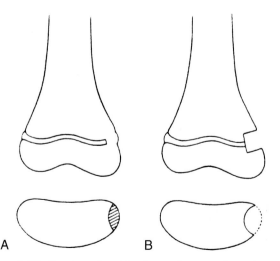

FIGURE **6–20.** Drawing of peripheral growth arrest shown in an anteroposterior view and transverse section through the physis below. *A,* Map of the bar composed from tomograms. *B,* Bar excised by a direct approach. (*A, B,* From Peterson, H.A. J Pediatr Orthop 4:246, 1984.)

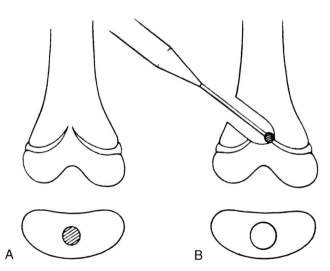

FIGURE **6–21.** *A,* A central bar with growth peripherally results in tenting of the physis. *B,* Excision of the central bone through a window in the metaphysis. (*A, B,* From Peterson, H.A. J Pediatr Orthop 4:246, 1984.)

FIGURE **6–22.** Contour of the cavity. *A,* The physis is exposed as usual. The adjacent metaphyseal bone surface should be smooth to help prevent the plug from staying with the metaphysis. *B,* Bone in the epiphysis is undermined in an attempt to allow the plug to stay with the epiphysis. A small rim of epiphyseal bone should be preserved to maintain viability of the physis *(arrow). C,* Undermining of bone away from the physis should be avoided because the protruding physis would be deprived of its blood supply and prevented from growing inward over the plug as the physis grows distally. *(A–C,* From Peterson, H.A. J Pediatr Orthop 4:246, 1984.)

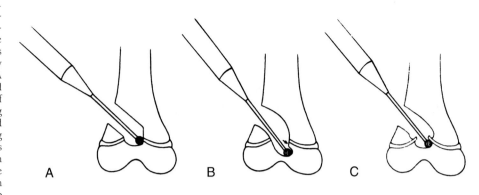

difficult. The entire circumference of the physis must be visualized to adequately remove the bar. Dental mirrors and the arthroscope have been used to better visualize the normal physis. To prevent migration, the material may be stabilized with a pin or the resection designed to create a cavity in the epiphysis so that the material is held within the substance of the epiphysis as the child grows (Fig. 6–22). An innovative suggestion is to use the Ilizarov apparatus to distract the epiphysis and cause epiphysiolysis, resect the bony bridge and fill it with methyl methacrylate, and correct any angular deformity at the same time.[161] These preliminary results are encouraging but need further investigation.[177] It is common to use metal markers for both the epiphysis and the metaphysis to facilitate documentation of continued growth in the postoperative period.

Angular deformity of up to 9° may correct spontaneously as a result of "catch-up" growth after bar resection.[173, 177] An accompanying corrective osteotomy is recommended when angular deformities are greater than 10° and whenever a significant deformity is present and the area of the bar is greater than 25%.[177] Near-normal longitudinal growth and correction of moderate angular deformities can be expected when the bridge is less than 25%; most poor results occur in those with very large growth arrest.[177] Williamson and Staheli recommend that resection be considered in all young children who have considerable growth remaining, even if the bar is large.[177] They reported resection of 48% in a 2-year-old and 54% in another that resulted in excellent growth for 2 years before recurrence.

Children should be monitored until maturity with scanograms; wire markers are helpful to assess growth. Successful results in resections as great as 50% have been reported, with 84% of anticipated growth achieved.[173, 177] All grow vigorously in the beginning, but some close prematurely and may require epiphysiodesis of the contralateral physis toward the end of growth.[173] Reporting on growth disturbances of the distal radial epiphysis after trauma, Zehntner and co-workers noted that corrective osteotomies work quite well.[178]

## NONUNION

Nonunion of long bone fractures is rare in children[193] (Fig. 6–23). In a large series from the Mayo Clinic, the tibia was involved most often (50%) and the femur, ulna, humerus, radius, and fibula less commonly.[193] Generally, nonunion is associated with high-energy trauma and open fractures with extensive soft tissue disruption and infection.[181–183, 189, 193] Cullen and associates found that communication and segmental injuries were the most significant predictors of delayed union.[181, 183] Deep infection increases the rate of nonunion.[200] Open reduction and internal fixation may contribute if the fixation is inadequate or holds the fracture fragments apart. Nonunion is more likely in an older child who is approaching maturation. An open fracture in children older than 11 or 12 years significantly increases the risk of nonunion when compared with the same injury in children younger than 6 years.[188, 200] Nonunion is usually associated with fractures of the shaft of long bones and only occasionally with distal metaphyseal injuries.[182] Nonunion of physeal fractures is commonly reported in children who are insensate, such as those with myelodysplasia or paraplegia.[187]

The same treatment techniques that have been successful in adults can be used here. To improve the endosteal response, the dense fibrous tissue and subchondral bone should be resected so that the marrow spaces are communicating. Internal fixation and an autogenous bone graft are recommended.[192, 193] Intramedullary fixation may be preferable for an unstable fracture.[182] Fixation plates provide more rigid fixation but need more extensive dissection and may further compromise blood flow to the bone.[185] The Ilizarov fixator may improve results in the lower extremities, in addition to treating the pseudarthrosis, and the discrepancy in length or angulation can be corrected at the same time.[185]

Nonunion of a displaced fracture of the lateral humeral condyle (Fig. 6–24) is a common problem. Initially, the nonunion may have only minimal separation; however, if the cartilage hinge is broken, the fracture fragments easily become displaced in the early period of cast immobilization. The fracture must be watched closely for displacement if nonoperative treatment is elected. If the fracture becomes displaced, it has a great propensity for nonunion because the fracture surface of the condyle rotates away from the metaphysis.[184] Flynn recommends that when the distance is 2 mm or greater, these fractures should be surgically reduced and pinned to prevent further displacement and nonunion.[186]

Early recognition of nonunion leads to salvage by early stabilization and bone grafting if the fragment is in an acceptable position and the growth plate of the condyle is open.[184, 186] Procrastination may allow the physis of the condylar fragment to close prematurely, with loss of a golden opportunity to salvage the elbow. If the fragment is not too rotated or displaced, removal of the fibrous tissue and bone grafting usually suffice.[184, 186, 191] Greater displacement requires reattachment of the fragment with a screw or threaded pin; however, some loss of elbow motion may occur.[191, 194] Every effort should be made to avoid further stripping of soft tissue to prevent avascular necrosis of the fragment.[197] It is imperative that the fragment be reduced because reduction may prevent a valgus unstable elbow and subsequent ulnar nerve palsy.[186, 194] In late cases in which anatomic reduction is not possible, the fragment is stabilized in the position that yields the greatest range of motion—"functional reduction." If necessary, supracondylar osteotomy can be performed to restore alignment.[197]

A pediatric carpal scaphoid nonunion is similar to that seen in an adult; usually, however, it occurs in adolescents in whom the injury was originally unrecognized. If the fracture is initially treated by cast immobilization, nonunion is rare.[201] Treatment of the nonunion is similar to that in an adult.[195, 196]

Traumatic loss, sepsis, or resection of the distal end of the fibula may lead to valgus angulation of the ankle as a result of loss of the buttressing effect of the fibula.[190] It is possible for the ankle ligaments to pull the fibular shaft down to compensate for fibular shortening of about 1 cm. If growth arrest occurs more than 2 years before skeletal maturity, distal movement of the fibula will be insufficient to compensate, and the talus will become displaced laterally into a valgus position.[186, 190] In a gap that is small, treatment with reduction and bone grafting has been helpful. If the gap is large, the fibula can be osteotomized and the distal fragment repositioned and fixed to the distal tibial epiphysis. This procedure should be done routinely if the fibula is used for a graft.[186] It has been reported that distal tibial growth arrest may retard growth of the distal end of the fibula, but such growth retardation has not been a consistent finding.

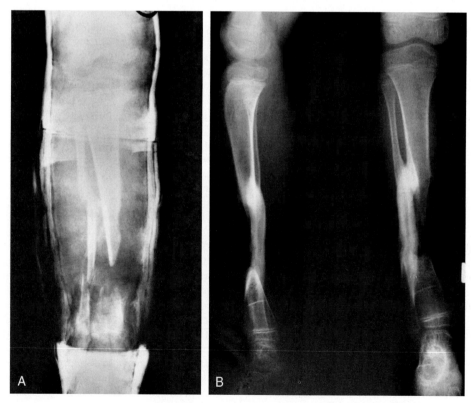

FIGURE 6–23. *A,* Nonunion of the tibia after a lawn mower injury with extensive soft tissue loss and infection. *B,* After the soft tissue problems and infection were resolved, adequate skin coverage was obtained and a bone graft from the fibula to the proximal and distal ends of the tibia was performed to achieve stability of the leg.

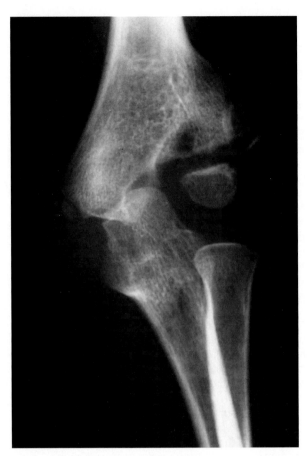

**FIGURE 6–24.** Nonunion of the lateral humeral condyle. The fracture fragment will easily become displaced if the cartilage hinge is broken. If cast immobilization is used, this fracture must be watched closely for displacement. Early recognition leads to salvage by early stabilization. This nonunion healed after bone grafting.

## REFRACTURE

Refracture is most common in young boys and suggests accidental repetition of the original injury—probably a combination of a fragile union and reckless physical activity.[179] Because healing is rapid in children, immobilization is often discontinued early. Schwarz and colleagues, in their review of 28 refractures, found that 84% were associated with incomplete healing of greenstick fractures.[198] Refracture can occur as late as 12 months after the original injury. In a review of 760 fractures, Bould and Bannister found a refracture rate of 4.9%, usually within the first 9 months.[180] The median for all fractures was 8 weeks after discontinuation of the cast and 16 weeks for midforearm fractures. Similarly, diaphyseal fractures were eight times more likely to refracture than metaphyseal fractures. Bould and Bannister found that cast immobilization of midforearm fractures for a minimum of 6 weeks reduced the risk of refracture by a factor of between 4 and 6.[180] A significant increase in deformity occurs after refracture. These fractures tend to be difficult to reduce by closed methods, and most authors believe that open reduction is

indicated.[179] Children who have osteopenic conditions such as osteogenesis imperfecta, myelodysplasia, paraplegia, or quadriplegia are at great risk for secondary fractures in the extremity that has been immobilized. In this group, immobilization should be of short duration and as little as necessary to keep the bone aligned, such as splints and soft dressings. Typically, exuberant callus formation splints the fracture and allows early removal of the cast.

Refracture can be a complication of external fixation of long bone fractures and has a reported rate of 12%,[199] most commonly at the original fracture site or less often through a pin site. Skaggs and associates found a correlation between refracture and the number of cortices demonstrating bridging callus on the anteroposterior and lateral views at the time of fixator removal.[199] Those with three or four cortices of bridging had a 4% refracture rate. Importantly, this rate was not influenced by dynamization, fracture configuration, or alignment.

## LIGAMENTOUS INSTABILITY

Although ligamentous injury can occur in any joint in children, certain problems are often undetected at the time of injury, particularly in the cervical spine and knee. In the cervical spine, teenagers seem to be particularly susceptible to soft tissue and ligamentous disruption between the posterior elements.[202] Such disruption frequently follows a hyperflexion injury. Typically, the initial radiographs appear satisfactory; however, with resolution of the pain and swelling, flexion views reveal posterior widening between the spinous processes. This widening is commonly associated with injuries in the lower portion (C4–C5, C5–C6, and C6–C7).[203] The lesion will not heal spontaneously, and the loose segments should be stabilized by a simple one-level or, occasionally, a two-level posterior spinal fusion.

Ligamentous injuries about the knee are frequently not recognized, particularly in those with an associated fracture of the femur or tibia, or both (the floating knee). Injury can occur to the collateral ligaments or the anterior cruciate and, less commonly, the posterior cruciate. Whether the incidence of this injury is increasing or recognition of it is improved is difficult to determine; however, it emphasizes the importance of early assessment of ligamentous integrity.[202] In children with an adjacent long bone fracture, examination of the knee may be difficult. If traction for a femur fracture is planned after insertion of a femoral pin, the knee can usually be examined adequately. Similarly, if an effusion is present, aspiration and inspection of the fluid for blood and fat can be helpful, and stress radiographs can be obtained (Fig. 6–25). Traction through the knee with the proximal tibial pin is contraindicated if a knee ligament injury is suspected. Similarly, if the ligamentous injury is reparable, the femur should be stabilized. Most authors recommend that the tibia be stabilized as well to facilitate knee ligament repair and subsequent rehabilitation. Although teenagers are the age group most often involved, the recommendations would be the same for a young child.

## NERVE INJURIES

Late development of neuropathy is often associated with fractures about the elbow, particularly the ulnar nerve. The ulnar nerve can be injured in the initial trauma, during reduction, or later as a result of progressive elbow deformity.[216] Childhood elbow injuries are believed to be responsible for up to half of all ulnar nerve palsies in adults. The ulnar nerve is often damaged acutely by posterior dislocation of the elbow, particularly if associated with a medial epicondylar fracture.[216] However, ulnar nerve damage has been reported with supracondylar, epicondylar, and condylar fractures.[216]

A valgus deformity that occurs after a lateral condylar fracture can lead to ulnar nerve problems. Varus deformity has also been reported, but less frequently, as a cause of ulnar nerve palsy secondary to impingement by the triceps tendon. Late ulnar nerve lesions at the elbow have been divided into three main categories: compression within the limited space of the cubital tunnel, traction such as occurs in a valgus deformity, and friction from bone fragments or osteophytes in close proximity to the nerve.[216] This condition is usually associated with ulnar nerve distribution symptoms, including paresthesias, intrinsic muscle weakness, and wasting.[216] An electromyogram can be helpful in establishing the diagnosis.

Treatment usually consists of surgical decompression of the nerve, correction of the angulatory deformity of the elbow, or both. Transposition is recommended if the ulnar nerve appears normal, if the symptoms are intractable, or if a valgus deformity of the elbow is present. If the condition has been of long duration, the pain and paresthesias should resolve, but weakness and muscle wasting may persist.[216]

Nerve injury is associated with approximately 12% to 16% of supracondylar fractures, most commonly injury to the ulnar and radial nerves and less often the median nerve.[205, 213, 214] Campbell and co-workers found that posterior lateral displacement of a type III supracondylar fracture was associated with a higher incidence of median nerve injuries (52%).[208] If the injury is closed and the reduction satisfactory, the child can be treated expectantly, and most will recover, usually in the first 2 months.[189, 207, 209, 214] One of the more subtle median nerve injuries is injury to the anterior interosseous branch from either traction or contusion.[209, 210] Physical findings are an inability to flex the distal phalanges of the thumb and index finger without associated sensory deficits (Fig. 6–26). This condition can be treated expectantly and usually resolves within 6 to 10 weeks.[210, 214]

In children, most nerves repaired within 1 year have a high rate of useful functional recovery because of their regenerative ability.[205] Bolitho and colleagues recommended early repair of ulnar nerve injuries in young children.[206] Distal injuries had a better outcome than proximal ones, but satisfactory function of the intrinsic hand muscles occurred in both groups. They found that repair of the transected nerve in young children (younger than 13 years) leads to good recovery, both motor and sensory.[232] The rate of clean-cut lesions from trauma in children is twice that from nerve compression.[205] Amillo and Mora assessed neural injuries associated with elbow fractures in 25 children (average age at injury, 9.4 years).[204] Eight had discontinuity of the nerve trunk and 17 had constrictive lesions around the nerve. In those with constrictive lesions, 80% had good results after neurolysis. In those who had disruption, 66% had good results after grafting. The prognosis was poor if surgery

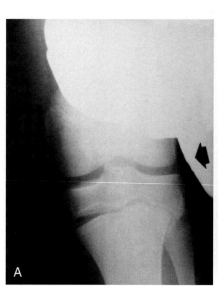
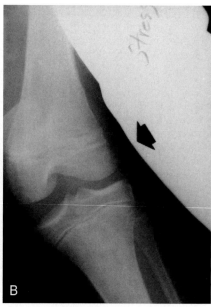

**FIGURE 6–25.** Two children who sustained injuries at the knee. *A,* A 13-year-old boy whose stress radiograph demonstrates a fracture of the proximal tibial epiphyseal plate. *B,* A 14-year-old boy whose stress radiograph demonstrates torn medial collateral ligaments and possible disruption of the anterior cruciate ligament.

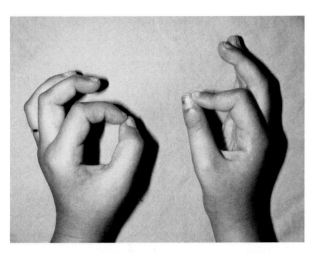

**FIGURE 6–26.** Supracondylar fracture in an 8-year-old girl that resulted in an anterior interosseous nerve palsy. Note the physical findings—inability to flex the distal phalanges of the thumb and index finger. The patient did not have an associated sensory deficit. She was treated expectantly, and the neurapraxia resolved in 6 weeks.

was performed more than a year after the injury. They recommended surgical exploration and neural lysis or repair with a graft for open neural injuries.[204] If it is closed, they recommend waiting 5 to 6 months before exploration. Grafts longer than 10 cm had a poor prognosis. In nerve injuries secondary to percutaneous pinning and open reduction and internal fixation, Brown and Zinar found that all deficits resolved spontaneously within 2 to 6 months.[207] They suggest waiting 6 months before performing electromyography to determine whether exploration is warranted.[207] Closed physeal fractures of the distal end of the radius are at risk for medial neuropathy because of either tenting of the nerve over the fracture or stretching or contusion of the nerve by internal or external forces at the time of injury.[218] Acute compartment syndrome may also complicate fractures of the distal end of the radius and lead to further confusion. Waters and associates recommend that if a patient has a normal neurologic examination but persistent neurologic symptoms and significant soft tissue swelling, closed reduction and percutaneous pinning may be indicated to eliminate the need for a constrictive cast.[218] The children who are most prone to compartment syndrome and nerve injury are those who have undergone repeated attempts at reduction.[217] Late open reduction may promote neurapraxia, compartment syndrome, or physeal arrest.[218]

Under very unusual circumstances, the median and ulnar nerves can become entrapped after dislocation of the elbow.[211, 215] When entrapment occurs, the diagnosis is often delayed. Early signs of entrapment are the presence of a lesion of the median nerve and pain greater than expected after reduction of the elbow dislocation.[211, 212] Later signs include a severe elbow flexion contracture and, radiographically, a bony depression in the distal medial humeral cortex corresponding to the location at which the median nerve travels posterior to the humerus and enters the elbow joint.[211, 212] In most children with median nerve injuries, the medial epicon-

dyle has been avulsed.[211] Green claims that every median nerve injury associated with an elbow dislocation should be viewed as representing probable nerve entrapment, particularly if more than mild hypesthesia is present.[211] Pain is a guideline if the neurologic deficit progresses; it should not be severe once the dislocation has been reduced. The presence of intense pain should alert one to the possibility of entrapment of the median nerve. The brachial artery and vein and the median nerve can be trapped between the fracture fragments in a widely displaced supracondylar fracture. Attempts at closed reduction usually lead to vascular compromise, which necessitates surgical reduction.

Secondary nerve injuries can result from simple positioning, particularly in children who are in coma or have head injuries.[212, 215] The ulnar nerve is very susceptible to compression at the elbow and the radial nerve at the midportion of the humerus if the arm is not properly positioned. If recognized early, these neurapraxias have good potential for recovery. The peroneal nerve may be compressed as it passes over the neck of the fibula. Frequent examination of the extremity for neurovascular status is essential, particularly in the immediate postinjury and early recovery periods or until the child is alert enough to report any changes. Obviously, in children with head injuries, casts should be well padded over these susceptible areas.

## REFLEX SYMPATHETIC DYSTROPHY

This condition is believed to be caused by dysfunction of the anatomic nervous system, usually after an injury to the ankle and foot, knee, or shoulder and hand.[219] It occurs more often in the lower extremities in children, in contrast to the shoulder and hand in adults.[221] Many terms have been used in the past to describe the condition, including causalgia, post-traumatic pain syndrome, shoulder-hand syndrome, and Sudeck's atrophy. The onset is heralded by severe pain and exquisite tenderness to light touch, including that of clothing.[219, 221, 233] Symptoms are intensified by weight bearing and relieved by keeping the involved areas as motionless as possible.[219] The extremity is usually swollen and exhibits vasomotor instability (83%), including skin discoloration, swelling with dependency, and decreased peripheral pulses; the skin temperature is usually warmer with increased sweating.[220, 221] The diagnostic criteria for reflex sympathetic dystrophy were suggested by Stanton and colleagues and include signs of vasomotor instability[231] (Table 6–1).

Dietz and associates found a helpful clinical sign of autonomic dysfunction (tache cerebrale) not previously described in the diagnosis of childhood reflex sympathetic dystrophy.[221] Tache cerebrale is elicited by stroking the skin in the affected area with a blunt object such as the head of a safety pin, and the contralateral limbs are used as a control. Autonomic dysfunction is demonstrated by the appearance of an erythematous line 15 to 30 seconds after the stimulus. It may persist as long as 15 minutes. The line was present in all five of the authors' patients.[221]

The onset of symptoms may follow a trivial injury, such as a simple twisted ankle or sprain (52%), or it may not be associated with a definite event.[221, 226] Reflex sympathetic dystrophy is usually seen in adolescents, most commonly preadolescent girls,[221, 230, 233] but it has been described in children as young as 3 years.[221] A variety of theories have been proposed, but no satisfactory explanation of its onset.[224]

Typically, the condition is present for an extended period before the diagnosis is made (average, 8 to 16 weeks; range, 1 week to 26 months).[226] The differential diagnosis includes juvenile rheumatoid arthritis, polymyositis, rheumatic fever, systemic lupus erythematosus, neoplasia, gout, and thrombophlebitis.[234] Symptoms may sometimes be confused with psychiatric conditions such as conversion disorder or malingering.[230] The results of laboratory studies are usually within normal limits.[219] Radiographs may reveal diffuse osteoporosis of the involved part. Bone scan findings have been inconsistent and show both increased uptake when the vasomotor phase is strong and decreased uptake with marked osteoporosis.[219, 228, 231]

Most pediatric patients are found to have psychologic problems, usually a pronounced indifference to the implications of the illness.[219, 230] Such children have a tendency to accept responsibility beyond their years and are very involved in school and extracurricular activities, sports, or social functions.[219, 229] They have difficulty expressing anger or being assertive on their own behalf.[219, 229] Their strength is in doing rather than saying; this manner of expression is consistent with how these children best approach their environment.[229] Typically, the condition serves a functional role by allowing them to slow down gracefully and affords a safe means of frustrating their parents' demands for performance without having to take responsibility for their behavior.[219] Most (83%) have emotional problems, and treatment must take these psychologic factors into account.[229, 231] Marital discord was present in about half the families of these patients, and the child often had the burden of keeping peace in the household. Many families show inappropriately high levels of enmeshment between parents and the child; because of high levels of stress in the parental relationship, the child consciously or unconsciously attempts to alleviate the problem.

The primary emphasis in management is to make the diagnosis and rule out other potential problems. Prompt diagnosis and therapy are directed at alleviating the symptoms quickly, thereby significantly improving the chance for permanent relief.[223, 230, 231, 233] Most authors suggest that narcotic analgesics be avoided in children.[224] A calcium channel blocker (nifedipine) and a sympathetic blocker (phenoxybenzamine) have been reported to be effective in children.[225] Vigorous active exercises, weight-bearing activities, and direct stimulation of the skin are usually successful.[221, 231] Corticosteroid therapy and sympathetic blockade are seldom necessary in children; most respond to continued positive reinforcement by a multidisciplinary team.[219, 221, 222, 230, 233] Recovery occurs in 7 to 8 weeks, but relapse is common (27%).[226, 227, 232]

The condition is more benign in children than in adults.[219, 227] Children seldom have the chronic atrophic changes that are found in adults.[219, 227] In follow-up, few children have long-term problems; most continue to function normally.[219, 227] Long-term problems are related to shortness of the limb or foot because of prolonged immobilization and osteoporosis.[228]

## REFERENCES

### Vascular Injuries

1. Bach, A.; Johansen, K. Limb salvage using temporary arterial shunt following traumatic near-amputation of the thigh. J Pediatr Orthop 2:187–190, 1982.
2. Bond, S.J.; Gotschall, C.S.; Eichelberger, M.R. Predictors of abdominal injury in children with pelvic fracture. J Trauma 31:1169–1173, 1991.
3. Campbell, C.C.; Waters, P.M.; Emans, J.B.; et al. Neurovascular injury and displacement in type III supracondylar humerus fractures. J Pediatr Orthop 15:47–52, 1995.
4. Clement, D.A.; Phil, D. Assessment of a treatment plan for managing acute vascular complications associated with supracondylar fractures of the humerus in children. J Pediatr Orthop 10:97–100, 1990.
5. Cole, W.G. Arterial injuries associated with fractures of the lower limbs in childhood. Injury 12:460–463, 1981.
6. Connolly, J. Management of fractures associated with arterial injuries. Am J Surg 120:331, 1970.
7. Copley, L.A.; Dormans, J.P.; Davidson, R.S. Vascular injuries and their sequelae in pediatric supracondylar humeral fractures: Toward a goal of prevention. J Pediatr Orthop 16:99–103, 1996.
8. Damron, T.; McBeath, A. Diagnosis and management of vascular injuries associated with skeletal trauma. Orthop Rev 19:1063–1070, 1990.
9. Dormans, J.P.; Squillante, R.; Sharf, H. Acute neurovascular complications with supracondylar humerus fractures in children. J Hand Surg [Am] 20:1–4, 1995.
10. Eren, N.; Ozgen, G.; Ener, B.K.; et al. Peripheral vascular injuries in children. J Pediatr Surg 26:1164–1168, 1991.
11. Fabian, T.C.; Turkleson, M.L.; Connelly, T.L.; Stone, H.H. Injury to the popliteal artery. Am J Surg 143:225–228, 1982.
12. Fainzilber, G.; Roy-Shapira, A.; Wall, M.J., Jr.; Mattox, K.L. Predictors of amputation for popliteal artery injuries. Am J Surg 170:568–571, 1995.
13. Friedman, J.; Fabre, J.; Netscher, D.; Jaksic, T. Treatment of acute neonatal vascular injuries—the utility of multiple interventions. J Pediatr Surg 34:940–945, 1999.
14. Friedman, R.J.; Jupiter, J.B. Vascular injuries and closed extremity fractures in children. Clin Orthop 188:112–119, 1984.
15. Garvin, K.L.; McCarthy, R.E.; Barnes, C.L.; Dodge, B.M. Pediatric pelvic ring fractures. J Pediatr Orthop 10:577–582, 1990.

**TABLE 6–1** • • • • • • • • • • • • • • • • • • • • • • • • • •

Pediatric Reflex Sympathetic Dystrophy: Diagnostic Criteria

Pain out of proportion to the inciting event
Evidence of neurovascular dysfunction as manifested by three or more of the following:
  Dependent edema
  Dependent rubor
  Mottling of the skin
  Hypersensitivity of skin to light touch
  Skin temperature changes
  Altered perspiration
  Changes in patterns of hair growth

• • • • • • • • • • • • • • • • • • • • • • • • • • • • • • • • •

*Source:* Stanton, R.P., et al. Orthopaedics 16:773–780, 1993.

16. Green, N.E.; Allen, B.L. Vascular injuries associated with dislocation of the knee. J Bone Joint Surg Am 59:236–239, 1977.
17. Ismail, N.; Bellemare, J.F.; Mollitt, D.L.; et al. Death from pelvic fracture: Children are different. J Pediatr Surg 31:82–85, 1996.
18. Johansen, K.; Bandyk, D.; Thiele, B.; Hansen, S.T. Temporary intraluminal shunts: Resolution of a management dilemma in complex vascular injuries. J Trauma 22:395–402, 1982.
19. Lange, R.H.; Bach, A.W.; Hansen, S.T.; Johansen, K.H. Open tibial fractures with associated vascular injuries: Prognosis for limb salvage. J Trauma 25:203–208, 1985.
20. McIntyre, R.C.; Bensard, D.D.; Moore, E.E.; et al. Pelvic fracture geometry predicts risk of life-threatening hemorrhage in children. J Trauma 35:423–429, 1993.
21. Navarre, J.R.; Cardillo, P.J.; Gorman, J.F.; et al. Vascular trauma in children and adolescents. Am J Surg 143:229–231, 1982.
22. Norman, J.; Gahtan, V.; Franz, M.; Bramson, R. Occult vascular injuries following gunshot wounds resulting in long bone fractures of the extremities. Am Surg 61:146–150, 1995.
23. Odland, M.D.; Gisbert, V.L.; Gustilo, R.B.; et al. Combined orthopedic and vascular injury in the lower extremities: Indications for amputation. Surgery 108:660–666, 1990.
24. O'Neill, P.A.; Riina, J.; Sclafani, S.; Tornetta, P., III. Angiographic findings in pelvic fractures. Clin Orthop 329:60–67, 1996.
25. Russo, V.J. Traumatic arterial spasm resulting in gangrene. J Pediatr Orthop 5:486–488, 1985.
26. Sabharwal, S.; Tredwell, S.J.; Beauchamp, R.D.; et al. Management of pulseless pink hand in pediatric supracondylar fractures of humerus. J Pediatr Orthop 17:303–310, 1997.
27. Samson, R.; Pasternak, B.M. Traumatic arterial spasm—rarity or nonentity? J Trauma 20:607–609, 1980.
28. Shaker, I.J.; White, J.J.; Signer, R.D.; et al. Special problems of vascular injuries in children. J Trauma 16:863–867, 1976.
29. Smith, P.L.; Lim, W.N.; Ferris, E.J.; Casali, R.E. Emergency arteriography in extremity trauma: Assessment of indications. AJR Am J Roentgenol 137:803–807, 1981.
30. Stanford, J.R.; Evans, W.E.; Morse, T.S. Pediatric arterial injuries. J Vasc Dis 27:1–7, 1976.
31. Starr, A.J.; Hunt, J.L.; Reinert, C.M. Treatment of femur fracture with associated vascular injury. J Trauma 40:17–21, 1996.
32. Vasli, L.P. Diagnosis of vascular injury in children with supracondylar fractures of the humerus. Injury 19:11–13, 1988.
33. Whitehouse, W.M.; Coran, A.G.; Stanley, J.C.; et al. Pediatric vascular trauma. Manifestations, management and sequelae of extremity arterial injury in patients undergoing surgical treatment. Arch Surg 111:1269–1275, 1976.
34. Zehntner, M.K.; Petropoulos, P.; Burch, H. Factors determining outcome in fractures of the extremities associated with arterial injuries. J Orthop Trauma 5:29–33, 1991.

### Compartment Syndromes

35. Aerts, P.; De Boeck, H.; Casteleyn, P.P.; Opdecam, P. Case report: Deep volar compartment syndrome of the forearm following minor crush injury. J Pediatr Orthop 9:69–71, 1989.
36. Bae, D.S.; Kadiyala, R.K.; Waters, P.M. Acute compartment syndrome in children: Contemporary diagnosis, treatment, and outcome. J Pediatr Orthop 21:680–688, 2001.
37. Chuang, D.C.; Carver, N.; Wei, F.C. A new strategy to prevent the sequelae of severe Volkmann's ischemia. Plast Reconstr Surg 98:1023–1031, 1996.
38. Clancey, G.J. Acute posterior compartment syndrome in the thigh. A case report. J Bone Joint Surg Am 67:1278–1280, 1985.
39. Hargens, A.R.; Akeson, W.H.; Mubarak, S.J.; et al. Fluid balance within the canine anterolateral compartment and its relationship to compartment syndromes. J Bone Joint Surg Am 60:499–505, 1978.
40. Hargens, A.R.; Romine, J.S.; Sipe, J.C.; et al. Peripheral nerve-conduction block by high muscle-compartment pressure. J Bone Joint Surg Am 61:192–200, 1979.
41. Heppenstall, R.B.; Scott, R.; Sapega, A.; et al. A comparative study of the tolerance of skeletal muscle to ischemia. Tourniquet application compared with acute compartment syndrome. J Bone Joint Surg Am 68:820–828, 1986.
42. Hernandez, J., Jr.; Peterson, H.A. Case report: Fracture of the distal radial physis complicated by compartment syndrome and premature physeal closure. J Pediatr Orthop 6:627–630, 1986.

43. Janzing, H.; Broos, P.; Romnens, P. Compartment syndrome as complication of skin traction, in children with femoral fractures. Acta Chir Belg 96:135–137, 1996.
44. Kline, S.C.; Moore, J.R. Neonatal compartment syndrome. J Hand Surg [Am] 17:256–259, 1992.
45. Langen, R.P.; Ruggieri, R. Acute compartment syndrome in the thigh complicated by a pseudoaneurysm. A case report. J Bone Joint Surg Am 71:762–763, 1989.
46. Mars, M.; Hadley, G.P. Failure of pulse oximetry in the assessment of raised limb intracompartmental pressure. Injury 25:379–381, 1994.
47. Mars, M.; Hadley, G.P. Raised compartmental pressure in children: A basis for management. Injury 29:183–185, 1998.
48. Matsen, F.A., III. Compartment syndrome: A unified concept. Clin Orthop 113:8–14, 1975.
49. Matsen, F.A., III; Veith, R.G. Compartmental syndromes in children. J Pediatr Orthop 1:33–41, 1981.
50. Mubarak, S.J.; Owen, C.A.; Hargens, A.R.; et al. Compartment syndromes: Diagnosis and treatment with the aid of the Wick catheter. J Bone Joint Surg Am 60:1091–1095, 1978.
51. Peters, C.L.; Scott, S.M. Compartment syndrome in the forearm following fractures of the radial head and neck in children. J Bone Joint Surg Am 77:1070–1074, 1995.
52. Ouellette, E.A.; Kelly, R. Compartment syndromes of the hand. J Bone Joint Surg Am 78:1515–1522, 1996.
53. Robertson, P.; Karol, L.A.; Rab, G.T. Open fractures of the tibia and femur in children. J Pediatr Orthop 16:621–626, 1996.
54. Rooser, B.; Bengtson, S.; Hagglund, G. Acute compartment syndrome from anterior thigh muscle contusion: A report of eight cases. J Orthop Trauma 5:57–59, 1991.
55. Schwartz, J.T.; Brumback, R.J.; Lakatos, R.; et al. Acute compartment syndrome of the thigh. A spectrum of injury. J Bone Joint Surg Am 71:392–400, 1989.
56. Silas, S.I.; Herzenberg, J.E.; Myerson, M.S.; Sponseller, P.D. Compartment syndrome of the foot in children. J Bone Joint Surg Am 77:356–361, 1995.
57. Turen, C.H.; Burgess, A.R.; Vanco, B. Skeletal stabilization for tibial fractures associated with acute compartment syndrome. Clin Orthop 315:163–168, 1995.

### Fat Embolism

58. Carty, J.B. Fat embolism in childhood. Review and case report. Am J Surg 94:970–973, 1957.
59. Chastre, J.; Fagon, J.-Y.; Soler, P.; et al. Bronchoalveolar lavage for rapid diagnosis of the fat embolism syndrome in trauma patients. Ann Intern Med 113:583–588, 1990.
60. Chuang, E.L.; Miller, F.S., III; Kalina, R.E. Retinal lesions following long bone fractures. Ophthalmology 92:370–374, 1985.
61. Drummond, D.S.; Salter, R.B.; Boone, J. Fat embolism in children: Its frequency and relationships to collagen disease. Can Med Assoc J 101:200–203, 1969.
62. Edwards, K.J.; Cummings, R.J. Case report: Fat embolism as a complication of closed femoral shortening. J Pediatr Orthop 12:542–543, 1992.
63. Fabian, T.C.; Hoots, A.V.; Stanford, D.S.; et al. Fat embolism syndrome: Prospective evaluation in 92 fracture patients. Crit Care Med 18:42–46, 1990.
64. Kotwica, Z.; Balcewicz, L.; Jagodzinski, Z. Head injuries coexistent with pelvic or lower extremity fractures—early or delayed osteosynthesis. Acta Neurochir 102:19–21, 1990.
65. Limbird, T.J.; Ruderman, R.J. Fat embolism in children. Clin Orthop 136:267–268, 1978.
66. Lozman, J.; Deno, D.C.; Feustel, P.J.; et al. Pulmonary and cardiovascular consequences of immediate fixation or conservative management of long-bone fractures. Arch Surg 121:992–999, 1986.
67. Mudd, K.L.; Hunt, A.; Matherly, R.C.; et al. Analysis of pulmonary fat embolism in blunt force fatalities. J Trauma 48:711–715, 2000.
68. Pell, A.C.; Christie, J.; Keating, J.F.; Sutherland, G.R. The detection of fat embolism by transoesophageal echocardiography during reamed intramedullary nailing. A study of 24 patients with femoral and tibial fractures. J Bone Joint Surg Br 75:921–925, 1993.

69. Pender, E.S.; Pollack, C.V., Jr.; Evans, O.B. Fat embolism syndrome in a child with muscular dystrophy. J Emerg Med 10:705–711, 1992.

70. Shulman, S.T.; Grossman, B.J. Fat embolism in childhood. Review with report of a fatal case related to physical therapy in a child with dermatomyositis. Am J Dis Child 120:480–484, 1970.

71. Svenninsen, S.; Nesse, O.; Finsen, V.; et al. Prevention of fat embolism syndrome in patients with femoral fractures—immediate or delayed operative fixation? Ann Chir Gynaecol 76:163–166, 1987.

72. ten Duis, H.J.; Nijsten, M.W.N.; Klasen, H.J.; Binnendijk, B. Fat embolism in patients with an isolated fracture of the femoral shaft. J Trauma 28:383–390, 1988.

### Hypercalcemia of Immobilization

73. Carey, D.E.; Raisz, L.G. Calcitonin therapy in prolonged immobilization hypercalcemia. Arch Phys Med Rehabil 66:640–644, 1985.

74. Claus-Walker, J.; Carter, R.D.; Campos, R.J.; Spencer, W.A. Hypercalcemia in early traumatic quadriplegia. J Chronic Dis 28:81–90, 1975.

75. Cristofaro, R.L.; Brink, J.D. Hypercalcemia of immobilization in neurologically injured children: A prospective study. Orthopaedics 2:485–491, 1979.

76. Henke, J.A.; Thompson, N.W.; Kaufer, H. Immobilization hypercalcemia crisis. Arch Surg 110:321–323, 1975.

77. Kaul, S.; Sockalosky, J.J. Human synthetic calcitonin therapy for hypercalcemia of immobilization. J Pediatr 126:825–827, 1995.

78. Little, J.A.; Dean, A.E., Jr.; Chapman, M. Immobilization hypercalcemia. South Med J 75:502, 1982.

79. Meythaler, J.M.; Tuel, S.M.; Cross, L.L. Successful treatment of immobilization hypercalcemia using calcitonin and etidronate. Arch Phys Med Rehabil 74:316–319, 1993.

80. Winters, J.L.; Kleinschmidt, A.G.; Frehsilli, J.J.; Sutton, M. Hypercalcemia complicating immobilization in the treatment of fractures. J Bone Joint Surg Am 48:1182–1184, 1966.

### Ectopic Bone Formation

81. Carlson, W.O.; Klassen, R.A. Myositis ossificans of the upper extremity: A long-term follow-up. J Pediatr Orthop 4:693–696, 1984.

82. De Smet, A.A.; Norris, M.A.; Fisher, D.R. Magnetic resonance imaging of myositis ossificans: Analysis of seven cases. Skeletal Radiol 21:503–507, 1992.

83. Ehara, S.; Shiraishi, H.; Abe, M.; Mizutani, H. Reactive heterotopic ossification. Its patterns on MRI. Clin Imaging 22:292–296, 1998.

84. Johnson, E.E.; Kay, R.M.; Dorey, F.J. Heterotopic ossification prophylaxis following operative treatment of acetabular fracture. Clin Orthop 305:88–95, 1994.

85. Kaplan, F.S.; Gannon, F.H.; Hahn, G.V.; et al. Pseudomalignant heterotopic ossification. Differential diagnosis and report of two cases. Clin Orthop 346:134–140, 1998.

86. Koch, B.M.; Wu, C.M.; Randolph, J.; Eng, G.D. Heterotopic ossification in children with burns: Two case reports. Arch Phys Med Rehabil 73:1104–1106, 1992.

87. Mital, M.A.; Garber, J.E.; Stinson, J.T. Ectopic bone formation in children and adolescents with head injuries: Its management. J Pediatr Orthop 7:83–90, 1987.

88. Moed, B.R.; Maxey, J.W. The effect of indomethacin on heterotopic ossification following acetabular fracture surgery. J Orthop Trauma 7:33–38, 1993.

89. Thompson, H.G.; Garcia, A. Myositis ossificans: Aftermath of elbow injuries. Clin Orthop 50:129–134, 1967.

90. Zagaja, G.P.; Cromie, W.J. Heterotopic bone formation in association with pelvic fracture and urethral disruption. J Urol 161:1950–1953, 1999.

### Superior Mesenteric Artery Syndrome (Cast Syndrome)

91. Amy, B.W.; Priebe, C.J.; King, A. Superior mesenteric artery syndrome associated with scoliosis treated by a modified Ladd procedure. J Pediatr Orthop 5:361–363, 1985.

92. Berk, R.N.; Coulson, D.B. The body cast syndrome. Radiology 94:303–305, 1970.

93. Philip, P.A. Superior mesenteric artery syndrome: An unusual cause of intestinal obstruction in brain-injured children. Brain Inj 5:351–358, 1992.

94. Walker, C.; Kahanovitz, N. Recurrent superior mesenteric artery syndrome complicating staged reconstructive spinal surgery: Alternative methods of conservative treatment. J Pediatr Orthop 3:77–80, 1983.

95. Warner, T.F.C.S.; Shorter, R.G.; McIlrath, D.C.; Dupree, E.L., Jr. The cast syndrome. An unusually severe case. J Bone Joint Surg Am 56:1263–1266, 1974.

### Traction-Induced Hypertension

96. Hamdan, J.A.; Taleb, Y.A.; Ahmed, M.S. Traction-induced hypertension in children. Clin Orthop 185:87–89, 1984.

97. Heij, H.A.; Ekkelkamp, S.; Vos, A. Hypertension associated with skeletal traction in children. Eur J Pediatr 151:543–545, 1992.

98. Linshaw, M.A.; Stapleton, F.B.; Gruskin, A.B.; et al. Traction-related hypertension in children. J Pediatr 95:994–996, 1979.

99. Talab, Y.A.; Hamdan, J.A.; Ahmed, M.S. Orthopaedic causes of hypertension in pediatric patients. Case report and review of the literature. J Bone Joint Surg Am 64:291–292, 1982.

100. Turner, M.C.; Ruley, E.J.; Buckley, K.M.; Strife, C.F. Blood pressure elevation with orthopaedic immobilization. J Pediatr 95:989–992, 1979.

### Spontaneous Deep Vein Thrombosis

101. Cullen, M.C.; Roy, D.R.; Giza, E.; Crawford, A.H. Complications of intramedullary fixation of pediatric forearm fractures. J Pediatr Orthop 18:14–21, 1998.

102. Horwitz, J.; Shenker, I.R. Spontaneous deep vein thrombosis in adolescence. Clin Pediatr (Phila) 16:787–790, 1977.

103. Joffe, S. Postoperative deep vein thrombosis in children. J Pediatr Surg 10:539–540, 1975.

104. Johari, A.N.; Sinha, M. Remodeling of forearm fractures in children. J Pediatr Orthop B 8:84–87, 1999.

105. Letts, M.; Lalonde, F.; Davidson, D.; et al. Atrial and venous thrombosis secondary to septic arthritis of the sacroiliac joint in a child with hereditary protein C deficiency. J Pediatr Orthop 19:156–160, 1999.

106. Manco-Johnson, M.J.; Nuss, R.; Hays, T.; et al. Combined thrombolytic and anticoagulant therapy for venous thrombosis in children. J Pediatr 136:446–453, 2000.

107. Nowak-Gottl, U.; Junker, R.; Hartmeier, M.; et al. Increased lipoprotein(a) is an important risk factor for venous thromboembolism in childhood. Circulation 100:743–748, 1999.

108. Wise, R.C.; Todd, J.K. Spontaneous, lower-extremity venous thrombosis in children. Am J Dis Child 126:766–769, 1973.

### Malunion-Synostosis

109. Bellemore, M.C.; Barrett, I.R.; Middleton, R.W.D.; et al. Supracondylar osteotomy of the humerus for correction of cubitus varus. J Bone Joint Surg Br 66:566–572, 1984.

110. Bohn, W.W.; Durbin, R.A. Ipsilateral fractures of the femur and tibia in children and adolescents. J Bone Joint Surg Am 73:429–439, 1991.

111. Carlson, C.S.; Rosman, M.A. Cubitus varus: A new and simple technique for correction. J Pediatr Orthop 2:199–201, 1982.

112. Creasman, C.; Zaleske, D.J.; Ehrlich, M.G. Analyzing forearm fractures in children. The more subtle signs of impending problems. Clin Orthop 188:40–53, 1984.

113. Davis, D.R.; Green, D.P. Forearm fractures in children. Pitfalls and complications. Clin Orthop 120:172–184, 1976.

114. Fowles, J.V.; Kassab, M.T.; Moula, T. Untreated intraarticular entrapment of the medial humeral epicondyle. J Bone Joint Surg Br 66:562–565, 1984.

115. Fuller, D.J.; McCullough, C.J. Malunited fractures of the forearm in children. J Bone Joint Surg Br 64:364–367, 1982.

116. Hoffer, M.M.; Garrett, A.; Brink, J.; et al. The orthopaedic management of brain-injured children. J Bone Joint Surg Am 53:567–577, 1971.

117. Kirby, R.M.; Winquist, R.A.; Hansen, S.T. Femoral shaft fractures in adolescents: A comparison between traction plus cast treatment and closed intramedullary nailing. J Pediatr Orthop 1:193–197, 1981.

118. Labelle, H.; Bunnell, W.P.; Duhaime, M.; Poitras, B. Cubitus varus deformity following supracondylar fractures of the humerus in children. J Pediatr Orthop 2:539–546, 1982.

119. Loder, R.T. Pediatric polytrauma: Orthopaedic care and hospital course. J Orthop Trauma 1:48–54, 1987.

120. Oppenheim W.L.; Clader, T.J.; Smith, C.; Bayer, M. Supracondylar humeral osteotomy for traumatic childhood cubitus varus deformity. Clin Orthop 188:34–39, 1984.

121. Price, C.T.; Scott, D.S.; Kurzner, M.E.; Flynn, J.C. Malunited forearm fractures in children. J Pediatr Orthop 10:705–712, 1990.

122. Roberts, J.A. Angulation of the radius in children's fractures. J Bone Joint Surg Br 68:751–754, 1986.

123. Rodgers, W.B.; Waters, P.M.; Hall, J.E. Chronic Monteggia lesions in children. J Bone Joint Surg Am 78:1322–1329, 1996.

124. Roy, D.R. Radioulnar synostosis following proximal radial fracture in a child. Orthop Rev 15:89–94, 1986.

125. Thomas, E.W.; Tuson, K.W.R.; Browne, P.S.H. Fractures of the radius and ulna in children. Injury 7:120–124, 1979.

126. Tredwell, S.S.; Peteghen, K.V.; Clough, M. Pattern of forearm fractures in children. J Pediatr Orthop 4:604–608, 1984.

127. Vince, K.G.; Miller, J.E. Cross-union complicating fracture of the forearm. Part II: Children. J Bone Joint Surg Am 69:654–661, 1987.

128. Vittas, D.; Larsen, E.; Torp-Pedersen, S. Angular remodeling of midshaft forearm fractures in children. Clin Orthop 265:261–264, 1991.

129. Ziv, I.; Rang, M. Treatment of femoral fracture in the child with head injury. J Bone Joint Surg Br 65:276–278, 1983.

**Late Angulation**

130. Balthazar, D.A.; Pappas, A.M. Acquired valgus deformity of the tibia in children. J Pediatr Orthop 4:538–541, 1984.

131. Green, N.E. Tibia valga caused by asymmetrical overgrowth following a nondisplaced fracture of the proximal tibial metaphysis. J Pediatr Orthop 3:235–237, 1983.

132. Jordan, S.E.; Alonso, J.E.; Cook, F.F. The etiology of valgus angulation after metaphyseal fractures of the tibia in children. J Pediatr Orthop 7:450–457, 1987.

133. Ogden, J.A.; Ogden, D.A.; Pugh, L.; et al. Tibia valga after proximal metaphyseal fractures in childhood: A normal biologic response. J Pediatr Orthop 15:489–494, 1995.

134. Robert, M.; Khouri, N.; Carlioz, H.; Alain, J.L. Fractures of the proximal tibial metaphysis in children: Review of a series of 25 cases. J Pediatr Orthop 7:444–449, 1987.

135. So, Y.C.; Fang, D.; Leong, J.C.Y.; Bong, S.C. Varus deformity following lateral humeral condylar fractures in children. J Pediatr Orthop 5:569–572, 1985.

136. Zionts, L.E.; Harcke, H.T.; Brooks, K.M.; MacEwen, G.D. Posttraumatic tibial valga: A case demonstrating asymmetric activity at the proximal growth plate on technetium bone scan. J Pediatr Orthop 7:458–462, 1987.

**Injury to the Triradiate Cartilage**

137. Bucholz, R.W.; Ezaki, M.; Ogden, J.A. Injury to the acetabular triradiate physeal cartilage. J Bone Joint Surg Am 64:600–609, 1982.

138. Fama, G.; Turra, S.; Bonaga, S. Traumatic lesions of the triradiate cartilage. Chir Organi Mov 77:247–256, 1992.

139. Hallel, T.; Salvati, E.A. Premature closure of the triradiate cartilage. A case report and animal experiment. Clin Orthop 124:278–281, 1977.

140. Harder, J.A.; Bobechko, W.P.; Sullivan, R.; Daneman, A. Computerized axial tomography to demonstrate occult fractures of the acetabulum in children. Can J Surg 24:409–411, 1981.

141. Heeg, M.; Klasen, H.J.; Visser, J.D. Acetabular fractures in children and adolescents. J Bone Joint Surg Br 71:418–421, 1989.

142. Heeg, M.; Visser, J.D.; Oostvogel, H.J.M. Injuries of the acetabular triradiate cartilage and sacroiliac joint. J Bone Joint Surg Br 70:34–37, 1988.

143. Scuderi, G.; Bronson, M.J. Triradiate cartilage injury. Report of two cases and review of the literature. Clin Orthop 217:179–189, 1987.

144. Valdiseri, L.; Bungaro, P.; D'Angelo, G. Traumatic lesions of the acetabular triradiate cartilage (presentation of four cases and considerations on treatment). Chir Organi Mov 81:361–367, 1996.

**Overgrowth and Undergrowth**

145. Aronson, J.; Tursky, E.A. External fixation of femur fractures in children. J Pediatr Orthop 12:157–163, 1992.

146. Beals, R.K. Premature closure of the physis following diaphyseal fractures. J Pediatr Orthop 10:717–720, 1990.

147. Beaty, J.H.; Austin, S.M.; Warner, W.C.; et al. Interlocking intramedullary nailing of femoral-shaft fractures in adolescents: Preliminary results and complications. J Pediatr Orthop 14:178–183, 1994.

148. Blasier, R.D.; Aronson, J.; Tursky, E.A. External fixation of pediatric femur fractures. J Pediatr Orthop 17:342–346, 1997.

149. Bowler, J.R.; Mubarak, S.J.; Wenger, D.R. Tibial physeal closure and genu recurvatum after femoral fracture: Occurrence without a tibial traction pin. J Pediatr Orthop 10:653–657, 1990.

150. Davids, J.R.; Maguire, M.F.; Mubarak, S.J.; Wenger, D.R. Lateral condylar fracture of the humerus following posttraumatic cubitus varus. J Pediatr Orthop 14:446–470, 1994.

151. de Pablos, J.; Franzreb, M.; Barrious, C. Longitudinal growth pattern of the radius after forearm fractures conservatively treated in children. J Pediatr Orthop 14:492–495, 1994.

152. Hunter, L.Y.; Hensinger, R.N. Premature monomelic growth arrest following fracture of the femoral shaft. A case report. J Bone Joint Surg Am 60:850–852, 1978.

153. Kohan, L.; Cumming, W.J. Femoral shaft fractures in children: The effect of initial shortening on subsequent limb overgrowth. Aust N Z J Surg 52:141–144, 1982.

154. Kregor, P.J.; Song, K.M.; Routt, M.L., Jr.; et al. Plate fixation of femoral shaft fractures in multiply injured children. J Bone Joint Surg Am 75:1774–1780, 1993.

155. Nork, S.E.; Bellig, G.J.; Woll, J.P.; Hoffinger, S.A. Overgrowth and outcome after femoral shaft fracture in children younger than 2 years. Clin Orthop 357:186–191, 1998.

156. Sahin, V.; Baktir, A.; Turk, C.Y.; et al. Femoral shaft fractures in children treated by closed reduction and early spica cast with incorporated supracondylar Kirschner wires: A long-term follow-up results. Injury 30:121–128, 1999.

157. Shapiro, F. Fractures of the femoral shaft in children. The overgrowth phenomenon. Acta Orthop Scand 52:649–655, 1981.

158. Staheli, L.T. Femoral and tibial growth following femoral shaft fracture in childhood. Clin Orthop 55:159, 1967.

159. Stephens, M.M.; Hsu, L.C.S.; Leong, J.C.Y. Leg length discrepancy after femoral shaft fractures in children. Review after skeletal maturity. J Bone Joint Surg Br 71:615–618, 1989.

**Growth Disturbances**

160. Aminian, A.; Schoenecker, P.L. Premature closure of the distal radial physis after fracture of the distal radial metaphysis. J Pediatr Orthop 15:495–498, 1995.

161. Bollini, G.; Tallet, J.M.; Jacquemier, M.; Bouyala, J.M. New procedure to remove a centrally located bone bar. J Pediatr Orthop 10:662–666, 1990.

162. Borsa, J.J.; Peterson, H.A.; Ehman, R.L. MR imaging of physeal bars. Radiology 199:683–687, 1996.

163. Bowler, J.R.; Mubarak, S.J.; Wenger, D.R. Case report—tibial physeal closure and genu recurvatum after femoral fracture: Occurrence without a tibial traction pin. J Pediatr Orthop 10:653–657, 1990.

164. Carlson, W.O.; Wenger, D.R. A mapping method to prepare for surgical excision of a partial physeal arrest. J Pediatr Orthop 4:232–238, 1984.

165. Cramer, K.E.; Limbird, T.J.; Green, N.E. Open fractures of the diaphysis of the lower extremity in children. Treatment, results and complications. J Bone Joint Surg Am 74:218–232, 1992.

166. Hresko, M.T.; Kasser, J.R. Physeal arrest about the knee associated with non-physeal fractures in the lower extremity. J Bone Joint Surg Am 71:698–703, 1989.

167. Jaramillo, D.; Hoffer, F.A.; Shapiro, F.; Rand, F. MR imaging of fractures of the growth plate. AJR Am J Roentgenol 155:1261–1265, 1990.

168. Karrholm, J.; Hansson, L.I.; Selvik, G. Changes in tibiofibular relationships due to growth disturbances after ankle fractures in children. J Bone Joint Surg Am 66:1198–1210, 1984.

169. Kling, T.F.; Bright, R.W.; Hensinger, R.N. Distal tibial physeal fractures in children that may require open reduction. J Bone Joint Surg Am 66:647–657, 1984.

170. Langenskiold, A. Surgical treatment of partial closure of the growth plate. J Pediatr Orthop 1:3–11, 1981.

171. Langenskiold, A.; Osterman, K.; Valle, M. Growth of fat grafts after operation for partial bone growth arrest: Demonstration by computed tomography scanning. J Pediatr Orthop 7:389–394, 1987.

172. Loder, R.T.; Swinford, A.E.; Kuhns, L.R. The use of helical computerized tomographic scan to assess body physeal bridges. J Pediatr Orthop 17:356–359, 1997.

173. Peterson, H.A. Partial growth plate arrest and its treatment. J Pediatr Orthop 4:246–258, 1984.

174. Porat, S.; Nyska, M.; Nyska, A.; Fields, S. Assessment of bony bridge by computed tomography: Experimental model in the rabbit and clinical application. J Pediatr Orthop 7:155–160, 1987.

175. Riseborough, E.J.; Barrett, I.R.; Shapiro, F. Growth disturbances following distal femoral physeal fracture-separations. J Bone Joint Surg Am 65:885–893, 1983.

176. Vocke, A.K.; Von Laer, L. Displaced fractures of the radial neck in children: Long-term results and prognosis of conservative treatment. J Pediatr Orthop B 7:217–222, 1998.

177. Williamson, R.V.; Staheli, L.T. Partial physeal growth arrest: Treatment by bridge resection and fat interposition. J Pediatr Orthop 10:769–776, 1990.

178. Zehntner, M.K.; Jakob, R.P.; McGanity, P.L.J. Growth disturbance of the distal radial epiphysis after trauma: Operative treatment by corrective radial osteotomy. J Pediatr Orthop 10:411–415, 1990.

**Nonunion and Refracture**

179. Arunachalam, V.S.P.; Griffiths, J.C. Fracture recurrence in children. Injury 7:37–40, 1975.

180. Bould, M.; Bannister, G.C. Refractures of the radius and ulna in children. Injury 30:583–586, 1999.

181. Buckley, S.L.; Smith, G.R.; Sponseller, P.D.; et al. Severe (type III) open fractures of the tibia in children. J Pediatr Orthop 36:627–634, 1996.

182. Cramer, K.E.; Limbird, T.J.; Green, N.E. Open fractures of the diaphysis of the lower extremity in children. Treatment, results and complications. J Bone Joint Surg Am 74:218–232, 1992.

183. Cullen, M.C.; Roy, D.R.; Crawford, A.H.; et al. Open fracture of the tibia in children. J Bone Joint Surg Am 78:1039–1047, 1996.

184. De Boeck, H. Surgery for non-union of the lateral humeral condyle in children: 6 cases followed for 1–9 years. Acta Orthop Scand 66:401–402, 1995.

185. Ebraheim, N.A.; Skie, M.C.; Jackson, W.T. The treatment of tibial nonunion with angular deformity using an Ilizarov device. J Trauma 38:111–117, 1995.

186. Flynn, J.A. Nonunion of slightly displaced fractures of the lateral humeral condyle in children: An update. J Pediatr Orthop 9:691–696, 1989.

187. Goldberg, B.A.; Mansfield, D.S.; Davino, N.A. Nonunion of a distal femoral epiphyseal fracture-separation. Am J Orthop 25:773–777, 1996.

188. Grimard, G.; Naudie, D.; Laberge, L.C.; Hamdy, R.C. Open fractures of the tibia in children. Clin Orthop 332:62–70, 1996.

189. Haasbeek, J.F.; Cole, W.G. Open fractures of the arm in children. J Bone Joint Surg Br 77:576–581, 1995.

190. Hsu, L.C.S.; O'Brien, J.P.; Hodgson, A.R. Valgus deformity of the ankle in children with fibular pseudarthrosis. J Bone Joint Surg Am 56:503–510, 1974.

191. Inoue, G.; Taumra, Y. Osteosynthesis for longstanding nonunion for the lateral humeral condyle. Arch Orthop Trauma Surg 112:236–238, 1993.

192. Ippolito, E.; Tudisco, C.; Farsetti, P.; Caterini, R. Fracture of the humeral condyles in children: 49 cases evaluated after 18–45 years. Acta Orthop Scand 67:173–178, 1996.

193. Lewallen, R.P.; Peterson, H.A. Nonunion of long bone fractures in children: A review of 30 cases. J Pediatr Orthop 5:135–142, 1985.

194. Masada, K.; Kawai, H.; Kawabata, H.; et al. Osteosynthesis for old, established non-union of the lateral condyle of the humerus. J Bone Joint Surg Am 72:32–40, 1990.

195. Maxted, M.J.; Owen, R. Two cases of non-union of carpal scaphoid fractures in children. Injury 13:441–443, 1982.

196. Mintzer, C.M.; Waters, P.M.; Simmons, B.P. Nonunion of the scaphoid in children treated by Herbert screw fixation and bone grafting. A report of five cases. J Bone Joint Surg Br 77:98–100, 1995.

197. Roye, D.P., Jr.; Bini, S.A.; Infosino, A. Late surgical treatment of lateral condylar fractures in children. J Pediatr Orthop 11:195–199, 1991.

198. Schwarz, N.; Pienaar, S.; Schwarz, A.F.; et al. Refracture of the forearm in children. J Bone Joint Surg Br 78:740–744, 1996.

199. Skaggs, D.L.; Leet, A.I.; Money, M.D.; et al. Secondary fractures associated with external fixation in pediatric femur fractures. J Pediatr Orthop 19:582–586, 1999.

200. Song, K.M.; Sangeorzan, B.; Benirschke, S.; Browne, R. Open fractures of the tibia in children. J Pediatr Orthop 16:635–639, 1996.

201. Wulff, R.N.; Schmidt, T.L. Carpal fractures in children. J Pediatr Orthop 18:462–465, 1998.

**Ligamentous Instability**

202. Buckley, S.L.; Sturm, P.F.; Tosi, L.L.; et al. Ligamentous instability of the knee in children sustaining fractures of the femur: A prospective study with knee examination under anesthesia. J Pediatr Orthop 16:206–209, 1996.

203. Pennecot, G.F.; Leonard, P.; Peyrot Des Gachons, S.; et al. Traumatic ligamentous instability of the cervical spine in children. J Pediatr Orthop 4:339–345, 1984.

**Nerve Injuries**

204. Amillo, S.; Mora, G. Surgical management of neural injuries associated with elbow fractures in children. J Pediatric Orthop 19:573–577, 1999.

205. Barrios, C.; de Pablos, J. Surgical management of nerve injuries of the upper extremity in children: A 15-year survey. J Pediatr Orthop 11:641–645, 1991.

206. Bolitho, D.G.; Boustred, M.; Hudson, D.A.; Hodgetts, K. Primary epineural repair of the ulnar nerve in children. J Hand Surg [Am] 24:16–20, 1999.

207. Brown, I.C.; Zinar, D.M. Traumatic and iatrogenic neurological complications after supracondylar humerus fractures in children. J Pediatr Orthop 15:440–443, 1995.

208. Campbell, C.C.; Waters, P.M.; Emans, J.B.; et al. Neurovascular injury and displacement in type III supracondylar humerus fractures. J Pediatr Orthop 15:47–52, 1995.

209. Dormans, J.P.; Squillante, R.; Sharf, H. Acute neurovascular complications with supracondylar humerus fractures in children. J Hand Surg [Am] 20:1–4, 1995.

210. Geutjens, G.G. Ischaemic anterior interosseous nerve injuries following supracondylar fractures of the humerus in children. Injury 26:343–344, 1995.

211. Green, N.E. Entrapment of the median nerve following elbow dislocation. J Pediatr Orthop 3:384–386, 1983.

212. Hallett, J. Entrapment of the median nerve after dislocation of the elbow. A case report. J Bone Joint Surg Br 63:408–412, 1981.

213. Kiyoshige, Y. Critical displacement of neural injuries in supracondylar humeral fractures in children. J Pediatr Orthop 19:816–817, 1999.

214. McGraw, J.J.; Akbarnia, B.A.; Hanel, D.P.; et al. Neurological complications resulting from supracondylar fractures of the humerus in children. J Pediatr Orthop 6:647–650, 1986.

215. Pritchett, J.W. Entrapment of the median nerve after dislocation of the elbow. J Pediatr Orthop 4:752–753, 1984.

216. Royle, S.G.; Burke, D. Ulna neuropathy after elbow injury in children. J Pediatr Orthop 10:495–496, 1990.

217. The, R.M.; Severijnen, R.S.V.M. Neurological complications in children with supracondylar fractures of the humerus. Eur J Surg 165:180–182, 1999.

218. Waters, P.M.; Kolettis, G.J.; Schwend, R. Acute median neuropathy following physeal fractures of the distal radius. J Pediatr Orthop 14:173–177, 1994.

## Reflex Sympathetic Dystrophy

219. Bernstein, B.H.; Singsen, B.H.; Kent, J.T.; et al. Reflex neurovascular dystrophy in childhood. J Pediatr 93:211–215, 1978.
220. Chelmisky, T.C.; Low, P.A.; Naessens, J.M.; et al. Value of autonomic testing in reflex sympathetic dystrophy. Mayo Clin Proc 70:1029–1040, 1995.
221. Dietz, F.R.; Mathews, K.D.; Montgomery, W.J. Reflex sympathetic dystrophy in children. Clin Orthop 258:225–231, 1990.
222. Doolan, L.A.; Brown, T.C.K. Reflex sympathetic dystrophy in a child. Anaesth Intensive Care 12:70–72, 1984.
223. Fermaglich, D.R. Reflex sympathetic dystrophy in children. Pediatrics 60:881–883, 1977.
224. Forster, R.S.; Fu, F.H. Reflex sympathetic dystrophy in children. A case report and review of the literature. Orthopaedics 8:475–477, 1985.
225. Muizelaar, J.P.; Kleyer, M.; Hertogs, I.A.; DeLange, D.C. Complex regional pain syndrome (reflex sympathetic dystrophy and causalgia): Management with the calcium channel blocker nifedipine and/or the alpha-sympathetic blocker phenoxybenzamine in 59 patients. Clin Neurol Neurosurg 99:26–30, 1997.
226. Murray, C.S.; Cohen, A.; Perkins, T.; et al. Morbidity in reflex sympathetic dystrophy. Arch Dis Child 82:231–233, 2000.
227. Ruggeri, S.B.; Athreya, B.H.; Doughty, R.; et al. Reflex sympathetic dystrophy in children. Clin Orthop 163:225–230, 1982.
228. Rush, P.J.; Wilmot, D.; Saunders, N.; et al. Severe reflex neurovascular dystrophy in childhood. Arthritis Rheum 25:952–956, 1985.
229. Sherry, D.D.; Weisman, R. Psychologic aspects of childhood reflex neurovascular dystrophy. Pediatrics 81:572–578, 1988.
230. Silber, T.J.; Majd, M. Reflex sympathetic dystrophy syndrome in children and adolescents. Report of 18 cases and review of the literature. Am J Dis Child 142:1325–1330, 1988.
231. Stanton, R.P.; Malcolm, J.R.; Wesdock, K.A.; Singsen, B.H. Reflex sympathetic dystrophy in children: An orthopedic perspective. Orthopedics 16:773–780, 1993.
232. Veldman, P.H.J.M.; Goris, R.J.A. Multiple reflex sympathetic dystrophy. Which patients are at risk for developing a recurrence of reflex sympathetic dystrophy in the same or another limb. Pain 64:463–466, 1996.
233. Wilder, R.T.; Berde, C.B.; Wolohan, M.; et al. Reflex sympathetic dystrophy in children. J Bone Joint Surg Am 74:910–919, 1992.
234. Wotring, K.; Mehn, J.; Stengem, C. Evaluation and treatment of the pediatric reflex neurovascular dystrophy patient. Arthritis Rheum 28(Suppl):143, 1985.

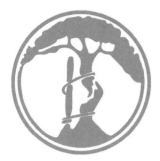

# 7

# Outcomes Assessment in Children with Fractures

James G. Wright, M.D., M.P.H., F.R.C.S.C.
Nancy L. Young, Ph.D.

Orthopaedic surgeons may ask what outcomes assessment has to do with pediatric fractures. When managing a child with a broken bone, orthopaedic surgeons need to choose the best treatment for that particular child with that particular fracture. Although the surgical literature has focused predominantly on radiographic and range-of-motion assessment, increasingly subjective patient assessment, often referred to as outcomes assessment, is being used both in clinical practice and in the literature to evaluate the effects of treatment.[78] Thus, surgeons need to understand these measures to decide whether they have any role in routine clinical practice and to appraise research that uses subjective patient measures to evaluate treatment.

Orthopaedic treatments can have one or more of the following aims: preserve life, treat symptoms or complaints (usually pain), restore function, and prevent future functional decline.[82, 85] The most common issue for children with fractures is restoration of normal function. Occasionally, the issue is prevention of future (often long-term) decline in function.[92] For example, patients with intra-articular incongruity or deformity from a fracture may have no complaints for many years, but treatment is intended to prevent the development of osteoarthritis.

Selection of a measure to evaluate orthopaedic treatment must be given careful consideration and must reflect the aims of treatment. A comparison of the outcomes between two treatments (or between treatment and no treatment) is used to make inferences about treatment effectiveness.[16] Selection of an inappropriate measure may lead to incorrect conclusions regarding fracture management. This chapter concentrates on the different measures that may be used to evaluate treatment options in children with musculoskeletal trauma. The chapter begins with a discussion of the relative advantages and disadvantages of various approaches to outcome measurement. Because the two most important outcomes of fracture treatment in children are arguably restoration of function and prevention of future func-

tional decline, the second section discusses the existing measures that have been described to measure health and physical function in children and provides a brief introduction to measurement development and evaluation by using as an example the Activities Scale for Kids (ASK).[90] The third section discusses some of the specific methodologic problems of measuring function in children, including the effect of age, growth, and development, and addresses the question of whether children can reliably and validly complete questionnaires, who the respondent should be (child, parent, or proxy), and the effect of context (capability or performance) on the measurement of disability.

## APPROACHES TO EVALUATION OF TREATMENT IN PEDIATRIC ORTHOPAEDICS

Fracture treatment can be evaluated by assessing both nonclinical and clinical outcomes. Outcome in the broadest sense refers to any effect of treatment. Nonclinical outcomes include data on the process of care, such as cost and length of stay. Clinical outcomes focus on mortality and morbidity and include complications of treatment and measures of impairment, disability, handicap, and quality of life.

This section begins with a discussion of nonclinical outcomes—specifically, different types of cost analyses—followed by a discussion of clinical outcomes.

### Cost Analysis

Nonclinical outcomes such as cost of treatment are primarily of interest to hospital administrators, third-party payers, and health policymakers. Approaches used to compare the relative costs and benefits of different treatments include cost-effectiveness, cost-benefit, and cost-utility analysis. Cost-effectiveness analysis is defined as the incremental cost divided by the incremental health benefit for patients.[10] Cost-benefit analysis translates the health benefits (to patients) into dollar values (e.g., cost per year of life gained). Cost-utility analysis assigns relative weights or importance values to the outcomes of treatment. These numeric weights, called utilities, refer to the subjective values associated with different health states.[63] Although the relative cost of different treatments is important, cost is particularly relevant when two treatments provide similar clinical outcomes.

Cost-effectiveness analysis has been used in many areas of medicine to compare treatments. If a new treatment both improves patient outcomes and saves money (such as polio immunizations), the treatment is deemed "dominant."[10] Dominant treatments should be adopted because they would both benefit patients and save money.[10] However, decisions in fracture management are rarely that simple because most new treatments are more expensive. Cost-effectiveness analysis, the most common form of cost analysis, allows comparisons between treatments by integrating information about both cost and clinical effectiveness. Cost-effectiveness analysis was used in Oregon to decide which services would be covered by Medicaid to maximize patient benefit when confronted with fixed resources.[73, 76] Arbitrary guidelines have been suggested whereby treatments with cost-effectiveness in excess of $100,000 per quality-adjusted life-year have relatively poor cost-effectiveness whereas those with less than $20,000 per quality-adjusted life-year have relatively good cost-effectiveness ratios.[45]

Cost-effectiveness analysis requires a determination of both the cost and the effectiveness of treatments. Accurate cost analysis requires complete cost accounting, including both direct costs (those directly attributable to the intervention, such as surgeon fees) and indirect costs (those not directly attributable to treatment, such as overhead cost to maintain the hospital facility and the cost borne by families).[8] The outcome (used to determine the effectiveness component of cost-effectiveness analysis) must be expressed in meaningful and appropriate units that allow comparisons between treatments. Treatment effectiveness is usually expressed in terms of clinical outcomes, which is discussed in the next section.

## Clinical Outcomes

Clinical outcomes are most relevant to surgeons and patients. Mortality is an infrequent outcome of most pediatric interventions. Thus, morbidity, including complications and measures of impairment, disability, handicap, and quality of life, should be the primary focus of most orthopaedic evaluations.[85]

When considering possible clinical outcomes to evaluate a surgical treatment, the framework of the World Health Organization International Classification of Impairment, Disability, and Handicap is helpful.[4, 79] Impairment, such as fracture deformity, refers to restrictions in physiologic or anatomic structure or function. Impairment is believed to result in disability (also called activity restriction), which in turn leads to handicap (also called participation restriction). Impairment measures can be physiologic (joint rotation or muscle strength), radiographic (adequacy of fracture reduction or limb alignment), or observational (gait analysis). Impairment measures are of major interest for orthopaedic surgeons because treatment is directed toward improving impairments, such as reducing a fracture. However, as discussed in further detail later, patients are more concerned with disability and handicap. Furthermore, improvement in impairment does not always lead to improvement in disability, and multiple factors other than treatment may affect children's functional status.[66, 80]

Objective measures of impairment, such as radiographic assessment, are tangible[83] and immediately relevant to surgeons. The major concern with objective measurements is that they may bear little relevance to patients' expectations of treatment and, more importantly, may not accurately represent changes in functional disability. For example, despite radiographic curve correction in children with spina bifida, walking ability may actually decline after scoliosis surgery.[52] Although objective outcomes such as radiographic measures and range of motion are important and must be measured, they are not sufficient alone. A complete assessment of treatment usually requires adding subjective patient reports.[85]

Subjective patient evaluation of treatment is generally performed with questionnaires or scales. Scales used to evaluate outcomes of fracture treatment can be disease specific or generic measures of health.[61] Disease-specific scales usually consider a single aspect (or domain) of health. Disease-specific measures most often focus on specific aspects of the disease or condition that are important to patients. Moreover, disease-specific measures generally attribute complaints to the specific condition, such as difficulty walking "because of a broken tibia." Generic health status measures have a broader perspective and attempt to measure all aspects of health; in addition to symptoms and physical function, mental, emotional, and social function is included.[77, 79] Finally, quality-of-life measures often consider aspects beyond health status, such as life satisfaction. A complete discussion of pediatric quality of life is beyond the scope of this chapter and can be found elsewhere.[71]

The primary advantage of generic measures of health is that they provide a relatively broad perspective that allows comparisons across different diagnostic groups. The primary advantage of disease-specific scales is that they tend to focus on aspects of the disease that are most relevant to children, their families, and clinicians. Both may be required for a complete assessment of treatment effectiveness.

Several activity-based physical functional disability scales are available to evaluate the effects of fracture treatment in children. However, these scales have not been widely used by orthopaedic surgeons. Surgeons' infrequent use of such scales may be attributed to lack of awareness of the existence of appropriate scales, difficulty obtaining the scales, or unfamiliarity with the factors to be considered when selecting scales.[92] In addition, because measurement of pediatric physical function has special problems (discussed in a later section) that few of the existing scales completely address, surgeons may have deemed these scales inadequate for inclusion in clinical practice or research. The next section addresses these issues and identifies the existing scales that may be appropriate for evaluating function in children.

Satisfaction with care is another element of treatment assessment. Provided that appropriate care has been delivered, family satisfaction with care should be maximized because it may affect compliance with treatment or increase the pursuit of additional health care services. Clinicians' assessment of satisfaction, however, generally differs from that of families.[62, 75] Furthermore, families' satisfaction may be affected by external factors in addition to their medical care.

Issues important to families that may affect satisfaction ratings include adequate communication and clinicians spending sufficient time with their children.[5, 6, 32, 54] Interestingly, one report suggests that parents' perceptions of improvement in their children may be more important than the actual clinical change.[41] In addition, for children in acute care situations, such as in emergency departments, the duration of waiting may be an important determinant of parental satisfaction.[7] Finally, external issues such as socioeconomic status,[81] parental health,[65] and family stress[3] may also affect satisfaction ratings.

## EXISTING PEDIATRIC OUTCOMES MEASURES

The purpose of this section is to aid surgeons in using outcomes measures by first cataloging pediatric physical function measures that have direct application to fracture patients and then explaining options relevant to the selection of an appropriate scale. Second, the processes of instrument development and evaluation will be described by using the example of the Activities Scale for Kids so that those who do not identify an appropriate measure have an understanding of the process involved in developing a new measure.

The first step in selecting an outcome measure is to determine the type of measure desired.[17, 82, 87] Because of the nature of orthopaedic interventions and the effects of most fractures, the physical function component of patient status is most likely to be affected and is therefore the focus of much of this section. Physical function is defined as the "ability to use the musculoskeletal system to interact with the environment in a purposeful way for the performance of activities of daily living, mobility (such as manual dexterity, transfers, ambulation), and leisure activities."[92] Physical function is a distinct subcomponent of more global health measures such as functional status, health status, and quality of life.

## Catalogue of Physical Function Scales

We previously performed a review of physical function measures appropriate for pediatric orthopaedics.[92] The primary intent of the scales shown in Table 7–1 was to quantify children's physical function. We did not include scales developed for adult populations without specific documentation of pediatric applications, developmental milestone inventories (see Ottenbacher and colleagues,[59] for example), or those directed primarily toward patients with neurologic conditions or arthritis.[56]

The scales listed in Table 7–1 are classified in column 7 by whether they are direct or indirect measures. *Direct measures* are scored on the basis of personal observation of the activity or behavior. *Indirect measures* are scored on the basis of reported activity or behavior. *Capability measures* assess what the child can do. *Performance measures* assess what the child does do. Indirect measures are further subdivided according to the method of administration, such as self-report scales or interviewer-administered scales.

Direct methods eliminate the biases of reported information but may be sensitive to environmental effects (such as different clinical settings). Furthermore, direct methods measure capability rather than performance and are quite expensive because they require more time to complete. Indirect methods are more feasible, may have greater consistency of administration (by minimizing environmental effects), and if self-administered, eliminate the biases caused by the presence of an interviewer. Self-report measures may have problems such as uncertain comprehension or interpretation of the questions and the biases of self-reporting.

Capability measures have the advantage of measuring all children in a consistent setting and being able to determine their best ability. However, capability measures may not relate to usual performance or community function. Performance measures may better reflect physical function in daily activities by taking into account the child's usual physical, social, and emotional setting. The distinction is important because improvement in performance often lags behind improvement in capability. For example, a child may have the required range of motion to climb stairs and be capable of doing so but not yet perform the activity at school.[93, 94]

Column 2 of Table 7–1 lists the intended use or purpose of the measures. Scales may be *discriminative* (distinguishing between groups of patients), *evaluative* (detecting change in patients), or *predictive* (forecasting the results of subsequent evaluations).[38] A scale developed for one purpose may not necessarily be valid if used for a different purpose or population.[17] In clinical practice, surgeons are most often interested in evaluating therapeutic efficacy and thus seek evaluative scales.

Other important aspects of choosing among scales are included in columns 3 to 6. Column 3 lists the construct or domains (e.g., physical, mental, social), the format of the question, and how the questions are scored and aggregated. Column 4 describes the clinical populations, such as age or disease group, for which they were developed. Column 5 describes the pragmatic details of administering the measure, including by whom (clinician or self-administered), how (observation or interview), to whom (parent, proxy, or child), the time required, and special equipment requirements.

Column 6 details the measurement properties (or standardization) for each of the scales. Standardization refers to the sensibility, reliability, validity, and responsiveness of a measure.[87] *Sensibility* is defined as

*Text continued on page 162*

**TABLE 7–1**

Physical Function Measures Appropriate for Pediatric Orthopaedics

| Scale Name | Purpose of Scale | Domains, Format, and Scoring | Population | Method of Administration | Standardization of Measure | Taxonomic Class |
|---|---|---|---|---|---|---|
| Functional Independence Measure for Children (WeeFIM)[1, 22, 23, 53, 60, 70] | Burden of care Discriminative Evaluative | Degree of assistance required (provided by a caregiver or assistive device) 7-point ordinal scale 6 subdomains: self-care, sphincter control, mobility, locomotion, communication, social cognition 18 questions derived from previous scales | Adult scale modified for children (0.5–7 yr old) Generic population | Trained clinician observation (different sections to be done by specialist clinicians) | No patient data reported Developers state that face validity and reliability were established in over 50 facilities, but no reference cited Stated to measure performance, but administration requires clinician observation of capability According to Gowland et al.[22]: adequate inter-rater and excellent intrarater reliability; validity information not reported Manual contains sufficient information for use, but no standardization data | Clinician observation of capability Direct measurement (clinical observation) Capability based (can do) |
| Motor Control Assessment (MCA)[72] | Motor control skills (not functional ability) Evaluative | 113 items | 2- to 5-yr-olds Mild to severe physical disability (n = 161, primarily neurologically impaired) | Clinician observation for 30–60 min | Validity: correlation with physical abilities score, 0.9 Reliability ICCs: intrarater = 0.99; inter-rater = 0.97 | Clinician observation of capability Direct measurement (clinical observation) Capability based (can do) |
| Tufts Assessment of Motor Performance (TAMP)[21, 28] | Physical function and motor performance Evaluative | 3 domains: mobility, ADL, and physical aspects of communication 32 items divided into 113 skills Scored on 4 dimensions: assistance (5-point ordinal scale), approach (2 points), pattern (2 points), and proficiency (3 points) | 6 yr and older, including adults (reliability study, n = 20 adults and 20 children[14]; item grouping study, n = 206 subjects 6 to 86 yr of age)[21] Neurologic and musculoskeletal disability | Clinician observation (1 hr) Standard equipment | Intrarater reliability using a videotaped assessment exceeded 0.85 (ICC) for all domain/dimension combinations Factor analysis of data on 206 subjects used to empirically determine item groupings: dynamic balance, fasteners, ambulation, manipulation, mat mobility, typing, grasp/release[21] | Clinician observation of capability Direct measurement (clinical observation) Capability based (can do) |

| Measure | Description | Population | Administration | Validity/Reliability | Method of Measurement |
|---|---|---|---|---|---|
| Klein-Bell ADL Scale[22, 39, 40, 46, 49, 50]<br>ADL function<br>Evaluative<br>Discriminative | 6 domains: dressing, bathing/hygiene, elimination, functional mobility, eating, emergency communication<br>170 skills items<br>Scores: able, unable, N/A<br>Includes age norms beside each question<br>More upper extremity function items than lower | All ages<br>Test population: 10 CP and 10 normal persons | Clinician observation<br>Approximately 1 hr to administer all items | Validity: discriminated between normal CP subjects, $P < .001$<br>Reliability for 5 children, inter-rater ICC = 0.99, test-retest ICC = 0.98<br>Responsiveness: greater change in normal persons than those with CP ($P = .08$) and agreement with parental ratings of change gave a corrected $\kappa$ of 0.77<br>According to Gowland et al.[22]: excellent content validity and reliability, adequate construct validity and responsiveness<br>These conclusions supported by Law and Letts[49] | Clinician observation of capability<br>Direct measurement (clinical observation)<br>Capability based (can do) |
| Barthel Index[22, 49, 51]<br>ADL<br>Discriminative<br>Predictive<br>Evaluative | ADL<br>Ordinal scale | Applied to adult and adolescent chronically disabled patients | Expert clinician observation<br>1 hr complete | According to Law and Letts[49]: excellent content validity, construct validity, inter-rater and intrarater reliability; good responsiveness; poor manual and internal consistency<br>According to Gowland et al.[22]: adequate content validity, criterion validity, inter-rater and intrarater reliability; poor manual; no normative data | Clinician observation of capability<br>Direct measurement (clinical observation)<br>Capability based (can do) |
| Karnofsky Scale[34, 37, 55]<br>Global rating of physical capacity<br>Evaluative<br>Predictive | Based primarily on mobility level<br>Scoring: 0–100 in 10-unit Guttman intervals | Undefined cancer population (generally poor description of samples) | Physician report<br>2 min | Weak evidence for validity demonstrated by comparing measure with other clinical criteria<br>Reliability: achieved 29% and 35% agreement between raters<br>Previous reviewers concluded that the scale is not appropriate for children, particularly preschoolers, and that it is unable to predict recurrence in brain tumor pediatric patients[4] | Physician report of capability<br>Direct measurement (clinical observation)<br>Capability based (can do) |

Continued

**TABLE 7–1**

Physical Function Measures Appropriate for Pediatric Orthopaedics *Continued*

| Scale Name | Purpose of Scale | Domains, Format, and Scoring | Population | Method of Administration | Standardization of Measure | Taxonomic Class |
|---|---|---|---|---|---|---|
| Vineland Adaptive Behavior Scales[22, 69] | Developmental assessment tool<br>Included as example of developmental scale classification | 4 domains: communication, daily living skills, socialization, and motor skills (impairment) | 0–18 yr<br>Normative data based on a large sample of disabled children | Trained clinician interview of parent 20–90 min | Reliability and validity reported by Gowland et al.[22] to be excellent | Interview measure of parent measure of performance<br>Indirect measurement (report of parent, patient, or proxy)<br>Interviewer-administered measure of performance |
| Quality of Well-being[36, 58] | Quality of life<br>Discriminative<br>Evaluative | 3 domains: mobility (5-level ordinal scale), social activity (5-level ordinal scale), physical activity (4-level ordinal scale)<br>Scores weighted according to population preferences<br>Similar to Rand Health Insurance Scale | Adult tool applied to children<br>25 males and 19 females with CF aged 7–36 yr, mean of 16.5 ± 6.9 yr | Interview administered to parents or patient, depending on age | Moderate construct validity assessed by comparing QWB with PFTs and exercise tolerance: QWB/FEV$_1$, $r = 0.6$; QWB/FEF$_{25\%-75\%}$, $r = 0.5$; QWB/PEFR, $r = 0.4$; QWB/Vo$_2$max, $r = 0.6$ | Indirect measurement (report of parent, patient, or proxy)<br>Interviewer administered |
| Canadian Occupational Performance Measure (COMP)[22, 47, 48] | Evaluative<br>Subjects generated their own items<br>Useful for comparison within individual patients rather than between patients | Domains: self-care, productivity, and leisure<br>Dimensions: importance of activities, level of performance, and satisfaction with performance<br>Scoring: 10-category ordinal scales | Not age specific<br>Developed for adults and applied to children | Clinician administered<br>Items spontaneously elicited from each patient<br>Interview of parent or child<br>Considers environmental demands | No evidence of validity or reliability included[22] | Interview measure of capability and performance<br>Indirect measurement (report of parent, patient, or proxy)<br>Interview administered and capability based (can do)<br>Independent/self-administered parent report of performance |

| Instrument | Purpose/Type | Concepts/Scoring | Population/Sample | Administration | Validity/Reliability | Measurement |
|---|---|---|---|---|---|---|
| Pediatric Evaluation of Disability Inventory (PEDI)[26,27] | Physical function and independence measure; Evaluative; Expert reviewers preferred to classify the tool as discriminative rather than evaluative | Domains: self-care, mobility, social function; Scoring dimensions: functional capability, caregiver assistance, environmental modifications; Scored able/unable for 197 functional skill items, 6 ordinal responses for 20 caregiver assistance items, 4 types of environmental modifications for 20 items | Chronically ill and disabled children 0.5–7 yr old | Parent report 20 min to 1 hr to complete | Concurrent validity: moderately high correlation with Battelle Development Screening Test for self-care and mobility domains but not social function domains; Significant differences between normal and disabled samples; Content validity and reliability studies are currently under way but unpublished; Normative data (sample of 412) not yet published; Manual includes a detailed report of standardization that is adequate in all areas of scaling methods discussed; describes calculation of standardized scores[2] | Indirect measurement (report of parent, patient, or proxy); Independent/self-administered |
| Play Performance Scale[43,44] | Play; Evaluative | Concepts based on Karnofsky Scale; Based on active play, quiet play, degree of physical limitation, degree of independence; Scored 0–100 in IQ point increments | 1 to 6 yr old; Brain tumors ($n = 98$ oncology patients $8 \pm 4.71$ yr of age, 29 siblings $8.76 \pm 4.42$ yr old, 40 normal persons $8.59 \pm 4.98$ yr)[44] | Parent report <5 min to complete | Inter-rater reliability (mother vs. father) $r = 0.71$, $n = 41$; Construct validity: detected significant difference between patients and siblings in global measure of performance from nurses and researchers ($r = 0.75$ and $n = 0.92$, respectively)[43] | Parent-reported measure of performance; Indirect measurement (report of parent, patient, or proxy); Independent/self-administered |
| Rand Health Insurance Study Scale (HIS)[13,14] | Physical activity; Discriminative | 4 domains: mobility, physical activity, role activity, and self-care; Children's tool similar to AIMS[7] | Ages 0–13 yr ($n = 2152$ children in 6 U.S. cities)[14] ($n = 3294$ Ontario children aged 4–16 yr)[1]; Healthy populations ($n = 156$ pediatric trauma survivors aged $8.7 \pm 4.4$ yr)[78]; JRA ($n = 62$) 1–19 yr old; Derived from an adult tool | Researcher administered; Parent report | Construct validity: comparison of HIS classification of able/disabled with 11 other scales showed that significant differences were small and the sample large; Found a 57/1000 prevalence of disability[14]; Wesson et al.[78] found the HIS not to be able to discriminate severity in a trauma population; Administered manually | Parent-reported measure of performance; Indirect measurement (report of parent, patient, or proxy); Independent/self-administered |

Continued

**TABLE 7–1**

Physical Function Measures Appropriate for Pediatric Orthopaedics *Continued*

| Scale Name | Purpose of Scale | Domains, Format, and Scoring | Population | Method of Administration | Standardization of Measure | Taxonomic Class |
|---|---|---|---|---|---|---|
| Childhood Health Assessment Questionnaire (CHAQ)[18, 19, 67, 68] | Functional status Evaluative | 8 domains: dressing and grooming, arising, eating, walking, hygiene, reach, grip, and activities 4-point ordinal scale for each item Unusual method of aggregation | JRA ($n = 62$) 1–19 yr old Derived from an adult tool | Parent or patient self-administered 10 min | No documentation of validity or reliability in children Responsiveness: CHAQ was a significant predictor of parents' global rating of change, $P = .02$ Report that "parents are reliable proxy reporters of their children's functional status," but no data or references are provided in support | Parent or self-report of capability Capability based (can do) Independent/self-administered |
| Activity Scale for Kids (ASK)[90–94] | Physical function Evaluative Discriminative | 2 versions: ASK performance and ASK capability 54 items 5-point ordinal scale Items equally weighted Scoring clearly described in manual | 5–15 yr old Musculoskeletal disorders Scale derived from interviews with children | Patient (or parent) self-report | Reliability: intrarater ICC >0.97 Validity: strong association with clinician-reported ASK scores ($r = 0.92$), concordance with parent report (ICC = 0.94) Responsiveness: standardized responses, mean = 1.2 | ASK capability: capability based (can do), independent/self-administered ASK performance: capability based (can do), interviewer administered |
| The POSNA Pediatric Musculoskeletal Functional Health Questionnaire[2, 9] | Health status Evaluative Discriminative | 7 domains: upper extremity, satisfaction, physical function, transfer/mobility, comfort, expectations, global function Ordinal responses | All ages Musculoskeletal disorders Scale derived by experts based on previous scales | Parent or adolescent (11–18 yr old) self-administered | All scales except happiness had internal reliability ≥0.8 for content and construct validity Responsive and sensitive to change | Parent or child report of performance Indirect measurement (report of parent, patient, or proxy) Independent/self-administered |

| Child Health Questionnaire (CHQ)[42] | Discriminative Evaluative | Three parent forms with 98, 50, and 28 items and 87-item child form considering physical functioning, role/social-emotional, role/social-behavioral, role/social-physical, bodily pain, general behavior, mental health, self-esteem, general health perception, change in health, parental impact—emotional, parental impact—time, family activities, family cohesion Families respond to different response categories | Children ≥5 yr | Self-administered | For items, established interval consistency (≥0.4 for 97% of items) and discriminant validity For scales, median reliability estimate of 0.84 Established constructive and discriminative validity | Indirect parent or child self-report of performance (does do) |
|---|---|---|---|---|---|---|

ADL, activities of daily living; AIMS, Arthritis Impact Measurement Scale; CF, cystic fibrosis; CP, cerebral palsy; FEF, forced expiratory flow; $FEV_1$, forced expiratory volume; ICC, intraclass correlation coefficient; JRA, juvenile rheumatoid arthritis; PEFR, peak expiratory flow rate; PFTs, pulmonary function tests; QWB, quality of well-being.
From Young NL et al. J Pediatr Orthop 15:249–251, 1995.

"a mixture of ordinary common sense plus a reasonable knowledge of pathophysiology and clinical reality."[17] *Reliability* (reproducibility or consistency) is the degree with which a scale yields similar answers when the measure is repeated.[84, 88] *Validity* (or accuracy) is the extent to which the scale measures what it is intended to measure.[17] *Responsiveness* (or sensitivity) is the ability of a scale to detect clinically important changes.[25] Some scales have been completely standardized on all criteria.

## Measurement Development and Evaluation

Table 7–1 was provided to aid orthopaedic surgeons in choosing an appropriate measure. Understanding the stages in measurement development may also aid surgeons in choosing among the available scales. The first step in the development of a new measurement or choosing among available measures is to define the purpose of the measurement and conceptualize the clinical domain or phenomenon to be measured.

*Measurement development* is generally performed in two stages: item generation and item reduction.[83, 87] The purpose of item generation is to assemble all potential items for a new scale to ensure an appropriate and comprehensive content. Items should be identified from some or all of the following sources: previous scales and relevant literature, discussion with clinicians, including health professionals, and consultation with families and patients.[17, 57, 74, 83] The second stage of development reduces the number of items by eliminating redundant or inappropriate items. Strategies of item reduction include clinical judgment,[20, 87] patient interviews,[24, 88] and statistical methods (e.g., logistic regression,[30] factor analysis,[57] and item characteristic analysis).[29]

*Measurement evaluation* (or standardization) includes documentation of sensibility, reliability, validity, and responsiveness.[87] The different stages in measurement development and evaluation are illustrated by using as an example a recently developed measure, the ASK.

The ASK focuses on physical disability.[89] It was developed after a comprehensive review of existing scales, and it addressed four deficiencies: few scales were appropriate for children aged 5 to 15 years with musculoskeletal disease; many were not self-report; few scales had documented reliability, validity, and responsiveness; and most important, practically all scales had failed to include children in the development process and therefore might not reflect disability in a child's usual community environments.

We chose a self-report format because abilities observed in the clinical setting often do not reflect abilities in the community. Self-reporting also provides a more feasible form of outcomes measurement that can be used in the home environment. Involvement of children in measurement development is important because the changes observed on scales developed exclusively with the input of clinicians may not reflect the changes that are important to children in their everyday lives in the community. A further justification for the inclusion of

children in the measurement of disability is that the process may help children take responsibility for their disability management.

The ASK was developed in four stages: item generation, item reduction, questionnaire development (formatting and pilot testings), and subsequent field testing (and questionnaire refinement).[90] In all stages the target group was children 5 to 15 years of age (experiencing physical difficulty of musculoskeletal origin). The lower age at which children can complete questionnaires is uncertain but appears to be at least as young as 5 to 7 years.[35, 94] Items for the ASK were generated from previous questionnaires, clinician input, and in-home interviews with children and their parents.[94] Including children is an important aspect of measurement development[64] that improves both the content and phrasing of questions. The number of items was reduced on the basis of input from families, by consensus of a multidisciplinary expert panel, and with the assistance of Rasch analysis.

The ASK has "excellent" test-retest reliability.[94] Validity was ascertained by comparison of the ASK scores with clinician ratings, by concordance with parent reporting, by correlation with the Childhood Health Assessment Questionnaire (CHAQ),[67, 68] and by direct clinician observation of children's function.[90, 91] The ASK has also been shown to be more responsive than the CHAQ.[90] In summary, the ASK currently contains 30 items with both capability and performance versions and serves as one example of a self-report measure of physical function useful for evaluating pediatric fracture treatment.

## METHODOLOGIC DIFFICULTIES OF MEASURING FUNCTION IN CHILDREN

Measuring physical function in children poses special challenges, including how to compensate for the effects of age, growth, and development on function. In addition, it has not been completely resolved whether children can reliably and validly complete questionnaires, who should be the respondent (child, parent, or proxy), and what the effect of context (capability or performance) is on the measurement of disability.[15, 93]

### Age, Growth, and Development

A prime consideration when evaluating the appropriateness of a pediatric scale for a specific population is the applicable age range of the scale and the effects of development on scores. Because of development, age may have a distinct impact on both children's ability to perform certain activities and their relative importance. For example, tricycle riding is an important part of physical function at age 4 but not at age 8, even though the motor skills required are still present.

At least two methods may accommodate for the effects of age.[92] First, a comprehensive scale can be developed that covers physical function across all age groups, such as the Rand Health Insurance Scale.[13, 14] This method is simple and feasible because only one scale is required. However, it has the potential to be less relevant for extreme age groups. For example, physical function scales developed for infants are not relevant to teens. A variation of this method is to have a single scale but to correct for age or stage of development by dividing the child's score by some maximal potential score specific for the child's age. The process of age-adjusted scores, however, requires normative data on the population in question and requires expected scores for disabled children that are not only rarely available but also quite difficult to define.

The second option is to use scales that are appropriate only for narrow age groups. This strategy, however, requires multiple scales to accommodate various age groups and makes measuring the effect of intervention in children who cross over into new age groups somewhat difficult. Thus, scales specific to narrow age ranges are not generally recommended unless a clear transition between scales for different age groups has been determined.

## Can Children Reliably and Validly Complete Questionnaires?

Children may be involved in both questionnaire development and questionnaire completion. Children's competence to participate in scale development depends on their understanding of the concept of disability and their ability to articulate that disability. Furthermore, children's competence to self-report their disabilities is contingent on the evidence that children's self-reports yield reliable and valid responses. Previous literature would suggest that children can provide reliable estimates of their disability.[11, 12] The literature suggests that children usually agree with their parents,[31, 33] particularly for observable behavior such as physical disability.[31, 33]

While developing the ASK, children were asked to identify activities in which they experienced problems or had not done recently because of their physical disability status. Children were as good as, if not better than, their parents at articulating their disability in open-ended interviews. Furthermore, a comparison of scores that children had given for different symptoms demonstrated that children were capable of distinguishing between the components of disability and did not simply give similar answers for their symptoms and disabilities.[94] Children have also been shown to complete the ASK reliably and validly.[94] Thus, children appear to be competent in both scale development and scale utilization.

## Who Should Be the Respondent?

If we accept that many children can competently participate in disability measurement, we must decide whether they should participate in the evaluative process. Clearly, parent reporting is required for children whose communicative capacity is impaired by age, illness, or cognitive ability. Proxy reporting, such as by teachers or health care providers, can be used and may be advantageous when strong parental bias is suspected. Based on the evidence of children's competency, however, children who are competent should probably become the preferred reporters of their physical disability for several reasons. First, children who participate in questionnaire completion may be motivated to become more involved in controlling their physical disability. Second, given the broad scope of environments experienced by children, the information provided by children may be more representative of their usual environments. Because parents (or proxies such as teachers) cannot be expected to know the qualitative aspects of their child's disability or the details of the disability in all environments, use of the child's report may improve the generalizability of results in community settings.

## What Is the Effect of Context on the Measurements of Disability?

Another methodologic issue relevant to measuring physical function in children is the context in which the measurement is performed. Environmental conditions are particularly important when measuring physical function because they define whether capability (what a child *can* do) or performance (what a child *does* do) is being measured and also because these conditions may affect the measurement, such as the degree of motivation or distraction in the presence of parents. Previous research has shown that children consistently report performance at a lower level than capability.[93] Thus, the evaluation of disability does depend on the context on which it is measured.

The decision to measure capability or performance depends somewhat on how the data will be used. Interventions may improve capability in the short term before such improvements have had sufficient time to be integrated into performance. Thus, capability may be favored when the objective is to detect the earliest clinically important change in disability. The primary advantages of performance measures are that they provide a direct assessment of community function and measure limitations of direct relevance to patients. Most musculoskeletal interventions are provided to improve, maintain, or delay deterioration of physical function in the patients' usual environments. Because home, school, and work environments are most meaningful to patients, the use of performance measures may be appropriate. By definition, performance measures are sensitive to changes in the circumstances and the environment of the individual. Because therapeutic interventions such as prescription of an assistive device can change not only the individual but also the environment, increases in performance scores associated with changes in the environment may lead to a reduction in disability. Thus, the goals of the intervention or how you define success and the timing of the outcome assessment must be considered when choosing between a capability measure and a performance measure.

In conclusion, standardized questionnaires are available to assess the effect of fracture treatment on injured children. The choice of a measure must consider the content of the scale and issues of feasibility. The content of the scale can be narrow, such as physical disability using the ASK, or assess multiple domains of health, such as the CHAQ. More feasible scales are those that are short and self-administered. We suggest that children have shown themselves to be competent reporters of their disability, and when age and cognitive abilities permit, they should be the preferred respondents.

## REFERENCES

1. Guide for Use of the Uniform Data Set for Medical Rehabilitation Including the Functional Independence Measure for Children (WeeFIM). New York, Research Foundation, 1991.
2. Pediatrics Outcomes Data Collection Package (Version 1.1). Chicago, American Academy of Orthopaedic Surgeons/Council of Musculoskeletal Specialty Societies, 1996.
3. Auslander, W. Mothers' satisfaction with medical care: Perceptions of racism, family stress, and medical outcomes in children with diabetes. Health Social Work 22(3):190–199, 1997.
4. Badley, E.M. An introduction to the concepts and classifications of the international classification of impairments, disabilities, and handicaps. Disabil Rehabil 15(4):161–178, 1993.
5. Baine, S.; Rosenbaum, P.; King, S. Chronic childhood illnesses: What aspects of caregiving do parents value? Child Care Health Dev 21:291–304, 1995.
6. Bradford, R. Staff accuracy in predicting the concerns of parents of chronically ill children. Child Care Health Dev 17:39–47, 1991.
7. Brown, K. Parent satisfaction with services in an emergency department located at a paediatric teaching hospital. J Paediatr Child Health 31:435–439, 1995.
8. Coyte, P.; Damji, Z.; Trerise, B.S.; et al. An economic evaluation of two treatments for paediatric femoral shaft fractures. Clin Orthop 336:205–215, 1997.
9. Daltroy, L.H.; Liang, M.H.; Fossel, A.H.; et al. The POSNA Pediatric Musculoskeletal Functional Health Questionnaire: Report of reliability, validity, and sensitivity to change. J Pediatr Orthop 18:561–571, 1998.
10. Detsky, A.; Naglie, I. A clinician's guide to cost-effectiveness analysis. Ann Intern Med 113:147–154, 1990.
11. Doherty, E.; Yanni, G.; Conroy, R.M.; et al. A comparison of child and parent ratings of disability and pain in juvenile chronic arthritis. J Rheumatol 20:1563–1566, 1993.
12. Duffy, C.M.; Arsenault, L.; Watanabe Duffy, K.N. Level of agreement between parents and children in rating dysfunction in juvenile rheumatoid arthritis and juvenile spondyloarthritis. J Rheumatol 20:2134–2139, 1993.
13. Eisen, M.; Donald, C.A.; Ware, J.E.J.; Brook, R.H. Conceptualization and Measurement of Health for Children in the Health Insurance Study. RAND R-2313-HEW, May 1980.
14. Eisen, M.; Ware, J.E.; Donal, C.A.; Brook, R.H. Measuring components of children's health status. Med Care 17:902–921, 1979.
15. Erling, A. Methodological considerations in the assessments of health-related quality of life in children. Acta Paediatr Suppl 428:106–107, 1999.
16. Feinstein, A.R. Clinical Epidemiology. The Architecture of Clinical Research. Philadelphia, W.B. Saunders, 1985.
17. Feinstein, A.R. Clinimetrics. Westford, MA, Yale University, 1987.
18. Feldman, A.B.; Haley, S.M.; Coryell, J. Concurrent and construct validity of the Pediatric Evaluation of Disability Inventory. Phys Ther 70:602–610, 1990.
19. Feldman, B.; Anne, A.; Luy, L.; et al. Measuring disability in juvenile dermatomyositis: Validity of the Childhood Health Assessment Questionnaire. J Rheumatol 22:326–331, 1995.
20. Fink, A.; Kosecoff, J.; Chassin, M.; et al. Consensus methods: Characteristics and guidelines for use. Am J Public Health 74:979–983, 1984.

21. Gans, B.M.; Haley, S.M.; Hallenborg, S.C.; et al. Description and interobserver reliability of the Tufts Assessment of Motor Performance. Am J Phys Med Rehabil 67:202–210, 1989.
22. Gowland, C.; King, G.; King, S.; et al. Review of selected measures in neurodevelopmental rehabilitation (a rational approach for selecting measures). In: Neurodevelopmental Clinical Research Unit. Hamilton, Ontario, Canada, Chedoke-McMaster Hospitals, 1991.
23. Granger, C.V.; Hamilton, B.B.; Kayton, R. Guide for Use of the Functional Independence Measure for Children (WeeFIM). New York, Research Foundation, State University of New York, 1989.
24. Guyatt, G.; Bombardier, C.; Tugwell P. Measuring disease-specific quality of life in clinical trials. Can Med Assoc J 134:889–895, 1986.
25. Guyatt, G.; Walter, S.; Norman G. Measuring change over time: Assessing the usefulness of evaluative instruments. J Chronic Dis 40:1129–1133, 1987.
26. Haley, S.M.; Coster, W.J.; Faas, R.M. A content validity study of the Pediatric Evaluation of Disability Inventory. Pediatr Phys Ther 3:177–184, 1991.
27. Haley, S.M.; Coster, W.J.; Ludlow, L.H.; et al. Pediatric Evaluation of Disability Inventory (PEDI). Development, Standardization and Administration Manual. Boston, New England Medical Center Hospitals, 1992.
28. Haley, S.M.; Ludlow, L.H.; Gans, B.M.; et al. Tufts assessment of motor performance: An empirical approach to identify motor performance categories. Arch Phys Med Rehabil 72:259–266, 1991.
29. Hambleton, R.; Swaminathan, H.; Rogers, J. Fundamentals of Item Response Theory. Sage Publications Inc., Newbury Park, CA, 1991.
30. Harrell F.; Lee, K. Regression modelling strategies for improved prognostic prediction. Stat Med 3:142–152, 1984.
31. Herjanic, B.; Reich, W. Development of a structured psychiatric interview for children: Agreement between child and parent on individual symptoms. J Abnormal Child Psychol 10:308–324, 1982.
32. Homer, C.; Fowler, F.; Gallagher, P.; et al. The Consumer Assessment of Health Plan Study (CAHPS) survey of children's health care. Jt Comm J Qual Improv 25:369–377, 1999.
33. Howe, S.; Levinson, J.; Shear, E.; et al. Development of a disability measurement tool for juvenile rheumatoid arthritis. Arthritis Rheum 34:873–880, 1991.
34. Hutchison, T.A.; Boyd, N.F.; Feinstein, A.R.; et al. Scientific problems in clinical scales, as demonstrated in the Karnofsky Index of Performance Status. J Chronic Dis 32:661–666, 1979.
35. Juniper, E.; Guyatt, G.; Feeny, D.; et al. Minimum skills required by children to complete health-related quality of life instruments for asthma: Comparison of measurement properties. Eur Respir J 10:2285–2294, 1997.
36. Kaplan, R.M.; Bush, J.W.; Berry, C.C. The Reliability, Stability, and Generalizability of a Health Status Index. Proceedings of the Social Statistics Sections. Alexandria, VA, American Statistical Association, 1978, pp. 704–709.
37. Karnofsky, D.A.; Burchenall, J.H. The clinical evaluation of chemotherapeutic agents in cancer. In: McLeod, C.M., ed. Evaluation of Chemotherapeutic Agents. New York, Columbia University Press, 1949, pp. 190–204.
38. Kirshner, B.; Guyatt, G. A methodological framework for assessing health indices. J Chronic Dis 38:27–36, 1985.
39. Klein, R.M.; Bell, B. The Klein-Bell ADL Scale Manual. Seattle, University of Washington Medical School, Health Sciences Resource Center/SB-56, 1979.
40. Klein, R.M.; Bell, B. Self-care skills: Behavioural measurement with the Klein-Bell ADL scale. Arch Phys Med Rehabil 63:335–338, 1982.
41. Lambert, W. Clinical outcome, consumer satisfaction, and ad hoc ratings of improvement in children's mental health. J Consult Clin Psychol 66:270–279, 1998.
42. Landgraf, J.M.; Abetz, L.; Ware, J.E.J. Child Health Questionnaire (CHQ): A user's manual. The Health Institute, New England Medical Center, Boston, 1996.
43. Lansky, L.L.; List, M.A.; Lansky, S.B.; et al. Toward the development of a Play Performance Scale for Children (PPSC). Cancer 56:1837–1840, 1985.

44. Lansky, S.; List, M.; Lansky, L.; et al. The measurement of performance in childhood cancer patients. Cancer 60:1651–1656, 1987.
45. Laupacis, A.; Feeny, D.; Detsky, A.; et al. How attractive does a new technology have to be to warrant adoption and utilization? Tentative guidelines for using clinical and economic evaluations. Can Med Assoc J 146:473–481, 1992.
46. Law, M. Copy of the Klein-Bell ADL Scale with Age Norms Applied. Hamilton, Ontario, McMaster University, 1992.
47. Law, M.; Baptiste, S.; Darswell-Opzoomer, A.; et al. The Canadian Occupational Performance Measure. Toronto, CAOT Publications, 1991.
48. Law, M.; Baptiste, S.; McColl, M.A.; et al. The Canadian Occupational Performance Measure: An outcome measure for occupational therapy. Can J Occup Ther 57:82–91, 1990.
49. Law, M.; Letts, L. A critical review of scales of activities of daily living. Am J Occup Ther 43:522–528, 1989.
50. Law, M.; Usher, P. Validation of the Klein-Bell Activities of Daily Living Scale for children. Can J Occup Ther 55:63–68, 1988.
51. Mahoney, F.I.; Barthel, D.W. Functional evaluation: The Barthel Index. Md State Med J 14:61–65, 1965.
52. Mazur, J.; Menelaus, M.B.; Dickens, D.R.; Doig, W.G. Efficacy of surgical management for scoliosis in myelomeningocele: Correction of deformity and alterations of functional status. J Pediatr Orthop 6:568–575, 1986.
53. McCabe, M.A.; Granger, C.V. Content validity of a pediatric functional independence measure. Appl Nurs Res 3:120–122, 1990.
54. McKay, M.; Hensey, O. From the other side: Parents' view of their early contacts with health professionals. Child Care Health Dev 16:373–381, 1990.
55. Milstein, J.; Cohen, M.; Sinks, L. The influence and reliability of neurologic assessment and Karnofsky performance score on prognosis. Cancer 56:1834–1836, 1985.
56. Murray, K. Functional measures in children with rheumatic diseases. Pediatr Rheumatol 42:1127–1154, 1995.
57. Nunnally, J.C. Psychometric Theory. New York, McGraw-Hill, 1978.
58. Orenstein, D.M.; Nixon, P.A.; Ross, E.A.; et al. The quality of well-being in cystic fibrosis. Chest 95:344–347, 1989.
59. Ottenbacher, K.; Msall, M.; Lyon, N.; et al. Measuring developmental and functional status in children with disabilities. Dev Med Child Neurol 41:186–194, 1999.
60. Ottenbacher, K.J.; Msall, M.E.; Lyon, N.R.; et al. Interrater agreement and stability of the Functional Independence Measure for Children (WeeFIM): Use in children with developmental disabilities. Arch Phys Med Rehabil 78:1309–1315, 1997.
61. Patrick, D.; Deyo R. Generic and disease-specific measures in assessing health status and quality of life. Med Care 27(Suppl):217–232, 1989.
62. Rey, J.; Plapp, J.; Simpson P. Parental satisfaction and outcome: A 4-year study in a child and adolescent mental health service. Aust N Z J Psychiatry 33:22–28, 1999.
63. Robinson, R. Economic evaluation and health care. Cost-utilization analysis. BMJ 307:859–862, 1993.
64. Ronen, G.; Rosenbaum, P.; Law, M.; Streiner, D. Health-related quality of life in childhood epilepsy: The results of children's participation in identifying the components. Dev Med Child Neurol 41:554–559, 1999.
65. Shaul, J. The impact of having parents report about both their own and their children's experiences with health insurance plans. Med Care 37(Suppl):59–68, 1999.
66. Simeonsson, R.; Lollar, D.; Hollowell, J.; Adams, M. Revision of the International Classification of Impairments, Disabilities, and Handicaps. J Clin Epidemiol 53:113–124, 2000.
67. Singh, G. Copy of Childhood Health Assessment Questionnaire and Guidelines. Stanford, CA, Stanford University School of Medicine, 1992.
68. Singh, G.; Athreya, B.; Fries, J.; Goldsmith, D. Measurement of health status in children with juvenile rheumatoid arthritis. Arthritis Rheum 37:1761–1769, 1994.
69. Sparrow, S.; Balla, D.; Cicchetti, D. Vineland Adaptive Behavior Scales, Interview Edition: Survey Form Manual. Circle Pines, MN, American Guidance Service, 1984.
70. Sperle, P.A.; Ottenbacher, K.J.; Braun, S.L.; et al. Equivalence reliability of the Functional Independence Measure for Children (WeeFIM) administration methods. Am J Occup Ther 51:35–41, 1997.
71. Spieth, L.E.; Harris, C.V. Assessment of health-related quality of life in children and adolescents: An integrative review. J Pediatric Psychol 21:175–193, 1995.
72. Steel, K.O.; Glover, J.E.; Spasoff, R.A. The motor control assessment: An instrument to measure motor control in physically disabled children. Arch Phys Med Rehabil 72:549–553, 1991.
73. Steinbrook, L.B.S.B. The Oregon Medicaid demonstration project—will it provide adequate medical care? N Engl J Med 326:340–344, 1992.
74. Streiner, D.L.; Norman, G.R. Health Measurement Scales. A Practical Guide to Their Development and Use. New York, Oxford University Press, 1995.
75. Thornton, N. Congruence between parent satisfaction with nursing care of their children and nurses' perceptions of parent satisfaction. Axone 18(2):27–37, 1996.
76. Ubel, P.; DeKay, M.; Baron, J.; et al. Cost-effectiveness analysis in a setting of budget constraints. Is it equitable? N Engl J Med 334:1174–1177, 1996.
77. Ware, J. Standards for validating health measures: Definition and content. J Chronic Dis 40:473–480, 1987.
78. Wesson, D.E.; Williams, J.I.; Spence, L.J.; et al. Functional outcome in paediatric trauma. J Trauma 29:589–592, 1989.
79. WHO. International classification of impairments, disabilities, and handicaps. Geneva, World Health Organization, 1980.
80. Wilson, I.B.; Cleary, P.D. Linking clinical variables with health-related quality of life. JAMA 273:59–65, 1995.
81. Wood, D. Are poor families satisfied with the medical care their children receive? Pediatrics 90:66–70, 1992.
82. Wright, J. New directions in orthopaedic clinical research: Outcomes research, clinical trials, and cost-effectiveness analysis. AAOS Bull 41(4):24–25, 1993.
83. Wright, J.; Feinstein, A. A comparative contrast of clinimetric and psychometric methods for constructing indexes and rating scales. J Clin Epidemiol 11:1201–1218, 1992.
84. Wright, J.; Treble, N.; Feinstein, A. The reliability of measurement of lower limb alignment using long radiographs. J Bone Joint Surg Br 73:721–723, 1991.
85. Wright, J.G. Quality-of-life in orthopaedics. In: Quality of Life and Pharmacoeconomics in Clinical Trials. Philadelphia, Lippincott-Raven, 1996, pp. 1039–1044.
86. Wright, J.G.; Feinstein, A.R. Improving the reliability of orthopaedic measurements. J Bone Joint Surg Br 74:287–291, 1992.
87. Wright, J.G.; McLeod, R.S.; Lossing, A.; et al. Measurement in surgical clinical research. Surgery 119:241–244, 1996.
88. Wright, J.G.; Rudicel, S.; Feinstein, A.R. Ask patients what they want. Evaluation of individual complaints before total hip replacement. J Bone Joint Surg Br 76:229–234, 1994.
89. Young, N.; Williams, J.; Yoshida, K.; Wright, J. Towards outcome assessment in paediatric orthopaedics: Introducing the Activities Scale for Kids (ASK). Paper presented at the Canadian Orthopaedic Association annual meeting, Quebec City, 1996.
90. Young, N.L.; Williams, J.; Yoshida, K.; Wright, J.G. Measurement properties of the Activities Scale for Kids (ASK). J Clin Epidemiol 53:125–137, 2000.
91. Young, N.L.; Williams, J.I.; Yoshida, K.K.; Wright, J.G. Methods of validity assessment for pediatric scales [abstract]. J Invest Med 44:309, 1996.
92. Young, N.L.; Wright, J.G. Measuring paediatric physical function in children. J Pediatr Orthop 15:244–253, 1995.
93. Young, N.L.; Yoshida, K.K.; Williams, J.I.; et al. The context of measuring disability. Does it matter whether capability or performance is measured? J Clin Epidemiol 49:1097–1101, 1996.
94. Young, N.L.; Yoshida, K.K.; Williams, J.I.; et al. The role of children in reporting their physical function. Arch Phys Med Rehabil 76:913–918, 1995.

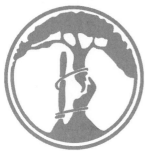

# CHAPTER 8

# Fractures of the Forearm, Wrist, and Hand

Peter F. Armstrong, M.D., F.R.C.S.(C.)
V. Elaine Joughin, M.D., F.R.C.S.(C.)
Howard M. Clarke, M.D., Ph.D., F.R.C.S.(C.), F.A.A.P., F.A.C.S.
R. Baxter Willis, M.D., F.R.C.S.(C.)

## FRACTURES OF THE FOREARM

Forearm fractures are common injuries in childhood. They account for 45% of all fractures in children and for 62% of upper limb fractures. The vast majority (81%) occur in children who are older than 5 years, with a peak incidence of distal forearm fractures occurring at ages 10 to 12 in girls and 12 to 14 in boys.[6, 82]

The most common cause of forearm fractures is a fall in or around the home. Sports-related injuries are next in frequency.[198] The peak incidence of these fractures occurs from April through September, when children are more likely to be playing outdoors.[44]

Approximately 75% to 84% of forearm fractures occur in the distal third, 15% to 18% in the middle third, and 1% to 7% in the proximal third.[13, 44] A small percentage are bilateral, and as many as 13% have an associated supracondylar fracture.[13, 44, 169] Just over 50% of these fractures are greenstick fractures.[198] Injuries to the distal growth plate of the radius occur in 14% to 18% of forearm fractures.[44, 198] In a study of 500 consecutive fractures in the pediatric age group, the site of a forearm fracture was likely to be more proximal with advancing skeletal age. In contrast, physeal fractures were primarily fractures of early adolescence rather than childhood.[178]

Historically, it has been the standard to treat most of these fractures in children by closed reduction and immobilization in a cast. It was thought that remodeling with growth would correct residual deformity, even if anatomic reduction could not be achieved or maintained. Although this standard is true in many instances, several studies have shown that complete remodeling does not always occur, especially in children older than 8

to 10 years. These children have insufficient growth and remodeling potential remaining to provide correction of significant residual deformity.[25, 27, 76, 107]

Rotation of the forearm is the motion most frequently lost after these fractures.[107] Residual rotational losses of greater than 20° have been found in 60% of patients who were treated for forearm fractures.[27, 33] Subjective results, however, are usually excellent, and decreased range of motion is often detectable only by special goniometric testing.[25, 27] Mild limitations in rotation are not noticeable to the patient because abduction and internal rotation at the shoulder adequately compensate for any loss in pronation and because adduction and external rotation of the shoulder may partially compensate for limitation in supination.[80] Therefore, even with stringent criteria, 85% of patients with displaced fractures achieve satisfactory results from closed reduction of the forearm.[25, 27]

Nevertheless, we believe that a number of important principles should be followed to achieve the ideal goal of fracture healing without deformity or dysfunction. It is important that every effort be made to achieve an adequate, but not necessarily anatomic reduction. In certain instances, open reduction and internal fixation may be required.[139]

## General Principles

As with all fractures, the basic principle is to accurately align, both axially and rotationally, the distal fracture fragments with the proximal fragments and maintain this position until the fracture has healed. Managing fractures of the forearm in children requires an understanding of several factors: (1) anatomy of the forearm, (2) deforming muscular forces, (3) the mechanism of injury, and (4) remodeling potential.

## ANATOMY

To accurately align fractures in the forearm, the basic anatomy of the forearm must be understood, including the normal shape of the forearm bones, the normal shape and importance of the interosseous space, and the anatomy of the proximal and distal radioulnar articulations. Children's fractures are different from fractures in adults in that growth and remodeling continue after the fracture has healed. This growth potential exists until the physes close at maturity. Thus, it is important to be aware of the timing of growth plate closure to determine the extent of remodeling capacity remaining.

**Development.** The radius and ulna ossify from primary ossification centers in the eighth week of gestation. At the wrist, the secondary ossification center of the distal radial epiphysis appears within the first year in girls and at just over 1 year of age in boys. A separate ossification center in the tip of the radial styloid process may be present and could be confused with a fracture. The distal ulnar epiphysis begins to ossify at 6 years in both girls and boys and often develops from two centers. The distal radial and ulnar physes contribute 75% to 80% of the total growth of the forearm.[31] Closure of the distal radial physis occurs at approximately 17 years of age in girls and 18 to 19 years in boys. The distal ulnar physis closes at between 16 and 17 years in girls and 17 and 18 years in boys.[53, 78, 125]

At the elbow, the proximal radial physis appears in the 5th to 7th year, and the proximal ulnar physis appears in the 9th to 10th year in both boys and girls. Both physes unite with the shaft between the ages of 16 and 18 years[78] (Fig. 8–1).

**Osteology.** The radius is a curved bone that is cylindrical in the proximal third and triangular in the middle third and flattens out in the lower end. The interosseous membrane attaches to the apex of the triangle on the radius. The bicipital tuberosity, which is the insertion point for the biceps tendon, is located just below the neck of the radius. In the supinated position, the shaft normally bows laterally distal to the bicipital tuberosity. In addition, the radius has a mild posterior bow, with the apex in the midshaft region. Distally and laterally, the radial styloid forms the insertion point for the brachioradialis.

The ulna has a triangular shape throughout the shaft, and the interosseous membrane attaches at its sharp lateral border. Like the radius, the ulna has a bow, but its apex is located posteriorly in the proximal third. In accurate reductions of fractures in the forearm, the anatomic contour of these bones must be restored to fully regain pronation and supination (Fig. 8–2).

**Radioulnar Articulations.** The radius is connected to the ulna via the proximal radioulnar articulation, the interosseous membrane, and the distal radioulnar articulation. Because the forearm is a two-bone complex, injury usually results in fracture of both bones or fracture of one bone associated with injury to one of the radioulnar articulations. Infrequently, especially with

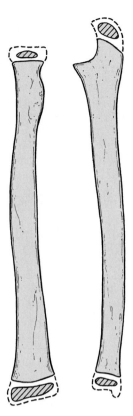

**FIGURE 8–1.** Ossification centers of the radius and ulna.

direct-blow injuries, a fracture to one bone may occur without any radiologic evidence of injury to the other bone. It is important to check radiographs carefully, including both the proximal and distal joints, to ensure that the other bone has not been injured.

Proximally, the radial head articulates with the capitellum and proximal end of the ulna. The annular ligament is the major structure responsible for maintaining stability of the proximal radioulnar joint. This joint is most stable in supination. In supination, the broadest portion of the articular surface of the radial head comes into contact with the proximal notch of the ulna, the interosseous membrane is most taut, and the anterior fibers of the quadrate ligament (a broad ligament between the lateral aspect of the ulna and medial portion of the radius) stabilize the radial head within the proximal radioulnar joint complex[166] (Fig. 8–3). In pronation and supination, the head of the radius pivots within the annular ligament, and the lower end of the radius swings around the head of the ulna, which is contained by the triangular fibrocartilage complex (TFCC).

The TFCC is composed of an articular disc, called the triangular fibrocartilage, that is joined by the volar and dorsal radiocarpal ligaments and by fibers of the ulnar collateral ligament at the wrist (Fig. 8–4). The triangular fibrocartilage is attached to the margin of the radius, and it separates the ulnar notch from the carpal articular surface. Its apex is fixed in the fossa at the base of the styloid process of the ulna. The triangular fibrocartilage measures about 1 cm and is thickest at the circumference, at which point it is connected with the articular

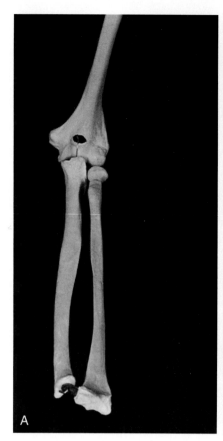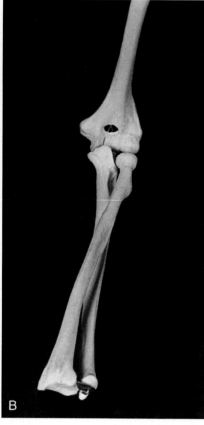

A    B

**FIGURE 8–2.** The appearance of the radius and ulna in supination (*A*) and pronation (*B*).

capsule. It firmly unites the distal ends of the bones. In addition, the triangular fibrocartilage limits the rotational movements of the radius and ulna and maintains congruity of the radioulnar joint against the torsional stresses of rotation of the forearm.[110, 146, 153] The distal radioulnar joint is stabilized by the ulnar collateral ligament, which originates from the distal portion of the styloid, by the anterior and posterior radioulnar ligaments, and by the pronator quadratus muscle.[110] The posterior distal radioulnar ligament has been shown to become taut in phase with pronation; the anterior becomes taut with supination.[153]

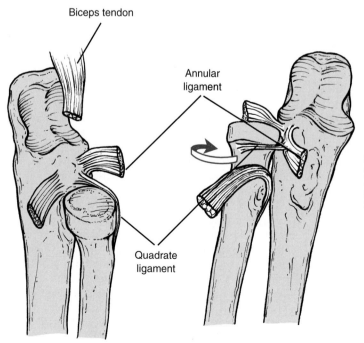

Biceps tendon

Annular ligament

Quadrate ligament

**FIGURE 8–3.** The annular ligament is the major stabilizing structure of the proximal radioulnar articulation. When the forearm is supinated, the anterior border of the quadrate ligament becomes taut and draws the radial head snugly against the radial notch of the ulna. (From Spinner, M.; Kaplan, E.B. Acta Orthop Scand 41:632–647, 1970.)

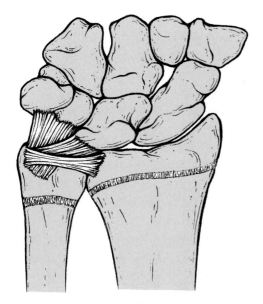

**FIGURE 8–4.** The triangular fibrocartilage complex consists of the triangular fibrocartilage and the ulnocarpal ligaments. It provides the articular surface for the carpus, provides a flexible mechanism for stable rotational movements of the radius and ulna, suspends the ulnar carpus from the radius, and cushions the forces transmitted through the ulnocarpal axis. (From Bowers, W.H. In: Green, D.P., ed. Operative Hand Surgery, 2nd ed., Vol. 2. New York, Churchill Livingstone, 1988, pp. 939–989.)

The distal and proximal radioulnar joints are interdependent for stability. With pronation and supination, movement occurs at each of these joints. Bado noted that with pronation, the radius "shortens" and, with supination, it "lengthens" relative to the ulna.[5] This interdependence may be the reason for late dislocation of the radial head in children who have had significant shortening of the ulna after an injury to its distal end. Similarly, excessive resection of the radial head before the end of growth can cause posterior dislocation of the distal part of the ulna.[153]

The radial and ulnar shafts are connected by the interosseous membrane (Fig. 8–5), and narrowing of the interosseous space has been shown to restrict rotation of the forearm. In a study of cadavers, it was demonstrated that the interosseous distance depends on the position of the forearm. With the forearm in the range of neutral to 30° of supination, the interosseous space forms an elongated ellipse that is widest in the middle third of the forearm. The interosseous membrane becomes increasingly relaxed with further supination or pronation. The narrowest distance was in pronation.[21] From this study it appears that in treating fractures of the forearm, restoring the interosseous distance with the forearm in neutral to 30° of supination is ideal for regaining full rotation.

**Bicipital Tuberosity.** Evans suggested that the bicipital tuberosity could be used as a landmark to determine the rotational position of the proximal fragment to which the distal fragment is aligned.[33] The "tuberosity view," an anteroposterior view of the elbow joint taken with the x-ray tube at an angle of 20° cephalad, was recommended by Evans for determining the position of the bicipital tuberosity relative to the shaft of the radius.[33] In

full supination, the bicipital tuberosity appears on the medial aspect of the radius; in midposition, it appears to be fully superimposed on the shaft of the radius[32] (Fig. 8–6); and in full pronation, it lies in the lateral position.[34] Unfortunately, the bicipital tuberosity is not always well visualized on radiographs of the forearm in children, so this view is less useful than it would first appear.[26, 186] Rotational malalignment can be easily recognized when the width and shape of the proximal and distal fragments do not match at the fracture site or when discontinuity of the normally smooth curvature of the bone is seen after trial reduction (Fig. 8–7). These factors, as well as the stability of the fracture in different positions of the forearm on trial reduction, are often more useful guides in determining the correct rotational alignment of the fracture.

**Forearm Rotation.** The forearm rotates through supination and pronation in an average total range of 150° to 180°.[5, 192] The mechanical axis of the forearm lies along a line connecting the rotational centers of the

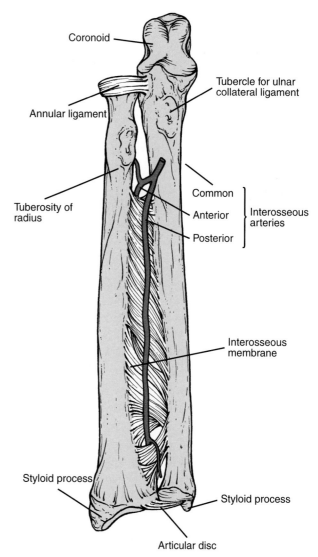

**FIGURE 8–5.** The interosseous membrane. (From Grant, J.C.B. An Atlas of Anatomy, 7th ed. Baltimore, Williams & Wilkins, 1988, Figure 6–51.)

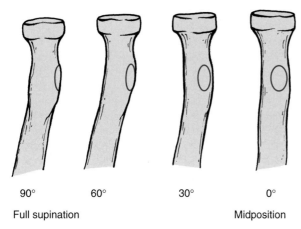

90°  60°  30°  0°

Full supination                    Midposition

FIGURE **8–6.** The radiologic position of the bicipital tuberosity from full supination (90°) to midposition (0°). (From Evans, E.M. J Bone Joint Surg Br 33:548–561, 1951.)

proximal end of the radius and distal end of the ulna (Fig. 8–8). Rotation of the radius about the ulna has been described as a half-cone.[5, 128]

Reduction of the interosseous space by any means results in limitation of the amplitude of the arc through which the radius swings around the ulna. Experimental fractures produced in cadavers and plated in 10° of malrotation create a 10° limitation in rotation. Ten degrees of angulation in the middle third of the shaft limits rotation by 20° to 27° because it produces widening and narrowing of the interosseous membrane during rotatory movements.[107, 173] Bayonet apposition, or overlapping, does not limit rotation as long as the interosseous space is maintained. In proximal fractures, narrowing of the interosseous distance may restrict rotation by causing the bicipital tuberosity to impinge on the ulna. Malalignment of fractures of the distal ulnar metaphysis may increase the tension on the articular disc

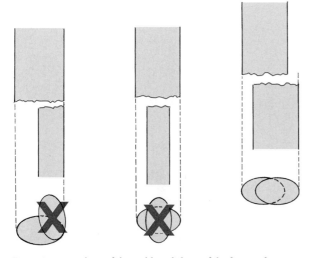

FIGURE **8–7.** Matching of the width and shape of the fracture fragments on radiographs is essential to ensure correct rotational alignment. (From King, R.E. In: Rockwood, C.A.J.; Wilkins, J.E.; King, R.E., eds. Fractures in Children, Vol. 3. Philadelphia, J.B. Lippincott, 1984, pp 301–362.)

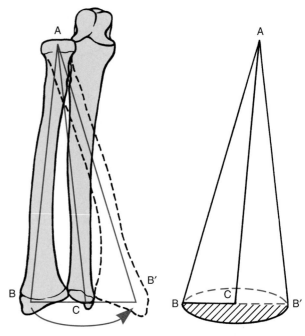

FIGURE **8–8.** The rotation of the radius on the ulna has a mechanical axis from the center of the radial head to the ulnar styloid. (From Ogden, J.A. In: Ogden, J.A., ed. Skeletal Injury in the Child, 2nd ed. Philadelphia, W.B. Saunders, 1990, pp. 451–526.)

so that the head of the ulna does not rotate freely.[142] Soft tissue tension (especially of the interosseous membrane) may be an important factor contributing to the limitation of rotation.[173]

These cadaver studies, of course, do not take into account any remodeling that may occur. Hogstrom and co-workers state that the residual angulation of these fractures coordinates poorly with the range of motion of the involved extremity after healing.[64] Even with fractures that heal in perfect alignment, some loss of forearm rotation may occur.[122]

Open reduction of forearm fractures is not without risk.[25] In children, rotational losses are likely to develop in fractures in the proximal third of the forearm that have been treated by open reduction and internal fixation, even though they have been restored to anatomic alignment.[180] In these cases, the residual impairment in function is probably caused by soft tissue scarring, which must be taken into account when surgical management of a proximal forearm fracture is being considered. Mild angular and rotatory deformities resulting from closed management may produce limitations in motion that are acceptable when compared with the limitations in motion generated by surgical management.[173]

One standard that is useful in assessing the results of fracture treatment is to compare the range of motion with that needed for most activities of daily living. Morrey and associates established that 30° to 130° of flexion at the elbow and 50° of pronation to 50° of supination are needed for most activities of daily living.[114]

Clinically, rotation of the injured forearm is usually compared with that of the opposite normal forearm. Unfortunately, forearm rotation is one of the most difficult clinical measurements to assess accurately and

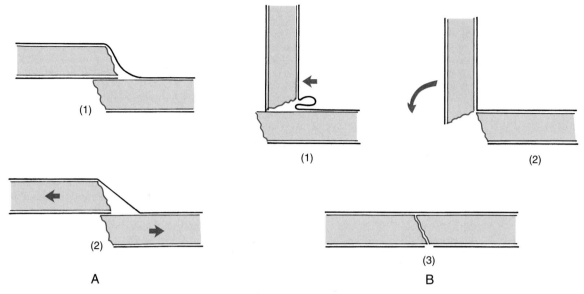

**FIGURE 8–9.** The technique of fracture reduction in children by opening of the periosteal hinge. *A,* Overlapping bone ends with an intact periosteum. Straight longitudinal traction does not reduce the fracture. *B,* The correct procedure for reduction of a fracture with intact periosteum.

reproducibly because the rotation of the carpus is difficult to exclude. Determining the total arc of forearm rotation rather than using separate measurements of pronation and supination is probably a more accurate method of assessing rotation after fracture healing.[114]

It is generally accepted that remodeling of rotational malalignment does not occur, although it has been shown that minor malrotation may spontaneously correct over a period of several years.[139] Experimental studies have shown that 10° of rotatory malalignment does not produce any significant clinical impairment. However, no studies are available that clinically compare supination and pronation at the time of healing with similar range-of-motion studies after remodeling has occurred.

**Periosteum.** Children's bones have very thick pluripotential periosteum. This property contributes to mechanical stability after fracture and rapid healing potential, which allows children to be treated in closed fashion as opposed to the adult treatment approach of open reduction and internal fixation. In the event of a fracture, the periosteum is usually disrupted on the convex, or tension, side at the fracture site, with a "hinge" of intact periosteum remaining on the concave, or compression, side. By applying tension forces on the appropriate side of the cast, the intact periosteum can help in the reduction of a fracture and in the stability and maintenance of the reduction. The pluripotential periosteum rapidly produces new bone to fill in the gap between the bone and the periosteal sleeve. This growth can be evident radiologically within a few weeks of the injury and provides early stabilization at the fracture site.

In a complete fracture with the fragments in bayonet apposition, applying traction to the forearm tightens the periosteal sleeve, locks the fragments in their relative positions, and thus prevents reduction of the fracture. By increasing the deformity and unlocking the hinge, the fracture can be reduced (Fig. 8–9). Once the fracture is reduced, the intact periosteum can be used to stabilize

the reduction by molding the cast appropriately with three-point fixation (Fig. 8–10).

## DEFORMING MUSCULAR FORCES

The muscular attachments in the forearm are important to consider in fracture management. Muscles influence the position of the fragments and create deforming forces that affect the position of both the proximal and the distal fragments within the cast (Fig. 8–11). In the proximal third of the radius, the biceps and the supinator cause flexion and supination of the forearm. The pronator teres inserts into the middle third of the radius and pronates the forearm. In the distal third of the forearm, the brachioradialis, which inserts on the lateral surface of the distal end of the radius above the radial styloid process, pulls the forearm into neutral. The pronator quadratus, the extensors of the wrist and thumb, the abductors of the thumb, and the flexor muscles of the forearm also contribute to fracture deformity; the magnitude of the deforming force depends on the configuration of the fracture.

Traditionally, positioning of the reduced forearm has been based on the location of the fracture in relation to the insertion of the pronator teres. Thus, fractures of the

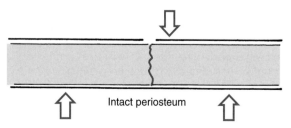

**FIGURE 8–10.** The technique of three-point fixation. Pressure is applied at the *arrows,* thus producing tension on the intact periosteum to stabilize the fracture.

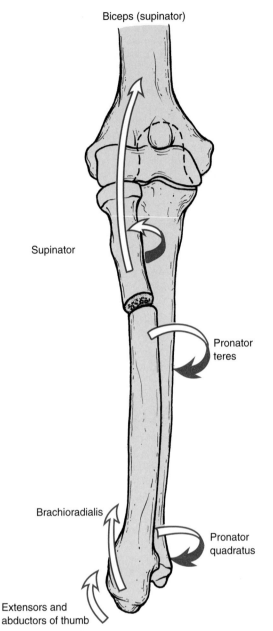

FIGURE **8–11.** Main deforming muscular forces of the forearm. (Redrawn from Cruess, R.L. Orthop Clin North Am 4:969, 1973.)

proximal third should be aligned in supination; in fractures of the middle third, the forearm should be in neutral; and in fractures of the distal third, the forearm should be pronated.[13] Evans disputed this idea and stated that fractures at a given location in the forearm do not necessarily present the same degree of rotational deformity. He found that in all cases, including fractures of the upper and lower thirds, the proximal fragments were supinated. Other factors that may influence the rotational position of the fracture fragments include variations in the direction and leverage of muscle pull at varying degrees of angulation of the fragments, variations in the tension of the biceps tendon with flexion and extension of the elbow, and the effect of the interosseous membrane.[33] Therefore, each fracture must be evaluated on an individual basis to determine the position of the

proximal fragments and, consequently, the best position in which to immobilize the forearm.

## MECHANISM OF INJURY

The most frequent mechanism of injury in forearm fractures is a fall on the outstretched hand.[95] The child automatically puts out the hand to break the fall, usually with the forearm pronated. On landing, the thenar eminence strikes first and places a sudden, supinational force on the pronated forearm. The hand becomes fixed on the ground, and above it, the momentum of the body continues to supinate the forearm. Although angular deformity is apparent on radiographs, in reality, rotational malalignment is present. Thus, reduction must be obtained by pronating the forearm in addition to correcting the angular deformity.[33]

Pronation and flexion are closely allied. A fracture occurring while the forearm is pronating tends to angulate posteriorly at the fracture site. Supination and extension are similarly related, and supination fractures angulate anteriorly (Fig. 8–12). In each case, vertical compression supplies the fracturing force, but the rotational element determines the direction of angulation. With rotational forces, the fractures of the two bones are likely to occur at different levels.

Forced pronation injuries include anterior dislocation of the head of the radius, Galeazzi fracture-dislocation with posterior dislocation of the lower end of the ulna, and anterior Monteggia fracture-dislocation.[33]

Other mechanisms of injury include a direct blow to the forearm and trapping the forearm between two objects (e.g., the bars on a crib). The fracture pattern in these cases is more likely to be a true angular deformity, without a rotational component, so the fractures of the two bones are usually at the same level. Frequently, the mechanism of injury in children cannot be obtained by history. In most cases, however, it can

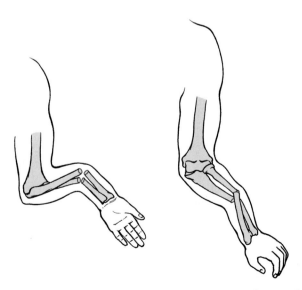

FIGURE **8–12.** Relationship of supination to anterior angulation and pronation to posterior angulation. (From Rang, M. Children's Fractures, 2nd ed. Philadelphia, J.B. Lippincott, 1982, p. 197.)

be deduced by observing the position of the forearm. The fracture is generally reduced by reversing the deformity.

## REMODELING POTENTIAL

Forearm fractures in children can be managed differently from adult fractures because of continuing growth in both the radius and ulna after the fracture has healed. As long as the physes are open, remodeling can occur. It is generally accepted that the amount of spontaneous correction is dependent on the age of the child, the amount of residual angulation at the fracture site, the distance between the fracture and the physes, and the relationship of the deformity to the plane of movement in an adjacent joint.[14, 200, 201]

The time between healing of the fracture and physeal plate closure is an important factor in determining the potential for correction of a deformity. Remodeling at the fracture site occurs by resorption of bone on the convex side and apposition of new bone on the concave side. Correction of angulation is brought about by an alteration in the direction and the amount of longitudinal growth that occurs at the physeal plate. The capacity for this correction is influenced by the degree of angulation of the fracture and the distance from the fracture to the physis[39, 40] (Fig. 8–13).

Friberg showed that fracture deformity at the distal end of the radius corrects at a rate of about 0.9° a month, or 10° a year, as a result of physeal growth. Volar and ulnar angulations result in a higher rate of correction than do dorsal angulations. This redistribution of growth in the physis induced by an abnormal inclination of the plate may be caused by a change in the direction and amplitude of the biomechanical forces acting on the plate.[39] The rate of correction follows an exponential course whereby increased correction takes place when the deformity is greater. Overcorrection by a few degrees has been shown to occur with remodeling.[39] The remodeling potential of fractures of the radius and ulna appears to be greater in the distal part of the shaft than in the midshaft. In their series, Younger and colleagues found that the mean angular correction for midshaft fractures was 4.4°, as compared with 8.6° for distal fractures.[201]

Unfortunately, although generalizations about the amount of remodeling potential can be made, only crude predictions of the amount of correction in a specific patient with a specific fracture are possible.[42] As discussed previously, it is generally believed that rotational deformities do not remodel[25, 27] (Fig. 8–14). A few authors have reported correction of malrotation in young children.[42, 139] These studies were long-term follow-ups of malunited fractures. Although it was not difficult to determine that the rotational malalignment had corrected, no actual measurements of the degree of correction were possible. In the absence of definitive studies concerning the remodeling potential of rotational deformities, it is recommended that rotational malalignment be completely corrected at the time of reduction.

Bayonet apposition is acceptable and will remodel in a child younger than 8 to 10 years if the rotation is correct,

if the interosseous space is preserved, and if the deformity is not angulated[142] (Fig. 8–15).

## Classification

Fractures of the radius and ulna in children can be classified according to fracture type: (1) plastic deformation, or bending of the bone without fracture (Fig. 8–16); (2) buckle, torus, or compression fracture, which appears as a buckling of the bone in the metaphysis (Fig. 8–17); (3) greenstick or incomplete fracture, which occurs through one side of the bone, with the cortex and periosteum intact on the opposite side (Fig. 8–18); and (4) complete fracture, which occurs through both cortices of the bone and is often associated with displacement.

They can also be classified according to the location of the fracture: shaft fractures are of the distal third, midshaft, or proximal third. Growth plate injuries are to the distal or proximal growth plate. Other special fracture patterns include fracture-dislocations (Monteggia and Galeazzi and their variants) and combination fractures (fractures of the humerus and forearm—"floating elbow").

Because the forearm is a two-bone complex, both bones are almost always injured. A single-bone fracture should raise suspicion of an injury to the proximal or distal joint. The only exception is an injury caused by a direct blow to the forearm. Commonly, the fracture types (e.g., plastic deformation, greenstick, buckle, or complete) in the radius and the ulna are different. A frequent combination is a greenstick fracture of the ulna with a complete fracture of the radius[95] (Fig. 8–19).

## Diagnosis

The mechanism of injury, the age of the child, and the presence of any associated injuries should be determined first. In very small children, the exact mechanism of injury may be unclear. On physical examination, the presence and location of swelling, deformity, and localized tenderness are noted. The skin is carefully inspected for the presence of open wounds, and any splints or bandages must be removed to fully expose the arm. A careful neurologic and vascular examination must be performed. One of the subtle signs of neurologic injury is the absence of sweating, which is indicative of sympathetic nerve disruption.

Adequate knowledge of the anatomy of the nerves of the forearm can help localize the site of nerve injury. In addition, the physical examination should be able to differentiate injury to the deep branches of the median and radial nerves, which are at risk of becoming caught within a fracture site.[45, 167, 188] The anterior interosseous nerve is a motor branch of the median nerve. It branches from the lateral side of the median nerve 5 to 8 cm distal to the lateral epicondyle. Then it passes through the arch of the deep head of the pronator teres. It continues on the interosseous membrane between the flexor pollicis longus and flexor digitorum profundus. It innervates the

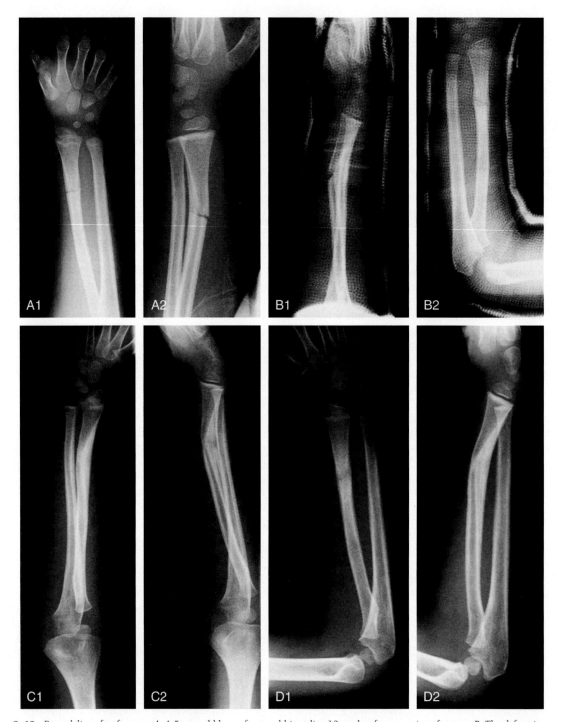

**FIGURE 8–13.** Remodeling after fracture. *A,* A 5-year-old boy refractured his radius 10 weeks after a previous fracture. *B,* The deformity was not reduced but was allowed to heal in the displaced position. *C,* Early remodeling with apposition of new bone along the deformity. *D,* Subsequent radiographs show increased new bone in the shaft, with early reorientation of the growth plate.

radial portion of the flexor digitorum profundus, flexor pollicis longus, and pronator quadratus. The sensory portion innervates the carpal joints and cannot be tested by clinical examination. Thus, to test for anterior interosseous nerve injury, one must check flexion of the interphalangeal (IP) joint of the thumb and, after stabilizing the proximal interphalangeal (PIP) joint, check flexion of the distal interphalangeal (DIP) joint

of the index finger. The posterior interosseous nerve is the motor branch of the radial nerve. It starts deep to the brachioradialis at the level of the elbow joint, enters the supinator from its posterior aspect, and passes laterally around the radial head between the two heads of the supinator. It then runs with the posterior interosseous vessels across the abductor pollicis longus and deep to the extensor digitorum communis and extensor pollicis longus. This nerve supplies all the extensors to the hand and wrist, except for the extensor carpi radialis longus. It does not supply sensation to the hand. Clinically, injury to the posterior interosseous nerve is detected by weak radial extension to the wrist and intact sensation to the dorsum of the hand.

All fractured limbs should be examined for the presence of a compartment syndrome. Despite the high incidence of forearm fractures in children, compartment syndrome is rare, but a high index of suspicion must be maintained.[61, 117, 119, 136, 155, 159] It is essential to examine the joints proximal and distal to the fracture clinically as well as radiographically to avoid missing associated dislocations or fractures. Radiologic studies should include adequate anteroposterior and lateral radiographs of the forearm, as well as both views of the wrist and elbow. They should be taken by changing the position of the x-ray tube rather than by rotating the forearm. The latter technique frequently changes the position through the fracture site.

## Management

When the child arrives in the emergency department, the extremity is splinted for both pain relief and prevention of further injury once a thorough clinical examination has been performed. The splint should be in place when the radiographs are taken to prevent the radiology technician from inadvertently injuring the extremity further by moving the limb instead of the x-ray tube.

Most displaced fractures of the forearm in children can be treated by closed reduction and maintenance in a well-molded long arm cast. If excessive swelling inside the cast is a concern, the cast can be split immediately to accommodate the soft tissue swelling while still controlling the fracture position. In some centers, a "sugar-tongs" splint is used initially instead of a circumferential cast (Fig. 8–20). Although the cast is applied longitudinally, the cast padding can be circumferential and may still need to be split if the soft tissue swelling is excessive.

The extent and type of deformity, the age of the child, and the child's medical history determine whether the reduction can be accomplished with conscious sedation, local anesthesia, or general anesthesia. Completely displaced fractures of the forearm require adequate closed reduction, which can only be accomplished with effective, yet safe levels of sedation and analgesia to minimize the child's apprehension and pain. Both these goals can usually be met in an emergency department without the need for general anesthesia. Cost savings of up to 70% can be expected with closed reduction in an ambulatory setting rather than the operating room.[109] A variety of safe and effective techniques are available to permit

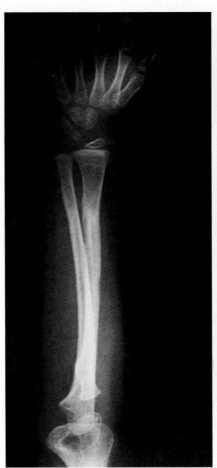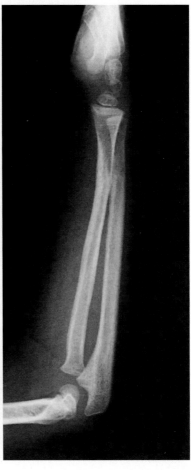

**FIGURE 8–14.** Malunion with a residual rotational deformity after reduction. This 4½-year-old girl was treated for a distal radial and ulnar fracture by closed reduction. The deformity recurred several weeks later and required re-reduction. These are her radiographs 6 months after the injury. Note that the proximal portion of the forearm appears pronated and the distal part appears supinated, thus indicating that the fracture has healed in a malrotated position. Clinically, she has 40° of excessive supination and 30° less pronation than in the opposite forearm.

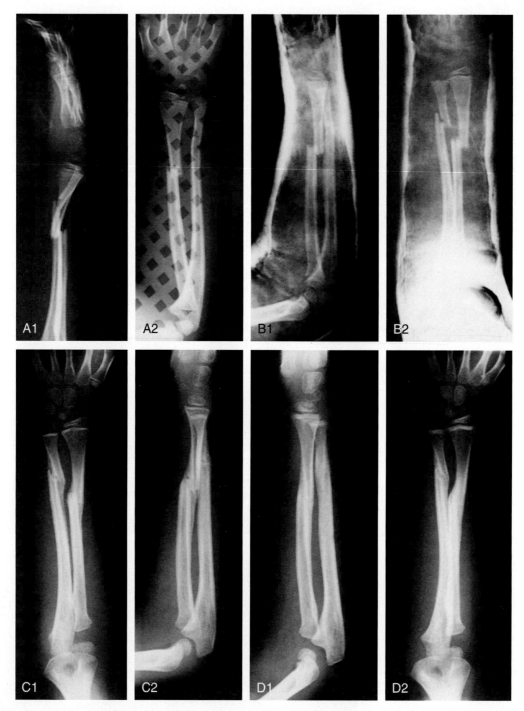

**FIGURE 8–15.** Bayonet apposition of the radius and ulna. *A,* A 6-year-old boy fell off a swing and sustained a complete fracture of the shaft of the radius and a greenstick fracture of the distal end of the ulna. Note that the distal fragment is volar to the proximal fragment, which differs from the usual dorsal displacement seen with this injury. This appearance is consistent with continued rotation of the forearm after the fracture occurred. *B,* With the patient under general anesthesia, the radius was manipulated so that the distal fragment was dorsal to the proximal fragment, and the usual reduction technique was then attempted. The greenstick fracture of the ulna was completed during the manipulation, thereby increasing the instability of the fracture. End-to-end reduction could not be achieved, and the fracture was casted in bayonet apposition. Note that the fracture ends of the distal and proximal fragments match in width and shape, an indication of correct rotatory alignment. *C,* The cast was removed at 6 weeks. *D,* On follow-up 1 month later, full supination and pronation are seen, as in the normal left forearm.

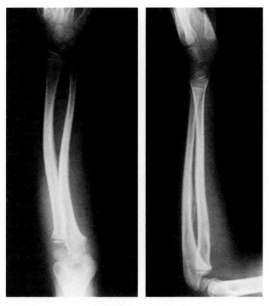

**FIGURE 8–16.** Plastic deformation of the radius and ulna in a 6-year-old boy.

adequate closed reduction in an emergency department or outpatient facility.[7, 14, 34, 61, 62, 109, 130] X-ray equipment or an image intensifier should be available to check alignment of the fracture after the reduction is performed.

Conscious sedation techniques are described in Chapter 18.

## UNDISPLACED FRACTURES

Undisplaced fractures may be treated in a cast or splint, mainly for comfort, until the fracture site is no longer painful.

## PLASTIC DEFORMATION

Pediatric bone is able to absorb more energy before it fractures than adult bone, primarily because it has greater capacity to undergo plastic deformation. In a review of the mechanism of plastic deformation in pediatric fractures, Mabrey and Fitch outlined the molecular, histologic, and biomechanical aspects of bone structure and the differences between pediatric and adult bone.[102] Bone is able to absorb a certain amount of energy under which it undergoes elastic deformation and recovers to its original length after the load is removed. When a material exceeds its elastic limit, it undergoes plastic deformation (Fig. 8–21). Microscopically, it appears as slip lines, parallel zones of disruption between fiber bundles, bent or wrinkled fiber bundles, and disruption of canaliculi between osteocytes.[15, 102] Macroscopically, plastic deformation appears as bowing of the affected bone, without an actual fracture. Unlike the situation in other pediatric fractures, minimal or no periosteal bone formation may be detected radiographically up to 4 weeks after injury.[15]

Plastic deformation of the forearm occurs in children

between the ages of 2 and 15 years.[102] Bowing of the radius and ulna can result in narrowing of the interosseous space, thereby limiting pronation and supination of the forearm.[15] In children younger than 4 years, angulations less than 20° usually remodel. Correction of plastic deformity is recommended when the deformity prevents reduction of a concomitant fracture or dislocation, prevents full rotation in children older than 4 years, or exceeds 20° in any age group.[102]

Bowing may be difficult to correct. Manipulation should always be done with the patient under general anesthesia because forces as great as 20 to 30 kg are usually necessary to correct the deformity.[96] The technique consists of placing the apex of the deformity over a wedge and applying a constant force at points proximal and distal to the apex of the bow over a period of 2 to 3 minutes (Fig. 8–22). Both rotational and angular components of the deformity must be corrected sequentially. Care should be taken to avoid placing force over the physes. Recurrence of the deformity is common, but its incidence can be reduced through the use of a well-fitting and carefully molded long arm cast. An average correction of 13°, or 85% of the prereduction deformity, can be expected.[102, 157]

It is common for one bone to undergo plastic deformation when the other bone fractures. During reduction, it is just as important to correct the plastic deformity as it is to reduce the fracture. Insufficient reduction may contribute to recurrent deformity or

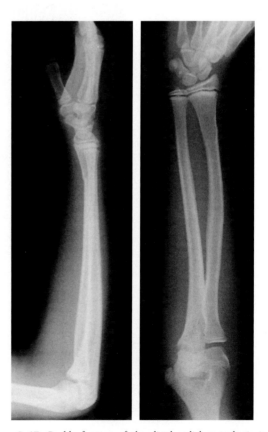

**FIGURE 8–17.** Buckle fracture of the distal radial metaphysis in a 12-year-old boy.

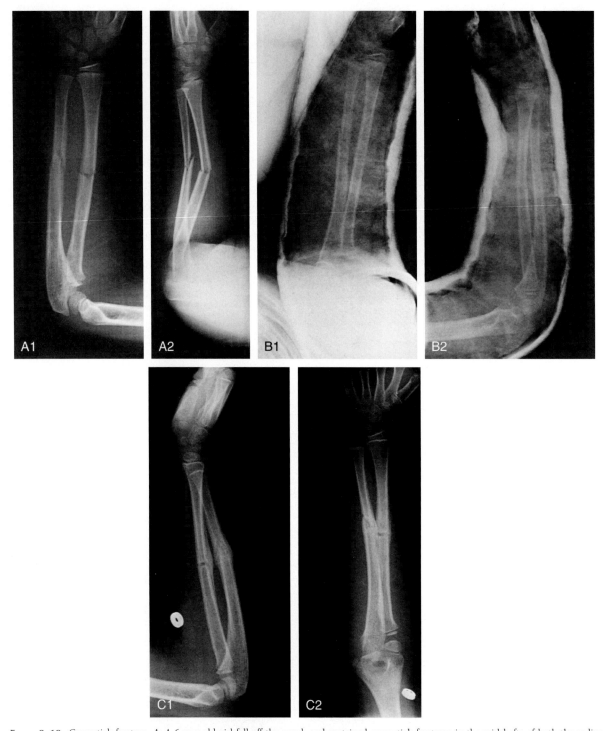

FIGURE 8–18. Greenstick fracture. *A,* A 6-year-old girl fell off the couch and sustained greenstick fractures in the midshafts of both the radius and the ulna. *B,* Manipulation with the patient under general anesthesia. On follow-up, no displacement is present. *C,* One month after cast removal, she had normal range of motion.

subsequent disruption of the distal radioulnar articulation. Unrecognized disruption of the distal radioulnar joint may result in long-term pain and disability.

## GREENSTICK FRACTURES

Greenstick fractures can usually be managed with closed reduction. It was traditionally thought that completing a greenstick fracture, by intentionally breaking the intact cortex during reduction, would decrease the risk for recurrence of the deformity.[13] Gruber reported that delayed consolidation could occur with some greenstick fractures. He suggested that the fracture be completed in an effort to avoid this phenomenon.[55]

However, valid arguments against this recommendation have been made. Deformity can recur not only in

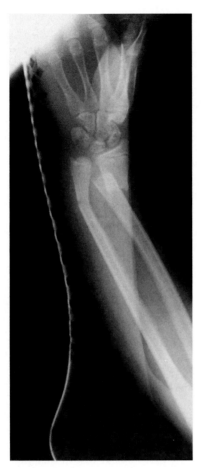

**FIGURE 8–19.** Complete fracture of the radius with a greenstick fracture of the ulna.

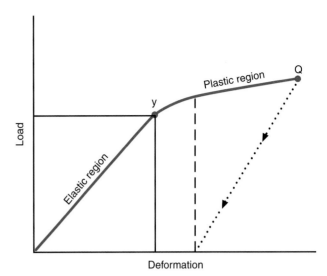

**FIGURE 8–21.** Load deformation curve. If a load is applied in the elastic region and then released, no permanent deformation will occur. If loading is continued past the yield point (y) and the load is released, plastic deformation will result. If loading continues, ultimate failure of the bone occurs at the failure point (Q). (From Frankel, V.H.; Nordin, M. Basic Biomechanics of the Skeletal System. Philadelphia, Lea & Febiger, 1980, pp. 15–16.)

## COMPLETE DISPLACEMENT

Complete fractures of the radius and ulna can be challenging to manage. The potential for malunion in the forearm is significant, primarily because of difficulties in obtaining and maintaining the reduction of two parallel bones that are subjected to angulatory and rotatory forces from muscular attachments. If the normal bow in a single bone is altered, its length relative to the other bone may decrease and cause disruption of either the proximal or the distal radioulnar joint. A change in angulation of greater than 10° and shortening of greater than 3 to 4 mm at the distal radioulnar joint necessitate remanipulation and correction of position.[25]

Fractures in patients older than 10 years, who have limited capacity for remodeling, and fractures in the proximal third of the forearm can be difficult to manage with closed manipulation and casting. Proximal fractures are challenging because the reduction is often difficult to

greenstick fractures but also in complete fractures. In addition, completion of the fracture can increase the displacement and instability of the fracture and thus make it more difficult to reduce and maintain. For this reason, some authors have recommended reversing the deformity and maintaining the arm in a well-molded cast without fracturing the intact cortex.[102] If care is taken while cracking the intact cortex, the stability of the fracture can be maintained.[128]

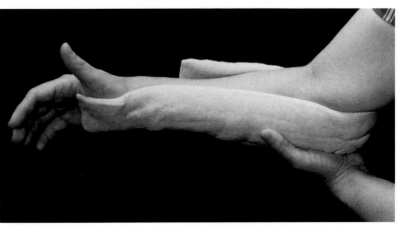

**FIGURE 8–20.** "Sugar-tongs" splint used to provide cast immobilization of the fracture yet allow room for soft tissue swelling.

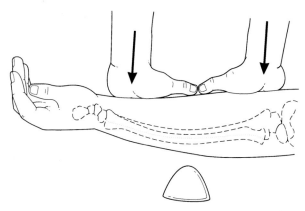

**FIGURE 8–22.** Method of reducing plastic deformity of forearm. (From Price, C. In: Letts, R., ed. Management of Pediatric Fractures. New York, Churchill Livingstone, 1994, p. 329.)

maintain, and redisplacement frequently results. These injuries therefore have a disproportionate share of problems at long-term follow-up.[25] Knight and Purvis stated over 50 years ago that to obtain satisfactory reduction, it is necessary to regain length and achieve apposition, axial alignment, and normal rotation of the fracture fragments.[80]

## TECHNIQUE OF CLOSED REDUCTION

Completely displaced fractures of the forearm are best reduced with adequate muscle relaxation. In most cases, the reduction can be accomplished with safe, conscious sedation techniques.[109] Occasionally, general anesthesia is required to obtain enough analgesia and muscle relaxation to achieve an acceptable reduction.[7, 15, 129] An image intensifier should be available to check the alignment of the fracture during reduction of the deformity.

The fracture deformity must first be increased to disengage the fracture fragments and open the periosteal hinge. It is often necessary to increase the deformity to greater than 90° to allow sufficient distraction of the fracture for reduction to be accomplished (Fig. 8–23). The radius and ulna are each reduced separately. With the operator applying traction in line with the angulated distal segment, the distal fragment is pushed with the operator's thumb onto the end of the proximal fragment. At the same time, the pronation or supination deformity is corrected. Once reduction has been achieved, maintaining pressure on the side of the intact periosteum stabilizes the reduction.

In a difficult reduction, finger traps with 10 to 15 lb of countertraction suspended from the upper part of the arm can be useful (Fig. 8–24). This technique requires time and patience as the soft tissues gradually stretch. The end result is often an acceptable reduction with correction of the angular and rotational deformity.

The position of immobilization is determined by the position and rotational alignment of the proximal fragment. The fracture is immobilized in the position in which the alignment is correct and the reduction feels stable.[142] The reduction is maintained in a well-molded circular cast that is lightly and evenly padded. The forearm portion should be oval, with a straight ulnar border (Fig. 8–25). Three-point molding is applied by (1) pushing with the palm of one hand on the side of the intact periosteum distal to the fracture site, (2) placing the other hand proximal to the fracture site on the opposite side of the forearm where the periosteum is not intact, and (3) placing the assistant's hand proximally on the arm on the same side as that of the operator's distal hand (i.e., the side of the intact periosteum) (Fig. 8–26). The elbow is immobilized at a right angle. The back of the above-elbow portion should be flat to prevent the elbow from slipping inside the cast. A loop is placed proximal to the site of the fracture to prevent "sagging" of the fracture fragments when the cast becomes loose from reduced swelling and atrophy of the forearm muscles[80, 142] (Fig. 8–27).

Most displaced fractures of the forearm are best

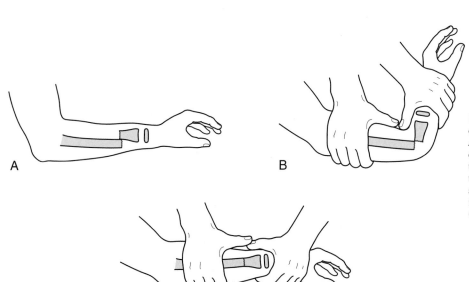

**FIGURE 8–23.** Technique of reduction of a complete fracture of the forearm. *A,* Initial fracture position. *B,* Hyperextend fracture to 100° to disengage the fracture ends. *C,* Push with the thumb on the distal fragment to achieve reduction. (*B, C,* Adapted from Levinthal, D.H. Surg Gynecol Obstet 57:790–799, 1933.)

The fracture is monitored carefully with weekly radiographs for the first 3 weeks after reduction. Such a follow-up schedule usually allows redisplacement to be detected before consolidation of the fracture. Redisplacement occurs in 7% to 13% of cases, usually within 2 weeks of the injury. As previously mentioned, greenstick fractures have a greater potential for redisplacement. There does not appear to be any correlation between the age of the patient or the severity of the initial displacement and the timing or severity of redisplacement.[185]

Recurrent deformity is frequently managed by applying a new, well-molded cast. Minor angulations with no rotational deformity can sometimes be corrected by wedging the cast. This procedure involves cutting half to two thirds of the circumference of the cast, centered at the apex of the deformity. The cast opening is spread, and a block is inserted. A radiograph is taken after the cast modification to ensure that the deformity has been adequately corrected. In some instances in which the deformity is too great to allow for correction by cast molding, the fracture must be remanipulated and recasted. In patients younger than 2 years, repeat manipulation is best performed within 1 week of the fracture because of the rapidity of fracture healing. In patients between 2 and 5 years of age, minor improvements can be made up to 2 weeks after the fracture. Generally, "good reductions last better than poor reductions, particularly in a well-molded cast."[142]

Younger and colleagues determined that axis deviation is the most important factor in determining outcome after pediatric forearm fractures.[201, 202] Axis deviation is an index that combines fracture position and angulation. It is defined as the distance between the fracture and the anatomic axes of the bone analyzed and is measured at the level of the fracture site[201] (Fig. 8–28). Axis deviation of 5 or less at the time of healing resulted in a good outcome. Their study also correlated true angulation and axis deviation, and an axis deviation of 5 correlated with a true angulation of 10° in the midshaft, 12.5° at the junction of the middle and distal thirds, 20° in the distal third, and 25° at the subphyseal level in the distal third.[200] These values correspond with those of others who have documented the remodeling

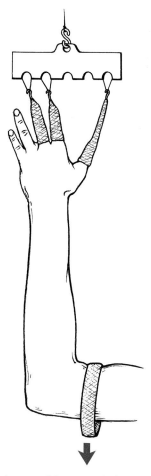

**FIGURE 8–24.** Application of traction with finger traps. (From King, R.E. In: Rockwood, C.A.J., et al., eds. Fractures in Children, Vol. 3. Philadelphia, J.B. Lippincott, 1984, pp. 301–362.)

maintained in a long arm cast to immobilize the elbow and neutralize the deforming forces of muscles that originate above the elbow. The above-elbow segment is usually applied after the forearm portion has been completed. To prevent the distal segment of the cast from digging into the forearm at the elbow, it is important to apply the padding in a continuous manner before either segment is applied.

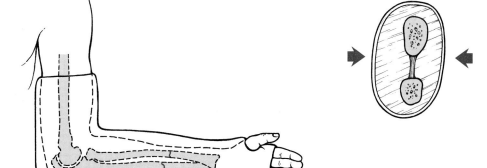

**FIGURE 8–25.** Ideal cast shape.

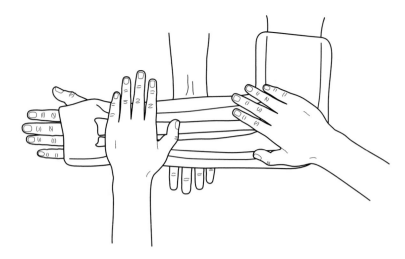

FIGURE 8–26. Molding technique. In this example, the intact periosteum is dorsal.

FIGURE 8–27. *A,* A loop placed distal to the fracture site will support the cast at the hand and not at the elbow; this design allows the cast to angle on the forearm and permits the fracture to sag. *B,* A loop placed proximal to the fracture site will create support for the cast so that no deforming force is directed at the fracture. (*A, B,* From Rang, M. Children's Fractures, 2nd ed. Philadelphia, J.B. Lippincott, 1982, p. 207.)

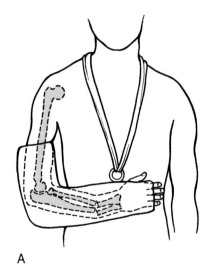

A

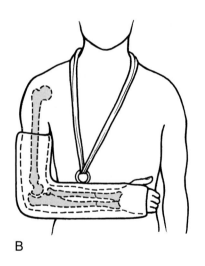

B

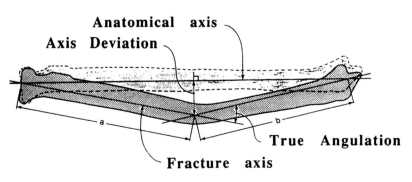

**Anatomical axis**
**Axis Deviation**
**True Angulation**
**Fracture axis**

FIGURE 8–28. The concept of axis deviation. The anatomic and fracture axes are represented. Axis deviation is measured at the level of the fracture site. Although the radius is curved, the representation is drawn as a straight line. Angulation is measured at the level of the fracture site by determining the angle between the cortex proximal and distal to the fracture. (From Younger, A., Tredwell, S.; MacKenzie, W.; et al. J Pediatr Orthop 14:200–206, 1994.)

potential of forearm fractures in children with residual angulation.[12, 27, 76, 107, 149]

## SURGICAL APPROACHES

In the reduction and stabilization of forearm fractures in children, many choices are available. Because of the rapid healing of pediatric fractures, solid fixation with plates and screws is not always necessary. K-wire fixation often provides enough stability for fracture healing to occur, usually in 3 to 4 weeks. In many cases, after closed reduction of an unstable fracture, percutaneous pin fixation can be quite useful, especially in a metaphyseal fracture. Alternatively, intramedullary fixation of the ulna can stabilize the forearm sufficiently to allow additional stabilization of the radius. Finally, intramedullary fixation of both the radius and ulna can be attempted. If none of these techniques are helpful or if stable fixation is essential for successful treatment (e.g., in proximal radial fractures), plate-and-screw fixation is the best choice (see the discussion under Fractures of the Shafts of the Radius and Ulna, Surgical Treatment).

Open reduction of the forearm in children may be necessary in one or both bones, depending on the configuration of the fracture. For example, an unstable, completely displaced fracture of the radius can be associated with a reducible greenstick fracture of the ulna, so open reduction of the radius is all that is required to achieve a stable adequate reduction. In other cases, the ulna is more unstable, and open reduction of the ulna with intramedullary fixation, along with closed reduction of the radius, is ideal. Finally, in completely unstable fractures, both the radius and the ulna must be approached surgically.

Open reduction for both bones of the forearm requires two separate surgical approaches. Open reduction for both-bone fractures through one incision is contraindicated because of the markedly increased risk of radioulnar synostosis. Two main approaches to the radius may be used—anterior and posterior. The ulna has only one approach for reduction, at its subcutaneous border. Normally, only part of the incision is required for any given operation, the part centered over the fracture site. The approach that is selected is based on the fracture deformity, the location in the forearm, and the safety of the approach in relation to possible nerve complications.

### Anterior Approach to the Radius

The anterior Henry approach is best used for fractures of the proximal third of the radius, especially when the bicipital tuberosity must be exposed; for fractures that have displaced in a volar direction; and for those in which soft tissue entrapment is suspected (Fig. 8–29). The entire approach is described from the elbow to the wrist, but for fracture reduction, only a portion of the approach is required.

Make the incision from the anterior flexor crease of the elbow, just lateral to the biceps tendon, down to the styloid process of the radius. Incise the deep fascia in line with the skin incision. Develop a plane between the medial border of the brachioradialis and flexor carpi radialis distally. More proximally, the plane is between the pronator teres and brachioradialis. Begin the dissection distally and work proximally. Just below the elbow joint is a leash of vessels from the radial artery that should be ligated to make it easier to move the brachioradialis laterally. Identify the superficial radial nerve, which is within the inferior fascia of the brachioradialis. The radial artery lies beneath the brachioradialis in the middle part of the forearm. This vessel is mobilized and retracted medially to expose the deeper muscular layer.

**Proximal Third.** Follow the biceps tendon to its insertion into the bicipital tuberosity of the radius. Just lateral to the tendon is a small bursa that must be incised to access the proximal part of the shaft of the radius. Because the radial artery is medial to the tendon, deepen the wound on the lateral side of the biceps tendon. The proximal third of the radius is covered by the supinator muscle, through which the posterior interosseous nerve passes into the posterior compartment of the forearm. To displace the nerve laterally, fully supinate the forearm. The supinator is incised along the line of its insertion into the anterior aspect of the radius. Continue the subperiosteal dissection. It is essential to avoid retraction of the posterior interosseous nerve, which recovers very slowly after neurapraxia. Do not place retractors on the posterior surface of the radial neck because the nerve comes into direct contact with the bone in approximately 25% of cases.[67]

**Middle Third.** After retracting the brachioradialis and the superficial branch of the radial nerve laterally (the radial artery is retracted medially), the pronator teres and flexor digitorum superficialis are exposed. Pronate the forearm to reach the insertion of the pronator teres on the lateral aspect of the radius. Then, subperiosteally strip the pronator teres and flexor digitorum superficialis from the anterior aspect of the radius.

**Distal Third.** The flexor pollicis longus and pronator quadratus arise from the anterior aspect of the distal third of the radius. After retracting the brachioradialis, supinate the forearm to expose the lateral origin of these muscles. The periosteum is then incised and stripped and the muscles retracted medially to expose the bone.

### Posterior Approach to the Radius

The posterior approach can also give access to the entire dorsal aspect of the radial shaft (Fig. 8–30). This approach exposes the tensile side of the bone, which may be a preferable location for plate fixation.

The incision runs from the lateral epicondyle of the humerus to Lister's tubercle. Lister's tubercle is about a third of the way across the dorsum of the wrist and feels like a small bony prominence. Incise the fascia in line with the skin. Identify the space between the extensor carpi radialis brevis and the extensor digitorum communis. The gap is more obvious where the abductor pollicis longus and extensor pollicis brevis emerge from between these two. Extend the dissection proximally.

**Proximal Third.** Identify the posterior interosseous nerve, which runs between the superficial and deep head of the supinator muscle, 1 cm proximal to the distal border. This nerve must be protected. Then fully supinate the arm to bring the anterior surface of the

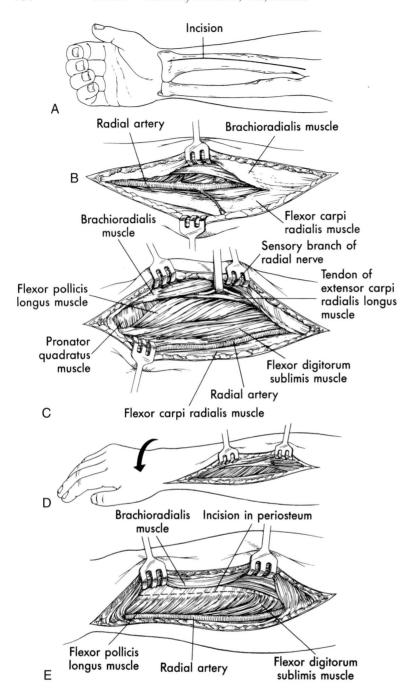

**FIGURE 8–29.** Anterior approach to the radius (Henry approach). *A,* Skin incision. *B,* Fascia is incised. The brachioradialis is retracted laterally and the flexor carpi radialis medially. *C,* The sensory branch of the radial nerve is within the fascia, beneath the brachioradialis. These structures are retracted together laterally. The radial artery deep to the brachioradialis is mobilized and retracted medially, along with the flexor carpi radialis. This maneuver exposes the flexor pollicis longus, the flexor digitorum sublimis, and distally, the pronator quadratus. *D,* The forearm is pronated to expose the radius lateral to the origins of the pronator quadratus and flexor pollicis longus. *E,* Periosteum is incised along the *broken line,* and the flexor pollicis longus and pronator quadratus are reflected by subperiosteal dissection. (*A–E,* From Crenshaw, A.H. In: Crenshaw, A.H., ed. Campbell's Operative Orthopedics, 8th ed. St. Louis, C.V. Mosby, 1992, pp. 108–109.)

radius into view. Detach the insertion of the supinator from the anterior aspect of the radius.

**Middle Third.** Retract the extensor carpi radialis longus and extensor digitorum communis. The abductor pollicis longus and extensor pollicis brevis are retracted by making an incision along their superior and inferior borders to reach the underlying radius.

**Distal Third.** Separate the extensor carpi radialis brevis from the extensor pollicis longus to expose the dorsal aspect of the bone.

### Approach to the Ulna

Fully pronate the arm. Make an incision over the subcutaneous border of the ulna (Fig. 8–31), and incise the deep fascia between the extensor carpi ulnaris and flexor carpi ulnaris. Proximally in the region of the olecranon, the anconeus is incised along the border of the flexor carpi ulnaris. Expose the bone subperiosteally. The ulnar nerve travels under the flexor carpi ulnaris on the flexor digitorum profundus. It is most vulnerable during very proximal dissections.

## Complications

Potential complications of forearm injuries in children include malunion, refracture, nonunion, nerve and arterial injuries, muscle or tendon entrapment, compartment syndrome, infection, and reflex sympathetic dystrophy. As each type of fracture is discussed, the specific complications associated with that fracture are presented in more detail. The following is a general discussion of complications that may be common to all.

## MALUNION

It is common for deformity to recur in any forearm fracture managed by closed manipulation. However, with careful follow-up, malunion is a potentially avoidable complication. Common causes of malunion are inadequate follow-up, improper positioning of the forearm in supination or pronation, failure to perform cast changes when appropriate, failure to correct an inadequate

reduction, and delay in diagnosis until after the fracture has united.[44, 142]

In studies of malunited fractures, the only patients who complained of any disability were those with severe restriction in forearm rotation.[27, 42, 122] Daruwalla found that loss of pronation was more common than loss of supination after forearm fractures in children.[27] In contrast, Knight and Purvis, in a study of adult fractures, found that supination was more frequently limited.[80] These authors agreed, however, that the main causes of limitation were residual angulatory deformity (especially if it resulted in narrowing of the interosseous space), residual posterior angulation of the ulnar fracture, residual rotational malalignment of the fracture fragments, and derangement of the inferior radioulnar joint

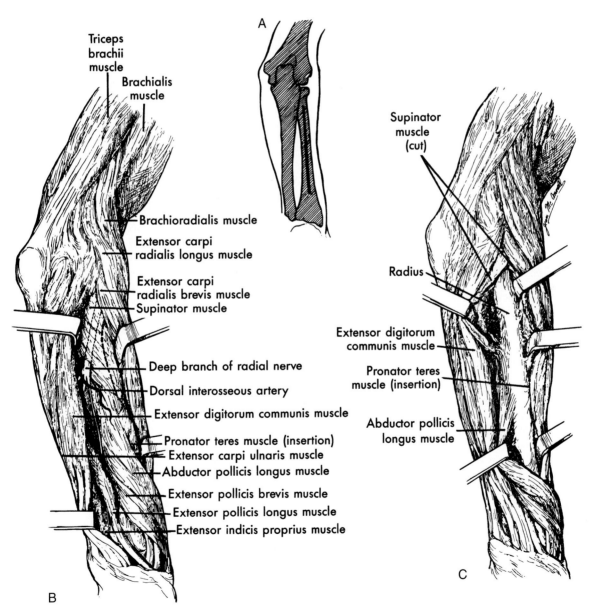

FIGURE 8–30. Posterior approach to the radius (Thompson approach). *A,* Skin incision along a line from the lateral epicondyle of the humerus to Lister's tubercle on the dorsal aspect of the radius. *B,* The fascia is incised between the extensor radialis brevis and extensor digitorum communis. The abductor pollicis longus and extensor pollicis brevis cross the plane of dissection in the distal third. *C,* The radius is exposed by reflecting the abductor pollicis longus and extensor pollicis brevis. (*A–C,* From Crenshaw, A.H. In: Crenshaw, A.H., ed. Campbell's Operative Orthopedics, 8th ed. St. Louis, C.V. Mosby, 1992, p. 105.)

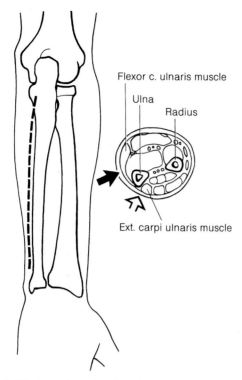

Flexor c. ulnaris muscle

Ulna

Radius

Ext. carpi ulnaris muscle

FIGURE 8–31. Approach to the ulna. The skin incision is made just lateral to the subcutaneous border of the ulna. The ulna is exposed longitudinally between the flexor carpi ulnaris and extensor carpi ulnaris. (From Schatzker, J.; Tile, M. The Rationale of Operative Fracture Care. Berlin, Springer-Verlag, 1987.)

as a result of relative shortening of the radius.[27, 80] It is interesting to note that inferior radioulnar instability is found infrequently, in spite of the fact that slight radial shortening is common.[80]

If a fracture has achieved early consolidation in an unsatisfactory position but is not yet solid, manual osteoclasis can be attempted (Fig. 8–32). With the child under general anesthesia, the fracture is manipulated with steady pressure at the fracture site. A wooden block in the shape of a wedge can be placed at the apex of the deformity to increase the pressure that can be applied (see Fig. 8–22). Once the fracture deformity is corrected, a long arm cast is applied with the forearm in the appropriate degree of rotation. The fracture is maintained in the cast for 4 to 6 weeks until the fracture is solid. In distal fractures, the cast can usually be changed at 4 weeks to a short arm cast, which is worn for the final 2 weeks.

If the fracture callus is mature, drill osteoclasis is a good method for correcting angular deformities. An incision is made over the apex of the deformity sufficiently large to introduce a drill guide to protect the soft tissues and to retract superficial cutaneous nerves and vessels. Several holes are made in the bone with a drill, guided by the image intensifier. A second incision is made over the apex of the other bony deformity, and the procedure is repeated. The bones are then manipulated to correct the deformity. A long arm cast is applied for 6 weeks until the fracture is solidly united. Unlike angular deformity, rotational malalignment cannot be corrected

with manual or percutaneous drill osteoclasis, and open techniques are necessary.

After the fracture is solidly united, a cosmetically poor result or malunion that is restricting more than 50% of normal forearm rotation and causing functional impairment can be treated by osteotomy (Fig. 8–33). Because of the variability among children in range of forearm rotation, it is important to measure rotation by comparing the fractured forearm with the opposite, normal forearm.[149] It is worthwhile, especially in younger children, to wait for 1 to 2 years after the fracture has healed to allow for maximal remodeling to occur. Comparable radiographs of the opposite forearm are obtained for preoperative planning of the osteotomy. Two-dimensional angular deformity noted on radiographs is usually a combination of rotational and angular malposition.[25] Angular correction is easier to plan for and perform than rotational correction is. Trial reductions with intraoperative radiographs help guide restoration of the normal anatomic contour. By placing the forearm through a range of motion before permanently fixing the plate, one can assess the amount of motion that has been regained. The osteotomy is secured with standard compression plating techniques or by intramedullary nails (Fig. 8–34).

Trousdale and Lindscheid reported on a series of 27 patients (aged 9 to 41 years) with malunited fractures of the forearm treated by osteotomy.[179] Seventeen of them had sustained their injuries during childhood, although only four had open growth plates at the time of osteotomy. Indications for the procedure included functional loss of rotation (average of 106°), an unstable and painful distal radioulnar joint, and a cosmetically unacceptable deformity (one patient). In patients treated for loss of rotation, they found that those managed early (within 12 months after injury) gained more than twice as much rotation as those who were treated more than 12 months after injury (average of 79°, versus an average of 30°). They thought that the difference may be the result of soft tissue scarring and contracture in the compartments of the forearm and interosseous membrane. Their recommendation was to treat significant malunion operatively within 12 months of injury.[179] It is important to note that none of the study patients were younger than 9 years at the time of injury. No guidelines for unacceptable angular and rotatory malalignment as an indication for surgery were included in the report.

The complication rate in the series of Trousdale and Lindscheid was 48%, and complications included degenerative disease in the proximal radioulnar joint, delayed union, infection, a retained drain, heterotopic ossification along the interosseous membrane, refracture through the site of the osteotomy, pain and dysesthesias along the radial nerve, subluxation of the ulnar head, loss of motion, and instability.[179] Even though most of the results in this group of mixed pediatric and adult patients were satisfactory, such significant complications cannot be discounted when planning an osteotomy.

Although it is unusual, derangement of the inferior radioulnar joint must be handled carefully in children. This problem is usually the result of excessive shortening of the radius secondary to fracture. Corrective osteotomy

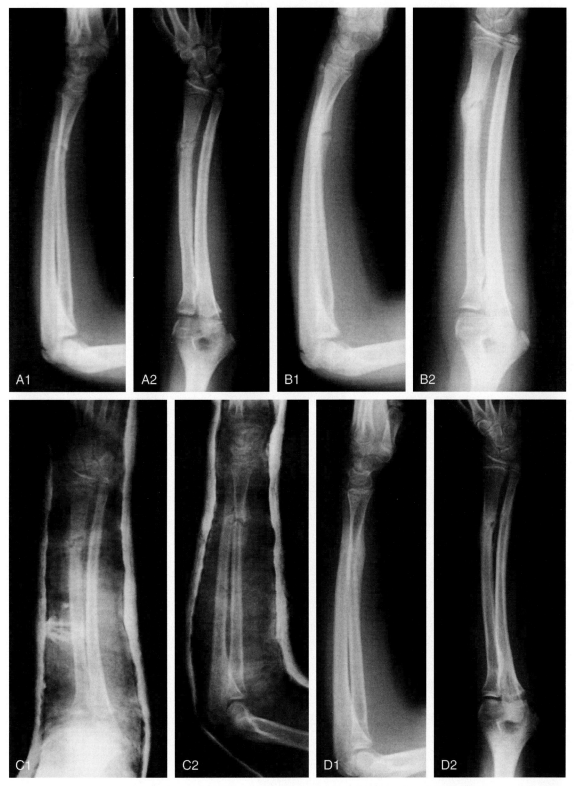

FIGURE **8–32.** Closed osteoclasis. An 11-year-old girl had an open, completely displaced fracture of the distal ends of the radius and ulna that was initially treated with débridement and open reduction without internal fixation. *A,* The cast was removed prematurely, 3 weeks after the injury. *B,* At 7 weeks, an unacceptable deformity developed at the fracture site. *C,* Manual osteoclasis was performed with the patient under general anesthesia. The cast was removed 6 weeks later. *D,* At follow-up, the patient had normal range of motion, with no clinical evidence of infection. The radiolucency at the fracture site seen on this radiograph resolved on further follow-up.

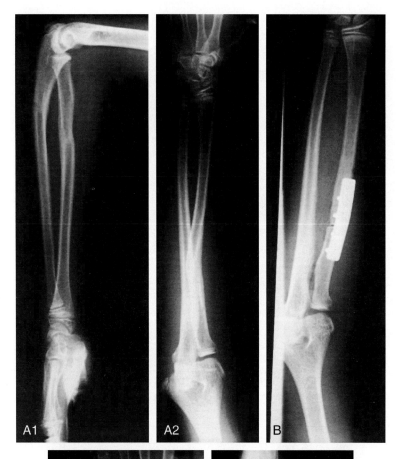

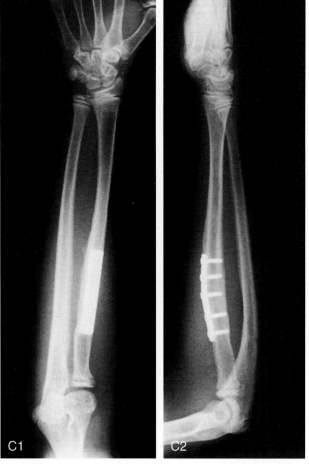

**FIGURE 8–33.** Malunion treated by osteotomy of the radius. *A,* A 14-year-old boy had a malunited fracture in the proximal third of both bones of the forearm after conservative treatment. The arm lacked 45° of pronation, thus preventing normal function. *B,* An osteotomy with plating of the radius was performed. *C,* Almost full motion was present 4 months postoperatively. The plate was removed 1 year after the osteotomy.

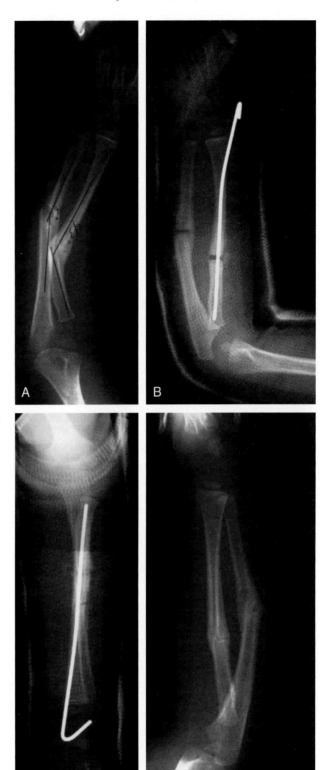

**FIGURE 8–34.** *A,* Malunion of a forearm fracture in a 2-year-old boy. Preoperative supination and pronation were markedly limited. *B,* After corrective osteotomy of both the radius and ulna with the use of a stainless steel intramedullary rod for fixation. *C,* Lateral radiograph. *D,* At completion of healing. The ulna has lost some alignment, but no loss of rotation occurred. At last follow-up, the child had 80° of supination and 80° of pronation.

of the distal end of the radius can be successful in achieving joint stability and relief of symptoms.[179] If instability is still present after securing the osteotomy with a plate and screws, the palmar capsule can be imbricated with nonabsorbable sutures and the joint temporarily stabilized with K-wires.[179] Creasman and

associates reported that the Darrach procedure (see under Dislocation of the Distal Radioulnar Joint, Management) seems to give an excellent outcome in terms of both restoring motion and abolishing pain in those with an unstable, painful distal radioulnar joint.[25] This procedure is not recommended before growth plate closure in the wrist. If it is done earlier, the proximal radioulnar joint can become secondarily unstable.[116]

## REFRACTURE

Recurrent fractures occur in 7% to 17% of cases.[89, 178] Refracture probably takes place because of either failure of the original fracture to unite solidly or a similar mechanism of injury (Fig. 8–35). Osteoporosis secondary to immobilization could contribute to the risk of refracture. Unfortunately, little can be done to completely avoid this complication, apart from recommending that the child refrain from participating in active sports for 1 month after removal of the cast. Tredwell and co-workers, in a study of 500 fractures in normal children, found that refractures occurred, on average, 6.5 months after the original injury.[178] They were more likely to occur in older children and in a region of the forearm more proximal to the usual pattern for the specific age group.[178] Refracture can occur as late as 1 year after the initial injury, but it is not reasonable to protect every child for this length of time. Warning the family of the possibility of refracture can help relieve anxiety should this complication occur.

## NONUNION

Delayed union in children is uncommon; nonunion in children is rare. They are more likely to occur as a result of high-energy trauma, after an open fracture, or in fractures associated with significant soft tissue loss or infection.[57] Open reduction and internal fixation may contribute to nonunion, particularly when the fixation is inadequate or when it distracts the fracture fragments.[13, 96] Repeated manipulation may also contribute to this complication.[96] If both bones are fractured, the ulna is more likely to be affected by delayed healing. With time and patience, most fractures will heal.

## NERVE AND VESSEL INJURIES

In closed forearm fractures, nerves and vessels are injured relatively infrequently, probably because the intervening layer of muscles surrounding the radius and ulna protects the nerves and vessels from injury.[142] However, injury to the anterior interosseous nerve secondary to a fracture of the radius has been reported,[45, 188] as has entrapment of the median nerve and ulnar nerve within a greenstick fracture.[3, 46, 140, 197] The anterior interosseous nerve is anatomically susceptible to injury in displaced fractures of the proximal third of the radius, especially those requiring open reduction.[45, 66] Injury to the posterior interosseous nerve may occur in Monteggia fractures, especially those with lateral dislocation of the radial head.[97, 167] Fractures of the distal part of the forearm that are completely displaced may be associated with compression of the median nerve at the wrist.[189]

## TENDON ENTRAPMENT

Tendons and muscles can also become entrapped at the fracture site. Entrapment is evident when full active and passive extension of the fingers or thumb is not possible during or after reduction of the fracture. Once the diagnosis is made, the solution is surgical exploration and release[81, 85, 144] (Fig. 8–36).

## COMPARTMENT SYNDROME

Compartment syndrome is uncommon after fracture of the forearm. Although it is more likely to develop after crush injuries of the forearm or with an associated supracondylar fracture of the humerus, it can also occur after a simple fracture. Compartment syndrome occurs when the pressure within an enclosed compartment of muscles is excessive and compromises the microvascular circulation and function of tissues. The two main causes are a relative decrease in compartment size because of external dressings and increased compartment content as a result of postinjury swelling. A limb with a vascular injury in which the repair has been delayed longer than 6 hours after injury is especially at risk for this complication.[152] Careful examination with monitoring while maintaining a high degree of suspicion is important to ensure that early treatment is initiated. Such vigilance is essential to avoid a potentially crippling result. Loss of reduction is insignificant when compared with the sequelae of an overlooked compartment syndrome.

The cardinal symptom of a compartment syndrome is pain that is frequently but not always out of proportion to the injury. It is usually aggravated by passive stretch of the muscles in the involved compartment. The pain is not usually relieved by splinting and tends to become progressively more severe. Other symptoms include numbness and tingling. The child's inability to actively move the fingers and severe pain with gentle passive extension of the fingers are classic features of an impending problem. The earliest physical finding is tenseness of the affected compartment. It is important to be aware that in younger children with abundant subcutaneous fat, a tense compartment can be difficult to feel. Casts or splints must be removed for thorough examination. The hand is often held stiffly, with the fingers relatively extended at the metacarpophalangeal (MP) joints and flexed at the IP joints. The child is reluctant to move the hand. Loss of the radial pulse, poor capillary refill, and pallor of the extremity occur late in the course of events and are not generally positive signs. If a peripheral pulse is absent, other causes of arterial obstruction must be considered, and arteriography is indicated.[122]

The first step in management of a suspected or incipient compartment syndrome is to remove constricting bandages and to widely split circular casts, including all the padding material under the cast. Bivalving a cast has been shown to be superior in reducing compartment pressure than has univalving the cast.[152] If the cast or bandage is the cause of the problem, relief of pain should be immediate. If the diagnosis cannot be made clinically, if the child is very young, uncooperative, or unconscious, or if an associated nerve injury is confounding the diagnosis, compartment pressure measurements should be performed. The techniques of compartment pressure measurement are well described.[172] Two commonly used

FIGURE **8–35.** Complete fracture of the distal end of the radius in association with a greenstick fracture of the distal part of the ulna. *A,* A 6-year-old boy sustained a fracture of the distal portion of the right forearm that healed in bayonet apposition. *B,* Two months later, he complained of wrist pain after a minor fall, and a new fracture line was seen at the site of the previous fracture. Note the change in orientation of the growth plate, as well as the cortical remodeling that has occurred.

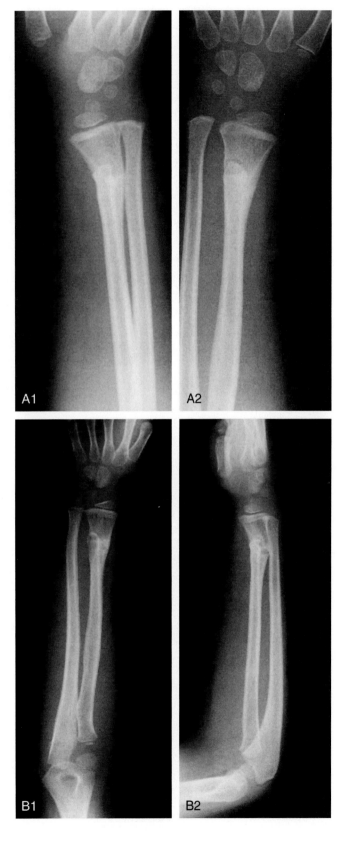

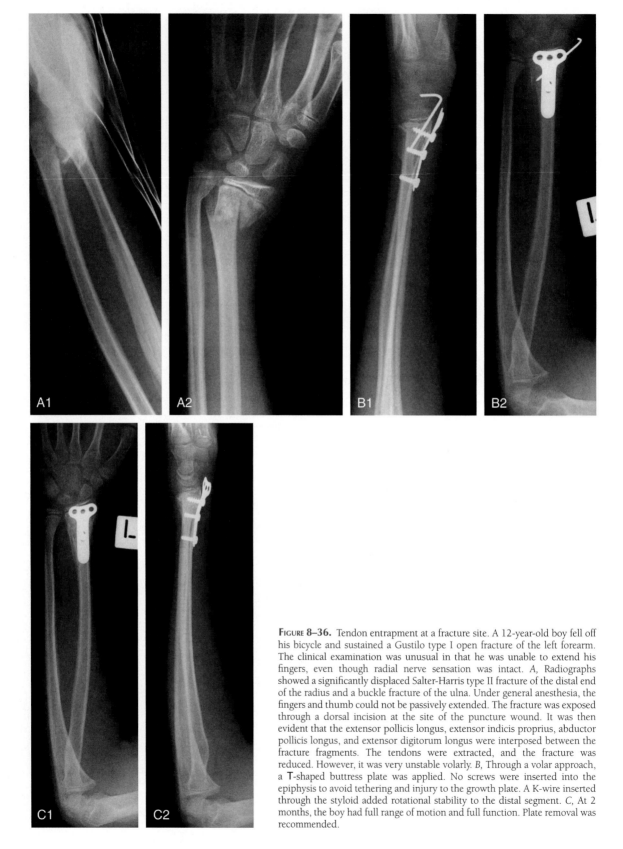

FIGURE 8–36. Tendon entrapment at a fracture site. A 12-year-old boy fell off his bicycle and sustained a Gustilo type I open fracture of the left forearm. The clinical examination was unusual in that he was unable to extend his fingers, even though radial nerve sensation was intact. A, Radiographs showed a significantly displaced Salter-Harris type II fracture of the distal end of the radius and a buckle fracture of the ulna. Under general anesthesia, the fingers and thumb could not be passively extended. The fracture was exposed through a dorsal incision at the site of the puncture wound. It was then evident that the extensor pollicis longus, extensor indicis proprius, abductor pollicis longus, and extensor digitorum longus were interposed between the fracture fragments. The tendons were extracted, and the fracture was reduced. However, it was very unstable volarly. B, Through a volar approach, a T-shaped buttress plate was applied. No screws were inserted into the epiphysis to avoid tethering and injury to the growth plate. A K-wire inserted through the styloid added rotational stability to the distal segment. C, At 2 months, the boy had full range of motion and full function. Plate removal was recommended.

methods are the slit catheter technique (Fig. 8–37) and the Stryker device, which directly measures tissue pressure with a convenient hand-held device.

Normal tissue pressure in a recumbent individual is 4 to 8 mm Hg. Physiologically, when the tissue fluid pressure within a compartment exceeds 30 mm Hg, capillary pressure is not sufficient to maintain muscle-capillary blood flow. Nerves within a compartment appear to be the most sensitive to excessive tissue pressure. A longer duration and higher magnitude of increased compartment pressure increase the chance for permanent nerve conduction changes.[58, 152] The ability of tissues to tolerate increased compartment pressure may vary with metabolic needs. Hypotension does not seem to affect local tissue pressure but can cause a greater degree of soft tissue ischemia and thus necessitate earlier decompression.[105] Although elevation of the extremity cannot reduce local venous pressure below the value of local tissue pressure, the limb should be kept at the level of the heart to promote arterial inflow.[151]

Matsen and Vieth reported on several clinical series in which surgical decompression was performed on clinical grounds alone. Compartment pressures were measured subsequent to the clinical diagnosis. In adults, the lowest pressure requiring decompression was 45 mm Hg, and in the pediatric series, it was 33 mm Hg.[105] Based on this evidence, we recommend immediate fasciotomy if the compartment pressure is greater than 30 mm Hg in a patient with clinical signs of a compartment syndrome or in a child in whom the diagnosis cannot be made clinically, as discussed earlier.

Fasciotomies of the forearm are performed with the patient under general anesthesia. The skin, fascia, and epimysium must all be opened. Most commonly, a volar fasciotomy is sufficient. One must be sure that an associated dorsal compartment syndrome is not present that has not been adequately decompressed by the volar fasciotomy. In these cases, a separate dorsal fasciotomy must be performed.

### Technique of Forearm Decompression

Volar forearm decompression is performed with a curvilinear volar incision beginning 1 cm proximal and 2 cm lateral to the medial epicondyle, proximal to the antecubital fossa (Fig. 8–38). The incision is carried obliquely across the antecubital fossa and over the volar aspect of the flexor group of muscles. It is continued distally to the proximal wrist crease, just ulnar to the palmaris longus tendon, obliquely across the crease, and along the thenar crease to the midpalm at a level even with the base of the thumb–index finger web. The fascia is incised in line with the skin incision. The lacertus fibrosus of the biceps tendon is divided proximally. The carpal tunnel is released under direct vision to avoid injuring the palmar cutaneous branch of the median nerve. Other areas of possible nerve compression are the proximal edge of the pronator teres and the proximal edge of the flexor digitorum superficialis. The deep flexor musculature should be adequately inspected and decompressed because it is frequently more severely involved.[196]

The dorsal compartment pressure is then remeasured. If it is still too high, the dorsal compartment must also be decompressed. The incision begins 2 cm lateral and 2 cm distal to the lateral epicondyle. It is extended straight distally toward the midline of the wrist. The dorsal fascia is incised in line with the skin incision.

An alternative approach has been recommended by Matsen and co-workers. It is an ulnar approach between the flexor carpi ulnaris and flexor digitorum sublimis. The incision can be extended distally to divide the carpal tunnel and medially and proximally to divide the lacertus

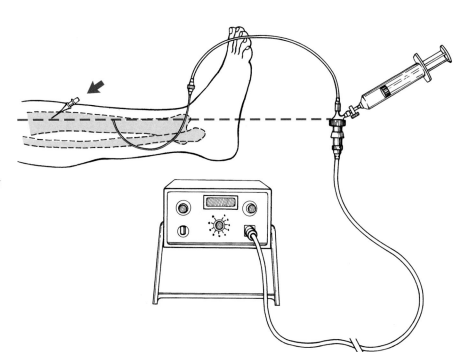

**FIGURE 8–37.** Slit catheter method of measuring compartment pressure.

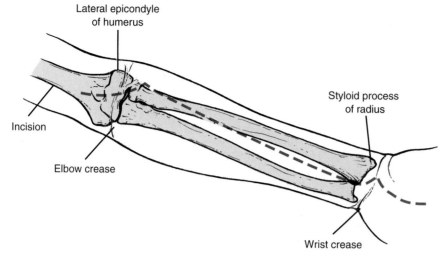

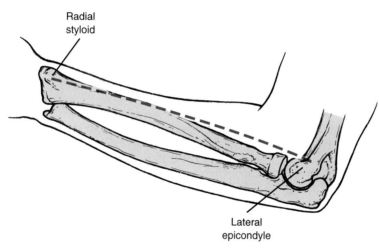

FIGURE 8–38. Incisions for forearm fasciotomy.

fibrosus. The deep compartment is exposed by retracting the flexor carpi ulnaris and flexor digitorum sublimis, with care taken to protect the ulnar artery and nerve lying on the flexor digitorum profundus.[106] This technique may be advantageous in producing a more cosmetic closure, although both approaches often require skin grafting.

In both instances, if the muscle appears necrotic, conservative débridement can be performed. If muscle viability is at all in question, it should be left and inspected again at a subsequent dressing change. The fascia and skin are left open, and a dressing is applied. Internal or external fixation techniques are often useful to stabilize the fracture for easier management of the soft tissue injury. Secondary closure or skin grafting is performed 7 to 10 days later.[172]

## INFECTION

Infection is a potential complication of open fractures and open reduction of closed fractures of the forearm. It can occur after a closed fracture but is rare.[20]

Management of an open fracture is directed toward preventing infection. Initially, prevention should include (1) swabbing the open wound for culture and sensitivity

studies, (2) covering the wound with a sterile dressing, (3) giving tetanus prophylaxis if it is not certain that the child's immunization is up to date, (4) administering intravenous broad-spectrum antibiotics effective against penicillin-resistant *Staphylococcus aureus,* (5) adequately débriding and irrigating the fracture wound within 8 hours of injury, and (6) providing appropriate stabilization of the fracture. Postdébridement cultures are also recommended. However, Kreder and Armstrong have questioned the value of routine cultures before and after débridement in determining the likelihood of infection and the probability of identifying an infecting organism in the pediatric age group.[84] If the wound is grossly contaminated, an aminoglycoside and penicillin should be added to the antibiotic regimen. The duration of antibiotic coverage after débridement is controversial, but 2 to 3 days of coverage is generally adequate for most wounds that do not become grossly infected. Management of open fractures is covered in more detail in Chapter 4.

Treatment of an infected fracture should include débridement of the fracture site and treatment with antibiotics that are effective against the organism that has been cultured. If possible, internal fixation should not be removed until the fracture has united.

## REFLEX SYMPATHETIC DYSTROPHY

Reflex sympathetic dystrophy is uncommon in children. The syndrome consists of continuous burning or aching pain in the involved extremity, hyperesthesia, excessive sweating, purple or reddish discoloration, swelling, and joint stiffness. Radiographically, patchy osteopenia may be evident 6 to 8 weeks later.

The pathophysiology of this syndrome is not well understood. It is hypothesized that chronic and excessive activity in the autonomic nervous system causes increased local blood flow to the affected limb. Chronic irritation of a peripheral sensory nerve may also lead to excessive autonomic nervous activity. The personalities of the child and the child's family are probably important factors in determining the risk or likelihood of this complication.

Management of this condition usually consists of aggressive physical therapy with emotional and psychologic counseling. Transcutaneous nerve stimulation has also been used with good results.[126] Pharmacologic therapy with corticosteroids or narcotics is not usually necessary and should be avoided. The condition generally resolves with time, typically within 6 to 12 months after injury.[126]

## OVERGROWTH

A broken bone usually grows faster for the first 6 to 8 months after the fracture has healed. In the forearm, overgrowth of one or both bones is likely to average about 6 to 7 mm and is therefore insignificant.[2, 13, 30, 121] Significant relative overgrowth of one bone may occur only after the other bone has sustained a physeal injury resulting in premature closure. Permanent growth plate injuries of both the radius and the ulna have been reported.[1, 13, 141, 191]

## Management of Specific Injuries

### GROWTH PLATE INJURIES TO THE DISTAL RADIUS AND ULNA

Fractures of the distal radial growth plate are the most common physeal plate injuries and account for 46% of all fractures of the physis. Of these, 75% occur in children between 10 and 16 years of age. Injuries to the distal radial growth plate are uncommon in children younger than 5 years.[156, 198]

Fifty-five percent of distal radial physeal injuries have an associated fracture of the distal end of the ulna, usually a fracture of the ulnar styloid. A greenstick or complete fracture or plastic deformation of the distal part of the ulna may also occur.[90, 91]

### Classification

Classification of growth plate injuries is presented in Chapter 1; in this discussion, the Salter-Harris classification is used[127, 156] (Fig. 8–39).

A Salter-Harris type II fracture is the most frequent type of physeal injury and accounts for 58% of fractures

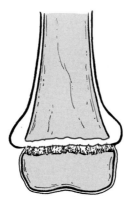 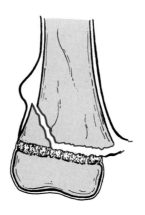 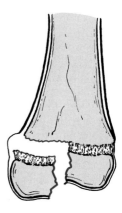

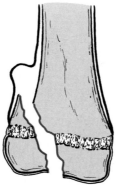 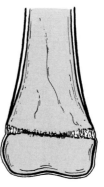

FIGURE **8–39.** Salter-Harris classification of growth plate injuries. (From Salter, R.B.; Harris, W.R. J Bone Joint Surg Am 45:587–622, 1963.)

of the distal radial epiphysis. The next most common are type I fractures of the distal end of the radius, which occur in 22% of cases. Type III, IV, and V fractures are rare and account for only 5% of cases.[90]

### Mechanism of Injury

As with most forearm fractures, the usual mechanism of injury is a fall on the outstretched hand. The physis is weaker than the fibrous joint capsule, tendons, and ligaments in children.[156] Shearing or avulsion forces are usually responsible for fractures through the physis.

### Diagnosis

As for all fractures of the forearm, the clinical examination should include a search for evidence of deformity, localization of tenderness and swelling, determination of the neurologic and vascular status of the forearm, and inspection of the skin. Finally, the examiner should check specifically for signs and symptoms suggestive of compartment syndrome because it can occur despite the distal nature of the injury.

Type I injuries occur in younger children, are seldom very displaced, and are diagnosed on clinical suspicion.[42, 140, 156] Children with these fractures have swelling and tenderness at the growth plate, despite normal radiographs. The correct diagnosis is made on clinical grounds and can be confirmed by the presence of periosteal new bone on radiographs taken after the fracture has healed.

### Management of Undisplaced Fractures

Undisplaced fractures are protected in a short arm cast for 2 weeks in children younger than 2 years and for 3 weeks in older children.

Salter-Harris type V fractures are frequently diagnosed retrospectively after growth arrest has occurred. At the time of the injury, these fractures are clinically similar to undisplaced type I fractures, with tenderness at the growth plate and normal radiographs. If the mechanism of injury involves a high compression load on the forearm, the possibility of a type V fracture should be considered. Because no fracture or displacement is usually evident, the injured forearm is splinted or casted for pain relief for 3 weeks. The child should be seen 6 months to 1 year after the injury for clinical examination and radiographs.

### Management of Displaced Fractures

**Salter-Harris Types I and II.** These fractures are usually displaced dorsally. The principles of reduction are similar to those for other completely displaced fractures of the forearm. The reduction is performed gently to avoid further injury to the physis.[90] The intact hinge of periosteum on the dorsal aspect of the radius usually prevents overcorrection with manipulation.[156] A long arm cast or a "sugar-tongs" splint with three-point molding is applied with the forearm pronated. Because the fracture occurs through the growth plate, healing is rapid,[156] and 3 weeks of immobilization is all that is usually necessary.

Some displaced Salter type II fractures may be difficult to reduce anatomically. Therefore, if 50% end-to-end apposition of the fracture fragments is achieved and the

angular and rotational malalignment has been corrected, repeated manipulation is not necessary (Fig. 8–40), especially in children with physeal remodeling potential of more than 2 years. Even with incomplete reduction, remodeling proceeds with minimal risk of growth arrest.[90, 91] The best time to reduce a physeal injury is the day of the injury. After 10 days, type I and II injuries are difficult to shift without excessive force. It is wiser to accept an imperfect reduction than to risk damage to the growth plate from either forceful manipulation or surgery.[156] In a study of fractures of the distal radial physis in children, premature growth arrest was noted in 27% of patients who underwent two or more attempts at closed reduction under general anesthesia. In contrast, none of the patients who had a single manipulation exhibited growth arrest. The remaining four patients who had a significant growth disturbance had experienced a compression type of injury that probably represented a Salter-Harris type V injury to the growth plate.[90]

Salter-Harris type II fractures have been encountered that were irreducible because of an invaginated periosteal flap on the tension side of the fracture[91] or because of displacement of the volar tendons, median nerve, and radial artery and veins.[103] These fractures require open reduction and, in some cases, internal fixation with smooth K-wires. Partial growth arrest has been reported after transphyseal pinning of similar fractures.[19, 68] However, these complications are rare, and it is more important to ensure maintenance of an adequate position. As for all growth plate injuries, these fractures should be reviewed clinically and radiologically for at least 1 year after the injury.

Abnormal growth of the distal part of the radius is rare and occurs mainly after physeal compression injuries or repeated forceful attempts at reduction.[90] Subsequent physeal growth is infrequently disturbed after fracture because the germinal layers of the physis remain attached to the epiphysis and the epiphyseal circulation is usually intact.[156] Even if the metaphyseal circulation is interrupted, the circulation is reestablished within 4 weeks; vascular invasion of the hypertrophic zone of the physis is resumed, with subsequent ossification of the zone of provisional calcification.[91] Invaginated periosteum between the hypertrophied and provisionally calcified zones is likely to undergo fibrous degeneration and resorption. Subsequent remodeling of metaphyseal bone then allows for correction of the deformity.[91] The length of time after injury during which the physis remains open limits the amount of growth and remodeling that can occur after a physeal fracture and must be taken into account when deciding how much deformity is acceptable.[39, 40]

A rare injury is a type II fracture that is displaced anteriorly. The most common mechanism of injury appears to be a fall on the palmar surface of the hand in association with high energy or forced flexion of the wrist. The anterior part of the articular surface of the radius is thus submitted to axial compression while traction is being placed on the posterior part. These fractures are easily reduced by closed manipulation but are very unstable and tend to redisplace. Seriat-Gautier and Jouve recommend open reduction and fixation with a volar buttress plate that is attached to the metaphysis by

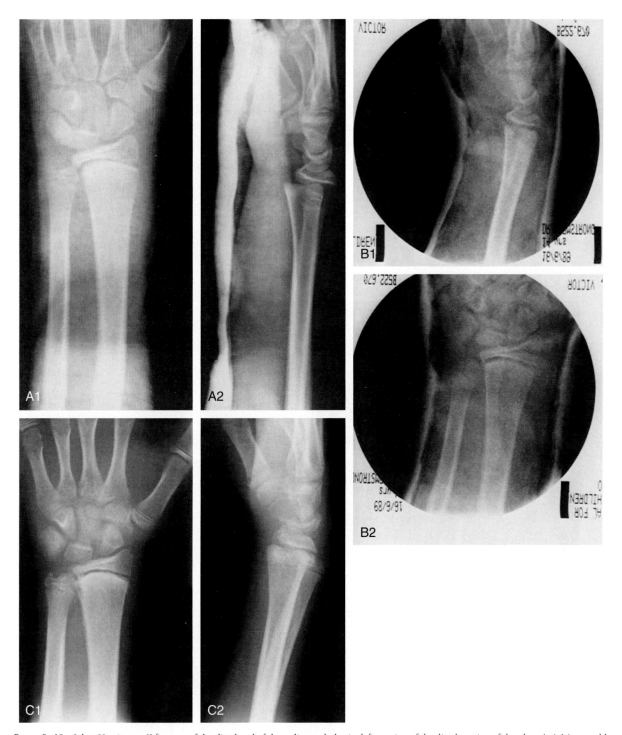

**FIGURE 8–40.** Salter-Harris type II fracture of the distal end of the radius and plastic deformation of the distal portion of the ulna. *A,* A 14-year-old boy fell while jumping. His initial radiographs appeared to show a type I injury to the distal radial growth plate. Note the plastic deformation of the distal end of the ulna. *B,* The fracture was reduced with the patient under general anesthesia. *C,* Follow-up radiographs show a small metaphyseal fragment, thus indicating that the injury was in fact a type II injury. The residual displacement did not need remanipulation because complete remodeling is expected.

screws, but without screws in the epiphysis; such treatment maintains anatomic reduction and avoids injury to the growth plate[161] (see Fig. 8–36).

**Salter-Harris Type III.** In children, type III fractures on the volar aspect of the distal end of the radius are analogous to the Barton type of fracture in adults. These fractures must be anatomically reduced to restore articular congruity and decrease the likelihood of growth

arrest. As with a Barton fracture, open reduction may be necessary to achieve the desired position. Internal fixation with pins or screws parallel to the physis is desirable, but if the fragment is too small, a smooth transphyseal pin may be inserted to stabilize it. This pin should be removed approximately 3 weeks after injury, once the fragment is stable.

**Salter-Harris Type IV.** Type IV fractures of the distal

part of the radius are quite rare. Anatomic reduction must be achieved, and open reduction is usually required in fractures with displacement (Fig. 8–41). If anatomic reduction is not achieved, growth disturbance secondary to formation of a bony bridge is likely.[156]

**Salter-Harris Type V.** Type V fractures are frequently diagnosed retrospectively after growth arrest has occurred. Because no fracture or displacement is usually evident, the injured forearm is splinted or casted for pain relief for 3 weeks.

### Follow-up

Up to 10% of fractures redisplace during the healing phase.[90] Careful weekly follow-up with adequate anteroposterior and lateral radiographs is recommended until new periosteal bone is seen.

It has been shown that fractures with an angular deformity of up to 30° will remodel satisfactorily, provided that the time to physeal closure is greater than 2 years.[90] As a result, for Salter-Harris type I and II physeal injuries in children younger than 10 years, angulation of up to 30° can be accepted. In children older than 10 years, up to 15° of angulation is generally acceptable, with complete remodeling expected.

### Complications

Complications of forearm fractures were discussed earlier. Growth disturbance is an additional complication of physeal injury.

**Malunion.** Unacceptable angular deformity after fracture union may require corrective osteotomy. Salter-Harris type I and II fractures frequently remodel

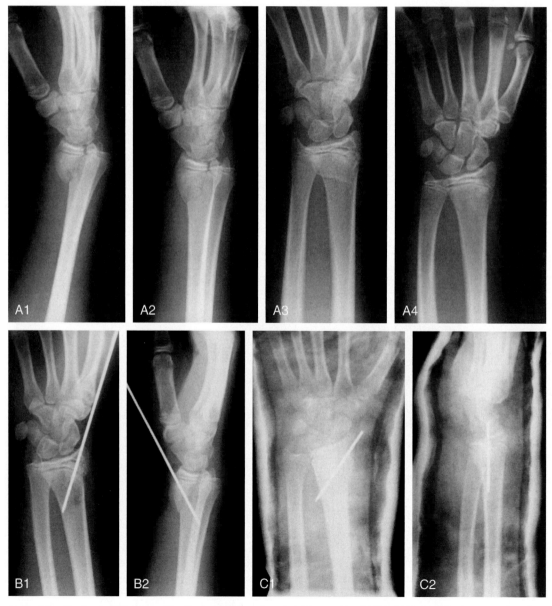

Figure 8–41. Salter-Harris type IV fracture of the distal end of the radius. *A,* A 12-year-old girl fell on her arm while playing soccer and sustained a type IV distal radial fracture. *B,* Closed reduction with the patient under general anesthesia failed, and open reduction plus fixation with a smooth K-wire was performed. *C,* The arm was immobilized in a short arm cast. The fracture healed without subsequent displacement.

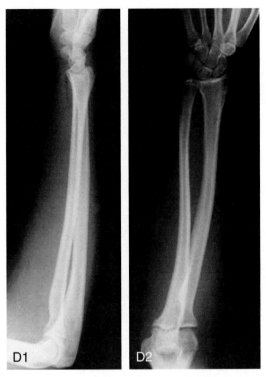

FIGURE **8–41** *Continued. D,* A follow-up radiograph 2 years later showed that the physes had closed without any growth abnormality.

significantly, so it is important to assess residual deformity, skeletal age, and the expected result after maturity. Corrective osteotomy should be performed proximal to the growth plate while ensuring that damage to the physis is avoided. Malunion of Salter-Harris type III injuries can result in post-traumatic arthritis. Once malunion has occurred, it is very difficult to correct. Reconstruction by osteotomy is indicated if gross deformity is present before the onset of symptoms. Malunion of Salter-Harris type IV injuries can result in growth disturbance secondary to formation of a bony bridge, as well as post-traumatic arthritis, in patients with significant joint incongruity.

**Growth Disturbance.** Significant growth disturbance occurs in 7% of physeal injuries and can result in progressive angulation or progressive shortening.[90] Premature closure of the growth plate is more common after compression injuries or repeated forceful attempts at reduction. Transphyseal pinning has also been shown to occasionally cause partial growth arrest.[19, 68] The growth plate injury may be discovered only when deformity begins to appear. Children who have sustained an injury to the growth plate should be monitored for a minimum of 1 year.[156] Prompt diagnosis can sometimes allow appropriate surgical intervention before a severe deformity develops.

After a physeal injury, the severity of the clinical problem depends on the site of the growth disturbance, the extent of involvement of the physeal plate, and the expected amount of growth remaining in the involved plate.[156] Some of the wrist deformities resemble Madelung's deformity, with premature fusion of the medial half of the radial physis, triangularization of the distal radial epiphysis with unequal growth of the

epiphysis, and ulnar and volar angulation of the distal radial articular surface associated with dorsal subluxation of the ulna and enlargement and distortion of the ulnar head.[141] This pseudo–Madelung's deformity, a rare occurrence, may cause limited painful wrist motion, wrist crepitus, a decrease in grip strength, and permanent disability.[202] However, post-traumatic deformity can be variable, depending on the degree and location of the partial growth arrest at the distal radial physis. Gross deformity develops if the discrepancy between radial and ulnar length is more than 4 mm.[90]

Investigations to detect growth arrest should include tomograms and computed tomography (CT) or magnetic resonance imaging (MRI) to map the extent of the bony bridge. If the bony bridge is less than 50% of the physis and the child has at least 2 years of growth remaining, resection of the bridge and interpositional grafting with fat or an artificial substance may be indicated. If the radius and ulna have a length discrepancy, this procedure should be accompanied by epiphysiodesis of the corresponding unaffected ulnar physis. These techniques are discussed extensively in Chapter 7.

If significant deformity is present and the bony bridge is extensive, other reconstructive surgery must be considered. The Darrach procedure is unacceptable in very young patients because of the loss of power and function that frequently results from it.[202] Simultaneous ulnar shortening and radial osteotomy to correct the radiocarpal angle give consistently better clinical results than does ulnar epiphysiodesis or the Darrach procedure.[90] Tricortical iliac grafts can be interposed into the radial osteotomy to restore the radiocarpal and radioulnar angles[113, 203] (Fig. 8–42). Newer techniques of correcting deformities, such as the Ilizarov technique, are being used more frequently.[193]

Rarely, growth arrest of the distal ulnar physis may occur after injury. It is best managed by radial shortening or ulnar lengthening with reconstruction of the distal radioulnar joint.

## DISTAL RADIAL AND ULNAR FRACTURES

Distal radial and ulnar fractures are most commonly seen in girls 11 to 13 years old and boys 13 to 15 years old,[5, 178] when it is postulated that the porosity of bone is temporarily increased during the period of most rapid linear growth.[5] The incidence of these fractures is lower in girls than boys.[6]

Fracture of the ulnar styloid frequently accompanies a distal radial fracture, possibly because a distal radial fracture is usually caused by a fall on a pronated hand, when the dorsal portion of the triangular fibrocartilage and the dorsal radiocarpal ligament tend to be taut.[128]

### Diagnosis

The mechanisms of injury for forearm fractures in general also apply to fractures in the distal ends of the radius and ulna. A "dinner-fork" type of deformity, which is the appearance of a dorsally displaced fracture of the distal end of the forearm, is seen after a supinatory force has been applied to the pronated hand. Dorsal angulation and volar displacement are seen after a pronation mechanism of injury.

## Management

The key to successful closed treatment of distal forearm fractures is recognition of the deforming forces and reversal of the deformity. It is acknowledged that most residual deformities of the distal third of the forearm with angulation as great as 35° will correct fully in 5 years in children who are still growing.[42, 44] Therefore, as with other fractures in the forearm, the length of time that the physis will remain open must be taken into account when deciding how much deformity is acceptable.

Although acceptable limits of reduction are widely disputed in the literature, the following guidelines have been recommended. In infants, up to 30° of angulation in the coronal plane can be accepted. Between the ages of 5 and 10 years, a good result can be expected if residual angulation is no greater than 15° to 20°. In children older than 10 years, the upper limit is 15° in the coronal plane and 10° of radial deviation.[27, 73, 123, 125, 128]

**Buckle Fractures.** Torus or buckle fractures can be immobilized in a short arm cast. These injuries are stable and are immobilized only for comfort while the fracture is healing. A period of 2 to 3 weeks is usually sufficient. After the cast is removed, the forearm should be checked clinically and resplinted if the fracture site remains tender.

**Greenstick Fractures.** Management of greenstick fractures of the forearm was discussed earlier. In the distal part of the forearm, we recommend that a well-molded cast extending above the elbow be used to limit pronation and supination. This cast is usually replaced after 3 to 4 weeks with a short arm cast for an additional 2 weeks, until the fracture is solid (Fig. 8–43).

**Complete Fractures.** These fractures can usually be reduced with closed manipulation (discussed under management of forearm fractures). For fractures of both the radius and the ulna, one fracture should be reduced first, then the other. If the ulnar segment is very short, it may be difficult to achieve perfect reduction of the ulna, but mild angulation will not be a problem (Fig. 8–44). Infrequently, adequate reduction cannot be achieved, and one must proceed with open techniques.

According to traditional teaching, fractures of the distal third of the forearm should be immobilized in pronation. Rang, however, cautions that if the fracture is put in either full pronation or full supination, one fragment will angulate anteriorly while the other angulates posteriorly.[142] Placing the fracture in each of these positions can be performed intraoperatively under image intensification to find the position in which it is most stable and in which the reduction is optimal. The arm should be immobilized in that position with a long arm cast.

The fracture should be monitored weekly for 3 weeks after reduction while redisplacement is still a possibility. Angulation that occurs in this postreduction period is usually corrected relatively easily with a cast change or modification. The procedure can be done without

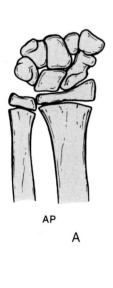
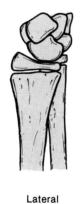

AP          Lateral

A

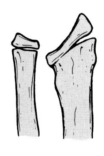

AP          Lateral

B

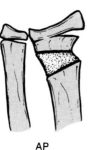
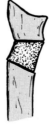

AP          Lateral

C

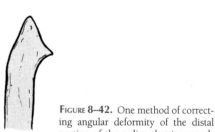

Figure **8–42.** One method of correcting angular deformity of the distal portion of the radius that is secondary to growth disturbance. *A,* Comparison with the normal wrist. *B,* Radiographic appearance of the distal ends of the radius and ulna. *C,* Appearance after insertion of a tricortical iliac crest bone graft designed to normalize the radiocarpal angles. (*A–C,* From Zehntner, M.K., Jakob, R.P.; McGanity, P.L. J Pediatr Orthop 10:411–415, 1990.)

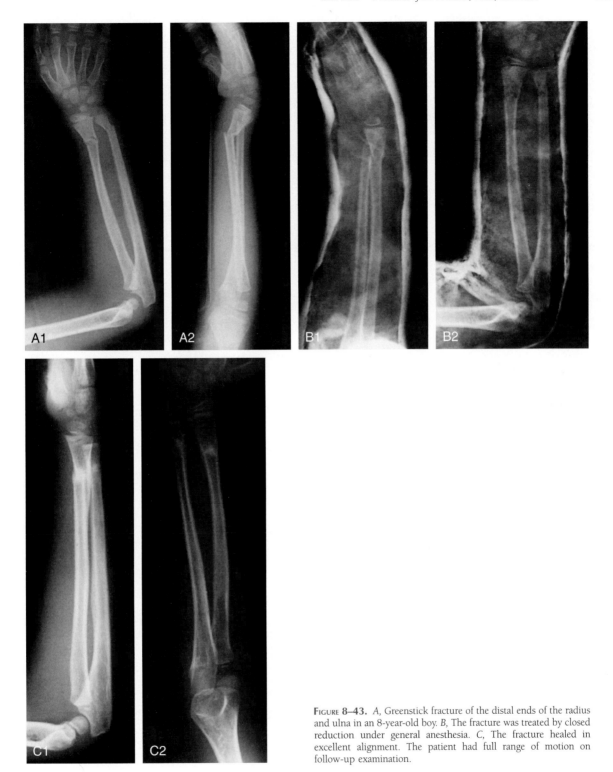

FIGURE 8–43. *A,* Greenstick fracture of the distal ends of the radius and ulna in an 8-year-old boy. *B,* The fracture was treated by closed reduction under general anesthesia. *C,* The fracture healed in excellent alignment. The patient had full range of motion on follow-up examination.

anesthesia if the deformity is mild and detected before the fracture is solid.

## FRACTURES OF THE DISTAL THIRD OF THE RADIUS

Fracture of the radius at the junction of the metaphysis and diaphysis with a supination deformity has been dubbed "the slipper" by Rang because of the tendency for

angulation to recur after reduction[142] (Fig. 8–45). This injury should be differentiated from a Galeazzi fracture, which is associated with disruption of the radioulnar TFCC. Fracture of the distal third of the radius occurs more frequently in patients older than 8 years. It is often an oblique fracture. The distal fragment is usually displaced medially secondary to the pull of the pronator quadratus, extensor pollicis longus, and abductor pollicis brevis. This fracture, alone or in association with a

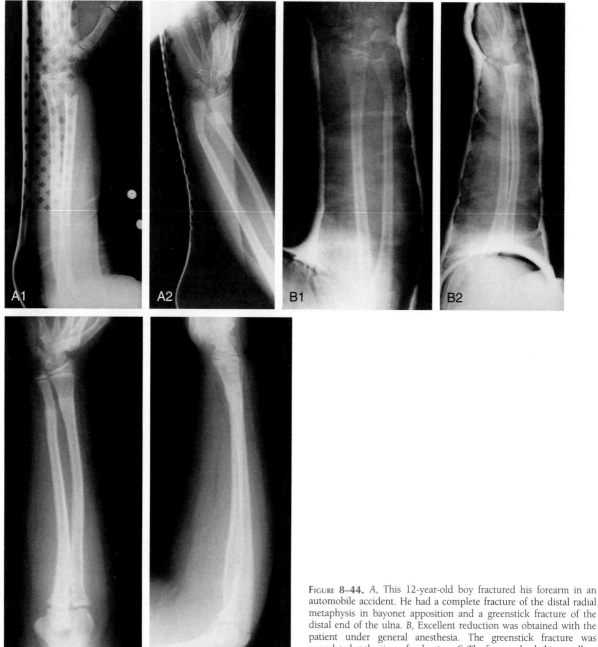

**FIGURE 8–44.** *A,* This 12-year-old boy fractured his forearm in an automobile accident. He had a complete fracture of the distal radial metaphysis in bayonet apposition and a greenstick fracture of the distal end of the ulna. *B,* Excellent reduction was obtained with the patient under general anesthesia. The greenstick fracture was completed at the time of reduction. *C,* The fracture healed in excellent position, and on follow-up examination, the child had regained full motion.

greenstick fracture or buckle fracture of the distal end of the ulna, is unstable and can be tricky to manage.

The fracture is reduced in the usual manner by first increasing the deformity and hooking the distal fragment onto the proximal fragment. Once the traction on the arm is released, however, the fracture tends to shorten and angulate because of its obliquity. Even by including the thumb in the cast, shortening is difficult to prevent (Fig. 8–46). According to traditional teaching, the fracture should be immobilized in pronation because it is distal to the insertion of the pronator teres. However, in pronation, the pull of the brachioradialis displaces the

fragment. The oblique thenar muscles and brachioradialis are relaxed in supination, thereby stabilizing the reduction (Fig. 8–47).

Gupta and Danielsson reported a randomized prospective trial of 60 patients with solitary greenstick fractures of the distal end of the radius that were immobilized in a position of pronation, neutrality, or supination. Before the study, they observed that minimally displaced fractures and fractures that required reduction had a tendency to angulate even if immobilized in an above-elbow cast. When the wrist was immobilized in pronation, the undisplaced fracture group had a lower

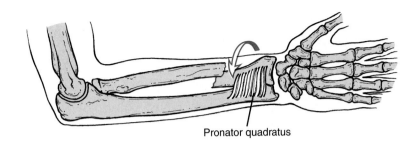

Pronator quadratus

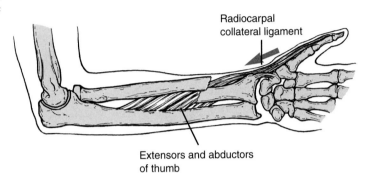

FIGURE 8–45. Deforming forces in fractures of the distal third of the radius. (From Hughston, J.C. J Bone Joint Surg Am 39:250, 1957.)

Radiocarpal collateral ligament

Extensors and abductors of thumb

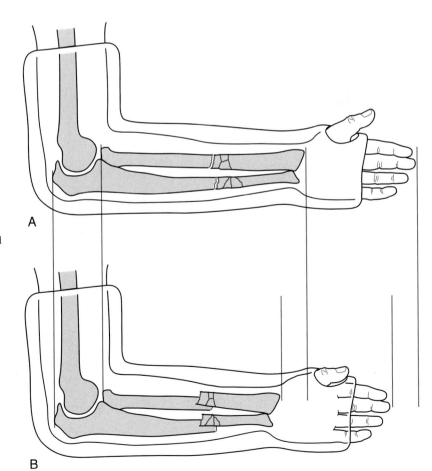

FIGURE 8–46. Shortening cannot be prevented by including the thumb in the cast.

A

B

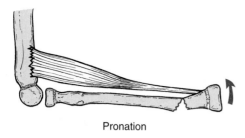

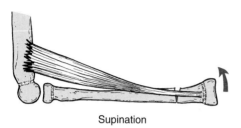

**Figure 8–47.** The role of the brachioradialis muscle, which tends to displace the fracture in pronation (*A*) and to "lock" the reduction in supination (*B*). (*A, B,* From Gupta, R.P.; Danielsson, L.G. J Pediatr Orthop 10:90–92, 1990.)

incidence of recurrent angulation than did patients who required closed reduction. In the fractures treated with the forearm in supination, the mean increase in dorsal angulation after initial treatment was less than in those treated in pronation and in a neutral position.[56] To maximize rotational control, it is recommended that distal radial fractures be immobilized in a long arm cast with the forearm in supination. The fracture is monitored carefully with weekly radiographs to detect early redisplacement, at which time cast changes or remanipulation can be performed. The cast should be removed at 6 weeks.

Some authors advocate pinning these frequently unstable fractures. Closed reduction is performed first. A K-wire is then inserted through a small incision in the skin at the lateral distal radial metaphysis (to prevent skewering of subcutaneous nerves or vessels) and advanced across the fracture site (Fig. 8–48). A long arm cast is applied for the first 4 weeks, followed by a short arm cast for another 2 weeks or until the fracture has healed. The pin is removed at approximately 6 weeks, when the radial fracture has healed.

Although reasonable alignment can usually be achieved with closed reduction, some shortening of the radius with respect to the ulna frequently occurs. Angulation up to 10° and shortening of the radius up to 5 mm are acceptable.[106] Slight displacement usually results in little or no functional disability, as evidenced by the paucity of reports on long-term disability from this type of fracture. If a reasonable position cannot be achieved, open reduction and plating or pinning of the distal end of the radius should be performed.

## FRACTURES OF THE SHAFTS OF THE RADIUS AND ULNA

Eighteen percent of all forearm fractures occur in the shafts of the radius and ulna. Whereas in older children the injury usually occurs in the metaphyseal region of the

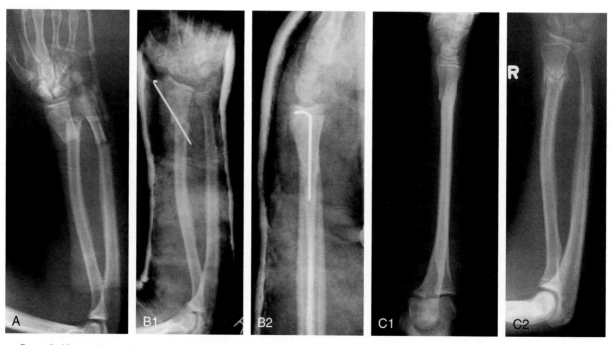

**Figure 8–48.** Distal-third fracture of the radius. *A,* A 14-year-old boy was hit into the boards while playing hockey. Along with a fracture of the distal third of the radius and a greenstick fracture of the ulna, he had a ½-cm puncture wound on the volar aspect. *B,* The skin edges and fracture fragments were débrided, and open reduction was performed. Through a short radial incision over the metaphysis, a K-wire was inserted. Postoperatively, numbness over the dorsum of the thumb was noted. The K-wire was removed at 6 weeks. *C,* At 3 months, the numbness had resolved. He had full supination and a lack of 10° pronation in comparison with the opposite forearm.

bone, in younger children, it occurs in the diaphysis.[165] Both bones of the forearm are usually injured unless the mechanism of injury is a direct blow to the arm, which may result in an isolated fracture of either the radius or the ulna. Isolated fractures of the ulna are uncommon.[180] A combination of complete fracture, greenstick fracture, or plastic deformation of the radius and ulna may occur at any location in the forearm. If only one bone appears to be injured, careful clinical and radiologic evaluation must be performed to eliminate the possibility of disruption at either the elbow or the wrist.

## Classification

Fractures of the shaft of the radius and ulna are classified according to the fracture types: plastic deformation, greenstick, and complete fractures. Complete fractures may be classified according to fracture configurations: transverse, oblique, spiral, butterfly, and comminuted fractures.

## Diagnosis

Careful examination for swelling, tenderness, and skin involvement must be undertaken and neurologic and vascular status ascertained. The most commonly injured nerves are the median nerve at the wrist and the anterior interosseous nerve at the elbow. Radiologic assessment must include the wrist and the elbow in both anteroposterior and lateral views.

## Management

General principles in the management of fractures of the forearm were enumerated earlier. Further guidelines specific to shaft fractures are presented next.

**Plastic Deformation.** Plastic deformation of both bones of the forearm is more common in children younger than 5 years. Provided that the angular deformity is less than 20°, little disability will result, even if the deformity is not corrected. In children older than 10 years, correction of the angular and rotatory deformity is essential to restore forearm rotation. The technique for reducing plastic deformities was described earlier.

**Greenstick Fractures.** Both angular and rotational components of the injury must be reduced. A well-molded long arm cast should be applied with good three-point molding. The cast should be removed at 4 to 6 weeks in children younger than 5 years and at 6 to 8 weeks in older children after checking to ensure that clinical union has occurred. Victor and colleagues recommend that athletes such as gymnasts be restricted from strenuous activity for 6 months because of the risk of refracture.[182]

**Complete Displacement.** If anatomic reduction is achieved, the fracture usually becomes relatively stable. Greater than 50% end-on apposition is desirable to achieve adequate stability of the fracture during closed treatment. The position of immobilization is determined by the position of the proximal fragment. The fracture should be immobilized in any position in which the alignment is correct and the reduction feels stable. A well-fitting long arm cast should be applied. Some authors suggest that if the radius is comminuted or tends

to shorten, the thumb may be included in the cast.[142] However, as mentioned previously, addition of the thumb does little to prevent shortening. If the fracture remains unstable in an unsatisfactory position, either internal or external fixation should be considered.

In the proximal third of the forearm, the bones are surrounded by a thick mass of muscles that make it difficult to attain perfect reduction. As the muscles atrophy during the period of immobilization, the cast becomes loose, and the effect of the three-point fixation within the cast is reduced. Angulation of 10° at this site is more likely to cause a restriction in motion than is a similar angulation in more distal fractures.[27] Several authors therefore recommend that fractures in the proximal third of the forearm be immobilized with the elbow extended to avoid angulation of the fracture secondary to slippage inside a loose, curved cast[43, 142] (Fig. 8–49). Rang suggested that all fractures of both bones of the forearm in children younger than 2 years be immobilized in extension. He believes that this practice provides better control of axial alignment in these smaller children.[142]

The child should be monitored weekly for 3 weeks after reduction of the fracture, during the time of greatest risk for redisplacement. This period is dependent on the age of the child because of the speed of fracture healing. In children younger than 2 years, remanipulation can correct angulation without excessive force within 1 week of the fracture. In patients between 1 and 5 years of age, minor improvements should be done within 2 weeks after the fracture.

Bayonet apposition in the forearm of a child younger than 10 years is acceptable, provided that the interosseous distance is maintained and the fracture is not malrotated or angulated (Fig. 8–50). In children older than 10 years, a fracture left in bayonet apposition will not remodel sufficiently to ensure maintenance of the interosseous distance, and permanent loss of motion will ensue.

In general, for children younger than 8 years, injuries with 20° of residual angulation will remodel sufficiently to obtain excellent results. In children older than 8 years, 10° of residual angulation at union will not result in a significant loss of pronation or supination. Difficulty arises when the immediate postreduction or 1-week radiographs show residual or secondary displacement. Kramhoft and Solgaard showed that 50% of fractures with 7° to 10° of dorsal angulation displaced further during healing.[83] By reducing significant residual angulation within the first 3 weeks, management is simpler, and the final result will be improved.

Price uses the following guidelines for acceptable alignment. For children 8 years or younger, one may accept complete displacement, angulation up to 15°, and malrotation up to 45°. For girls 9 to 14 years and boys 9 to 16 years old, distal fractures have a better prognosis than proximal shaft fractures do. Therefore, distal fractures may be treated closed in the presence of complete displacement and up to 15° of angulation and 30° of malrotation. Proximal shaft fractures in the older age group will have a satisfactory result with complete

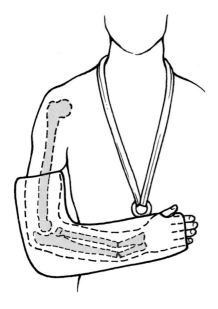

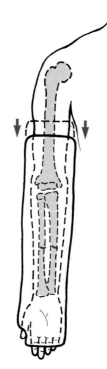

FIGURE 8–49. Slippage of the arm in a straight cast does not cause redisplacement of the fracture. (From Rang, M. Children's Fractures, 2nd ed. Philadelphia, J.B. Lippincott, 1982, p. 209.)

displacement and up to 10° of angulation and 30° of malrotation.[138]

### Surgical Treatment

In general, treatment of forearm fractures in children is nonoperative because of the rapid healing of these fractures and the potential for considerable remodeling of residual deformity.[73, 123, 138] Acceptable parameters for continued closed management of pediatric forearm fractures include the following. In children younger than 9 years, complete displacement (bayonet apposition), angulation up to 15°, and malrotation up to 45° are acceptable. In children 9 years and older, 10° of angulation for proximal fractures and 15° degrees for distal fractures are acceptable along with 30° of malrotation. As long as the child has at least 2 years of growth remaining, complete bayonet apposition is acceptable.[123, 138]

Indications for operative treatment of pediatric forearm fractures include (1) open fractures, (2) failure to obtain or maintain adequate closed reduction, (3) displaced fractures in children approaching skeletal maturity, and (4) certain pathologic fractures that are unstable. The criteria developed by Noonan and Price and by Younger and others are critical in deciding whether continued closed treatment methods will be acceptable.[123, 201, 202]

Techniques of operative intervention include open reduction and internal fixation with plates and screws and intramedullary fixation by either closed or open methods.[4, 37, 54, 101, 131, 148, 163, 200]

The technique of intramedullary nailing of pediatric forearm fractures by either closed or open methods is becoming increasingly popular. Either elastic titanium nails or stainless steel pins (Rush rods, Steinmann pins,

K-wires) are used. In some cases, single-bone fixation of both-bone forearm fractures can be performed while the other bone is rotated into a reduced position, and external cast immobilization is then instituted until the fractures have healed.[37]

Advantages of intramedullary fixation over open reduction and plate fixation include the possibility of a closed rather than open technique. In some cases of acute unstable fractures in which satisfactory reduction cannot be obtained or maintained, closed intramedullary nailing has been used successfully. However, in many cases, it is necessary to perform a minimal open reduction to clear soft tissue from the fracture ends in order to obtain satisfactory reduction (see Fig. 8–51).

The radial rods are introduced in a retrograde manner through a dorsoradial approach. Branches of the superficial radial nerve are dissected free and protected during the procedure. A small oblique drill hole is placed in the distal radial metaphysis and an appropriately sized intramedullary nail selected for insertion. Elastic intramedullary nails are available in incremental sizes from 2.0 up to 4.0 mm. In most cases, a diameter of 2.0 or 2.5 mm is selected for diaphyseal forearm fractures in children. The elastic intramedullary nails have a prebent end and a smooth straight end. The prebent end is inserted through the oblique drill hole and attempts made to reduce the fracture and pass the nail into the proximal fragment similar to closed nailing of femoral or tibial fractures. If it is not possible to reduce the fracture and pass the nail, open reduction is performed through an anterior Henry approach or dorsal Thompson approach. The surgical approach may be less extensive than the approach used for plate fixation. Soft tissue interposition is corrected and the nail passed into the proximal fragment. If the radius is nailed first, a decision is then

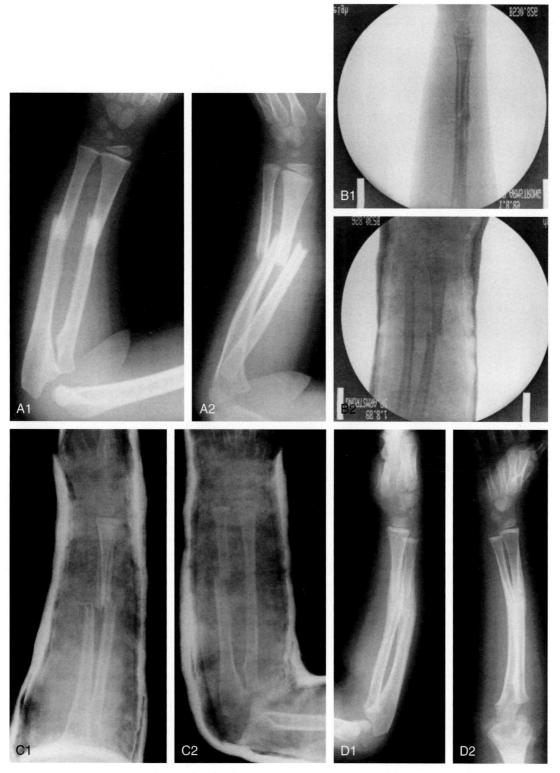

**FIGURE 8–50.** Complete midshaft fractures of the radius and ulna with bayonet apposition. *A,* A 5-year-old boy fell at camp and fractured the midshafts of both forearm bones. *B,* With the patient under general anesthesia, the fractures were reduced, with 50% cortical end-on apposition of the radius. *C,* Subsequent displacement occurred, but the position was thought to be acceptable. *D,* The cast was removed 5 weeks later. After 1 month, the forearm lacked 30° of supination and 15° of pronation. At 5 years of age, future remodeling is expected and will result in improved motion. Therefore, no further treatment is planned.

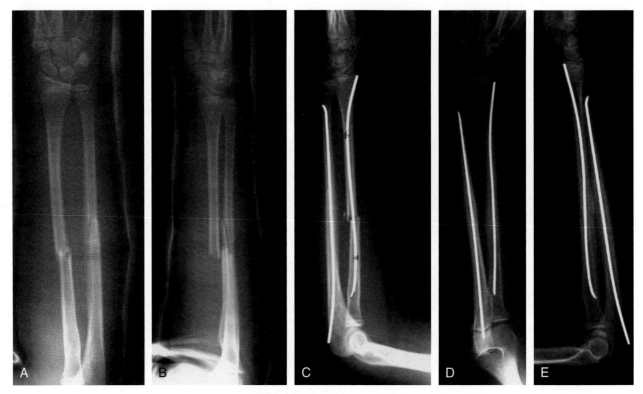

**Figure 8–51.** *A,* Anteroposterior (AP) radiograph of a both-bone forearm fracture in a 12-year-old boy with shortening of the radius. *B,* Lateral radiograph. *C,* After closed intramedullary nailing of both bones with flexible titanium nails. *D,* AP radiograph after 3 months. *E,* Lateral radiograph after 3 months.

made regarding the need for stabilization of the ulna (Fig. 8–52).

A recent study by Richter and colleagues demonstrated that if both the radius and ulna were stabilized with intramedullary nails, external immobilization was not generally required. However, cast immobilization is recommended for 6 to 8 weeks to ensure rotational stability of the fractures.

An alternative method is to perform closed nailing of the ulna fracture through the olecranon apophysis. In most cases, the fractured ulna can be reduced and the flexible titanium nail introduced by closed techniques. Prebending of the nail is not necessary. If needed, the

fracture can be exposed through a small incision on the subcutaneous border and the nail passed into the distal fragment. The forearm may then be manipulated in an attempt to reduce the radial fracture. If stable, a long arm cast is applied and single-bone fixation only used (Fig. 8–53). However, if the radius is unstable or the reduction is unacceptable, a radial nail is introduced.

Richter and associates inserted the ulnar nail distal to the proximal apophysis, which requires that the nail be prebent.[148] However, no accounts of growth disturbance of the proximal part of the ulna have been reported with the insertion of a smooth pin across the olecranon

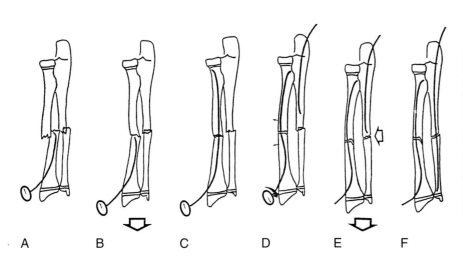

**Figure 8–52.** Intramedullary pinning of both bones of the forearm. *A,* Introduction of the radial nail through a 1-cm incision on the lateral aspect of the radius. *B,* Manipulation of the fracture. *C,* Advancement of the nail to the proximal end of the radius. *D,* Rotation of the nail to reduce the fracture and insertion of the ulnar nail just distal to the olecranon apophysis. *E,* Manipulation of the fracture. *F,* Advancement of the ulnar pin (and rotation). (*A–F,* From Lascombes, P.; Prevot, J.; Ligier, J.N.; et al. J Pediatr Orthop 10:167–171, 1990.)

A         B         C         D         E         F

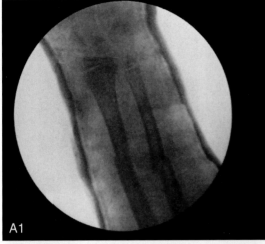

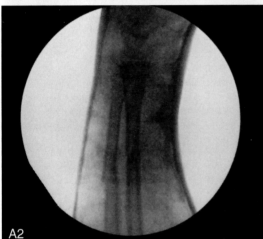

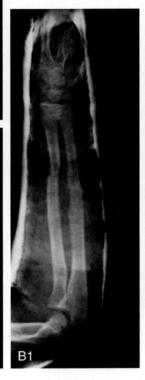

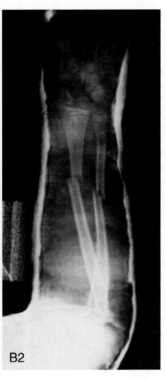

**FIGURE 8–53.** Ulnar intramedullary pin fixation for fractures of both bones of the forearm. *A,* A 10-year-old boy fell off his bicycle and fractured the midshafts of both bones of his forearm. Initially, excellent alignment was achieved by closed reduction with the patient under general anesthesia. Note the obliquity of the fractures, which predisposes this fracture to redisplacement. *B,* The fracture started to displace 1 week later.

*Illustration continued on following page*

apophysis. It is therefore safe and easier to introduce the ulnar nail by this approach.

Some authors advocate intramedullary fixation of the ulna alone, with the fracture pattern converted to a greenstick equivalent. Stabilization of the ulna allows correction and stabilization of the angulatory and rotational malalignment of the radius by closed technique. This method is often satisfactory for younger patients (between 6 and 12 years), but for older patients (>12 years) or for fractures with extensive soft tissue disruption and periosteal stripping, fixation of both the radius and ulna is recommended[163] (see Fig. 8–54).

Intramedullary fixation converts the shear stress at the fracture to compression and allows the formation of external callus.[4] Although this method is not as biomechanically rigid as plate-and-screw fixation, it is sufficient to permit rapid bony union in children. The micromotion that occurs at the fracture is minimal and probably clinically insignificant. Benefits of intramedullary fixation include stable fixation, rapid union, small scars, relatively short operative time, excellent clinical results, and ease of hardware removal.

Caution should be emphasized when the intramedullary rods are removed. Refracture has been reported up to 6 months after implant removal. It is advantageous to leave the intramedullary nails in place for at least 3 months if possible. To avoid refracture, it is advisable to place the patient in a long arm cast or a well-molded short arm cast for a period of 4 to 6 weeks after rod removal.

Complications of intramedullary fixation occur in 0% to 50% of patients[4, 89] and include hardware migration, loss of reduction, infection, nerve injury, loss of motion, and radioulnar synostosis and refracture. For the most part, complications associated with the surgical technique can be brought to acceptable levels with meticulous attention to detail. Most recent studies evaluating intramedullary fixation have reported very low complication rates.[54, 101, 131, 148, 163, 200]

Equally effective results can be expected with nonelastic stainless steel nails. The radial nail needs to be prebent to accommodate the normal radial bow. The blunt end of the nail should be introduced to avoid having the nail impinge on the endosteal surface.

In studies comparing plate-and-screw fixation with intramedullary nailing for pediatric forearm fractures, functional results were equal 12 to 24 months after fracture union.[200] With use of the modified grading system of Price, excellent results can be expected to occur 80% to 85% of the time and good results for the remainder.[138] An excellent result is one in which the patient has no complaints during strenuous physical

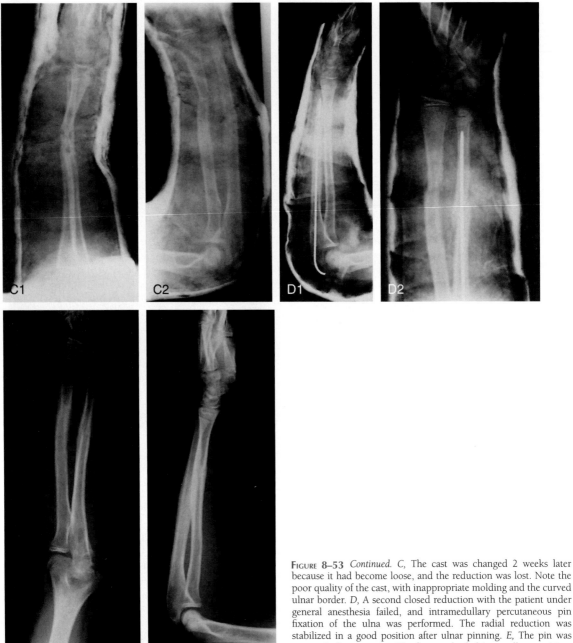

FIGURE **8–53** *Continued. C,* The cast was changed 2 weeks later because it had become loose, and the reduction was lost. Note the poor quality of the cast, with inappropriate molding and the curved ulnar border. *D,* A second closed reduction with the patient under general anesthesia failed, and intramedullary percutaneous pin fixation of the ulna was performed. The radial reduction was stabilized in a good position after ulnar pinning. *E,* The pin was removed after 6 weeks. The fracture healed in excellent position, and normal range of motion was achieved.

activity or in which 10° or less of forearm rotation is lost (or both). A result is considered good in those with only mild complaints during vigorous physical activity or in those with an 11° to 30° loss of forearm rotation (or both). Forearm rotation loss of 31° to 90° and mild subjective complaints during daily activities constitute a fair result. All other results are considered poor.[138]

In older children (>12 years) and in fractures with significant comminution and soft tissue stripping, open reduction and internal fixation with plates and screws will provide better fracture stability. In most cases, the AO 3.5-mm dynamic compression plate is used for fixation of the radius and a small-fragment one-third tubular plate for fixation of the ulna. Stability is obtained

with six cortices of fixation proximal and distal to the fracture site. Each bone should be approached through separate incisions to avoid synostosis. This technique usually allows enough stability to permit early range of motion although the technique does not seem to have any advantage over intramedullary nailing and cast immobilization in terms of loss of motion[123, 200] (Fig. 8–55).

Controversy still exists regarding the need for hardware removal. In the case of intramedullary nails, the nails are left in a subcutaneous position for ease of subsequent removal. With the exception of pathologic fractures (osteogenesis imperfecta), it is recommended that all intramedullary nails be removed after solid bony

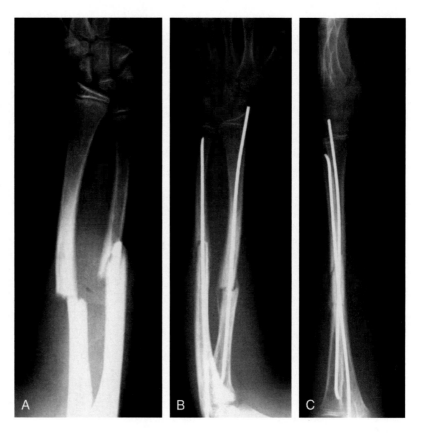

FIGURE **8–54.** *A,* Anteroposterior radiograph of fracture of both bones of the forearm with a Grade I open ulna fracture. *B,* The fracture was grossly unstable, and after irrigation and débridement, stabilization was achieved with flexible intramedullary titanium nails. *C,* Lateral radiograph.

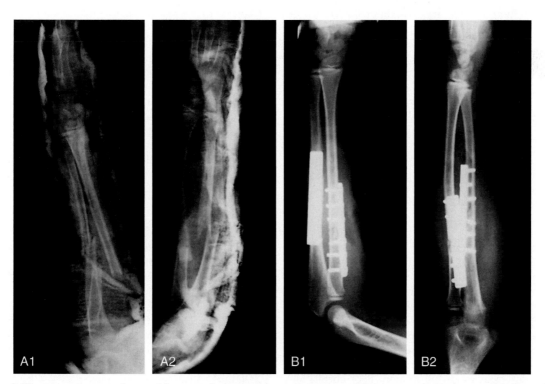

FIGURE **8–55.** Open reduction and internal fixation with plates and screws. *A,* A 12-year-old boy was assaulted and sustained fractures of the radius and ulna. This fracture configuration can also be classified as a Monteggia equivalent. *B,* With the patient under general anesthesia, the fractures were manipulated, but because satisfactory position could not be achieved, open reduction was performed with two separate incisions.

union has occurred, usually in at least 3 months. If the nails are left protruding through the skin, irritation and local infection can occur at the pin-skin interface and necessitate their removal before complete union. If this technique is used, a protective cast will need to be applied after nail removal to obviate refracture. For this reason, it is recommended that the nails be cut off in a subcutaneous position and left in place for approximately 3 months before removal. To prevent refracture, a long arm or short arm cast is applied for 4 to 6 weeks.

In the case of plates and screws, elective removal is highly controversial. Reasons given to justify operative removal include a stress riser effect at the end of the plate leading to fracture and the unknown effects of retained stainless steel or titanium over many years. Enough reports have appeared in the literature of iatrogenic injury to nerves and vessels, especially with removal of a radial plate, that we would recommend that an ulnar plate be removed only if it becomes symptomatic.[83] Pain and refracture are so rare that routine removal of a radial plate is not justified.

### Follow-up Care and Rehabilitation

**Closed Reduction.** The parents should be warned at the initiation of treatment that several cast changes may be necessary to ensure that alignment is maintained. If a minor change in alignment is observed, a cast change to one that is well fitting and well molded and that corrects the position of alignment is recommended. If the angulation is uniplanar, the cast can also be wedged.[77]

In midshaft fractures of the forearm that are undisplaced, 6 weeks in a long arm cast is recommended. If the fracture site is still tender after 6 weeks, the child is treated in a short arm cast for an additional 2 weeks. In children younger than 5 years who have undisplaced fractures, 4 weeks in a long arm cast followed by 2 weeks in a short arm cast may be sufficient.

After removal of the cast, the child is encouraged to practice range-of-motion exercises of the elbow and forearm. The child is reviewed clinically and radiologically after 4 weeks. In most children, physiotherapy is not necessary. However, if range of motion has not returned by 8 weeks after fracture and a mechanical block is not suspected, physiotherapy can be initiated. The child is discouraged from returning to contact sports for 1 month after removal of the cast because of the risk of refracture.

### Complications

The potential complications of shaft fractures of the forearm were discussed earlier. The following are some additional points that are specific to these fractures.

Malunion is the most frequent complication and results in loss of supination or pronation of the forearm. Price and colleagues reviewed 39 patients with forearm shaft fractures treated by closed reduction who had malunion at the completion of treatment. In their series, age at the time of injury did not correlate with the prognosis for recovery of full motion. Poor correlation was noted between radiographic remodeling and loss of motion. They believed that loss of motion may be caused by soft tissue scarring producing tension on the interos-

seous membrane. Mild degrees of malrotation corrected with remodeling. The combination of a proximal shaft fracture with angulation, malrotation, and encroachment carried the greatest risk for loss of motion. All patients were satisfied with their cosmetic appearance and function. The current practice of these authors is to accept up to 10° of angulation, 45° of malrotation, and complete displacement before considering remanipulation or resorting to open reduction.[139]

If less than 45° of supination or pronation is present 2 years after union of the fracture, surgical correction may be considered. An osteotomy should be planned preoperatively by comparing the radiographic appearance of the radius and ulna with that of the normal side. Solid fixation with plates and screws is recommended to ensure that the intraoperative correction is maintained. Range-of-motion exercises are then initiated in the early postoperative period.

Nonunion is an infrequent problem in children. Most reported nonunions followed either open fractures or open reduction and internal fixation in patients with severe comminution or bone loss. These injuries are treated with bone grafting and solid compression and fixation with AO dynamic compression plate and screws (Fig. 8–56). Alternatively, external fixation techniques with compression can be used.

Cross union of the radius and ulna is a potential complication of fractures of the radius and ulna at the same level[144]; in the pediatric age group, this complication is rare, however. The risk of cross union is significantly increased after repeated manipulations, severe comminution and displacement of the fragments, surgical trauma, application of onlay bone grafts (especially with narrowing of the interosseous space), and closed head injury.[144] Although a single incision doubtless increases the likelihood of cross union, surgery through two incisions does not necessarily prevent it. Disabling loss of pronation and supination is an indication for excision of the cross union, which should await bone scan confirmation that bone formation is quiescent. Interposed fat is inserted to prevent recurrence of the cross union. However, the results after excision are not as good in children as in adults, possibly because of the growth potential of immature periosteum or soft tissue contractures that preclude the regaining of full motion.[184]

### Conclusions

The vast majority of displaced pediatric forearm fractures can be managed by closed reduction under an appropriate conscious sedation protocol in an emergency department setting. It is mandatory that follow-up radiographs be taken once weekly for the first 2 to 3 weeks to ensure that satisfactory fracture alignment is maintained.

In the event that satisfactory reduction cannot be obtained or maintained, internal fixation should be undertaken. Intramedullary nail fixation has proved to be an effective method of stabilizing pediatric forearm fractures. Advantages over plate-and-screw fixation include the possibility of fracture stabilization by a closed technique or relatively limited surgical exposure and ease of implant removal. Plate-and-screw fixation is an

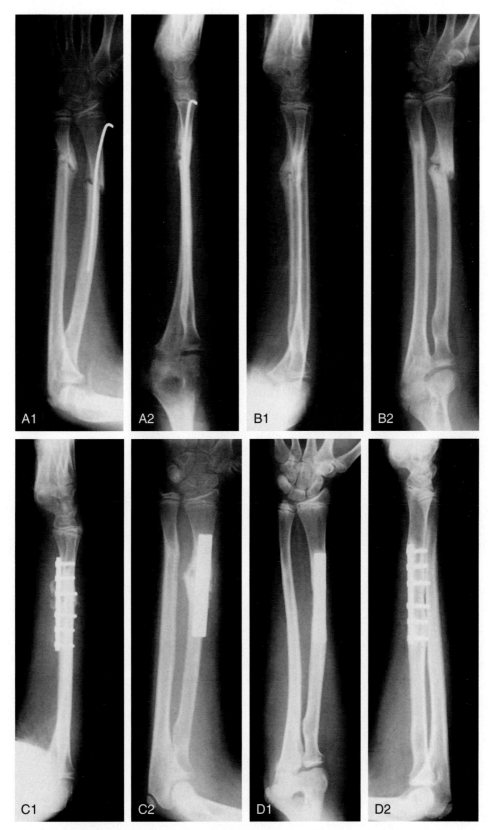

**FIGURE 8–56.** Nonunion of the radius. *A,* A 13-year-old boy who had a grade I open fracture of the distal ends of the radius and ulna was treated with débridement and immobilization in a cast. After the reduction was lost, open reduction and fixation with an intramedullary pin were performed. *B,* The radial fracture did not unite. *C,* Bone grafting and compression plating of the radius were done 4 months after the fracture. *D,* The fracture united, and the plate was removed.

equally acceptable method of fracture fixation in this age group.

## IPSILATERAL FRACTURES OF THE UPPER EXTREMITY

In approximately 4% to 13% of elbow fractures in children, a fracture of the ipsilateral forearm may be present.[133] Some of the frequently seen combinations include (1) fracture of the forearm in association with a supracondylar fracture of the humerus (Fig. 8–57), (2) fracture of the distal radial physis with a supracondylar fracture of the humerus, (3) dislocation of the elbow in association with a fracture of the forearm, (4) fracture of the olecranon with an injury to the distal radial physis, (5) fracture of the forearm in association with a lateral condylar fracture of the humerus,[128] (6) fracture of the distal part of the forearm in association with type I or equivalent Monteggia lesions,[5] and (7) transcarpal injuries associated with distal radial fractures.[24, 49, 79]

Ipsilateral fractures of the elbow and forearm have been called "floating elbow." They usually occur in

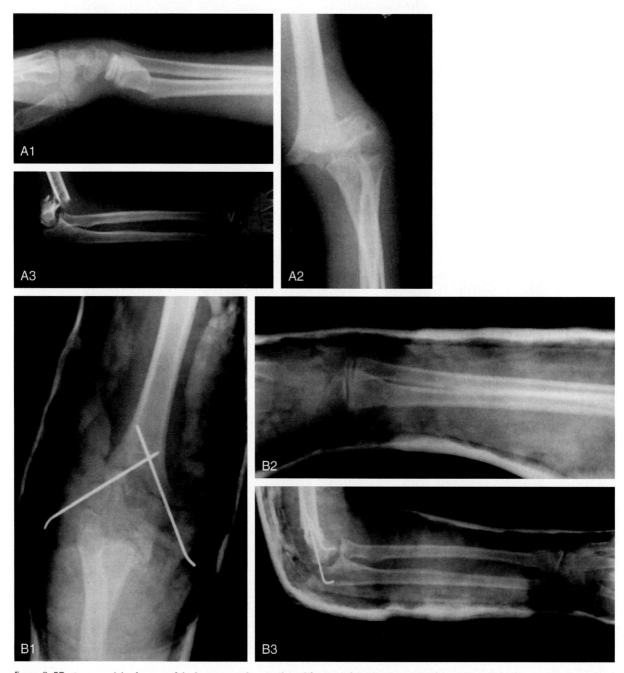

FIGURE **8–57.** Supracondylar fracture of the humerus with an ipsilateral fracture of the distal portion of the radius. *A,* An 8-year-old boy sustained a supracondylar fracture of the humerus and fracture of the distal ends of the radius and ulna. *B,* The supracondylar fracture was first reduced and pinned. The distal radial and ulnar fractures were then reduced, and the arm was immobilized in a long arm cast.

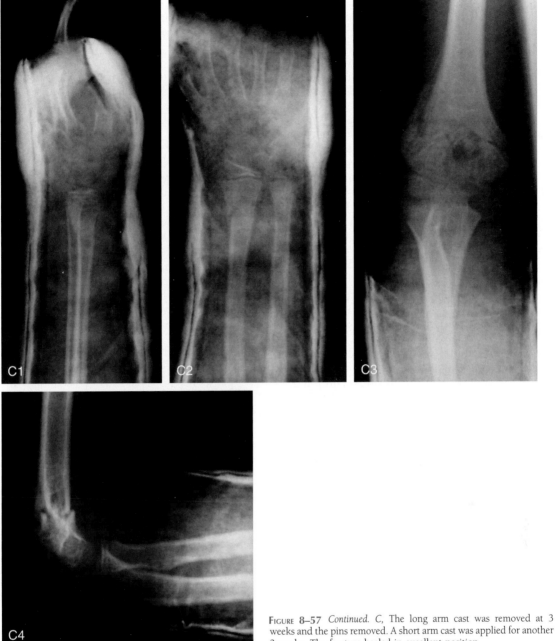

FIGURE 8–57 *Continued. C,* The long arm cast was removed at 3 weeks and the pins removed. A short arm cast was applied for another 3 weeks. The fracture healed in excellent position.

children between the ages of 6 and 12 years. The mechanism of injury is frequently a fall from a height onto the outstretched hand; less frequently, these fractures result from traffic accidents.[133] The segmental nature of the injuries increases the risk of significant compromise of arterial flow and venous return and therefore increases the potential for the development of compartment syndrome.[169] Similar to the management of a "floating knee," it is recommended that one or both of these fractures be reduced and stabilized with internal fixation.

If an associated supracondylar fracture of the humerus is present, the first step consists of closed reduction and percutaneous fixation of this fracture to provide a stable base for management of the associated forearm in-jury.[169, 195] Similarly, lateral condylar fractures should be pinned, even if the fracture is not initially displaced, before dealing with the distal fracture.[133]

## Open Fractures

Open fractures should always be treated with careful débridement of soft tissues and bones, copious irrigation of the wound and fracture fragments, and then reduction of the fracture. Appropriate intravenous antibiotic therapy for 2 to 3 days and tetanus prophylaxis (when indicated) are initiated. Internal fixation is an option in patients with extensive soft tissue damage or if the fracture is not stable. In the event that internal fixation is required in a grossly contaminated wound, the actual fixation can be delayed until subsequent wound inspections and dressing changes result in a clean wound. Intramedullary fixation is preferred because of the limited exposure required for insertion of the nails and because of the ease of soft tissue coverage of the bone. Alternatively, external fixation can be an option in these cases but is used infrequently.[160]

Haasbeek and Cole reviewed 61 cases of open fractures involving the humerus, radius, and ulna in children.[57] Forty-six (75%) involved the forearm. Treatment of the midshaft fractures included a cast (9), intramedullary rods or K-wires (10), plates (8), or external fixation (1). Complications in fracture healing occurred in 10 of 28 children (36%) with midshaft fractures of the radius and ulna. Nerve injuries occurred in 11% and compartment syndrome in 20%. No cases of osteomyelitis occurred. At late review, 87% of the children with open forearm fractures had good or excellent results.

## Monteggia Fractures

In 1814, Giovanni Battista Monteggia first described an injury consisting of fracture of the proximal third of the ulna and anterior dislocation of the proximal epiphysis of the radius. Bado redefined the Monteggia lesion as a group of traumatic lesions having in common dislocation of the radiohumeroulnar joint in association with a fracture of the ulna at various levels or with lesions at the wrist.[5] Although in 60% to 70% of cases the ulnar fracture is at the junction of the proximal and middle thirds, Bado included in his classification fractures at any location in the ulna.[5] Of all forearm fractures in children, 0.4% are the Monteggia type.[44] The peak incidence occurs between the ages of 4 and 10 years.[129]

### CLASSIFICATION

Bado's classification was originally devised to include lesions in both children and adults. Because the relative frequency of the various Monteggia fractures differs in children and adults, some authors dispute the usefulness of this classification in children.[93] However, because Bado's classification includes all the lesions that do occur in children, with modification, it is still useful (Fig. 8–58). Most importantly, it includes the Monteggia equivalents, which occur frequently in children, especially ulnar fractures associated with Salter-Harris type II fractures of the proximal end of the radius.

#### Monteggia Lesions

Type I—anterior dislocation of the radial head and fracture of the ulnar diaphysis at any level with anterior angulation

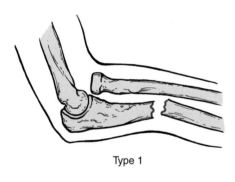

Type 1

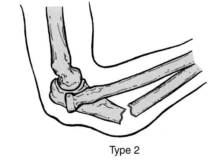

Type 2

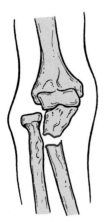

Type 3

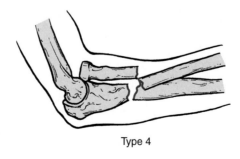

Type 4

**FIGURE 8–58.** Monteggia fracture classification. (From Olney, B.W.; Menelaus, M.B. J Pediatr Orthop 9:219–223, 1989.)

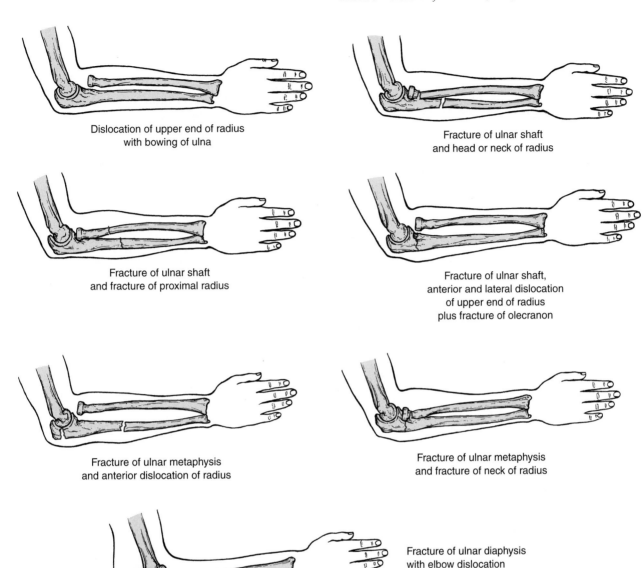

Dislocation of upper end of radius
with bowing of ulna

Fracture of ulnar shaft
and head or neck of radius

Fracture of ulnar shaft
and fracture of proximal radius

Fracture of ulnar shaft,
anterior and lateral dislocation
of upper end of radius
plus fracture of olecranon

Fracture of ulnar metaphysis
and anterior dislocation of radius

Fracture of ulnar metaphysis
and fracture of neck of radius

Fracture of ulnar diaphysis
with elbow dislocation

FIGURE 8–59. Monteggia type I–equivalent fractures. (From Olney, B.W.; Menelaus, M.B. J Pediatr Orthop 9:219–223, 1989.)

Type II—posterior or posterolateral dislocation of the radial head and fracture of the ulnar diaphysis with posterior angulation

Type III—lateral or anterolateral dislocation of the radial head with fracture of the ulnar metaphysis

Type IV—anterior dislocation of the radial head with fracture of the proximal third of the radius and fracture of the ulna at the same level.

*Monteggia Equivalents—Type I* (Fig. 8–59)

Anterior dislocation of the radial head with plastic deformation of the ulna

Fracture of the ulnar diaphysis with fracture of the neck of the radius

Fracture of the ulnar diaphysis along with fracture of the proximal third of the radius proximal to the ulnar fracture

Fracture of the ulnar metaphysis with anterior dislocation of the radius (not included by Bado)

Fracture of the ulnar diaphysis with anterior dislocation of the radial head and fracture of the olecranon

Fracture of the ulnar metaphysis along with fracture of the neck of the radius (not included by Bado)

Posterior dislocation of the elbow and fracture of the ulnar diaphysis, with or without fracture of the proximal end of the radius

Letts and colleagues proposed a different classification in children that reclassifies the Bado type I into three categories: anterior dislocation of the radial head with (A) an anterior bend of the ulnar shaft, (B) an anterior greenstick fracture of the ulnar shaft, and (C) a complete fracture of the ulna with the apex of angulation being anterior. Type D is a posterior dislocation with an ulnar fracture, and type E is a lateral dislocation with an ulnar fracture.[93] The Monteggia equivalents in Bado's classification were not included.

Bado included fracture of the neck of the radius in his classification, but this injury is not commonly accepted as a Monteggia fracture. Simple anterior dislocation of the radial head was also included (Fig. 8–60). Most isolated traumatic dislocations of the radial head are probably Monteggia equivalents in which the ulna has undergone plastic deformation.[5, 93]

Bado type I fractures are the most common in both children and adults. Type II fractures occur rarely in children but are the second most frequent lesion in adults. Rarely seen in adults, type III fractures are the second most common Monteggia lesions in children, followed by Monteggia equivalents.[93] The most common Monteggia equivalent is a fracture of the ulnar diaphysis with a more proximal fracture in the radius,[134] although not all authors recognize this entity as a Monteggia fracture.[129]

## MECHANISM OF INJURY

**Type I.** The classic type I Monteggia fracture may result from direct trauma, from a bending force as in hyperextension, or from forced hyperpronation.[145] Evans in 1949 experimentally reproduced the most common mechanism of injury—forced hyperpronation of the forearm from a fall on the outstretched hand. After the hand strikes the ground, a rotational force is added to the downward momentum of the falling body when a twisting of the trunk causes external rotation of the arm. If this force continues, the ulna fractures, and the radius is forced into extreme pronation and is levered forward until the radial head dislocates. The radius crossing the

ulna at the junction of the middle and proximal thirds acts as a fulcrum to force the radial head to dislocate anteriorly.[33, 146]

**Type II.** This lesion is thought to be caused by direct trauma with the forearm in supination or by a rotational force in supination.[146] Frequently, the fracture is open. This injury is rare in children.

**Type III.** These injuries are unusual, and all reported cases have occurred in children.[118] The mechanism of injury may be direct trauma over the inner aspect of the elbow, with or without rotation.[146] This mechanism provides an adduction force, but both angulation and rotational forces are likely to be involved. The final position of the displaced radial head may be either anterolateral or posterolateral, depending on the rotational position of the forearm at the time of the primary adduction injury.[118] The metaphyseal fracture of the ulna usually occurs just below the coronoid process. An associated radial nerve injury can occur but generally resolves spontaneously within 6 to 8 weeks.

**Type IV.** A type IV lesion is caused by forced pronation.[136]

**Monteggia Equivalents.** These entities are discussed in more detail under management of the specific injuries. Generally, Monteggia equivalents are the result of a fall that creates a hyperpronation force on the extended, outstretched arm. They account for 5% of all injuries to the elbow and forearm in children,[134] with the highest incidence between the ages of 5 and 10 years.

In children, the ulnar fracture is often a greenstick fracture. The angulation of the fracture may have been greater at the instant of injury than when the radiographs are made. In children, the radial head may pull out of the intact annular ligament, whereas in adults, the injury tears the ligament. In less severe injuries with minimal

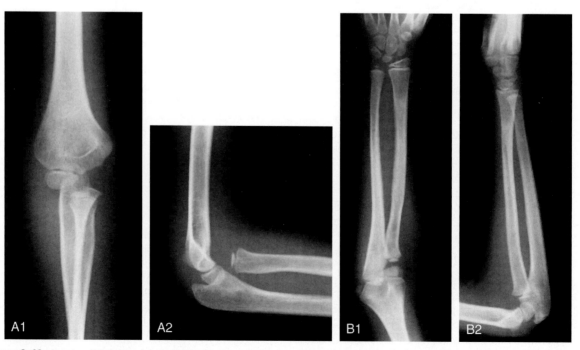

**FIGURE 8–60.** Anterior dislocation of the radial head without fracture or plastic deformation of the ulna. *A*, A 5-year-old girl fell from a height of 4 feet. *B*, No evidence of fracture could be seen in her forearm on initial or subsequent films.

angulation of the ulnar fracture, the dislocation may be missed, with late recognition of the dislocation of the radial head more than a month after the injury.[74]

**Combined Injuries.** Rarely, Monteggia-type injuries have an associated distal radial and ulnar injury.[10, 38, 85, 150, 164]

## DIAGNOSIS

Unfortunately, the diagnosis of this injury is frequently missed. Gleeson and Beattie reported that the diagnosis of Monteggia fracture-dislocations was missed in 50% of cases by senior emergency medicine residents and by 25% of senior radiologists.[50] It is essential in all injuries of the forearm to obtain both anteroposterior and lateral radiographs of the elbow and wrist. When one bone of the forearm is fractured, the presence of any shortening of that bone means that the proximal or distal radioulnar joint has dislocated.[145, 146] Clinical signs and symptoms include pain, an inability to move the elbow, and deformity, with fixed pronation of the forearm and hand.

Reduction of the radial head is best assessed on a true lateral view. A line drawn through the center of the radial head should pass through the center of the capitellum.[96] On the anteroposterior view, with the forearm in supination, a line is drawn tangentially to the bicipital tuberosity and head of the radius; another line is drawn tangentially to the other border of the radial head. These lines should encompass the entire capitellum. Before 10 years of age, the bicipital tuberosity is not sufficiently ossified to use this technique. In younger children, a line drawn through the center of the radial neck and head should pass through the center of the capitellum in any view.[158]

Lincoln and Mubarak challenged the existence of an "isolated" traumatic radial head dislocation. After demonstrating a new radiographic sign—the "ulnar bow sign" (Fig. 8–61)—they showed that all their patients with previously diagnosed isolated radial head dislocation had coexisting slight ulnar bows. This injury may be more accurately described as a minimal Monteggia fracture-dislocation.[98] The slight ulnar bow does not need to be specifically treated to reduce the radial head.[98]

If an open wound is associated with a type I lesion, it is usually located anteriorly over the ulna. In type II lesions, the dislocated radial head frequently perforates the skin in the posterolateral aspect of the elbow joint.[5]

One has to be careful in the evaluation of unusual patterns of injury. Posterior dislocation of the radial head can be congenital, and the usual deformity of the radial head may not be obvious on radiographs in young children. A decrease in range of motion at the elbow and forearm may not always be recognized by the parents before the injury; therefore, the history can be misleading. Examination of the opposite elbow may be helpful, although congenital dislocation can be unilateral. Unfortunately, if the diagnosis is missed, surgical intervention usually results in failure, with recurrence of the dislocated radial head (Fig. 8–62). A knowledge of the usual patterns of injury and a high index of suspicion might be helpful in avoiding unnecessary surgery.

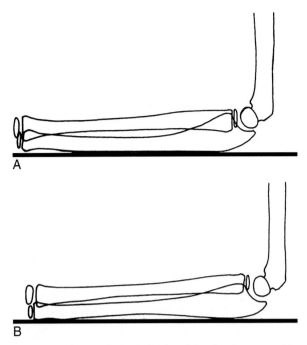

FIGURE 8–61. *A,* Normal straight border of the ulna demonstrated by the ulnar bow line. *B,* Minimal Monteggia fracture-dislocation with radial head subluxation and a positive ulnar bow sign. (*A, B,* From Lincoln, T.; Mubarak, S. J Pediatr Orthop 14:454–457, 1994.)

## MANAGEMENT OF ACUTE INJURIES

Approximately 90% of children with this injury have good to excellent results. In patients younger than 13 years who are treated by initial closed reduction, the long-term results are excellent.[94] Open reduction is required if adequate closed reduction cannot be achieved. It is more frequently necessary in older children or after a delay in diagnosis or treatment.

### Type I Fractures

Traction is applied with the forearm extended and supinated. The ulnar angulation is reduced, which frequently allows spontaneous reduction of the radial head. If spontaneous reduction does not occur, the elbow is gently flexed while pressure is applied anteriorly over the head of the radius. Once reduction is achieved, the elbow is immobilized in a long arm cast in full supination and flexion to 100° or as much flexion as the swollen elbow will tolerate.

In children, most of these injuries can be reduced with closed manipulation. If the child has an oblique fracture of the ulna (especially an obliquity that courses in a distal posterior–to–proximal anterior direction), the reduction may be difficult to maintain. Often, these fractures redisplace and cause late redislocation of the radial head. In this situation, fixation of the ulnar fracture is recommended. We have found that intramedullary fixation of the ulna is a satisfactory method of fixation that decreases the need for later extensive hardware removal, as well as the risk of refracture after hardware removal (Fig. 8–63). If the fracture can be reduced by closed manipulation, a K-wire or Rush rod can be inserted percutaneously through the tip of the olecranon and across the fracture site. Intramedullary fixation with flexible intramedullary nails would be an ideal choice for this clinical setting. If the fracture cannot be reduced by closed manipulation, the ulnar fracture is exposed and the fragments are pinned with a retrograde pinning technique.[176] Once the ulnar fracture is reduced, the radial head reduction is usually stable. This technique was described in the section on diaphyseal fractures of the radius and ulna. An alternative is plate-and-screw fixation of the ulnar fracture.

Occasionally, the radial head does not reduce after anatomic reduction of the ulnar fracture because of interposition of the annular ligament. Ogden states that the interposition is of three types: (1) partial; (2) complete, in which the radial head pulls out of the intact ligament (most frequent); and (3) secondary to the presence of osteocartilaginous fragments.[128]

In this instance, open reduction of the radial head is performed by using the posterior approach to the elbow or the Boyd approach[17] (Fig. 8–64). The advantage of the Boyd approach is that both components of the Monteggia lesion can be accessed through one incision. However, this approach has been criticized for increasing the chance of cross union. Another alternative is the use of two separate incisions. The portion of capsule and adjacent annular ligament is removed, and the annular

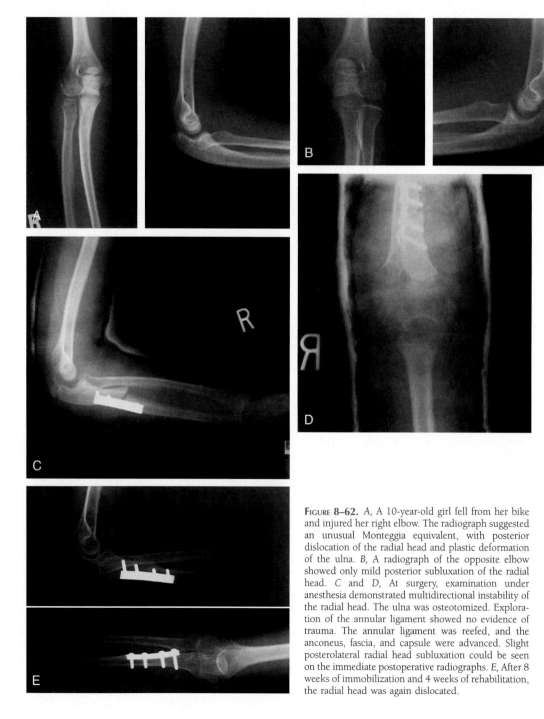

FIGURE 8–62. *A,* A 10-year-old girl fell from her bike and injured her right elbow. The radiograph suggested an unusual Monteggia equivalent, with posterior dislocation of the radial head and plastic deformation of the ulna. *B,* A radiograph of the opposite elbow showed only mild posterior subluxation of the radial head. *C* and *D,* At surgery, examination under anesthesia demonstrated multidirectional instability of the radial head. The ulna was osteotomized. Exploration of the annular ligament showed no evidence of trauma. The annular ligament was reefed, and the anconeus, fascia, and capsule were advanced. Slight posterolateral radial head subluxation could be seen on the immediate postoperative radiographs. *E,* After 8 weeks of immobilization and 4 weeks of rehabilitation, the radial head was again dislocated.

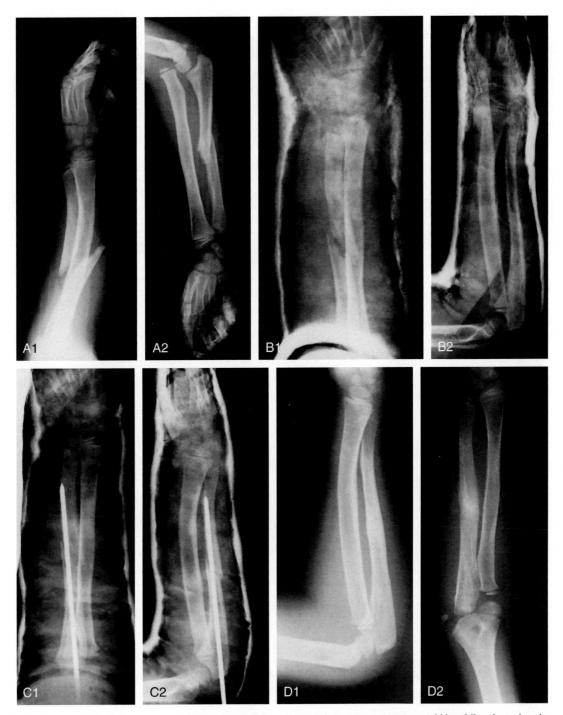

**FIGURE 8–63.** Compound Monteggia type I fracture that required intramedullary ulnar pinning. *A,* A 7-year-old boy fell in the park and sustained this injury with an open wound on the volar aspect of the forearm caused by protrusion of the proximal ulnar fragment. A deformity of the distal ends of the radius and ulna seen radiographically showed evidence of a previous fracture. Formal débridement was done by extending the anterior wound, and the fracture was reduced under direct vision. *B,* The fracture had displaced when reexamined at the time of secondary wound closure. *C,* Retrograde pinning of the ulna was performed, which was difficult because of the bowing in the ulna from the previous fracture. *D,* Follow-up radiograph at 2 months (the patient had fractured his medial epicondyle after another fall).

ligament is repaired. If it cannot be repaired, it is reconstructed with the Bell-Tawse procedure, which is described later under the heading entitled Complications.

Once reduction has been obtained, it is usually stable and internal fixation is not necessary. Some authors recommend insertion of a transcapitellar pin into the

radial head to maintain the reduction.[12] We strongly advise against this technique because of the risk of pin breakage.[93, 192] Alternatively, the radius may be held in position by a K-wire passed through the radius into the ulna.[93] However, the potential for cross union exists with this technique.

Careful follow-up is essential, and adequate radio-

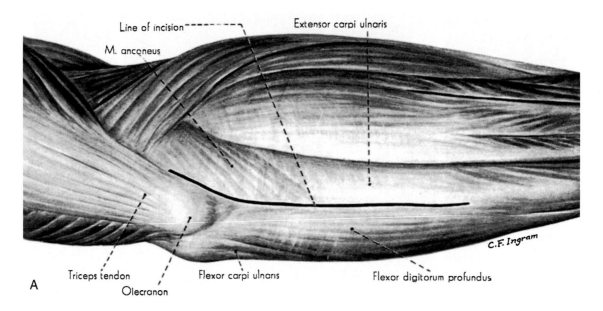

A

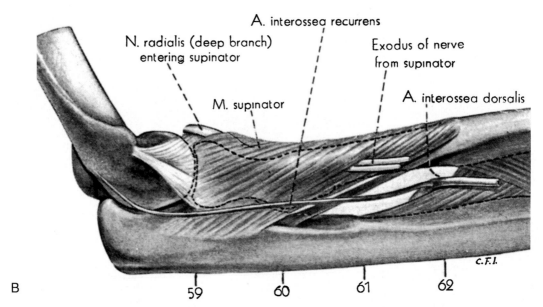

B                    59        60        61        62

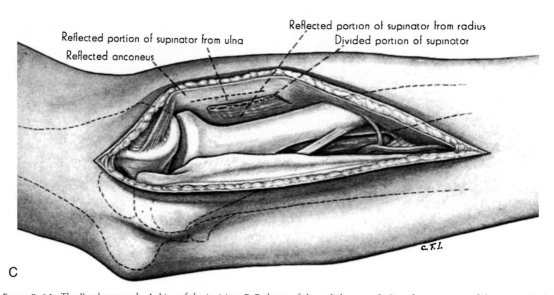

C

FIGURE 8–64. The Boyd approach. *A*, Line of the incision. *B*, Pathway of the radial nerve. *C*, Complete exposure of the upper third of the ulna, upper fourth of the radius, and radiohumeral articulation. (From Boyd, H.B. Surg Gynecol Obstet 71:81–88, 1940.)

graphs of the elbow and forearm need to be taken in both lateral and anteroposterior views. The arm is maintained in a long arm cast for 6 weeks; alternatively, at 4 weeks the cast can be changed to a cast brace for an additional 2 weeks. The intramedullary pin is extracted after the cast is removed, usually on an outpatient basis with a local anesthetic. Range-of-motion exercises are then initiated. The child is cautioned to not participate in contact sports for 1 month after cast removal to avoid the possibility of refracture (Fig. 8–65).

### Type II Fractures

Closed reduction under general anesthesia is usually successful. This technique is performed by extending the child's elbow with the forearm in supination, correcting the angulation of the ulna, and pushing with the thumb over the posterior aspect of the radial head. Alternatively, Bado suggests placing the elbow in 90° of flexion and

applying gentle traction and pronation.[5] The arm is then immobilized for 4 weeks in a long arm cast with the elbow in sufficient extension to obtain stability. The cast is changed to a long arm cast with elbow flexed for another 2 weeks. Careful follow-up is essential. As for type I fractures, if reduction of the ulna cannot be maintained, internal fixation may be necessary.

### Type III Fractures

Closed reduction is performed by applying traction and putting abduction strain on the fully extended elbow and supinating the forearm while direct ulnarward pressure is applied over the dislocated radial head. Once the lateral angulation is corrected, supination of the forearm tends to reduce the dislocation of the radial head because of tightening of the interosseous ligament between the radius and the ulna.[111] The arm is then immobilized in flexion for 6 weeks. If the reduction is unsuccessful or

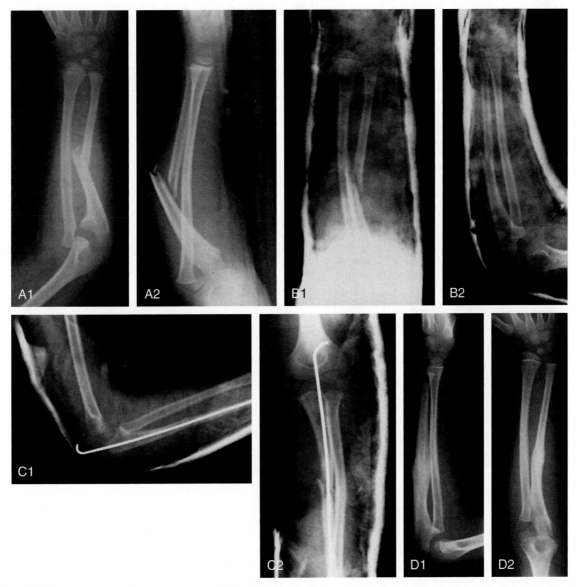

**FIGURE 8–65.** Monteggia type I fracture. *A,* A 5-year-old boy fell from a bicycle onto his left arm. The fracture was treated by closed reduction under general anesthesia. *B,* In 2 weeks, the fracture had redisplaced. Note the obliquity of the ulnar fracture, a finding predisposing to recurrent deformity. *C* and *D,* Closed reduction and percutaneous pinning of the ulna were undertaken, and the fracture subsequently healed in good position.
*Illustration continued on following page*

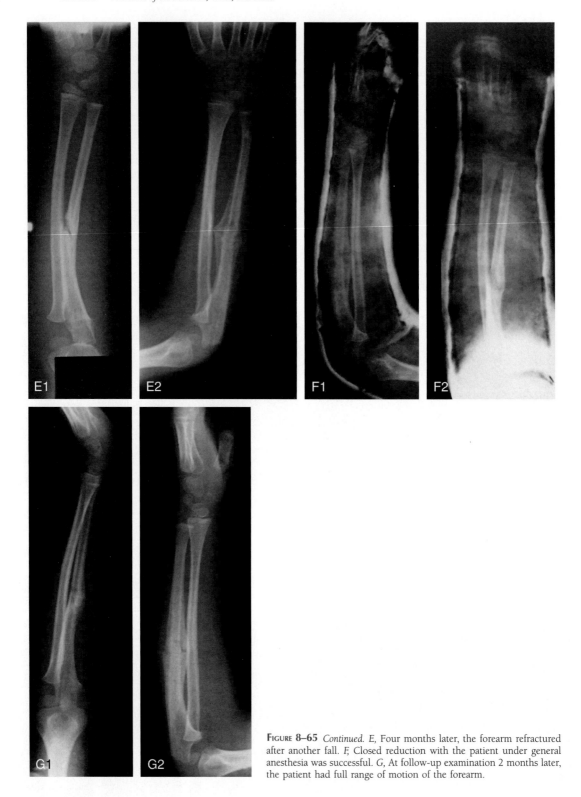

FIGURE 8–65 *Continued.* E, Four months later, the forearm refractured after another fall. F, Closed reduction with the patient under general anesthesia was successful. G, At follow-up examination 2 months later, the patient had full range of motion of the forearm.

cannot be maintained, open reduction of the ulnar fracture is performed.

## Type IV Fractures

Type IV fractures are extremely rare, so little has been written on the management of these injuries. Closed manipulation should consist of restoring the alignment of the ulnar fracture and strong supination in an attempt to

reduce both the radial head dislocation and the radial fracture.[78] These fractures are difficult to reduce by closed manipulation. As with other Monteggia fractures, the first step is accurate reduction of the ulna and fixation with the techniques described previously. If the ulnar fracture is unstable, plate fixation or an intramedullary pin should be used.[48, 150] It is important to achieve and maintain stable and accurate reduction, which means that the ulna must be kept out to length and the angulation corrected. Often, this objective can be accomplished only by open reduction and internal fixation.

If closed manipulation of the radius fails, the radial shaft fracture should be exposed carefully. The posterior or Boyd approach to the radius should be used, with care taken to avoid injury to the posterior interosseous nerve. Generally, the radial head dislocation can be reduced easily at the same time that the radius is reduced, but annular ligament interposition may interfere with the reduction. For this reason, an extensile approach is recommended so that both the radial head and the radial shaft can be exposed, if necessary. Ideally, separate incisions should be used for exposure to the radial and ulnar fractures to reduce the risk of cross union, but this technique is not always possible. The radial fracture should be fixed with a plate of the appropriate size. The intramedullary rod techniques that were described under the management of radial shaft fractures can be used in young children if the fracture is not too far proximal.

### Monteggia Equivalents

In general, Monteggia-equivalent fractures are more difficult to reduce by closed manipulation than type I fracture-dislocations are.

**Anterior Dislocation of the Radial Head with Plastic Deformation of the Ulna.** As discussed earlier, a significant number of missed anterior dislocations are associated with plastic deformation of the ulna.[93] If the deformity in the ulna is not adequately corrected, recurrent dislocation may result.

The technique of reduction of the ulna was discussed earlier. With the patient under general anesthesia, the ulna is reduced, the forearm is supinated, and pressure is applied over the anterior aspect of the radial head. A long arm cast is applied with the forearm supinated for 4 weeks. In patients with recurrence of the dislocation, an osteotomy of the ulna may be necessary. Because of the possibility of recurrence,[134] follow-up should be extended to 1 year after the injury.

**Fracture of the Shaft of the Ulna with a Fracture of the Radial Neck.** The most common mechanism of injury is a fall onto the outstretched hand with the forearm in any position of rotation and with a valgus strain on the extended elbow. The radial head is firmly secured against the radial notch of the ulna and the capitellum during valgus stress. The compression force fractures the radius at a relatively weak site at the neck or near the physis, and a Salter-Harris type II fracture is created. The pull of the biceps tendon displaces the distal radial fragment anteriorly and can cause the radial head to dislocate or subluxate posteriorly.[36]

Three basic types of proximal radial fractures are observed: (1) fractures of the neck with the head and shaft of the radius remaining in contact, (2) fractures through the radial neck or proximal physis with complete dislocation of the radial head, and (3) fractures through the radial neck or physis with the radial head remaining intact.[129]

Closed reduction may be performed with traction and varus stress. While the forearm is rotated in alternating pronation-supination movements, the displaced radial

fragment is reduced by applying direct pressure with the thumb. Reduction and internal fixation of the ulna often allow adequate closed reduction of radial neck fractures (Fig. 8–66). Up to 30° of angulation in the radial neck is acceptable in younger children because of the bone's potential for remodeling. Although closed reduction may be achieved, it is frequently difficult to maintain, and open reduction is then indicated. Among children with fractures of the radial neck and head, 71% require operative treatment.[129] Open reduction of radial neck fractures usually results in long-term elbow stiffness and should be avoided except for specific indications (see Fig. 8–66).

If the radial neck fracture cannot be reduced satisfactorily and the child has loss of pronation and supination of the forearm, manipulation of the fracture can be performed by percutaneous insertion of a small Steinmann pin into the radial head. The Steinmann pin is used to guide the head into an acceptable position while trying to avoid the necessity of opening the fracture. Usually, it can be positioned in an acceptable manner, though often not anatomic. In the rare instance that an unacceptable position of the proximal radial head fragment persists, open reduction through either an extended Kocher or posterior approach is performed. The stability of the reduction determines the necessity for fixation of the radial neck fracture and should be determined at the time of surgery. If necessary, K-wires should transfix the radial neck and head but should not enter the joint space. Because of the high risk of elbow stiffness, the elbow should be immobilized no longer than 3 weeks; a cast brace is applied for an additional 2 weeks to allow early controlled motion. Unfortunately, even with open treatment, results are frequently poor because of significant loss of motion or cross union.[36]

**Fracture of the Shaft of the Ulna with a Proximal Fracture of the Radius.** This fracture pattern, the most common of the Monteggia variants, is not always differentiated from other shaft fractures of the radius and ulna. These fractures can usually be reduced by closed manipulation, but the reduction can be difficult to maintain.[134] The fracture is manipulated by traction, with the elbow flexed in a right angle and the forearm in full supination. Over 50% of these injuries may require a second reduction.[134] Intramedullary fixation or plate fixation of the ulnar fracture can be used to maintain the ulnar reduction. If satisfactory alignment of the radius cannot be achieved, open reduction and fixation of the radial fracture should be undertaken through a separate incision from the ulnar incision. The posterior interosseous nerve must be protected in this surgical approach.

Papavasiliou and Nenopoulos reported that in all patients with 15° of residual angulation of the ulna, 20° of pronation was lost.[134] Residual angulation should therefore be less than 15° to produce an acceptable result.

**Fracture of the Ulnar Metaphysis in Association with Anterior Dislocation of the Radial Head.** In this injury, fracture of the olecranon is the result of a hyperextension injury to the elbow, and forward dislocation of the radial head is produced by concomitant pronation of the forearm.[69] Alternatively, the child may

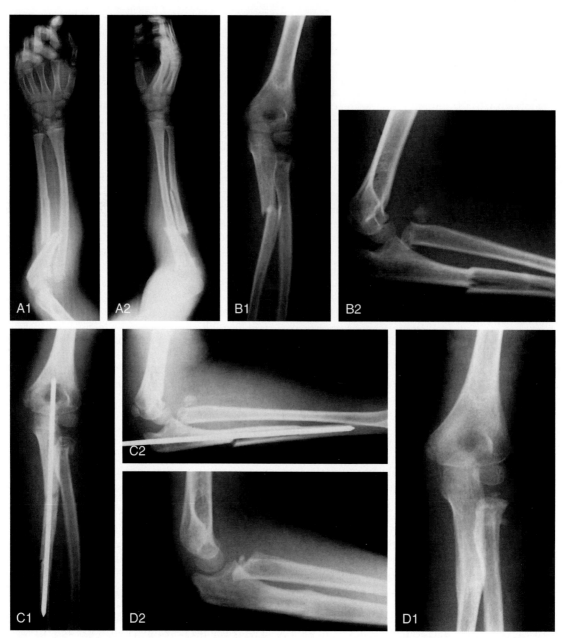

FIGURE **8–66.** Monteggia-equivalent fracture. *A*, An 8-year-old girl fell from a tree and sustained a displaced segmental fracture of the ulna and a displaced fracture of the radial neck. An anterior interosseous nerve palsy was noted. *B*, With the patient under general anesthesia, closed reduction was attempted, but the alignment could not be maintained. Fixation of the ulna by intramedullary pinning was performed. Examination using the image intensifier with the patient under anesthesia indicated that the radial head was stable and that the radial neck fracture ends were in an acceptable position. *C*, The early postoperative course was complicated by a compartment syndrome requiring fasciotomies. At the time of secondary wound closure under anesthesia, the radial head was inspected and the forearm put through a range of motion. The cortical fragment noted anteriorly was thought to be metaphyseal in origin, and it did not appear to contribute to the stability of the radial head and neck. At 4 weeks, the above-elbow cast was replaced by a short arm cast, which was worn for an additional 2 weeks. The patient was then referred to physiotherapy for range-of-motion exercises. *D*, At radiologic follow-up 1 year later, the anterior deformity indicates that the previously noted fragment was in fact a portion of the radial head, thus indicating a Salter-Harris type IV fracture that had been misdiagnosed. The forearm remained stable, however, and the patient had nearly full range of motion. The anterior interosseous nerve injury was completely resolved. Further follow-up is indicated.

have had a sideways fall onto the outstretched hand[174] or a fall onto the outstretched hand with the forearm supinated. The direction of angulation of the ulna is likely to be determined by the direction of the fall, which may produce varus, valgus, or hyperextension strain on the forearm.[199] Wright reported a fracture of the medial epicondyle in association with this variant.[199] These fractures are frequently comminuted or oblique and are consequently very unstable. Often difficult to reduce by closed means, they are equally difficult to stabilize with open reduction.

Some fractures can be managed by placing an intramedullary pin in the ulna and using the K-wire as a "joystick" to manipulate the fracture. Unfortunately, most of these fractures are located very proximally in the metaphyseal bone of the ulna, so the pin cannot securely control the proximal fragment and the reduction fails. If the fracture is oblique with little comminution, small-fragment lag screws can be used to secure the reduction. Otherwise, a combination of screws, plates, and K-wires may be necessary. The radial head dislocation is usually easily reduced once the ulnar fracture is reduced. The arm should be immobilized postoperatively with the forearm in supination and the elbow flexed to maximize stability. Four weeks in a long arm cast or splint is recommended. Range of motion of the elbow is encouraged after cast removal despite lack of complete healing of the ulna.

**Fracture of the Ulnar Diaphysis with Anterior Dislocation of the Radial Head and Fracture of the Olecranon.** The most probable mechanism is a fall onto the outstretched hand with the forearm supinated, along with a varus, valgus, or hyperextension strain on the forearm. The basic principles of treatment are the same as for other Monteggia type I fracture-dislocations; that is, once adequate reduction of the ulnar fractures has been obtained, the radial head dislocation can be reduced.

Management of ulnar fractures includes closed reduction of the ulnar shaft in addition to the ulnar metaphysis. If the olecranon or metaphyseal fracture is not stable, internal fixation should be considered. Frequently, an intermedullary pin in the ulna can control both fractures. Closed reduction of the radial neck fracture may be attempted, and if adequate reduction cannot be achieved, closed percutaneous manipulation with a Steinmann pin or open reduction is indicated.

**Fracture of the Ulnar Metaphysis with Fracture of the Neck of the Radius.** A fracture of the neck of the radius in children is most often a Salter-Harris type II fracture. As with other anteriorly displaced Monteggia-equivalent fractures, the probable mechanism is a fall onto the outstretched hand during which the forearm is held supinated, as though the child were falling backward.[199]

If the fracture is undisplaced, it usually heals well with simple immobilization (Fig. 8–67). A displaced fracture that was recognized late or one that had inadequate treatment or loss of reduction during follow-up is at significant risk for loss of pronation and supination and a poor result.[199]

**Posterior Dislocation of the Elbow and Fracture of the Ulnar Diaphysis, with or without Fracture of the Proximal Radius.** The posterior dislocation of the elbow is reduced first by using traction and applying direct pressure posteriorly over the olecranon and flexing the elbow. The forearm is then gently supinated.[5] The arm is immobilized in a long arm cast with the forearm in supination for 6 weeks. Alternatively, a cast brace may be applied at 4 weeks so that controlled range-of-motion exercises can be started earlier.

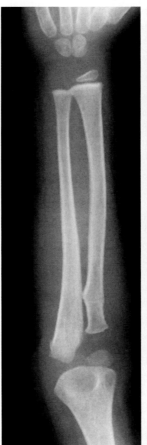
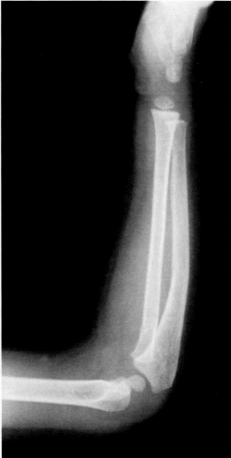

FIGURE 8–67. Monteggia type I–equivalent fracture. A 3-year-old boy fell off the bed and sustained a greenstick fracture of the ulnar shaft and a buckle fracture of the proximal third of the radius.

Ravessoud suggested that a displaced ulnar shaft fracture in association with a displaced lateral condylar fracture and intact radiohumeral articulation is a type III Monteggia equivalent.[143] He recommends open reduction and internal fixation of the lateral condylar fracture, as well as open reduction and internal fixation of the ulnar shaft fracture, to permit earlier mobilization of the elbow.[143] We recommend that the lateral condylar fracture be treated by open reduction and internal fixation with smooth K-wires. Depending on the location and degree of displacement of the ulnar fracture, the ulna is internally stabilized with an intramedullary pin or a plate and screws. The elbow is immobilized for 3 weeks, after which time the smooth K-wires in the elbow are removed. The child is then allowed to move the elbow, either with or without a cast brace, depending on the child's age and the stage of the healing process in the ulna. The cast is removed at approximately 6 weeks, followed by further range-of-motion exercises.

## FOLLOW-UP AND REHABILITATION

Careful follow-up with adequate radiologic evaluation of reduction of the radial head is essential. Comparison views of the opposite elbow can be helpful because in the anteroposterior view, lateral subluxation of the radial head can be difficult to evaluate. Displacement of the radial head frequently recurs, with loss of reduction of the ulna. If open reduction of the radial head was necessary, aggressive physiotherapy should be undertaken after cast removal because of the high risk of elbow stiffness. Prolonged immobilization beyond 3 to 4 weeks is discouraged.

## COMPLICATIONS

Factors leading to poor results include failure to obtain anatomic reduction of the ulna; persistence or recurrence of dislocation of the radial head; heterotopic ossification, including synostosis of the proximal parts of the radius and ulna; nerve injury; and compartment syndrome.[129, 145]

### Late Diagnosis or Redislocation

A Monteggia fracture-dislocation that was diagnosed late or redisplaced after treatment can cause pain, decreased elbow range of motion, decreased forearm rotation, and unstable cubitus valgus.[70, 97] Persistent dislocation in a child is rarely painful, and although it may limit pronation, it does not usually interfere with motion of the elbow.[74] However, because of continued growth of the radius in the dislocated position, the cubitus valgus may increase and the radial head may enlarge and cause distortion of the supinator muscle and pressure on the posterior interosseous or radial nerve, with the possible late development of progressive radial nerve palsy.[70, 97] For this reason, it is recommended that all such lesions in children be reduced.

The classic treatment was to leave the radial head dislocated and excise it at skeletal maturity, if necessary. However, it is generally agreed that the radial head should never be excised in children.[12] The resultant loss

of growth in the radius would inevitably produce progressive radial deviation at the wrist joint and progressive valgus deformity at the elbow.[156]

Old Monteggia fracture-dislocations should be treated with open reduction of the persistently dislocated radial head and reconstruction of the annular ligament. Recurrence of radial head subluxation after reduction has been linked to insufficient correction of the ulnar deformity.[74] Therefore, to achieve reduction of the radial head, corrective ulnar osteotomy is usually necessary.[171] In children with marked limitation of flexion because of severe, long-standing anterior dislocation of the radial head, an osteotomy of the radius with angular correction or shortening may also be required.[141] The annular ligament, in most instances, has become a mass of fibrous tissue and scar that must be excised to allow reduction of the radial head. Reconstruction of the annular ligament with a fascial graft is necessary (Fig. 8–68). If the annular

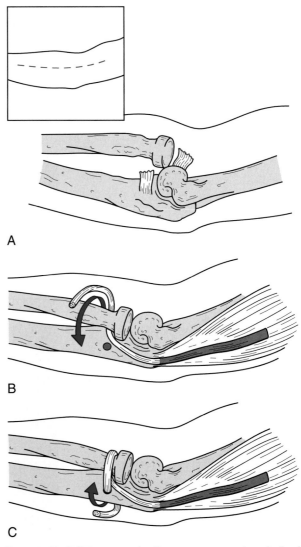

**FIGURE 8–68.** Bell-Tawse annular ligament reconstruction. *A,* Boyd approach to the proximal ends of the radius and ulna. *B,* A strip of triceps fascia is passed between the ulna and radial head at the level of the annular ligament. *C,* It is then passed around the neck of the radius, through a drill hole in the ulna, and pulled around to be sutured to itself. (From Bell-Tawse, A.J.S. J Bone Joint Surg Br 47:718–723, 1965.)

ligament is found to be intact, transection and repair may be sufficient to restore stability without resorting to fascial graft reconstruction. The likelihood of postoperative stiffness may be decreased with the simpler procedure.[74]

This procedure can be recommended only for children who have no major intra-articular injury, no damage to the epiphyseal centers, and only mild adaptive changes of the radial head. A preoperative arthrogram or MRI of the elbow is advised to determine the shape of the radial head, especially if the radial head has been dislocated for a prolonged period.[171] If significant overgrowth of the radius as well as secondary changes in the proximal and distal radioulnar joints is present, anatomic reduction of the radial head will not provide good articulation of those joints and is contraindicated.[74] In this situation, the classic treatment of late excision after skeletal maturity or interposition arthroplasty may be considered only in those with clinical indications for intervention.

**Procedure (Bell-Tawse Annular Ligament Reconstruction with Lloyd-Roberts Modification).** The patient is positioned prone on the operating table with the upper extremity resting on a hand table (see Fig. 8–68). A Boyd approach is recommended (see Fig. 8–64). The elbow joint is entered through a lateral capsular incision. The interposed soft tissues, which may include the joint capsule and annular ligament, are carefully removed, with care taken to avoid injury to the articular cartilage. Usually, the radial head can be reduced with anterior pressure and supination of the forearm. If the reduction cannot be obtained in this manner, osteotomy of the ulna should be considered and performed at this stage. The osteotomy should correct the angular deformity and increase the length of the ulna to allow reduction of the dislocated radial head.[171] The radial head, once reduced, is often stable. A 1- × 7-cm strip of fascia is then dissected from the lateral portion of the triceps tendon, with its distal attachment on the olecranon preserved. A subperiosteal tunnel is fashioned so that the strip can be passed medial to the olecranon at a point opposite the origin of the annular ligament. The strip is then passed around the neck of the radius and sutured to itself or secured through a drill hole in the ulna.[66] If the triceps tendon is unsuitable, a free tendon graft as recommended by Watson-Jones should be used.[9]

Lloyd-Roberts and Bucknill recommended passing a K-wire percutaneously through the capitellum and into the proximal end of the radius to stabilize the reduction.[100] As discussed previously, we do not recommend this procedure because of the frequency of complications, including pin breakage and irreversible joint stiffness.[93, 192] The arm should be immobilized in a long arm cast with the forearm in supination and the elbow flexed to 80°. We believe that immobilizing the elbow in a position less than 90° may allow room inside the cast for some swelling and decrease the possibility of development of a compartment syndrome. Once the swelling has subsided, a new snug long arm cast is applied. Six weeks after the surgery, range-of-motion exercises are begun. The complication of cross union of the proximal ends of the radius and ulna has been encountered with this technique[184]; therefore, early motion with continuous passive motion and subsequent cast bracing could be used in the immediate postoperative period if the radial head is sufficiently stable intraoperatively.

### Malunion

Varus angulation of the ulna is the most common residual deformity; unlike posterior angulation, it is not associated with redislocation of the radial head. In the study by Olney and Menelaus, up to 25° of angulation was still consistent with full range of motion of the elbow and forearm.[129]

### Nerve Injuries

Nerve palsies secondary to Monteggia fracture-dislocation occur in 11% to 20% of cases.[5, 129] The posterior interosseous nerve is most frequently injured in type III lesions with lateral dislocation of the radial head; however, this injury can also occur in type I lesions[129] (Fig. 8–69). The injury may be caused by direct pressure from the radial head, compression at the proximal edge of the arcade of Frohse, or entrapment between the radial head and the ulna, or it may be caused by traction.[115, 167, 191] Surgical exploration of the nerve is not indicated because the radial nerve usually undergoes spontaneous recovery within 6 months of the injury.[18, 129] If early recovery of the nerve is not apparent on electromyographic evaluation within 3 months of the injury, surgical exploration is warranted.

Ulnar nerve injury can also occur from compression within the cubital tunnel. If recovery does not take place spontaneously, surgical decompression is frequently successful.[170] Injuries to the radial and median nerves have also been reported in association with Monteggia lesions. Recovery occurred in all cases within 6 months of injury.[129]

## Galeazzi Fractures

Although first described by Sir Astley Cooper in 1822, this fracture pattern was named after Riccardo Galeazzi, who in 1934 described his experience with fracture of the distal end of the radius accompanied by disruption of the distal radioulnar joint. This injury is rare in children, with the peak incidence between 9 and 12 years of age.[110, 187]

## CLASSIFICATION

The classic type is a fracture of the shaft of the radius in association with dislocation of the distal radioulnar joint. The fracture occurs most frequently at the junction of the middle and distal thirds of the radius, but it may occur within the distal third of the radius[187] (Fig. 8–70). Other variations of this lesion include fractures of both the radius and ulna or double fractures of the radius in association with dislocation of the distal radioulnar joint.[110] The fracture can be displaced anteriorly or posteriorly.[187]

In children, the Galeazzi-equivalent injury, which is a fracture of the radius associated with a fracture of the distal ulnar physis, is more likely to occur because of the relative weakness of the physis in comparison to the ligamentous attachments of the articular disc.[88, 94, 145, 187] In this case, the distal radioulnar joint is not disrupted because the ulnar epiphysis remains attached to the distal end of the radius. Instead, a type I or II fracture of the distal part of the ulna occurs. Letts and Rowhani developed a classification of Galeazzi and Galeazzi-equivalent fractures in children[94] (Fig. 8–71, Table 8–1). By appropriately identifying these injuries, the risk of future growth plate arrest at the ulnar physis will be appreciated, and accurate reduction of the distal end of the ulna to ensure stability of the distal radioulnar joint will be achieved.

The Essex-Lopresti fracture, which is a fracture of the radial neck or head associated with dislocation of the distal radioulnar joint, is not generally considered to be a Galeazzi fracture.[110] The mechanism of injury is a longitudinal force on the outstretched hand that creates a compressive force through the radial head into the capitellum. It has not been reported in children. However, we have encountered a variant of this fracture in a 12-year-old girl (Fig. 8–72).

## MECHANISM OF INJURY

The usual mechanism of injury is a fall on the outstretched hand, combined with extreme pronation of the forearm. In the classic type, the articular disc tears or becomes detached at the extremes of pronation and

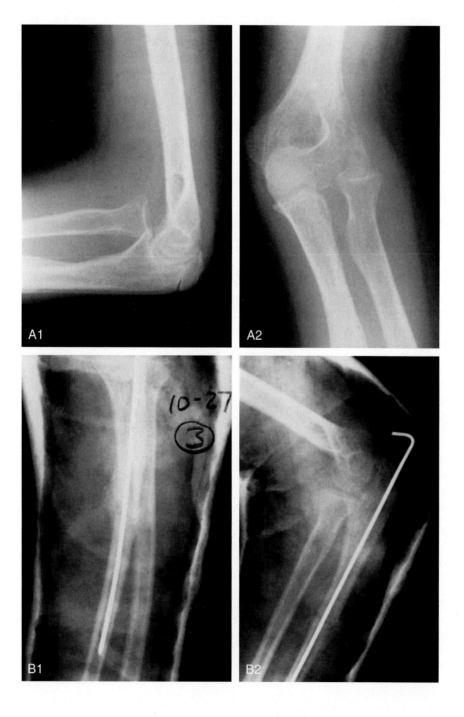

**Figure 8–69.** Recurrent radial head dislocation after a Monteggia fracture-dislocation. *A,* An 11-year-old girl fell and sustained a Monteggia fracture-dislocation. She was treated by closed manipulation and casting in hyperflexion. After 5 weeks the cast was removed, and she was found to have redislocated her radial head. *B,* With the patient under general anesthesia, osteoclasis of the ulna and intramedullary fixation were performed. Initial radiographs showed that the radial head seemed to be reduced. Full range of motion of the forearm was achieved in the operating room. The patient was immobilized in a long arm cast. Postoperatively, she had a posterior interosseous palsy.

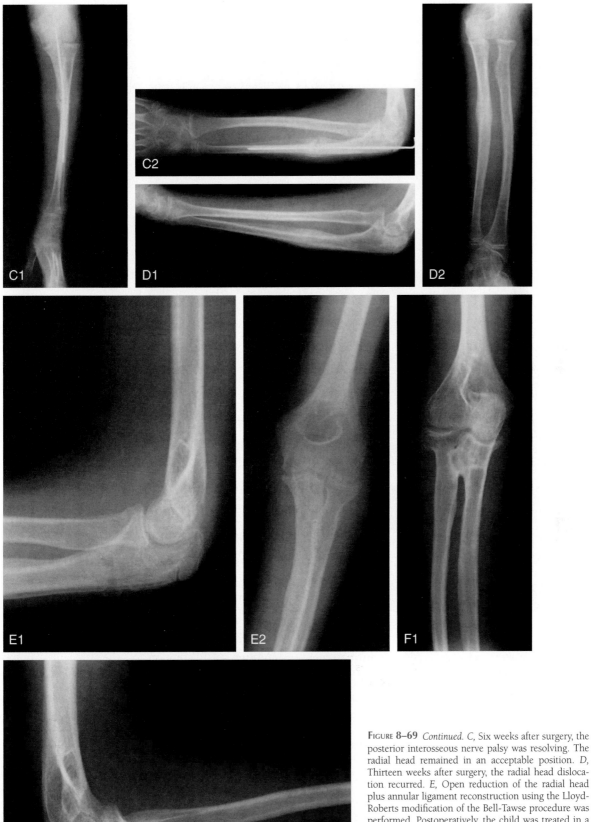

FIGURE **8–69** *Continued. C,* Six weeks after surgery, the posterior interosseous nerve palsy was resolving. The radial head remained in an acceptable position. *D,* Thirteen weeks after surgery, the radial head dislocation recurred. *E,* Open reduction of the radial head plus annular ligament reconstruction using the Lloyd-Roberts modification of the Bell-Tawse procedure was performed. Postoperatively, the child was treated in a continuous passive-motion machine. *F,* Three months after the operative procedure, a proximal radioulnar synostosis had developed. Her forearm is fixed in slight supination, and she may ultimately require a repositioning osteotomy.

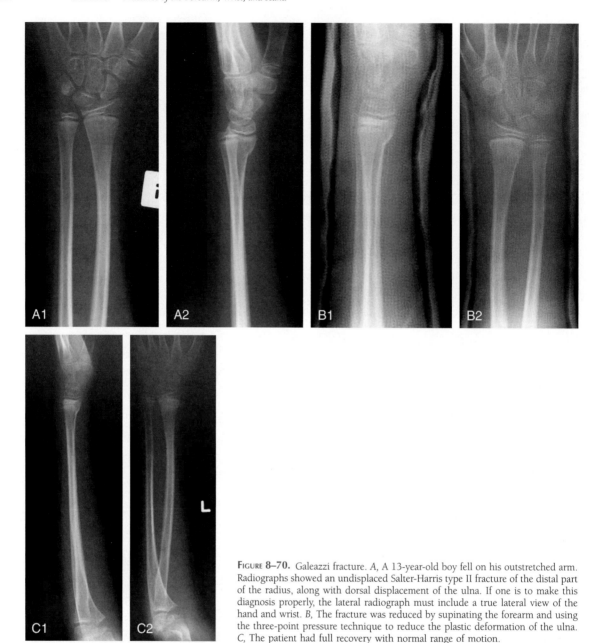

**FIGURE 8–70.** Galeazzi fracture. *A*, A 13-year-old boy fell on his outstretched arm. Radiographs showed an undisplaced Salter-Harris type II fracture of the distal part of the radius, along with dorsal displacement of the ulna. If one is to make this diagnosis properly, the lateral radiograph must include a true lateral view of the hand and wrist. *B*, The fracture was reduced by supinating the forearm and using the three-point pressure technique to reduce the plastic deformation of the ulna. *C*, The patient had full recovery with normal range of motion.

extension of the wrist, with dislocation occurring secondary to the rotational forces. A direct blow may be responsible in a minority of cases.[110] More distal fractures in the radius tend to be associated with more severe trauma than seen with proximal injuries and are frequently the result of a fall from a height.[187]

Complete dislocation of the distal radioulnar joint always involves rupture of the articular disc and the associated dorsal and volar distal radioulnar ligaments. The Galeazzi fracture-dislocation is unstable as a result of disruption of the TFCC and mechanical factors acting on the distal fragment of the radius. The most important stabilizing force is provided by the triangular fibrocartilage.[110, 146] The question of whether the triangular fibrocartilage is ruptured is the crucial one in determining the presence of a Galeazzi lesion. Some authors believe that avulsion of the ulnar styloid process is an indication of disruption of the triangular fibrocartilage.[110]

The mechanical factors acting on the distal fragment of the radius contribute to the instability of this fracture. The brachioradialis tends to shorten the radius by means of its insertion into the radial styloid, the pronator quadratus rotates the distal radial fragment toward the ulna, and the force of the thumb abductors and extensors tends to relax the radial collateral ligament and shorten the radial side of the wrist. The weight of the hand also acts as a strong volar-displacing force.[110, 146]

Pediatric Galeazzi fractures have less distal radioulnar soft tissue injury or tearing of the interosseous membrane. In this case, the firm attachment of the articular disc to the distal ends of the radius and ulna and the ulnar collateral ligament to the epiphysis results in a concentration of forces at the physis during hyperpronation.[94, 145]

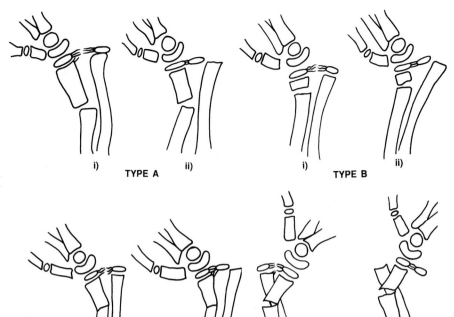

**FIGURE 8–71.** Classification of Galeazzi and Galeazzi-equivalent injuries in children. (From Letts, M.; Rowhani, N. J Pediatr Orthop 13:561–566, 1993.)

TYPE A    TYPE B    TYPE C    TYPE D

## DIAGNOSIS

The clinical appearance is an angular concave deformity on the radial side of the forearm, which seems shortened. The distal radioulnar joint may be deformed, swollen, and painful. The ulnar head may seem to protrude and may be slightly more mobile than usual. An apparently solitary fracture of the radius should raise clinical suspicion of disruption of the distal radioulnar joint. Adequate anteroposterior and lateral radiographs are important in making the correct diagnosis. Care should be taken to get a true lateral view of the wrist. Walsh and co-workers found that the diagnosis had been missed in 41% of cases.[187] They reported that arthrography of the radioulnar joint has been useful in investigating uncertain clinical instability. A positive examination shows contrast injected into the wrist joint appearing in the distal radioulnar joint.[110]

## MANAGEMENT

Most of these fractures in children can be managed with closed treatment.[94, 110, 145, 187] If the radial fracture is accurately reduced and the forearm is immobilized in full supination, the torn articular disc and associated ligaments will be approximated and heal in an appropriate position.[94, 145, 146, 187] The arm should be immobilized in an above-elbow plaster cast with the forearm in supination for about 6 weeks. Such treatment applies to both anterior and posterior displacement of the radial fracture.[187] An inability to reduce either the distal radioulnar joint or the distal ulnar physis suggests the possibility of entrapment of the extensor tendons.[10, 72, 75, 132] Follow-up should occur on a weekly basis until fracture healing is apparent radiographically.

An oblique fracture pattern in the radius is relatively unstable. If the distal radial fracture cannot be maintained in less than 10° of angulation and without shortening of greater than 4 mm, stabilization of the distal end of the radius with closed pinning or with open reduction and fixation should be considered.

## COMPLICATIONS

Malunion with recurrent radioulnar subluxation can occur, but this complication is uncommon in the pediatric age group. Poorer results are seen if the diagnosis is delayed and if the forearm has been

---

**TABLE 8–1**  · · · · · · · · · · · · · · · · · · · · · · · · · · · · ·

Letts and Rowhani Classification of Pediatric Galeazzi Fracture Patterns

---

Type A: Fracture of the radius at the junction of the middle and distal thirds with:
1. Dorsal dislocation of distal ulna.
2. Epiphyseal fracture of distal ulna with dorsal displacement of ulnar metaphysis.

Type B: Fracture of the distal third of the radius with:
1. Dorsal dislocation of distal ulna.
2. Epiphyseal fracture of distal ulna with dorsal displacement of ulnar metaphysis.

Type C: Greenstick fracture of the radius with dorsal bowing and:
1. Dorsal dislocation of distal ulna.
2. Epiphyseal fracture of distal ulna with displacement of ulnar metaphysis.

Type D: Fracture of distal radius with volar bowing and:
1. Volar dislocation of distal ulna.
2. Epiphyseal fracture of distal ulna with volar displacement of ulnar metaphysis.

· · · · · · · · · · · · · · · · · · · · · · · · · · · · · · · · · · · ·

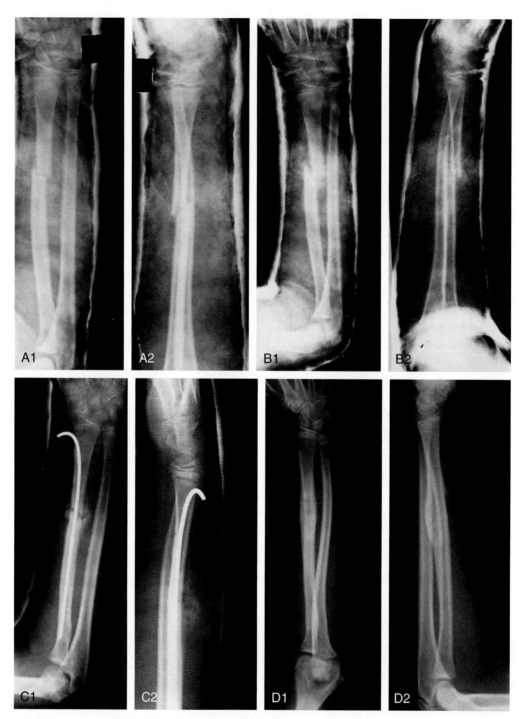

FIGURE 8–72. Essex-Lopresti variant. *A,* A 12-year-old girl tripped and fell onto her outstretched arm. She complained of pain in her elbow and wrist. Undisplaced fractures of the radial neck and olecranon are visible. Note the soft tissue swelling over the dorsal aspect of the wrist, widening of the distal radioulnar joint, and dorsal dislocation of the distal end of the ulna. *B,* Radiographs of the opposite forearm taken for comparison confirmed that the distal radioulnar joint in the injured forearm was abnormal. The anatomic configuration of the radius was identical to that of the injured forearm, thus ruling out previous injury as a cause of the apparently excessive bowing of the radius. *C,* The patient was treated in a long arm cast with the forearm in supination. The distal radioulnar joint was reduced in this position. The cast was maintained for 4 weeks. *D,* It was replaced by a short arm splint for 2 additional weeks. At follow-up examination, the patient remained asymptomatic, with full range of motion of the forearm.

immobilized in an incorrect position or in a below-elbow cast.[187] If recurrent subluxation becomes a clinical problem after completion of treatment, surgical reconstruction of the distal radioulnar joint should be considered, in combination with distal radial osteotomy (Fig. 8–73).

Rarely, nerve injuries have been described in association with a Galeazzi fracture, including injuries to the ulnar nerve at the distal end of the ulna and interosseous nerve palsy.[110, 147] In the Galeazzi-equivalent injury with an injury to the distal ulnar physis, growth arrest can occur.[94, 120]

# WRIST INJURIES

## Dislocation of the Distal Radioulnar Joint

Isolated dislocations of the distal radioulnar joint are uncommon but are more likely to occur in older children who are approaching maturity. This injury is actually a dislocation of the radiocarpal complex from the ulna, although it is commonly described as a dorsal or volar dislocation of the distal portion of the ulna.[26, 47, 60, 133] With this injury, the damage is to the TFCC in association with the dorsal or volar radioulnar ligaments.

The head of the ulna is seated within the sigmoid notch of the radius. The base of the styloid is the attachment area for the triangular fibrocartilage and ulnocarpal ligaments, which together make up the TFCC

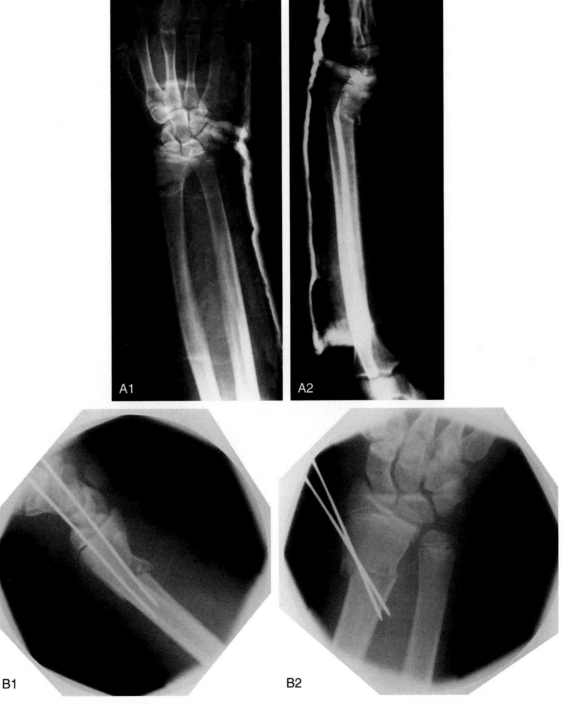

FIGURE 8–73. Galeazzi-equivalent injury. *A,* A 15-year-old boy fell from a motorcycle onto his left arm. This Galeazzi-equivalent fracture was initially treated by closed reduction. Note the Salter-Harris type IV fracture fragment of the ulnar styloid. *B,* Within 24 hours, repeat radiographs showed recurrence of the deformity. Closed reduction was repeated, with pinning of the radial metaphysis.

*Illustration continued on following page*

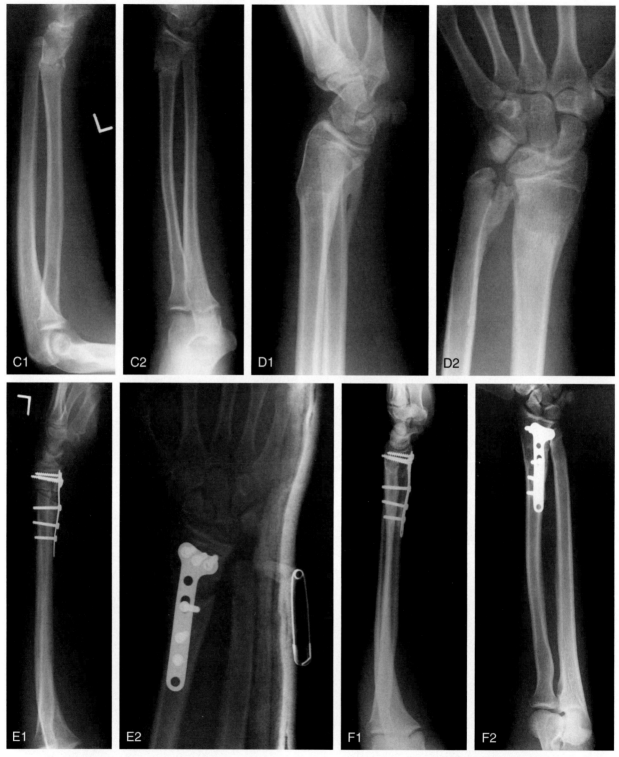

FIGURE **8–73** *Continued. C,* The pins were removed at 6 weeks, and range-of-motion exercises were prescribed. Recurrent volar and ulnar tilt of the distal end of the radius, as well as dorsal subluxation of the ulna, were not appreciated. *D,* At 4 months, the radial angulation had increased. A bony exostosis had formed in the interim and extended proximally from the Salter-Harris type IV fragment. Total active motion was from 20° pronation to 20° supination. No volar-dorsal movement was detectable passively at the distal radioulnar joint. *E,* Five months after the fracture, late reconstruction of the wrist was undertaken. The pronator quadratus and dorsal carpal ligament were found to be extending into the radioulnar joint. The radial tilt was restored by performing an opening wedge osteotomy with a tricortical iliac crest bone graft, and the exostosis was excised. At the end of the procedure, supination was 90° and pronation, 75°. *F,* After 2½ years, the patient has only 10° supination and 30° pronation. He is satisfied with the result, although activities such as weightlifting and receiving change are difficult.

(Fig. 8–74). The TFCC provides a continuous gliding surface across the entire distal face of the ulna for carpal movements, suspends the ulnar carpus from the dorsal ulnar face of the radius, cushions the forces transmitted through the ulnar-carpal axis, and solidly connects the ulna to the volar carpus.[16]

## MECHANISM OF INJURY

The mechanism of injury is usually a fall on the outstretched hand. Hypersupination injuries can result in a tear of the volar radioulnar ligament and as a consequence can cause volar displacement of the distal end of the ulna. Injury to the dorsal radioulnar ligament occurs with hyperpronation injuries and results in dorsal dislocation of the distal part of the ulna[125, 153] (Fig. 8–75).

## DIAGNOSIS

The distal portion of the ulna is usually tender, and pain can be elicited with compression of the distal ends of the radius and ulna. Any attempt to pronate or supinate the forearm is painful. With dorsal dislocation of the ulna—the more common distal radioulnar joint injury—careful physical examination reveals a dorsal prominence of the distal end of the ulna, along with fixed pronation of the forearm. With volar dislocation, the normal dorsal prominence of the distal part of the ulna may disappear, and a slight prominence may be evident on the anterior aspect of the wrist. Frequently a marked furrow is located on the medial side of the distal extensor aspect of the forearm. The distal part of the forearm has a narrowed appearance and is fixed in supination.[153]

Adequate anteroposterior and lateral views of the wrist are important to make the correct diagnosis. The standard zero position of the wrist with the forearm in neutral rotation is used on both anteroposterior and lateral views, with the ulnar styloid placed in the center of the ulna and the radius superimposed on the lateral view.[16] Comparison views of the opposite forearm are frequently necessary. Volar displacement of the ulna in relation to the radius is best seen on the lateral radiograph. On the anteroposterior view, the ulna and

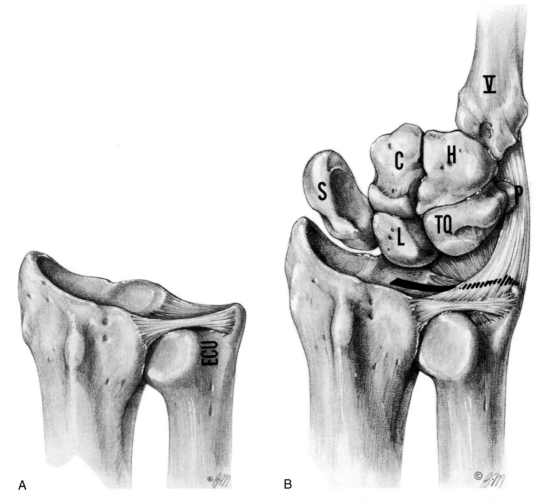

A                    B

**FIGURE 8–74.** The triangular fibrocartilage complex. *A,* The combined triangular fibrocartilage and ulnocarpal V ligament. *B,* Meniscal reflection that extends from the radius, over the triangular fibrocartilage, and distally to the base of the fifth metatarsal. The *arrow* shows access to the prestyloid recess. C, capitellum; ECU, extensor carpi ulnaris; H, hamate; L, lunate; S, scaphoid; TQ, triquetrum; V, 5th metacarpal. (*A, B,* From Bowers, W.H. In: Green, D.P., ed. Operative Hand Surgery, 2nd ed, Vol 2. New York, Churchill Livingstone, 1982, pp. 945–946.)

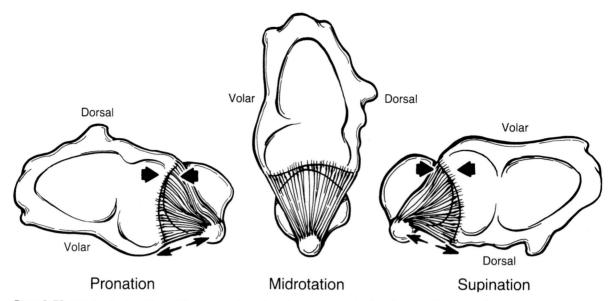

**FIGURE 8–75.** Distal radioulnar joint stability in pronation is dependent on tension developed in the volar margin of the triangular fibrocartilage (TFC) plus compression between the contact areas of the radius and ulna (volar surface of the ulnar articular head and dorsal margin of the sigmoid notch). A tear of the volar TFC therefore allows dorsal displacement of the ulna in pronation. The reverse is true in supination, where a tear of the dorsal margin of the TFC allows volar displacement of the ulna relative to the radius as this rotation extreme is reached. (From Bowers, W.H. In: Green, D.P., ed. Operative Hand Surgery, 2nd ed. New York, Churchill Livingstone, 1982, p. 948.)

radius may appear to be overlapping. Commonly, the ulnar styloid process is broken at its base.[153] If the diagnosis cannot be made with standard radiographs of the wrist, fluoroscopy with provocative stress testing and arthrography will be helpful. These imaging methods may be combined with a localized anesthetic block, also useful in localizing the pathology. Bone scans and three-dimensional CT scans may also be useful.[16]

## MANAGEMENT

The dislocation is reduced by reversing the mechanism of injury and applying direct pressure over the distal end of the ulna. The more common mechanism of injury is a pronation force that results in disruption of the volar triangular fibrocartilage and dorsal dislocation of the ulna. As described earlier, reduction and stabilization of the radioulnar joint would occur with the forearm in supination. The ulnocarpal ligaments and the passive contribution of the pronator quadratus supply additional stabilizing forces in this position. For volar dislocations, the dorsal triangular fibrocartilage is torn, and immobilization in pronation is necessary.

If the dislocation has been missed and the ulna cannot be passively reduced, symptomatic injuries can be treated by soft tissue reconstructive procedures. Symptoms include pain at the distal end of the ulna, with associated instability of the distal radioulnar joint. Many variants of the soft tissue procedures may be used for reconstruction, including rerouting of the tendon of the extensor carpi ulnaris, flexor carpi ulnaris, or pronator quadratus or the use of a fascial sling[16, 153] (Fig. 8–76). One example is a dorsal approach between the extensor carpi ulnaris and extensor digiti minimi. The forearm is

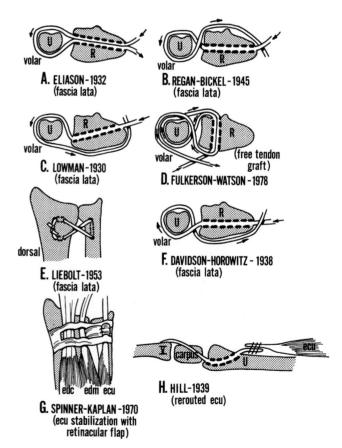

**FIGURE 8–76.** A sampling of soft tissue reconstructions suggested in the literature for an unstable distal radioulnar joint. ecu, extensor carpi ulnaris; edc, extensor digitorum communis; edm, extensor digitorum minimus; r, radius; u, ulna. (From Bowers, W.H. In: Green, D.P., ed. Operative Hand Surgery, 2nd ed. New York, Churchill Livingstone, 1982, p. 971.)

pronated, and the dorsal ulnar sensory nerve is protected. The extensor digiti minimi is retracted. The capsule is sharply detached and reflected toward the ulna. The dorsal radiotriquetral ligament is incised to reveal the dorsal margin of the sigmoid notch and the triangular fibrocartilage. Soft tissues are then repaired directly or reinforced with the extensor carpi ulnaris or a fascial sling. A temporary K-wire can be placed across the joint for extra stabilization during the healing process.

Unfortunately, soft tissue surgery alone is not always effective. Chronic symptoms can be relieved by the Darrach procedure (i.e., excision of the distal portion of the ulna). However, this procedure should be avoided in growing children to prevent the late complication of dislocation of the radial head. Once the physes in the wrist and the elbow are closed, excision of the distal end of the ulna can be considered.[125]

The Darrach procedure involves resecting about 2.5 cm of the distal part of the ulna. The ulnar styloid is divided at its base and left attached to the ulnar collateral ligament. The periosteal envelope and ligament are plicated to stabilize the end of the bone. Many modifications of this procedure are used and entail tendinous or fascial stabilizers to improve the stability of the wrist while relieving the radioulnar pain.

A fracture at the base of the styloid, because of its major attachments to the triangular fibrocartilage and ulnocarpal ligaments, is really an avulsion fracture of the major stabilizing ligaments of the distal end of the ulna. Minimally displaced fractures can be treated by immobilization in a well-fitting below-elbow cast with the wrist in neutral rotation and slight ulnar deviation. It has been suggested that moderately or severely displaced fractures be managed by accurate closed reduction or by open reduction and fixation through a dorsal ulnar incision.[52]

In children, the epiphysis encompasses the entire distal part of the ulna (see Fig. 8–1). Elsewhere in the forearm, most physeal fractures are Salter-Harris type I and II injuries. If a styloid fracture occurs, it is considered a nonarticular type III fracture and is usually treated conservatively without known sequelae. It is important, however, to remember that this fracture is really an avulsion fracture of the ulnocarpal ligaments and triangular fibrocartilage, and if the injury involves significant displacement in an unstable fracture, reduction and pinning may be an option.

## Carpal Fracture-Dislocations

Carpal fracture-dislocations are rare in children.[24, 28, 65, 135] They are more likely to occur in those who are approaching skeletal maturity and can hence be treated as adult fractures (Fig. 8–77). The mechanism of these injuries is usually a crush or extreme hyperextension caused by violent trauma that may or may not be associated with a fall.[52, 125] Several classifications of these injuries take into account the fact that the line of injury crosses the carpus transversely, which can cause ligamentous or bony injury through or around each of the bones in the wrist. The two rows of the carpus are bridged by the scaphoid, so if a midcarpal dislocation occurs between the two rows, the scaphoid must either rotate or fracture.

### MANAGEMENT

Undisplaced fractures can be treated in a short arm cast for 6 weeks. Closed reduction of displaced fractures can be difficult. Traction is best applied with finger traps (see Fig. 8–24), and with the aid of the image intensifier to check the reduction, the wrist is manipulated into radial or ulnar deviation, dorsiflexion, and palmar flexion until an adequate position is achieved. Usually, these fractures are unstable, and percutaneous pinning with one to three K-wires must be performed (Fig. 8–78). Weekly radiographic follow-up is recommended because these fractures may redisplace, even with K-wire fixation. A short arm cast is maintained for 6 weeks, at which time the pins are removed. If adequate closed reduction cannot be obtained, open reduction is performed through a dorsal or volar approach (or both).[28]

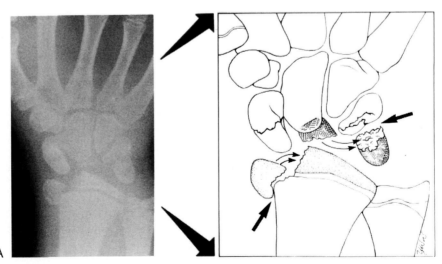

**FIGURE 8–77.** *A,* Posteroanterior radiograph of a transcarpal fracture-dislocation in a 10-year-old boy. *B,* Line drawing of the injury highlighting the specific pattern of fractures and displacement. (*A, B,* From DeCoster, T.A.; Faherty, S.; Morris, A.L. J Orthop Trauma 8:76–78, 1994.)

A                                                                                                    B

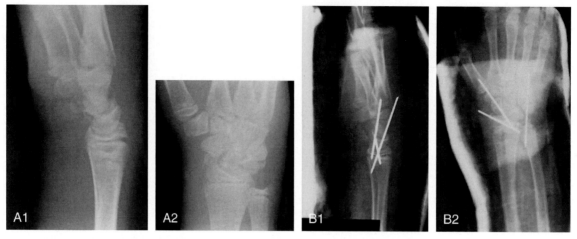

**FIGURE 8–78.** Proximal row carpal fracture-dislocation. *A,* A 12½-year-old girl suffered a fracture when a metal railing fell on her right wrist. *B,* Closed reduction was performed with the patient under general anesthesia, and pronation and radial deviation of the wrist were used to reduce the scaphoid and radial styloid fractures. The fractures were pinned percutaneously and a short arm thumb spica cast applied. The fracture was carefully monitored with weekly radiographs to ensure that the reduction was maintained.

## Fractures of the Carpal Bones

The lunate, scaphoid, and pisiform frequently have more than one center of ossification, which may be mistaken for a fracture. The developing carpus is mostly cartilage, and because of its cushioning effect, fracture or dislocation of the carpus is extremely rare in children.[116] The scaphoid is the most commonly injured carpal bone, with the majority of fractures occurring in children between the ages of 10 and 15 years. Although fractures of the lunate, capitate, pisiform, and triquetrum have been reported, they are rare.[92, 125]

### MECHANISM OF INJURY

Fractures of the scaphoid constitute 0.45% of children's upper limb fractures. Like most pediatric forearm injuries, they usually result from a fall on the outstretched hand (Fig. 8–79). The fractures occur most frequently in the distal pole (59%) and mainly at the scaphoid tuberosity, presumably the result of an avulsion injury. Fractures of the waist of the scaphoid are less common (33%).[23] In contrast, Stanciu and Dumont found a different distribution in adolescents, with 57% of fractures occurring in the middle third.[168]

### DIAGNOSIS

Similar to adult scaphoid fractures, swelling is seen over the dorsal aspect of the radiocarpal joint and especially over the anatomic snuffbox. Wrist motion is limited by pain, and the area over the anatomic snuffbox and scaphoid tuberosity is tender. These fractures are best visualized radiographically on an oblique or pronated view. Fracture displacement is rare. Incomplete or single-cortex fractures occur in 23% of pediatric cases.[23]

### MANAGEMENT

Initial radiographs may be normal in 12% of cases.[23] Scintigraphy has been recommended as part of the workup of an individual with symptoms of a scaphoid fracture without radiographic confirmation.[162, 177] MRI has also been used with good results.[71] In contrast, ultrasonography is unsuitable for the early diagnosis of scaphoid fractures.[22] If a scaphoid fracture is clinically suspected, the wrist should be immobilized in a thumb spica cast for 2 weeks, at which time the radiographs are repeated. If no evidence of fracture can be found at that time, the cast can be safely removed. If a scaphoid fracture is detected, the cast is reapplied for another 4 weeks. The only indication for acute open reduction and internal fixation is the presence of severe displacement that is at risk for nonunion.[111]

Most scaphoid fractures in children heal within 6 weeks of injury, and nonunion is rare. The prime cause of delayed union or nonunion is a delay in diagnosis or displacement of the fracture. Almost all nonunions occur at the waist of the scaphoid.[112] Continued immobilization usually results in fracture union. If union is not obtained by 6 months after the injury, autogenous bone grafting performed through a volar approach to the scaphoid is indicated. Other operative approaches have been reported, such as use of the dorsal approach and fixation with a Herbert screw.[112, 190]

## Fractures of the Triquetrum

Fractures of the triquetrum are a more common cause of post-traumatic wrist pain in children than was previously recognized. Letts and Esser reported on 15 children who sustained triquetral fractures.[92] The injury was most common in the group aged 11 to 13 years. A fall on the outstretched hand was the most frequent cause. Three had been missed at first. Multiple views, including a 45° oblique radiograph, are recommended in patients with significant wrist injuries. Most of the fractures seen were flake avulsion or impingement fractures (Fig. 8–80), although two complete fractures of the body were encountered (Fig. 8–81).

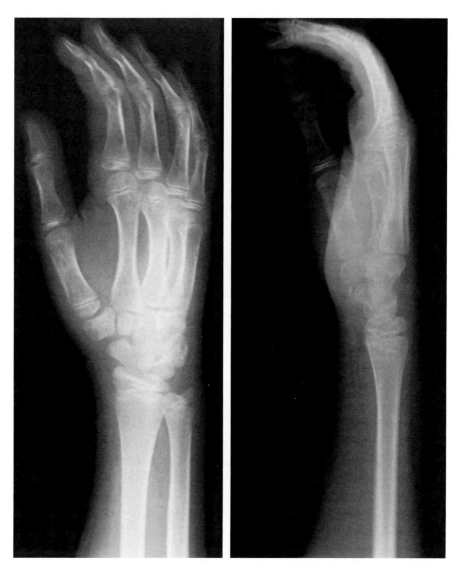

FIGURE 8–79. Fracture of the scaphoid tuberosity. A 12-year-old boy slipped in the schoolyard and landed on his extended right hand. He was treated in a thumb spica cast for 6 weeks, and the fracture healed uneventfully.

## MANAGEMENT

Letts and Esser's patients were all treated in below-elbow casts or volar splints for 3 weeks. They found that most patients healed satisfactorily, both radiologically and functionally. However, 2 of 10 patients complained of persistent discomfort with hyperextension of the wrist on long-term follow-up.[92]

## Carpometacarpal Dislocations

Carpometacarpal (CMC) dislocations are rare in children and are usually the result of violent trauma. They most frequently occur in combination with fractures of the adjoining metacarpal. CMC dislocation of the thumb is especially uncommon because the stress causes a growth plate injury in the adjacent physis.

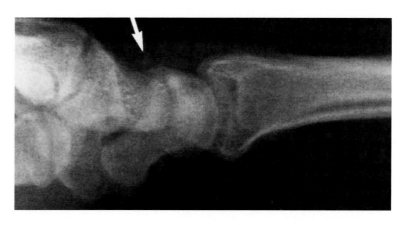

FIGURE 8–80. Small flake fracture of the triquetrum, evident on a lateral view of the wrist. (From Letts, M.; Esser, D. J Pediatr Orthop 13:228–231, 1993.)

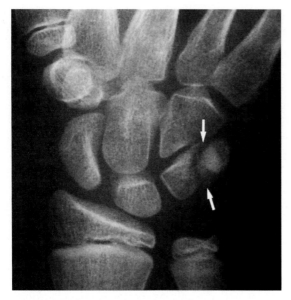

**FIGURE 8–81.** Fracture of the body of the triquetrum. (From Letts, M.; Esser, D. J Pediatr Orthop 13:228–231, 1993.)

## MANAGEMENT

After closed reduction, pin fixation to the adjacent metacarpals and carpus is recommended because these fracture-dislocations tend to be unstable. If adequate closed reduction cannot be accomplished, open reduction through a dorsal approach should be undertaken.[59, 79, 158, 193] The hand and wrist are immobilized in a short arm cast with the hand in the "position of safety" (i.e., with the MP joints immobilized at 90° and the IP joints extended) for 4 weeks. The child then commences exercises to recover range of motion in the hand. The pins are removed 6 weeks after the injury.

## FRACTURES AND DISLOCATIONS OF THE HAND

### Incidence

Hand trauma is common in childhood, both early, as toddlers begin to explore the world around them, and later, as young teenagers assert their independence. The epidemiology of these injuries reflects the changing patterns of activity throughout the growing years. Hastings and Simmons undertook a retrospective review of 354 pediatric hand fractures with a minimal 2-year follow-up.[211] All patients were younger than 18 years. The peak incidence of fractures was in the early teenage years, possibly related to contact sports. A smaller peak was seen in infancy, related mostly to crush injuries in doors. The etiology varies with age, but overall, Hastings and Simmons found that the mechanisms included torque and angulation (34%), crush (21%), direct blow (10%), axial compression (9.5%), unknown (24%), and in one case, a pathologic fracture.[211] The little finger is involved most commonly (30%), and the thumb is involved in 20%; the other fingers are involved in nearly equal distributions (index, 16%; middle, 16%; and ring, 18%). Fractures of the proximal phalanx account for nearly half the injuries seen (43%), and fractures of the metacarpals and remaining phalanges are evenly distributed.

## Principles of Treatment

### ANESTHESIA

Anesthesia both for closed reduction of phalangeal fractures and for the treatment of open injuries of the fingertip is best accomplished with a digital nerve block at the base of the affected digit. Infants and small children are bundled in a sheet or secured in a papoose-like wrap before the part is prepared. A 1% solution of lidocaine without epinephrine is instilled with a 3-mL syringe and a 27- or 30-gauge needle. A small bead of anesthetic is placed under the dorsal skin on the radial side of the digit; the needle is advanced through this area almost to the palmar skin along the shaft of the proximal phalanx. After the plunger is withdrawn to ensure that a vessel has not been punctured, the anesthetic is instilled while the needle is slowly withdrawn. A line of solution is then deposited along the dorsal surface of the digit, and finally, the ulnar side is injected. No more than 1 mL of anesthetic should be used for one finger because a greater amount poses a risk of vascular compromise by compression. Median nerve blocks at the wrist or ulnar nerve blocks at the cubital tunnel can be used for metacarpal fractures, but we prefer hematoma blocks to reduce the risk of direct injection into the nerve. General anesthesia is rarely required for closed fractures in children, but it is frequently necessary in dislocations and open fractures with soft tissue injuries.

### MANIPULATION

Manipulation of fractures and dislocations can prove quite difficult in children, given their small size. Adequate anesthesia is the key. An assistant who can both comfort and control the child is invaluable. Flexion of the MP or IP joints of the finger usually aids in securing sufficient purchase, as well as in improving control of the reduction. Occasionally, it is necessary to use a fulcrum to manipulate fractures at the base of the proximal phalanx. A pencil or smooth pen barrel—being a familiar, nonthreatening object—is effective.

### IMMOBILIZATION

Because most hand fractures in children can be satisfactorily treated with immobilization alone,[213] an understanding of the attendant principles is warranted. The immobilization position commonly used in adults—wrist and IP joint extension and MP joint flexion—is not satisfactory for small children. Children can further extend the wrist and flex their short fingers until they are fisted in the splint, or they can slide the whole hand out of the splint if it is not secured above the elbow. To reduce these risks, the wrist and MP and IP joints are all maintained in straight extension against a flat splint. Securing the bandage over the MP joints reduces the child's ability to extend the wrist or flex the fingers and reduces the risk of escape. Extending the bandage above the elbow provides additional security.

Immobilization of a small child's hand requires a more thorough effort than may be necessary in an adult. Plaster casts for children younger than 6 years should routinely extend above the flexed elbow, even to splint fingers or metacarpals. Skin glue can be used to enhance the security of the bandage. In older children, a forearm plaster slab is sufficient. Our preference is to use a volar or dorsal slab—or both, as necessary—in the first few days after injury. On follow-up examination, the bandage is removed, repeat radiographs are taken, and if the reduction is satisfactorily maintained, a circumferential plaster cast is applied. If the fracture is not sufficiently stable to remain reduced during the period required for films, it probably requires at least pin fixation, if not open reduction.

Although plates and screws have become a standard method of fixation in adult hand fractures, such fixation is possible only occasionally in children's hand fractures.[219] The extensive dissection and periosteal stripping required for internal fixation increase the risk of devascularizing the epiphyses of small bones. In addition, the bulk of the hardware often precludes its use. In contrast to adults, the thick periosteum of children's bones can be used to advantage in providing a strong hinge against which to reduce a fracture. K-wires in sizes of 0.028, 0.035, and 0.045 inch are easily used to provide secure fixation. K-wires can be allowed to protrude through the skin with no untoward effects,[213] and if they are left in place less than 4 weeks, pin tract infection is rare.

Many methods are available to facilitate elevation of a child's hand after reduction. We prefer a stockinette bandage with the proximal end split and tied around the chest and the opposite end suspended from an intravenous pole. Alternatively, the bandage can be secured to an overhead line of twill tape running from one end of the crib to the other.[221]

## Fractures

In most cases, fractures of a child's hand can be treated successfully by closed means. Leonard and Dubravcik reviewed a large series of 263 hand fractures in children younger than 17 years.[213] Treatment consisted of splinting alone in 75% of cases, manipulation and splinting in 15%, and open reduction in 10%. Their particular indications for open reduction included open wounds and fractures of the phalangeal neck.

Fracture healing in a child is very rapid and occurs in about half the time required for an adult. Nonunion is extremely rare.[223] For these reasons, immobilization can often be limited to 3 weeks, particularly when the metaphysis or epiphysis is involved. Overtreatment may be a major source of complications.[223]

Malalignment may be corrected by remodeling with growth.[218] In general, fractures displaced within the plane of joint motion remodel quite satisfactorily (Fig. 8–82), whereas those deviating laterally from the joint plane do less well. Rotational deformity does not correct with further growth and may not be acceptable. Therefore, limited indications exist for the operative treatment of fractures of the hand in a child (see later). When surgery is undertaken, however, particular care is required to manage delicate tissues and small bones.

Physeal injury is a common finding in fractures in a child's hand. Hastings and Simmons found that 34% of their cases involved the physis, with fractures through closing or recently closed physes seen up to the age of 17 years.[211] The Salter-Harris classification of physeal fracture[218] is described elsewhere (see Fig. 8–39). Salter-Harris type II injuries predominate (78.7%), with Salter-Harris type III (13.1%) and I (7.4%) injuries being less common and Salter-Harris types IV (1.8%) and V being rare. Salter-Harris type II injuries peak in the early teenage years. These fractures occurred in the proximal phalanx in 69% of cases, with the border digits predominating; injury to the little finger was the most common single fracture[209, 211] and usually resulted from an abduction injury. Growth disturbance arising from injury to the physis is rare but is always a concern.[207, 209]

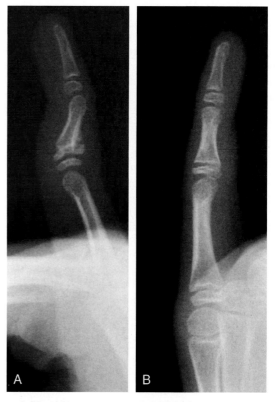

**FIGURE 8–82.** This 10-year-old jammed her little finger while playing a ball game at school. She was treated with a splint, but no reduction was undertaken initially. *A,* When she was first evaluated at our center, a fracture of the base of the middle phalanx in 45° of dorsal angulation was seen. The fracture was clinically and radiologically united. The finger was treated with aggressive mobilization. *B,* On follow-up examination over 1 year later, the middle phalanx had remodeled satisfactorily, with complete correction of the dorsal angulation.

In general, Salter-Harris type I and II injuries can be treated by closed reduction and immobilization and carry a favorable prognosis. Salter-Harris type III and IV fractures are, by definition, intra-articular and should be opened and reduced anatomically to lessen the resulting joint incongruity and subsequent risk of late osteoarthritis. Clearly, it is necessary to assess the size of the intra-articular fragment and the feasibility of securing adequate fixation before proceeding. Type III and IV injuries have a worse prognosis. Treatment in the rare type V injury is dictated by the usually open nature of the wound and must be individualized. The prognosis for normal growth in patients with type V injuries is very guarded.

## DISTAL PHALANX

Salter-Harris type I and II fractures are the childhood equivalent of the mallet finger.[206] The flexor remains attached to the distal fragment and angulates it volarward, and the extensor is attached to the epiphysis and holds it in extension. The nail bed stays with the distal fragment. In an adolescent, a mallet finger is usually manifested as a Salter-Harris type III injury with a small intra-articular fragment. Usually, it can be treated with splinting in extension, which should produce good or excellent results in 80% of patients.[216] This treatment can be used in open injuries as well, in which even the skin need not be closed.[216]

Recommendations for the operative treatment of displaced fragments vary widely. Campbell[206] favors anatomic reduction. McFarlane and Hampole[216] believe that surgery is justified in an avulsion fracture of more than one third of the articular surface of the distal phalanx. One K-wire is placed to hold the fragment and another to hold the DIP joint in extension for 3 weeks. Splinting is maintained for 6 weeks. Niechajev[217] suggests that surgery be reserved for those with subluxation of the distal phalanx or with fragments displaced more than 3 mm. He uses a pull-out wire to hold the already reduced fragment in place.

In fractures of the volar aspect of the DIP joint, an avulsion injury of the profundus tendon must always be considered. These injuries are seen in teenagers and involve the ring finger in 75% of cases.[212] Although in most of these injuries either no fracture or a small flake fracture is seen, in unusual cases, a large bony fragment may represent an intra-articular component sufficient to require K-wire fixation.[212] In small children, a 25- or 27-gauge hypodermic needle may be a suitable substitute for achieving fixation. Avulsions of the profundus tendon occur without fracture as well; in these cases, surgery for the tendon injury is required, with either direct tendon repair or fixation with a pull-out wire.

Open fractures of the distal phalanx are often accompanied by injury to the nail bed. Although a full discussion of these injuries is beyond the scope of this chapter, some points bear emphasis. Zook and co-workers[225] studied 290 consecutive nail bed injuries over a 5½-year period. After reviewing their results, they concluded that nail bed lacerations should be repaired under tourniquet control and loupe magnification after removing the nail plate. For the nail bed, *7–0 chromic*

sutures were used, and 5–0 or 6–0 nylon sutures were used for the skin component of the lacerations. If a fracture of the distal phalanx is associated with a nail bed injury, it is important to reduce the fracture as accurately as possible to achieve a flat nail bed.[224] A K-wire may sometimes be necessary to maintain the reduction. In multiply comminuted fractures, the fragments should be reduced as much as possible and the nail plate used as a splint.[224] These authors prefer to use the original nail for splinting the eponychial fold open rather than a piece of gauze because postoperative discomfort is reduced.[225] Wood[223] prefers to leave the nail plate attached in fractures of the distal phalanx to further splint the fracture and levers it back into position under the eponychial fold.

## MIDDLE PHALANX

Fractures of the middle phalanx usually result from forces applied directly to the bone, whereas loads applied to the whole digit commonly injure the base of the proximal phalanx. Transverse fractures of the shaft of the middle phalanx can be treated in a fashion comparable to that for the proximal phalanx (see later), with unstable fractures requiring pinning. Longitudinal crush injuries are often stable and minimally displaced and, if not intra-articular, can be treated with protective immobilization alone.

Oblique fractures of the distal middle or proximal phalanx should be carefully assessed radiographically because they are often intra-articular, with the fracture splitting the two articular condyles (Fig. 8–83). Treatment of this injury, once diagnosed, is controversial. Campbell[206] recommends monitoring undisplaced fractures radiographically for evidence of slippage and intervening if necessary. Our preference is to pin these fractures with a single oblique K-wire to obviate the later displacement that can occur. This procedure is done percutaneously, if possible. The K-wire is inserted into the condylar fragment, which can be manipulated, if necessary, before the K-wire is passed into the distal end of the shaft of the middle phalanx. Mobilization is undertaken after 3 weeks.

Physeal injuries in the middle phalanx are uncommon. Most laterally directed forces cause injury to the physis of the proximal phalanx. Closed reduction and appropriate immobilization should prove adequate.

## PROXIMAL PHALANX

Salter-Harris type II fractures of the base of the proximal phalanx are extremely common injuries, and almost all can be treated by closed reduction and splinting[206] (Fig. 8–84). A digital nerve block is used. The MP joint is flexed, and a finger or pencil is placed in the appropriate web to provide a fulcrum on which the fracture can be reduced. Postreduction radiographs are taken to confirm the reduction, and the finger is loosely buddy-taped to its neighbor. Plaster immobilization for 3 weeks with radiologic review after 3 to 7 days is undertaken.

A rare complication of fracture of the proximal phalanx is entrapment of the flexor tendon within the fracture site. Harryman and Jordan described a case in

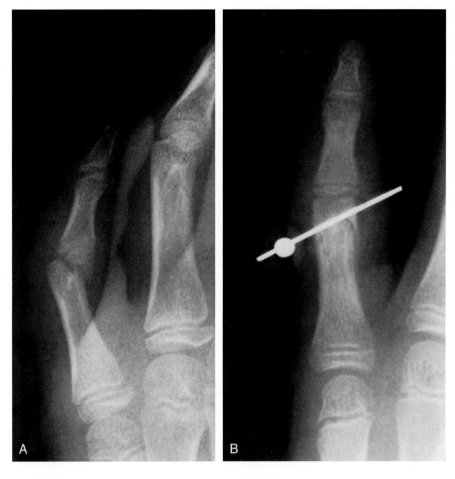

FIGURE 8–83. After falling from his bicycle, this 13-year-old was found to have an oblique fracture of the distal proximal phalanx. *A,* The fracture splits the two condyles. *B,* Closed reduction was successful, with a single oblique K-wire being used to hold the fracture. The pin was left in place for 16 days before mobilization.

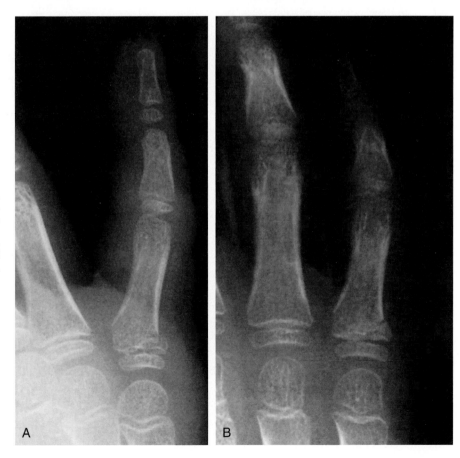

FIGURE 8–84. This 9-year-old boy fell down the stairs at home. *A,* He sustained a Salter-Harris type II injury to the proximal phalanx of his little finger. Reduction was undertaken under digital blockade. *B,* Good maintenance of the reduction was seen at 3 weeks, when the finger was mobilized.

which a markedly displaced Salter-Harris type II fracture was irreducible by closed means.[210] On volar exploration, the metaphysis had penetrated the flexor sheath, and the flexor tendons were wound around it and trapped in the fracture site.

In older children, Salter-Harris type III or IV fractures may be seen, often as the physis is beginning to close. These injuries are intra-articular and, given a fracture fragment of sufficient size to allow purchase with a K-wire, should be reduced anatomically (Fig. 8–85). Open reduction is usually required to provide adequate mobilization of the fracture, but care must be taken to not strip the periosteum and hence the blood supply to the epiphysis. The patient or family should be warned that these injuries may result in premature closure of the physis, with subsequent growth disturbance.

Hyperextension injuries to the MP joint can cause tears of the volar plate that are seen radiographically as small avulsion fractures of the volar base of the proximal phalanx. These injuries usually occur after the physeal plates are closed. Tenderness and swelling are noted over the volar aspect of the joint, but without ligament instability. Treatment consists of immobilization with the MP joint in flexion for 10 days, followed by gradual mobilization.

Transverse phalangeal shaft fractures are usually stable and can be treated by immobilization alone.[213] If the fracture is unstable (meaning that adequate reduction cannot be obtained or maintained), percutaneous pinning is performed.[206] In particular, pinning or open reduction may be required in spiral fractures of the proximal phalanx, which are often very unstable[223] (Fig. 8–86). The use of plates for fixation may be considered in teenagers of adult size with closed physes.

Fractures of the head or neck of the proximal phalanx must be examined carefully. Truly undisplaced fractures of the neck of the proximal phalanx (supracondylar fractures) can be treated with splinting.[206] Rotation of the fragment in distal fractures of the proximal phalanx in children can easily be missed, however, particularly if true lateral radiographs are not obtained.[208] The distal fragment, which is small, may be rotated dorsally by as much as 180°, with the intact collateral ligaments acting as the pivot point. On casual inspection, the radiograph appears to reveal a minimally displaced fracture, but the articular surface of the proximal phalanx may be facing directly into the fracture site. Open reduction is mandatory.[208] In cases in which dorsal angulation of distal fractures of the proximal phalanx has been missed or ignored, little remodeling is likely to occur because no physis is present. A volar surgical approach, with removal of the bone causing the block to flexion, is described as a late reconstruction.[220]

## METACARPALS

The degree of acceptable apex dorsal angulation in a fracture of the fifth metacarpal neck is controversial. Authors vary in their opinions, with some stating that 35° of apex dorsal angulation of a boxer's fracture is acceptable[204] and others recommending reduction of fractures at the neck of the metacarpal only if they are

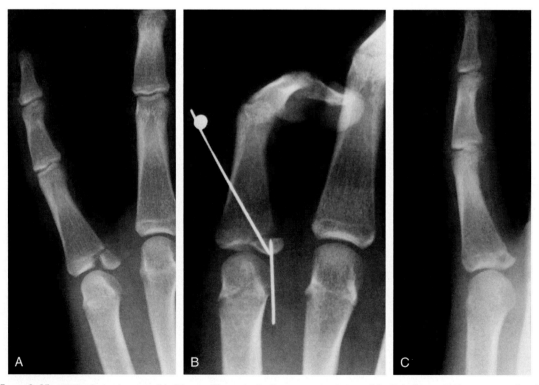

**FIGURE 8–85.** While playing lacrosse, this 17-year-old sustained a hyperextension injury of the little finger. *A,* The injury produced a Salter-Harris type III fracture of his almost-closed physis. Open reduction was undertaken by splitting the extensor tendon and rotating the small fragment through 90°. *B,* Two K-wires were used for fixation. *C,* Two months later, consolidation of the fracture is seen, with little articular deformity.

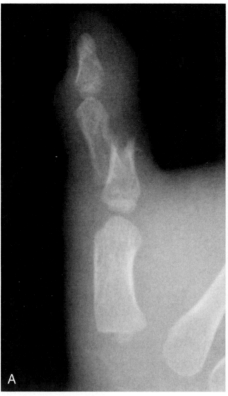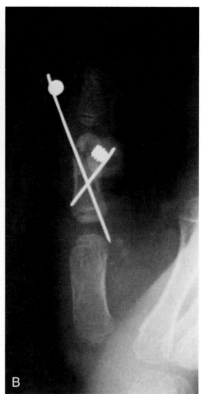

**Figure 8–86.** This 4-year-old fell on his outstretched hand. *A,* A spiral fracture of the proximal phalanx of the thumb is seen; closed reduction was not possible. At open reduction, the extensor tendon was found to be torn away from the bone, with the ragged periosteum at the fracture site preventing reduction. *B,* Two K-wires were used to secure the reduced fracture fragments.

angulated more than 40° into the palm or are unstable.[219] Our recommendation is to first attempt closed reduction under local anesthesia, followed by plaster fixation. If on subsequent views taken 3 to 7 days later angulation greater than 30° is seen, the patient is taken to the operating room, where a single longitudinal K-wire is placed after further closed reduction. This recommendation is based on the observation that most of these injuries occur in teenagers nearing the end of growth and that power grip may be affected if the fifth ray is angulated. In addition, inadequately treated or reduced fractures may be seen late with a tender lump in the palm. Reduction is achieved by holding the MP joint in 90° of flexion, applying longitudinal traction, and pushing firmly over the dorsal convexity of the fracture. A K-wire is passed retrograde through the metacarpal head. Long-term follow-up of these injuries often reveals loss of the normal prominence of the fifth metacarpal head, and the patient and family should be made aware of this possible outcome.

Physeal injuries of the metacarpal head are uncommon. Four were seen in a series of 103 fractures in 100 patients of all ages.[199] All were Salter-Harris type III injuries that were treated with splinting and careful mobilization at 3 weeks, and all did well.

Avascular necrosis of the metacarpal head has been seen after blunt trauma. This lesion is difficult to diagnose because in the early stages, radiographs may be normal. This injury should be considered in cases with traumatic effusion of the MP joint.[215] The joint should be aspirated and the hand splinted. Late follow-up reveals stiffness, pain, and radiologic evidence of collapse of the metacarpal head.

Fractures of the bases of the second through fifth metacarpals are frequently stable, and if so, reduction is not required. Splinting in a forearm plaster cast is sufficient treatment.[219] If significantly malaligned, these fractures can be fixed with percutaneous K-wires.

Fractures of the shaft of the metacarpals can be treated by closed means in most cases. In the isolated situation of late displacement and unacceptable angulation, rotation, or both, open reduction plus internal fixation with small-fragment plates and screws is recommended.

## THUMB

Most fractures of the thumb metacarpal occur at its base. Unlike in adults, the ligaments and capsule at the base of the thumb are extremely strong, with the weakest point at the physis and the proximal metaphysis. Salter-Harris type II fractures are seen, but commonly, the shaft of the metacarpal is fractured just distal to the epiphysis. The intra-articular fractures seen so often in adult practice are extremely uncommon in children.

Wood[223] accepts 30° of angulation in fractures of the base of the thumb metacarpal that are angulated in a radial direction. In ulnar angulation, open reduction is often required, and redisplacement may occur if closed treatment is used.[223] Translocation of the fragments relative to one another is often more of a concern than angular deviation. Of particular note, the distal fragment can become lodged into the cleft between the bases of the first and second metacarpals. Such fractures require careful reduction to remove the potential bony block that might reduce the mobility of the CMC joint of the thumb (Fig. 8–87).

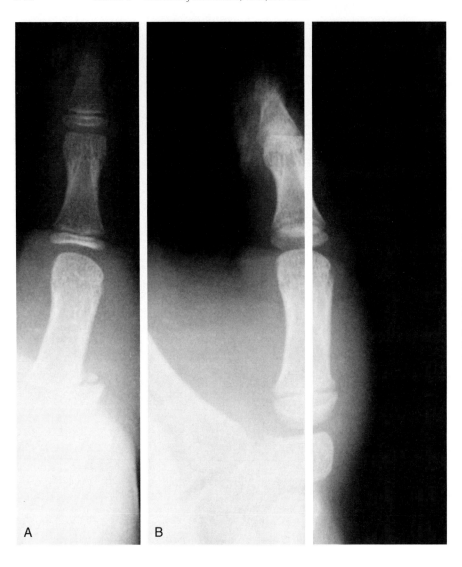

FIGURE **8–87.** This 12-year-old fell from his bicycle and sustained a Salter-Harris type II fracture of the thumb metacarpal. *A,* Of note, displacement of the proximal end of the distal fragment toward the base of the second metacarpal is a potential bony block to unimpeded movement of the thumb carpometacarpal joint. *B,* Closed reduction was not possible immediately, but 5 days later, after the swelling had subsided, manipulation achieved an excellent position that was fixed with a single axial K-wire.

Closed reduction of proximal shaft fractures of the thumb is made difficult by the inability to obtain sufficient control of the metacarpal fragment through the swollen thenar mass. In some cases, it may be of benefit to attempt reduction after several days have elapsed to allow resolution of the swelling. Open reduction, when indicated, is best approached through an incision between the glabrous and nonglabrous skin along the radial aspect of the thumb. Unlike in adult fracture-dislocations, exposure of the CMC joint is not required.

## Dislocations

### INTERPHALANGEAL JOINTS

Dorsal dislocation of the DIP joint is rare in childhood[206] and is usually produced by a direct blow to the end of the finger (Fig. 8–88). Initial treatment is by closed reduction under local or, if necessary, general anesthesia. The finger is then immobilized for 10 days before gentle range of motion is encouraged. Failure of closed reduction requires an open dorsal approach with possible division of the collateral ligament.[206]

Dislocations of the PIP joint are also rare in children. When they occur, the displacement is usually dorsal. Closed manipulation should be sufficient treatment, with immobilization as described earlier. Irreducible injuries with an interposed volar plate or those that are unstable after reduction as a result of collateral ligament injury[206] should be opened and repaired directly. Volar dislocation of the PIP joint is sometimes seen, but irreducible volar dislocation has never been reported.[206]

### METACARPOPHALANGEAL JOINT

Dislocation of the MP joints of digits other than the thumb and index finger is uncommon but has been reported[205] and can be treated by using the principles described later.

### INDEX FINGER

Dislocation of the MP joint of the index finger may be either reducible or not. These injuries are characteristically caused by a hyperextension injury to the joint. With sufficient force, the volar plate is torn and becomes

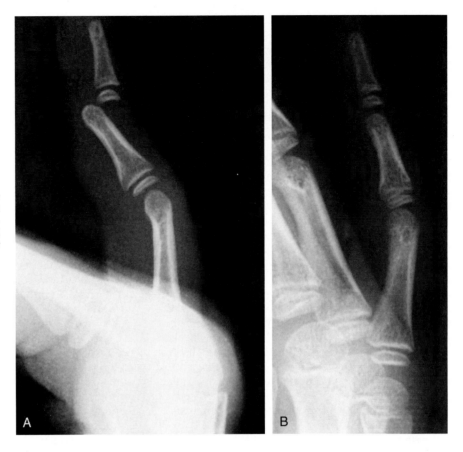

FIGURE 8–88. *A,* A hyperextension injury dislocated the distal interphalangeal joint of this 7-year-old's little finger. *B,* Reduction was undertaken with use of a digital block and was followed by splinting for 10 days.

interposed in the joint, and the lumbrical and flexor tendons cinch the neck of the metacarpal on its radial and ulnar sides, respectively. This combination renders the dislocation irreducible and sometimes occurs as a result of force applied to an otherwise reducible dislocation during attempted reduction. If gentle closed reduc-

tion fails, a volar zigzag surgical approach is recommended[214] (Fig. 8–89). Division of the A1 pulley may be sufficient to release the flexor noose; however, the volar plate usually requires an axial incision to achieve adequate release. The joint is immobilized in 60° of flexion for 10 days before gradual movement is begun.

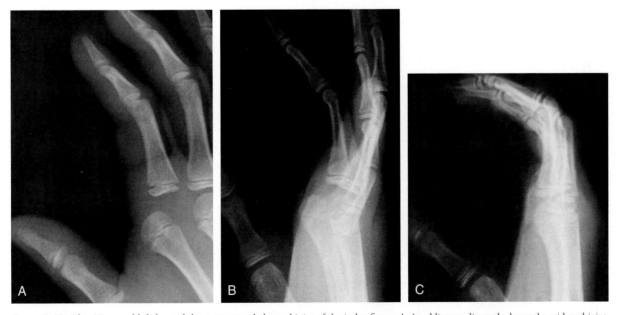

FIGURE 8–89. This 11-year-old dislocated the metacarpophalangeal joint of the index finger. *A,* An oblique radiograph shows the widened joint space produced by the interposition of the volar plate. *B,* On the lateral view, the dorsal dislocation can be seen, with the second metacarpal head appearing unsatisfied in the palm. *C,* An open approach with division of the A1 pulley was required to achieve reduction in this case.

Dislocation of the MP joint of the index metacarpal in a child may be complicated by vascular compromise of the physis of the metacarpal head or by an osteochondral fracture, with either leading to subsequent deformity with growth. In addition, the vascular supply may be compromised by the operative exposure.[214]

### THUMB

Irreducible dislocation of MP joints other than in the index finger is rare.[206] In the thumb, ligament injury or fracture is much more commonly seen. Mild cases of forcible abduction and extension of the thumb usually produce a sprain of the ulnar collateral ligament of the MP joint. Stronger force results in a Salter-Harris type II fracture of the base of the proximal phalanx or a proximal metacarpal shaft fracture. Ulnar collateral ligament avulsion without fracture is rare,[190] but if it should occur, Stener[222] observed that the ligament ruptures at its distal attachment to the proximal phalanx. As the now-unrestrained thumb is abducted farther, the proximal edge of the adductor expansion passes over the torn end of the ligament. When the thumb returns to its rest position, the proximal stump of the ligament folds back on itself, and the adductor aponeurosis becomes interposed between the two torn ends. This displacement renders nonoperative treatment of the lesion impossible.

Accurate descriptions of the pathologic anatomy of dislocation of the MP joint of the thumb are not new. Barnard[205] believed that the rent in the capsule supporting the volar plate entrapped the head of the metacarpal.

He went on to describe in some detail a comparable dislocation of the MP joint of the little finger. Closed reduction of a dorsal MP dislocation should be attempted under appropriate anesthesia. The thumb is flexed at the CMC and IP joints and adducted. This maneuver usually allows sufficient relaxation of the tight structures around the neck of the metacarpal to permit reduction (Fig. 8–90). If closed treatment fails, open reduction usually reveals the head of the metacarpal protruding through the joint capsule and the flexor pollicis brevis,[223] which must be repaired.

## SUMMARY

Trauma to a child's hand is common, with large numbers of fractures and some dislocations being seen in the emergency department. Most injuries can be treated in the emergency room setting, except for those with associated injuries to nerves or tendons, which require general anesthesia for adequate management.

Early and frequent follow-up is key in the closed management of fractures to confirm the adequacy of both the reduction and the splint. Immobilization can be maintained in infants and children for 3 weeks without risking the development of significant residual stiffness. Injuries to the physis are common because the ligaments and periosteum are strong and the epiphyses are relatively weak. These injuries heal rapidly and without growth disturbance if appropriately treated.

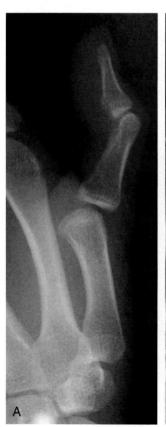
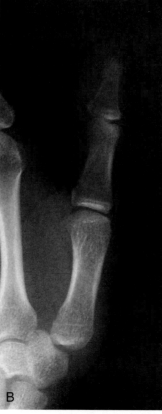

FIGURE **8–90.** This 15-year-old complained of a swollen, tender thumb after playing basketball. *A,* Dorsal dislocation of the thumb metacarpophalangeal joint was found radiographically. *B,* After closed reduction, in this case under general anesthesia, congruity of the joint was achieved.

# REFERENCES

## Forearm and Wrist

1. Abram, L.J.; Thompson, G.H. Deformity after premature closure of the distal radial physis following a torus fracture with a physeal, compression injury: Report of a case. J Bone Joint Surg Am 69:1450–1453, 1987.
2. Aitken, A.P. The end results of the fractured distal radial epiphysis. J Bone Joint Surg 17:302–308, 1935.
3. al-Qattan, M.M.; Clarke, H.M.; Zimmer, P. Radiological signs of entrapment of the median nerve in forearm shaft fractures. J Hand Surg Br 19:713–719, 1994.
4. Amit, Y.; Salai, M.; Chechik, A.; et al. Closing intramedullary nailing for the treatment of diaphyseal forearm fractures in adolescence: A preliminary report. J Pediatr Orthop 5:143–146, 1985.
5. Bado, J.L. The Monteggia lesion. Clin Orthop 50:71–86, 1967.
6. Bailey, D.A.; Wedge, J.H.; McCulloch, R.G.; et al. Epidemiology of fractures of the distal end of the radius in children as associated with growth. J Bone Joint Surg Am 71:1225–1231, 1989.
7. Barnes, C.; Blasier, R.; Dodge, B. Intravenous regional anesthesia: A safe and cost effective outpatient anesthetic for upper extremity fracture treatment in children. J Pediatr Orthop 11:717–720, 1991.
8. Bednar, D.W.G. Complications of forearm-plate removal. Can J Surg 35:428–431, 1992.
9. Bell-Tawse, A.J.S. The treatment of malunited anterior Monteggia fractures in children. J Bone Joint Surg Br 47:718–723, 1965.
10. Biyani, A. Ipsilateral Monteggia equivalent injury and distal radial and ulnar fracture in a child. J Orthop Trauma 8:431–433, 1994.
11. Biyani, A.; Bhan, S. Dual extensor tendon entrapment in Galeazzi fracture dislocation: A case report. J Trauma 29:1295–1297, 1989.
12. Blount, W.P. Forearm fractures in children. Clin Orthop 51:93–107, 1967.
13. Blount, W.; Shaefer, A.; Johnson, J. Fractures of the forearm in children. JAMA 120:111, 1942.
14. Bolte, R.; Stevens, P.; Scott, S.; Schunk, J. Mini-dose Bier block intravenous regional anesthesia in the emergency department treatment of pediatric upper-extremity injuries. J Pediatr Orthop 14:534–537, 1994.
15. Borden, S., IV. Traumatic bowing of the forearm in children. J Bone Joint Surg Am 56:611–616, 1974.
16. Bowers, W.H. The distal radioulnar joint. In: Green, D.P., ed. Operative Hand Surgery, 2nd ed., Vol 2. New York, Churchill Livingstone, 1988, pp. 939–989.
17. Boyd, H.B. Surgical exposure of the ulna and proximal third of the radius through one incision. Surg Gynecol Obstet 71:81–88, 1940.
18. Boyd, H.B.; Boals, J.C. The Monteggia lesion. Clin Orthop 66:94–100, 1969.
19. Boyden, E.M.; Peterson, H.A. Partial premature closure of the distal radial physis associated with Kirschner wire fixation. Orthopedics 14:585–588, 1991.
20. Canale, S.T.; Puhl, J.; Watson, F.M.; Gillespie, R. Acute osteomyelitis following closed fractures. J Bone Joint Surg Am 57:415–418, 1975.
21. Christensen, J.B. A study of the interosseous distance between the radius and ulna during rotation of the forearm. J Bone Joint Surg Br 46:778–779, 1964.
22. Christiansen, T.G.; Rude, C.; Lauridsen, K.K.; Christensen, O.M. Diagnostic value of ultrasound in scaphoid fractures. Injury 22:397–399, 1991.
23. Christodoulou, A.G.; Colton, C.L. Scaphoid fractures in children. J Pediatr Orthop 6:37–39, 1986.
24. Compson, J.P. Trans-carpal injuries associated with distal radial fractures in children: A series of three cases. J Hand Surg Br 17:311–314, 1992.
25. Creasman, C.; Zaleske, D.J.; Ehrlich, M.G. Analyzing forearm fractures in children: The more subtle signs of impending problems. Clin Orthop 188:40–53, 1984.
26. Dameron, T.B. Traumatic dislocation of the distal radioulnar joint. Clin Orthop 83:55–63, 1972.
27. Daruwalla, J.S. A study of radioulnar movements following fractures of the forearm in children. Clin Orthop 139:114–120, 1979.
28. DeCoster, T.A.; Faherty, S.; Morris, A.L. Case report: Pediatric carpal fracture dislocation. J Orthop Trauma 8:76–78, 1994.
29. Deluca, P.; Lindsey, R.; Ruwe, P. Refracture of bones of the forearm after the removal of compression plates. J Bone Joint Surg Am 70:1372–1376, 1988.
30. de Pablos, J.; Franzreb, M.; Barrios, C. Longitudinal growth pattern of the radius after forearm fractures conservatively treated in children. J Pediatr Orthop 14:492–495, 1994.
31. Digby, K. The measurement of diaphyseal growth in proximal and distal directions. J Anat Physiol 50:187, 1915.
32. Evans, E.M. Fractures of the radius and ulna. J Bone Joint Surg Br 33:548–561, 1951.
33. Evans, E.M. Rotational deformity in the treatment of fractures of both bones of the forearm. J Bone Joint Surg 27:373–379, 1945.
34. Evans, J.K.; Buckley, S.L.; Alexander, A.H.; Gilpin, A.T. Analgesia for the reduction of fractures in children: A comparison of nitrous oxide with intramuscular sedation. J Pediatr Orthop 15:73–77, 1995.
35. Evans, M.C.; Graham, H.K. Radial neck fractures in children: A management algorithm. J Pediatr Orthop B 8:93–99, 1999.
36. Fahmy, N.R.M. Unusual Monteggia lesions in children. Injury 12:399–404, 1980.
37. Flynn, J.M.; Waters, P.M. Single bone fixation of both-bone forearm fractures. J Pediatr Orthop 16:655–659, 1996.
38. Frazier, J.L.; Buschmann, W.R.; Insler, H.P. Monteggia type I equivalent lesion: Diaphyseal ulna and proximal radius fracture with a posterior elbow dislocation in a child. J Orthop Trauma 5:373–375, 1991.
39. Friberg, K.S.I. Remodelling after distal forearm fractures in children. I. The effect of residual angulation on the spatial orientation of the epiphyseal plates. Acta Orthop Scand 50:537–546, 1979.
40. Friberg, K.S.I. Remodelling after distal forearm fractures. II. The final orientation of the distal and proximal epiphyseal plates of the radius. Acta Orthop Scand 50:731–739, 1979.
41. Friberg, K.S.I. Remodelling after distal forearm fractures in children. III. Correction of residual angulation in fractures of the radius. Acta Orthop Scand 50:741–749, 1979.
42. Fuller, D.J.; McCullough, C.J. Malunited fractures of the forearm in children. J Bone Joint Surg Br 64:364–367, 1982.
43. Gainor, B.J.; Olson, S. Combined entrapment of the median and anterior interosseous nerves in a pediatric both-bone forearm fracture. J Orthop Trauma 4:197–199, 1990.
44. Gandhi, R.K.; Wilson, P.; Mason Brown, J.J.; Macleod, W. Spontaneous correction of deformity following fractures of the forearm in children. Br J Surg 50:5–10, 1962.
45. Geissler, W.B.; Fernandez, D.L.; Graca, R. Anterior interosseous nerve palsy complicating a forearm fracture in a child. J Hand Surg Am 15:44–47, 1990.
46. Genelin, F.; Karlbauer, A.F.; Gasperschitz, F. Greenstick fracture of the forearm with median nerve entrapment. J Emerg Med 6:381–385, 1988.
47. Gibson, A. Uncomplicated dislocation of the inferior radio-ulnar joint. J Bone Joint Surg 7:180–188, 1925.
48. Gibson, W.K.; Timperlake, R.W. Operative treatment of a type IV Monteggia fracture-dislocation in a child. J Bone Joint Surg Br 74:780–781, 1992.
49. Giddins, G.E.; Shaw, D.G. Lunate subluxation associated with a Salter-Harris type 2 fracture of the distal radius. J Hand Surg Br 19:193–194, 1994.
50. Gleeson, A.P.; Beattie, T.F. Monteggia fracture-dislocation in children. J Accid Emerg Med 11:192–194, 1994.
51. Gonzales-Herrang, P.; Alvarez-Romera, A.; Burgos, J.; et al. Displaced radial neck fractures in children treated by closed intramedullary pinning (Metaizeau technique). J Pediatr Orthop 17:325–331, 1997.
52. Green, D.P. Carpal dislocations and instabilities. In: Green, D.P., ed. Operative Hand Surgery, 2nd ed. New York, Churchill Livingstone, 1982, pp. 875–938.
53. Greulich, W.W.; Pyle, S.I. Radiographic Atlas of Skeletal Development of the Hand and Wrist, 2nd ed. Stanford, CA, Stanford University Press, 1964.
54. Griffet, J.; Fe Hayek, T.; Baby, M. Intramedullary nailing of forearm fractures in children. J. Pediatr Orthop B 8:88–89, 1999.

55. Gruber, R. The problem of relapse fracture of the forearm in children. In: Chapchal, G., ed. Fractures in Children. New York, Thieme, 1981, p. 154.

56. Gupta, R.P.; Danielsson, L.G. Dorsally angulated solitary metaphyseal greenstick fractures in the distal radius: Results after immobilization in pronated, neutral, and supinated position. J Pediatr Orthop 10:90–92, 1990.

57. Haasbeek, J.F.; Cole, W.G. Open fractures of the arm in children. J Bone Joint Surg Br 77:576–581, 1995.

58. Hargens, A.R.; Romine, J.S.; Sipe, J.C.; et al: Peripheral nerve conduction block by high muscle compartment pressure. J Bone Joint Surg Am 61:192–200, 1979.

59. Hazlett, J.W. Carpometacarpal dislocations other than the thumb: A report of 11 cases. Can J Surg 11:315–322, 1968.

60. Heiple, K.G.; Freehafer, A.A. Isolated traumatic dislocation of the distal end of the ulna or distal radio-ulnar joint. J Bone Joint Surg Am 44:1387–1394, 1962.

61. Hennrikus, W.L.; Simpson, R.B.; Klingelberger, C.E.; Reis,. M.T. Self-administered nitrous oxide analgesia for pediatric fracture reductions. J Pediatr Orthop 14:538–542, 1994.

62. Hennrikus, W.L.; Shin, A.Y.; Klingelberger, C.E. Self-administered nitrous oxide and a hematoma block for analgesia in the outpatient reduction of fractures in children. J Bone Joint Surg Am 77:335–339, 1995.

63. Hernandez, J., Jr.; Peterson, H. Case report: Fracture of the distal radial epiphysis complicated by compartment syndrome and premature physeal closure. J Pediatr Orthop 6:627–630, 1986.

64. Hogstrom, H.; Nilsson, B.E.; Willner, S. Correction with growth following diaphyseal forearm fracture. Acta Orthop Scand 47:299–303, 1976.

65. Hokan, R.; Bryce, G.M.; Cobb, N.J. Dislocation of scaphoid and fractured capitate in a child. Injury 24:496–497, 1993.

66. Hope, P.G. Anterior interosseous nerve palsy following internal fixation of the proximal radius. J Bone Joint Surg Br 70:280–282, 1988.

67. Hoppenfield, S.; De Boer, P. Surgical Exposures in Orthopaedics: The Anatomic Approach. Philadelphia, J.B. Lippincott, 1984, p. 115.

68. Horii, E.; Tamura, Y.; Nakamura, R.; Miura, T. Premature closure of the distal radial physis. J Hand Surg Br 18:11–16, 1993.

69. Hume, A.C. Anterior dislocation of the head of the radius associated with undisplaced fracture of the olecranon in children. J Bone Joint Surg Br 39:508–512, 1957.

70. Hurst, L.C.; Dubrow, E.N. Surgical treatment of symptomatic chronic radial head dislocation: A neglected Monteggia fracture. J Pediatr Orthop 3:227–230, 1983.

71. Imaeda, T.; Nakamura, R.; Miura, T.; Makino, N. Magnetic resonance imaging in scaphoid fractures. J Hand Surg Br 17:20–27, 1992.

72. Itoh, Y.; Horirichi, Y.; Takahashi, M.; et al. Extensor tendon involvement in Smith's and Galeazzi's fractures. J Hand Surg Am 12:535–540, 1987.

73. Jones, K.; Weiner, D.S. The management of forearm fractures in children: A plea for conservatism. J Pediatr Orthop 19:811–815, 1999.

74. Kalamchi, A. Monteggia fracture-dislocation in children: Late treatment in two cases. J Bone Joint Surg Am 68:615–619, 1986.

75. Karlsson, J.; Appelguist, R. Irreducible fractures of the wrist in a child: Entrapment of the extensor tendons. Acta Orthop Scand 58:280–281, 1987.

76. Kay, S.; Smith, C.; Oppenheim, W.L. Both-bone midshaft forearm fractures in children. J Pediatr Orthop 6:306–310, 1986.

77. Keenan, W.; Clegg, J. Intraoperative wedging of casts: Correction of residual angulation after manipulation. J Pediatr Orthop 15:826–829, 1995.

78. King, R.E. Fractures of the shafts of the radius and ulna. In: Rockwood, C.A.J.; Wilkins, K.E.; King, R.E., eds. Fractures in Children, Vol. 3. Philadelphia, J.B. Lippincott, 1984, pp. 301–362.

79. Kleinman, W.B.; Grantham, S.A. Multiple volar carpometacarpal dislocation. J Hand Surg 3:377–382, 1978.

80. Knight, R.A.; Purvis, G.D. Fractures of the forearm in adults. J Bone Joint Surg Am 31:755–764, 1949.

81. Kolkman, K.A.; van Niekerk, J.L.; Rieu, P.N.; Festen, C. A complicated forearm greenstick fracture: Case report. J Trauma 32:116–117, 1992.

82. Kramhoft, M.; Bodtker, S. Epidemiology of distal forearm fractures in Danish children. Acta Orthop Scand 59:557–559, 1988.

83. Kramhoft, M.; Solgaard, S. Displaced diaphyseal forearm fractures in children: Classification and evaluation of the early radiographic prognosis. J Pediatr Orthop 9:586–589, 1989.

84. Kreder, H.; Armstrong, P. The significance of perioperative cultures in open pediatric lower-extremity fractures. Clin Orthop 302:206–212, 1994.

85. Kristiansen, B.; Eriksen, A.F. Simultaneous type II Monteggia lesion and fracture-separation of the lower radial epiphysis. Injury 17:51–52, 1986.

86. Lahoti, O.; Wong, J.; Regan, B.; et al. Fracture of the scaphoid associated with volar displacement of a lower radial epiphyseal fracture: Case report. Scand J Plast Reconstr Surg Hand Surg 27:155–156, 1993.

87. Landfried, M.J.; Stenclik, M.; Susi, J.G. Variant of Galeazzi fracture-dislocation in children. J Pediatr Orthop 11:332–335, 1991.

88. Langkamer, V.G.; Ackroyd, C.E. Removal of forearm plates (a review of the complications). J Bone Joint Surg Br 72:601–604, 1990.

89. Lascombes, P.; Prevot, J.; Ligier, J.N.; et al. Elastic stable intramedullary nailing in forearm shaft fractures in children: 85 cases. J Pediatr Orthop 10:167–171, 1990.

90. Lee, B.S.; Esterhai, J.L.; Das, M. Fracture of the distal radial epiphysis. Clin Orthop 185:90–96, 1984.

91. Lesko, P.D.; Georgis, T.; Slabaugh, P. Irreducible Salter-Harris type II fracture of the distal radial epiphysis. J Pediatr Orthop 7:719–721, 1987.

92. Letts, M.; Esser, D. Fractures of the triquetrum in children. J Pediatr Orthop 13:228–231, 1993.

93. Letts, M.; Locht, R.; Weins, J. Monteggia fracture-dislocations in children. J Bone Joint Surg Br 67:724–727, 1985.

94. Letts, M.; Rowhani, N. Galeazzi-equivalent injuries of the wrist in children. J Pediatr Orthop 13:561–566, 1993.

95. Levinthal, D.H. Fractures in the lower one-third of both bones of the forearm in children. Surg Gynecol Obstet 57:790–799, 1933.

96. Lewallen, R.P.; Peterson, H.A. Nonunion of long bone fractures in children: A review of 30 cases. J Pediatr Orthop 5:135–142, 1985.

97. Lichter, R.L.; Jacobsen, T. Tardy palsy of the posterior interosseous nerve with a Monteggia fracture. J Bone Joint Surg Am 57:124–125, 1975.

98. Lincoln, T.; Mubarak, S. "Isolated" traumatic radial-head dislocation. J Pediatr Orthop 14:454–457, 1994.

99. Lindsey, R.W.; Fenison, A.T.; Doherty, B.J.; et al. Effects of retained diaphyseal plates on forearm bone density and grip strength. J Orthop Trauma 8:462–467, 1994.

100. Lloyd-Roberts, G.C.; Bucknill, T.M. Anterior dislocation of the radial head in children. J Bone Joint Surg Br 59:402–407, 1977.

101. Luhmann, S.J.; Gordon, J.E.; Schoenecker, P.L. Intramedullary fixation of unstable both-bone forearm fractures in children. J Pediatr Orthop 18:451–456, 1998.

102. Mabrey, J.D.; Fitch, R.D. Plastic deformation in pediatric fractures: Mechanism and treatment. J Pediatr Orthop 9:310–314, 1989.

103. Manoli, A. Irreducible fracture-separation of the distal radial epiphysis. J Bone Joint Surg Am 64:1095–1096, 1982.

104. Matsen, F.A., III. A practical approach to compartment syndromes. Part I: Definition, theory, and pathogenesis. Instr Course Lect 32:88–91, 1983.

105. Matsen, F.A., III; Vieth, R.G. Compartmental syndromes in children. J Pediatr Orthop 1:33–41, 1981.

106. Matsen, F.A., III; Winquist, R.A.; Kurgmire, R.D. Diagnosis and management of compartmental syndromes. J Bone Joint Surg Am 62:286–291, 1980.

107. Matthews, L.S.; Kaufer, H.; Garver, D.F.; Sonstegard, D.A. The effect on supination-pronation of angular malalignment of fractures of both bones of the forearm. J Bone Joint Surg Am 64:14–17, 1982.

108. Mayfield, J.; Johnson, R.; Kilcoyne, R. The ligaments of the human wrist and their functional significance. Anat Rec 186:417–428, 1976.

109. McCarty, E.C.; Mencio, G.A.; Green, N.E. Anesthesia and analgesia for ambulatory management of fractures in children. J Am Acad Orthop Surg 7:81–91, 1999.

110. Mikic, Z.D. Galeazzi fracture-dislocations. J Bone Joint Surg Am 57:1071–1080, 1975.

111. Mintzer, C.; Waters, P.M. Acute open reduction of a displaced scaphoid fracture in a child. J Hand Surg Am 19:760–761, 1994.

112. Mintzer, C.M.; Waters, P.M.; Simmons, B.P. Nonunion of the scaphoid in children treated by Herbert screw fixation and bone grafting: A report of five cases. J Bone Joint Surg Br 77:98–100, 1995.

113. Moore, T.M.; Lester, D.K.; Sarmiento, A. The stabilizing effect of soft-tissue constraints in artificial Galeazzi fractures. Clin Orthop 194:189–194, 1985.

114. Morrey, B.F.; Askew, L.J.; An, K.; Chao, E.Y. A biomechanical study of normal functional elbow motion. J Bone Joint Surg Am 63:872–877, 1981.

115. Morris, A.H. Irreducible Monteggia lesion with radial-nerve entrapment. J Bone Joint Surg Am 56:1744–1746, 1974.

116. Mubarak, S.J. A practical approach to compartment syndromes. Part II: Diagnosis. Instr Course Lect 32:92–102, 1983.

117. Mubarak, S.; Carroll, N. Volkmann's contracture in children: Aetiology and prevention. J Bone Joint Surg Br 61:285–293, 1979.

118. Mullick, S. The lateral Monteggia fracture. J Bone Joint Surg Am 59:543–545, 1977.

119. Naito, M.; Ogata, K. Acute volar compartment syndrome during skeletal traction in distal radius fracture: A case report. Clin Orthop 241:234–237, 1989.

120. Nelson, O.A.; Buchanan, J.R.; Harrison, C.S. Distal ulnar growth arrest. J Hand Surg Am 9:164–171, 1984.

121. Nielsen, A.B.; Simonsen, O. Displaced forearm fractures in children treated with AO plates. Injury 15:393–395, 1984.

122. Nilsson, B.E.; Obrant, K. The range of motion following fracture of the shaft of the forearm in children. Acta Orthop Scand 48:600–602, 1977.

123. Noonan, K.J.; Price, C.T. Forearm and distal radius fractures in children. J Am Acad Orthop Surg 6:146–156, 1998.

124. Nork, S.E.; Hennrikus, W.L.; Loncarich, D.P.; et al. Relationship between ligamentous laxity and the site with upper extremity fractures in children: Extension supracondylar fracture versus distal forearm fracture. J Pediatr Orthop B 8:90–92, 1999.

125. O'Brien, E.T. Fractures of the hand and wrist region. In: Rockwood, C.A.; Wilkins, K.E.; Kin, R.E., eds. Fractures in Children, Vol. 3. Philadelphia, J.B. Lippincott, 1984, pp. 229–299.

126. Ogden, J.A. Complications. In: Ogden, J.A., ed. Skeletal Injury in the Child, 2nd ed. Philadelphia, W.B. Saunders, 1990, pp. 247–248.

127. Ogden, J.A. Injury to the growth mechanisms. In: Ogden, J.A., ed. Skeletal Injury in the Child, 2nd ed. Philadelphia, W.B. Saunders, 1990, pp. 97–174.

128. Ogden, J.A. Radius and ulna. In: Ogden, J.A., ed. Skeletal Injury in the Child, 2nd ed. Philadelphia, W.B. Saunders, 1990, pp. 451–526.

129. Olney, B.W.; Menelaus, M.B. Monteggia and equivalent lesions in childhood. J Pediatr Orthop 9:219–223, 1989.

130. Olney, B.; Lugg, P.; Turner, P. Outpatient treatment of upper extremity injuries in childhood using intravenous regional anesthesia. J Pediatr Orthop 8:576–579, 1988.

131. Ortega, R.; Loder, R.T.; Louis, D.S. Open reduction and internal fixation of forearm fractures in children. J Pediatr Orthop 16:651–654, 1996.

132. Paley, D.; McMurtry, R.Y.; Murray, J.F. Dorsal dislocation of the ulnar styloid and extensor carpi ulnaris tendon into the distal radioulnar joint: The empty sulcus sign. J Hand Surg Am 12:1029–1032, 1987.

133. Papavasiliou, V.; Nenopoulos, S. Ipsilateral injuries of the elbow and forearm in children. J Pediatr Orthop 6:58–60, 1986.

134. Papavasiliou, V.A.; Nenopoulos, S.P. Monteggia-type elbow fractures in childhood. Clin Orthop 233:230–233, 1988.

135. Peiro, A.; Martos, F.; Mut, T.; Aracil, J. Trans-scaphoid perilunate dislocation in a child: A case report. Acta Orthop Scand 52:31–34, 1981.

136. Peters, C.L.; Scott, S.M. Compartment syndrome in the forearm following fractures of the radial head or neck in children. J Bone Joint Surg Am 77:1070–1074, 1995.

137. Posman, C.L.; Little, R.E. Radioulnar synostosis following an isolated fracture of the ulnar shaft. Clin Orthop 213:207–210, 1986.

138. Price, C. Fractures of the midshaft radius and ulna. In: Letts, R., ed. Management of Pediatric Fractures. New York, Churchill Livingstone, 1994, p. 329.

139. Price, C.T.; Scott, D.S.; Kurzner, M.E.; Flynn, J.C. Malunited forearm fractures in children. J Pediatr Orthop 10:705–712, 1990.

140. Prosser, A.J.; Hooper, G. Entrapment of the ulnar nerve in a greenstick fracture of the ulna. J Hand Surg Br 11:211–212, 1986.

141. Ranawat, C.S.; Defiore, J.; Straub, L.R. Madelung's deformity: An end-result study of surgical treatment. J Bone Joint Surg Am 57:772–775, 1975.

142. Rang, M. Children's Fractures, 2nd ed. Philadelphia, J.B. Lippincott, 1982, p. 197.

143. Ravessoud, F.A. Lateral condylar fracture and ipsilateral ulnar shaft fracture: Monteggia equivalent lesions? J Pediatr Orthop 5:364–366, 1985.

144. Rayan, G.M.; Hayes, M. Entrapment of the flexor digitorum profundus in the ulna with fracture of both bones of the forearm: Report of a case. J Bone Joint Surg Am 68:1102–1103, 1986.

145. Reckling, F.W. Unstable fracture-dislocations of the forearm (Monteggia and Galeazzi lesions). J Bone Joint Surg Am 64:857–863, 1982.

146. Reckling, F.W.; Cordell, L.D. Unstable fracture-dislocations of the forearm. Arch Surg 96:999–1007, 1968.

147. Reckling, F.W.; Peltier, L.F. Riccardo Galeazzi and Galeazzi's fracture. Surgery 58:2453–2459, 1965.

148. Richter, D.; Ostermann, P.A.W.; Ekkernkamp, A; et al. Elastic intramedullary nailing: A minimally invasive concept in the treatment of unstable forearm fractures in children. J Pediatr Orthop 18:457–461, 1998.

149. Roberts, J.A. Angulation of the radius in children's fractures. J Bone Joint Surg Br 68:751–754, 1986.

150. Rodgers, W.B.; Smith, B.G. A type IV Monteggia injury with a distal diaphyseal radius fracture in a child. J Orthop Trauma 7:84–86, 1993.

151. Rorabeck, C.H. A practical approach to compartment syndromes. Part III: Management. Instr Course Lect 32:102–113, 1983.

152. Rorabeck, C.H.; Clarke, K.M. The pathophysiology of the anterior tibial compartment syndrome: An experimental investigation. J Trauma 18:299–304, 1978.

153. Rose-Innes, A.P. Anterior dislocation of the ulna at the inferior radio-ulnar joint. J Bone Joint Surg Br 42:515–521, 1960.

154. Roy, D.R.; Crawford, A.H. Operative management of fractures of the shaft of the radius and ulna. Orthop Clin North Am 21:245–250, 1990.

155. Royle, S.G. Compartment syndrome following forearm fracture in children. Injury 21:73–76, 1990.

156. Salter, R.B.; Harris, W.R. Injuries involving the epiphyseal plate. J Bone Joint Surg Am 45:587–622, 1963.

157. Sanders, W.E.; Heckman, J.D. Traumatic plastic deformation of the radius and ulna: A closed method of correction of deformity. Clin Orthop 188:58–67, 1989.

158. Sandzen, S.C. Fracture of the fifth metacarpal resembling Bennett's fracture. Hand 5:49–51, 1973.

159. Santoro, V.; Mara, J. Compartmental syndrome complicating Salter-Harris type II distal radius fracture. Clin Orthop 233:226–229, 1988.

160. Schuind, F.; Andrianne, Y.; Burny, F. Treatment of forearm fractures by Hoffman external fixation: A study of 93 patients. Clin Orthop 266:197–204, 1991.

161. Seriat-Gautier, B.; Jouve, J.L. Les decollements-fractures de l'extremite inferieure du radius a deplacement anterieur chez l'enfant. Chir Pediatr 29:265–268, 1988.

162. Shewring, D.J.; Savage, R.; Thomas, G. Experience of the early use of technetium 99 bone scintigraphy in wrist injury. J Hand Surg Br 19:114–117, 1994.

163. Shoemaker, S.D.; Comstock, C.P.; Mubarak, S.J.; et al. Intramedullary Kirschner wire fixation of open or unstable forearm fractures in children. J Pediatr Orthop 19:328–337, 1999.

164. Shonnard, P.Y.; DeCoster, T.A. Combined Monteggia and Galeazzi fractures in a child's forearm: A case report. Orthop Rev 23:755–759, 1994.

165. Southcott, R.; Rosman, M.A. Non-union of carpal scaphoid fractures in children. J Bone Joint Surg Br 59B:20–23, 1977.

166. Spinner, M.; Kaplan, E.B. The quadrate ligament of the elbow—its relationship to the stability of the proximal radio-ulnar joint. Acta Orthop Scand 41:632–647, 1970.

167. Spinner, M.; Freundlich, B.D.; Teicher, J. Posterior interosseous nerve palsy as a complication of Monteggia fractures in children. Clin Orthop 58:141–145, 1968.

168. Stanciu, C.; Dumont, A. Changing patterns of scaphoid fractures in adolescents. Can J Surg 37:214–216, 1994.

169. Stanitski, C.L.; Micheli, L.J. Simultaneous ipsilateral fractures of the arm and forearm in children. Clin Orthop 153:218–222, 1980.

170. Stein, F.; Grabias, S.L.; Deffer, P.A. Nerve injuries complicating Monteggia lesions. J Bone Joint Surg Am 53:1432–1436, 1971.

171. Stoll, T.M.; Willis, R.B.; Patterson, D.C. Treatment of the missed Monteggia fracture in the child. J Bone Joint Surg Br 74:436–440, 1992.

172. Sullivan, C.M.; Mubarak, S.J. Diagnosis and treatment of upper extremity compartment syndrome. Tech Orthop 4:30–37, 1989.

173. Tarr, R.R.; Garfinkel, A.I.; Sarmiento, A. The effects of angular and rotational deformities of both bones of the forearm. J Bone Joint Surg Am 66:65–70, 1984.

174. Theodorou, S.D. Dislocation of the head of the radius associated with fracture of the upper end of the ulna in children. J Bone Joint Surg Br 51:700–706, 1969.

175. Thomas, W.G.; Kershaw, C.J. Entrapment of extensor tendons in a Smith's fracture: Brief report. J Bone Joint Surg Br 70:491, 1988.

176. Thompson, H.A.; Hamilton, A.T. Monteggia fracture: Internal fixation of the fractured ulna with intramedullary Steinmann pin. Am J Surg 79:579–584, 1950.

177. Tiel-van Buul, M.M.; van Beek, E.J.; Broekhuizen, A.H.; et al. Radiography and scintigraphy of suspected scaphoid fracture. A long-term study in 160 patients. J Bone Joint Surg Br 75:61–65, 1993.

178. Tredwell, S.; Van Peteghem, K.; Clough, M. Patterns of forearm fractures in children. J Pediatr Orthop 4:604–608, 1984.

179. Trousdale, R.T.; Linscheid, R.L. Operative treatment of malunited fractures of the forearm. J Bone Joint Surg Am 77:894–902, 1995.

180. Vainionpaa, S.; Bostman, O.; Batiala, H.; Rokkanen, P. Internal fixation of forearm fractures in children. Acta Orthop Scand 58:121–123, 1987.

181. Vender, M.I.; Watson, H.K. Acquired Madelung-like deformity in a gymnast. J Hand Surg Am 13:19–21, 1988.

182. Victor, J.; Mulier, T.; Fabry, G. Refracture of radius and ulna in a female gymnast: A case report. Am J Sports Med 21:753–754, 1993.

183. Villa, A.; Paley, D.; Catagni, M.A.; et al. Lengthening of the forearm by the Ilizarov technique. Clin Orthop 250:125–137, 1990.

184. Vince, K.G.; Miller, J.E. Cross-union complicating fracture of the forearm. Part II: Children. J Bone Joint Surg Am 69:654–661, 1987.

185. Voto, S.J.; Weiner, D.S.; Leighley, B. Redisplacement after closed reduction of forearm fractures in children. J Pediatr Orthop 10:79–84, 1990.

186. Voto, S.J.; Weiner, D.S.; Leighley, B. Use of pins and plaster in the treatment of unstable pediatric forearm fractures. J Pediatr Orthop 10:85–89, 1990.

187. Walsh, H.P.J.; McLaren, C.A.N.; Owen, R. Galeazzi fractures in children. J Bone Joint Surg Br 69:730–733, 1987.

188. Warren, J.D. Anterior interosseous nerve palsy as a complication of forearm fractures. J Bone Joint Surg Br 45:511–512, 1963.

189. Waters, P.M.; Kolettis, G.J.; Schwend, R. Acute median neuropathy following physeal fractures of the distal radius. J Pediatr Orthop 14:173–177, 1994.

190. Watson, H.K.; Pitts, E.C.; Ashmead, D.T.; et al. Dorsal approach to scaphoid nonunion. J Hand Surg Am 18:359–365, 1993.

191. Watson, J.A.; Singer, G.C. Irreducible Monteggia fracture: Beware nerve entrapment. Injury 25:325–327, 1994.

192. Wedge, J.H.; Robertson, D.E. Displaced fractures of the neck of the radius. J Bone Joint Surg Br 64:256, 1982.

193. Whitson, R.O. Carpometacarpal dislocation: A case report. Clin Orthop 6:189–195, 1955.

194. Wilkins, K. Operative Management of Upper Extremity Fractures in Children. Rosemont, IL, American Academy of Orthopaedic Surgeons, 1994.

195. Williamson, D.M.; Cole, W.G. Treatment of ipsilateral supracondylar and forearm fractures in children. Injury 23:159–161, 1992.

196. Willis, R.B.; Rorabeck, C. Treatment of compartment syndrome in children. Orthop Clin North Am 21:401–412, 1990.

197. Wolfe, J.S.; Eyring, E.J. Median-nerve entrapment within a greenstick fracture. J Bone Joint Surg Am 56:1270–1272, 1974.

198. Worlock, P.; Stower, M. Fracture patterns in Nottingham children. J Pediatr Orthop 6:656–660, 1986.

199. Wright, P.R. Greenstick fracture of the upper end of the ulna with dislocation of the radio-humeral joint or displacement of the superior radial epiphysis. J Bone Joint Surg Br 45:727–731, 1963.

200. Wyrsch, B.; Mencio, G.A.; Green, N.E. Open reduction and internal fixation of pediatric forearm fractures. J Pediatr Orthop 16:644–650, 1996.

201. Younger, A.; Tredwell, S.; MacKenzie, W.; et al. Accurate prediction of outcome after pediatric forearm fracture. J Pediatr Orthop 14:200–206, 1994.

202. Younger, A.S.W.; Tredwell, S.J.; MacKenzie, W.G. Factors affecting fracture position at cast removal after pediatric forearm fracture. J Pediatr Orthop 17:332–336, 1997.

203. Zehntner, M.K.; Jakob, R.P.; McGanity, P.L. Growth disturbance of the distal radial epiphysis after trauma: Operative treatment by corrective radial osteotomy. J Pediatr Orthop 10:411–415, 1990.

**Hand**

204. Almquist, E.E. Hand injuries in children. Pediatr Clin North Am 33:1511–1522, 1986.

205. Barnard, H.L. Dorsal dislocation of the first phalanx of the little finger: Reduction by Faraboeuf's dorsal incision. Lancet 1:88–90, 1901.

206. Campbell, R.M., Jr. Operative treatment of fractures and dislocations of the hand and wrist region in children. Orthop Clin North Am 21:217–243, 1990.

207. Culp, R.; Osgood, J. Posttraumatic physeal bar formation in the digit of a child: A case report. J Hand Surg Am 18:322–324, 1993.

208. Dixon, G.L.; Moon, N.F. Rotational supracondylar fractures of the proximal phalanx in children. Clin Orthop 83:151–156, 1972.

209. Fischer, M.; McElfresh, E. Physeal and periphyseal injuries of the hand: Patterns of injury and results of treatment. Hand Clin 10:287–301, 1994.

210. Harryman, D.; Jordan, T. Physeal phalangeal fracture with flexor tendon entrapment: A case report and review of the literature. Clin Orthop 250:194–196, 1990.

211. Hastings, H., 2nd; Simmons, B.P. Hand fractures in children: A statistical analysis. Clin Orthop 188:120–130, 1984.

212. Leddy, J.P.; Packer, J.W. Avulsion of the profundus tendon insertion in athletes. J Hand Surg 2:66–69, 1977.

213. Leonard, M.H.; Dubravcik, P. Management of fractured fingers in the child. Clin Orthop 73:160–168, 1970.

214. Light, T.R.; Ogden, J.A. Complex dislocation of the index metacarpophalangeal joint in children. J Pediatr Orthop 8:300–305, 1988.

215. McElfresh, E.C.; Dobyns, J.D. Intra-articular metacarpal head fractures. J Hand Surg Am 8:383–393, 1983.

216. McFarlane, R.M.; Hampole, M.K. Treatment of extensor tendon injuries of the hand. Can J Surg 16:366–375, 1973.

217. Niechajev, I.A. Conservative and operative treatment of mallet finger. Plast Reconstr Surg 76:580–585, 1985.

218. Salter, R.B.; Harris, W.R. Injuries involving the epiphyseal plate. J Bone Joint Surg Am 45:587–622, 1963.

219. Segmuller, G.; Schonenberger, F. Fractures of the hand. In: Weber, B.G.; Bruner, C.; Freuler, F., eds. Treatment of Fractures in Children and Adolescents. New York, Springer-Verlag, 1980, pp. 218–225.
220. Simmons, B.P.; Peters, T.T. Subcondylar fossa reconstruction for malunion of fractures of the proximal phalanx in children. J Hand Surg Am 12:1079–1082, 1987.
221. Stalter, K.; Smoot, E.C.; Osler, T. Method for elevating the pediatric hand. Plast Reconstr Surg 81:788, 1988.
222. Stener, B. Displacement of the ruptured ulnar collateral ligament of the metacarpo-phalangeal joint of the thumb: A clinical and anatomical study. J Bone Joint Surg Br 44:869–879, 1962.
223. Wood, V.E. Fractures of the hand in children. Orthop Clin North Am 7:527–542, 1976.
224. Zook, E.G. Nail bed injuries. Hand Clin 1:701–716, 1985.
225. Zook, E.G.; Guy, R.J.; Russell, R.C. A study of nail bed injuries: Causes, treatment, and prognosis. J Hand Surg Am 9:247–252, 1984.

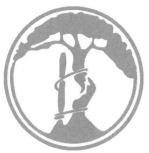

# CHAPTER 9

# *Fractures and Dislocations about the Elbow*

Neil E. Green, M.D.

Fractures about the elbow are extremely common. Hanlon and Estes estimated that upper extremity injuries account for 65% of all fractures and dislocations in children.[88] Lichtenburg claimed that fractures about the distal end of the forearm are the most common injuries and that fractures and dislocations about the elbow are next in frequency.[115] Cheng and colleagues found that supracondylar fractures of the distal end of the humerus account for 16.6% of all childhood fractures. In the age group 0 to 7 years, they account for about 30% of all limb fractures.[35] Elbow injuries occur more often in the skeletally immature than they do in adults.[29, 166]

## DISTAL HUMERAL FRACTURE

### Anatomy

#### OSSIFICATION

Ossification of the distal end of the humerus progresses with age. At birth, the distal humeral metaphysis is ossified; however, none of the structures that constitute the epiphysis are ossified. The capitellum is the first structure to ossify and may be seen radiographically as early as 6 months of age according to Silberstein and coworkers.[185] Haraldsson, in his classic article in 1959,[89] stated that the capitellum may ossify as early as 1 month of age; however, 6 months is probably the youngest age at which this ossification center is seen (Fig. 9–1). Although ossification of the capitellum may not take place until as late as 2 years of age, Silberstein and associates state that it is invariably present by that time.[185]

The medial epicondyle is the next ossification center to appear. It may be seen radiographically as early as 5 years of age in some but may not appear until 9 years in others. The medial epicondyle forms its own ossification center in the distal end of the humerus, whereas the capitellum, the trochlea, and the lateral epicondyle fuse

to form a single ossification center. The trochlea, which appears next, may become ossified as early as 7 years of age, but more commonly it begins to ossify between the ages of 9 and 10 years. The lateral epicondyle is the last portion of the distal humeral epiphysis to ossify. It may be identified radiographically as early as 8 to 9 years of age.

The capitellum and trochlea may fuse as early as the age of 10 years, but fusion usually begins by 12 years of age. This combined ossification center fuses to the lateral epicondyle at the same time to form the main body of the distal humeral epiphysis. The epiphysis fuses to the metaphysis of the humerus as early as 12 to 13 years of age, which signals the end of longitudinal growth of the distal humeral physis. Finally, the medial epicondyle fuses to the distal end of the humerus between 14 and 17 years of age.

#### VASCULAR ANATOMY

The collateral circulation about the elbow is rich and is usually sufficient to maintain adequate circulation to the forearm and hand even if the main blood supply from the brachial artery is interrupted (Fig. 9–2). Although interruption of the brachial artery may not result in loss of the limb, it usually produces some signs of ischemia, such as claudication and cold intolerance.[105, 107, 116, 120, 214]

#### JOINT ANATOMY

The entire articular surface of the distal end of the humerus is intra-articular; however, the medial and lateral epicondyles are both extra-articular. The elbow capsule attaches the ulna distal to the olecranon and coronoid process, so these structures are intra-articular. In addition, the entire radial head is located within the capsule, thus making it intra-articular. Two elbow fat pads are located between the capsule and the distal end of the humerus, one anterior and the other posterior. The

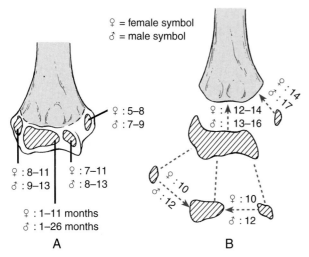

**FIGURE 9–1.** Ossification and fusion of the growth centers of the distal end of the humerus. *A,* Appearance of the distal humeral ossification centers in the early years. If wear of the ossification center begins before the age of 1 year, the designation is noted with the letter "m" for months. *B,* Fusion of the distal humeral ossification centers. (*A, B,* Adapted from Haraldsson, S. Acta Orthop Scand 38 (Suppl), 1959.)

radiographic appearance of these fat pads may aid in diagnosing injuries about the elbow; with an elbow effusion, one or both may become elevated from the distal humeral surface as seen on a lateral radiograph[145] (Fig. 9–3).

The appearance of an elevated fat pad, indicative of elbow joint effusion after trauma, in the absence of a radiographically visible fracture does not mean that an occult fracture is present. De Beaux and associates analyzed 45 cases of elbow trauma in children with one or two elevated fat pads and no radiographic evidence of fracture. Only 6% of those who underwent repeat radiographs 2 weeks after injury were found to have sustained a fracture. They concluded that routine repeat radiographic examination is not necessary in these cases. If the children remain symptomatic, however, repeat radiographic examination is required.[49]

## RADIOGRAPHIC ANATOMY

Different radiographic lines have been described to help in the radiographic diagnosis of distal humeral fractures. Baumann's angle may be helpful in determining the adequacy of reduction of a supracondylar fracture of the distal part of the humerus.[10] This angle is defined as the angle created by the intersection of a line drawn along the physis of the capitellum and a line perpendicular to the longitudinal axis of the humerus as seen on anteroposterior radiographs (Fig. 9–4).

Unfortunately, Baumann's angle is dependent on the position of the elbow when the radiograph is taken.[57, 171] Variations of humeral rotation are especially likely to alter this angle, which reduces its reliability. One can reduce this variability by obtaining a true anteroposterior radiograph of the elbow (Fig. 9–5). If the elbow can be fully extended, an anteroposterior radiograph of the distal end of the humerus and an anteroposterior radiograph of the elbow are identical. However, if the elbow cannot be fully extended, an anteroposterior

radiograph of the distal end of the humerus results in a tangential distal humeral view. It has been shown that a tangential view of the distal part of the humerus results in exaggeration of the rotational effect on Baumann's angle. When using Baumann's angle, one must therefore obtain a true anteroposterior view of the distal end of the humerus with the x-ray beam perpendicular to the humerus and to the radiographic plate. This position is least sensitive to humeral rotation. If a true anteroposterior radiograph cannot be taken because of pin placement, radiographs of the distal ends of each humerus should be obtained in matched rotation and flexion to attempt to negate the distortion of Baumann's angle associated with humeral rotation.[30]

The medial epicondylar epiphyseal angle may also be useful in determining the accuracy of reduction of supracondylar humeral fractures. This angle is formed by the intersection of a line drawn along the medial epicondylar growth plate with the longitudinal axis of the humerus. In younger children, in whom the medial epicondyle is not yet ossified, one may still use this angle. In these young children, a line is drawn along the straight medial and distal border of the lower humeral metaphysis[23] (Fig. 9–6).

Silberstein and associates[185] defined other lines to facilitate the diagnosis of distal humeral fractures as viewed on a lateral radiograph. The anterior coronoid line is drawn along the coronoid and continued proximally. It should just touch the capitellum anteriorly in a normal elbow. If the capitellum is angled or displaced anteriorly, this line intersects or lies posterior to the capitellum.

The anterior humeral line is drawn along the anterior cortex of the humerus.[174] It should pass through the middle of the ossified capitellum as seen on a lateral radiograph. If this line passes anterior to the middle of

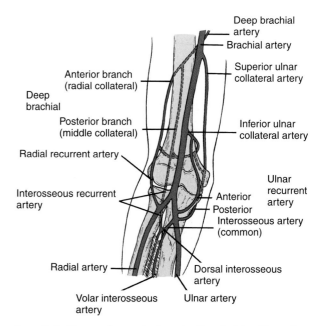

**FIGURE 9–2.** The vascular supply about the elbow is rich, with excellent collateral circulation. The collateral circulation is usually sufficient to maintain viability of the extremity in the event of occlusion of the brachial artery.

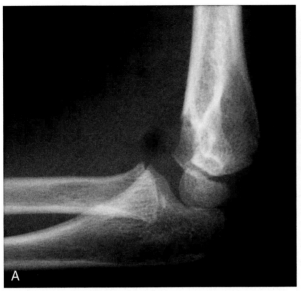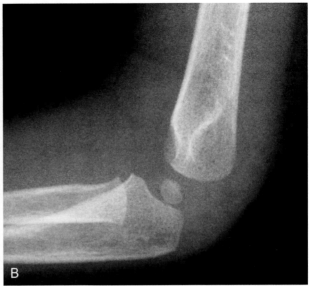

**FIGURE 9–3.** Elevated fat pads anteriorly and posteriorly about the elbow indicate the presence of an elbow effusion. *A*, This lateral radiograph of the elbow in a child who sustained a nondisplaced supracondylar fracture shows a markedly displaced anterior fat pad. *B*, A lateral elbow radiograph of a different child shows no obvious fracture, but both an anterior and a posterior elevated fat pad can be noted. The child was treated for a supracondylar fracture that became evident 3 weeks later after observation of the periosteal reaction and fracture line.

the capitellum, the capitellum or the distal end of the humerus has been displaced posteriorly. Conversely, if it passes posterior to the middle of the capitellum, the distal end of the humerus has been displaced anteriorly

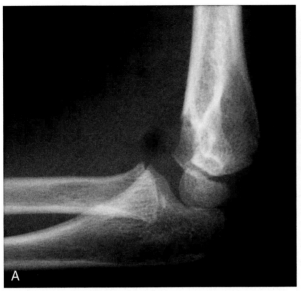

**FIGURE 9–4.** Baumann's angle is formed by the intersection of a line that follows the metaphysis of the lateral aspect of the distal end of the humerus (i.e., the physis of the capitellum) and a line perpendicular to the axis of the humerus.

(Fig. 9–7). This line is not accurate if a lateral radiograph of the distal part of the humerus is not a true lateral radiograph. Skibo and Reed showed that if the humerus is rotated and not perfectly lateral to the radiographic plate, the anterior humeral line is not reliable and in many instances is falsely positive.[186]

Silberstein and colleagues noted that the physis of the capitellum is wider posteriorly than anteriorly when viewed on a lateral radiograph. This appearance may be mistaken for an injury to the physis if one is not familiar with the normal radiographic anatomy (Fig. 9–8).

Comparison radiographs of the elbow have been advocated to assist in the diagnosis of subtle elbow trauma in children. A recent study of elbow trauma was designed to evaluate the efficacy of comparison elbow radiographs. Radiographs of children's injured and contralateral elbows were evaluated by orthopaedic residents, emergency physicians, and a pediatric radiologist. They concluded that comparison radiographs of the uninjured elbow did not improve the diagnostic accuracy of elbow trauma in the pediatric emergency department.[34]

Other means of evaluating elbow trauma have become popular. Magnetic resonance imaging (MRI) may be used to better outline the extent of articular fractures about the elbow. When one is unsure whether an elbow fracture extends into the articular surface, MRI has been shown to better demonstrate the extent of the fracture.[20] Ultrasonography may also help evaluate trauma to an immature elbow. It is especially useful when trauma occurs in very young children, in whom ossification of the distal end of the humerus is minimal.[48]

## CARRYING ANGLE OF THE ELBOW

The carrying angle of the elbow is the clinical measurement of varus-valgus angulation of the arm with the

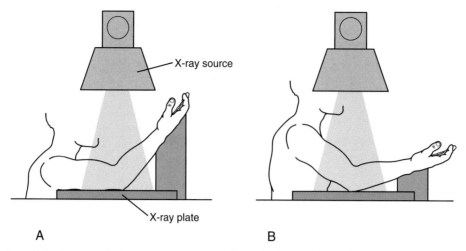

A                                    B

FIGURE 9–5. One must obtain a true anteroposterior radiograph of the distal part of the humerus to accurately assess the anatomy of the bone. *A*, Because children with acute elbow injuries are unable to fully extend their elbow, one must instruct the radiology technician to obtain an anteroposterior radiograph of the distal portion of the humerus that will demonstrate it accurately. If the elbow can be fully extended, the anteroposterior radiograph of the distal end of the humerus and an anteroposterior radiograph of the elbow will be identical. *B*, If the elbow cannot be fully extended, the anteroposterior radiograph of the elbow will include the distal portion of the humerus tangentially, thereby distorting the bony architecture. (*A, B*, Redrawn from Camp, J.; et al. J Pediatr Orthop 13:522, 1993.)

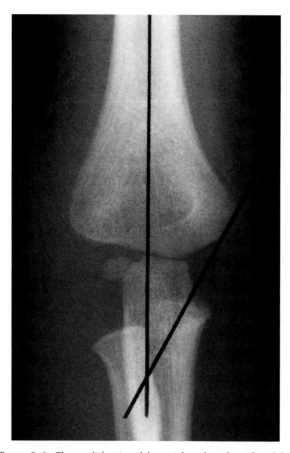

FIGURE 9–6. The medial epicondylar epiphyseal angle is found by drawing a line along the medial epicondylar growth plate that intersects the longitudinal axis of the humerus. In this radiograph, the medial epicondyle is not yet ossified; therefore, the line is drawn along the medial border of the distal humeral metaphysis.

elbow fully extended and the forearm fully supinated. The intersection of a line along the midaxis of the upper part of the arm and a line along the midaxis of the forearm defines this angle. Beals has shown that the carrying angle varies widely among individuals.[16] The angle increases with age, and no consistent difference is seen between males and females. The carrying angle of a given elbow is best evaluated by comparing that angle with the carrying angle of the contralateral elbow.

## SUPRACONDYLAR FRACTURE

### Anatomy

The distal end of the humerus is unique in design. Although the medial and lateral columns are strong, they are connected by a thin wafer of bone that is only 1 mm thick in the central portion.[10, 46] This central thin area of the distal part of the humerus is produced by the olecranon fossa posteriorly and the coronoid fossa anteriorly (Fig. 9–9). It is because of this distinct distal humeral anatomy that a supracondylar fracture is so unstable. If the distal fragment rotates even slightly, the medial column of the distal fragment does not line up with the medial column of the proximal fragment, and only the thin bone between the two columns abuts. Dameron[46] compared this circumstance to attempting to balance the blades of two knives on each other. Because this feat is impossible, the two fragments invariably rotate and then tilt to produce an angular deformity of the elbow.

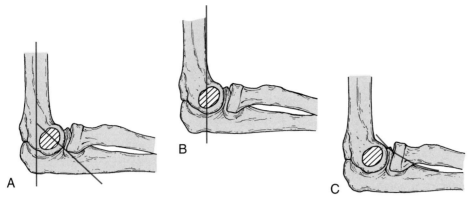

**FIGURE 9–7.** Radiographic lines that may be demonstrated on a lateral radiograph of the elbow. *A,* The capitellum of the distal end of the humerus is angulated anteriorly approximately 30°. This angle may be demonstrated by drawing a line parallel to the midpoint of the distal humeral shaft; where that line intersects with a line drawn through the midpoint of the capitellum indicates the anterior inclination of the capitellum. *B,* The anterior humeral line is drawn down the outer edge of the anterior cortex of the distal end of the humerus. As the line is drawn distally through the capitellum, it should pass through the middle of the capitellum. *C,* The anterior coronoid line is drawn along the coronoid fossa of the proximal portion of the ulna and is then continued proximally. It should just touch the capitellum anteriorly. The line lies posterior to the most anterior portion of the capitellum if the capitellum is angulated anteriorly. If the capitellum is angulated posteriorly, the line no longer touches the capitellum.

## Incidence

Supracondylar fractures occur most often in immature skeletons and are usually seen in the first decade of life. They have been shown to account for about 30% of all limb fractures in children younger than 7 years.[36, 61, 92, 217] Supracondylar fractures are the most common fractures about the elbow in children and account for about 60% of the total.[62, 129] Two types of supracondylar fractures may result, depending on the mechanism of injury. The extension type occurs in over 96% of supracondylar fractures, whereas the flexion type constitutes less than 4% of these injuries.

## Mechanisms of Injury

Supracondylar fractures of the distal end of the humerus may be produced by either a hyperextension or a flexion injury. An injury that results from a fall on the outstretched hand with the elbow hyperextended causes the more common extension type of fracture. If the injury occurs from a fall on the olecranon with the elbow flexed, the less common flexion type of supracondylar fracture results.

Various investigators have been able to produce the flexion type of supracondylar fracture in both immature cadavers and monkeys.[3, 11, 166] Henrikson[92] studied children who had sustained supracondylar fractures of the humerus and found that their uninjured opposite elbows were capable of more than the average amount of hyperextension. Others have also confirmed that the

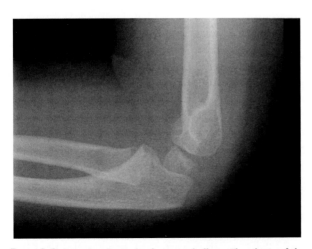

**FIGURE 9–8.** Lateral radiograph of a normal elbow. The physis of the capitellum is slightly wider posteriorly than anteriorly. This finding should not be confused with an injury to the physis.

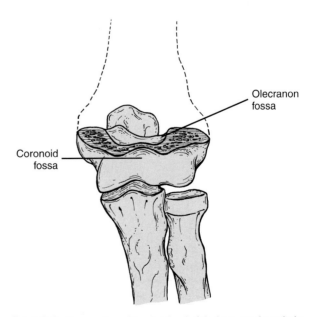

**FIGURE 9–9.** Cross section of the distal end of the humerus through the region of the coronoid fossa. Note that the midportion of the humerus is extremely thin at this level whereas the medial and lateral sides (columns) are thicker.

opposite elbow will hyperextend in children who have sustained a supracondylar fracture of the humerus.[35, 150] They concluded that children who fall on an outstretched hand will most commonly sustain either a distal radial fracture or a supracondylar fracture of the humerus. Children with ligamentous laxity and whose elbows demonstrate hyperextension will more commonly sustain a supracondylar humeral fracture, whereas children without hyperextension of the elbow will be more likely to sustain a distal humeral fracture. McLauchlan has been the only researcher who has not found increased hyperextension of the elbow in this group of patients.[134] The ability to hyperextend the elbow is believed to direct the force from a fall on the outstretched hand to the anatomically weak olecranon fossa and result in a fracture. Because ligamentous laxity is greatest in the young, the peak incidence of this fracture is in the first decade of life.

## Consequences of Injury

The hyperextension force produces the fracture, which begins as a crack in the anterior cortex of the supracondylar area of the humerus. As the hyperextension moment progresses, the anterior periosteum stretches over the fracture of the anterior cortex. This injury has been termed a stage I fracture by Abraham and colleagues.[3] If at this point the hyperextension force ceases, a nondisplaced or minimally angulated fracture occurs. Radiographically, one may see a decrease in the normal anterior inclination of the capitellum on a lateral view.

A stage II fracture is the result of continued hyperextension of the elbow. Hence, the distal fragment continues to angle posteriorly but does not become displaced. In a stage III injury, the anterior periosteum is completely torn, and the distal fragment is displaced posteriorly. Although the anterior periosteum is completely torn in a stage III fracture, the posterior periosteum is usually intact and is used as a hinge to assist in closed reduction of the fracture. If the fracture is displaced posteromedially, which is generally the case, a medial periosteal hinge usually exists in addition to the posterior periosteum.

## Associated Injuries

### NERVE INJURIES

A supracondylar fracture of the distal end of the humerus in children is associated with a relatively high risk of nerve injury (between 7% and 15.5%) according to published reports of all supracondylar fractures, although Campbell and associates found that in 59 patients with type III supracondylar fractures, 24 (41%) had acute nerve injuries.* Older reports showed that 45% of nerve injuries involved the radial nerve and 32% involved the median nerve. Campbell and colleagues found that median nerve injury was associated with posterolateral displacement 87% of the time. The radial nerve was

---

*See references 14, 31, 44, 59, 67, 73, 102, 116, 118, 132, 192.

injured when the fracture became displaced in a posteromedial direction.[31] The ulnar nerve is less commonly involved in that it is injured about 23% of the time.[191] Ulnar nerve injury is more often associated with the flexion type of supracondylar fracture of the humerus. Although radial nerve injury was the most commonly reported injury in the older literature, more recent investigators have found the anterior interosseous to be the most commonly injured nerve.[31, 44, 59] Because this nerve is purely a motor nerve, diagnosis of injury to it requires specific examination of the flexor pollicis longus and flexor digitorum profundus of the index finger. As the proximal fragment is displaced anteriorly, the median nerve, with its associated anterior interosseous nerve, is stretched anteriorly. Such stretching puts the anterior interosseous branch especially at risk because it is tethered under the fibrous arch that arises from the deep head of the pronator teres.[102, 192]

### VASCULAR INJURIES

Although the consequences of vascular injury associated with supracondylar humeral fractures may be significant, permanent vascular compromise of the extremity occurs in less than 1% of all such fractures.[159, 214] The brachial artery is usually protected by the brachialis muscle. If the displacement of the fracture is great, the brachialis muscle may be torn and the protection it provides to the brachial artery lost.

The proximal fragment of the supracondylar fracture is usually displaced anteriorly. If the brachialis muscle is torn, the anterior spike of the proximal fragment is displaced significantly. The brachial artery may become tethered and occluded by this spike of bone because the artery is tethered to the distal fragment by the supratrochlear artery.[177] This occlusion is usually relieved by reducing the fracture. The artery may also become entrapped within the substance of the fracture.[197] In this instance, the circulation is usually satisfactory until one attempts reduction of the fracture with manipulation or traction. Reduction of a fracture with an entrapped brachial artery results in loss of the radial pulse and possibly compromise of the circulation of the extremity. An entrapped brachial artery may be accompanied by the median nerve. These structures, if entrapped in the fracture, will prevent one from achieving anatomic reduction of the fracture. If this inability to reduce the fracture perfectly is accompanied by absence of the radial pulse, one should be aware of the strong possibility that the artery and possibly the median nerve are entrapped in the fracture. Such entrapment necessitates open reduction of the fracture with removal of the neurovascular structures from within the fracture.

## Classification

Supracondylar humeral fractures may be classified by the direction of displacement of the proximal fragment. If a child falls on an outstretched hand with the elbow extended, an extension type of supracondylar fracture results. In this type, by far the most common, the proximal fragment of the humerus is displaced anteriorly.

The flexion type of supracondylar fracture of the distal end of the humerus occurs from a fall on the olecranon with the elbow flexed. This injury is much less common and constitutes less than 4% of all supracondylar fractures.[214]

Extension-type supracondylar fractures are usually classified according to the amount of displacement of the two fragments. This classification was originally proposed by Gartland and is still the most useful.[75] Type I is a nondisplaced fracture. The fracture line may be easily visible or indistinct. Good lateral views and observation of fat pad elevation help identify this fracture radiographically.

A type II fracture is an angulated fracture with an intact posterior cortex. On a lateral radiograph, one can identify the posterior angulation of the distal fragment by the position of the capitellum. Normally, the capitellum is angulated anteriorly about 30°. This angulation may also be documented radiographically by observation of the anterior humeral line, which normally crosses the middle of the capitellum on a lateral radiograph of the elbow. If this line runs anterior to the middle of the capitellum, one must suspect a type II supracondylar fracture of the distal end of the humerus (see Fig. 9–7). Abraham and colleagues[3] have shown that the anterior periosteum is torn in a type II fracture; however, it is not completely torn and maintains some continuity anteriorly.

A type III supracondylar fracture is completely displaced, with all continuity of the two distal humeral fragments lost. The fracture is most often displaced posteromedially, although it may infrequently be displaced posterolaterally. Much has been written about displacement of the distal fragment. Posteromedial displacement is thought to be best held reduced with pronation of the forearm because the soft tissues help close the lateral side of the fracture with the forearm in pronation. Conversely, if the fracture is displaced posterolaterally, supination is the position of choice for immobilization of the reduced fracture.

## EXTENSION-TYPE SUPRACONDYLAR FRACTURE

### History

Children who are old enough to provide an adequate history complain of pain in the elbow region and an inability to move the elbow after having fallen on an outstretched hand with the elbow extended. These consequences are the rule for type II and III fractures; children who sustain type I injuries, however, may not have the total restriction of movement that is seen in more displaced fractures.

### Physical Examination

The results of physical examination of a patient with a supracondylar humeral fracture depend on the type of fracture sustained. If the fracture is nondisplaced, the swelling may not be great, but point tenderness will be noted in the supracondylar region of the distal end of the humerus.

Children who sustain a type II fracture have pain with attempted movement of the elbow but may be able to initiate a small amount of elbow motion because of the stability of the fracture.

Those who have sustained type III fractures have the most pain and swelling. These children are unable to initiate any movement of the elbow because of pain. When such a child is seen in an emergency department, the elbow is usually splinted in extension, which is the position of the elbow at the time of injury. Generally, significant swelling has occurred in the elbow, mostly about the distal part of the humerus. With significant displacement of the fracture, ecchymosis of the skin may be observed in the antecubital region of the elbow. When the proximal fragment of the humerus has penetrated the brachialis muscle, the skin in front of the elbow may be puckered and indicate the severity of the fracture displacement. Little else can be discerned about the fracture itself because of the amount of pain and swelling with this injury. The forearm is generally pronated because the distal fragment is usually internally rotated. This internal rotation must be corrected at the time of closed reduction.

A complete neurovascular evaluation of the arm is essential because this fracture is notorious for producing some form of neurovascular damage. It is not uncommon for the radial pulse to be absent at the time of initial evaluation. This lack of a pulse may be secondary to tethering of the artery over the anterior surface of the proximal fragment of the distal end of the humerus. If the pulse is absent, one should attempt gentle reduction to relieve the pressure on the artery, if possible. Although absence of the radial pulse causes concern, the pulse usually returns, and rarely is the artery torn. Arterial spasm may be differentiated from arterial rupture or occlusion with the use of a Doppler probe. The extensive collateral circulation around the elbow allows for sufficient circulation to the arm in most instances to maintain viability, even if the artery is damaged. This situation is different from the circulation around the knee, where the popliteal artery is crucial, because the collateral circulation in this area is insufficient to maintain viability of the lower part of the leg.[81]

Examination of the forearm is critical to determine the status of the circulation to the forearm and hand. Even if the pulse is absent, the limb will be viable if the collateral circulation is adequate; however, signs of ischemia are common. Adequacy of the collateral circulation is determined by examination of perfusion and function of the forearm and hand and by the presence of a pulse on Doppler examination. Volkmann's ischemia has been associated with this fracture, and one must look carefully for signs of impending ischemia: pain, compartment tightness, and decreasing motor and sensory function. The classic finding is pain out of proportion to the injury, especially pain with passive extension of the fingers. In patients with any question of compartment ischemia, the compartment pressures of the forearm should be measured.

The neurologic examination should include a motor

and sensory assessment of the median, ulnar, and radial nerves. In addition, one should look carefully for injury to the anterior interosseous nerve. This branch of the median nerve is a pure motor nerve. It supplies motor function to the flexor pollicis longus and the flexor digitorum profundus to the index finger. An inability to flex the distal joints of the thumb and index finger indicates injury to this nerve.

## Radiographic Evaluation

Accurate radiographic diagnosis of a type III fracture of the supracondylar region of the distal end of the humerus is not usually difficult. Accurate diagnosis of a type I or even a type II fracture may pose more difficulty. As previously mentioned, use of the fat pad signs on lateral radiographs is helpful in localizing the trauma to the region of the elbow joint. In addition, on a lateral radiograph one should look for any alteration in the intersection of the capitellum with the anterior humeral line; if this line crosses anterior to the middle of the capitellum, a type I or II supracondylar fracture is likely to be present.

## Management

### TYPE I FRACTURE

Although a type I fracture is nondisplaced, the distal fragment may be angulated posteriorly as seen on a lateral radiograph. Treatment depends on the extent of posterior angulation of the distal fragment. Rang[166] states that reduction is not required if the posterior angulation is 20° or less. Normally, the capitellum is angulated anteriorly about 30°. Even if the capitellum is in a straight line with the longitudinal axis of the humerus, remodeling of the injury should be able to correct this amount of angulation if the growth potential is sufficient. For some time, however, children with this injury will have more than normal elbow extension and less than normal elbow flexion because of the extension angulation of the distal fragment.

In general, this fracture requires immobilization for comfort and protection. The immobilization should not be circular, even though this injury does not generally swell as much as a displaced supracondylar fracture does. It is usually better to apply a long posterior splint with medial and lateral side splints to immobilize the elbow. The elbow should be placed in about 90° of flexion unless enough swelling is present to suggest possible compromise of the circulation. In that case, the elbow should be extended until comfort and circulation are optimal. Three weeks of immobilization is usually sufficient for healing. At that time, the splints are removed, and if healing is judged to be adequate radiographically, the child is allowed unrestricted motion of the elbow.

One pitfall in treating a type I fracture lies in not recognizing associated medial angulation of the fracture; if left uncorrected, this angulation will produce a cubitus

varus deformity that will not be corrected with growth. Although rare in a type I fracture, medial compression may be identified (Fig. 9–10). The use of Baumann's angle on an anteroposterior radiograph may be helpful to identify the varus deformity caused by the medial compression. Mohammad and colleagues assessed the Baumann angle and reaffirmed the opinion of others that the Baumann angle is not an accurate measure of the carrying angle of the elbow.[144] This angle is complex and is very dependent on the position of the arm while undergoing radiographic examination. Arm rotation will alter the measurement, and therefore its use is not always accurate and one may miss a cubitus varus deformity. Therefore, if one suspects compression of the medial column of the distal end of the humerus in association with a type I fracture, it is best identified clinically by inspecting the arm with full elbow extension to compare the carrying angle with that of the normal uninjured elbow. De Boeck and colleagues identified 13 patients with medial compression of the distal end of the humerus in an innocent-looking fracture that produced a varus deformity. Most of the fractures were type I fractures that looked benign on initial radiographs, but on close inspection, medial compression and medial comminution could be identified.[50]

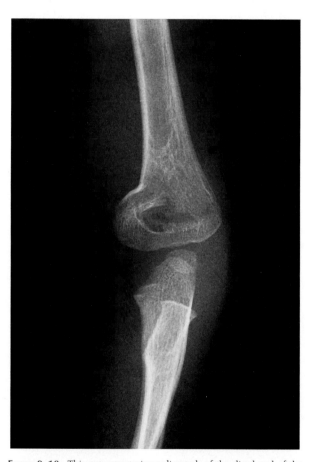

FIGURE 9–10. This anteroposterior radiograph of the distal end of the humerus and elbow shows a nondisplaced supracondylar fracture. Note the compression of the metaphysis on the medial side. The lateral side is straight and has not been compressed. This injury has produced a cubitus varus deformity that should be corrected.

A type I fracture with medial compression must be reduced to prevent a cubitus varus deformity. If one is uncertain whether a varus deformity of the distal end of the humerus will result from this fracture, examination under anesthesia allows visual inspection of the fully extended elbow. If the fracture is in varus, the fracture is reduced by applying longitudinal traction with the elbow in full extension. An assistant applies countertraction to the upper part of the arm. Valgus correction is obtained by using the forearm as a lever. Once it is reduced, the fracture should be stabilized with two crossed K-wires because the fracture is inherently unstable. The medial comminution of the distal end of the humerus causes the fracture to drift back into a varus position if the fracture is not stabilized with pin fixation. Once the fracture is stabilized with crossed pins, the elbow may be flexed to 80° to 90° and immobilized for 3 weeks.

## TYPE II FRACTURE

Type II fractures are similar to type I fractures, although the severity of the angulation of the distal fragment is greater. In type II fractures, the anterior cortex is broken, but the posterior cortex remains intact. In addition to posterior angulation, some rotation of the distal fragment may be present.

Authorities disagree about the need for reduction of these fractures. Gartland[75] believes that even if the distal fragment has lost all its anterior angulation, as seen on a lateral radiograph, reduction of the fracture is not necessary because the deformity will remodel. Mann[121] is even more optimistic about the remodeling of these fractures in children. He states that remodeling should be expected to be complete even if the fracture is angulated posteriorly 10°. A significant amount of remodeling is possible about the distal end of the humerus because of the proximity to the elbow joint. In addition, the younger the child at the time of injury, the greater the amount of remodeling potential. One must remember, however, that remodeling is possible only in the plane of motion of the elbow joint. In other words, only anterior or posterior angulation may remodel; varus or valgus angulation will not correct with growth. Varus compression of the medial side of the fracture is even more likely in a type II than a type I fracture. Varus angulation of the elbow may be assessed in the same way as for a type I fracture. Both Baumann's angle and the medial epicondylar epiphyseal angle on the injured side may be compared with their counterparts on the opposite uninjured side. However, clinical examination of the fully extended elbow is the best means of accurately assessing the carrying angle, although this maneuver may not be possible without anesthesia because of pain. If varus deformity is a possibility, the patient should be anesthetized so that the arm can be thoroughly examined.

Fractures with medial compression should be corrected with a valgus force as described in the section on type I fractures (see Fig. 9–10). If reduction is necessary, the fracture will probably be unstable because of the likelihood of medial comminution of a type II fracture. The technique of reduction is similar to the description of reduction of type III fractures as described later in this chapter. The fracture should be reduced with the patient under general or regional anesthesia and with fluoroscopic control of the reduction. After the medial compression has been corrected with a valgus force on the extended elbow, the elbow is flexed maximally and the olecranon is pushed anteriorly to reduce the posterior angulation. In this case, pin fixation with K-wires should be performed to maintain the reduction and to prevent cubitus varus deformity. A type II fracture is inherently more stable than a type III fracture. Therefore, fixation with two lateral pins is recommended for type II fractures. The arm is then immobilized with the elbow in 80° to 90° of flexion if swelling allows. Pronation of the forearm used to be popular to help maintain fracture reduction and decrease the tendency to varus deformity, but it is not necessary once the fracture is stabilized with K-wires.

Reduction of the posterior angulation is also necessary, with or without medial comminution, if the distal fragment is angulated too far posteriorly (i.e., if the longitudinal axis of the capitellum is angulated posterior to the longitudinal axis of the shaft of the humerus). Another pitfall in the treatment of type II fractures is to disregard the rotational deformity that may be present. If uncorrected, this rotational malalignment will lead to tilt of the distal fragment and varus angulation. Thus, this rotation should be corrected, along with posterior tilt and medial compression, if present, and the fracture should then be stabilized with pin fixation (Fig. 9–11). If correction of the posterior angulation, medial compression, or rotational deformity of the distal fragment is not necessary, simple immobilization may be sufficient; however, one must be certain that no underlying deformity exists, and careful examination of the anesthetized arm is the best way of ensuring the absence of such deformity.

## TYPE III FRACTURE

A type III fracture is defined as a completely displaced supracondylar fracture in which both the anterior and the posterior cortices have lost contact with each other. In most instances, the proximal and distal bone fragments are not in contact. This fracture carries the greatest risk of neurovascular injury. At present, closed reduction with percutaneous pinning is accepted as the best method of treatment. The same treatment is preferred for a fracture that is not reducible and for one in which the neural or vascular status changes during fracture reduction.

## Treatment

### SKIN TRACTION

Because of the risk of vascular compression resulting in Volkmann's ischemia of the forearm, traction became a popular mode of treatment of this fracture. Both skin and skeletal traction have been used.

Dunlop's traction is skin traction applied to the arm with the child supine.[57, 60] Traction straps are applied to

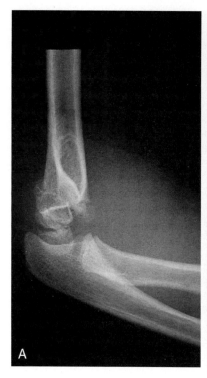
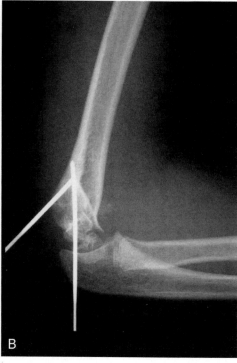

**FIGURE 9–11.** Type II supracondylar fracture of the distal end of the humerus. *A,* A lateral radiograph of the distal part of the humerus demonstrates posterior angulation of the distal humeral fragment. Note that if one drew the anterior humeral line, it would no longer intersect the capitellum, nor would the coronoid line lie on the anterior aspect of the capitellum. In addition, the capitellum has lost its normal 30° of angulation. *B,* Postreduction radiograph of the distal end of the humerus.

the forearm with the arm supinated. A counterweight is hung from the upper part of the arm to help pull the proximal fragment of the humerus posteriorly to approximate the distal fragment. Longitudinal traction is then applied to the supinated forearm with the elbow flexed about 45°. Several modifications of this technique have been described. Ingebrightsen's method involved skin traction that was applied as overhead traction.[57, 214] Traction applied to the upper portion of the arm pulled vertically, and traction applied to the forearm pulled horizontally, with the elbow flexed close to a right angle. Graham advocated extension skin traction applied to the arm with the elbow in full extension.[77, 78]

Regardless of the type of skin traction used, the results were about the same, despite isolated reports of excellent outcomes. Although the problem of compartment ischemia seemed to be lessened with the use of skin traction, the incidence of cubitus varus was unacceptably high in most series. For example, Piggot reported good results with extension skin traction,[162] as did Dodge with Dunlop's traction.[57] In contrast, D'Ambrosia and Zink found an unacceptably high incidence of cubitus varus with skin traction,[45] as did Prietto.[163] Because of the risk of cubitus varus, the use of skin traction for the treatment of this fracture has essentially been abandoned in the United States.

## SKELETAL TRACTION

Skeletal traction has been the most popular contemporary traction treatment of supracondylar humeral fractures. In general, traction is applied to the fracture through the proximal end of the ulna with the elbow in flexion. Initially, traction was accomplished through the use of a Steinmann pin placed transversely through the

proximal part of the ulna with the child sedated. An axillary block may be used, although some prefer general anesthesia for fracture reduction and application of traction because it allows continuous monitoring of compartment function.[112] The pin must be inserted under sterile conditions. The point of insertion is important because of the proximity of the ulnar nerve. Therefore, the pin is inserted from the medial side of the arm at about the level of the coronoid process of the ulna, which is about 2.5 cm distal to the tip of the olecranon.[81, 187, 188, 190] For placement of the pin, the elbow should be flexed to allow the nerve to move anteriorly and to enhance the surgeon's ability to feel the landmarks. A smooth pin rather than a threaded pin is used because nerve injury is more likely if the pin is placed too close to the nerve. Once the pin has been inserted in the ulna, the arm is placed in traction.

Because of the risk of injury to the ulnar nerve, a winged screw is preferred by some authors.[62, 81, 133, 153, 157] The screw is inserted into the proximal end of the ulna at the same distance from the tip of the olecranon as used for insertion of the traction pin. Instead of being inserted transversely, it is inserted into the ulnar cortex in line with the longitudinal axis of the humerus (Fig. 9–12). Another advantage of the screw is the existence of multiple holes in its wing so that the direction of pull of the traction can be altered to adjust for varus or valgus deformity.

Although some advocate sidearm traction, most authors prefer overhead traction because it elevates the elbow, thereby helping to reduce swelling.[45, 87, 113] In addition, D'Ambrosia and Zink point out that with the arm overhead, the forearm rotates into pronation, which is the preferred position of the forearm in fractures that are displaced posteromedially.[45] Pronation is believed to close the lateral side of the fracture, which decreases the risk of cubitus varus.

For the application of sidearm traction, after the pin or screw is inserted, the child is placed supine on the edge of the bed with the fractured arm overhanging the side of the bed. The elbow is flexed to a right angle with the hand pointing to the ceiling. Skin traction straps are placed on the forearm and connected to a pulley and weights sufficient to support the arm. The skeletal traction is also connected to weights through a separate pulley. Additional weights may be suspended from the upper part of the arm to help pull the proximal fragment of the humerus posteriorly.

For the application of overhead skeletal traction, the direction of the traction is vertical through a series of pulleys. The forearm is suspended in a sling. Because this fracture usually has an internal rotation deformity, the hand is directed to the opposite upper corner of the bed (for example, if the right humerus is fractured, the hand is pointed toward the upper left corner) (see Fig. 9–12).

Radiographs of the distal end of the humerus are important to assess the efficacy of the traction; however, the anteroposterior view is difficult to obtain. One must extend the elbow to obtain an adequate anteroposterior view, and this motion in itself may alter the position of the reduction of the fracture.

Kramhoft and associates[112] reduced the fracture

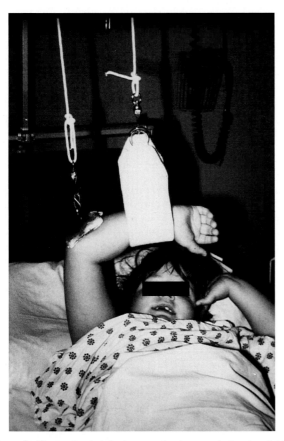

FIGURE **9–12.** Overhead skeletal traction has been applied to this child's arm with a supracondylar humeral fracture. A winged screw was inserted into the proximal end of the ulna at about the level of the coronoid process. Skeletal traction was then applied through the screw.

under general anesthesia and placed the extremity in traction with the patient still in the operating room. Frequently, the fracture was remanipulated under anesthesia one or more times during the traction treatment. Other authors placed the arm in skeletal traction, with the expectation that the traction itself will reduce the fracture acceptably.[45, 62] Traction was usually maintained for 2 to 3 weeks. Hammond recommended 2 weeks of traction, after which the arm was placed in a cast.[87] Others, such as Fahey,[62] left the patient in traction for 2½ to 3 weeks and then placed the arm in a sling.

The use of skeletal traction for the treatment of this fracture has generally had better results than the use of skin traction.[45, 65, 112, 156] Nevertheless, the use of any kind of traction poses problems. The long hospital stay required for completion of traction care is not generally acceptable as long as alternative methods are available that provide equivalent or better treatment. Sutton and colleagues evaluated the cost of treatment and the outcomes of 65 children with supracondylar humeral fractures treated either with skeletal traction or with closed reduction and percutaneous pinning. The results were basically equivalent in the two groups, with 90% of the results satisfactory. The cost of treatment was significantly different, however, depending on the type of treatment. The cost of treatment was lowest in patients whose fractures were reduced and pinned in the operating room and the pins subsequently removed in the office. The cost of treatment was 117% greater for patients treated by skeletal traction if the skeletal traction pin was inserted in the emergency room. The cost increased by 142% for those treated by olecranon traction with the olecranon pin inserted in the operating room.[198]

## CLOSED REDUCTION AND CAST TREATMENT

Closed reduction with cast treatment of supracondylar humeral fractures was the preferred means of management in many centers. Reduction of the fracture is generally accomplished with the patient under general anesthesia. With the elbow extended, gentle longitudinal traction is applied to the supinated forearm, with countertraction applied to the upper part of the arm by an assistant. The medial or lateral displacement is then corrected with finger pressure over the medial or lateral epicondyle. Most of these fractures are displaced posteromedially, and they are also internally rotated. To bring the medial column of the distal fragment anterior to meet the medial column of the proximal fragment, the distal fragment is externally rotated.[45] At this point, the fracture is reduced by flexing the elbow while maintaining the longitudinal traction. In addition, the thumb of the surgeon pushes the olecranon forward to eliminate the posterior displacement of the distal fragment. The elbow must be flexed maximally to hold the fracture reduced while radiographs are obtained to assess the quality of the reduction.

A lateral radiograph is relatively easy to obtain, but the arm should not be rotated to obtain this view. Instead, the placement of the arm should be maintained and the machine moved to the cross-table position. Because an anteroposterior view is not possible, one must obtain the so-called Jones view, which is a transcondylar one. This view is achieved by placing the upper part of the subject's arm on the radiographic cassette. The elbow is maximally flexed with the forearm pronated. The radiographic tube is placed over the distal end of the humerus and directed perpendicular to it. In essence, one is obtaining an anteroposterior radiograph of the distal end of the humerus through the overlying forearm. This radiograph is understandably difficult to interpret because of the overlying bone and soft tissue. The medial epicondylar angle is also useful and may assist in evaluation of the reduction as viewed on a transcondylar radiograph.[23]

The position of the elbow is critical for maintaining reduction of the fracture. To control the reduction, acute flexion of the elbow is necessary. This position tightens the posterior periosteum of the distal end of the humerus and also tightens the triceps muscle, which tends to lock the reduction in place. Many authors recommend pronation of the forearm for fractures that are postero-medially displaced; such pronation also prevents cubitus varus. Rang and colleagues[167] believe that the fracture fragment has an intact medial periosteal hinge that becomes taut with the forearm in pronation and the fracture reduced. Griffin[82] also endorses this concept. They all agree that the fracture must be reduced first. Acute elbow flexion is required to tighten the posterior periosteal hinge. Once the posterior periosteal hinge is tight, with maximal elbow flexion, the pronation of the elbow tightens the medial periosteum; this maneuver closes the lateral fracture surfaces and thereby reduces the degree of varus. Arnold and coworkers[9] recommend pronation as the position of stability for this fracture after reduction. They believe that the brachioradialis and the wrist extensors become tight with pronation of the forearm, which tends to close the fracture on the lateral side and thereby reduce the amount of varus deformity.

Thus, regardless of the rationale, all authors agree that acute flexion of the elbow with pronation of the forearm is required to stabilize a displaced fracture of the supracondylar region of the distal end of the humerus. The problem with this position of the elbow is that acute flexion increases the tension in an already swollen elbow, thus increasing the risk of vascular compromise by reducing arterial flow to the forearm and venous outflow from the forearm. Such circulatory compromise has been documented clinically by Mapes and Hennrikus. They found that the Doppler pulse became weaker and possibly disappeared in patients with supracondylar humeral fractures when the elbow is flexed. The more the elbow was flexed, the weaker the pulse became.[123] Less than acute flexion is frequently required to maintain adequate circulation to the distal portion of the arm in patients with displaced supracondylar fractures. Unfortunately, anything less than acute flexion risks loss of fracture reduction because with even minor degrees of extension of the elbow, the posterior periosteum becomes lax and permits fracture displacement. For this reason, closed reduction with cast immobilization is not recommended as treatment of this fracture.

This dilemma led to the currently accepted methods of treatment of this fracture. It became obvious that because acute flexion was necessary to maintain reduction, another means of maintaining the reduction was needed to reduce the risk of vascular compromise. This realization led to the development of internal fixation of these fractures, an approach that is accepted as the standard today.

## AUTHOR'S PREFERRED TREATMENT

### Closed Reduction and Percutaneous Pinning

One of the major problems with supracondylar humeral fractures is the risk of development of cubitus varus. This deformity is not the result of a growth disturbance but rather the direct result of malreduction of the fracture or loss of reduction. When one looks at the distal end of the humerus, where this fracture occurs, it becomes evident that the width of the humerus is only 2 to 3 mm, at most, across the olecranon fossa. Therefore, if a supracondylar fracture is not anatomically reduced, the medial column of the proximal and distal fragments will not line up. The medial column of the distal fragment is posterior to the proximal portion of the medial column because of malrotation of the fracture fragments. Thus, the proximal fragment is balancing on a fragment of bone 2 mm thick. As one can imagine, it is impossible to maintain varus-valgus alignment unless the medial columns of the two fragments are opposing. Hence, the reduction must not only be accurate but must also be maintained, for any rotation of the distal fragment displaces the medial column of the distal fragment posterior to the medial column of the proximal fragment. Such displacement leads to tilting of the distal fragment into varus, with the development of cubitus varus.

The modern era of treatment of this fracture began in 1948 with a description by Swenson of percutaneous pinning of distal humeral fractures in adults.[199] In 1961, Casiano reported the use of this technique in children.[32] Since this description, multiple reports of the use of percutaneous pinning for the maintenance of reduction of a displaced supracondylar fracture have appeared.[62, 65, 66, 82] Some authors recommend the use of two lateral pins to avoid the ulnar nerve. Others advise using a very small incision on the medial side to allow palpation of the medial condyle so that the nerve can be avoided. This technique may be helpful in a very swollen elbow. The drawback to the use of two lateral pins is that the fixation provided is less secure biomechanically than that provided by crossed pins. Two lateral pins may still allow rotation of the fracture, thereby enabling the medial column to rotate posteriorly, unless the starting points of the two pins are widely separated, which is difficult because of the small size of the distal fragment. Once medial column support is lost, the fracture may tilt into varus.[215] Kallio and associates recommended two lateral pins for fracture stabilization, but they achieved good results in only 68% of patients. They stated that the two lateral pins must cross outside the lateral cortex of the distal fragment and that they must diverge and pass the fracture well apart from each other as they penetrate the medial cortex.[104] Most of the more recent reports of pin fixation of this fracture recommend crossed medial and lateral pin fixation.[26, 136, 158] Zionts and coworkers studied the torsional strength of different pin configurations for the stabilization of displaced supracondylar humeral fractures. They found that the torque required to produce 10° of rotation was 37% less with the use of two lateral pins than with the use of medial and lateral pins. In addition, 80% less torque was necessary to produce the same amount of rotation with the use of two crossed lateral pins as compared with the use of crossed medial and lateral pins.[218]

The reduction must be anatomic before the fracture is stabilized with pins. Some authors believe that malrotation of the fracture is not significant because the malrotation can be compensated for by the shoulder, which has such wide rotational motion. Although this concept is true, the problem with a malrotated supracondylar fracture is that if it is not adequately reduced, the fracture surfaces that oppose each other are the very thin proximal and distal portions of the olecranon fossa. As mentioned, trying to maintain reduction of this fracture in this circumstance is difficult at best; it is easy for the fracture to tilt medially without medial column support and result in cubitus varus. If the pin fixation is very secure, maintenance of the reduction is possible; however, most authors who reported their results of closed pinning of this fracture also recorded a variable incidence of cubitus varus. Nevertheless, a 1992 study by France and Strong showed that the results of closed reduction and percutaneous pinning were significantly better than the results of closed reduction with casting and traction.[70]

Aronson and Prager[10] have used Baumann's angle to determine the adequacy of reduction of this fracture intraoperatively. They recommend the use of two lateral pins to stabilize the fracture. If Baumann's angle is within 4° of that of the opposite uninjured elbow, the reduction is accepted. If the angle is greater, a repeat reduction is performed and a radiograph of the distal end of the humerus obtained. This treatment is repeated until Baumann's angle lies within a satisfactory range. With this attention to reduction, these authors reported no instances of cubitus varus. This result points out the need for excellent reduction of this fracture to decrease the incidence of a cubitus varus deformity.

Although Aronson and Prager[10] supported the use of Baumann's angle for determining the adequacy of reduction, others have not found this angle to be beneficial. Nacht and colleagues[146] found that the precise margin of the lateral condyle was not distinct, thus making measurement of Baumann's angle difficult. They also stated that this angle was not helpful in children younger than 3 years because it is impossible to define bony landmarks in the elbow at that age. Mohammad and associates compared Baumann's angle with the carrying angle of the elbow and found that the angle is very complex and not an accurate indicator of the carrying angle.[144] Use of the medial epicondylar epiphyseal angle, however, may be helpful.[23]

**Technique.** The timing of reduction of the fracture has in the past been as soon as technically possible. It has been thought that early reduction plus pin fixation

increases the chance of obtaining an anatomic reduction and reduces the risk of complications such as vascular compromise. Two separate reports have documented that delaying reduction of this fracture does not lead to increased complications. Mehlman and colleagues reviewed 115 patients with supracondylar fractures of the distal end of the humerus.[135] They delayed treatment of the fracture so that reduction and pinning could be undertaken during the normal operative time. They did not detect any increased incidence of cubitus varus, pin tract infection, or vascular complications. They also did not have an increased need for open reduction in the delayed-treatment group. Iyengar and associates also found similar results.[80, 98, 135] The attitude of trauma surgeons toward the need for immediate treatment of fractures in children and adults has changed. Operating in the middle of the night does not always guarantee that all of the participants are at their best. In addition, the personnel who are available for assistance may not be familiar with the procedure. The equipment necessary is usually easily found in the day by the normal orthopaedic operating room personnel; however, the evening and night teams may have difficulty locating all the necessary instruments. Radiology technicians who work during the day will have no trouble with the C-arm, but night technologists may find the procedure challenging.

The concerns that have prevented our group from delaying the treatment of these fractures has been the possible higher rate of complications such as an increased risk for the need for open reduction, nerve injury, and the possible occurrence of compartment ischemia. The results presented by these two authors were excellent. They did not find any difference in the two groups in the need for open reduction. Ten failures of closed reduction occurred in the early group; seven required open reduction. They performed only five open reductions in the late group. The authors likewise found no other differences between the two groups. It may therefore be advisable to delay reduction of this fracture until one is able to treat it during normal operating time. The child should be admitted to the hospital while awaiting fracture reduction, during which time the circulation and neurologic status of the arm are continuously monitored.

Flynn and associates[65] have used a special bracket over which the elbow is flexed to help stabilize the elbow during the pinning procedure; however, I prefer to keep the patient in the supine position and suspend the injured elbow over the edge of the table. The child is placed on a radiolucent operating table and put under general anesthesia. The patient is positioned supine with the involved extremity completely free. The shoulder of the involved extremity is positioned at the edge of the table so that the remainder of the arm can hang free over the edge. This position allows free access to the C-arm, which is placed directly under the arm, and the tube of the C-arm serves as the operating table. The main tube of the C-arm is sterilely draped so that the upper part of the arm and elbow lie on the C-arm (Fig. 9–13).

The arm is sterilely prepared, and the fracture is reduced by first extending the elbow with longitudinal traction applied to the forearm. An assistant places

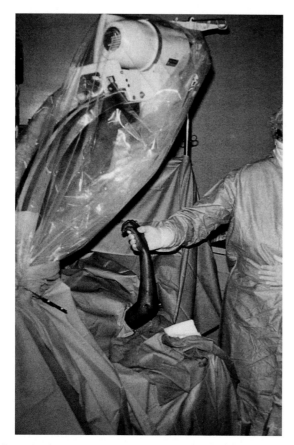

Figure 9–13. The C-arm machine is draped sterilely so that it can be used as the operating table for reduction and pinning of supracondylar humeral fractures.

countertraction on the upper part of the arm. Medial or lateral displacement is corrected, and the arm is externally rotated to correct the internal rotation deformity. The elbow is then flexed maximally, with traction maintained. The surgeon's thumb is used to push the olecranon forward, which assists in the reduction. Maximal elbow flexion is maintained with the arm fully externally rotated. Most fractures can be reduced with this technique, but if the posterior periosteum is torn, the fracture will be totally unstable and the hinge that the posterior periosteum provides for reduction is lost, thereby making reduction of the fracture difficult. If the spike of the proximal fragment penetrates the brachialis muscle, the muscle must be removed to obtain fracture reduction. Peters and colleagues described a technique for dislodgment of the entrapped brachialis muscle. While countertraction is applied through the axilla, the anterior musculature of the arm is grasped as close to the axilla as possible. This musculature is gradually "milked" in a proximal-to-distal direction off the spike of the proximal fragment. Pressure is placed primarily on the lateral side to avoid injury to the medial neurovascular structures. Freeing of the entrapped muscle is accompanied by an audible "pop." Once the brachialis muscle is removed from between the fracture fragments, the reduction is easier[160] (Fig. 9–14). Rasool and Naidoo[169] found that the neurovascular bundle was just anterior to the anterior edge of the fracture in 18 patients, behind

the fracture edge in 5, and separated by the fracture spike in 4. All these patients had a supracondylar humeral fracture with posterolateral fracture displacement. In addition, the brachialis muscle was buttonholed by the proximal fragment. They caution against manipulation of a supracondylar humeral fracture that is displaced in a posterolateral direction with buttonholing of the brachialis muscle because of the risk of neurovascular injury.

The reduction is assessed with the fluoroscope. A lateral projection is easy to obtain; however, it is important to move the radiographic machine rather than the elbow because rotation of the arm, especially internal rotation, may cause loss of reduction of the fracture. An anteroposterior projection is more difficult to obtain because extension of the elbow before pinning results in loss of the reduction; the Jones (transcondylar) view may be used. If, however, the reduction appears to be satisfactory as seen on the lateral projection, the fracture should be pinned. Once stabilized, the elbow may be extended to view the fracture on the anteroposterior projection. The carrying angle is also observed with the elbow extended.

It is debatable whether a medial pin is required or whether two lateral pins are sufficient. It has been shown that crossed pins are more stable biomechanically; however, authors who believe that two lateral pins are adequate state that the stability afforded by these two lateral pins will maintain the reduction.[203]

Smooth 0.062-inch pins are used to lessen the risk of injury to the physis and the ulnar nerve. In large children, a slightly larger pin may be used. Biodegradable pins made of polyglycolic acid have been used for fracture stabilization and theoretically offer an attractive alternative to metal pins, which must be removed. A recent report, however, by the authors of numerous articles on this technique warn about the use of biodegradable pins in supracondylar fractures. They reported an unacceptable incidence of pin breakage and fracture displacement with these pins.[25]

The pins should be inserted with the assistance of a power drill and the C-arm. The patient's arm is held fully externally rotated with the elbow maximally flexed once the reduction has been obtained. The lateral radiograph on the C-arm demonstrates the status of the reduction. The lateral pin is inserted first. The patient's arm can be rotated to the neutral position to insert this pin; however, stability is insufficient to allow full internal rotation of the arm. With the arm in neutral rotation, the lateral pin has to be inserted somewhat blindly because the C-arm image shows only the transcondylar view. This pin can also be inserted with the arm left in external rotation. To do so, the upper part of the arm is elevated on several towels and the elbow placed as close as possible to the far edge of the C-arm. The lateral pin may then be inserted into the lateral epicondyle from below, with cephalad angulation at about 35° to 45°, as for the medial pin.

The medial pin is inserted through the medial epicondyle. The elbow is left in the same position with the arm externally rotated. Care must be taken to avoid injury to the ulnar nerve, which can usually be palpated in its groove behind the epicondyle. Because the fracture has been partially stabilized with the lateral pin, the elbow can be extended to 80°, which allows the ulnar nerve to move posteriorly away from the medial epicondyle and affords more protection from iatrogenic injury with the medial pin. With the elbow fully flexed, the ulnar nerve is drawn tightly to the ulnar groove of the distal end of the humerus, where it is closely approxi-

mated to the medial epicondyle. Therefore, with the elbow extended to about 80°, the surgeon places the thumb of one hand on the ulnar nerve to protect it and inserts the pin into the medial epicondyle with the other hand. If significant swelling obscures the landmarks,

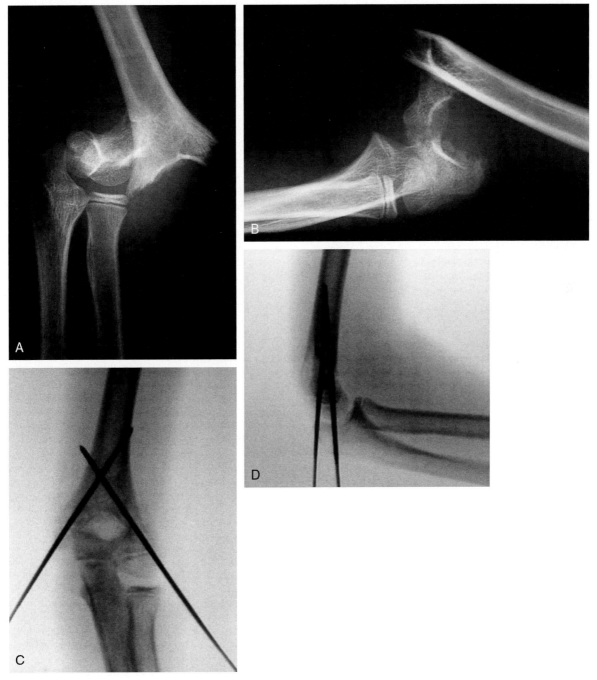

FIGURE 9–14. Markedly displaced extension-type supracondylar humeral fracture. The anterior spike of the distal fragment was tenting the skin on the anterior surface of the distal part of the arm in the antecubital fossa. The neurovascular examination of the extremity was normal. The fracture was reducible by closed means. The distal end of the humerus had penetrated through the brachialis muscle, but the muscle was massaged off the bone to allow the proximal humeral fragment to be brought posterior to the body of the brachialis. The fracture was pinned percutaneously. *A*, An anteroposterior radiograph of the distal portion of the humerus demonstrates the marked displacement of the fracture. Note that the proximal part of the forearm is in a lateral position because of the amount of rotation of the fracture. *B*, A lateral radiograph of the distal end of the humerus demonstrates the marked anterior displacement of the distal fragment, which penetrated the brachialis muscle and almost penetrated the skin in the antecubital fossa. The distal fragment and the forearm are in an anteroposterior position, the extent of which indicates the amount of rotation of the fracture. *C*, An intraoperative anteroposterior view of the elbow shows the anatomic reduction in this plane. The two crossed pins cross the fracture and were inserted percutaneously. Note that the medial pin enters the medial epicondyle laterally to avoid injuring the ulnar nerve. *D*, A lateral intraoperative radiograph demonstrates anatomic restoration of the anatomy of the distal end of the humerus. Both pins cross through the middle of the humerus.

manual pressure may help decrease the swelling locally. If this technique is unsuccessful, a small incision may be made over the medial epicondyle to assist in pin placement. To avoid nerve injury, Michael and Stanislas recommend using a nerve stimulator on a needle to locate the ulnar nerve when inserting the medial pin.[138] The pin is directed toward the lateral cortex of the humerus, proximal to the fracture site. To increase stability, the far cortex of the humerus must be just engaged by both pins (Fig. 9–15).

Once the medial pin is across the fracture and has engaged the opposite cortex of the humerus and the fracture is stabilized, the elbow can be extended to enable one to view the carrying angle and obtain a true anteroposterior radiograph. The pins are bent outside the skin, and the arm is splinted with the elbow in 80° to 90° of flexion. To prevent compression, the plaster should not be circular. The exact amount of elbow flexion is dictated by the amount of swelling and by the radial pulse.

The child should be hospitalized until it is certain that the risk of circulatory compromise is past. The arm is placed in a sling. Follow-up requires repeat radiographs in about a week to be certain that the reduction has not been lost. Three weeks of immobilization is usually all that is required. At that time, the splint and pins are removed if radiographs demonstrate sufficient healing. Unprotected motion, with activities restricted, is allowed to encourage use of the arm and movement of the elbow.

### Open Reduction and Internal Fixation

Open reduction plus internal fixation of supracondylar humeral fractures was once thought to be indicated only in rare circumstances because of concern about loss of motion, myositis ossificans, and infection. Later reports, however, showed excellent results with the use of open reduction.[15, 183, 210] Two relatively recent reports showed excellent results in most patients.[7, 43] Cramer and associates compared the results of open reduction and pin fixation with those of closed reduction and percutaneous pin fixation.[43] The results of the two groups were comparable in spite of the fact that the fractures in the open reduction group were more severe and were unable to be reduced by closed means. Open reduction is indicated for open fractures, in those with circulatory compromise or neurologic loss during or after closed reduction, and when adequate closed reduction cannot be obtained. The last reason is the least well defined, but almost all reports of closed reduction and pinning cite a risk of development of cubitus varus.[8, 62, 67, 145, 215] To decrease this risk, anatomic reduction of the fracture should be sought because such reduction prevents the medial tilt of the medial column that causes the cubitus varus deformity. Open reduction is indicated if excellent closed reduction cannot be achieved. The cause of the inability to achieve anatomic reduction is variable. Fleuriau-Chateau and colleagues performed 41 open reductions. Their most common indication for open reduction was buttonholing of the brachialis muscle by the distal end of the proximal fragment. They also found

tethering of the median or radial nerve (or both), with or without the brachial artery, that was not predicted on preoperative testing.[64] Another indication for open reduction of a supracondylar fracture is for a comminuted fracture. Occasionally, one may encounter a supracondylar fracture in which the distal fragment is also broken into fragments. In this instance, one must openly reduce the fracture to achieve anatomic reduction (Fig. 9–16).

**Technique.** A longitudinal 3- to 4-cm incision is made over the medial side of the distal end of the humerus and elbow. Once the skin and subcutaneous fat have been incised, the fracture hematoma and the fracture are encountered. The ulnar nerve is protected but does not have to be visualized. The periosteum over the proximal fragment will have been stripped by the injury. The fracture is explored to be certain that no neural or vascular structure is trapped. My colleagues and I have treated three patients whose fractures could not be reduced by closed means because the brachial artery, the median nerve, or both were trapped in the fracture.[43] Less than 1 mm of periosteum is elevated from the distal fragment to prevent circulatory embarrassment of this fragment. Adequate visualization of the fracture is necessary to ensure anatomic reduction. The fracture is then reduced and cross-pinned. If anatomic reduction is not possible, a lateral approach is made to ensure a perfect reduction. The lateral incision is also a longitudinal incision over the lateral condyle of the distal end of the humerus; such an incision allows exposure of the lateral side of the fracture. The pins are left protruding from the skin and are bent (Fig. 9–17).

Another surgical approach to the distal end of the humerus is a posterior triceps-dividing approach, which is used in adults if an olecranon osteotomy is not used. Concern about loss of motion, loss of triceps strength, or both has caused resistance to the adoption of this surgical approach. Two studies showed that this technique did not result in any increased loss of motion when compared with children treated by closed reduction and percutaneous pinning.[184] Kasser and colleagues also found no loss of motion in elbows operated on through a triceps-splitting approach. They documented a 3% deficit in strength, which they did not consider significant, and recommended this approach for complex distal humeral fractures.[106, 175] Gruber and Healey also recommended the posterior approach to the elbow for open reduction of this fracture. One of 20 patients did not regain full flexion and 2 of 20 did not regain full extension. They had no nerve injuries, loss of strength, or angular deformities.[83]

One is always amazed at the minimal discomfort that these children experience with decompression of the hematoma. They can usually be discharged from the hospital the day after surgery. Their follow-up is the same as that for closed pinning. The pins are generally removed and motion begun 3 weeks after surgery. The risk of myositis ossificans, which discouraged surgery on these fractures in the past, has not been a problem in my experience, nor has it been reported as a complication in the published series.[7, 15, 43, 82, 164, 183, 210]

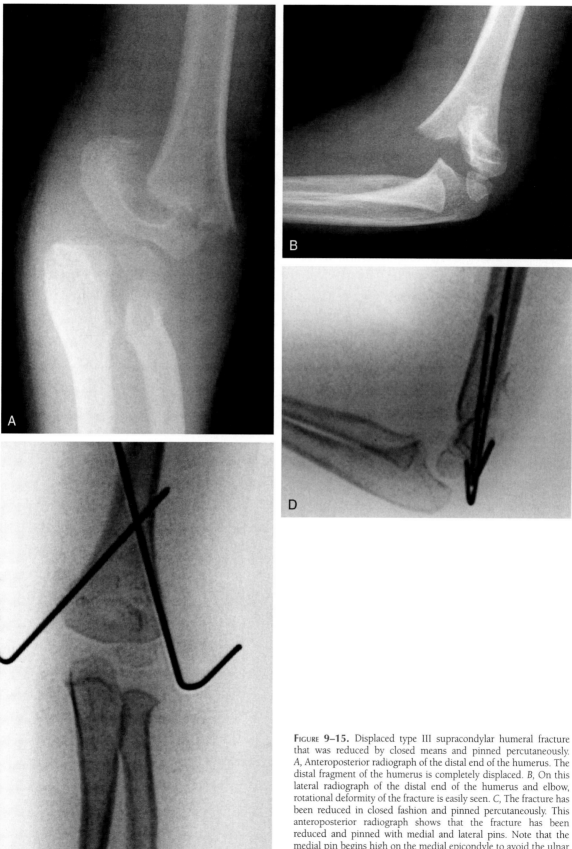

FIGURE 9–15. Displaced type III supracondylar humeral fracture that was reduced by closed means and pinned percutaneously. *A,* Anteroposterior radiograph of the distal end of the humerus. The distal fragment of the humerus is completely displaced. *B,* On this lateral radiograph of the distal end of the humerus and elbow, rotational deformity of the fracture is easily seen. *C,* The fracture has been reduced in closed fashion and pinned percutaneously. This anteroposterior radiograph shows that the fracture has been reduced and pinned with medial and lateral pins. Note that the medial pin begins high on the medial epicondyle to avoid the ulnar nerve. *D,* Reduction of the fracture is complete, as seen on this lateral radiograph.

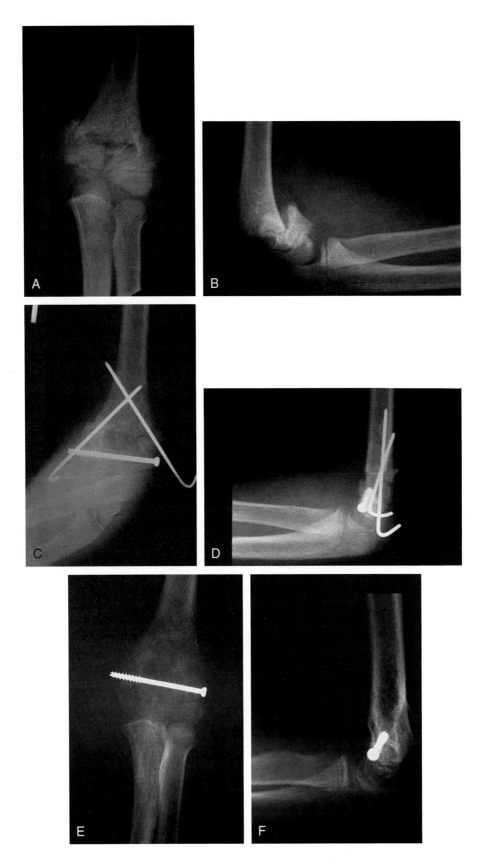

**FIGURE 9–16.** Comminuted displaced supracondylar fracture of the distal end of the humerus in a 9-year-old boy. *A,* Anteroposterior radiograph of the distal part of the humerus demonstrating a supracondylar fracture with a "T" fracture of the distal fragment. Separation of the capitellum and the trochlea is evident. *B,* Lateral radiograph of the elbow. The distal fragments are flexed anteriorly. *C,* Postoperative anteroposterior radiograph of the elbow. The elbow was approached posteriorly by a triceps-splitting approach, and the two distal fragments were reduced and stabilized with a cannulated screw first, which converted the fracture into a simple two-part supracondylar fracture that could be stabilized in the normal manner with two crossed pins. *D,* Lateral radiograph of the elbow demonstrating reduction of the fracture. Note that the flexed distal fragment is now reduced anatomically. *E,* Follow-up anteroposterior radiograph after pin removal and fracture healing 6 months postinjury. Complete healing has been achieved with no evidence of growth disturbance or avascular necrosis. The boy clinically demonstrates a full painless elbow range of motion. *F,* Lateral radiograph of the healed supracondylar fracture.

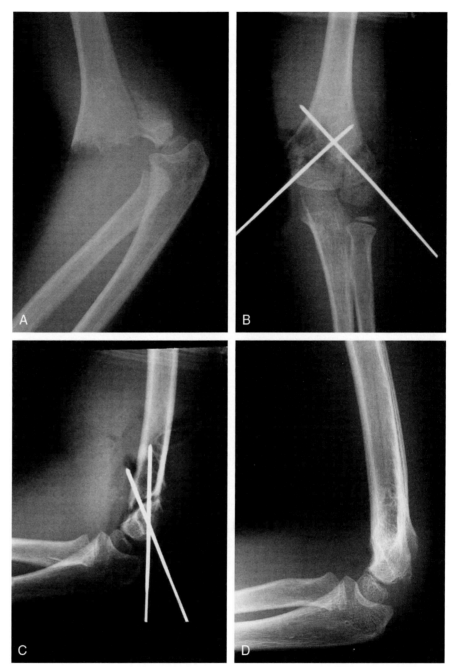

FIGURE 9–17. Displaced extension-type supracondylar fracture. The spike of the distal end of the humerus penetrated through the brachialis muscle, and the fracture could not be reduced anatomically by closed means. Open reduction was performed through both a medial and a lateral approach. *A,* Anteroposterior radiograph of a supracondylar fracture of the distal end of the humerus. *B,* Intraoperative postreduction anteroposterior radiograph demonstrating good reduction of the fracture. The lateral pin was withdrawn several millimeters. *C,* Intraoperative lateral radiograph of the fracture showing correction of the posterior displacement and restoration of the architecture of the distal part of the humerus. *D,* A lateral radiograph of the elbow 6 months after injury demonstrates normal distal humeral anatomy.

## Complications

### VASCULAR COMPROMISE

Vascular problems can be grouped into two types: acute, from interruption of the blood supply to the arm, and subacute, or Volkmann's ischemia. Fortunately, acute vascular insufficiency is uncommon. The vascular status of the extremity is judged by skin color, temperature of the extremity, functioning of the arm, amount of pain, and radial pulse. The elbow has excellent collateral circulation that usually provides sufficient blood flow to the arm even if the brachial artery is damaged.[105, 116, 118, 175, 212, 214] The mere absence of the radial pulse on palpation is not an indication of vascular insufficiency. In fact, the radial pulse may be absent because of spasm, only to return after reduction of the fracture. Loss of the pulse during reduction may indicate obstruction from too much elbow flexion or entrapment of the artery in the fracture. Absence of the pulse on palpation and by Doppler is significant and means that an arterial injury is probably present. Some authors believe that absence of pulse with the use of Doppler is an indication for arterial exploration.

Campbell and associates studied 59 children with supracondylar humeral fractures.[31, 209] They found a higher incidence (19%) of vascular abnormality than others have, although 5 of the 11 children had absent pulses that returned after fracture reduction and required no further treatment. The other six patients underwent exploration of the brachial artery. The artery was interposed in the fracture in one patient and lacerated in one, and one had an intimal tear. The other three patients were found to have spasm that resolved without other treatment. They recommend vascular exploration if the radial pulse is absent after reduction of the fracture.

Copley and coworkers reviewed 128 children with grade III supracondylar fractures of the humerus.[38] Seventeen of the children had absent or diminished (detected on Doppler but not on palpation) radial pulses on initial examination.[38, 213] Fourteen of the 17 recovered pulses after fracture reduction, but the remaining 3 had persistent absence of the radial pulse. These patients underwent arterial exploration of the brachial artery immediately, and a significant vascular injury requiring repair was found in each. In 2 of the 14 patients whose pulses returned after fracture reduction, progressive postoperative deterioration in their circulation developed during the first 24 to 36 hours after reduction, with loss of the radial pulse. Both had arteriograms that identified arterial injuries, and both underwent exploration and vascular repair. These investigators found that absence of the radial pulse after immediate reduction of a supracondylar humeral fracture indicated the existence of a significant arterial injury requiring surgical exploration and vascular repair. They stated that arteriography is not indicated because the location of the arterial injury is always at the level of the fracture. Although arterial spasm may have the same clinical appearance as true vascular injury, the signs and symptoms should improve significantly within 1 to 3 hours after reduction of the

fracture. The flow chart that they used when deciding how to treat these injuries when the vascular status is not completely normal probably represents treatment that is more aggressive than necessary (Fig. 9–18). If the vascular status of the injured extremity is normal before and after reduction of the fracture, only splinting and observation are necessary. If the pulse is absent (i.e., not palpable and not detectable on Doppler) after fracture reduction, they state that vascular repair is necessary. As seen in the following paragraphs, other authors have shown that arterial repair is not necessary even if the radial pulse remains absent after fracture reduction as long as the distal circulation of the arm is normal.

Schoenecker and colleagues agreed with these other authors in recommending arterial exploration in the absence of a Doppler-detectable radial pulse.[181] They explored seven patients without a radial pulse after a supracondylar fracture and found that four arteries were either kinked or entrapped in the fracture. They repaired three of the arteries. On the other hand, Garbuz and associates reviewed 326 patients with supracondylar fractures of the distal end of the humerus and found 22 patients with absence of the radial pulse on examination.[74] Fifteen of the radial pulses returned after fracture reduction, and they were monitored without exploration of the brachial artery. Seven patients had persistent absence of the radial pulse after reduction together with a dysvascular hand, and all underwent arterial exploration with arterial repair. They recommend that patients with an absent radial pulse but good circulation to the hand need only observation after fracture reduction because the collateral circulation around the elbow is

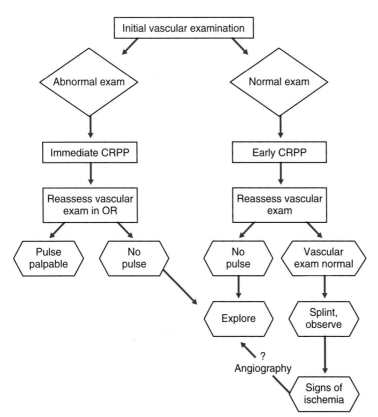

**FIGURE 9–18.** Flow chart to guide decision making in cases in which a possible vascular injury is associated with a displaced supracondylar humeral fracture. CRPP, closed reduction and percutaneous pinning; OR, operating room. (Redrawn from Copley, L.A., et al. J Pediatr Orthop 16:99–103, 1996.)

excellent and will provide the arm and hand with excellent blood flow.[74, 181, 186, 208]

Sabharwal and colleagues reviewed patients with supracondylar fractures of the distal end of the humerus and found that 13 of 410 fractures did not have a radial pulse.[178] All the patients without a radial pulse had adequate collateral circulation as demonstrated by magnetic resonance angiography, duplex scanning, or both. They performed arterial exploration in all these patients and found an arterial injury in all of them. Arterial repair was performed in all patients; however, asymptomatic reocclusion and residual stenosis were observed in these patients in follow-up. They recommend observation of patients with supracondylar humeral fractures and an associated absent radial pulse. They reason that the collateral circulation is adequate for the normal survival and use of the upper extremity and they further state that if the brachial artery is repaired, it is likely to become occluded as a result of insufficient flow.[78, 178]

The first step in the management of supracondylar fractures of the humerus with an absent radial pulse and adequate distal circulation is closed reduction under general anesthesia. If the circulation remains good, the fracture is pinned and splinted and then merely observed. The only indication for arterial exploration is restricted to those with a truly dysvascular arm after fracture reduction. An arteriogram may be performed in the operating room before repair of the artery is undertaken; however, the location of the lesion is at the level of the fracture and an arteriogram will probably not reveal anything that is not already known. Ligation of the artery to eliminate spasm, though once popular, is not indicated. Open reduction and pin fixation of the fracture are also performed.

Some authors have recommended the use of traction in the face of vascular insufficiency.[81, 154, 181] If the circulation improves, they advise continuing the entire treatment of the fracture with the use of traction. If the circulation does not improve within 1 hour of initiation of traction, however, arterial exploration is recommended. Such management is no longer considered appropriate treatment of a supracondylar humeral fracture. Reduction plus pin fixation is the treatment of choice, and as seen earlier, arterial exploration is indicated only in the event of a truly dysvascular extremity. Simple absence of the radial pulse with good peripheral circulation is not an indication for arterial exploration and repair.

Volkmann's ischemia is most common in fractures treated with the elbow flexed acutely. Fortunately, it is much less frequent with the use of traction, percutaneous pinning, or open reduction and pinning. For that reason, closed reduction and flexion treatment of this fracture are not recommended. Pinning of the fracture allows the elbow to be extended sufficiently to decrease the risk of ischemia.

The signs and symptoms of forearm ischemia are well known. Pain should alert one to its presence, and pain with passive finger extension is an early sign.[81, 152] Measurement of compartment pressure and early fasciotomy if the pressure is high help reduce the risk of permanent damage. Pain is the hallmark of an impending

compartment syndrome; however, I had one referral patient and was told of another in whom complete Volkmann's ischemia developed without pain. I reviewed the medical record of the referred child, and all the nurses' and physicians' notes documented that the child was comfortable and required no pain medication. However, progressively deteriorating neurologic status was documented and was the only clinical sign of compartment ischemia. Although such instances are undoubtedly very rare, they alert one to the possibility of a so-called silent compartment syndrome.

## NEUROLOGIC INJURY

The incidence of neurologic injury varies greatly in published reports, with some authors reporting few, if any, and others reporting an incidence as high as 15%.[14, 41, 67, 71, 102, 118, 132, 192] It has been shown that the risk of nerve injury is increased with increasing fracture displacement.[81, 111, 152] Most series report that radial nerve injury is the most common, followed by median nerve injury; ulnar nerve injury is the least common. Brown and Zinar[28] found 19 patients with 23 nerve injuries in 162 supracondylar humeral fractures. Twelve radial, 6 ulnar, and 5 median neuropathies were detected. They believed, however, that four of the ulnar nerve injuries and one radial nerve injury were iatrogenic and resulted from both percutaneous pinning and open reduction and internal fixation. Michael and Stanislas have recommended using a nerve stimulator on a needle when performing percutaneous pinning through the medial epicondyle to avoid injury to the ulnar nerve.[138] Spinner and Schreiber[192] reported a high incidence of injury to the anterior interosseous nerve with supracondylar fracture of the distal end of the humerus. My colleagues and I also found that injury to this nerve is the most common with supracondylar fractures.[44] Our study identified 15 nerve injuries in 101 patients. Of these 15 injuries, 6 were isolated to the anterior interosseous nerve, and 4 others involved anterior interosseous nerve injury in combination with another nerve injury. Because this nerve is purely a motor nerve, injury to it can be detected only if flexion of the distal joints of the thumb and index fingers is tested; it is therefore possible to miss such an injury. The incidence of anterior interosseous nerve injury seems to be greater than has been appreciated in the past, and it may be the most common nerve injury as a result of this fracture.

Spinner and Schreiber[192] found that the nerve passes through a fibrous arch 2 to 3 cm below the joint. This fibrous arch, which arises from the deep head of the pronator teres, may tether the nerve and cause it to stretch with anterior displacement of the proximal fragment of the distal end of the humerus. The relatively ulnar position of the anterior interosseous nerve suggests that fractures with posterolateral displacement are more likely to cause tethering of the nerve with subsequent nerve injury.[59]

Regardless of the nerve injured, almost all reports found that these nerves recover spontaneously.[28, 39, 41, 44, 59, 71, 95, 102] Routine nerve exploration was not recommended by these authors unless no nerve recovery at all occurred within 3 months. Jones and Louis[102] reported recovery beginning as late as 4 to 5 months after injury. It is recommended, however, that nerve exploration be performed if nerve function deteriorates during or after closed reduction of the fracture because of the likelihood of nerve entrapment in the fracture site.[71, 117] Amillo and Mora recommended that if nerve recovery is not seen within a reasonable period, nerve exploration should be undertaken as early as possible because in their experience nerve recovery was less predictable if nerve exploration was performed after 1 year postinjury.[5]

## CUBITUS VARUS

Cubitus varus is the most common persistent deformity resulting from malreduction or loss of reduction of supracondylar fractures. The reported incidence of this deformity varies widely, from a low of 0% to a high of 60%.[8, 10, 42, 54, 81, 121, 133] This deformity is not the result of growth arrest of the distal humeral physis, although some authors have clung to this belief.[92, 96] Some believe that lateral growth stimulation resulting from the fracture produces the varus deformity.[13, 27, 96, 156] Medial tilt of the distal fragment producing varus deformity is almost universally accepted as the cause, however.[57, 67, 75, 113, 187, 189] Because of the anatomy of the distal end of the humerus, with its very thin metaphysis, nearly anatomic reduction is necessary to allow the proximal and distal medial columns of the humerus to abut and provide fracture stability. Lack of contact of the two medial columns, which results from persistent posterior rotation of the medial side of the distal fragment, allows the fracture to tilt into varus. Therefore, this deformity is best prevented by obtaining anatomic reduction of the fracture and then stabilizing it with medial and lateral pins. If anatomic reduction cannot be obtained, open reduction and pin fixation are necessary to obtain stable anatomic reduction.

Detection of this deformity requires full elbow extension, which may help explain the impression that this deformity occurs after the fracture has healed. If the fracture is immobilized for a prolonged period, loss of elbow extension may persist. The deformity may not be recognized until full elbow extension is finally achieved.

Although the cubitus varus, or gunstock, deformity may be unsightly, it does not limit function,[9, 57] and because it is the result of malunion, it does not progress. It has long been thought that this deformity was of cosmetic importance alone; however, Abe and associates reported on 15 patients with tardy ulnar nerve palsy caused by cubitus varus deformity. The mean interval between fracture and the onset of symptoms was 15 years. Their operative findings suggest that the main cause of the palsy was compression by a fibrous band running between the two heads of the flexor carpi ulnaris. Surgical treatment included release of the fibrous band in 14 patients, with anterior subcutaneous transfer of the ulnar nerve in 5 of them. Eleven also underwent corrective osteotomy.[2] Another theory regarding the cause of tardy ulnar palsy associated with cubitus varus deformity was mentioned in a study by Mitsunari and colleagues.[142] They found internal rotation deformity associated with cubitus varus in five patients with tardy ulnar nerve palsy. Although an association can undoubtedly be found between cubitus varus and internal rotation deformity—because it has been shown that the internal rotation position of the fracture allows medial tilt of the fracture into varus—these authors have not proved a cause and effect. Spinner and colleagues have also noticed an association between cubitus varus and ulnar neuropathy.[193] They found that varus deformity of the distal end of the humerus leads to snapping of the medial portion of the triceps and the ulnar nerve, which results in the nerve injury. They treated the deformity with valgus osteotomy with or without lateral translation of the medial portion of the triceps. They also performed medial epicondylectomy on some of the patients.

Davids and associates identified six cases of lateral condyle fracture of the humerus in children with preexisting cubitus varus caused by malunion of a previous supracondylar humeral fracture. They stated that both the torsional moment and the shear force generated across the capitellar physis by a routine fall are increased by varus malalignment.[47] It therefore appears that a cubitus deformity may predispose a child to subsequent lateral condylar fracture. Takahara and Sasaki have also found an increased incidence of fracture of the lateral condyle or fracture of the distal humeral physis in patients with a cubitus varus deformity.[200]

Correction of the deformity is easiest when the child is approaching skeletal maturity because solid fixation can be achieved without concern for the distal humeral physis. Ippolito and associates[97] found that the correction deteriorated with continued growth in patients who underwent osteotomy to correct cubitus varus. Most patients and their families desire correction when the deformity is noticed. Several methods of correction have been proposed. King and Secor[110] proposed a medial opening wedge osteotomy that is fixed with Steinmann pins and a Riedel clamp. Coventry and Henderson[41] prefer a lateral closing wedge osteotomy for correction. Other authors are concerned about both loss of correction and undercorrection with this approach.[170, 201] If this type of osteotomy is stabilized with K-wires, the arm should be immobilized in extension to better control the correction. Oppenheim and associates[153] believe that a critical angle must be achieved for insertion of the lateral pin. If the angle is too acute, the pin will slide off the opposite cortex of the humerus; if the angle is too obtuse, the pin will not cross the osteotomy site.

Gaddy and colleagues reported good or excellent results in 12 children who underwent osteotomy for correction of cubitus varus deformity of the distal end of the humerus.[72] They performed closing wedge, laterally based distal humeral osteotomies through a lateral incision. They determined the preoperative carrying angle by measuring the angle formed by the intersection of the longitudinal axis of the upper part of the arm and the forearm with the elbow in full extension and the forearm in supination. They also measured the radiographic humerus-elbow-wrist angle, which was compared with the same angle of the opposite normal arm. The size of the laterally based wedge is plotted on preoperative radiographs. The osteotomy is then planned with the wedge proximal to the olecranon fossa. The osteotomies are stabilized with crossed medial and lateral K-wires.

Others have been concerned about loss of correction of the cubitus varus deformity when the fixation consists of percutaneous pins. Hernandez and Roach reported on 23 patients who underwent osteotomy for correction of cubitus varus and found that 10 had poor results because of loss of correction secondary to the instability of internal fixation with crossed pins. They recommended the use of a lateral two-hole plate plus a medial pin for internal fixation, although they did not report their results with this technique.[85] Devnani also used a two-hole plate to stabilize the osteotomy. In addition, he recommended completion of the osteotomy to enable medial displacement because a prominent lateral condyle will result if the distal fragment is displaced medially.[55]

Because of the risk of loss of correction with pin fixation, French[71] described fixation of a lateral closing wedge osteotomy with the use of two screws linked with a wire. The screws are placed on either side of the osteotomy. To help correct the rotational deformity, the two screws may be offset. With the elbow extended, the osteotomy is closed and a wire is placed around the two screws and then tightened. Correction of the carrying angle can then be checked with the elbow extended and the forearm supinated. Bellemore and colleagues[19] also used this technique and obtained better results than with pin fixation.

DeRosa and Graziano[54] described an osteotomy that they attribute to Lloyd-Roberts in which the inferior cut of the osteotomy does not reach the lateral cortex; instead, it stops 0.5 cm short and is connected to the proximal cut with a vertical cut. This approach leaves a lateral spike of bone attached to the distal fragment. Once the osteotomy is closed, it can be stabilized with a single screw placed from the lateral spike across the osteotomy (Fig. 9–19). Others have recommended a step-cut osteotomy but recognize that this technique should be used only for small deformities of less than 30°; otherwise, a prominent lateral condyle will result.[109]

Most of the published techniques to correct cubitus varus have focused on the angular deformity alone. As has been shown, cubitus varus results from an initial uncorrected internal rotation deformity of the distal fragment that allows the fracture to tilt into varus. Wong and Balasubramaniam measured humeral torsion in patients with a cubitus varus deformity and found that the arm with the deformity had 30° more internal rotation of the distal end of the humerus than did the normal side. Nevertheless, they corrected the deformity with a simple laterally based closing wedge osteotomy and stated that correction of the humeral torsion was not essential for correction of the deformity.[216]

A three-dimensional osteotomy to correct the varus, internal rotation, and extension deformity has been proposed. The authors of this technique state that this osteotomy achieves wider bony contact and is more stable than a simple lateral closing wedge osteotomy.[205, 206]

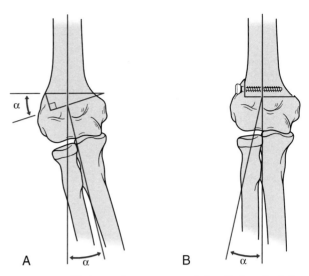

**FIGURE 9–19.** Closing wedge osteotomy of the distal end of the humerus. *A,* The osteotomy is designed to correct the varus deformity of the distal part of the humerus; a small buttress of metaphysis is left to allow for screw fixation of the osteotomy. *B,* The appearance of the osteotomy after the wedge of bone has been removed and the osteotomy has been stabilized with a screw.

Regardless of the type of osteotomy performed and the type of fixation used, one may approach the distal end of the humerus either laterally or posteriorly. The lateral approach allows direct access to the lateral aspect of the distal part of the humerus. The humerus is then exposed subperiosteally. The advantage of this approach is that the elbow may be visualized both clinically and by radiography anteriorly. Some have recommended the posterior triceps-splitting approach to the distal end of the humerus.[24] The ulnar nerve is easily protected, and the deformity is visualized directly. The disadvantage of this approach is the inability to visualize the elbow anteriorly.

### Author's Preferred Method of Treatment

The osteotomy is performed by creating a laterally based closing wedge through the supracondylar region of the distal end of the humerus. The distal portion of the humerus may be approached laterally through the interval between the brachioradialis and extensor carpi radialis longus muscles anteriorly and the triceps posteriorly. The radial nerve is protected anteriorly in this muscle wad; however, too much retraction must be avoided to prevent stretching of the radial nerve. The periosteum is split and the humerus is exposed subperiosteally both anteriorly and posteriorly. The size of the wedge to be removed can be determined preoperatively as shown by Oppenheim and colleagues.[152] They recommend making a tracing of an anteroposterior radiograph of the normal arm and then reversing it and placing it over the anteroposterior radiograph of the affected arm. The humerus-elbow-wrist angle is determined for both arms. A cutout simulating the laterally based closing wedge is then performed, with the desired angle arranged so that it is 2 cm above the olecranon fossa. The two limbs of the osteotomy should be of equal length. If the lower limb is longer than the upper limb, the prominence of the lateral epicondyle will be accentuated. Pin fixation may be used. Both the medial and lateral pins may be inserted to the level of the lower limb of the osteotomy before completion of the osteotomy if one prefers. If one leaves the medial cortex intact but very thin, it can be "cracked" as the closing wedge is closed. This technique creates a fairly stable osteotomy. Unfortunately, in patients with a moderately severe deformity, this type of osteotomy will leave a prominent lateral condyle, which can be eliminated by completing the osteotomy and translating the distal fragment medially (Fig. 9–20).

## Flexion-Type Supracondylar Fracture

Flexion-type fractures are much less common than the extension type. Wilkins[214] estimated the incidence to be about 2.5% of all supracondylar fractures; Fowles and Kassab[67] found the incidence to be slightly higher. This fracture is the result of a fall on the point of the flexed elbow. When children with this injury are seen in an emergency department, the elbow is held flexed, in contrast to the extended elbow seen with the extension type of supracondylar fracture. These fractures are more stable in extension than flexion because the anterior periosteum is intact. However, a long arm cast with the elbow extended is cumbersome.

Rang[166] found that this type of cast would not stay on, and he attached a pelvic band to help keep the cast in place.

Treatment of this fracture is similar to treatment of the extension type. If the fracture is nondisplaced, simple immobilization is all that is necessary. If the distal fragment is merely angulated anteriorly, reduction and immobilization with the elbow in extension are usually successful (Fig. 9–21). If the fracture is displaced, closed reduction and pinning should be performed. Fowles and Kassab[67] had better results with open reduction and pin fixation. They found that the distal fragment had become buttonholed through the triceps in fractures that were not reducible.

## FRACTURE-SEPARATION OF THE DISTAL HUMERAL PHYSIS

### Incidence

The exact incidence of this injury is not known because it has been underdiagnosed.[46] DeLee and colleagues[53] reviewed three cases of infantile supracondylar fractures that had been reported by MacAfee and concluded that these were actually fracture-separations of the distal humeral physis. At one time, this injury was thought to

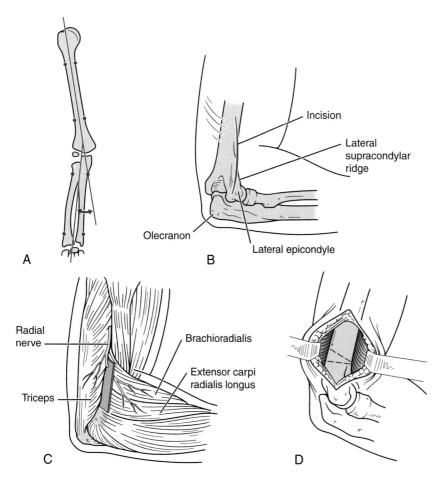

FIGURE 9–20. Author's preferred method of a closing wedge osteotomy of the distal end of the humerus for correction of cubitus varus. *A,* The best method of measuring the true cubitus varus of the distal end of the humerus. The humerus-elbow-wrist (HEW) angle is measured by drawing a line along the longitudinal axis of the humerus. This line intersects a line drawn from the middle of the distal end of the humerus to the ulnar aspect of the distal end of the radius. *B,* The incision is longitudinal over the lateral supracondylar ridge of the humerus. *C,* The interval between the triceps and the brachioradialis is developed to reflect the brachioradialis and the extensor radialis longus and brevis anteriorly and the triceps posteriorly. The radial nerve is protected anteriorly under the brachioradialis. *D,* The distal portion of the humerus is exposed laterally and the base of the osteotomy is outlined on the lateral cortex of the distal end of the humerus.

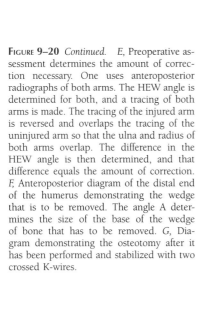

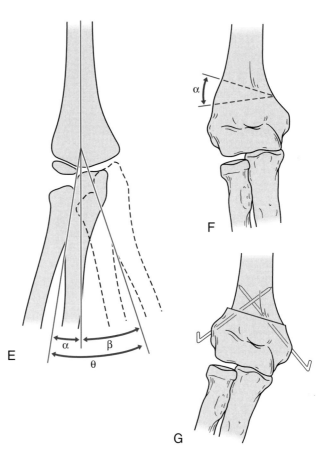

FIGURE **9–20** *Continued.* *E,* Preoperative assessment determines the amount of correction necessary. One uses anteroposterior radiographs of both arms. The HEW angle is determined for both, and a tracing of both arms is made. The tracing of the injured arm is reversed and overlaps the tracing of the uninjured arm so that the ulna and radius of both arms overlap. The difference in the HEW angle is then determined, and that difference equals the amount of correction. *F,* Anteroposterior diagram of the distal end of the humerus demonstrating the wedge that is to be removed. The angle A determines the size of the base of the wedge of bone that has to be removed. *G,* Diagram demonstrating the osteotomy after it has been performed and stabilized with two crossed K-wires.

be very rare; however, it is now seen and recognized more frequently.

## Mechanisms of Injury

Three clear mechanisms of injury seem to be the cause of this fracture. It may be the result of birth trauma. One must be able to differentiate this injury from brachial plexus palsy because neonates frequently do not move a painful extremity, thereby mimicking paralysis. Holda and coworkers[94] reported that after the neonatal period, a fall from a height was the cause of the fractures in their series. However, three of their seven patients were younger than 1½ years old, which makes child abuse more likely. DeLee and colleagues reported that child abuse was proved or suspected in six of their sixteen patients.[53] One must therefore strongly suspect the possibility of child abuse if this fracture is seen in a young child.

## Classification

DeLee and colleagues[53] based their classification of this injury on the age of the child and the presence or absence of ossification of the capitellum. Type A occurs in infants from birth to 9 months of age. No ossification center is present in the capitellum at this age, and no metaphyseal bony fragment is attached to the distal fragment. Type B

occurs in children 7 months to 3 years of age. The ossification center of the capitellum is present radiographically, and a fragment of the metaphysis (Thurston-Holland sign) may or may not be displaced with the epiphysis. Type C occurs in children 3 to 7 years of age. The capitellum is well ossified, and a large Thurston-Holland metaphyseal fragment is seen on the radiograph. This latter injury must be distinguished from a lateral condylar fracture.

## Diagnosis

These children present with marked swelling about the elbow; the physical appearance of the joint resembles that of an elbow dislocation. Gentle manipulation of the elbow reveals a muffled crepitus that is thought to be diagnostic of epiphyseal separation. It is the result of two cartilaginous surfaces rubbing together and should be distinguished from bony crepitus.

On anteroposterior radiographs, the radius and ulna are displaced in relation to the humerus. However, the radius and ulna are in their normal relationship to each other. This injury must be distinguished radiographically from an elbow dislocation, a displaced fracture of the lateral condyle of the humerus, and a supracondylar fracture of the distal end of the humerus.

On an anteroposterior radiograph of a normal elbow, a line drawn along the longitudinal axis of the radius

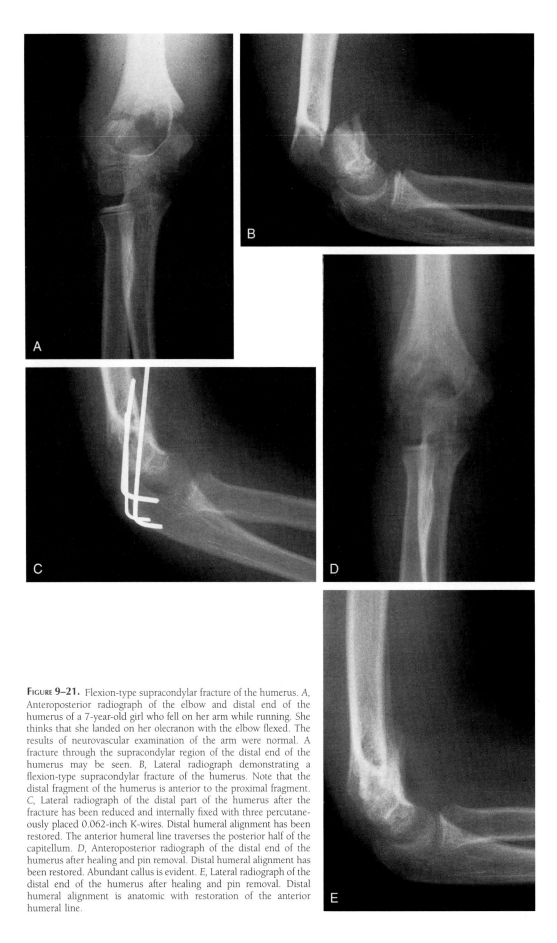

**FIGURE 9–21.** Flexion-type supracondylar fracture of the humerus. *A*, Anteroposterior radiograph of the elbow and distal end of the humerus of a 7-year-old girl who fell on her arm while running. She thinks that she landed on her olecranon with the elbow flexed. The results of neurovascular examination of the arm were normal. A fracture through the supracondylar region of the distal end of the humerus may be seen. *B*, Lateral radiograph demonstrating a flexion-type supracondylar fracture of the humerus. Note that the distal fragment of the humerus is anterior to the proximal fragment. *C*, Lateral radiograph of the distal part of the humerus after the fracture has been reduced and internally fixed with three percutaneously placed 0.062-inch K-wires. Distal humeral alignment has been restored. The anterior humeral line traverses the posterior half of the capitellum. *D*, Anteroposterior radiograph of the distal end of the humerus after healing and pin removal. Distal humeral alignment has been restored. Abundant callus is evident. *E*, Lateral radiograph of the distal end of the humerus after healing and pin removal. Distal humeral alignment is anatomic with restoration of the anterior humeral line.

passes through the capitellum regardless of the position of the elbow. If this line does not pass through the capitellum, dislocation of the radius, elbow dislocation, or a displaced fracture of the lateral condyle of the distal end of the humerus is present. In a fracture-separation of the distal humeral physis, the relationship of the radius to the capitellum remains intact; however, the radius and ulna lose their normal relationship with the distal end of the humerus. In addition, the capitellum is displaced medially with the radius and ulna because a fracture-separation of the distal humeral physis is usually displaced medially, whereas an elbow dislocation is generally displaced laterally (Fig. 9–22).

A displaced fracture of the lateral condyle of the distal part of the humerus may be distinguished by the fact that the radius and ulna retain their normal relationship with the humerus; however, because the capitellum is displaced, the radius does not retain its normal relationship with it. A supracondylar fracture is uncommon in the very young. Furthermore, a fracture line should be seen above the epiphysis.

In the very young (before the capitellum has ossified), a fracture-separation is most easily confused with elbow dislocation. Elbow dislocation is very uncommon in this age group, however. In addition, the forearm is displaced laterally with dislocation of the elbow. The radius and ulna are displaced medially in relation to the epiphysis of the distal end of the humerus with a fracture-separation of the distal humeral physis. Arthrography of the elbow joint may assist with the diagnosis, especially when the capitellum has not yet ossified (Fig. 9–23). Others have shown that arthrography may be necessary to distinguish a lateral condylar fracture from a Salter-Harris type II fracture of the distal humeral physis.[1, 52] Ultrasonography may also be used to help identify this injury[125] (Fig. 9–24).

## Treatment

Unlike a supracondylar fracture, this fracture is usually stable because it occurs through the thicker distal end of the humerus below the thin supracondylar region. It would appear that cubitus varus deformity is less likely to develop as a complication of this fracture than it is after a supracondylar fracture.[46] Nevertheless, Holda and coworkers[94] found that a cubitus varus deformity developed in five of their seven patients. Two other articles that reviewed the results of treatment of this fracture found a high and unacceptable rate of cubitus varus deformity.[1, 52] The conclusion of these authors was that accurate reduction and pin fixation are necessary to prevent cubitus varus deformity.

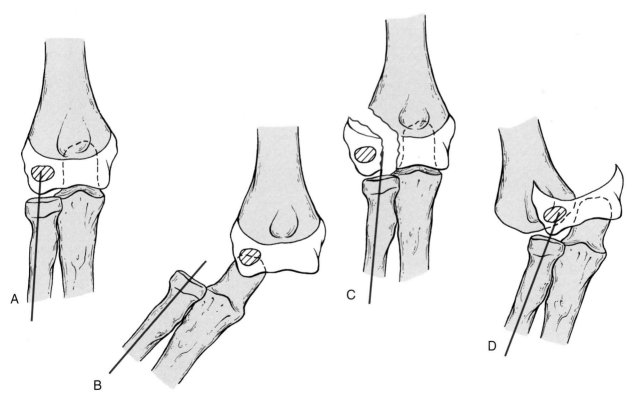

**FIGURE 9–22.** Comparison of injuries about the distal end of the humerus. *A,* Normal distal humeral relationships. *B,* Dislocation of the elbow. A line drawn along the longitudinal axis of the radius no longer intersects the capitellum. The capitellum, however, maintains its normal relationship to the distal end of the humerus. *C,* Displaced fracture of the lateral condyle. The longitudinal axis of the proximal part of the radius does not intersect the capitellum, and the capitellum is displaced from its normal position on the distal metaphysis of the humerus. *D,* Fracture-separation of the distal humeral physis. Note that the capitellum is displaced from its normal position on the lateral side of the distal humeral metaphysis but maintains its normal relationship with the radial head. (Adapted from DeLee, J.C.; et al. J Bone Joint Surg Am 62:46, 1980.)

DeLee and colleagues[53] recommend closed reduction if the fracture is fresh; however, if the fracture is old, they recommend splinting the arm until the fracture is solid, with no attempt at reduction. The findings of Holda and coworkers[94] tend to corroborate this strategy because

their results with more aggressive treatment were poor. Mizuno and associates[143] obtained good results with open reduction through a posterior approach.

With this injury, my preference is to first investigate the possibility of child abuse. If necessary, the child can

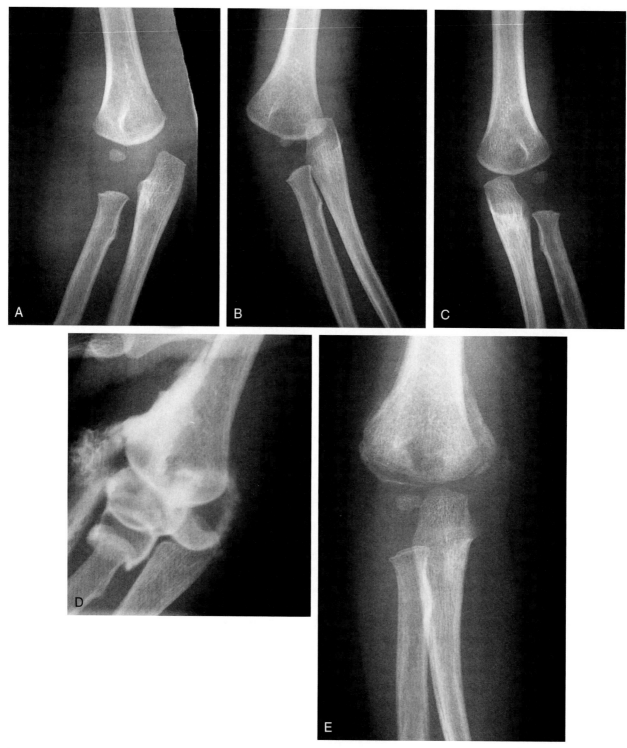

FIGURE 9–23. Fracture-separation of the distal humeral physis. *A,* Anteroposterior radiograph of the injured extremity. The capitellum is displaced medially. *B,* Anteroposterior stress view of the same elbow demonstrating the marked instability and further displacement of the capitellum medially. *C,* Anteroposterior view of the opposite normal extremity showing the normal relationship between the capitellum and the distal humeral metaphysis. *D,* Arthrogram of the elbow showing that the capitellum and proximal end of the radius are well aligned and that the capitellum is displaced medially. *E,* An anteroposterior radiograph of the same elbow 3 weeks after injury shows healing of the fracture. The capitellum remains slightly displaced medially.

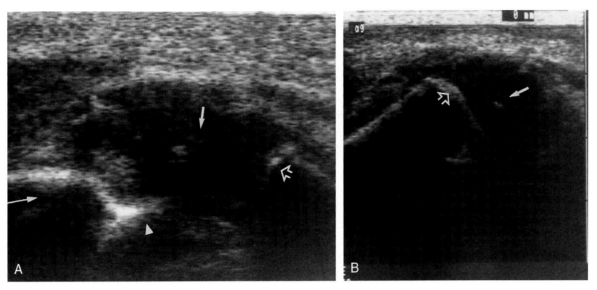

**FIGURE 9–24.** Ultrasound images of the elbow of a 17-month-old infant with a type I distal humeral fracture. *A,* A sagittal posterior sonogram shows a fracture *(triangle)* through the physis. The *thin arrow* on the left points to the distal end of the humerus. The *vertical arrow* points to the displaced capitellum. Ossification of the capitellum can be seen. The head of the radius is articulating with the capitellum *(open arrow).* *B,* Posterolateral sonogram after reduction of the fracture. The *open arrow* points to the distal humeral physis. The capitellum can be seen in its normal position *(closed arrow).* The distal end of the humerus is seen just underneath the *open arrow.* (Courtesy of Dr. R. S. Davidson.)

be admitted to the hospital to facilitate this inquiry. Admission may also be warranted to observe for circulatory change. If the fracture is not recent and the child has radiographic evidence of healing, simple immobilization is indicated (Fig. 9–25). If reduction is required, closed reduction and percutaneous pinning are probably warranted because of the reported high incidence of cubitus varus deformity resulting from simple

immobilization of this fracture. Closed reduction is performed by placing gentle traction on the forearm. The medial displacement of the distal fragment is then corrected. Any malrotation is corrected, and the elbow is flexed to 90° and then pinned as one does for a supracondylar fracture of the distal end of the humerus. The arm is splinted for 3 weeks, after which the pins are removed and unrestricted motion is allowed.

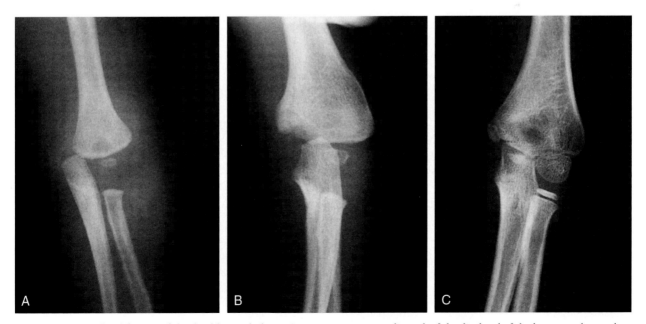

**FIGURE 9–25.** Displaced fracture of the distal humeral physis. *A,* An anteroposterior radiograph of the distal end of the humerus taken at the time of injury demonstrates medial displacement of the capitellum. Note that the longitudinal axis of the radius intersects the capitellum. *B,* Anteroposterior radiograph of the elbow 3 months after injury. The displacement was not corrected at the time of immobilization. *C,* A follow-up radiograph 5 years after injury demonstrates remodeling of the distal end of the humerus. Clinically, the patient had full mobility in the elbow.

# FRACTURE OF THE LATERAL CONDYLE OF THE HUMERUS

## Incidence

This fracture is relatively common and occurs in 12% to 16.8% of fractures about the elbow in children.[66, 139]

## Mechanisms of Injury

Two theories on the cause of this fracture have been proposed. Avulsion of the lateral condyle of the humerus may result from a fall on the outstretched hand with the forearm supinated. A varus force on the arm transmits the force through the forearm extensor musculature to its attachment on the lateral condyle of the humerus and results in avulsion of the condyle.[99, 165, 174] Using a similar mechanism, Jakob and colleagues were able to reproduce this injury in young cadavers, thus confirming this force as a possible etiology[99] (Fig. 9–26). Both Stimson[196] and Fahey,[62] however, believed that this fracture was the result of a compression injury. Stimson[196] produced this fracture in cadavers with a force directed to the outstretched hand with the elbow flexed. Undoubtedly, both mechanisms of injury are possible.

## Classification

Milch[139] classified this fracture according to the location of the fracture line through the distal part of the

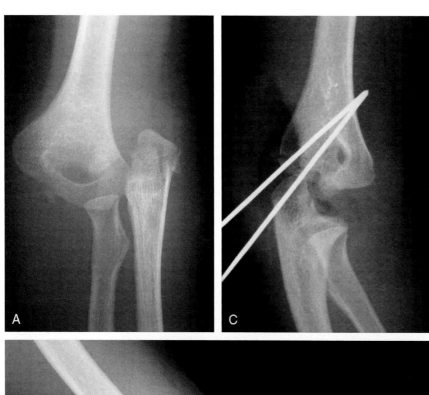

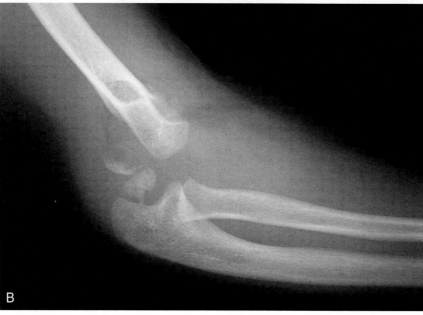

FIGURE 9–26. Displaced fracture of the lateral condyle of the distal end of the humerus with a nondisplaced fracture of the olecranon. *A,* An anteroposterior radiograph demonstrates the fracture of the olecranon and medial displacement of the capitellum. From this radiograph one can appreciate that the injury occurred with a varus force with the elbow in extension. The capitellum was therefore avulsed. *B,* Lateral radiograph showing the injury to be a fracture of the lateral condyle, including the entire capitellum and a portion of the distal humeral metaphysis. *C,* Postreduction intraoperative radiograph of the distal end of the humerus showing reduction and pinning of the fracture.

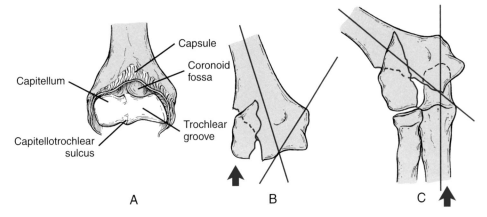

FIGURE 9–27. *A,* Drawing of the distal end of the humerus showing the trochlear groove and the capitellotrochlear sulcus. *B,* Type I fracture of the lateral condyle. The fracture line is lateral to the trochlear groove. The relationship between the proximal portion of the forearm and distal end of the humerus remains intact. The capitellum may be displaced partially or totally. *C,* The fracture line goes through the trochlear groove and is making the elbow joint unstable. The radius and ulna may therefore become displaced laterally.

humerus. If the fracture line is lateral to the trochlear groove, the fracture may or may not become displaced; however, the elbow joint does not dislocate (Fig. 9–27). As long as some or all of the trochlea remains unfractured, it serves as a lateral buttress for the coronoid-olecranon ridge of the ulna and prevents lateral displacement of the ulna. This fracture, termed type I by Milch, may cross through the ossification center of the capitellum (Fig. 9–28), or it may go through a portion of the trochlea and leave the capitellum intact (Fig. 9–29). The fracture line in a type II fracture lies at or medial to the trochlear groove. As a consequence of the loss of trochlear abutment, the ulna and radius are displaced laterally (Fig. 9–30). Mirsky and associates reviewed their experience with lateral condylar fractures in children and

found that the classic Milch classification is not accurate.[141] They stated that 52% of fractures classified as type II were in reality not type II fractures. Eight percent of the fractures were either through the capitellotrochlear groove or beyond it through the trochlear epiphysis. The remaining 20% of the fractures actually exited through the distal humeral physis medially.

Salter and Harris[179] classified these fractures as type IV fractures because the fracture line begins in the metaphysis, crosses the physis, and enters into the epiphysis. Some believe that because the trochlea is not ossified at the age when this fracture usually occurs, the fracture does not actually cross the physis and should therefore be called a type II fracture in the Salter-Harris classification.[22] Although this point is technically correct

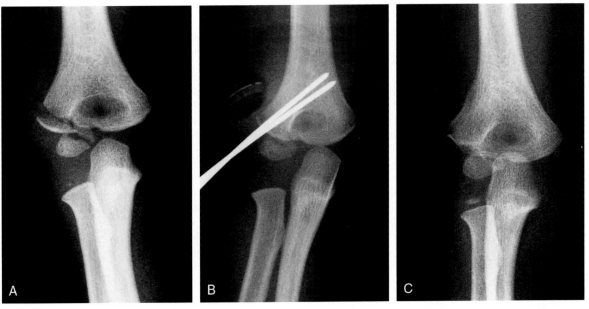

FIGURE 9–28. Milch type I fracture of the lateral condyle of the distal end of the humerus. *A,* An anteroposterior radiograph of the distal end of the humerus demonstrates a lateral condylar fracture. Note that the fracture line crosses the distal humeral physis and then crosses the center of ossification of the capitellum. *B,* Intraoperative anteroposterior radiograph with two pins holding the fracture reduced in an anatomic position. *C,* Seven months after surgery, the fracture is healed, as seen on this radiograph, and the patient has full elbow function.

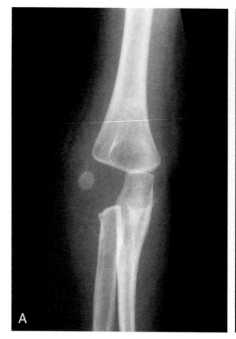
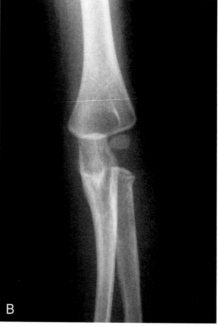

FIGURE 9–29. *A,* Anteroposterior radiograph of the distal end of the humerus in a child who sustained a displaced type I fracture of the lateral condyle. Note that the capitellum is displaced laterally but that the radius and ulna have maintained their normal relationship with the distal end of the humerus. *B,* Anteroposterior radiograph of the opposite elbow for comparison. The capitellum is in its normal position in relation to the distal end of the humerus, and the head of the radius articulates with the capitellum.

and the risk of growth arrest of the physis is probably less when the trochlea is not ossified, the fracture does indeed fulfill the Salter-Harris criteria for a type IV fracture.

Jakob and colleagues[99] also classified this fracture according to the amount of displacement of the capitellum seen radiographically (Fig. 9–31). A type I fracture is actually a partial fracture that is nondisplaced. The fracture line does not go through the entire cartilaginous epiphysis, and therefore the joint surface is intact. This fracture may be able to be treated without surgical reduction. A type II fracture is a complete fracture that extends completely through the articular surface. The capitellum may be laterally displaced, but it is not rotated (Fig. 9–32). A type III fracture is completely displaced, and the capitellum is rotated out of the joint. The normal relationship of the proximal end of the radius to the capitellum is completely lost (see Fig. 9–28). Finnbogason and associates also classified nondisplaced or minimally displaced lateral condylar fractures (2-mm or less displacement) into three categories according to the amount of displacement.[63] Type A fractures have a minimal or no fracture gap on the radial or dorsal radial aspect of the fracture. In addition, the fracture line does not continue all the way to the epiphyseal cartilage (Fig. 9–33). Type B fractures are identical to type A fractures, except that the fracture line can be followed all the way to the epiphyseal cartilage. The lateral fracture gap is larger than the medial gap (Fig. 9–34). Type C fractures demonstrate a fracture line that extends all the way to the epiphyseal cartilage and is as wide medially as it is laterally (Fig. 9–35).

## Diagnosis

Clinically, swelling of the elbow that is most marked laterally is noted. Most of the tenderness is localized here

as well. The fracture is usually easily identified radiographically if the capitellum is well ossified and if it is displaced. Oblique radiographs of the elbow may assist in the diagnosis of a nondisplaced or minimally displaced fracture. It may be difficult to differentiate this fracture from a type I fracture of the distal humeral physis or from dislocation of the elbow if the fracture is lateral to the trochlear groove and if the capitellum is not ossified. Although arthrography will be helpful, it should be borne in mind that a fracture of the lateral condyle is very rare in this age group whereas fracture-separation of the entire physis is more common.

## Treatment

Nondisplaced type I fractures may be treated with immobilization only. It has been my experience that nondisplaced fractures are less common than displaced fractures. One must be absolutely certain that the fracture is truly nondisplaced before electing to treat it nonoperatively. Frequent radiographs out of plaster must be obtained to ensure that displacement does not occur during the 3 weeks of immobilization. Finnbogason and associates[63] stated that their type A fractures could be treated with simple immobilization and that all the type A fractures that they treated this way healed without displacement. Type B and C fractures are potentially unstable. The investigators were unable to determine which of these fractures would become displaced if treated nonoperatively. Therefore, it is prudent to pin these fractures to reduce the risk of subsequent displacement. Pinning of the fracture may be performed percutaneously in type B and C fractures. One must be certain that a type C fracture is truly nondisplaced and that the articular surface is anatomically reduced. Mintzer and associates recommend percutaneous pinning of these

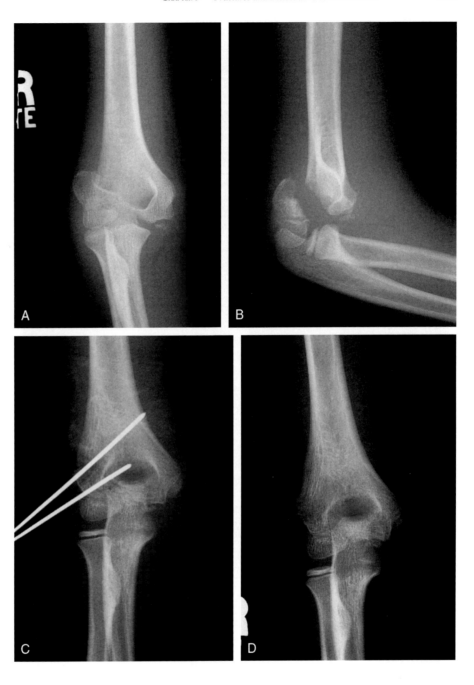

FIGURE 9–30. Displaced Milch type II fracture of the lateral condyle. *A,* An anteroposterior radiograph demonstrates a fracture of the lateral condyle with lateral displacement of the fracture along with lateral displacement of the proximal ends of the radius and ulna. The fracture line travels through the trochlear groove or medial to it. Because of the loss of elbow stability, the radius and ulna are displaced laterally. *B,* A lateral radiograph of the distal end of the humerus demonstrates the large fragments of the lateral condyle. *C,* Postreduction anteroposterior radiograph showing the fracture to be reduced and pinned. *D,* A follow-up radiograph 1 year later shows healing of the fracture.

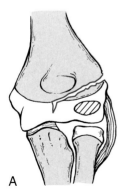
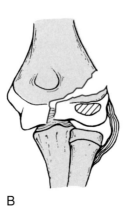
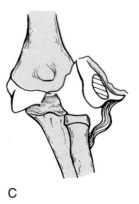

FIGURE 9–31. Classification of lateral condylar fractures according to the amount of displacement. *A,* Type I fracture. Note that the fracture line enters the cartilaginous surface of the distal end of the humerus between the capitellum and trochlea but that the fracture is not complete into the articular surface and is therefore nondisplaced. *B,* Complete fracture (type II). The fracture is complete through the articular surface but is not displaced out of the elbow joint. *C,* Complete fracture with complete displacement of the lateral condyle (type III).

A                    B                    C

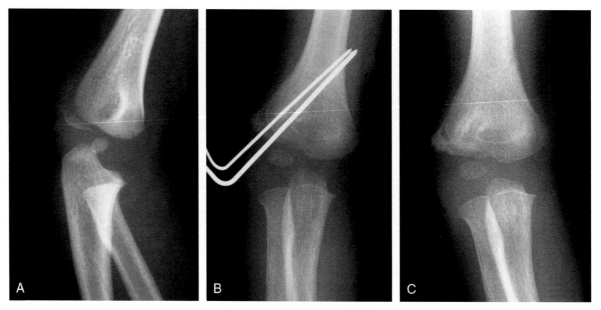

FIGURE 9–32. Type II lateral condyle fracture. *A,* The fracture is displaced, but the capitellar fragment is not rotated. *B,* The fracture was reduced by open means and pinned with two smooth pins. *C,* Three months later, the fracture is healed.

fractures if the articular surface is not disrupted.[140] To determine the status of the articular surface, they recommend arthrography. If the articular surface is intact, percutaneous pinning is performed. If the articular surface shows that the fracture line has extended into the joint and the articular surface is separated, open reduction and pinning are necessary. Once the fracture is stabilized, the elbow is immobilized for 4 weeks. The pins are then removed and motion is begun.

Type II fractures can occasionally be reduced in closed fashion and then secured by percutaneous pins. One must be certain, however, that anatomic reduction has been obtained; otherwise, a poor result will ensue.[89, 217] Because the fracture is intra-articular, the joint surface must be reconstituted perfectly to prevent the development of an irregular articular surface (see Fig. 9–32). Nonunion is another problem seen with this fracture and is common in displaced fractures treated nonoperatively. The third reason for obtaining perfect reduction is that this injury is a Salter-Harris type IV fracture, which usually results in growth arrest if not reduced perfectly. In this fracture, however, because the epiphyseal portion of the fracture usually goes through the cartilaginous portion of the epiphysis, growth arrest is less likely.[80, 89]

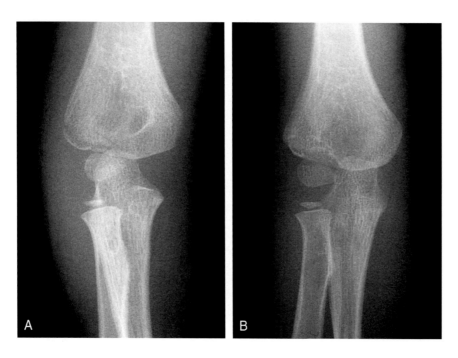

FIGURE 9–33. Type A nondisplaced lateral condylar fracture of the distal end of the humerus according to Finnbogason. *A,* Anteroposterior radiograph of the elbow of a child who sustained a nondisplaced fracture of the lateral condyle. The fracture line through the capitellum has a minimal gap laterally, and the fracture line cannot be followed to the epiphyseal cartilage. *B,* One month later, the fracture has healed after nonoperative cast treatment.

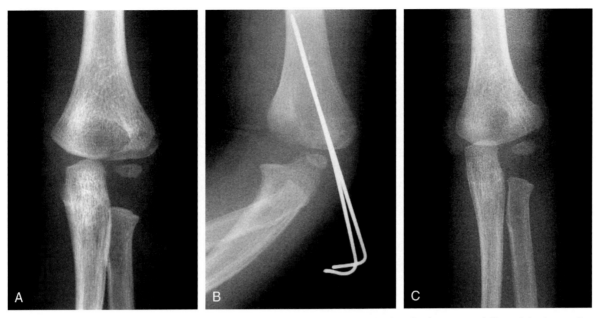

FIGURE 9–34. *A,* Type B nondisplaced lateral condylar fracture. The fracture gap is wider laterally than it is medially, and the fracture line extends to the epiphyseal cartilage. *B,* The fracture was pinned percutaneously. *C,* Two months after surgery, the fracture is well healed.

In general, displaced type II and all type III fractures must be reduced perfectly, which usually requires open reduction with pin fixation.*

A Kocher approach to the lateral side of the distal end of the humerus is used. Once the fracture is exposed, the periosteum of the distal end of the humerus is elevated a few millimeters to visualize it. The periosteum on the distal fragment must be elevated no more than 1 to 2 mm from the fracture surface to protect

_____

*See references 61, 63, 65, 66, 89, 99, 101, 133, 177, 190, 209.

the blood supply to this fragment. However, it is imperative that the entire fracture be visible. One must see the anterior joint surface to be certain that anatomic reduction has been obtained. The fracture is secured with two smooth Kirschner pins. Intraoperative radiographs are obtained to ascertain the quality of the reduction (Fig. 9–36). The elbow is immobilized for 4 weeks, after which the pins are removed and motion is begun. Some authors have recommended suture fixation, but such fixation is not secure enough and nonunion may result.[42, 217]

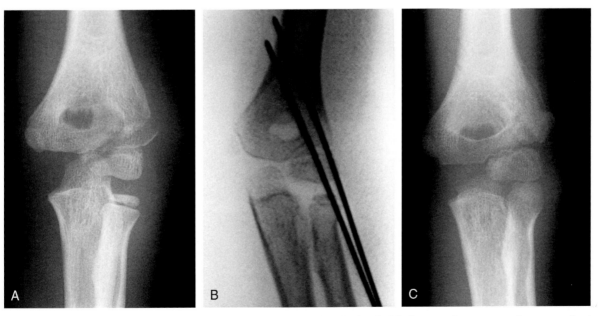

FIGURE 9–35. *A,* This type C nondisplaced fracture of the lateral condyle of the distal end of the humerus demonstrates a fracture gap that is as wide laterally as it is medially. *B,* The fracture was pinned percutaneously with two smooth pins. *C,* Two months later, the fracture is well healed.

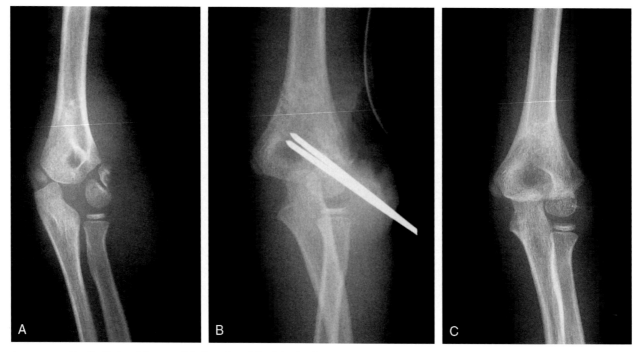

FIGURE **9–36.** Totally displaced fracture of the lateral condyle of the distal end of the humerus. *A,* An anteroposterior radiograph of the distal end of the humerus shows a displaced and rotated fracture of the lateral condyle. *B,* Intraoperative anteroposterior radiograph of the distal humeral fracture. *C,* Anteroposterior radiograph 7 months after the fracture.

## DELAYED OPEN REDUCTION

Some authors believe that if fractures of the lateral condyle are seen late, open reduction should not be performed.[89, 99, 136, 165] They reported a high incidence of avascular necrosis, probably because of the extensive soft tissue stripping necessary to mobilize the fracture. Jakob and colleagues[99] recommend no treatment if the fracture is seen after 3 weeks. Dhillon and associates[56]

recommend that these fractures be left alone if not treated within 6 weeks of the time of injury. Such has not been my experience in four patients seen between 6 and 12 weeks after injury. They all underwent open reduction with pin fixation. One was a Milch type I fracture in which the fracture line went directly through the ossification center of the capitellum and would have resulted in growth arrest if not reduced (Fig. 9–37). All

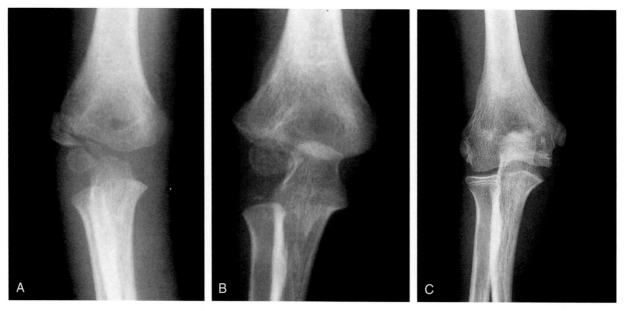

FIGURE **9–37.** *A,* Milch type I fracture of the lateral condyle. The fracture line crosses through the midportion of the ossification center of the capitellum. This fracture was originally treated with cast immobilization; when the patient was referred 6 weeks after injury, the fracture was still displaced. Open reduction and internal fixation of the fracture were performed. *B,* Four months after reduction, the fracture is healed. *C,* Seven years after reduction, the distal end of the humerus appears normal.

these fractures united without avascular necrosis or growth arrest, and all patients regained and maintained full elbow motion. The surgical approach to the lateral condyle is the same as one would use for an acute injury—a direct lateral incision. The delayed union is identified from proximal on the humeral shaft distally. The fracture is exposed in a proximal-to-distal direction to avoid stripping soft tissue from the lateral condylar fragment. It is important to not injure the blood supply to this fracture fragment to avoid avascular necrosis of the lateral condyle. Once the fracture is identified, the fibrous nonunion is opened carefully with a scalpel, and an osteotome is used to help strip the fibrous tissue from the fracture surface. The soft tissue is not stripped from the fracture fragment, and only the soft tissue at the edge of the fracture is sharply removed to allow perfect visualization of both sides of the fracture. Once mobilization of the fracture is complete and the two fracture surfaces have been débrided of soft tissue with raw bony surfaces remaining, the fracture is reduced and internally fixed. If the child is young and the metaphyseal fragment is small, the fracture is stabilized with smooth K-wires. On the other hand, if the child is older and the metaphyseal fragment is large enough, the fracture is stabilized with one or two screws inserted into the metaphysis of the fracture.

Roye and associates also found that delayed open reduction and internal fixation of these fractures could result in an excellent outcome.[176] Gaur and colleagues lengthened the aponeurosis of the common forearm extensor musculature because they believed that this muscle became contracted and was the main cause of difficulty in the late reduction of lateral condylar fractures.[76]

Because of these results, it is recommended that lateral condylar fractures be reduced even if seen late because the results of nonunion are poor and the results of open reduction, if performed carefully, are good. It is not known how old a fracture can be openly reduced. Roye and coworkers[176] openly reduced ununited fractures more than 2 years old, although they would be better classified as true nonunion. My experience with fractures 12 weeks old suggests that the chance of a satisfactory result is good up to this time if the fracture is accurately reduced and internally fixed and allowed to heal.

## Complications

### NONUNION AND CUBITUS VALGUS

Nonunion is usually the result of inadequate internal fixation or failure to perform it. Suture fixation of this fracture was popular for a time.[42] However, the incidence of nonunion has led most authors to abandon this technique in favor of pin fixation. Nonunion may also result from misdiagnosis of this fracture. If the displacement is minimal and the metaphyseal fragment is small, it is possible that the fracture may not be correctly identified. Because this fracture is intra-articular, nonunion is believed to be the result of synovial fluid bathing the fracture and preventing union.[89]

Treatment of established nonunion is controversial. Some recommend no treatment or a delay in treatment until the child is close to skeletal maturity.[89, 99] Flynn and associates[66] recommend grafting to obtain union in order to prevent valgus and tardy ulnar nerve palsy. Some patients with nonunion have pain, especially if the dominant extremity is involved; the pain is usually secondary to the elbow instability. The lateral condylar fragment is most often completely mobile, which allows increased valgus stress to the elbow.

Internal fixation and grafting of these mobile nonunions generally result in loss of some elbow motion; however, the tradeoff may be beneficial if the pain can be relieved.[126] The metaphyseal fragment should be stabilized to the main portion of the metaphysis with compression screws, and a bone graft should be added (Fig. 9–38).

## FRACTURE OF THE CAPITELLUM IN ADOLESCENTS

Fracture of the capitellum in adolescents that does not involve the entire lateral condyle is a rare injury, and treatment has been controversial. These fractures are seen more commonly in adults, but when present in children, they are almost always seen in adolescents and teenagers older than 12 years. Letts and colleagues have shown that operative reduction of these fractures is usually successful in restoring normal elbow function.[114] They reviewed capitellar fractures in seven adolescents with an average age of $14\frac{1}{2}$ years. Six of the seven fractures were type I fractures with a large anterosuperior fragment that required operative reduction and internal fixation in five cases. They used a variety of fixation devices, including K-wires, Herbert screws, and cannulated screws. De Boeck and Pouliart also reported on six children between the ages of 11 and 15 years with this fracture, all of which were type I.[51] All underwent operative reduction and internal fixation with one screw. Their results were excellent; no patients had avascular necrosis and all had normal function. The surgical approach to the capitellum was by a lateral incision. The fragment was reduced and held in position while it was stabilized with a screw that entered the humerus posteriorly and was then directed anteriorly into the capitellar fragment. I have also found that this fragment requires operative reduction and internal fixation. My approach to the fracture is through a lateral incision, but I have internally fixed the fragment transversely in a lateral-to-medial direction with a cannulated screw (Fig. 9–39).

## FRACTURE OF THE MEDIAL CONDYLE OF THE HUMERUS

Fracture of the medial condyle is very uncommon and accounts for less than 2% of all elbow fractures in children.[21, 214] Two mechanisms of injury have been proposed, as is the case for lateral condylar fractures.[33, 68, 108, 208] The fracture may occur from a fall on the outstretched hand with the elbow extended, with subsequent avulsion of the medial condyle.[68, 208] Varma and Srivastava[208] stated that their two patients sustained their injuries by falling on the olecranon, which was driven into the trochlea and fractured the medial condyle.

## Classification

Kilfoyle[108] devised a classification identical to the one used for lateral condylar fractures. A type I fracture is nondisplaced, and the fracture line does not go into the articular surface. The fracture line in a type II fracture goes through the articular surface, but the fracture is essentially nondisplaced. A type III fracture is totally

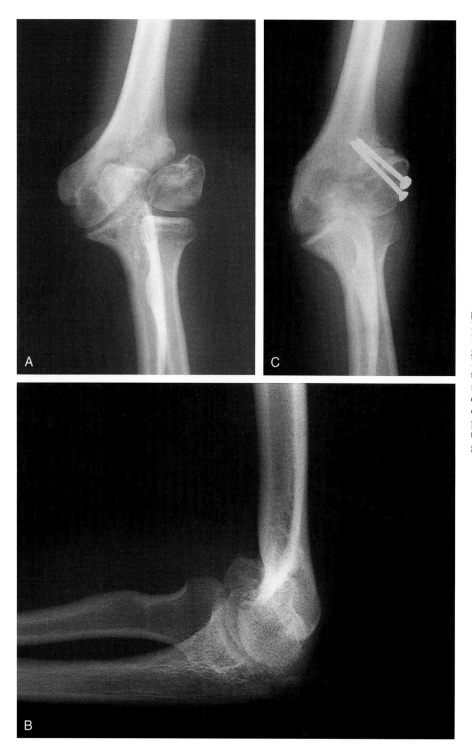

FIGURE 9–38. Nonunion fracture of the lateral condyle of the distal end of the humerus. *A,* An anteroposterior radiograph demonstrates nonunion of the lateral condyle. *B,* Lateral radiograph of the elbow. The lateral condyle is freely mobile and moves proximally with elbow flexion and distally and posteriorly with elbow extension. *C,* Anteroposterior radiograph after open reduction and internal fixation with bone grafting of the nonunion.

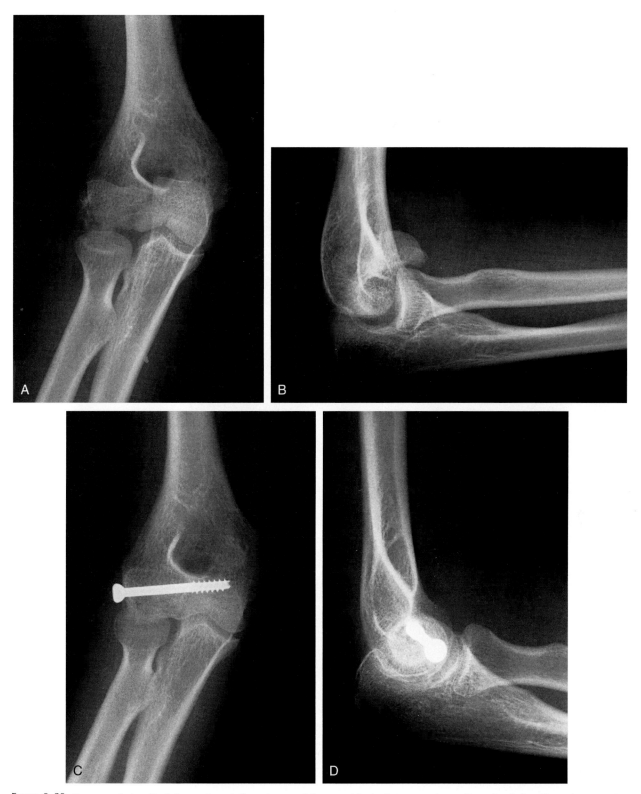

**FIGURE 9–39.** Fracture of the distal humeral capitellum in an adolescent girl. *A,* Anteroposterior radiograph of the elbow demonstrating the anteriorly displaced fracture of the capitellum. *B,* Lateral radiograph of the elbow demonstrating the displaced fracture of the capitellum. The capitellum is displaced anteriorly. *C,* Anteroposterior radiograph of the elbow 6 months after open reduction of the fracture of the capitellum. The capitellum has been reduced and internally fixed with a screw. The capitellum is normal in appearance without evidence of avascular necrosis. *D,* Lateral radiograph of the elbow demonstrating anatomic reduction of the capitellum with reduction of the radiocapitellar joint.

displaced and rotated. Bensahel and coworkers,[21] using a similar classification, claimed that these different injuries occur in different age groups. A type I injury occurs in children younger than 5 years, a type II fracture may be seen in any age group, and a type III fracture occurs in somewhat older children. In their series, this fracture was seen in children with an average age of 7 years.

## Diagnosis

This fracture may be difficult to diagnose because it is frequently seen before ossification of the trochlea begins.

Clinically, the child has a swollen, painful elbow, with most of the pain and swelling on the medial side. This injury is most commonly mistaken for a fracture of the medial epicondyle. Clinically, examination of the two injuries yields different results. Avulsion of the medial epicondyle in a young child is usually accompanied by elbow dislocation. The elbow is likely to be unstable with a valgus force. In contrast, with a fracture of the medial condyle of the humerus, varus instability results because the medial side of the elbow joint is fractured (Fig. 9–40).

Radiographically, a fracture is suggested if the medial condyle is markedly displaced. One should also look for

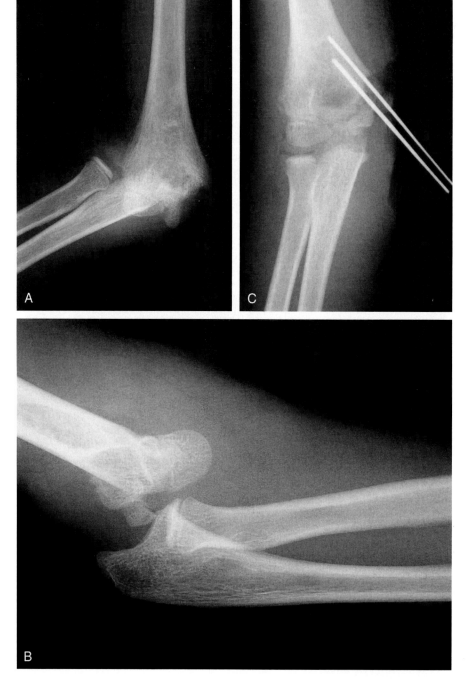

**FIGURE 9–40.** Displaced fracture of the medial condyle of the distal end of the humerus. *A,* Anteroposterior radiograph of the elbow. Note the displacement of the medial epicondyle. Note also that the trochlea has been displaced but is positioned behind the distal humeral metaphysis and is therefore difficult to visualize. *B,* A lateral radiograph of the elbow shows that the injury includes both the epicondyle and the trochlea. This injury is therefore a fracture of the entire lateral condyle. *C,* Intraoperative anteroposterior radiograph demonstrating reduction and internal fixation with smooth pins.

a fleck of bone avulsed from the metaphysis. An arthrogram of the elbow may be necessary to confirm the diagnosis.

## Treatment

Type I fractures heal with simple immobilization; however, type II fractures should be stabilized with percutaneous pinning if the reduction is anatomic. If adequacy of the reduction is in question, open reduction and pinning of the fracture should be performed. A type III fracture must undergo open reduction and pin fixation. The elbow should be immobilized for 3 weeks, followed by pin removal and mobilization.

## FRACTURE OF THE MEDIAL EPICONDYLE

### Incidence

Fracture of the medial epicondyle is a relatively common injury that occurs in about 10% of children's elbow fractures.[133, 214] Most are seen in adolescents (between 10 and 14 years of age)[13, 73, 143, 166] and in males (more than 75%).[189]

### Mechanisms of Injury

This injury is the result of avulsion of the medial epicondyle caused by a valgus force combined with contraction of the forearm flexor muscles.[108, 189, 217] If the valgus force is great enough, an elbow dislocation results in addition to avulsion of the medial epicondyle. In many series of medial epicondylar fractures, most occur with elbow dislocation.[108, 133, 189, 217]

### Classification

Most systems of classification of this fracture are similar and based on the amount of displacement of the fragment and whether it is entrapped in the elbow joint[17, 189, 214] (Table 9–1). Woods and Tullos[217] have also classified this injury, but their classification pertains to teenagers who are very near the age of closure of the apophysis of the medial epicondyle.

### Diagnosis

Diagnosis of this fracture is generally easy. The child has a history of a valgus injury to the arm, with pain and swelling localized to the medial side of the elbow. In the case of an elbow that also dislocated but spontaneously reduced, generalized pain and swelling are present, but the point tenderness is greatest medially. Radiographically, the apophysis of the medial epicondyle may appear

| **TABLE 9–1** |
| --- |
| Classification of Fractures of the Medial Epicondyle |

I. Undisplaced
II. Minimally displaced (<5 mm)
III. Displaced (>5 mm)
 Elbow not dislocated or reduced
 Epicondyle not in joint
 Epicondyle in joint
 Elbow dislocated

wider than normal in a nondisplaced fracture. Frequently, a comparison radiograph of the opposite elbow is of benefit.

The diagnosis may be difficult if the fracture occurs in a young child and the medial epicondyle is not fully ossified. A high level of suspicion and a careful physical examination should alert the physician to the true injury. Woods and Tullos[217] recommend that a stress radiograph be performed to determine the amount of instability (Fig. 9–41). They perform the stress test with the patient supine and the elbow flexed to a right angle. The shoulder is externally rotated with the upper part of the arm resting on the table; the elbow and forearm are suspended over the edge of the table. If the elbow is unstable, the medial side of the elbow will widen, which can be demonstrated with an anteroposterior radiograph of the elbow taken in this position.

### Treatment

Treatment of this fracture depends on the amount of displacement of the epicondyle. For nondisplaced and minimally displaced (less than 5 mm) fractures, most recommend immobilization of the elbow in 90° of flexion for 5 to 7 days for comfort.[22] Elbow motion is then begun to prevent stiffness. Treatment of fractures that are displaced more than 5 mm remains controversial. In 1950, Smith[188] stated that even displaced fractures healed, although with a fibrous union, and that no disability resulted from this fibrous union. He claimed that the loss of motion seen as a result of this fracture could be prevented with early motion. Bernstein and colleagues[22] also recommend closed treatment of displaced fractures of the medial epicondyle. Peterson, however, recommends open reduction and internal fixation for fractures that are displaced more than 2 mm or are rotated.[161]

Others believe that valgus instability of the elbow is an indication for open reduction and pin fixation, especially in the dominant arm of an athlete.[166, 167, 217] Woods and Tullos[217] showed that medial elbow stability depends on the medial collateral ligament of the elbow and the forearm flexor muscles. They demonstrated the three bands of the medial collateral ligament. The eccentric position of the epicondyle ensures that one of the bands of the ligament will remain taut throughout the range of elbow motion. However, when the medial epicondyle is displaced, the entire collateral ligament is displaced with it. The ligament loses its tightness, which leads to medial instability of the elbow (Fig. 9–42). It therefore seems reasonable to openly reduce and internally fix a displaced fracture with valgus instability (Fig. 9–43).

Ulnar nerve symptoms were once thought to be an indication for exploration of the fracture.[37, 108, 201] Bernstein and colleagues,[22] however, found no permanent ulnar nerve injuries as a result of this fracture and recommended observation. Median nerve injury, though very uncommon, is an indication for nerve exploration. This nerve may rarely become entrapped in the elbow joint as a result of elbow dislocation with an associated fracture of the medial epicondyle. The elbow dislocation may have reduced spontaneously and left the medial epicondyle trapped within the elbow joint. Therefore, if one detects median nerve symptoms in a patient with a displaced fracture of the medial epicondyle, the median nerve should be explored because of the high probability that the nerve is trapped within the elbow joint[77, 127, 164, 172] (Fig. 9–44).

## AUTHOR'S PREFERRED METHOD OF TREATMENT

Evaluation of a fracture of the medial epicondyle includes the amount of displacement, rotation of the fragment, and stability of the joint. If the fracture is displaced more than 2 mm and the elbow is unstable, open reduction

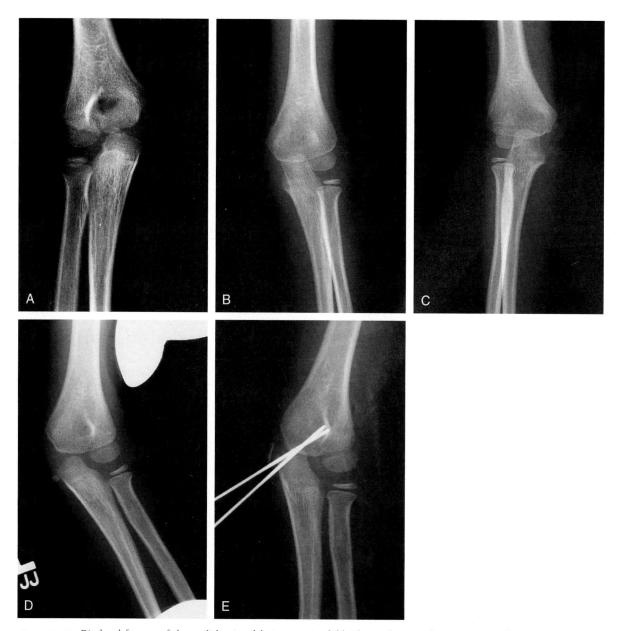

**FIGURE 9–41.** Displaced fracture of the medial epicondyle in a young child. The mechanism of injury was an elbow dislocation with spontaneous reduction. The treating physician splinted the elbow for comfort, but the child sustained recurrent episodes of elbow dislocation with spontaneous reduction. *A,* Initial radiograph of the elbow at the time of injury. The radiograph is dark, and the ossification center of the medial epicondyle, which is very small at this age, cannot be visualized. *B,* Four months later, the child was seen because of recurrent instability of the elbow. One can see the faint outline of the displaced medial epicondyle. *C,* The normal opposite elbow reveals the medial epicondyle in its normal position. *D,* A stress radiograph demonstrates the amount of elbow instability. The medial epicondyle is markedly displaced. *E,* The patient underwent open reduction and internal fixation of the medial epicondyle 5 months after injury. Two years later, the child has full elbow function and has had no further episodes of instability.

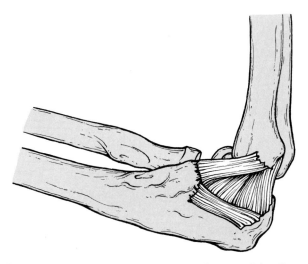

**FIGURE 9–42.** Drawing of the ulnar collateral ligament of the elbow. Note the anterior band, posterior band, and oblique band.

and internal fixation should be performed. Evaluation of stability may be done radiographically, as suggested by Woods and Tullos,[217] but in patients with acute fractures, pain may limit the ability to obtain a reliable evaluation of medial elbow stability. Anesthesia may be necessary to accurately determine medial elbow stability. The fracture is approached with an incision placed directly over the medial epicondyle. The ulnar nerve should be identified and protected throughout the surgical procedure. The medial epicondyle is reduced and held in place with a towel clamp while the fracture is stabilized. In a very skeletally immature patient, the fracture may be fixed with two smooth pins. The pins are left exposed through the skin and are either bent or capped to prevent pin migration. The pins are removed in about 4 weeks and motion is begun. In an adolescent or teenage patient who is very near the end of growth, the fracture may be internally fixed with a screw (Fig. 9–45).

A displaced medial epicondyle may become entrapped in the elbow joint when the dislocation is reduced. This fragment must be removed from the joint. Roberts[173] recommended using a closed maneuver. He placed a valgus stress on the elbow joint with the forearm supinated to try to dislodge the epicondyle. Fowles and associates stated that open reduction plus internal fixation is indicated for medial epicondylar fractures when the medial epicondyle is trapped in the joint.[69] Although one may be able to dislodge the medial epicondyle with this maneuver, because open reduction plus internal fixation is the treatment of choice for this injury, it is probably best to dislodge the medial epicondyle at the time of open reduction. These fractures are unstable when tested and are best treated by internal fixation for that reason (Fig. 9–46).

## FRACTURE OF THE LATERAL EPICONDYLE

Fracture of the lateral epicondyle is an extremely uncommon injury. It is probably the result of an avulsion

of the epicondyle along with the attachment of the forearm extensor muscles. Treatment is immobilization for comfort and early mobilization.

## T-CONDYLAR FRACTURE

### INCIDENCE AND CLASSIFICATION

Although rare in the pediatric age group, T-condylar fractures are seen in teenagers. Usually, the distal humeral physis is closed or very near the end of growth. Jarvis and D'Astous[100] reported on 16 patients with this injury; the average age of their patients was 12 years, 9 months. These authors also classified the fractures into three groups. Type I is a nondisplaced fracture (however, they had no type I fractures in their series). Type II fractures are displaced, with displacement defined as greater than 1 mm of separation or step-off of the articular surface. A type III fracture is a fracture-dislocation; it occurred only once in their series.

### TREATMENT

T-condylar fractures must be treated as one would treat any intra-articular fracture. A minimally displaced fracture can be reduced and stabilized with a percutaneous screw.[105, 184] If the joint surface is displaced, open reduction and internal fixation should be performed. Most recommend a posterior approach through the triceps, which provides the best visualization of the fracture. An olecranon osteotomy may be performed in a skeletally mature patient. The internal fixation devices used depend on the type of fracture and the degree of instability. In some relatively stable fractures, as seen in younger teenagers, lag screws provide excellent fracture stability (see Fig. 9–46). Reduction of the displaced articular surface is imperative. Even displaced fractures are stable when reduced if comminution of the fracture is minimal, and lag screw fixation provides stable fixation (Fig. 9–47).

Comminuted distal humeral fractures require more extensive exposure and greater fixation. One must restore the articular surface to its anatomic position and correct any angular deformity.

## FLOATING ELBOW

Floating elbow injuries (distal humeral fractures with fractures of the forearm) are severe injuries that require fixation of both fractures if they are displaced.[90] Frequently, one or both of the fractures will require open reduction (Figs. 9–48 and 9–49).

## PROXIMAL RADIAL FRACTURE

### Incidence

Fractures about the proximal end of the radius occur in about 8% of all elbow fractures in children.[62, 214]

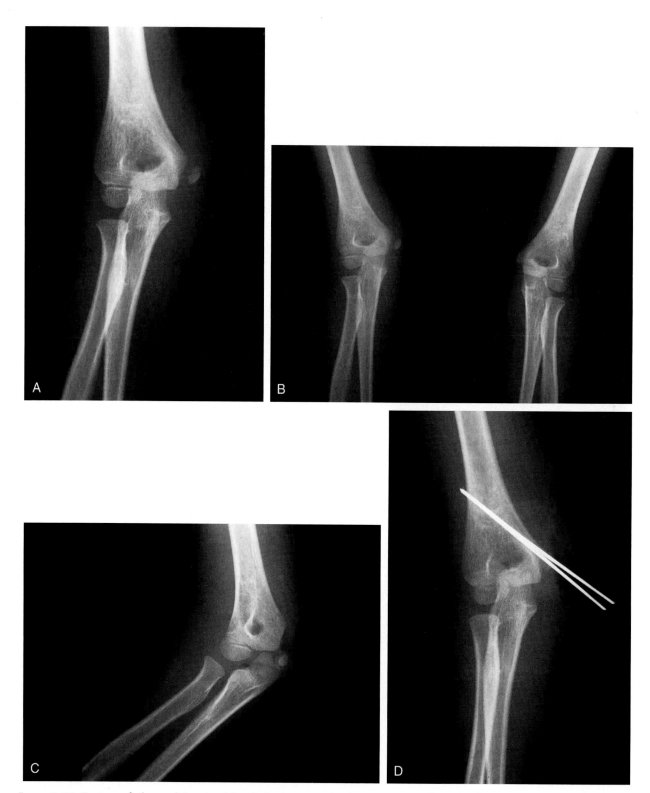

**FIGURE 9–43.** Fracture of the medial epicondyle of the humerus. *A,* Anteroposterior radiograph of the distal end of the humerus demonstrating a fracture with more than 5 mm of displacement. *B,* Anteroposterior radiographs of both elbows demonstrating the displacement of the medial epicondyle of the elbow on the right. *C,* Stress anteroposterior radiograph of the elbow demonstrating the instability of the medial epicondyle. Note that the medial epicondyle has become displaced significantly distally with valgus stress of the elbow. *D,* A postoperative radiograph of the elbow shows that the medial epicondyle has been reduced and fixed with two smooth K-wires.

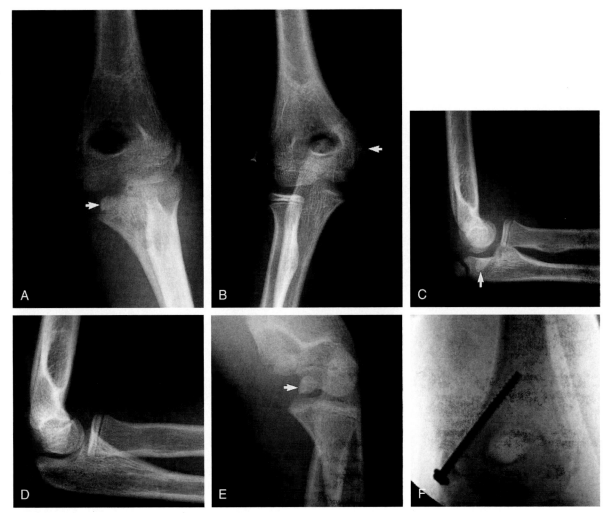

**FIGURE 9–44.** Fracture of the medial epicondyle with entrapment in the elbow joint secondary to elbow dislocation. This 9-year-old boy presented with a painful elbow after an injury. The elbow had dislocated and reduced spontaneously. *A,* An anteroposterior radiograph of the injured elbow shows absence of the medial epicondyle. The *arrow* points to the medial epicondyle entrapped within the elbow joint. *B,* An anteroposterior radiograph of the opposite elbow shows the medial epicondyle *(arrow)* in its normal position. *C,* A lateral radiograph of the injured elbow demonstrates widening of the elbow joint. The medial epicondyle can be seen within the elbow joint. It is overlying the olecranon *(arrow).* *D,* A comparison lateral radiograph of the opposite elbow shows that the elbow joint is not widened as it is on the opposite side. *E,* An oblique radiograph of the injured elbow again demonstrates the medial epicondyle within the elbow joint *(arrow).* *F,* Anteroposterior radiograph of the injured elbow after open reduction of the fracture. The medial epicondyle was removed from the joint, replaced in its normal position, and stabilized with a screw.

These fractures are different from those seen in adults because in children, most involve the neck of the radius and the physis rather than the head.[92] The majority occur in children between the ages of 9 and 12 years.[92, 149, 170, 204, 208]

## Anatomy

The normal proximal end of the radius angulates close to the head of the radius. It may be mistaken for a fracture if one is not aware of this normal angulation. A normal lateral angulation of up to 15° is seen on an anteroposterior radiograph. On a lateral radiograph, the normal angulation is about 5°.[207]

## Mechanisms of Injury

Proximal radial fractures in a mature patient frequently involve an injury to the head of the radius. In a skeletally immature patient, however, the head of the radius is mostly cartilage, and the force is directed to the physis and the metaphysis. A fracture of the neck of the radius in children may occur in one of two ways. A fall on the outstretched hand with the elbow extended transmits a valgus force to the neck of the radius and results in a fracture. If the fracture involves the proximal radial physis, any of the four types of fractures of the physis described by Salter and Harris may occur.[179] In addition, the fracture line may involve only the metaphysis of the radius, without injury to the physis.

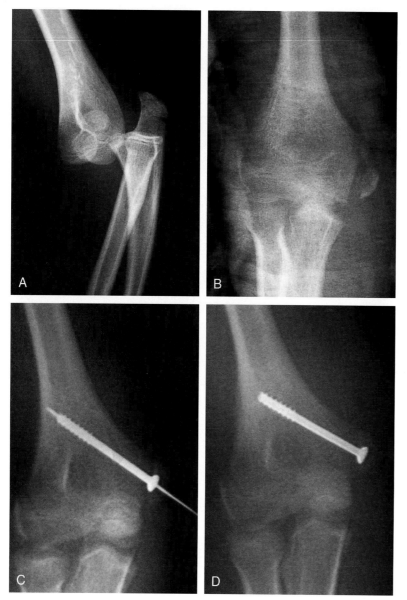

FIGURE 9–45. Fracture of the medial epicondyle that is displaced 5 mm. The elbow dislocated, and after reduction it was unstable on stress testing. Because of the instability, open reduction and screw fixation were indicated. *A,* This 15-year-old boy sustained an elbow dislocation on his dominant extremity, as seen on this radiograph. *B,* An anteroposterior radiograph of the elbow after reduction of the dislocation demonstrates a fracture of the medial epicondyle with 5 mm of displacement. *C,* Intraoperative radiograph showing the insertion of a cannulated screw across the reduced fracture. *D,* Postoperative radiograph of the elbow showing early union of the fracture of the medial epicondyle.

The proximal end of the radius may also be fractured in association with posterior dislocation of the elbow. The injury that results is usually a fracture through the physis. Jeffrey[101] described displacement of the epiphysis of the radius posteriorly. This fracture occurs when the elbow dislocation spontaneously reduces after posterior dislocation. The capitellum fractures the radial epiphysis as the elbow is reduced, with the epiphysis pushed posteriorly. Newman[149] later showed that the radial epiphysis may also be fractured through the physis at the time of posterior elbow dislocation. Because the injury occurs at the time of the dislocation rather than during the reduction, the radial epiphysis is displaced anteriorly[101, 149] (Fig. 9–50).

## Classification

Authors have classified proximal radial fractures in children in different manners.[100, 149, 151, 214] Wilkins, relying heavily on the classification of Jeffrey[101] and Newman,[149] combined these groupings to produce his own classification.[214] He divided valgus injuries into three types according to the location of the fracture line. The injuries resulting from posterior elbow dislocation are divided into two groups according to whether the radial head is displaced anteriorly or posteriorly (Table 9–2).

## Diagnosis

The diagnosis of a displaced fracture of the neck of the radius is usually easily made radiographically. Some nondisplaced fractures may be difficult to visualize radiographically, however, and rotational views of the proximal end of the radius may be helpful. The clinical examination of the patient should alert one to the diagnosis. The child has tenderness over the radial head, and rotation of the forearm produces pain in the lateral aspect of the elbow that may radiate distally into the forearm.

## Management

Authors disagree about the need for reduction of angulated fractures of the radial neck in children. It is known that these fractures remodel and that this remodeling may be considerable because of the degree of movement of the radiohumeral and radioulnar joints. Nevertheless, the literature is replete with articles recommending treatment of angulated radial neck fractures. Some, such as Salter and Harris[179] and Jones and Esah,[103] favor anatomic positioning and recommend accepting no more than 15° of angulation. Fahey[62] accepts 25° of angulation, whereas Rang[166] and Jeffrey[101] accept 30° of angulation, as do Tibone and Stoltz.[202] Henrikson[92] finds 35° of angulation acceptable, as do McBride and Monnet.[130] However, Vahvanen[207] believes that only 10° of proximal radial angulation will correct spontaneously with growth.

No clearly documented indication has therefore been proposed for the need to reduce these fractures. Most currently believe that up to 30° of angulation may be accepted if sufficient growth remains to expect remodeling. If the angulation is greater, closed reduction of the fracture should be attempted. Patterson[159] described a maneuver used for reduction of this fracture. With an assistant providing countertraction on the upper part of the arm, the surgeon supinates the forearm and applies longitudinal traction. At the same time, the elbow is forced into varus by the assistant. Before reduction, the forearm should be rotated until the position of maximal tilt of the radial head is directed laterally.[101] The thumb of the surgeon then pushes the radial head back into place.

In 1981, Angelov[6] described a method of percutaneous reduction of the angulated radial neck. A double-pronged instrument is inserted percutaneously and is used to push the head of the radius into the correct position. Others have reported on the successful use of this technique[58, 194] (Fig. 9–51). Dormans[58] used intraoperative arthrography to help determine the amount of angulation when reducing this fracture percutaneously. He used a percutaneously introduced Steinmann pin to push the fracture of the radial neck back into position. The displaced fracture of the neck of the radius may also be reduced with the use of an elastic intramedullary nail as described by Metaizeau and colleagues.[137, 182] The elastic intramedullary nail is inserted into the radius through an insertion hole in the distal radial metaphysis. The nail is advanced proximally in the radial canal until the fracture of the neck of the radius is reached. The bent tip of the nail is used to lever the head of the radius back into position. The nail is rotated with a "T-handle chuck," and once the bent tip of the nail enters the neck of the radius, it is advanced proximally enough to permit a secure hold. The elbow is manually stressed into valgus, and the T-handle is rotated while observing the procedure on the fluoroscope machine. The radial head is rotated back into place as the nail is rotated. Once

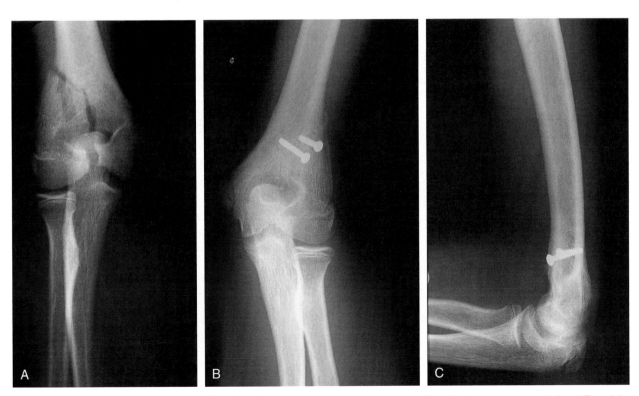

**FIGURE 9–46.** T-condylar fracture of the distal end of the humerus. *A,* An anteroposterior radiograph demonstrates the displaced T-condylar fracture. *B,* Anteroposterior radiograph after open reduction and internal fixation with two lag screws. *C,* Lateral radiograph after open reduction of the fracture.

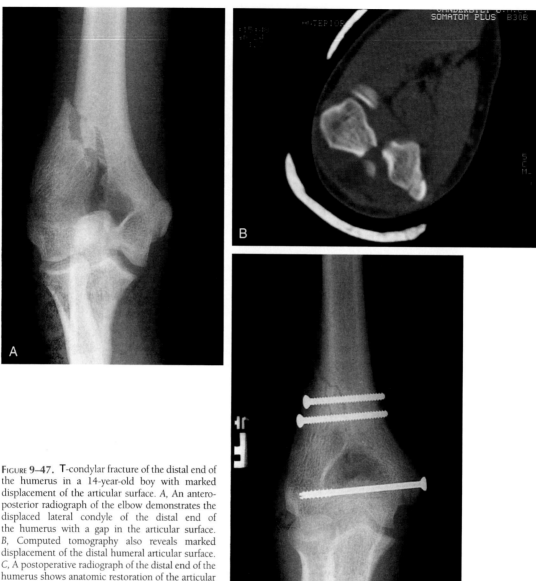

FIGURE 9–47. T-condylar fracture of the distal end of the humerus in a 14-year-old boy with marked displacement of the articular surface. *A,* An antero-posterior radiograph of the elbow demonstrates the displaced lateral condyle of the distal end of the humerus with a gap in the articular surface. *B,* Computed tomography also reveals marked displacement of the distal humeral articular surface. *C,* A postoperative radiograph of the distal end of the humerus shows anatomic restoration of the articular surface. The fracture was stabilized with three lag screws. Early motion was begun, and full function returned.

reduced, the fracture is stable; however, most authors recommend leaving the nail in place for internal fixation[137, 182] (Fig. 9–52).

Open reduction is indicated if the fracture cannot be reduced satisfactorily by either closed or percutaneous means. However, stiffness and avascular necrosis of the radial head may occur.[58, 195, 202] The radial head and neck should be approached through a lateral Kocher approach to the elbow. Care is taken to avoid injury to the radial nerve, which may be exposed to protect it.[103] Rang[166] advocates pronation of the forearm to avoid injury to the nerve. Some authors prefer to use no means of internal fixation after reduction of this fracture in the belief that the fracture is inherently stable.[151, 167, 172] Most authors, however, recommend the use of pin fixation to ensure maintenance of reduction.[103, 166] The

pin should be inserted into the edge of the radial head and should cross the fracture obliquely (Fig. 9–53). A pin through the capitellum that crosses the elbow joint and then enters the radial head should not be used because the pin is likely to break.[149] Open reduction of a displaced fracture of the radial neck should not be avoided because of the fear of avascular necrosis. One should make every effort to reduce the fracture by closed means with percutaneous manipulation or manipulation with a flexible intramedullary nail. If these attempts fail, one should not hesitate to operate on the displaced fracture and reduce it into an anatomic position (Fig. 9–54).

The length of immobilization of the elbow depends on the nature of the fracture and the type of reduction used. If the fracture is minimally angulated and no reduction is necessary, the elbow should be immobilized for comfort for 5 to 7 days only. Elbow mobilization is then begun to avoid loss of motion. If the fracture has been reduced, immobilization for 3 weeks is sufficient. The elbow should be immobilized in 90° of flexion because if significant elbow motion is lost as a result of the injury, elbow function will be best if the motion that remains is at the neutral or functional position.

## OLECRANON FRACTURE

### Incidence

Olecranon fractures are relatively uncommon and constitute 5% of all fractures about the elbow.[62, 129, 214] Newell[148] reported on 40 cases seen over a 40-year period, most of which were minimally displaced.

Wilkins[214] stated that less than 20% require surgical treatment.

## Mechanisms of Injury

Fracture of the olecranon may be the result of a fall on the olecranon with the elbow flexed. An intra-articular fracture is the usual result. It may be nondisplaced, or it may be displaced enough to require reduction. Olecranon fractures in children may also result from a fall on the outstretched hand with the elbow extended. If the elbow does not hyperextend but the fall is accompanied by a varus or valgus force, a fracture of the olecranon may result. These injuries are usually greenstick fractures. Bado[12] classified them as Monteggia fractures because a valgus force that produces a fracture of the olecranon usually fractures the neck of the radius. A varus-directed force may result in dislocation of the head of the radius.

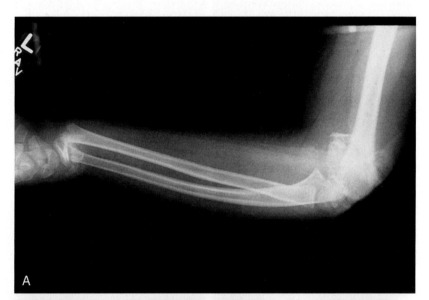

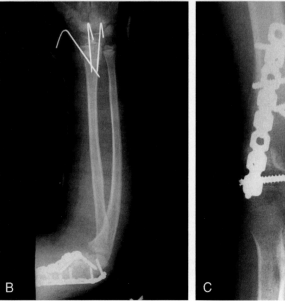

FIGURE 9–48. Floating elbow. *A*, This child sustained a very comminuted distal humeral fracture associated with an open fracture of the distal ends of the radius and ulna. *B*, The humeral fracture was reduced by open means and internally fixed. The forearm fracture was débrided and stabilized with pins. *C*, An anteroposterior view of the distal end of the humerus demonstrates restoration of the articular surface of the elbow.

## Classification

The most commonly used classification is that of Matthews,[128] although others have described these fractures as a variant of the Monteggia fracture-dislocation (Table 9–3) (see Chapter 8).

## Treatment

Most of these fractures are nondisplaced and require no reduction. Extension injuries associated with a dislocation of the head of the radius require treatment (see Chapter 8). Occasionally, flexion injuries of the olecra-

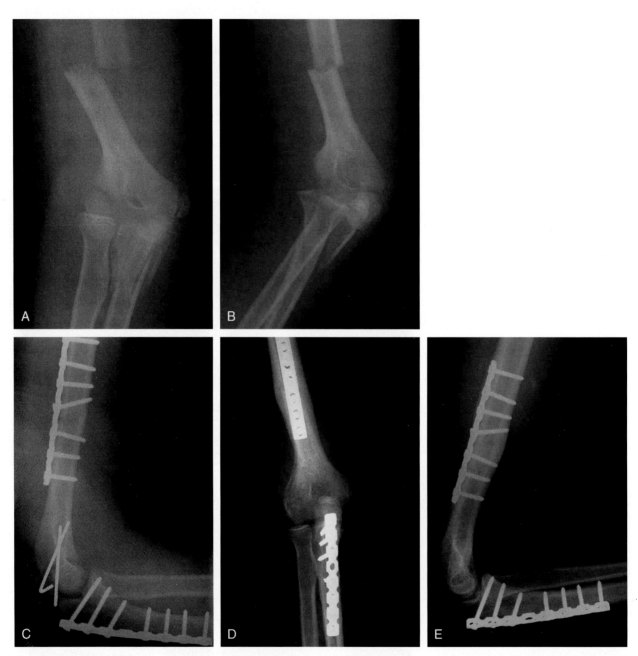

FIGURE 9–49. Floating elbow in a 9-year-old boy involved in a motor vehicle accident. *A,* Anteroposterior radiograph of the elbow demonstrating a transverse fracture of the humerus at the junction of the middle and distal thirds. In addition, a comminuted fracture of the olecranon is present. One is also able to see a transverse supracondylar fracture. *B,* Lateral radiograph of the elbow. The three fractures are also seen. *C,* Lateral radiograph of the elbow 3 weeks after open reduction of the fractures. The humeral fracture was exposed through a posterior triceps-splitting incision. It was reduced and internally fixed with a seven-hole compression plate. The supracondylar fracture was stabilized with two lateral 0.062-inch pins. The olecranon fracture was also reduced openly through a directly posterior incision. The fracture was stabilized with an eight-hole reconstruction plate and seven screws. *D,* Anteroposterior radiograph of the elbow 6 months after the injury. The fractures have all healed and the percutaneous pins have been removed (removed 3 weeks postoperatively). The patient has full flexion and extension of the elbow and also has full pronation and supination of the forearm. *E,* Lateral radiograph of the elbow 6 months postinjury demonstrating complete union of all of the fractures.

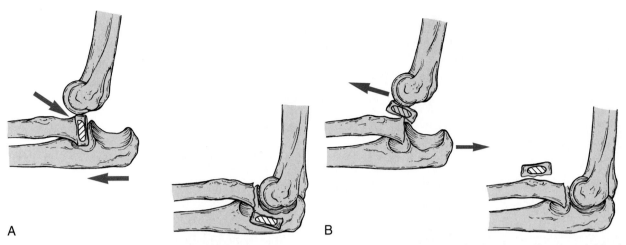

**FIGURE 9–50.** Displaced fracture of the radial neck. *A,* The neck is fractured as an elbow dislocation is reduced and is pushing the radial head posteriorly. *B,* Displacement of the radial head and neck anteriorly. At the time of elbow dislocation, the radial head and neck remain anterior to the radius through the metaphysis of the radius. (*A,* From Jeffrey, C.C. J Bone Joint Surg 40:396, 1958. *B,* From Newman, J.H. Injury 9:114, 1977.)

non are displaced and require open reduction. The type of fixation used depends on the type of fracture sustained. This fracture is most commonly seen in teenagers, and the fracture should be treated as one would treat the same fracture in an adult (Fig. 9–55). More complex fractures require different means of fixation (Fig. 9–56).

## DISLOCATION OF THE ELBOW JOINT

### Incidence

Dislocation of the elbow is a rare injury in children. Henrikson found 45 elbow dislocations among 1579 elbow injuries in children, an incidence of about 3%.[92] Although these injuries may occur at almost any age, the peak incidence is during the second decade of life.[118, 147, 214]

### Mechanisms of Injury

Two likely mechanisms may be responsible for dislocation of the elbow joint, and both probably require a

posteriorly directed force. If this force is directed in a posterior direction only, a straight posterior dislocation of the elbow occurs (Fig. 9–57). Authorities disagree about whether the elbow is in flexion or hyperextension at the time of injury.[101, 155] If an initial valgus force is combined with a posteriorly directed force, the medial epicondyle is avulsed in skeletally immature patients (Fig. 9–58).

### Classification

Elbow dislocations in adults have been classified by Stimson.[196] This classification is dependent on the direction of displacement of the ulna; for example, if the ulna is displaced posteriorly, it is classified as a posterior dislocation. The two main groups are based on the proximal radioulnar joint. If that joint is intact, a pure dislocation of the elbow joint is present. The dislocation may be posterior, which is by far the most common, or it may be in a medial or lateral direction. Stimson also described an anterior dislocation, which is extremely rare.[117, 147, 173] His second main group includes elbow dislocations in which the proximal radioulnar joint is also disrupted.

### Treatment

Closed reduction of the dislocation should be performed as soon as possible. Before any treatment, a complete evaluation of the neurovascular status of the extremity must be made because injury to the brachial artery and the median and, less commonly, the ulnar nerves may occur at the time of dislocation. Anesthesia to reduce discomfort and relax the musculature about the elbow greatly facilitates the reduction. Although general anesthesia can be used, an axillary block usually provides both pain control and muscle relaxation. Self-administered nitrous oxide may also be used.

Regardless of the method of anesthesia, reduction of the dislocation requires traction to dislodge the coronoid

---

**TABLE 9–2**

Classification of Proximal Radial Fractures

> I. Valgus fractures
> Type A: Salter-Harris types I and II
> Type B: Salter-Harris type IV
> Type C: Fracture of the radial metaphysis only
> II. Fractures secondary to posterior elbow dislocation
> Type D: Reduction injuries
> Type E: Dislocation injuries

From Wilkins, K.E. Fractures and dislocations of the elbow region. In: Rockwood, C.H.; Wilkins, K.E.; King, R.E., eds. Fractures in Children. Philadelphia, J.B. Lippincott, 1984.

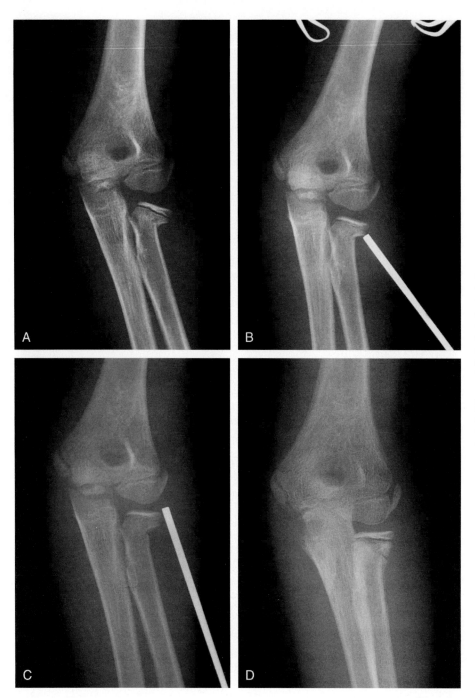

FIGURE **9–51.** Angulated fracture of the radial neck. *A,* An anteroposterior radiograph of the elbow shows a fracture of the radial neck that is angulated 45°. *B,* Anteroposterior radiograph with a percutaneously inserted Steinmann pin. The blunt end of the Steinmann pin has been inserted against the head and neck of the radius proximal to the fracture. *C,* The fracture has been reduced by general pressure with the blunt end of the Steinmann pin against the radial head. *D,* An anteroposterior radiograph shows complete correction of the angulation of the fracture.

process and the radial head from their posterior position. Before applying traction, one must first correct any lateral displacement to try to prevent entrapment of the median nerve within the elbow joint.[77] Once the medial or lateral displacement has been corrected, the forearm should be supinated. Distal and longitudinal traction is then applied with the patient's elbow flexed while an assistant holds the upper part of the arm to provide countertraction. The assistant stabilizes the upper part of the arm, and traction with the elbow in flexion may effect the reduction. The surgeon may also use the thumb and fingers to push the olecranon forward while continuing the traction.

The stability of the elbow should be checked. Usually, the elbow is stable, and if the elbow is stable after reduction, 1 week of immobilization to allow for resolution of pain and swelling is sufficient. It is important to begin range-of-motion exercises at that point to reduce the risk of loss of elbow motion, which is a known complication of elbow dislocation. If the elbow is unstable at the time of reduction, it should be immobilized in the position of stability for a minimum of 3 weeks and possibly longer. After that time, a removable splint should be worn. Although motion is encouraged, full extension is not attempted until 6 weeks after the injury.

Instability of the dislocation may also result from entrapment of the medial epicondyle within the elbow joint. Careful inspection of the radiographs reveals the position of the medial epicondyle. If it is within the elbow joint after reduction, it must be removed either by manipulation or, more commonly, by open reduction, after which it is internally fixed with pins (Fig. 9–59).

## Complications

### VASCULAR COMPROMISE

Disruption of the brachial artery has been reported in association with elbow dislocation, but fortunately, it is rare.[91, 107, 120] Brachial artery injury is more common with open elbow dislocation.[91, 120] Louis and associates[120] stated that with brachial artery laceration in association with elbow dislocation, the collateral circulation about the elbow is disrupted and severe ischemia of the forearm results. This complication requires immediate arterial exploration and vascular repair.

### NEUROLOGIC INJURY

Both ulnar and median nerve injuries have been reported to occur with dislocation of the elbow. Injuries to the ulnar nerve have been associated with valgus dislocation and avulsion of the medial epicondyle. These nerve lesions are transient.[71] Median nerve lesions are uncommon; when they do occur, however, they may produce profound nerve damage because the nerve may become entrapped within the elbow joint as a result of the elbow dislocation.[77, 78, 84, 122, 128, 164, 166, 172]

Hallett[85] described three mechanisms by which the median nerve may become entrapped within the elbow joint. In the first type, the nerve becomes entrapped

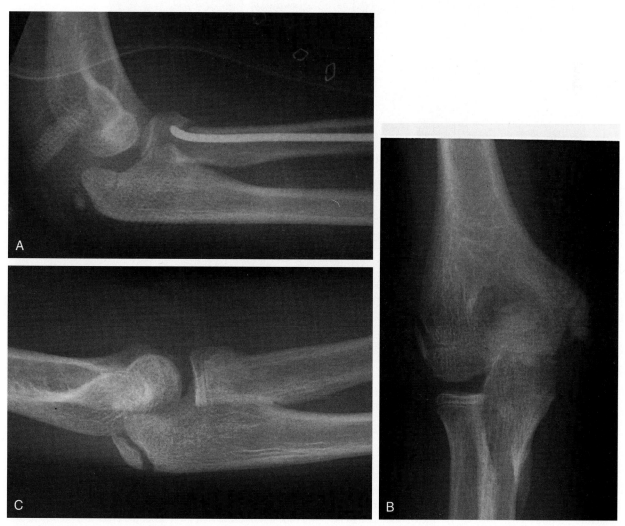

**FIGURE 9–52.** Displaced fracture of the neck of the radius with an associated nondisplaced olecranon fracture in a 6-year-old girl. In addition to the fractures, she also had an impending forearm compartment syndrome. She presented with marked pain and decreased neurologic function after transfer from another hospital. Compartment pressures were significantly elevated. She underwent immediate anterior forearm compartment release in addition to reduction and stabilization of the radial neck fracture with an elastic intramedullary nail. *A,* Lateral radiograph of the elbow after reduction of the radial neck. A titanium elastic nail has been used to reduce the radial neck fracture, and it was left in place to help stabilize the fracture. *B,* Anteroposterior radiograph of the elbow 1½ years after fracture. The fracture has healed with no evidence of avascular necrosis of the head of the radius. In addition, the physis of the radius is open. *C,* Lateral radiograph also demonstrating a healed fracture and an open proximal radial physis.

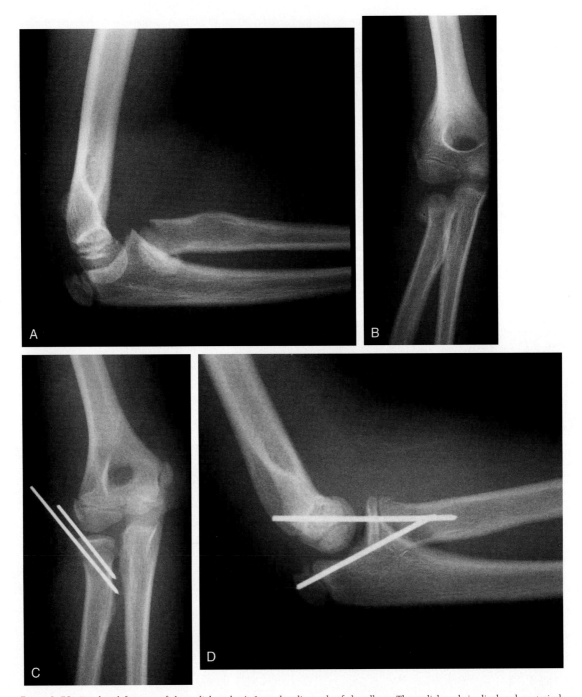

FIGURE 9–53. Displaced fracture of the radial neck. *A*, Lateral radiograph of the elbow. The radial neck is displaced posteriorly. *B*, Anteroposterior radiograph. The radial head and neck are displaced posteriorly and angulated laterally. *C*, Anteroposterior radiograph of the elbow after open reduction and internal fixation with two smooth Steinmann pins. The pins have been placed along the edge of the radial head and neck across the metaphysis and physis. *D*, Postoperative lateral radiograph.

within the joint after a valgus dislocation. The medial epicondyle is avulsed, or the forearm flexor muscles are detached, along with tearing of the ulnar collateral ligaments. The nerve slips behind the humerus during the dislocation and becomes entrapped within the joint after the reduction. In the second type, the nerve is caught in the healing fracture of the medial epicondyle. In the third type, the nerve becomes looped anteriorly in the joint.

Hallett considered the diagnosis of this injury to be difficult because of the absence of pain. My experience has been otherwise.[79] I encountered a 7-year-old girl who had dislocated her elbow 4 months previously. After the dislocation she complained of pain in her arm, and because of her refusal to extend her elbow, she was referred for physical therapy. In spite of this therapy, the patient never regained elbow extension and continued to complain of elbow pain. By the time that she was seen by

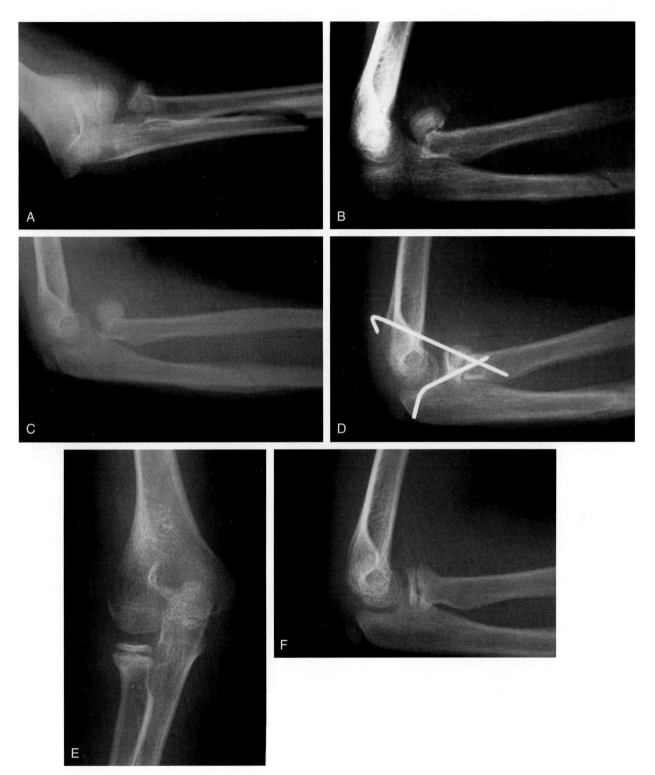

FIGURE **9–54.** Monteggia variant fracture with a displaced fracture of the neck of the radius in a 9-year-old girl. *A,* Lateral radiograph of the elbow and forearm demonstrating a fracture of the ulna and an angulated fracture of the neck of the radius. *B,* The ulnar fracture is healing 1 month after injury, but the fracture of the neck of the radius is significantly angulated anteriorly. *C,* Seven weeks after injury the ulnar fracture is healed; the fracture of the neck of the radius is also healed but is angulated anteriorly 90° with dislocation of the radiocapitellar joint. Although the fractures have healed, the patient has very limited forearm rotation and elbow flexion. *D,* Lateral radiograph of the elbow after osteotomy of the neck of the radius with reduction of the head of the radius. *E,* An anteroposterior radiograph of the elbow 9 months after osteotomy of the radius demonstrates reduction of the radiocapitellar joint and normal growth of the proximal radial physis. *F,* Lateral radiograph of the elbow demonstrating reduction of the radiocapitellar joint with a normal proximal radial contour and normal growth of the proximal radial physis.

**TABLE 9–3** ....................................

Classification of Fractures of the Olecranon

| | |
|---|---|
| Type I: | Undisplaced; no associated injury |
| Type II: | Undisplaced with proximal radial fracture or supracondylar fracture |
| Type III: | Undisplaced but with soft tissue damage (e.g., neurovascular damage) |
| Type IV: | Displaced fracture |

....................................

me, she had a complete median nerve lesion. The nerve was found to be looped around the posterior of the humerus and entered the elbow joint posteriorly. Radiographically, she had a cortical depression in the ulnar side of the distal end of the humerus caused by the nerve, as described by Matev[127] (Fig. 9–60). The nerve required resection and anastomosis because the portion within the joint was found to be nothing but scar. The patient

regained nearly total normal motor function and almost normal sensation in the median nerve distribution.

Median nerve injury is uncommonly associated with elbow dislocation. If, however, a patient with an elbow dislocation, especially if accompanied by a fracture of the medial epicondyle, has a lesion of the median nerve, medial nerve exploration should be undertaken because the nerve is probably trapped in the elbow joint.[80, 168]

## Recurrent Dislocation

Because recurrent dislocation of the elbow is uncommon, few reports of this complication are available. Osborne and Cotterill[155] believed that recurrence was the result of failure of reattachment of the posterolateral capsule and ligaments of the elbow joint. If an elbow dislocation is produced by a valgus injury to the elbow, the medial epicondyle and medial collateral ligaments are avulsed.

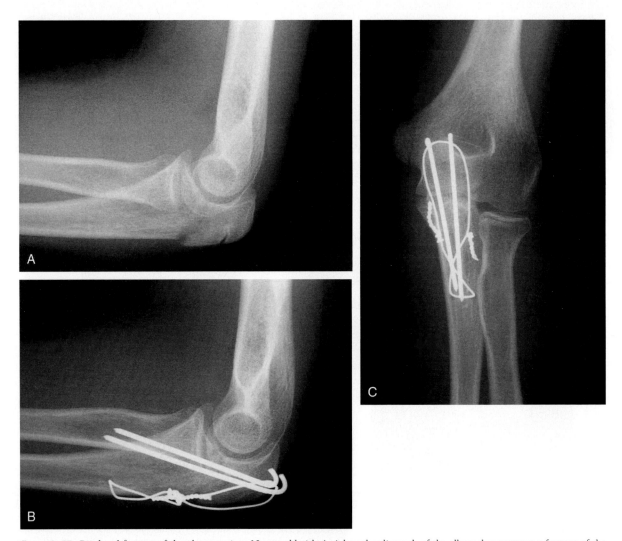

**FIGURE 9–55.** Displaced fracture of the olecranon in a 13-year-old girl. *A,* A lateral radiograph of the elbow demonstrates a fracture of the olecranon with 3 mm of displacement. *B,* A lateral radiograph of the elbow 4 weeks after surgery shows union of the fracture. The fracture was stabilized with two pins and a tension band. Early active elbow motion was begun, and the patient had nearly full elbow flexion and extension at the time of this radiograph. *C,* Anteroposterior radiograph of the fracture 4 weeks after open reduction of the fracture. Note the tension band, which has been placed in a figure 8 and locked proximally by the bent K-wires and is traveling distally through a coronal drill hole in the ulna distal to the fracture.

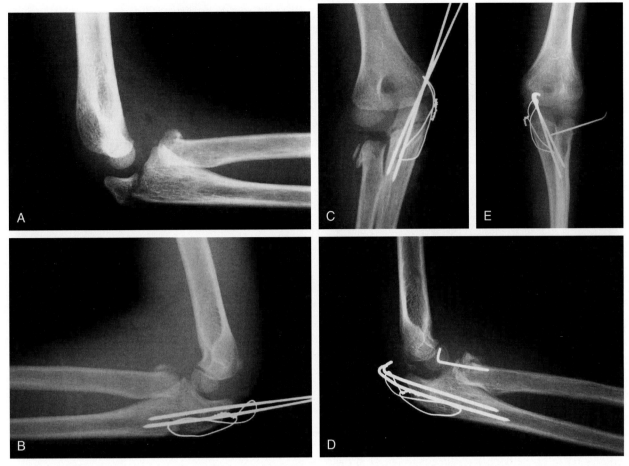

**FIGURE 9–56.** Fracture of the olecranon and radial neck. *A,* Lateral radiograph of the elbow showing a displaced fracture of the olecranon with anterior displacement of the distal ends of the ulna and radius. Note the displaced fracture of the radial neck. *B,* Intraoperative lateral radiograph of the elbow after open reduction and internal fixation of the olecranon with two smooth pins and a tension band wire. *C,* Anteroposterior radiograph of the elbow after reduction of the olecranon. The radial head and neck are still displaced out of the elbow joint. *D,* Lateral radiograph after open reduction of the radial head. *E,* Anteroposterior radiograph after open reduction of the radial head. The radial head is fixed with a smooth pin that enters the edge of the radial head and crosses the metaphysis and physis.

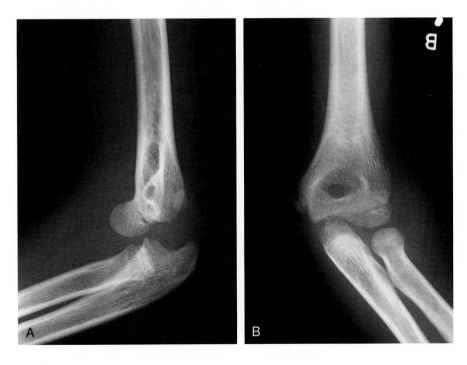

**FIGURE 9–57.** Posterior dislocation of the elbow. *A,* Lateral radiograph of the elbow. The ulna and radius are displaced posteriorly. *B,* Anteroposterior radiograph of the posterior dislocation of the elbow.

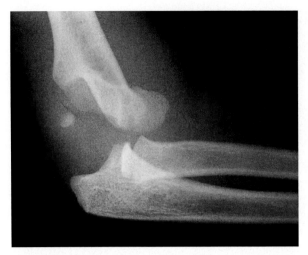

**FIGURE 9–58.** Lateral radiograph demonstrating dislocation of the elbow with avulsion of the medial epicondyle. The mechanism of injury was a valgus force.

In the cases of recurrent dislocation described, the instability was on the lateral rather than the medial side.[204] These dislocations, therefore, most likely result from a posteriorly directed force rather than a valgus injury. Some authors have observed avulsion of the capsule and lateral collateral ligaments along with a small piece of bone and cartilage from the lateral side of the elbow.[154, 204]

Treatment of recurrent dislocation of the elbow requires repair of the lax posterolateral structures of the elbow. Osborne and Cotterill[155] described a method of reattachment of the capsule and lateral collateral ligaments to restore elbow stability. These structures are incised in line with their fibers, beginning at the humeral epicondylar ridge. The incision is continued distal to the annular ligament. The bone of the lateral epicondyle is roughened, and the capsule and collateral ligament are reattached to the bone with sutures.

## Divergent Elbow Dislocation

This type of elbow dislocation is uncommon.[53, 91, 93] The probable mechanism is an axial load on the elbow with the forearm pronated, which results in both elbow dislocation and disruption of the proximal radioulnar articulation[93] (Fig. 9–61). The elbow joint is reduced first; the divergence of the radius and ulna is then reduced by pronation of the forearm.

## RADIAL HEAD DISLOCATION

### Incidence

Isolated traumatic dislocation of the head of the radius is extremely rare. This injury is most frequently associated with fracture of the ulna, thus being a type of Monteggia fracture-dislocation.[133] Hamilton and Parkes[86] stated

that suspected isolated radial head dislocations in children were most likely associated with bending of the ulna. If the ulna did not appear bent on the radiographs, they concluded that it had regained its normal shape. Weisman and colleagues reported two patients with reduced radial heads on original radiographs; however, the radial head was dislocated on follow-up radiographs 10 and 21 days after injury.[211] They also believed that the radial head had dislocated initially but had reduced spontaneously when seen radiographically and then dislocated again in the cast.

The annular ligament stabilizes the head of the radius and prevents dislocation. This ligament may be torn with the forearm in pronation.[212, 213]

## Differentiation from Congenital Dislocation of the Radius

Frequently, congenital radial head dislocation is not noticed by the patient or the family because arm function is normal. Usually, when a child sustains a relatively minor injury to the elbow, radial head dislocation is observed. Differentiation from a true acute injury may be made by careful examination of the extremity. Although a child with a congenital dislocation and recent trauma may have pain, it is usually less severe than one would expect with traumatic dislocation. The elbow motion, especially in rotation, is most likely greater than expected.

Radiographs demonstrate dysplasia of the radiohumeral joint (Fig. 9–62). The capitellum may be hypoplastic. The radial head is usually dome shaped, without the central depression that one would see with traumatic dislocation of a normal radial head.[4, 124, 131]

## Management

Surgical treatment of true congenital dislocation of the head of the radius is not warranted in children because attempts at reduction have not been rewarding. A child with essentially normal elbow function will probably lose elbow motion and function after surgical reduction. Neglected traumatic dislocation, in contrast, has been treated with open reduction with good results, even when the interval between the trauma and the surgical reduction has been more than 3 years.[18, 119] Use of a strip of the triceps tendon to reconstruct the annular ligament has been advocated.[18, 119]

## SUBLUXATION OF THE RADIAL HEAD

### Incidence

Although subluxation of the radial head is the most accurate description of this injury, it is also known by the terms "pulled elbow" and "nursemaid's elbow." It is probably the most common traumatic elbow injury in

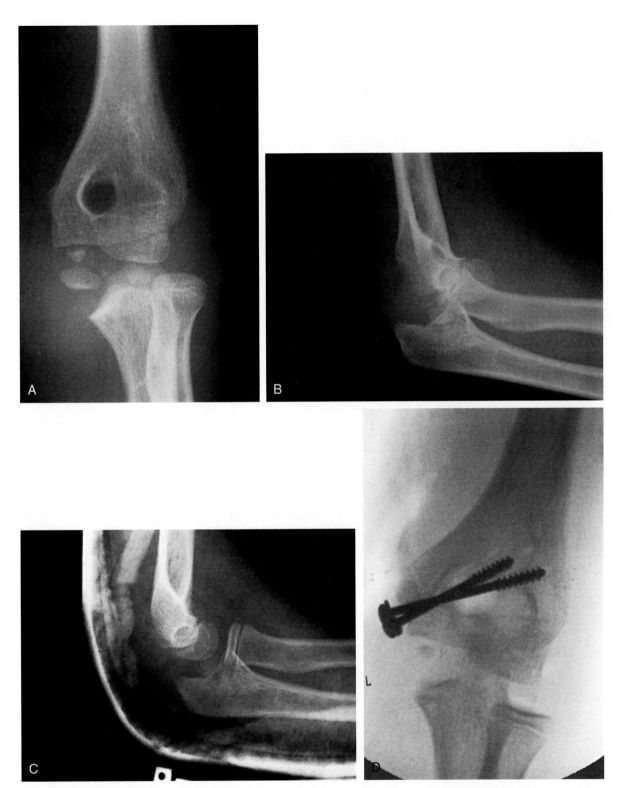

**FIGURE 9–59.** Posterior elbow dislocation in a 13-year-old boy with a medial epicondylar fracture. The medial epicondyle is entrapped in the elbow joint. *A,* Anteroposterior radiograph of the elbow demonstrating the dislocation of the elbow. Note that the medial epicondyle is displaced and is in the elbow joint. It can be seen anterior to the ossification center of the trochlea. *B,* Lateral radiograph of the dislocated elbow. The medial epicondyle is seen in the elbow joint. *C,* Lateral radiograph of the elbow after reduction. The elbow joint space is wider than normal, and the medial epicondyle is located within the elbow joint. It is seen lying between the capitellum and the olecranon on this radiograph. *D,* Anteroposterior radiograph of the elbow after open reduction of the displaced fracture of the medial epicondyle. The elbow was approached surgically with an incision along the medial side of the elbow. The medial epicondyle was removed from the elbow joint with a valgus force on the elbow. The epicondyle was repositioned into its normal position and internally fixed with two screws.

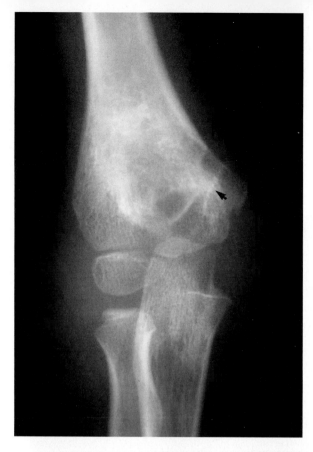

FIGURE 9–60. Anteroposterior radiograph taken 4 months after dislocation of the elbow. Note the cortical depression in the distal end of the humerus just proximal to the medial epicondyle (arrow). This depression marks the location of the median nerve that became entrapped in the elbow joint after dislocation.

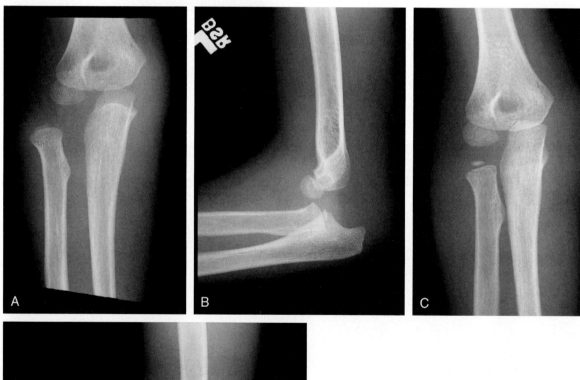

FIGURE 9–61. Divergent dislocation of the elbow. A, An anteroposterior radiograph of the elbow demonstrates the separation between the radius and the ulna. B, Lateral radiograph of the elbow. The radius and ulna are posteriorly dislocated. C, An anteroposterior radiograph after closed reduction demonstrates restoration of the normal anatomy of the elbow. D, Lateral radiograph of the elbow after reduction. (From Holbrook, J.L.; Green, N.E. Clin Orthop 234:72, 1988.)

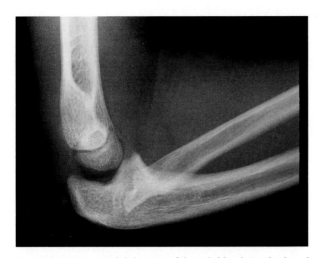

**FIGURE 9–62.** Congenital dislocation of the radial head. On this lateral radiograph, the radial head is displaced posteriorly and has migrated proximally. The radial neck is narrow and dysplastic, indicative of a long-standing dislocation.

children. Radial head subluxation has been estimated to occur in 15% to 27% of all elbow injuries in children younger than 10 years.[40, 191] Even though the average age at injury is between 2 and 4 years, I have encountered this injury in children up to age 8 years.

## Mechanism of Injury

This injury is produced with the forearm in pronation. With longitudinal traction and the forearm in pronation, the annular ligament tears at its attachment to the radius. The head of the radius moves distally, and as the traction is released, the annular ligament becomes caught between the radial head and the capitellum.[40, 180, 199] The tear in the annular ligament may be small, with only a small portion of it caught between the radial head and the capitellum. With a large tear, more of the annular ligament becomes entrapped, and reduction of the subluxation is more difficult.

This injury is not seen in older children; Salter and Zaltz claim that this injury is rare after the age of 5 years because the ligament becomes thicker with age and resists tearing.[180] The shape of the radial head is oval rather than circular. The sagittal diameter in supination is greater than the coronal diameter of the radial head; therefore, the subluxation can be reduced with the forearm in supination.

Radial head subluxation results from a pull on the child's extended arm. Typically, the arm is pulled by a parent or a person walking with the child who helps the child step up onto a sidewalk. However, the injury may occur whenever someone pulls on the child's extended and pronated forearm. Children may even produce the injury themselves. If the child grabs something to break a fall, radial head subluxation may result.

## Management

A child with radial head subluxation holds the arm flexed at the elbow with the forearm pronated. The initial pain quickly subsides, and the child may return to play but will not use the injured extremity. An infant may hold the arm limp. This pseudoparalysis may cause concern that brachial plexus stretch has occurred.

Careful examination of the arm reveals pain in the elbow only. Radiographs should be obtained to rule out another injury. The subluxation is then reduced by forcefully supinating the forearm with the elbow in 60° to 90° of flexion. With the forearm forcefully supinated, the elbow is fully flexed maximally.[191] The surgeon's thumb is placed over the radial head. As the radial head reduces, one is usually (but not always) able to palpate and hear the click of reduction. The greater the tear in the annular ligament, the more forceful the supination that is required. The child begins to use the arm quickly after the subluxation is reduced and should be observed until the arm is used. Immobilization of the arm is not necessary. It is important for the family to observe the child's use of the arm. If use of the arm is not normal, the family should bring the child back for reevaluation.

### REFERENCES

1. Abe, M.; Ishizu, T.; Nagaoka, T.; Onomura, T. Epiphyseal separation of the distal end of the humeral epiphysis: A follow-note. J Pediatr Orthop 15:426–434, 1995.
2. Abe, M.; Ishizu, T.; Shirai, H.; et al. Tardy ulnar palsy caused by cubitus varus deformity. J Hand Surg [Am] 20:5–9, 1995.
3. Abraham, E.; Powers, T.; Witt, P.; Ray, R.D. Experimental hyperextension supracondylar fractures in monkeys. Clin Orthop 171:309–318, 1982.
4. Almquist, E.E.; Gordon, L.H.; Blue, A.I. Congenital dislocation of the head of the radius. J Bone Joint Surg Am 51:1118–1127, 1969.
5. Amillo, S.; Mora, G. Surgical management of neural injuries associated with elbow fractures in children. J Pediatr Orthop 19:573–577, 1999.
6. Angelov, A. A new method for treatment of the dislocated radial neck fracture in children. In: Chapchal, G., ed. Fractures in Children. New York, Georg Thieme, 1981, pp. 192–194.
7. Archibald, D.A.; Roberts, J.A.; Smith, M.G. Transarticular fixation for severely displaced supracondylar fractures in children. J Bone Joint Surg Br 73:147–149, 1991.
8. Arino, V.L.; Lluch, E.E.; Ramirez, A.M.; et al. Percutaneous fixation of supracondylar fractures of the humerus in children. J Bone Joint Surg Am 59:914–916, 1977.
9. Arnold, J.A.; Nasca, R.J.; Nelson, C.L. Supracondylar fractures of the humerus. J Bone Joint Surg Am 59:589–595, 1977.
10. Aronson, D.D.; Prager, B.I. Supracondylar fractures of the humerus in children. A modified technique for closed pinning. Clin Orthop 219:174–184, 1987.
11. Ashhurst, A.P.C. An Anatomical and Surgical Study of Fractures of the Lower End of the Humerus. Philadelphia, Lea & Febiger, 1910.
12. Bado, J.L. The Monteggia lesion. Clin Orthop 50:71–86, 1967.
13. Bakalim, G.; Wilppula, E. Supracondylar humeral fractures in children. Acta Orthop Scand 43:366–374, 1972.
14. Banskota, A.; Volz, R.G. Traumatic laceration of the radial nerve following supracondylar fracture of the elbow. A case report. Clin Orthop 184:150–155, 1984.
15. Basom, W.C. Supracondylar and transcondylar fractures in children. Clin Orthop 1:43–48, 1953.
16. Beals, R.K. The normal carrying angle of the elbow. Clin Orthop 19:194–196, 1976.
17. Bede, W.B.; Lefebure, A.R.; Rostman, M.A. Fractures of the medial humeral epicondyle in children. Can J Surg 18:137–142, 1975.

18. Bell Tawse, A.J. The treatment of malunited anterior Monteggia fractures in children. J Bone Joint Surg Br 47:718–723, 1965.
19. Bellemore, M.C.; Barret, I.R.; Middleton, R.W.; et al. Supracondylar osteotomy of the humerus for correction of cubitus varus. J Bone Joint Surg Br 66:566–572, 1984.
20. Beltran, J.; Rosenberg, Z.S.; Kawelblum, M.; et al. Pediatric elbow fractures: MRI evaluation. Skeletal Radiol 23:277–281, 1994.
21. Bensahel, H.; Csukonyi, Z.; Badelon, D.; Badaoui, S. Fractures of the medial condyle of the humerus in children. J Pediatr Orthop 6:430–433, 1986.
22. Bernstein, S.M.; King, J.D.; Sanderson, R.A. Fractures of the medial epicondyle of the humerus. Contemp Orthop 12:637–641, 1981.
23. Biyani, A.; Gupta, M.S.; Sharma, M.S. Determination of medial epicondylar epiphyseal angle for supracondylar humeral fractures in children. J Pediatr Orthop 13:94–97, 1993.
24. Blasier, R.D. The triceps-splitting approach for repair of distal humeral malunion in children. A report of a technique. Am J Orthop 25:621–624, 1996.
25. Bostman, O.; Makela, E.A.; Sodergard, J.; et al. Absorbable polyglycolic pins in internal fixation of fractures in children. J Pediatr Orthop 13:242–245, 1993.
26. Boyd, D.W.; Aronson, D.D.; Prager, B.I. Supracondylar fractures of the humerus: A prospective study of percutaneous pinning. J Pediatr Orthop 12:789–794, 1992.
27. Brewster, A.H.; Karp, M. Fractures in the region of the elbow in children. An end-result study. Surg Gynecol Obstet 71:643–649, 1940.
28. Brown, I.C.; Zinar, D.M. Traumatic and iatrogenic neurological complications after supracondylar humerus fractures in children. J Pediatr Orthop 15:440–443, 1995.
29. Buhr, A.J.; Cooke, A.M. Fracture patterns. Lancet 1:531–536, 1959.
30. Camp, J.; Ishizue, K.; Gomez, M.; et al. Alteration of Baumann's angle by humeral position: Implications for treatment of supracondylar humerus fractures. J Pediatr Orthop 13:521–525, 1993.
31. Campbell, C.C.; Waters, P.M.; Emans, J.B.; et al. Neurovascular injury and displacement in type III supracondylar fractures. J Pediatr Orthop 15:47–52, 1995.
32. Casiano, E.; Reduction and fixation by pinning "banderillero." Mil Med 125:262–264, 1961.
33. Chacha, P.B. Fracture of medial condyle of humerus with rotational displacement. J Bone Joint Surg Am 52:1453–1458, 1970.
34. Chacon, D.; Kissoon, N.; Brown, T.; Galpin, R. Use of comparison radiographs in the diagnosis of traumatic injuries of the elbow. Ann Emerg Med 21:895–899, 1992.
35. Cheng, J.C.; Lam, T.P.; Shen, W.Y. Closed reduction and percutaneous pinning for type III displaced supracondylar fractures of the humerus in children. J Orthop Trauma 9:511–515, 1995.
36. Cheng, J.C.; Shen, W.Y. Limb fracture pattern in different pediatric age groups: A study of 3,350 children. J Orthop Trauma 7:15–22, 1993.
37. Collins, R.; Lavine, S.A. Fracture of the medial epicondyle. Clin Proc Child Hosp (Wash) 20:274–277, 1964.
38. Copley, L.A.; Dormans, J.P.; Davidson, R.S. Vascular injuries and their sequelae in pediatric supracondylar humeral fractures: Toward a goal of prevention. J Pediatr Orthop 16:99–103, 1996.
39. Corkery, P.H. The management of supracondylar fractures in the humerus in children. Br J Clin Pract 18:583–591, 1964.
40. Corrigan, A.B. The pulled elbow. Med J Aust 2:187–189, 1965.
41. Coventry, M.B.; Henderson, C.C. Supracondylar fractures of the humerus: 49 cases in children. Rocky Mt Med J 53:458–465, 1956.
42. Crabbe, W.A. Treatment of fracture separation of the capitular epiphysis. J Bone Joint Surg Br 45:722–726, 1963.
43. Cramer, K.; Devito, D.P.; Green, N.E. Comparison of closed reduction and percutaneous pinning versus open reduction and percutaneous pinning in displaced supracondylar fractures of the humerus in children. J Orthop Trauma 6:407–412, 1992.
44. Cramer, K.E.; Green, N.E.; Devito, D.P. Incidence of anterior interosseous nerve palsy in supracondylar humerus fractures in children. J Pediatr Orthop 13:502–505, 1993.
45. D'Ambrosia, R.; Zink, W. Fractures of the elbow in children. Pediatr Ann 11:541–548, 1982.
46. Dameron, T.B. Transverse fractures of distal humerus in children. Instr Course Lect 30:224–235, 1981.
47. Davids, J.R.; Maguire, M.F.; Mubarak, S.J.; Wenger, D.R. Lateral condylar fracture of the humerus following posttraumatic cubitus varus. J Pediatr Orthop 14:466–470, 1994.
48. Davidson, R.S.; Markowitz, R.I.; Dormans, J.; Drummond, D.S. Ultrasonographic evaluation of the elbow in infants and young children after suspected trauma. J Bone Joint Surg Am 76:1804–1813, 1994.
49. De Beaux, A.C.; Beattie, T.; Gilbert, F. Elbow fat pad sign: Implication for clinical management. J R Coll Surg Edinb 37:205–206, 1992.
50. De Boeck, H.; De Smet, P.; Penders, W.; De Rydt, D. Supracondylar elbow fractures with impaction of the medial condyle in children. J Pediatr Orthop 15:444–448, 1995.
51. De Boeck, H.; Pouliart, N. Fractures of the capitellum humeri in adolescents. Int Orthop 24:246–248, 2000.
52. De Jager, L.T.; Hoffman, E.B. Fracture-separation of the distal humeral epiphysis. J Bone Joint Surg Br 73:143–146, 1991.
53. DeLee, J.C.; Wilkins, K.E.; Rogers, L.F.; Rockwood, C.A. Fracture-separation of the distal humerus epiphysis. J Bone Joint Surg Am 62:46–51, 1980.
54. DeRosa, G.P.; Graziano, G.P. A new osteotomy for cubitus varus. Clin Orthop 236:160–165, 1988.
55. Devnani, A.S. Lateral closing wedge supracondylar osteotomy of humerus for post-traumatic cubitus varus in children. Injury 28:643–647, 1997.
56. Dhillon, K.S.; Sengupta, S.; Singh, B.J. Delayed management of fracture of the lateral humeral condyle in children. Acta Orthop Scand 59:419–424, 1988.
57. Dodge, H.S. Displaced supracondylar fractures of the humerus in children: Treatment by Dunlop's traction. J Bone Joint Surg Am 54:1408–1418, 1972.
58. Dormans, J.P. Arthrographic-assisted percutaneous manipulation of displaced and angulated radial neck fractures in children. J Orthop Techn 2:77–81, 1994.
59. Dormans, J.P.; Squillante, R.; Sharf, H. Acute neurovascular complications with supracondylar humerus fractures in children. J Hand Surg [Am] 20:1–4, 1995.
60. Dunlop, J. Transcondylar fractures of the humerus in childhood. J Bone Joint Surg Am 21:59–73, 1939.
61. Eliason, E.L. Dressing for supracondylar fractures of the humerus. JAMA 82:1934–1935, 1924.
62. Fahey, J.J. Fractures of the elbow in children. Instr Course Lect 17:13–46, 1960.
63. Finnbogason, T.; Karlsson, G.; Lindberg, L.; Mortensson, W. Nondisplaced and minimally displaced fractures of the lateral condyle in children: A prospective radiographic investigation of fracture stability. J Pediatr Orthop 15:422–425, 1995.
64. Fleuriau-Chateau, P.; McIntyre, W.; Letts, M. An analysis of open reduction of irreducible supracondylar fractures of the humerus in children. Can J Surg 41:112–118, 1998.
65. Flynn, J.C.; Matthews, J.G.; Benoit, R.L. Blind pinning of displaced supracondylar fractures of the humerus in children. J Bone Joint Surg Am 56:263–273, 1974.
66. Flynn, J.C.; Richards, J.F., Jr.; Saltzman, R.I. Prevention and treatment of non-union of slightly displaced fractures of the lateral humeral condyle in children. An end-result study. J Bone Joint Surg Am 57:1087–1092, 1975.
67. Fowles, J.V.; Kassab, M.T. Displaced supracondylar fractures of the elbow in children. A report on the fixation of extension and flexion fractures by two lateral percutaneous pins. J Bone Joint Surg Br 56:490–500, 1974.
68. Fowles, J.V.; Kassab, M.T. Displaced fractures of the medial humeral condyle in children. J Bone Joint Surg Am 62:1159–1163, 1980.
69. Fowles, J.V.; Slimane, N.; Kassab, M.T. Elbow dislocation with avulsion of the medial humeral epicondyle. J Bone Joint Surg Br 72:102–104, 1990.
70. France, J.; Strong, M. Deformity and function in supracondylar fractures of the humerus in children variously treated by closed reduction and splinting, traction, and percutaneous pinning. J Pediatr Orthop 12:494–498, 1992.

71. French, P.R. Varus deformity of elbow following supracondylar fractures of the humerus in children. Lancet 2:439–441, 1959.

72. Gaddy, B.C.; Manske, P.R.; Pruitt, D.L.; et al. Distal humeral osteotomy for correction of posttraumatic cubitus varus. J Pediatr Orthop 14:214–219, 1994.

73. Galbraith, K.A.; McCullough, C.J. Acute nerve injury as a complication of closed fractures or dislocations of the elbow. Injury 11:159–164, 1979.

74. Garbuz, D.S.; Leitch, K.; Wright, J.G. The treatment of supracondylar fractures in children with an absent radial pulse. J Pediatr Orthop 16:594–596, 1996.

75. Gartland, J.J. Management of supracondylar fractures of the humerus in children. Surg Gynecol Obstet 109:145–154, 1959.

76. Gaur, S.; Varma, A.N.; Swarup, A. A new technique for old ununited lateral condyle fractures of the humerus in children. J Trauma 34:68–69, 1993.

77. Graham, H.A. Supracondylar fractures of the elbow in children. 1. Clin Orthop 54:85–91, 1967.

78. Graham, H.A. Supracondylar fractures of the elbow in children. 2. Clin Orthop 54:93–102, 1967.

79. Green, N.E. Entrapment of the median nerve following elbow dislocation. J Pediatr Orthop 3:384–386, 1983.

80. Green, N.E. Overnight delay in the reduction of supracondylar fractures of the humerus in children. J Bone Joint Surg Am 83:321–322, 2001.

81. Green, N.E.; Allen, B.A. Vascular injuries associated with dislocation of the knee. J Bone Joint Surg Am 59:236–239, 1977.

82. Griffin, P.P. Supracondylar fractures of the humerus. Pediatr Clin North Am 22:477–486, 1975.

83. Gruber, M.A.; Healey, W. The posterior approach to the elbow revisited. J Pediatr Orthop 16:215–219, 1996.

84. Haddad, R.J., Jr.; Saer, J.K.; Riordan, D.C. Percutaneous pinning of displaced supracondylar fractures of the elbow in children. Clin Orthop 71:112–117, 1970.

85. Hallett, J. Entrapment of the median nerve after dislocation of the elbow. J Bone Joint Surg Br 63:408–412, 1981.

86. Hamilton, W.; Parkes, J.I. Isolated dislocation of the radial head without fracture of the ulna. Clin Orthop 97:94–96, 1973.

87. Hammond, G. The management of supracondylar fractures of the humerus in children. Surg Clin North Am 22:747–762, 1952.

88. Hanlon, C.; Estes, W. Fractures in childhood: A statistical analysis. Am J Surg 87:312–323, 1954.

89. Haraldsson, S. On osteochondrosis deformans juvenilis capituli humeri including investigation of intra-osseous vasculature in distal humerus. Acta Orthop Scand Suppl 38, 1959.

90. Harrington, P.; Sharif, I.; Fogarty, E.E.; et al. Management of the floating elbow injury in children. Simultaneous ipsilateral fractures of the elbow and forearm. Arch Orthop Trauma Surg 120:205–208, 2000.

91. Harvey, S.; Tchelebi, H. Proximal radio-ulnar translocation. J Bone Joint Surg Br 61:447–449, 1979.

92. Henrikson, B. Supracondylar fracture of the humerus in children. Acta Chir Scand Suppl 369, 1966.

93. Holbrook, J.; Green, N.; Allen, B. Divergent pediatric elbow dislocation. Clin Orthop 234:72–74, 1988.

94. Holda, M.; Manolia, A.; LaMont, R. Epiphyseal separation of the distal end of the humerus with medial displacement. J Bone Joint Surg Am 62:52–57, 1980.

95. Holmerg, L. Fractures in the distal end of the humerus in children. Acta Chir Scand Suppl 103, 1945.

96. Hoyer, A., Treatment of supracondylar fracture of the humerus by skeletal traction in an abduction splint. J Bone Joint Surg Am 34:623–637, 1952.

97. Ippolito, E.; Moneta, M.; D'Arrigo, C. Post-traumatic cubitus varus: Long-term follow-up of corrective humeral osteotomy in children. J Bone Joint Surg Am 72:757–765, 1990.

98. Iyengar, S.R.; Hoffinger, S.A.; Townsend, D.R. Early versus delayed reduction and pinning of type III displaced supracondylar fractures of the humerus in children: A comparative study. J Orthop Trauma 13:51–55, 1999.

99. Jakob, R.; Fowles, J.V.; Rang, M.; Kassab, M.T. Observations concerning fractures of the lateral humeral condyle in children. J Bone Joint Surg Br 57:430–436, 1975.

100. Jarvis, J.; D'Astous, J. The pediatric T-supracondylar fracture. J Pediatr Orthop 4:697–699, 1984.

101. Jeffrey, C. Nonunion of epiphysis of the lateral condyle of the humerus. J Bone Joint Surg 40:396–405, 1958.

102. Jones, E.; Louis, D. Median nerve injuries associated with supracondylar fractures of the humerus in children. Clin Orthop 150:181–186, 1980.

103. Jones, T.; Esah, M. Displaced fracture of the neck of the radius in children. J Bone Joint Surg Br 53:429–439, 1971.

104. Kallio, P.; Foster, B.; Paterson, D. Difficult supracondylar elbow fractures in children: Analysis of percutaneous pinning technique. J Pediatr Orthop 12:11–15, 1992.

105. Kamal, A.; Austin, R. Dislocation of the median nerve and brachial artery in supracondylar fractures of the humerus. Injury 12:161–164, 1980.

106. Kasser, J.; Richards, K.; Millis, M. The triceps-dividing approach to open reduction of complex distal humeral fractures in adolescents: A Cybex evaluation of triceps function and motion. J Pediatr Orthop 10:93–96, 1990.

107. Kilburn, P.; Sweeney, J.; Silk, F. Three cases of compound posterior dislocation of the elbow with rupture of the brachial artery. J Bone Joint Surg Br 44:119–121, 1982.

108. Kilfoyle, R. Fractures of the medial condyle and epicondyle of the elbow in children. Clin Orthop 41:43–50, 1965.

109. Kim, H.S.; Jahng, J.S.; Han, D.Y.; et al. Modified step-cut osteotomy of the humerus. J Pediatr Orthop B 7:162–166, 1998.

110. King, D.; Secor, C. Bow elbow (cubitus varus). J Bone Joint Surg Am 33:572–576, 1951.

111. Kiyoshige, Y. Critical displacement of neural injuries in supracondylar humeral fractures in children. J Pediatr Orthop 19:816–817, 1999.

112. Kramhoft, M.; Keller, I.; Solgaard, S. Displaced supracondylar fractures of the humerus in children. Clin Orthop 221:215–220, 1987.

113. Lagenskiold, A.; Kivilaakso, R. Varus and valgus deformity of the elbow following supracondylar fracture of the humerus. Acta Chir Scand Suppl 38:313–320, 1967.

114. Letts, M.; Rumball, K.; Bauermeister, S.; et al. Fractures of the capitellum in adolescents. J Pediatr Orthop 17:315–320, 1997.

115. Lichtenburg, R. A study of 2532 fractures in children. Am J Surg 87:330–338, 1954.

116. Liddell, W. Neurovascular complications in widely displaced supracondylar fractures of the humerus. J Bone Joint Surg Br 49:806, 1967.

117. Linscheid, R.; Wheeler, D. Elbow dislocations. JAMA 194:113–118, 1965.

118. Lipscomb, P.; Burselson, R. Vascular and neural complications in supracondylar fractures of the humerus in children. J Bone Joint Surg Am 37:487–492, 1955.

119. Lloyd-Roberts, G.; Bucknill, T. Anterior dislocation of the radial head in children. J Bone Joint Surg Br 59:402–407, 1979.

120. Louis, D.; Ricciardi, J.; Spengler, D. Arterial injury: A complication of posterior elbow dislocation. J Bone Joint Surg Am 56:1631–1636, 1974.

121. Mann, T. Prognosis in supracondylar fractures. J Bone Joint Surg Br 45:516–522, 1963.

122. Mannerfelt, L. Median nerve entrapment after dislocation of the elbow. J Bone Joint Surg Br 50:152–155, 1968.

123. Mapes, R.; Hennrikus, W.L. The effect of elbow position on the radial pulse measured by Doppler ultrasonography after surgical treatment of supracondylar elbow fractures in children. J Pediatr Orthop 18:441–444, 1998.

124. Mardam-Bey, T.; Ger, E. Congenital radial head dislocation. J Hand Surg [Am] 4:316–320, 1979.

125. Markowitz, R.; Davidson, R.S.; Harty, M.P.; et al. Sonography of the elbow in infants and children. AJR Am J Roentgenol 159:829–833, 1992.

126. Masada, K.; Kawai, K.; Kawabata, H.; et al. Osteosynthesis for old established non-union of the lateral condyle of the humerus. J Bone Joint Surg Am 72:32–40, 1990.

127. Matev, I. A radiological sign of entrapment of the median nerve in the elbow joint after posterior dislocation. J Bone Joint Surg Br 58:353–355, 1976.

128. Matthews, J. Fractures of the olecranon in children. Injury 12:207–212, 1980.

129. Maylahn, D.; Fahey, J. Fractures of the elbow in children. JAMA 166:220–228, 1958.

130. McBride, E.; Monnet, J. Epiphyseal fracture of the head of the radius in children. Clin Orthop 16:264–271, 1960.
131. McFarland, B. Congenital dislocation of the head of the radius. Br J Surg 24:41–49, 1936.
132. McGraw, J.J.; Akbarnia, B.A.; Hanel, D.P.; et al., Neurological complications resulting from supracondylar fractures of the humerus in children. J Pediatr Orthop 6:647–650, 1986.
133. McKeever, P.; et al. Percutaneous reduction of angulated radial neck fractures in children: A report of 15 cases. Paper presented at the American Association of Orthopaedic Surgeons annual meeting, New Orleans, 1990.
134. McLauchlan, G.J.; Walker, C.R.; Cowan, B.; et al. Extension of the elbow and supracondylar fractures in children. J Bone Joint Surg Br 81:402–405, 1999.
135. Mehlman, C.T.; Strub, W.M.; Roy, D.R.; et al. The effect of surgical timing on the perioperative complications of treatment of supracondylar humeral fractures in children. J Bone Joint Surg Am 83:323–327, 2001.
136. Mehserle, W.; Meehan, P. Treatment of the displaced supracondylar fracture of the humerus (type III) with closed reduction and percutaneous cross-pin fixation. J Pediatr Orthop 11:705–711, 1991.
137. Metaizeau, J.P.; Lascombes, P.; Lemelle, J.L.; et al., Reduction and fixation of displaced radial neck fractures by closed intramedullary pinning. J Pediatr Orthop 13:355–360, 1993.
138. Michael, S.P.; Stanislas, M.J. Localization of the ulnar nerve during percutaneous wiring of supracondylar fractures in children. Injury 27:301–302, 1996.
139. Milch, H. Fractures and fracture-dislocations of humeral condyles. J Trauma 4:592–607, 1964.
140. Mintzer, C.; Walters, P.M.; Brown, D.J.; Kasser, J.R. Percutaneous pinning in the treatment of displaced lateral condyle fractures. J Pediatr Orthop 14:462–465, 1994.
141. Mirsky, E.C.; Karas, E.H.; Weiner, L.S. Lateral condyle fractures in children: Evaluation of classification and treatment. J Orthop Trauma 11:117–120, 1997.
142. Mitsunari, A.; Muneshige, H.; Ikuta, Y.; Murakami, T. Internal rotation deformity and tardy ulnar nerve palsy after supracondylar humeral fracture. J Shoulder Elbow Surg 4:23–29, 1995.
143. Mizuno, K.; Hirohata, K.; Kashiwagi, D. Fracture-separation of the distal humeral epiphysis in young children. J Bone Joint Surg Am 61:570–573, 1979.
144. Mohammad, S.; Rymaszewski, L.A.; Runciman, J. The Baumann angle in supracondylar fractures of the distal humerus in children. J Pediatr Orthop 19:65–69, 1999.
145. Murphy, W.; Siegel, M. Elbow fat pad with new signs and extended differential diagnosis. Radiology 124:659–665, 1977.
146. Nacht, J.; Ecker, M.L.; Chung, S.M.; et al. Supracondylar fractures of the humerus in children treated by closed reduction and percutaneous pinning. Clin Orthop 177:203–209, 1983.
147. Neviaser, J.; Wickstrom, J. Dislocation of the elbow: A retrospective study of 115 patients. South Med J 70:172–173, 1977.
148. Newell, R. Olecranon fractures in children. Injury 7:33–36, 1975.
149. Newman, J. Displaced radial neck fractures in children. Injury 9:114–121, 1977.
150. Nork, S.E.; Hennrikus, W.L.; Loncarich, D.P.; et al. Relationship between ligamentous laxity and the site of upper extremity fractures in children: Extension supracondylar fracture versus distal forearm fracture. J Pediatr Orthop B 8:90–92, 1999.
151. O'Brien, P. Injuries involving the radial epiphysis. Clin Orthop 41:51–58, 1965.
152. Oppenheim, W.; Clader, T.J.; Smith, C.; Bayer, M. Supracondylar humeral osteotomy for traumatic childhood cubitus varus deformity. Clin Orthop 188:34–39, 1984.
153. Oppenheim, W.; Davlin, L.B.; Leipzig, J.M.; Johnson, E.E. Concomitant fractures of the capitellum and trochlea. J Orthop Trauma 3:260–262, 1989.
154. Ormandy, L. Olecranon screw for skeletal traction of the humerus. Am J Surg 127:615–616, 1974.
155. Osborne, G.; Cotterill, P. Recurrent dislocation of the elbow. J Bone Joint Surg Br 48:340–346, 1966.
156. Ottolengthi, C. Acute ischemic syndrome: Its treatment; prophylaxis of Volkmann's syndrome. Am J Orthop 2:312–316, 1960.

157. Palmer, E.; Niemann, K.M.; Vesely, D.; Armstrong, J.H. Supracondylar fracture of the humerus in children. J Bone Joint Surg Am 60:653–656, 1978.
158. Paradis, G.; Lavallee, P.; Gagnon, N.; Lemire, L. Supracondylar fractures of the humerus in children. Technique and results of crossed percutaneous K-wire fixation. Clin Orthop 297:231–237, 1993.
159. Patterson, R. Treatment of displaced transverse fractures of the neck of the radius in children. J Bone Joint Surg 16:695–698, 1934.
160. Peters, C.; Scott, S.; Stevens, P. Closed reduction and percutaneous pinning of displaced supracondylar humerus fractures in children: Description of a new closed reduction technique for fractures with brachialis muscle entrapment. J Orthop Trauma 9:430–434, 1995.
161. Peterson, H. Physeal injuries of the distal humerus. Orthopedics 15:799–808, 1992.
162. Piggot, J. Supracondylar fractures of the humerus in children. Analysis at maturity of fifty-three patients treated conservatively [letter]. J Bone Joint Surg Am 68:1304, 1986.
163. Prietto, C. Supracondylar fractures of the humerus. J Bone Joint Surg Am 61:425–428, 1979.
164. Pritchard, D.; Linscheid, R.L.; Svien, H.J. Intra-articular median nerve entrapment with dislocation of the elbow. Clin Orthop 90:100–103, 1973.
165. Ramsey, R.; Griz, J. Immediate open reduction and internal fixation of severely displaced supracondylar fractures of the humerus in children. Clin Orthop 90:130–132, 1973.
166. Rang, M. Children's Fractures. Philadelphia, J.B. Lippincott, 1983.
167. Rang, M.; Moseley, C.F.; Roberts, J.M.; et al. Symposium: Management of displaced supracondylar fractures of the humerus. Contemp Orthop 18:497–535, 1989.
168. Rao, S.B.; Crawford, A.H. Median nerve entrapment after dislocation of the elbow in children. A report of 2 cases and review of literature. Clin Orthop 312:232–237, 1995.
169. Rasool, M.N.; Naidoo, K.S. Supracondylar fractures: Posterolateral type with brachialis muscle penetration and neurovascular injury. J Pediatr Orthop 19:518–522, 1999.
170. Reidy, J.; Van Gorden, G. Treatment of displacement of the proximal radial epiphysis. J Bone Joint Surg Am 45:1355, 1963.
171. Reinaerts, H.; Cheriex, E. Assessment of dislocation in supracondylar fracture of the humerus treated by overhead traction. Reconstr Surg Traumatol 17:92–99, 1979.
172. Roaf, R. Foramen in the humerus caused by the median nerve. J Bone Joint Surg Br 39:748–749, 1957.
173. Roberts, P. Dislocation of the elbow. Br J Surg 56:806–815, 1969.
174. Rogers, L.; Malove, S., Jr.; White, H.; Tachdjian, M.O. Plastic bowing, torus and greenstick supracondylar fractures of the humerus: Radiographic clues to obscure fractures of the elbow in children. Radiology 128:145–150, 1978.
175. Rowell, P. Arterial occlusion in juvenile humeral supracondylar fracture. Injury 6:254–256, 1974.
176. Roye, D.; Bini, S.; Infosino, A. Late treatment of lateral condylar fractures in children. J Pediatr Orthop 11:195–199, 1991.
177. Rutherford, A. Fractures of the lateral humeral condyle in children. J Bone Joint Surg Am 67:851–856, 1985.
178. Sabharwal, S.; Tredwell, S.J.; Beauchamp, R.D.; et al. Management of pulseless pink hand in pediatric supracondylar fractures of humerus. J Pediatr Orthop 17:303–310, 1997.
179. Salter, R.; Harris, W. Injuries involving the epiphyseal plate. J Bone Joint Surg Am 45:587–592, 1963.
180. Salter, R.; Zaltz, C. Anatomic investigations of the mechanism of injury and pathologic anatomy of "pulled elbow" in young children. Clin Orthop 77:134–143, 1971.
181. Schoenecker, P.L.; Delgado, E.; Rotman, M.; et al. Pulseless arm in association with totally displaced supracondylar fracture. J Orthop Trauma 10:410–455, 1996.
182. Sessa, S.; Lascombes, P.; Prevot, J.; Gagneux, E. Fractures of the radial head and associated elbow injuries in children. J Pediatr Orthop B 5:200–209, 1996.
183. Shifrin, P.; Gehring, H.; Iglesias, L. Open reduction and internal fixation of displaced supracondylar fractures of the humerus in children. Orthop Clin North Am 7:573–581, 1976.

184. Sibly, T.; Briggs, P.; Gibson, M. Supracondylar fractures of the humerus in childhood: Range of movement following posterior approach to open reduction. Injury 22:456–458, 1991.

185. Silberstein, M.J.; Brodeur, A.E.; Graviss, E.R.; Luisiri, A. Some vagaries of the medial epicondyle. J Bone Joint Surg Am 63:524–528, 1981.

186. Skibo, L.; Reed, M. A criterion for a true lateral radiograph of the elbow. Can Assoc Radiol J 45:287–291, 1994.

187. Smith, F. Displacement of the medial epicondyle of the humerus into the elbow joint. Ann Surg 124:410–425, 1946.

188. Smith, F. Medial epicondyle injuries. JAMA 142:396–402, 1950.

189. Smith, F. Children's elbow injuries: Fractures and dislocations. Clin Orthop 50:7–30, 1967.

190. Smith, F.; Joyce, J. Fractures of lateral condyle of humerus in children. Am J Surg 7:224–239, 1954.

191. Snellman, O. Subluxation of the head of the radius in children. Acta Orthop Scand 28:311–315, 1959.

192. Spinner, M.; Schreiber, S. Anterior interosseous nerve paralysis as a complication of supracondylar fractures of the humerus in children. J Bone Joint Surg Am 51:1584–1590, 1969.

193. Spinner, R.J.; O'Driscoll, S.W.; Davids, J.R.; Goldner, R.D. Cubitus varus associated with dislocation of both the medial portion of the triceps and the ulnar nerve. J Hand Surg [Am] 24:718–726, 1999.

194. Steele, J.; Graham, H. Angulated radial neck fractures in children. A prospective study of percutaneous reduction. J Bone Joint Surg Br 74:760–764, 1992.

195. Steinberg, E.L.; Golomb, D.; Salama, R.; Wientroub, S. Radial head and neck fractures in children. J Pediatr Orthop 8:35–38, 1988.

196. Stimson, L. A Practical Treatise on Fractures and Dislocations. Philadelphia, Lea Brothers, 1900.

197. Stone, J. Fractures of the elbow in children. J Orthop Surg 3:395–400, 1921.

198. Sutton, W.R.; Greene, W.B.; Georgopoulos, G.; Dameron, T.B., Jr. Displaced supracondylar humeral fractures in children. A comparison of results and costs in patients treated by skeletal traction versus percutaneous pinning. Clin Orthop 278:81–87, 1992.

199. Swenson, A. The treatment of supracondylar fractures of the humerus by Kirschner wire transfixion. J Bone Joint Surg Am 30:993–997, 1948.

200. Takahara, M.; Sesaki, I.; Kimura, T.; et al. Second fracture of the distal humerus after varus malunion of a supracondylar fracture in children. J Bone Joint Surg Br 80:791–797, 1998.

201. Theodorou, S.; Ierodiaconou, M.; Roussis, N. Fracture of the upper end of the ulna associated with dislocation of the head of the radius in children. Clin Orthop 228:240–249, 1988.

202. Tibone, J.; Stoltz, M. Fracture of the radial head and neck in children. J Bone Joint Surg Am 63:100–106, 1981.

203. Topping, R.E.; Blanco, J.S.; Davis, T.J. Clinical evaluation of crossed-pin versus lateral-pin fixation in displaced supracondylar humerus fractures. J Pediatr Orthop 15:435–439, 1995.

204. Trias, A.; Comeau, Y. Recurrent dislocation of the elbow in children. Clin Orthop 100:74–77, 1974.

205. Uchida, Y.; Ogata, K.; Sugioka, Y. A new three-dimensional osteotomy for cubitus varus deformity after supracondylar fracture of the humerus in children. J Pediatr Orthop 11:327–331, 1991.

206. Usui, M.; Ishii, S.; Miyano, S.; et al. Three-dimensional corrective osteotomy for treatment of cubitus varus after supracondylar fracture of the humerus in children. J Shoulder Elbow Surg 4:17–22, 1995.

207. Vahvanen, V. Fracture of the radial neck in children. Acta Orthop Scand 49:32–38, 1978.

208. Varma, B.; Srivastava, T. Fracture of the medial condyle of the humerus in children: A report of 4 cases including the late sequelae. Injury 4:171–174, 1972.

209. Wadsworth, T. Premature epiphyseal fusion after injury of the capitulum. J Bone Joint Surg Br 46:46–49, 1964.

210. Weiland, A.; Meyer, S.; Tolo, V.T.; et al. Surgical treatment of displaced supracondylar fractures of the humerus in children. Analysis of fifty-two cases followed for five to fifteen years. J Bone Joint Surg Am 60:657–661, 1978.

211. Weisman, D.; Rang, M.; Cole, W.G. Tardy displacement of traumatic radial head dislocation in childhood. J Pediatr Orthop 19:523–526, 1999.

212. Wiley, J.; Galey, J. Monteggia injuries in children. J Bone Joint Surg Br 67:728–731, 1985.

213. Wiley, J.J.; Pegington, J.; Horwich, J.P. Traumatic dislocation of the radius at the elbow. J Bone Joint Surg Br 56:501–507, 1974.

214. Wilkins, K.E. Fractures and dislocations of the elbow region. In: Rockwood, C.H.; Wilkins, K.E; King, R.E., eds. Fractures in Children. Philadelphia, J.B. Lippincott, 1984, pp. 363–450.

215. Wilson, P.D. Fractures and dislocations in the region of the elbow. Surg Gynecol Obstet 56:335–359, 1933.

216. Wong, H.K.; Balasubramaniam, P. Humeral torsional deformity after supracondylar osteotomy for cubitus varus: Its influence on the postosteotomy carrying angle. J Pediatr Orthop 12:490–493, 1992.

217. Woods, G.M.; Tullos, H.G. Elbow instability and medial epicondyle fracture. Am J Sports Med 5:23–30, 1977.

218. Zionts, L.E.; McKellop, H.A.; Hathaway, R. Torsional strength of pin configuration used to fix supracondylar fractures of the humerus in children. J Bone Joint Surg Am 76:253–256, 1994.

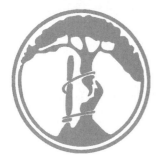

# CHAPTER 10

# Fractures and Dislocations about the Shoulder

Lawrence X. Webb, M.D.
James F. Mooney III, M.D.

## CLAVICLE

### Relevant Anatomy

The clavicle, or collar bone, is an **S**-shaped bone at the anterior base of the neck. Through articulations with the sternum medially and with the scapula at the acromion process laterally, it serves as an osseous connection between the axial skeleton and the upper extremity. In cross section, the medial portion of the clavicle is rounded or prismatic, and the lateral third is flattened. The anterosuperior aspect of the clavicle is subcutaneous.

The clavicle acts as an origin for the pectoralis major on the medial two thirds of its anterior surface and for the deltoid on the lateral third of its anterior surface. Inferiorly, through its middle two fourths, it affords an attachment for the subclavius muscle and its enveloping clavipectoral fascia while providing an attachment for both portions of the coracoclavicular ligament and the acromioclavicular ligament laterally and for the costoclavicular ligament medially. Posteriorly, the clavicle provides an attachment in its lateral third for the trapezius and for the clavicular head of the sternocleidomastoid muscle medially. The subclavian vessels and brachial plexus lie posterior to the junction of the medial two thirds and the lateral third of the bone.[42]

### Developmental Anatomy

The clavicle is the first bone to begin to ossify, which it does from two primary ossification centers that appear during the fifth or sixth week of fetal life.[37, 81] In contradistinction, it is one of the last to completely ossify, with its medial physis not closing completely until 24 to 26 years of age.[58]

## MEDIAL CLAVICULAR FRACTURES AND PSEUDOSTERNOCLAVICULAR JOINT DISLOCATIONS

### Incidence

Fracture of the medial portion of the clavicle occurs infrequently in children, in whom it accounts for only about 5% of all clavicular fractures.[103] Medial physeal fractures are more common than medial shaft fractures, and the former can mimic sternoclavicular joint dislocations in adults.[90]

### MECHANISM

The capsule of the sternoclavicular joint is more resistant to injury than the metaphysis of the medial part of the clavicle. Because the physeal plate does not close until about 24 or 25 years of age,[42, 58] medial-injuring forces in children and adolescents usually produce a physeal injury rather than pure dislocation of the sternoclavicular joint.[90] The most common mechanism of injury is thought to be compression of the shoulder toward the midline. Whether displacement occurs anterior or posterior to the sternum is determined by the secondary force vectors of this intershoulder compression.[29] In addition, a direct anterior force can also fracture the medial segment of the clavicle; in this case, displacement is always posterior.

### DIAGNOSIS

The patient has a history of either a blow to the medial part of the clavicle or the sternal area or an indirect mechanism such as occurs when the shoulder is used to butt against another player in a contact sport or a fall on the shoulder. Physical examination reveals local swelling

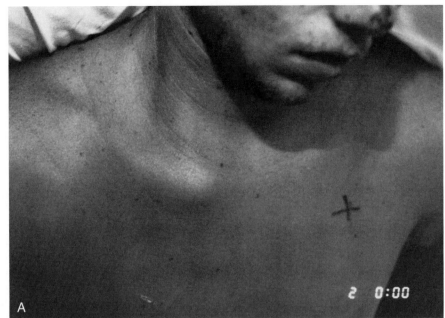

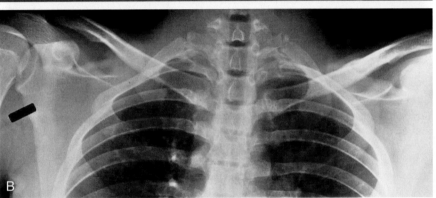

FIGURE **10–1.** Fracture of the medial portion of the clavicle. *A,* This patient sustained multiple injuries; the prominence of the right medial clavicle is obvious. *B,* A chest radiograph shows the asymmetry consistent with a medial physeal injury (the epiphysis is unossified). Incidental note is made of a contralateral first-rib fracture.

and tenderness about the medial part of the clavicle (Fig. 10–1). When the displacement is posterior, symptoms of respiratory embarrassment, dysphagia, dysphonia, or distended neck veins from compression of the neighboring trachea, esophagus, recurrent laryngeal nerve, or great vessels, respectively, may be present. X-rays angled to minimize the effect of obscuring overlying tissues—for example, the "serendipity" view of Rockwood[29] (Fig. 10–2) or the Hobbs view,[51] with the medial part of the clavicles and the sternoclavicular joints visualized bilaterally for comparison—usually confirm the diagnosis. Computed tomography (CT) of the sternoclavicular joint

is extremely helpful in more clearly delineating the direction and extent of displacement and the relationship of the displaced clavicle to neighboring structures (see Fig. 10–3).

## TREATMENT

Nondisplaced fractures of the medial portion of the clavicle can be managed symptomatically and have a good prognosis. A "bump" should be expected and will remodel to some extent with time, especially in a younger child. Respiratory distress secondary to a posteriorly

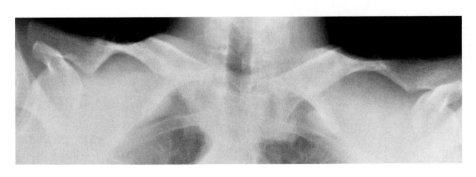

FIGURE **10–2.** A "serendipity" or cephalic tilt radiograph of a 14-year-old child. No fractures or dislocations are noted. The film is obtained by placing a nongrid cassette behind the supine patient's head and neck and angling the beam cephalad 40° from a distance of 45 to 60 inches.

displaced medial clavicular fracture may be life threatening, and an adequate airway should be secured as part of the patient's initial treatment.[1]

Generally, anteriorly displaced fractures require little treatment. Closed reduction can be attempted with longitudinal traction and direct pressure over the fracture. Usually, reduction is easily obtained but difficult to maintain, with redisplacement common. A posteriorly displaced medial clavicular fracture can sometimes be reduced by drawing the patient's shoulder posteriorly and into abduction; this maneuver is sometimes easier when the patient is supine and a folded towel is placed between the shoulder blades to abduct the shoulder girdles. Longitudinal traction on the involved upper extremity may be beneficial. Posterior displaced fractures that fail to reduce with closed techniques may be amenable to percutaneous reduction. After suitable anesthesia and skin preparation, a sterile towel clip is used to grab the medial part of the clavicle and manipulate it to its reduced position. A thoracic surgeon should be available when such a reduction is undertaken.

Maintenance of reduction is common if the displacement is posterior. The displacing forces can be negated successfully by a figure-of-eight plaster wrap and an arm sling. Such immobilization should be maintained for a month. The medial clavicular physis has great remodeling capacity, and late pain and deformity are rarely seen after displaced medial clavicular fractures.

Open reduction should be reserved for open injuries requiring débridement, for posterior displacements that are adversely affecting neighboring vital structures, and for significant displacements that cannot be reduced (and maintained) by closed techniques.[8, 34, 90] Internal fixation with metal implants is inadvisable and has been associated with potentially grave complications.[20] Alternatively, sutures placed strategically through drill holes in the outer portion of the neighboring sternum or sternoclavicular ligament and the medial section of the clavicle should suffice to stabilize the reduction until it heals.[90] One additional, albeit rare, indication for open reduction is scapulothoracic dissociation. In this situation, anatomic reduction helps "set" the scapula in the correct position on the thoracic wall and facilitates repair

of the torn scapular suspensory musculature close to its correct resting length.

## Fractured Clavicular Shaft at Birth

### INCIDENCE

The clavicle is the most commonly fractured bone in the newborn.[106] The incidence of clavicular birth fractures ranges from 2.8 to 7.2 per 1000 term deliveries, and clavicular fractures account for 84% to 92% of all obstetric fractures.[21, 35, 82, 106]

### MECHANISM AND DIAGNOSIS

Clavicular injury at birth has been shown to correlate with birth weight, inexperience of the delivering physician, and midforceps delivery.[21] The mechanism of fracture production is indirect: axial compression on the shoulder girdle during passage through a narrow birth canal. The most common fracture site is at the junction of the lateral and middle thirds of the bone. The fracture is usually nondisplaced or only minimally displaced; often, it is unappreciated initially and discovered as a lump over the clavicle about 10 days after birth. This lump is the most definitive sign of the fracture; earlier than 10 days, an asymmetric Moro reflex has been reported to be fairly specific for a clavicular fracture in the newborn.[112] Occasionally, the fracture is manifested by pseudoparalysis of the arm[21, 71] (Fig. 10–4). In this instance, the differential diagnosis includes fracture of the proximal end of the humerus, brachial plexus palsy, and sepsis of the shoulder joint, clavicle, scapula, or proximal part of the humerus.[71, 106, 112] It should be kept in mind that two of these diagnoses can coexist, for example, fracture with brachial plexus palsy or fracture with infection.[18, 131]

### TREATMENT

In a patient in whom upper extremity movements elicit tenderness or in those with pseudoparalysis, splinting the

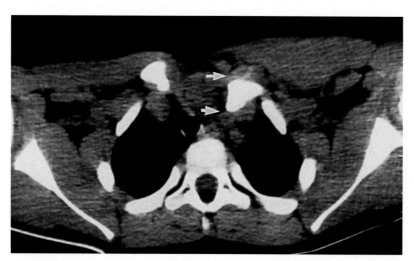

FIGURE 10–3. Shown is a computed tomographic scan of an adolescent with a left posterior sternoclavicular dislocation. Note the impingement on the posterior structures.

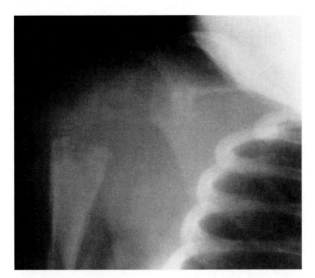

FIGURE **10–4.** Pseudoparalysis of the shoulder. This 4-week-old infant with pseudoparalysis after injury was treated for a clavicular fracture. The child was seen again in follow-up at 2½ weeks, at which time a "sucked candy" appearance of the proximal humeral metaphysis was apparent. Aspiration confirmed osteomyelitis. The differential diagnosis of pseudoparalysis in such a case is clavicular, proximal humeral, or scapular trauma; brachial plexus palsy; or sepsis of the joint, neighboring bone, or both.

upper extremity to the chest wall with a stockinette stretch bandage or a similar soft, expandable bandage for approximately 10 days is appropriate.[14, 29, 60] Anecdotally, it may be helpful to clip the sleeve of the affected side to the front of the infant's shirt or gown to avoid the potential problems of interference with loose and shifting bandages in this age group.

## Fractured Clavicular Shaft in Childhood

### INCIDENCE

Fracture of the clavicle is the most frequent childhood fracture.[120] The most common portion of the bone to fracture is the shaft, and such fractures account for approximately 85% of all childhood clavicular fractures.[79]

### MECHANISM

The most common mechanism of a clavicular shaft fracture is a fall onto the shoulder. This mechanism accounted for 87% of the 150 prospectively studied cases carefully documented in the report by Stanley and coworkers.[120] Often, the bone breaks where it changes shape (concave to convex and cross-sectionally from round to flat). Less commonly, the bone is fractured by a direct blow; this mechanism accounted for 7% of Stanley and colleagues' cases, with the remaining 6% of patients having fallen on their outstretched hands.[120]

## ASSOCIATED INJURIES

High-energy trauma is associated with a larger number of fragments and greater fragment displacement and with a consequently higher likelihood of injury to surrounding nonosseous structures such as the brachial plexus, neighboring vessels, or apex of the lung.[55, 79, 92, 127]

## DIAGNOSIS

Characteristically, the child holds the elbow of the affected limb with the opposite hand and tilts the head toward the affected side to minimize the displacing pull by the sternocleidomastoid and trapezius muscles. Radiographs are confirmatory, although for nondisplaced fractures, they may initially be read as negative. The use of good soft tissue technique and careful attention to the periclavicular soft tissue shadow may detect subtle nondisplaced fractures. Overlying structures may obscure a medial physeal injury, and a Rockwood "serendipity" view[29] (40° cephalad-directed tube angle) or Hobbs projection[51] may be helpful. Children with appropriate histories and point tenderness over the clavicle but negative primary radiographs usually have callus at the site of injury on follow-up radiographs obtained 2 or 3 weeks later.

## TREATMENT

More than 200 methods of nonoperative management of a clavicular shaft fracture have been described.[62] Most commonly, these fractures are managed with an apparatus that draws the shoulder backward (e.g., a figure-of-eight plaster wrap or a figure-of-eight bandage or strap). Patient comfort can be enhanced by placing the ipsilateral arm in a sling for the first couple of weeks.

A common residuum of the injury is a knot or bump at the point where the fracture heals. The child and parents should be made aware of this possibility at the initial visit. Characteristically, the knot or bump becomes less distinct as the bone remodels over the next 6 to 9 months.[90] Long-term impairment as a consequence of a childhood closed clavicular fracture managed by closed methods is rare.

Débridement followed by open reduction is indicated for an open clavicular shaft fracture. Internal fixation is best avoided but may be necessary to prevent impingement of displaced sharp bone ends on neighboring vital structures or to prevent them from protruding through the wound.[123] A 3.5- or 2.7-mm reconstruction plate is appropriate internal fixation; one should avoid using smooth pins because of concern regarding migration. Delayed wound closure and support in a figure-of-eight bandage and a sling are appropriate. Open reduction may also be indicated for significantly displaced, irreducible fractures (e.g., those that have buttonholed through the trapezius or the fascia, with secondary tenting of the skin).[69] We have also plated the clavicle in an older adolescent who had a clavicular fracture associated with multiple rib fractures and a flail chest that needed to be managed by thoracotomy and rib stabilization (Fig. 10–5). In this patient, stabilization of the clavicle

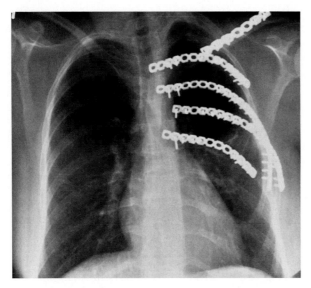

FIGURE **10–5.** One infrequent indication for operative fixation of the clavicle is in an older adolescent with concomitant ipsilateral multiple rib fractures requiring stabilization. In this case, anatomic repositioning of the clavicle fracture fragments permits accurate "setting" of the scapula on the chest wall.

contributed to stabilization of the chest wall and set the scapulothoracic articulation at the correct point on the thoracic wall. This indication for clavicular osteosynthesis is seen infrequently, even at major trauma centers (personal communication, J.W. Meredith, Wake Forest University Medical Center; B. Claudi, Technical University of Munich, 1992).

## Distal Clavicular Fracture

### RELEVANT ANATOMY

Two anatomic facts greatly enhance our understanding of trauma to the distal end of the clavicle in children. The first is that the secondary ossification center at the distal end of the clavicle remains unossified until shortly before it unites with the diaphysis at approximately 19 years of age.[126] The second is that the thick periosteal sleeve surrounding the distal part of the clavicle and its epiphysis provides a strong attachment for the acromioclavicular and coracoclavicular ligaments.[99] These anatomic relationships make it easier to understand why a fracture in this region is much more common than dislocation of the acromioclavicular joint. When the distal end of the clavicle fractures in a child, it creates a rent in the periosteal sleeve, and with displacement, the ossified lateral metaphysis herniates through the rent while the unossified epiphysis is retained in the sleeve. Because the epiphysis is cartilage and is radiolucent, it gives the radiographic appearance of what is, in an adult, an acromioclavicular joint dislocation.

### INCIDENCE

The lateral aspect of the clavicle, including the acromioclavicular joint, accounts for 10% of fractures of the

clavicle; these fractures occur with greater frequency than do fractures at the medial end of the bone.[2, 29, 79]

## MECHANISM OF INJURY

This injury is produced by a force on the point of the shoulder—a fall or a blow. The patient presents with pain and tenderness over the apex of the shoulder. If the fracture is displaced, deformity of the shoulder and tenting of the skin may also be noted. Radiographs of the shoulder demonstrate a high-riding lateral clavicular metaphysis in relation to the neighboring acromion. Occasionally, an associated fracture of the base of the coracoid process may be present.[33, 138]

## CLASSIFICATION

Distal clavicular fractures have been classified into three types by Dameron and Rockwood,[29] with type I being a fracture without displacement; type II, a displaced fracture, nonarticular; and type III, a fracture involving the acromioclavicular joint (Fig. 10–6). However, it should be noted that these classifications were formulated to describe fractures occurring in adults, and for the reasons just discussed, fractures involving the joint are a rarity.

## TREATMENT

In view of the tremendous remodeling potential (i.e., the osteogenic capacity of the retained periosteal sleeve), these injuries should be managed nonoperatively. Treatment usually consists of a simple sling or shoulder Velpeau immobilization for 3 weeks, followed by gentle functional shoulder exercises. Several reports have described Y-shaped distal clavicular anatomy or distal clavicular duplication and ascribed them to developmental causes.[40, 128] Ogden suggested a traumatic etiology as well, with one limb of the Y being the original, now upwardly displaced, lateral clavicular metaphysis[90] (Fig. 10–7) and the second limb being the bone that forms in the retained (nondisplaced) periosteal sleeve. The condition is asymptomatic and does not require treatment. As a rule, one should expect a normal-appearing and normally functioning shoulder after a distal clavicular fracture in a child.

## ACROMIOCLAVICULAR JOINT INJURY

A true injury to the acromioclavicular joint is rare in children but is seen in older adolescents.[29] The mechanism of injury is the same as in adults: a blow to or a fall on the point of the shoulder. Allman[2] classified these injuries into three types: type I, a mild sprain of the acromioclavicular ligaments without subluxation of the joint; type II, a sprain of the acromioclavicular ligaments with subluxation of the joint but no disruption of the coracoclavicular ligament; and type III, dislocation of the joint with disruption of both ligaments, which is seen on

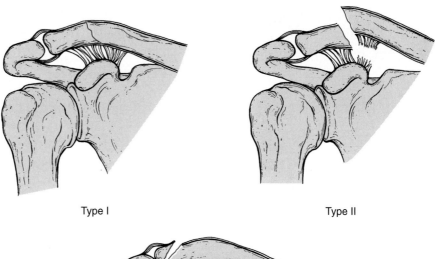

FIGURE 10–6. Distal clavicular fractures classified into three types by Dameron and Rockwood.[29] Type I is nondisplaced and nonarticular, type II is displaced and nonarticular, and type III is intra-articular.

Type I

Type II

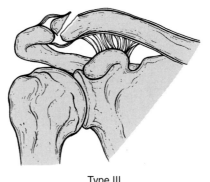

Type III

anteroposterior (AP) radiographs as an increase in the coracoclavicular distance (Fig. 10–8).

Treatment of types I and II injuries consists of a simple form of immobilization such as a sling or shoulder Velpeau dressing for 3 to 4 weeks. The immobilization should be followed by functional shoulder exercises, with gradual progression of movement dictated by patient comfort. Type I injuries do well as a rule. Type II injuries are occasionally accompanied by late sequelae such as weakness and pain with shoulder movement. Affected individuals may be candidates for a reconstruc-

tion procedure in their early adult years, such as a Weaver-Dunn reconstruction.

The best method of managing type III injuries has been abundantly discussed in the literature on adult acromioclavicular fractures. Indications for open treatment include acromioclavicular joint injuries in conjunction with scapulothoracic dissociation,[3, 87] irreducible injuries wherein the clavicle becomes subcutaneous and buttonholed through the fibers of the trapezius,[88, 95] open injuries requiring débridement and irrigation, and patient preference for early stabilization and mobiliza-

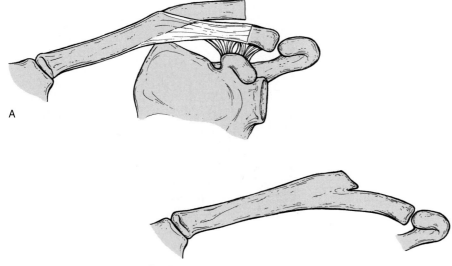

A

B

FIGURE 10–7. *A*, Distal clavicular fracture in an immature child with upward displacement. *B*, Healing occurs within the retained periosteal sleeve.

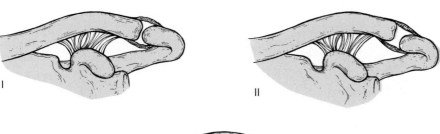

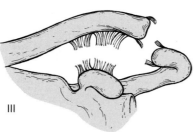

FIGURE **10–8.** Allman's three types of acromioclavicular joint injury.

tion. Early operative fixation may be most appropriate in high-level throwing or lifting athletes. These uncommon indications notwithstanding, nonoperative management[65, 124] is the treatment of choice for this injury in adolescents and should be conducted as outlined earlier.

## SCAPULA

### Developmental Anatomy

The scapula begins to ossify from a single center at the eighth week of fetal life.[135] The center for the middle of the coracoid process forms at 1 year of age and that for the base of the coracoid/upper portion of the glenoid at 10 years.[60] At puberty, two to five centers form in the acromion and fuse by 22 years of age; failure of fusion of any of these centers gives rise to the variant os acromiale[68] (Fig. 10–9). A horseshoe-shaped secondary center at the inferior rim of the glenoid, a center for the medial border, and a center for the inferior angle form and later fuse with the remainder of the bone by 22 years of age.[42, 75, 111]

### Anatomy

The scapula is a flat bone richly invested in muscle over the posterosuperolateral aspect of the chest wall; it is richly invested with muscle attachments ($n = 17$) on both its superficial and deep aspects, with only the dorsal edge of its spine and acromion being subcutaneous. It articulates with the clavicle at the acromioclavicular joint, with the humerus at the glenohumeral joint, and functionally with the chest wall at the scapulothoracic articulation (not a true joint). The muscles that house the scapula participate in shoulder movements by rotating as well as translating the scapula on the chest wall.[53, 56] The articular surface of the glenoid is pear shaped; a fibrocartilaginous labrum on its rim helps center the humeral head in the glenoid during function. The bony

projections (i.e., the acromion and coracoid process) are oriented at 120° to each other and to the axillary border of the scapula when viewed from the true lateral aspect of the bone[107] (the so-called **Y** view of the scapula; Fig. 10–10).

### Incidence and Classification

Fractures of the scapula are rare in children[4, 30] and are classified according to the portion of the bone that is fractured—the body, glenoid, acromion, or coracoid.[27]

#### BODY FRACTURES

Scapular body fractures occur as a result of direct, significant trauma. With the large amount of surrounding muscle, deformity is rarely evident. Clues on physical examination include abrasions, ecchymoses, neighboring

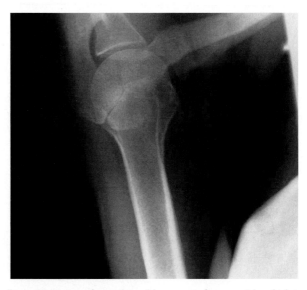

FIGURE **10–9.** One of several possible patterns of os acromiale, which in this case was discovered incidentally on an axillary lateral projection of the glenohumeral joint.

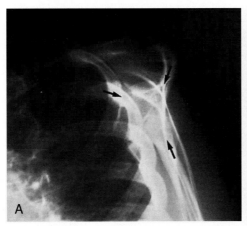

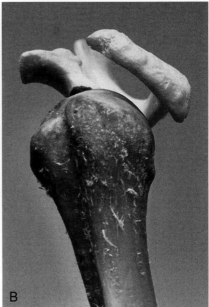

FIGURE **10–10.** A Y view (*A*) of the glenohumeral joint, with a corresponding view of the dry bony scapula and overlying humerus (*B*).

wounds, swelling, and tenderness. True AP and lateral radiographic views are usually diagnostic, but opposite-side comparison views are often necessary to detect subtle injuries in children.

In general, body fractures, like scapulothoracic dissociations, imply a large amount of force, and associated injury to the underlying chest as well as injury to neighboring structures (subclavian and axillary vessels, brachial plexus) should be searched for. These fractures are managed by sling immobilization of the shoulder for 2 to 3 weeks, followed by gentle mobilization (e.g., pendulum exercises) and progression over a period of several weeks to full activity in accord with patient comfort and findings on physical and radiographic examination.

Scapulothoracic dissociation can be diagnosed on an AP view of the chest[32] (Fig. 10–11). A search for associated injury to the brachial plexus,[32, 101] vascular

structures,[3] and chest wall[3] should be conducted. Scapulothoracic dissociation has not been reported in newborns or very young children but has occurred in two older children aged 8 and 11 years.[3, 87] Both children underwent operative repair of the detached suspensory muscles and open restoration of the articulation with the clavicle.

## GLENOID FRACTURES

Generally, fractures of the glenoid may be the result of a direct force on the lateral aspect of the shoulder.[15] Some fractures of the glenoid are caused by forces transmitted by a fall on a flexed elbow.[69] Whether a posterior or an anterior rim fragment is associated with a corresponding subluxation of the head is determined by the position of the arm at the time of injury. CT scanning is especially useful in assessing the size and significance of these fractures. If the fragment is large, the humeral head may sublux; in cases with associated glenohumeral dislocation, significant displacement of an associated glenoid rim fragment may be apparent.[69]

For minimally displaced glenoid fragments not associated with humeral head subluxation or dislocation, the recommended treatment is sling immobilization for 3 weeks, followed by gentle functional exercises. For the uncommon situation of a large fragment associated with humeral head subluxation or dislocation, operative anatomic reduction with a lag screw (Fig. 10–12) or a small "hook"[139] or "spring"[74] plate and repair of associated capsular tears are indicated. Careful preoperative planning is strongly recommended, and the surgical approach is dictated by the location of the fragment to be fixed. Postoperatively, the patient's arm is immobilized in a sling for 3 weeks, followed by gentle functional exercises. Screws or plates may be removed after 3 months.[69] No unanimity of opinion has been reached

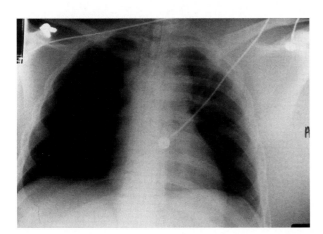

FIGURE **10–11.** Scapulothoracic dissociation. The main radiographic finding is asymmetry of the shoulder girdle, with the affected side (*left*) being laterally displaced.

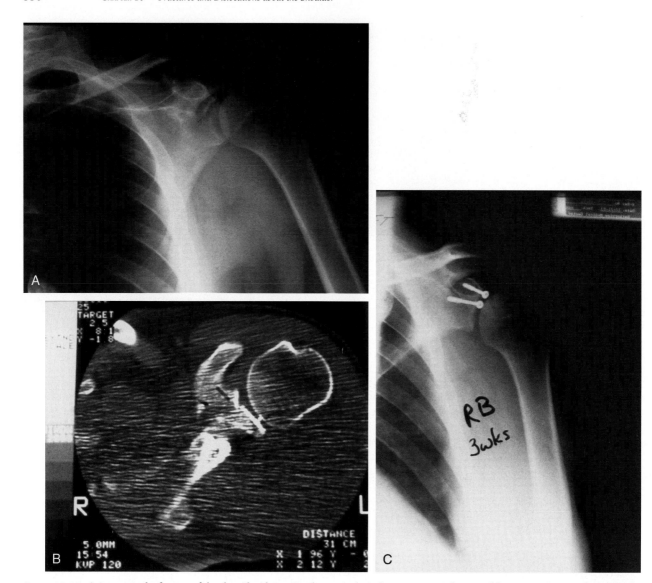

FIGURE **10–12.** *A,* Intra-articular fracture of the glenoid with associated acromioclavicular separation and acromial fracture. *B,* Computed tomography demonstrates the step-off displacement in the joint. *C,* The articular fragment was repositioned anatomically via an anterior approach. The fragment was held in place by two lag screws.

regarding the issue of hardware removal in this setting.[69, 114] The severity of symptoms ascribed to retained hardware may warrant their removal, but the symptoms should outweigh the risks associated with additional surgery.

## ACROMION FRACTURES

Fractures of the acromion are rare but can result from a direct force on the point of the shoulder.[76] Failure of one of the several acromial epiphyses to fuse[68] (i.e., os acromiale; see Fig. 10–9) should not be mistaken for a fracture. Opposite-side comparison radiographs may be helpful, as may reference to an appropriate skeletal radiographic atlas of normal variants.[59, 61] The usual treatment consists of sling immobilization for 3 weeks, followed by early functional shoulder exercises.

## CORACOID FRACTURES

Fracture of the coracoid process is uncommon in children.[90] The two fracture patterns seen when the injury does occur represent an avulsion by the pull of either the acromioclavicular ligaments or the conjoined tendon of the coracobrachialis and short head of the biceps brachii.[9] The first type of fracture occurs through the physis at the base of the coracoid and the upper quarter of the glenoid,[49, 63, 138] and the second type occurs through the tip of the coracoid.[27] Coracoid fractures can accompany distal clavicular fractures, apparent acromioclavicular joint injuries, and shoulder dislocations.[12, 125, 136] The injury can be demonstrated by the Stryker notch view[46] or by an axillary lateral view when the gantry is widened to include the coracoid on the film (Fig. 10–13). Treatment usually consists of sling immobilization of the shoulder for 3 weeks, followed by gentle functional shoulder exercises.

# GLENOHUMERAL JOINT DISLOCATION

## Developmental Anatomy

Between 4½ and 7 weeks of gestation, the proximal upper limb bud blastema differentiates into the scapula, the humerus, and an interzone.[39] This interzone and its surrounding mesenchyme give rise to the capsule and intra-articular structures of the glenohumeral joint.[36] Differentiation of these structures is complete by 7 to 8 weeks after fertilization; thereafter, the joint cavity and its surrounding structures, as well as supporting elements such as the rotator cuff muscles and tendons, increase in absolute dimensions while maintaining relative size.[36]

## Anatomy

The glenohumeral articulation is a true synovial joint of the ball-and-socket variety. The joint comprises the rather shallow, pear-shaped glenoid and the spherical head of the humerus. The closely related capsule, its

associated glenohumeral ligaments, and its overlying rotator cuff tendons provide a mobile and dynamic extension of the glenoid cavity that centers the humeral head within that cavity and enables it to pass through a greater arc of motion than any other joint in the body.[56] However, the glenohumeral joint's major reliance on soft tissue support makes it susceptible to injury with resultant subluxation or dislocation.[89]

## Incidence

During childhood, because of the relative strength of the surrounding soft tissue structures, the open proximal humeral physis is mechanically the weakest link in the glenohumeral articulation. Thus, skeletal trauma here is most often manifested as a Salter-Harris type II proximal humeral fracture.[109] During the adolescent years, as the proximal humeral growth plate begins to close, the incidence of glenohumeral dislocation and associated capsular injuries rises. In the series reported by Rowe and colleagues of some 500 glenohumeral dislocations seen over a 20-year period, only 8 (1.6%) occurred in children younger than 10 years of age, whereas 99 (19.8%) occurred in patients aged 10 through 20 years.[102] Approximately half the injuries in the 10- to 20-year-old group (48 of 99) were recurrent dislocations.[102] Recurrence rates ranged from 20%[105] to 100%[4] in children

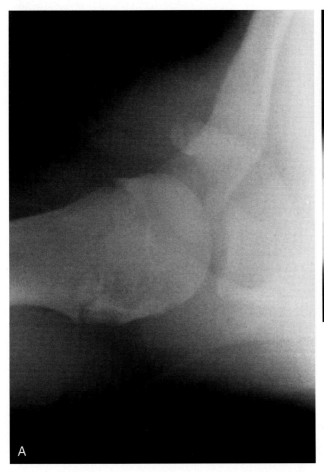

A

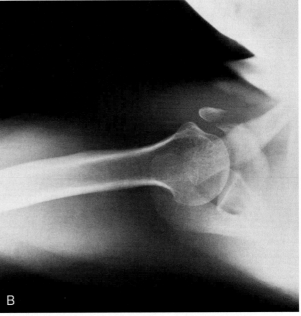

B

FIGURE **10–13.** *A,* The coracoid is adequately visualized on the axillary lateral projection when the gantry is wide. *B,* The tip of the coracoid has been avulsed in this mature individual.

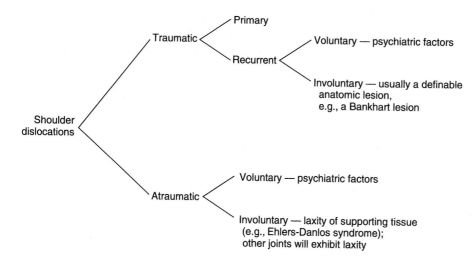

FIGURE **10–14.** Etiologic classification of glenohumeral dislocations.

younger than 10 years of age and from 48%[105] to 90%[4] in patients between the ages of 10 and 20 years. Dislocation of the shoulder during infancy is very rare but has been reported in association with brachial plexus palsy,[66, 67] sepsis,[43] and congenital deformity.[25, 44, 45]

## Classification

Glenohumeral dislocations may be classified according to the direction of the dislocation: anterior, posterior, or inferior (the last two are much less common). They may also be classified according to etiology, as shown in Figure 10–14.

## Mechanism of Injury

Anterior glenohumeral dislocation is usually produced by a force on the outstretched hand with the shoulder in abduction, external rotation, and elevation, a position that causes anterior levering of the humeral head and secondary stretching of the anterior and inferior capsular tissues. Eighty-five percent have anterior and inferior capsular detachment from the glenoid neck—the so-called Bankhart lesion.[7] Posterior dislocation can accompany epileptic seizures and convulsions from electroshock therapy and is explained by the powerful override of the internal rotators, which lever the humeral head in the opposite (posterior) direction.[111, 129]

Many patients with a history of atraumatic dislocation can voluntarily sublux or dislocate their shoulders. Those who perform this atraumatic, voluntary type of dislocation are more likely to be children or adolescents than adults.[104] In the initial report by Rowe and coworkers on the subject,[104] 20 of 26 patients (77%) were 16 years or younger; psychiatric factors were found to play an important role in these voluntary dislocations. Whether this ability is spontaneous or acquired after an initial minimally traumatic injury is unclear. In Rowe's series,[104] 11 patients could recall no specific episode of initial trauma; the remaining 15 could recall a minor twist or a fall.

## Diagnosis

Traumatic dislocation causes pain and swelling about the shoulder. The attitude of the arm depends on the type of dislocation. With an anterior dislocation, the arm is held abducted and slightly externally rotated; with a posterior dislocation, it is fixed in adduction and internal rotation; and with an inferior dislocation, it is held in abduction with the forearm lying on or behind the patient's head (the so-called luxation erecta position). Atraumatic dislocation causes little or minimal pain and swelling.

A careful neurovascular examination should be performed routinely. Injury to the axillary nerve and tears of the rotator cuff tendons are sometimes seen in association with glenohumeral dislocation and should be assessed. In their series of 226 anterior dislocations, Pasila and associates[91] reported an 11% incidence of brachial plexus injuries, 8% incidence of axillary nerve injuries, and 11% incidence of rotator cuff tears. The neighboring axillary artery and vein are also at risk for injury secondary to excessively forceful reduction.[16]

When chronic instability is suspected, the examiner can demonstrate glenohumeral laxity by manually stabilizing the scapula and exerting gentle anterior-to-posterior, posterior-to-anterior, or inferior-to-superior force on the humeral head with the opposite hand and comparing the response with that of the opposite side. Alternatively, the examiner can elicit an apprehension sign by checking the limits of comfortable external rotation in varying degrees of abduction for both shoulders or by conducting the Feagan test.[97] Radiographic evaluation should include a "trauma series"[98] consisting of an AP and lateral view in the plane of the scapula. Because the overlying humeral head and chest wall can obscure subtle rim fractures (as well as a fracture of the lesser humeral tuberosity), an axillary lateral view or a modified axillary lateral view[13] should also be obtained.

## Treatment

Reduction of an acute, traumatic dislocation can usually be accomplished safely by any of several classic methods. For immediate reduction of an acute dislocation (as in those witnessed and clinically apparent as dislocations and treated on an athletic field), slight abduction and derotation of the affected arm with minimal traction can be attempted as described by O'Brien and associates.[89] The Hippocratic method[50] consists of slow and gentle traction on the affected arm with gentle internal and external rotation to disengage the humeral head. With this technique, the physician applies countertraction by placing a stockinged foot on the patient's chest wall (Fig. 10–15A), but not in the axilla. Alternatively, one can use a modification of this technique by placing a twisted sheet around the upper part of the patient's chest and having an assistant pull on the sheet to provide the desired countertraction (see Fig. 10–15B).

The Stimson method[121] calls for positioning the patient prone and allowing the affected arm to hang from the edge of the table with a weight (5 to 10 pounds) suspended from the end of the arm (see Fig. 10–15C). Numerous other methods have been described by Milch,[78] Lacey and Crawford,[64] Russell and coworkers,[108] Janecki and Shahcheragh,[57] Mirick and associates,[80] and White.[133]

After reduction, the neurovascular examination should be repeated and documented. A sling should be applied, followed by early motion; progression is dictated by patient comfort. A period of enforced shoulder immobilization was shown in Hovelius' large prospective series to not influence the recurrence rate.[54] Both the patient and the parents should be informed of the high likelihood of recurrence, the maneuver that is likely to trigger it (for an anterior dislocation, it would be elevation with external rotation), and which sports are high risk (for an anterior dislocation, it might be tennis or other overhead racquet sports). Patients with recurring dislocations, especially if the dislocations are brought about by trivial activities of daily living that are hard to modify, are candidates for a repair directed toward the specifically implicated disorder, such as a Bankart repair[102] for a lax anterior capsule secondary to capsular avulsion from the anterior inferior glenoid neck. Currently, such management can be performed by either open or arthroscopic techniques. Evaluation is continuing regarding recurrence and other sequelae for each type of approach.[23, 38]

Patients who are voluntary dislocators are best managed initially by nonoperative means consisting of a rehabilitation program aimed at strengthening the rotator cuff and deltoid muscles[47, 84, 103] and, when indicated, specific counseling directed toward modifying any underlying attention-seeking behavior pattern.[104] If this treatment is successful, any recurring dislocations are often of the involuntary variety and may be multidirectional. Surgical treatment with an appropriate capsular

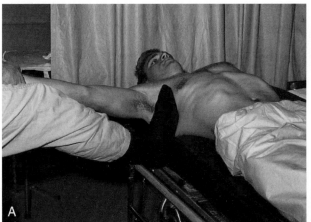
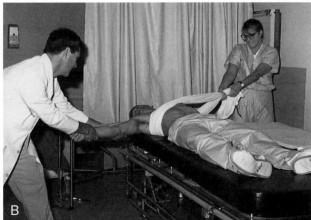
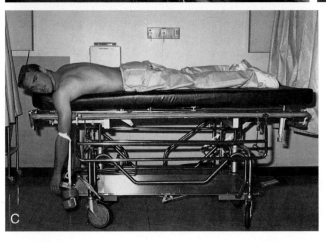

FIGURE **10–15.** Glenohumeral reduction techniques. *A,* Hippocratic method. *B,* Modified Hippocratic method. *C,* Stimson's method.

shift to correct this problem, as described by Neer and Foster,[86] would then be indicated.

## PROXIMAL HUMERAL FRACTURES

### Developmental Anatomy

The primary ossification center for the humerus appears at about the sixth week of fetal life.[41] The ossification center for the humeral head appears at about the time of birth, that for the greater tuberosity between 7 months and 3 years, and that for the lesser tuberosity 2 years later. These proximal secondary ossification centers coalesce at about 5 to 7 years of age.[42, 96, 100, 110] The growth plate[100] closes between 14 and 17 years of age in females and between 16 and 18 years of age in males.[42, 96, 98, 110]

### Anatomy

The proximal physis is tent shaped, its apex being located in the posteromedial aspect of the proximal end of the humerus on cross section[90] (Fig. 10–16). A small portion of the posterior proximal and medial metaphysis is intracapsular and extracartilaginous. The capsular attachment provides a strong tether just distal to this structure.[42] This anatomic characteristic, in addition to

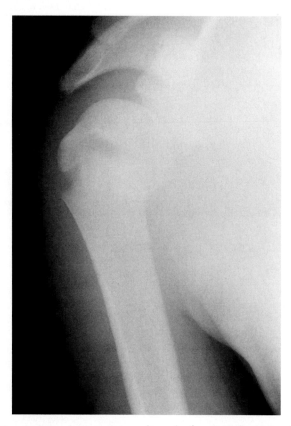

FIGURE 10–16. Anteroposterior radiograph of a minimally displaced Salter I fracture in a 14-year-old boy.

the relative thickness of the posteromedial periosteum and thinness of the anterolateral periosteum,[28] may help explain the tendency for the metaphyseal fragment to buttonhole the periosteum anterolaterally when the proximal end of the humerus is fractured and (in Salter-Harris type II injuries) for a small posteromedial piece of metaphysis to stay with the proximal fragment.

It should be noted that physeal fractures pass through the zone of hypertrophy adjacent to the zone of provisional calcification with sparing of the zone of embryonal cartilage, thereby retaining the growth potential of the physis.[9, 28, 109] The proximal humeral physis contributes 80% of the longitudinal growth of the humerus; thus, fractures at that site have great remodeling potential.[9, 31, 84, 100]

### Incidence

Fractures involving the proximal humeral growth plate represent approximately 0.45% of all childhood fractures[100] and approximately 3% of all epiphyseal fractures.[85] Salter-Harris type I injuries predominate in neonates and children younger than 5 years,[27] metaphyseal fractures predominate in those between 5 and 11 years, and Salter-Harris type II injuries predominate in those older than 11 years of age.[27]

### Mechanism of Injury

Injury in the newborn is usually attributable to the position of the arm during vaginal delivery. Hyperextension and excessive external rotation have been implicated.[26, 46, 113] The forces that bring about a proximal humeral fracture in children are most commonly indirect and result from a fall on the outstretched arm,[52, 72, 118] although a direct force, such as a blow on the posterolateral aspect of the upper part of the arm, was implicated as the most prevalent mechanism in one series.[85]

### Diagnosis

Diagnosis can be difficult in a newborn. The findings may be subtle, such as irritability with arm movements, or more pronounced, such as pseudoparalysis, in which case they should be distinguished from entities such as septic arthritis (see Fig. 10–4), brachial plexus palsy, and distal clavicular injuries.[29, 41, 52] A history of prematurity, maternal sepsis, umbilical artery catheterization, or an abnormal erythrocyte sedimentation rate or white blood cell count may necessitate further workup to rule out joint sepsis or osteomyelitis. Plain films of the proximal end of the humerus should be obtained, along with comparison views of the opposite limb. In addition, arthrography, ultrasonography,[137] and magnetic resonance imaging have been used to outline the position of the proximal (largely cartilaginous) fragment.[6, 17, 24, 29, 85, 134]

In older children, pain, splinting, and arm dysfunction are evident. Ecchymosis and swelling are variably present, and in displaced fractures, the arm may be shortened and the proximal metaphysis bulging beneath the anterior aspect of the shoulder. Diagnostic plain radiographs at 90° to each other should be obtained, as in the assessment of glenohumeral injury.

## Classification

The Salter and Harris classification of epiphyseal injuries has been applied to physeal injuries of the proximal end of the humerus.[109] Most of these fractures in children younger than 5 years are type I; 75% of fractures in children older than 11 years are type II, with most of the remainder being type I. Metaphyseal fractures predominate between 5 and 11 years of age.[27] Salter-Harris types III, IV, and V injuries are rarely seen.[27, 72] The single reported case of a Salter-Harris type III injury was associated with a dislocation in a 10-year-old child.[22]

Fracture stability (either before or after closed reduction) is also a means of classifying these fractures (stable versus unstable) and can be used to guide treatment.

Salter-Harris type II fractures were further subdivided into four grades by Neer and Horwitz, who used the extent of fracture displacement as the criterion for their grades[84] (Table 10–1). It should be noted that grades III and IV are associated with varus angulation. In Neer and Horwitz's series,[84] shortening of 1 to 3 cm was reported in 11% of group I and group II patients and in 33% of group IV patients; no shortening resulted at the time of injury in any patient younger than 11 years of age. Thus, the remodeling potential (in years) may play more of a role in determining the final outcome than the extent of displacement.

## Treatment

In general, proximal humeral fractures are managed by closed techniques. The need for reduction is determined by the extent of displacement and remodeling capacity. Nondisplaced fractures can be managed by sling-and-swathe immobilization followed by protected motion. Displaced fractures (1 cm or angulation greater than 45°) in patients older than 12 years of age should be reduced and then managed as described later. When adequate reduction cannot be achieved or when the reduction achieved is lost as the arm is brought to the chest wall, a

**TABLE 10-1** ...........................................

Neer-Horwitz Classification of Proximal Humeral Fractures

| Grade | Displacement |
|---|---|
| I | <5 mm |
| II | <1/3 shaft width |
| III | 2/3 shaft width |
| IV | >2/3 shaft width |

From Neer, C.S., II; Horwitz, B.S. Clin Orthop 41:24, 1965.

**TABLE 10-2** ...........................................

Acceptable Alignment of Pediatric Proximal Humeral Fractures

| Patient Age (yr) | Allowable Displacement and/or Angulation |
|---|---|
| <5 | Up to 70-degree angulation, 100% displacement |
| 5–12 | Up to 40- to 70-degree angulation |
| >12 | Up to 40-degree angulation, 50% displacement |

Based on Beaty, J.H. Fractures of the proximal humerus and shaft in children. Instr Course Lect 41:369–372, 1992.

decision must be made regarding whether to accept this malposition (usually varus with or without displacement), to make further attempts at reduction, or to use more elaborate immobilization methods (which potentially entail greater morbidity). This decision should take into account the age of the patient (and thus the remodeling potential of the bone), as well as the fact that a functional shoulder can be expected regardless of the method used.[9, 28, 118] With the more severely displaced varieties of growth plate injury in an older child (older than 11 years of age), one can anticipate 1 to 3 cm of arm shortening and some loss of glenohumeral motion (abduction).[86]

Sherk and Probst[117] set up minimal guidelines for an acceptable reduction: angulation of less than 20° and displacement of less than 50%. When these criteria are met, an acceptable outcome can be expected.[19, 117] More recently, Beaty delineated basic guidelines for acceptable alignment of pediatric proximal humeral fractures.[10] Allowable displacement and angulation decrease with increasing patient age because of the tremendous remodeling potential in younger patients (Table 10–2).

The choices for treatment of displaced fractures include closed reduction with olecranon pin traction, a "salute" cast, closed reduction with percutaneous pinning,[11] or open reduction with internal fixation (usually percutaneous pinning). For a ventilator-dependent child or a child whose other injuries require enforced recumbency, olecranon pin[96] or percutaneous winged screw[72] skeletal traction is well suited. For a child who is otherwise mobile, a salute cast is one alternative, but it can be associated with skin breakdown, abduction contracture, and brachial plexus injury.[11, 52, 96] Alternatively and perhaps preferentially,[70] for a child with injuries requiring monitoring of the abdomen or chest, fixation with percutaneous Steinmann or small (2.5 mm) Schanz pins can be performed coincident with reduction. By using an image intensifier and with the child appropriately anesthetized,[11] two or three smooth K-wires or small-diameter Steinmann or Schanz pins are directed obliquely cephalad from the lateral metaphysis across the reduced physis and into the proximal epiphysis. Stability of the fixation can then be evaluated under fluoroscopy (Fig. 10–17). The pins are cut and bent (in a J or L shape) at the ends outside or just under the skin, and a sterile dressing is applied. Simple sling-and-swathe or collar-and-cuff immobilization is then applied to support the limb until the fracture heals.

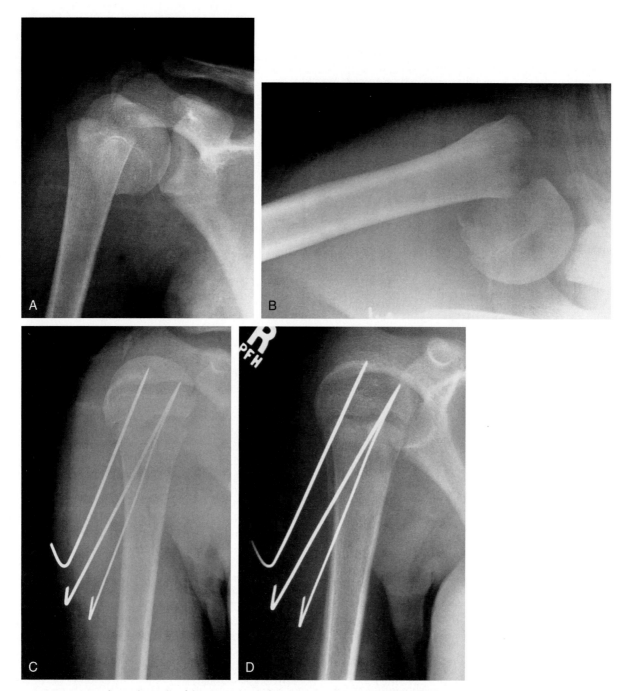

**FIGURE 10–17.** *A* and *B*, Radiographs of the proximal end of the humerus of a 14-year-old girl after a four-wheeler accident during which she sustained multiple trauma. *C*, The fracture was managed with closed reduction and percutaneous pinning. *D*, At follow-up 4 weeks later, the pins were removed; the patient quickly regained normal use of her shoulder.

The pins are usually removed in 2 to 3 weeks, at which time gentle pendulum exercises can be started.

Open reduction should be reserved for special circumstances, such as an open injury requiring surgical débridement, associated glenohumeral dislocation (in which forceful attempts at closed reduction may be hazardous to neighboring neurovascular soft tissue structures), associated vascular injuries, or the rare circumstance when the fracture is irreducible because of an interposed biceps tendon[130] buttonholing the distal fragment. Skeletal stabilization (usually percutaneous

pinning) is generally necessary in a fracture with concomitant glenohumeral dislocation because it enables one to control the position of the humeral head within the glenoid by positioning the arm against the chest wall. Reestablishing skeletal continuity also enables one to better assess the stability of the joint reduction.

If skeletal traction, a salute cast, or percutaneous pins are used, the type of immobilization can be changed at about 3 weeks, when the fracture is "sticky," to a simpler form such as a collar-and-cuff or sling-and-swathe immobilization (Fig. 10–18). Periods of gentle motion out of the sling can start at that time. The fracture is usually healed by 4 to 6 weeks, at which point light activities are permitted. Vigorous activities involving the shoulder can be resumed in a gradual, stepwise fashion after completing a series of intermediate goals along the way. The timetable depends on the individual and that person's healing capacity, the severity of the injury, and the type of stressful activity to be resumed (e.g., pole vaulting versus kite flying).

## HUMERAL SHAFT FRACTURES

### Developmental Anatomy

The humeral diaphysis begins to ossify during the sixth or seventh week of fetal life and is completely ossified by birth.[41] On cross section, the shaft is cylindrical proximally and flattened distally in the coronal plane.[42] The posterior aspect of the bone provides the origin for the lateral head of the triceps (superolaterally) and for its medial head (inferomedially), with the "spiral groove" lying in between. The radial nerve and its accompanying artery have a close relationship to the bone along this

groove. Just proximal to its midpoint, the lateral aspect of the shaft provides the insertion for the deltoid muscle. Medially at this level is the attachment for the coracobrachialis. More proximally, the pectoralis major inserts into the lateral ridge of the intertubercular groove. The brachialis muscle has its origin from the distal half of the anterior aspect of the humeral shaft.[42] An appreciation of these muscle attachments is essential for understanding the deforming forces acting on humeral fracture fragments (Fig. 10–19).

### Incidence

The humeral shaft is fractured less frequently in children than in adults. Among the humeral shaft fractures of childhood, diaphyseal fractures are more common in children older than 12 years or younger than 3 years of age.[110] For children younger than 10 years, the incidence of shaft fractures is approximately 26 per 100,000 per year.[100] Overall, shaft fractures account for 2% to 5% of all fractures in children.[77] Traditionally, such fractures in patients 3 years or younger have correlated highly with child abuse. However, a recent review demonstrated that only 18% of humeral shaft fractures in a group of patients

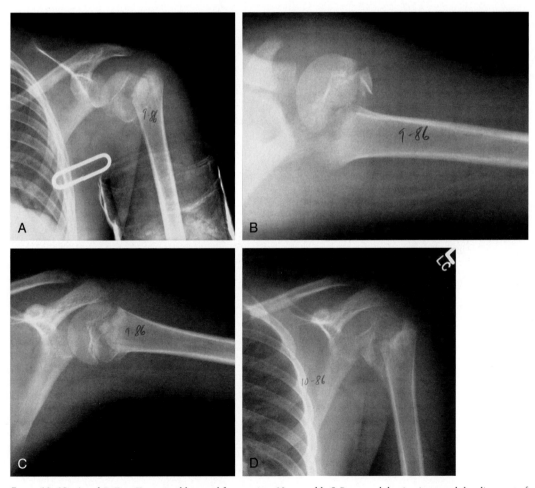

**FIGURE 10–18.** *A* and *B,* Type II proximal humeral fracture in a 12-year-old. *C,* Because abduction improved the alignment of the fracture, the patient was treated in abduction. *D,* One month later, early healing is evident.

*Figure continued on following page*

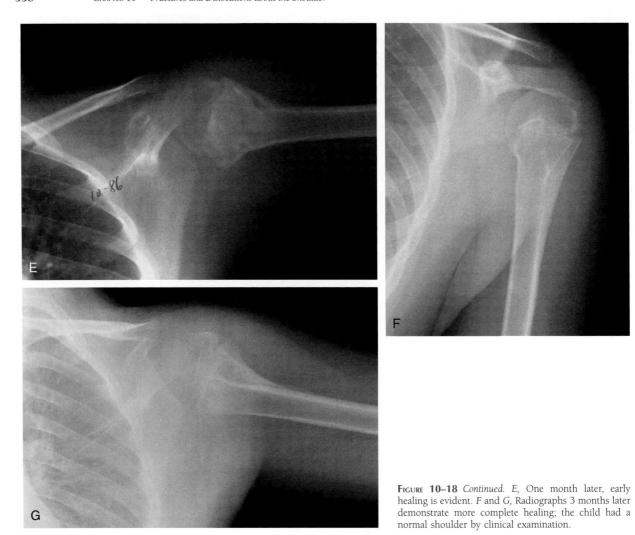

FIGURE 10–18 *Continued. E,* One month later, early healing is evident. *F* and *G,* Radiographs 3 months later demonstrate more complete healing; the child had a normal shoulder by clinical examination.

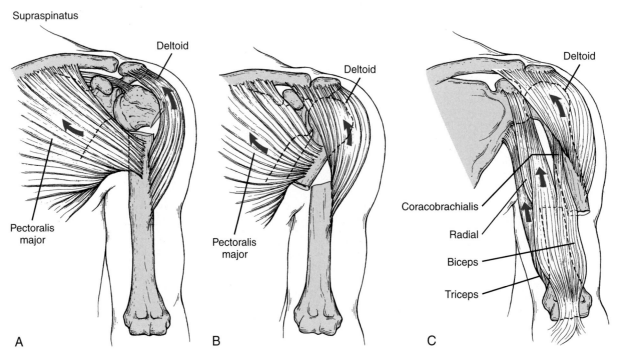

FIGURE 10–19. Muscle attachments (*A* to *C*) that direct deforming forces in proximal humeral fractures.

younger than 3 years could be classified as probable abuse.[115]

## Mechanism of Injury

Transverse or short oblique fracture patterns are the result of direct trauma to the arm, which is the most common mechanism of injury. Indirect trauma (e.g., violent twisting) results in a spiral or long oblique fracture pattern; this pattern is the one commonly seen when child abuse is the cause,[96] but the appearance of other patterns does not rule out this etiology. Minor trauma may cause a humerus with an underlying unicameral bone cyst to fracture at the level of the cyst[85] (Fig. 10–20), which is the most common manifestation of this entity.[119] Symptomatic unicameral cysts are located most frequently in the proximal end of the humerus and the humeral shaft.

Fracture at the junction of the middle and distal thirds of the shaft may be associated with injury to the closely related radial nerve.[96] This injury should always be tested for by asking the patient to extend the ipsilateral metacarpophalangeal joints or the thumb (or both).

## Diagnosis

Similar to proximal humeral fractures in neonates, humeral shaft fractures in this age group may also be manifested as pseudoparalysis. Brachial plexus palsy, clavicular fracture, proximal humeral fracture, and infection should be differentiated.[113] A child with a greenstick fracture may have minimal symptoms and tenderness. An older child with a displaced humeral shaft fracture usually has a history of trauma to the arm. The exception to this rule is a child with a fracture through a unicameral bone cyst that is brought about by otherwise trivial use of the arm[85] (see Fig. 10–20). Obvious deformity of the arm may be evident if it has not already been splinted, and palpation elicits tenderness and crepitus over the arm. Plain radiographs in two views are confirmatory.

## Treatment

Isolated closed injuries are best managed by closed methods. One can take advantage of the stout surrounding periosteum by several methods, including a hanging cast,[94] traction through an olecranon pin[73] or winged screw,[72] or the weight of the arm in a shoulder Velpeau dressing[39] or a collar-and-cuff bandage.[132] Fracture in a newborn can be managed by splinting the arm to the chest wall.[5]

Remodeling in newborns and very young children is robust. Maintenance of alignment is more important for fractures of the distal half of the humerus, where remodeling is less active. As a guideline, one should strive to maintain alignment within 15° of anatomic.[52] Bayonet apposition is not a problem; usually, some overgrowth of the humerus takes place.[48]

Most fractures are "sticky" by 3 to 4 weeks (2 to 3 weeks in newborns and very young children), and

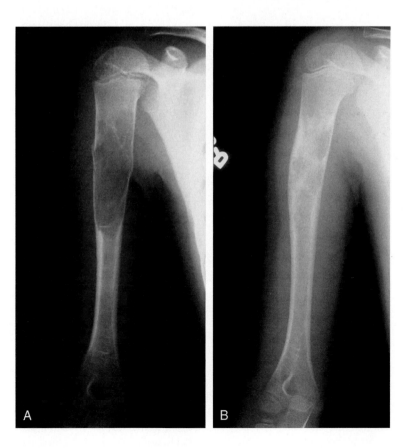

**FIGURE 10–20.** *A,* Anteroposterior radiograph at initial evaluation of a fracture through a unicameral (simple) bone cyst in the proximal end of the humerus of a 6-year-old girl. *B,* Anteroposterior and lateral radiographs 6 months after direct methylprednisolone injection reveal complete healing of the fracture and nearly complete resolution of the cyst.

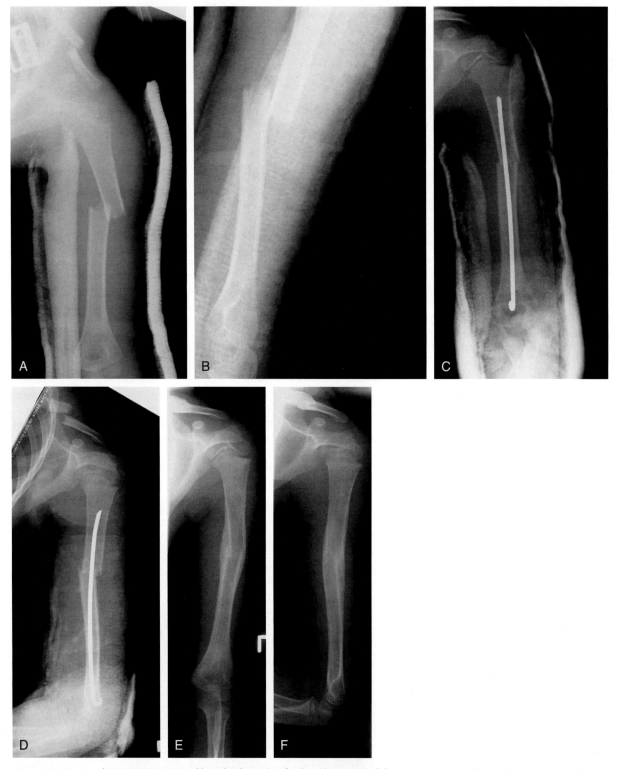

**Figure 10–21.** *A* and *B,* Anteroposterior and lateral radiographs of a closed humeral shaft fracture in a 5-year-old boy with an ipsilateral clavicle fracture, bilateral femur fractures, severe closed head injury, and pulmonary contusion. *C* and *D,* Anteroposterior and lateral radiographs immediately after intramedullary fixation of the humeral fracture with a Rush rod performed at the time of external fixation of the femoral fractures. *E* and *F,* Anteroposterior and lateral radiographs 6 months after fixation and subsequent removal of the Rush rod. The patient had full active and passive range of motion of the elbow and shoulder.

protected motion can then be started with brief periods out of the Velpeau dressing or collar-and-cuff bandage. By 6 to 8 weeks (3 to 6 weeks in newborns and very young children), most fractures have healed well enough to go without support. Subsequent rehabilitation of the upper extremity is tailored to the demands of the individual. For a young child, rehabilitation can consist simply of the resumption of light play, with avoidance of activities that would risk a fall (e.g., skateboarding, climbing) until the humerus has remodeled sufficiently.

Associated radial nerve injuries should be observed for 16 to 20 weeks.[122] The exception to this rule is a child who has radial nerve function at initial evaluation but loses it during an attempt at reduction. Under these circumstances, the radial nerve should be explored.[116] In patients with no sign of return of function (the earliest returning motor function is that of the brachioradialis), the nerve should be explored, with neurolysis or neurorrhaphy if indicated.

Open fractures require surgical débridement and irrigation. One should not close a traumatic wound primarily; coverage should be delayed until one is confident that the wound is clean (usually at day 5). Subsequent to the application of a sterile dressing, the fracture fragments can be stabilized with a shoulder Velpeau dressing or similar technique. Alternatively, an external fixator can be used for an open fracture with significant soft tissue injury or stripping when frequent dressing changes are needed. Internal fixation (Fig. 10–21), adroitly applied by a surgeon familiar with the method to minimize further local devascularization of wounded tissue, has a number of advantages in a polytraumatized child, especially one with associated chest or severe head trauma.[70] These advantages include early functional use of the extremity, easier nursing care of the patient, and greater ease in mobilizing the patient. These advantages must be weighed against the enhanced potential for local infection and the need for later implant removal. Such internal fixation methods include rigid plate fixation and intramedullary stabilization (see Fig. 10–21). Although seldom necessary in children, internal fixation may be necessary in those with an associated vascular injury requiring repair or with nonunion of a shaft fracture. In the latter instance, bone grafting and rigid fixation with compression plating should be undertaken and elbow and shoulder motion initiated in the immediate postoperative period.

*Acknowledgments*

The authors wish to thank Drs. Thomas Sumner and Robert Bechtold, Department of Radiology, Bowman Gray School of Medicine, Wake Forest University, Winston-Salem, NC; Dr. Richard Lange, Department of Orthopaedic Surgery, University of Wisconsin Hospital, Madison, WI; John Faris, Forsyth Radiologic Associates, Winston-Salem, NC; and Dr. Paul Rush, Laurinburg, SC, for their help in compilation of the figures for this chapter and Barbara Crouse for her help in preparation of this manuscript.

## REFERENCES

1. ACS Committee on Trauma. Advanced Trauma Life Support Manual. Chicago, American College of Surgeons, 1988.
2. Allman, F.L., Jr. Fractures and ligamentous injuries of the clavicle and its articulation. J Bone Joint Surg Am 49:774–784, 1967.
3. An, H.S.; Vonderbrink, J.P.; Ebraheim, N.A.; et al. Open scapulothoracic disassociation with intact neurovascular status in a child. J Orthop Trauma 2:36–38, 1988.
4. Asher, M.A. Dislocations of the upper extremity in children. Orthop Clin North Am 7:583–591, 1976.
5. Asted, B. A method for the treatment of humerus fractures in the newborn using the S. von Rosen splint. Acta Orthop Scand 40:234–236, 1969.
6. Aufranc, O.E.; Jones, W.N.; Bierbaum, B.E. Epiphysial fracture of the proximal humerus. JAMA 207:727–729, 1969.
7. Bankart, A.S. Recurrent or habitual dislocation of the shoulder-joint. Clin Orthop 291(June):3–6, 1993.
8. Barth, E.; Hagen, R. Surgical treatment of dislocations of the sternoclavicular joint. Acta Orthop Scand 54:746–747, 1983.
9. Baxter, M.P.; Wiley, J.J. Fractures of the proximal humeral epiphysis: Their influence on humeral growth. J Bone Joint Surg Br 68:570–573, 1986.
10. Beaty, J.H. Fractures of the proximal humerus and shaft in children. Instr Course Lect 41:369–372, 1992.
11. Beebe, A.; Bell, D.F. Management of severely displaced fractures of the proximal humerus in children. Tech Orthop 4(4):1–4, 1989.
12. Bernard, T.N.; Brunet, M.E.; Haddad, R.J. Fractured coracoid process in acromioclavicular dislocations, report of our cases and review of the literature. Clin Orthop 175:227–232, 1983.
13. Bloom, M.H.; Obata, W.G. Diagnosis of posterior dislocation of the shoulder with use of Velpeau axillary and angle-up roentgenographic views. J Bone Joint Surg Am 49:943–949, 1967.
14. Blount, W.P. Fractures in children. In: Fractures in Children. Baltimore, Williams & Wilkins, 1954.
15. Butters, K.P. Fractures and dislocations of the scapula. In: Rockwood, C.A., Jr; Green, D.P.; Bucholz, R.W., eds. Fractures in Adults. New York, J.B. Lippincott, 1991, pp. 990–1019.
16. Calvet, J.; LeRoy, M.L.L. Luxations de l'epaule et lesions vasculaires. J Chir (Paris) 58:337–346, 1942.
17. Campbell, J.; Orth, M.C.; Almond, H.G.A. Fracture-separation of the proximal humeral epiphysis. J Bone Joint Surg Am 59:262–263, 1977.
18. Canale, S.T. Fractures of shaft and proximal end of humerus. In: Crenshaw, A.H., ed, Campbell's Operative Orthopaedics. Toronto, C.V. Mosby, 1987, pp. 1886–1887.
19. Canale, S.T.; Puhl, J.; Watson, F.M.; Gillespie, R. Acute osteomyelitis following closed fractures. Report of three cases. J Bone Joint Surg Am 57:415–418, 1975.
20. Clark, R.L.; Milgram, J.W.; Yawn, D.H. Fatal aortic perforation and cardiac tamponade due to a Kirschner wire migrating from the right sternoclavicular joint. South Med J 67:316–318, 1974.
21. Cohen, A.W.; Otto, S.R. Obstetric clavicular fractures. J Reprod Med 25:119–122, 1980.
22. Cohn, B.T.; Froimson, A.I. Salter 3 fracture dislocation of glenohumeral joint in a 10-year old. Orthop Rev 15:97–98, 1986.
23. Cole, B.J.; L' Insalata, J.; Irrgang, J.; Warner, J.J. Comparison of arthroscopic and open anterior shoulder stabilization. A two- to six-year follow-up study. J Bone Joint Surg Am 82:1108–1114, 2000.
24. Conwell, H.E. Fractures of the surgical neck and epiphyseal separations of upper end of humerus. J Bone Joint Surg 8:508–516, 1926.
25. Cozen, L. Congenital dislocation of the shoulder and other anomalies. Arch Surg 35:956–966, 1937.
26. Cumming, W.A. Neonatal skeletal fractures. Birth trauma or child abuse? J Can Assoc Radiol 30:30–33, 1979.
27. Curtis, R.J.; Rockwood, C.A. Fractures and dislocations of the shoulder in children. In: Rockwood, C.A., Jr.; Matsen, F.A.I., eds. The Shoulder. Philadelphia, W.B. Saunders, 1990, pp. 991–1032.
28. Dameron, T.B.; Reibel, D.B. Fractures involving the proximal humeral epiphyseal plate. J Bone Joint Surg Am 51:289–297, 1969.
29. Dameron, T.B.; Rockwood, C.A., Jr. Fractures and dislocations of the shoulder. In: Rockwood, C.A., Jr., ed. Fractures in Children. Philadelphia, J.B. Lippincott, 1984, pp. 577–682.
30. DePalma, A.F. Surgery of the Shoulder. Philadelphia, J.B. Lippincott, 1973.
31. Digby, K.H. Measurement of diaphyseal growth in proximal and distal directions. J Anat Physiol (Lond) 50:187–188, 1915.
32. Ebraheim, N.A.; An, H.S.; Jackson, W.T.; et al. Scapulothoracic dissociation. J Bone Joint Surg Am 70:428–432, 1988.
33. Eidman, D.K.; Siff, S.J.; Tullos, H.S. Acromioclavicular lesions in children. Am J Sports Med 9:150–154, 1981.
34. Eskola, A. Sternoclavicular dislocation: A plea for open treatment. Acta Orthop Scand 57:227–228, 1986.
35. Farkas, R.; Levine, S. X-ray incidence of fractured clavicle in vertex presentation. Am J Obstet Gynecol 59:204–206, 1950.
36. Gardner, E. The prenatal development of the human shoulder joint. Surg Clin North Am 43:1465–1470, 1963.

37. Gardner, E. The embryology of the clavicle. Clin Orthop 58:9–16, 1968.

38. Gartsman, G.M.; Roddey, T.S.; Hammerman, S.M. Arthroscopic treatment of anterior-inferior glenohumeral instability. Two- to five-year follow-up. J Bone Joint Surg Am 82:991–1003, 2000.

39. Gilchrist, D.K. A stockinette-Velpeau for immobilization of the shoulder-girdle. J Bone Joint Surg Am 49:750–751, 1967.

40. Golthamer, C.R. Duplication of the clavicle ("os subclaviculare"). Radiology 68:576–578, 1957.

41. Gray, D.J.; Gardner, E. The prenatal development of the human humerus. Am J Anat 124:431–446, 1969.

42. Gray, H. Anatomy of the Human Body. Philadelphia, Lea & Febiger, 1985.

43. Green, N.E.; Wheelhouse, W. Anterior subglenoid dislocation of the shoulder in an infant following pneumococcal meningitis. Clin Orthop 135:125–127, 1978.

44. Greig, D.M. True congenital dislocation of the shoulder. Edin Med J 30:157–175, 1923.

45. Haliburton, R.; Barber, J.R.; Fraser, R.L. Pseudodislocation: An unusual birth injury. Can J Surg 10:455–462, 1967.

46. Hall, R.H.; Isaac, F.; Booth, C.R. Dislocations of the shoulder with special reference to accompanying small fractures. J Bone Joint Surg 41:489–494, 1959.

47. Hawkins, R.J.; Koppert, G.; Johnston, G. Recurrent posterior instability (subluxation) of the shoulder. J Bone Joint Surg Am 66:169–174, 1984.

48. Hedstrom, O. Growth stimulation of long bones after fracture or similar trauma. A clinical and experimental study. Acta Orthop Scand Suppl 122:1–134, 1969.

49. Heyse-Moore, G.H.; Stoker, D.J. Avulsion fractures of the scapula. Skeletal Radiol 9:27–32, 1982.

50. Hippocrates. The Genuine Work of Hippocrates. Baltimore, Williams & Wilkins, 1939.

51. Hobbs, D.W. Sternoclavicular joint: A new axial radiographic view. Radiology 90:801, 1968.

52. Hohl, J.C. Fractures of the humerus in children. Orthop Clin North Am 7:557–571, 1976.

53. Hollinshead, P.D. The back and limbs. In: Hollinshead, P.D., ed. Anatomy for Surgeons. Philadelphia, Harper & Rowe, 1982, pp. 259–340.

54. Hovelius, L. Anterior dislocation of the shoulder in teenagers and young adults. J Bone Joint Surg Am 69:393–399, 1987.

55. Howard, F.M.; Shafer, S.J. Injuries to the clavicle with neurovascular complications. J Bone Joint Surg Am 47:1335–1346, 1965.

56. Inman, V.T.; Saunders, J.B.d.M.; Abbott, L.C. Observations on the function of the shoulder joint. J Bone Joint Surg 26:1–30, 1944.

57. Janecki, C.J.; Shahcheragh, G.H. The forward elevation maneuver for reduction of anterior dislocations of the shoulder. Clin Orthop 164:177–180, 1982.

58. Jit, I.; Kulkarni, M. Times of appearance and fusion of epiphysis at the medial end of the clavicle. Indian J Med Res 64:773–782, 1976.

59. Keats, T.E. Atlas of Normal Roentgen Variants That May Simulate Disease. Chicago, Mosby–Year Book, 1996.

60. Key, J.A.; Conwell, H.E. The management of fractures, dislocations, and sprains. In: Key, J.A.; Conwell, H.E., eds. Fractures of the Clavicle. St. Louis, Mosby, 1946, pp. 495–512.

61. Koehler, A. Borderlands of Normal and Early Pathologic Findings in Skeletal Radiography. New York, Thieme, 1993.

62. Kreisinger, V. Sur le traitment des fratures de la clavicule. Rev Chir 65:396–407, 1927.

63. Kuhns, L.R.; Sherman, M.P.; Poznanski, A.; Holt, J.A. Humeral head and coracoid ossification in the newborn. Radiology 107:145–149, 1973.

64. Lacey, T.; Crawford, H.B. Reduction of anterior dislocations of the shoulder by means of the Milch abduction technique. J Bone Joint Surg 34:108–109, 1952.

65. Larsen, E.; Bjerg-Nielsen, A.; Christensen, P. Conservative or surgical treatment of acromioclavicular dislocation. J Bone Joint Surg Am 68:552–555, 1986.

66. Laskin, R.S.; Sedlin, E.D. Luxatio erecta in infancy. Clin Orthop 80:126–129, 1971.

67. Lemperg, R.; Liliequist, B. Dislocation of the proximal epiphysis of the humerus in newborns. Acta Paediatr Scand 59:377–380, 1970.

68. Liberson, F. Os acromiale: A contested anomaly. J Bone Joint Surg 19:683–689, 1937.

69. Liechti, R. Fractures of the clavicle and scapula. In: Weber, B.G.; Brenner, C.; Freuler, F., eds. Treatment of Fractures in Children and Adolescents. New York, Springer-Verlag, 1980, pp. 87–95.

70. Loder, R.T. Pediatric polytrauma: Orthopaedic care and hospital course. J Orthop Trauma 1:48–54, 1987.

71. Madsen, E.T. Fractures of the extremities in the newborn. Acta Obstet Gynecol Scand 34:41–74, 1955.

72. Magerl, F. Fractures of the proximal humerus. In: Weber, B.G.; Brenner, C.; Freuler, F., eds. Treatment of Fractures in Children and Adolescents. New York, Springer-Verlag, 1980, pp. 88–117.

73. Magnuson, P.B. Fractures. Philadelphia, J.B. Lippincott, 1933.

74. Mast, J.W.; Jakob, R.P.; Ganz, R. Planning and Reduction Technique in Fracture Surgery. New York, Springer-Verlag, 1988.

75. McClure, J.G.; Raney, R.B. Anomalies of the scapula. Clin Orthop 110:22–31, 1975.

76. McGahan, J.P.; Rab, G.T.; Dublin, A. Fractures of the scapula. J Trauma 20:880–883, 1980.

77. Mehmann, P. Fractures of the shaft of the humerus. In: Weber, B.G.; Brenner, C.; Freuler, F., eds. Treatment of Fractures in Children and Adolescents. New York, Springer-Verlag, 1980, pp. 118–129.

78. Milch, H. Treatment of dislocation of the shoulder. Surgery 3:732–740, 1938.

79. Miller, D.S.; Boswick, J.A., Jr. Lesions of the brachial plexus associated with fractures of the clavicle. Clin Orthop 64:144–149, 1969.

80. Mirick, M.J.; Ruiz, E.; Clinton, J.E. External rotation method of shoulder dislocation reduction. J Am Coll Emerg Physicians 8:528–531, 1979.

81. Moseley, H.F. The clavicle: Its anatomy and function. Clin Orthop 58:17–27, 1968.

82. Nasso, S.V.A. La frattura della clavicola del neonato. Minerva Pediatr 6:593–597, 1954.

83. Neer, C.S.; Francis, K.C.; Marcov, R.C. Treatment of unicameral bone cyst. A follow-up study of 175 cases. J Bone Joint Surg 48:731–745, 1966.

84. Neer, C.S.; Horwitz, B.S. Fractures of the proximal humeral epiphyseal plate. Clin Orthop 41:24–31, 1965.

85. Neer, I.C.S. Involuntary inferior and multidirectional instability of the shoulder: Etiology, recognition, and treatment. Instr Course Lect 34:232–238, 1985.

86. Neer, I.C.S.; Foster, C.R. Inferior capsular shift for involuntary inferior and multidirectional instability of the shoulder. J Bone Joint Surg Am 62:897–908, 1980.

87. Nettrour, L.F.; Krufky, E.L.; Mueller, R.E.; Raycroft, J.F. Locked scapula: Intrathoracic dislocation of the inferior angle. A case report. J Bone Joint Surg Am 54:413–416, 1972.

88. Neviaser, R.J. Injuries to the clavicle and acromioclavicular joint. Orthop Clin North Am 18:433–438, 1987.

89. O'Brien, S.J.; Warren, R.F.; Schwartz, E. Anterior shoulder instability. Orthop Clin North Am 18:395–408, 1987.

90. Ogden, J.A. Skeletal Injury in the Child. Philadelphia, W.B. Saunders, 1900.

91. Pasila, M.; Jaroma, H.; Kiviluoto, O.; Sundholm, A. Early complications of primary shoulder dislocation. Acta Orthop Scand 49:260–263, 1978.

92. Penn, I. The vascular complications of fractures of the clavicle. J Trauma 4:819–831, 1964.

93. Pollack, R.G. Operative results of the inferior capsular shift. J Bone Joint Surg Am 82:919–928, 2000.

94. Pollen, A.G. Fractures and Dislocations in Children. Baltimore, Williams & Wilkins, 1973.

95. Powers, J.A. Acromioclavicular separations: Closed or open treatment? Clin Orthop 104:213–223, 1974.

96. Rang, M. Injuries of the shoulder and humeral shaft. In: Children's Fractures. Philadelphia, J.B. Lippincott, 1983, pp. 143–151.

97. Rockwood, C.A. Subluxations and dislocations about the shoulder. In: Rockwood, C.A., Jr.; Green, D.P., eds. Fractures in Adults. Philadelphia, J.B. Lippincott, 1984, pp. 758–759.

98. Rockwood, C.A.; Szalay, E.A.; Curtis, R.J. X-ray evaluation of shoulder problems. In: Rockwood, C.A., Jr.; Matsen, F.A., III, eds. The Shoulder. Philadelphia, W.B. Saunders, 1990, pp. 178–207.

99. Rockwood, C.A. Fractures of the outer clavicle in children and adults [abstract]. J Bone Joint Surg Br 64:642, 1982.

100. Rose, M.D.; Melton, I.; Morrey, M.D.; et al. Epidemiologic features of humeral fractures. Clin Orthop 168:24–30, 1982.

101. Rounds, R.C. Isolated fracture of the coracoid process. J Bone Joint Surg 31:662–663, 1949.

102. Rowe, C.R.; Pierce, D.S.; Clark, J.G. Anterior dislocations of the shoulder: Prognosis and treatment. Surg Clin North Am 43:1609–1614, 1973.

103. Rowe, C.R.; Zarins, B.; Ciullo, J.V. Recurrent anterior dislocation of the shoulder after surgical repair. J Bone Joint Surg Am 66:159–168, 1984.

104. Rowe, C.R.; Pierce, D.S.; Clark, J.G. Voluntary dislocation in the shoulder. A preliminary report on a clinical, electromyographic, and psychiatric study of 26 patients. J Bone Joint Surg Am 55:455–460, 1973.

105. Rowe, C.R.; Zarins, B.; Ciullo, J.W. Recurrent anterior dislocation of the shoulder after surgical repair. Apparent causes of failure and treatment. J Bone Joint Surg Am 66:159–168, 1984.

106. Rubin, A., Birth injuries: Incidence, mechanisms, and end results. Obstet Gynecol 23:218–221, 1964.

107. Rubin, S.A.; Gray, R.L.; Green, W.R. The scapular "Y": A diagnostic aid in shoulder trauma. Radiology 110:725–726, 1974.

108. Russell, J.A.; Holmes, E.M., III; Keller, D.J.; Vargas, J.H.I. Reduction of acute anterior shoulder dislocations using the Milch technique: A study of ski injuries. J Trauma 21:802–804, 1981.

109. Salter, R.B. Fractures, dislocations and soft tissue injuries. In: Textbook of Disorders & Injuries of the Musculoskeletal System. Baltimore, Williams & Wilkins, 1970, pp. 438–439.

110. Salter, R.B.; Harris, W.R. Injuries involving the epiphyseal plate. J Bone Joint Surg 45:587–622, 1963.

111. Samilson, R.L. Congenital and developmental anomalies of the shoulder girdle. Orthop Clin North Am 11:219–231, 1980.

112. Sanford, H.N. Moro reflex as a diagnostic aid in fracture of the clavicle in the newborn infant. Am J Dis Child 41:1304–1306, 1992.

113. Scaglietti, O. The obstetrical shoulder trauma. Surg Gynecol Obstet 66:868–877, 1938.

114. Schmalzried, T.P.; Grogan, T.J.; Neumeier, R.P.A.; Dorey, P.F.J. Metal removal in a pediatric population: Benign procedure or necessary evil? J Pediatr Orthop 11:72–76, 1991.

115. Shaw, B.A.; Murphy, K.M.; Shaw, A.; et al. Humerus shaft fractures in young children. Accident or abuse? J Pediatr Orthop 17:293–297, 1997.

116. Shaw, J.L.; Sakellarides, H. Radial-nerve paralysis associated with fractures of the humerus. A review of 45 cases. J Bone Joint Surg 49:899–902, 1967.

117. Sherk, H.H.; Probst, C. Fractures of the proximal humeral epiphysis. Orthop Clin North Am 6:401–413, 1975.

118. Smith, F.M. Fracture-separation of the proximal humeral epiphysis. Am J Surg 91:627–635, 1956.

119. Spjut, H.J.; Dorfman, H.D.; Fechner, R.E.; Ackerman, L.V. Tumors of bone and cartilage. In: Atlas of Tumor Pathology, Fasc. 5. Washington, D.C., Armed Forces Institute of Pathology, 1971, pp. 347–390.

120. Stanley, D.; Trowbridge, E.A.; Norris, S.H. The mechanism of clavicular fracture. A clinical and biomechanical analysis. J Bone Joint Surg Br 70:461–464, 1988.

121. Stimson, L.A. An easy method of reducing dislocations of the shoulder and hip. Med Rec 57:356–357, 1900.

122. Szalay, E.A.; Rockwood, C.A., Jr. The Holstein-Lewis fracture revisited [abstract]. Orthop Trans 7:516, 1983.

123. Tachdjian, M.D. Fractures involving the proximal humeral physis (fracture-separation of upper epiphysis of humerus). In: Pediatric Orthopedics. Philadelphia, W.B. Saunders, 1972, pp. 1555–1560.

124. Taft, T.N.; Wilson, F.C.; Oglesby, J.W. Dislocation of the acromioclavicular joint: An end-result study. J Bone Joint Surg Am 69:1045–1051, 1987.

125. Taga, I.; Yoneda, M.; Ono, K. Epiphyseal separation of the coracoid process associated with acromioclavicular sprain. Clin Orthop 207:138–141, 1986.

126. Todd, T.W.; D'Errico, J., Jr. The clavicle epiphyses. Am J Anat 41:25–50, 1928.

127. Tse, D.H.W.; Slabaugh, P.B.; Carlson, P.A. Injury to the axillary artery by a closed fracture of the clavicle: A case report. J Bone Joint Surg Am 62:1372–1374, 1980.

128. Twigg, H.L.; Rosenbaum, R.C. Duplication of the clavicle. Skeletal Radiol 6:281, 1981.

129. Vastamaki, M.; Solonen, K.A. Posterior dislocation and fracture-dislocation of the shoulder. Acta Orthop Scand 51:479–484, 1980.

130. Visser, J.D.; Rietberg, M. Interposition of the tendon of the long head of biceps in fracture separation of the proximal humeral epiphysis. Neth J Surg 32:12–15, 1980.

131. Watson, F.M., Jr.; Whiteside, T.E., Jr. Acute hematogenous osteomyelitis complicating closed fractures. Clin Orthop 117:296–302, 1976.

132. Watson-Jones, R. Fractures and Joint Injuries. Baltimore, Williams & Wilkins, 1955.

133. White, A.D.N. Dislocated shoulder—a simple method of reduction. Med J Aust 2:726–727, 1976.

134. White, P.G.; Mah, J.Y.; Friedman, L. Magnetic resonance imaging in acute physeal injuries. Skeletal Radiol 23:627–631, 1994.

135. Wilber, M.C.; Evans, E.B. Fractures of the scapula. An analysis of forty cases and a review of the literature. J Bone Joint Surg Am 59:358–362, 1977.

136. Wong-Pack, W.K., Bobechko, P.E.; Becker, E.J. Fractured coracoid with anterior shoulder dislocation. J Can Assoc Radiol 31:278–279, 1980.

137. Zieger, M.; Dorr, U.; Schulz, R.D. Sonography of slipped humeral epiphysis due to birth injury. Pediatr Radiol 17:425–427, 1987.

138. Zilberman, Z.; Rejovitzky, R. Fracture of the coracoid process of the scapula. Injury 13:203–206, 1982.

139. Zuelzer, W.A. Fixation of small but important bone fragments with a hook plate. J Bone Joint Surg 33:430–436, 1951.

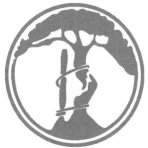

# CHAPTER 11

# Fractures of the Spine in Children

J. Andy Sullivan, M.D.

Fractures of the spine in children are uncommon. Once recognized, most are easy to manage. Unrecognized or improperly managed, they may become catastrophic or fatal. Proper management depends on knowledge of normal development of the spine and the normal radiographic variants that accompany this development.

## DEVELOPMENTAL ANATOMY OF THE SPINE

The first two cervical vertebrae vary in their development from the remaining cervical vertebrae and from the thoracic and lumbar vertebrae. The atlas (C1) usually develops from three ossification centers, one for the body and one for each of the neural arches[1, 4] (Fig. 11–1A). Occasionally, the body may be formed from two centers or may completely fail to appear, and the neural arches may extend forward and fuse.[4] Failure of the body to appear results in failure of anterior fusion, and a cleft is left. The ossification center for the anterior arch is present in approximately 20% of individuals at birth and appears in the remainder during the first year of life. The anterior arch is occasionally bifid. Closure of the posterior arch of C1 is usually completed by the third year. Variations include an absent ring of C1 or failure to completely ossify. The ring of C1 reaches its normal adult size by 4 years of age. The body joins the neural arches by a neurocentral synchondrosis that usually closes by the seventh year.

The axis (C2) develops from four separate centers (see Fig. 11–1B): one for each of the neural arches, one for the center or body, and one for the odontoid. All the ossification centers are present at birth,[1, 4] and fusion occurs by 3 years of age. Before this time, these synchondroses may be mistaken for fractures (Fig. 11–2). According to Freiberger and co-workers,[34] odontoid development occurs in the fifth fetal month by ossification of two longitudinal primary centers, which

fuse at birth. The tip of the odontoid usually appears above the V-shaped shaft at around 6 to 7 years of age and fuses by the 12th year. Failure to fuse may leave a small ossicle known as the ossiculum terminale. The dens, or odontoid process, sits on the centrum, or body, and is joined by the neural arches. It is separated from the centrum of the axis by a region of growth cartilage that disappears at 5 to 7 years of age. In children, fractures can occur through this cartilaginous center. Fusion of the odontoid through the neural arches and the body of the axis occurs between the ages of 3 to 6 years.[1]

The facet joint changes in orientation with maturity. The angle of the C1–C2 facet is 55° in newborns and increases to 70° at maturity.[71] In the lower cervical spine, the angle of the facet joints is 30° at birth and 60° to 70° at maturity. These angles, coupled with the greater ligamentous laxity in young children, explain the increased translational motion that is present.

C3–C7 and the thoracic and lumbar spine develop in a similar manner[1] (see Fig. 11–1C). Each is formed from three ossification centers: one for each neural arch and one for the vertebral centrum. A neurocentral synchondrosis joins them and disappears at around 3 to 6 years of age. Ordinarily, the arches fuse between the age of 2 and 4 years. In the cervical and thoracic vertebrae, five secondary ossification centers are present, including one each for the spinous processes, transverse processes, and vertebral end-plate (the ring apophyses). In the lumbar spine, the mammillary processes each develop from two ossification centers. These secondary ossification centers appear during puberty and fuse to the vertebrae by 25 years of age. A child's spine has usually assumed adult characteristics and is near adult size by the age of 8 to 10 years, so the radiologic characteristics of the spine, except for the apophyses, are comparable to those in adults.

Each vertebra grows in height by endochondral ossification in each of the end-plates. Increase in width occurs by perichondrial and periosteal appositional growth.

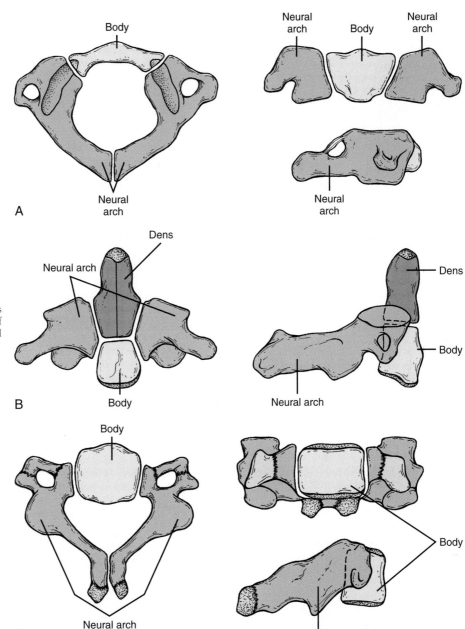

FIGURE 11–1. *A,* Ossification centers of C1. *B,* Ossification centers of C2. *C,* Ossification centers typical of C3-L5.

## RELEVANT ANATOMY

The skull articulates with the atlas through the two occipitoatlantal joints.[1] The predominant motion that occurs here is flexion and extension, with almost no rotation. The spine has four atlantoaxial joints—one anterior and one posterior to the odontoid and the remaining two between the atlas and axis articular processes. The transverse ligament is the first line of defense to prevent atlantoaxial dislocation.[33, 97] The stability of the articulation of the skull to the spine is enhanced by additional ligaments from the axis to the occiput. These ligaments include the alar ligaments (which serve as checkreins to limit rotation and prevent the odontoid from impinging on the cord), the apical dental ligament, and the cruciate ligament. Once the

odontoid has moved its transverse diameter, the alar, or check, ligaments are taut.

Steel[97] analyzed lateral flexion and extension cervical spine films of 50 normal adults and 50 normal children (aged 12 to 15 years). He also performed stress tests of the cervical spine. The first structure to fail in stress testing was the transverse ligament, followed by the accessory ligaments. Once the transverse ligament ruptures, the alar ligaments are insufficient to prevent catastrophic movement of the odontoid with further stress. When the transverse ligament fails, it ruptures near its attachment to the arch. The elasticity in the ligament causes it to shorten, and therefore it may fail to heal. Although the alar ligaments may heal after injury, they are not strong enough to prevent injury to the cord with additional stress.[33, 97]

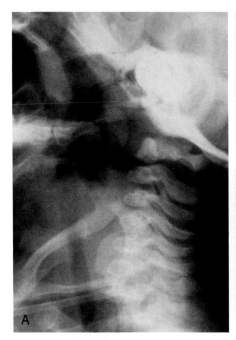
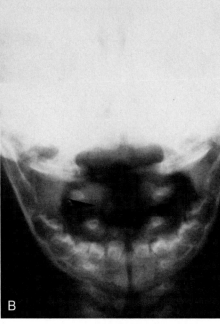

FIGURE **11–2.** Axis ossification centers and synchondroses of C2. *A*, Lateral cervical spine radiograph in an infant. The *arrowhead* points to an apparent cleft at the base of C2, which is the synchondrosis at the base of the odontoid. *B*, Anteroposterior radiograph of an infant. Note the bifid appearance and cleft at the top of the odontoid.

In a review of radiographs, Steel found that the maximal translation of the odontoid in relation to the atlas was 3 mm in adults (20% of the transverse diameter of the odontoid) and 4 mm in children (30% of the transverse diameter of the odontoid).[97] Displacement of 3 to 5 mm is considered to be in the normal range in children. When this distance is exceeded, the transverse ligament is presumed to have ruptured. When the distance exceeds 10 to 12 mm, all ligaments have failed. Steel based the rule of thirds on the finding that at the level of the atlantoaxial articulation, one third of the space in the spinal canal is occupied by the odontoid and one third by the cord, with one third left as the so-called space available for the cord (SAC) (Fig. 11–3).

The anatomy of C3–C7 is similar. C7 has a very long, stout, nonbifid spinous process (vertebra prominens). The transverse processes of C7 are also very large, and the transverse process of the foramen is small. The vertebral artery passes anterior to the transverse process of C7, not through the foramina. Occasionally, a cervical rib may occur in place of the transverse process of C7. The thoracic vertebrae are unique in that they have costal

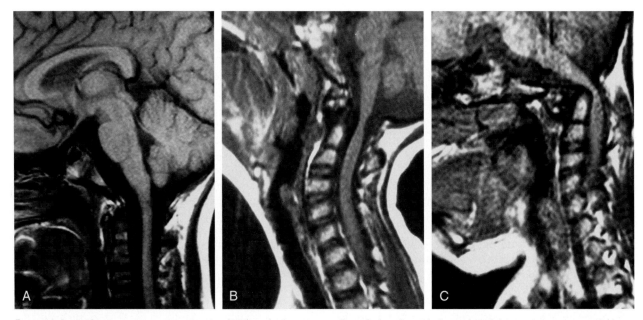

FIGURE **11–3.** *A*, This magnetic resonance imaging (MRI) study shows a normal canal, the odontoid, the cord, and the remaining space available to the cord. *B*, Extension MRI scan in a patient with Down syndrome demonstrating the odontoid, mild constriction of the cord at that level, and the space available to the cord. *C*, Flexion MRI scan demonstrating forward translation of C1 relative to the odontoid and tenting of the cord over the odontoid as the space available to the cord is compromised.

processes for articulation with the ribs. The lumbar vertebrae are the largest of all the vertebrae.

## ANOMALIES OF THE SPINE

### Cervical

Cervical spine anomalies can include failure of formation or failure of segmentation. C1 can fail to segment from the skull, with subsequent narrowing of the foramen magnum and neurologic symptoms. Wedge-shaped vertebrae, bifid vertebrae, or a combination of these abnormalities can also occur. Klippel and Feil[55] described a patient with a short neck, a low posterior hairline, and severe restriction of motion of the neck because of complete fusion of the cervical vertebrae. This combination is now known as the Klippel-Feil syndrome. Hensinger and colleagues[44] reviewed 50 patients with this classic triad of findings and added to these a constellation of associated anomalies that occur frequently in these patients, including congenital scoliosis, renal anomalies, Sprengel's deformity, impaired hearing, synkinesis, and congenital heart disease.

Hensinger and associates[44] reported on congenital anomalies of the odontoid process, including aplasia (complete absence), with absence of the base; hypoplasia (partial absence), in which a stubby peg is located at the base of the odontoid above the C1 articulation; and the most common anomaly, os odontoideum. The incidence of these anomalies is unknown because they are frequently discovered incidentally.

### Thoracolumbar

Thoracolumbar anomalies include failure of segmentation and failure of formation. These anomalies can lead to block vertebrae, wedge vertebrae, bifid vertebrae, and the most common, spina bifida occulta. The resultant spinal deformity depends on the severity, orientation, and location of the anomaly.

## RADIOLOGY OF THE SPINE

In children, the epiphyseal centers mentioned earlier and normal variants are often mistaken for fractures. The epiphyseal plates should be distinguished by their distinctive smooth appearance and their proper anatomic location. Normally, bifid structures are similarly distinguished from fractures, which have more irregular lines and sclerosis.

The articulation of the skull with the cervical spine can be difficult to evaluate radiographically. Anomalies of the odontoid can be confused with acute injury. In the cervical spine, one must be aware of the phenomenon of pseudosubluxation and the normal values for the soft tissue spaces.

Wholey and co-workers[109] reviewed the relationship of the odontoid to the basion. The middle half of the odontoid lies directly beneath the basion (the midsagittal point of the anterior lip of the foramen magnum) and is an average distance of 5 mm from the basion (see Fig. 11–6). In infants and young children, this distance may be as much as 1 cm. These investigators stated that a variation greater than 1 to 2 cm in the relationship of the odontoid to the basion requires further evaluation. They believed that this relationship was much more reproducible than the drawing of McGregor's or Chamberlain's line.

In another series of radiographs in children, an increased distance between the odontoid process and the anterior arch of the atlas was noted during flexion.[14] Movement of 3 mm or more was observed on radiographs made with the neck in flexion in 14 children (20%) in this age group. With extension, the anterior arch of the atlas overrode the odontoid in 14 of 70 patients (20%). In this study, overriding was present when more than two thirds of the viable anterior arch of the atlas lay above the superior margin of the odontoid process.

Dolan[24] reviewed the many ways in which the cervicobasilar relationship can be evaluated. Cervicobasilar abnormalities can be caused by occipital hypoplasia, trauma, tumor, infection, abnormal cranial ossification, and generalized bone disease.

The radiographic finding for odontoid agenesis or hypoplasia is usually a slight depression between the superior articular facets of C1 and C2.[41, 44] Lateral laminagrams or computed tomography (CT) may be helpful. Regardless of the method used, views in flexion and extension must be obtained. In os odontoideum, a wide radiolucent gap is demonstrable between the fragments[32, 34, 35] (see Fig. 11–13C). The os odontoideum moves anteriorly with the ring of C1. This motion, normally less than 3 mm, is up to 1 cm in most symptomatic patients. Mach bands are an optical phenomenon that can be mistaken for a fracture. These dark and light lines appear at the borders of structures with different radiodensity. They are known to occur across the base of the dens, where they may mistaken for a fracture[18] (Fig. 11–4).

Wholey and co-workers[109] reviewed 600 lateral cervical spine radiographs in children and looked at the retropharyngeal and retrotracheal spaces and the diameter of the cervical canal. They concluded that a retropharyngeal space greater than 7 mm and a retrotracheal space greater than 14 mm were abnormal in a child. The cervical canal diameter is 22 mm at C1 and 18 mm at C7. Between the ages of 3 and 6 years, the child's spine gradually approaches adult dimensions. Prevertebral soft tissues are rather uniform in adults, but in young children, they vary in thickness and shape and are more difficult to evaluate. Crying, position changes in an uncooperative patient, and the amount of adenoid lymphoid tissue may lead to the false impression of a widened prevertebral soft tissue space.[8]

The effect of trauma on the measurement of prevertebral soft tissues was studied retrospectively by Matar

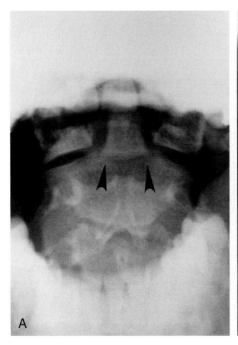

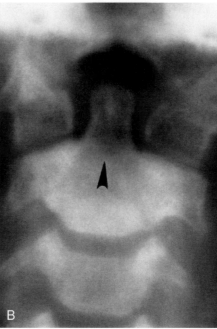

FIGURE 11–4. Mach bands. *A,* Note the apparent radiolucent line at the base of the odontoid *(arrowheads),* which could be mistaken for a fracture. *B,* Tomogram demonstrating that no fracture is present.

and Doyle.[64] Two independent observers, one of whom was blinded, measured the prevertebral soft tissue spaces at C2–C3 and determined the upper limit of normal to be 7 mm; at C6–C7, 21 mm was considered to be the upper limit of normal. With these measurements, a true-positive rate of 53% and a false-positive rate of 5% were observed. These figures are statistically significant. Routine measurement of prevertebral soft tissue spaces is a simple procedure that may provide an important clue to subtle cervical spine injury.

Pseudosubluxation is a condition in which one cervical vertebra is apparently displaced on another on the lateral cervical spine radiograph, especially with flexion (Fig. 11–5). Cattell and Filtzer[15] obtained lateral flexion and extension radiographs in 160 randomly selected children between the ages of 1 and 16 years (10 per year). They stated that anterior subluxation of C2 on C3 was difficult to measure in young children because of poor bony landmarks or reference points. By using the posterior corners of C2 and C3, they were able to demonstrate striking anterior displacement as a result of combined forward shift and flexion of C2 on C3. This displacement was described as marked in 9% (15 patients) and moderate in 15% (24 patients). Forty percent of patients younger than 8 years had anterior displacement. Based on this and other studies, pseudosubluxation of up to 4 mm is acceptable in a child.[4, 15, 79, 98, 104] The most common level is C2–C3, but displacement occurs at C3–C4 as well. Swischuk[100] described a line that can be used to evaluate pseudosubluxation. It is drawn along the posterior arch of C1, C2, and C3. The line should pass within 1.5 mm of the posterior arch of C2 (Fig. 11–6); a distance greater than 1.5 mm is considered nonphysiologic.

Shaw and co-workers[91] evaluated pseudosubluxation of C2 on C3 in polytraumatized children to determine its

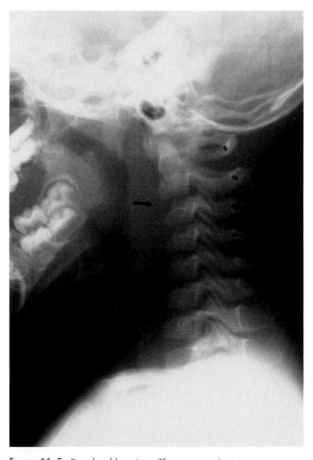

FIGURE 11–5. Pseudosubluxation. The *arrow* points to an apparent subluxation of C2 on C3, which in reality is within normal limits. This child was subsequently found to be normal. The *arrow* is in the retropharyngeal space, which also appears widened but is normal. The *dots* on the posterior spines are to draw Swischuk's line, which revealed that this spine was normal (see text). (Courtesy of Dr. Teresa Stacy.)

prevalence and significance. Normal and C2–C3 pseudosubluxation groups were defined by using standard criteria in their study. Pseudosubluxation of C2 on C3 was present in 21.7% of patients on admission radiographs. They showed that pseudosubluxation had no significant association with intubation status, injury severity, or outcome. They concluded that C2–C3 pseudosubluxation can be considered a benign variant even in the setting of polytrauma.[91]

Other radiographic variations also occur in children. In very young children, reversal of a normal smooth anterior curve can be seen on a lateral projection. Cervical vertebrae are also noted to be wedge-shaped early in life and gradually achieve their adult shape on lateral views by 8 years of age.[98] In the thoracic and lumbar spines of young children, well-defined anterior and posterior indentations in the vertebral bodies are seen on lateral radiographs.[106] Posteriorly, these indentations result from the passage of vascular structures. Anteriorly, they are created by a difference in density caused by the growth plates and vascular structures. The posterior notch is present at all ages but becomes less prominent with age. The anterior arch disappears with normal development of the marrow space. Persistent synchondroses can simulate fracture.[95]

Woodring and Lee reviewed 216 consecutive patients with cervical injuries to determine the use and limitations of CT and whether complex motion tomographic studies were needed.[111] Although CT was better than plain films

in detecting most types of cervical fractures, plain films were better than CT in detecting fractures of the vertebral body, dens, and spinous process and significantly better than CT in detecting subluxation and dislocation. When plain films and CT were combined, they identified 98% of the fractures and 99% of the subluxations and dislocations; 100% of patients with abnormalities were identified.

In the 20 patients who had both CT scanning and complex motion tomographic studies, the motion studies detected more fractures, subluxations, and dislocations than CT scanning did. In particular, complex motion tomographic studies were better than CT in detecting atlantoaxial dislocation and subluxation and fractures of the spinous processes, lateral masses, articular processes, vertebral bodies, and dens. These authors concluded that although more routine use of CT scanning in evaluating cervical spine trauma should increase the rate of detection, complex motion tomographic studies remain the gold standard for the diagnosis of atlantoaxial dislocation, subluxation of vertebral bodies, and fracture of the lateral masses, articular processes, vertebral bodies, and dens.

Davis and associates studied a series of 32,117 trauma patients.[21] Cervical spine injuries were identified in 740, and cervical spine trauma was misdiagnosed in 34. They particularly wanted to know what had caused the delay in clinical diagnosis and to determine whether it was a result of fundamental problems or lack of advanced diagnostic skill or equipment. The single most common

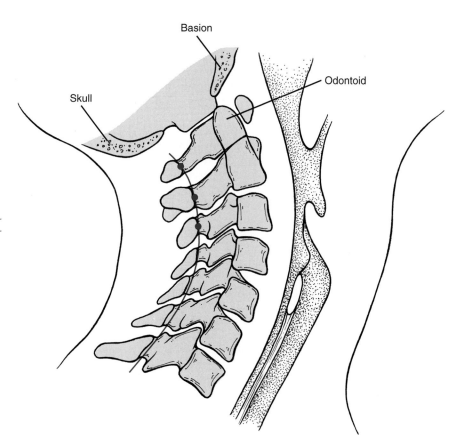

**FIGURE 11–6.** Line drawing of the cervical spine illustrating the basion, odontoid, and Swischuk's line.

error was the failure to obtain an adequate series of cervical spine radiographs. Delayed diagnosis could have been avoided in 31 of 34 patients by the appropriate use of a standard three-view spine series and careful interpretation.

Dwek and Chung reviewed 247 children with a history of trauma who had routine cervical spine radiographs followed by flexion-extension radiographs.[25] Review of the static cervical spine radiographs revealed normal findings in 224 patients (91%), and the flexion-extension radiographs confirmed the normal findings in all patients with normal results on the cervical spine radiographs. Of 23 children (9%) with abnormal findings on static cervical spine radiographs, 7 (30%) had congenital abnormalities that were visible on flexion-extension radiographs; 10 (43%) had traumatic injuries, including fracture, subluxation, or soft tissue swelling; 2 (9%) had instability; and 6 (26%) had questionable abnormalities that were noted on static cervical spine radiographs. They concluded that in children with a history of trauma and normal findings on static cervical spine radiographs, additional flexion-extension radiographs are of questionable use. Baker and colleagues showed that a three-view radiographic series had a sensitivity of 94% in patients with cervical spine injury.[5]

Link and colleagues reviewed a series of 202 patients with substantial cranial trauma.[57] Routine radiography was performed in all patients, as was CT of the head. Twenty-eight patients (14%) had C1 or C2 fractures. Plain radiographs did not demonstrate cervical fractures in 11 of them. Nine patients (4.4%) had fractures of the occipital condyles. These authors concluded that routine CT of the craniocervical junction is useful in patients with substantial cranial trauma because of detection of occipital condyle fractures and fractures of C1 and C2 not seen on plain films. Three-dimensional reconstruction of the occipital-cervical junction and the cervical spine is useful in special cases (see Fig. 11–10B).

Green and Mencio (personal communication, 1999) prospectively studied 150 children younger than 8 years who sustained trauma and had cervical spine radiographs taken. They developed a protocol for evaluation of the cervical spine in children who are either obtunded or too young to cooperate with an examination (Fig. 11–7). The original reason for the study was to help determine when the cervical immobilization that is in place when the child arrives at the emergency department may be safely removed. Anteroposterior (AP), lateral, and oblique radiographs are obtained. If they are abnormal, appropriate treatment is undertaken. If, on the other hand, the radiographs are normal, a CT scan from the occiput through C2 is obtained. If all studies are normal, the cervical collar is removed. All the patients in the study were found on subsequent review to be free of any cervical spine injury. The study has continued for another 5 years and more than 300 additional patients have been seen and evaluated. One 19-month-old child did have a C1–C2 ligament injury that was not detected on either plain radiographs or CT scan.

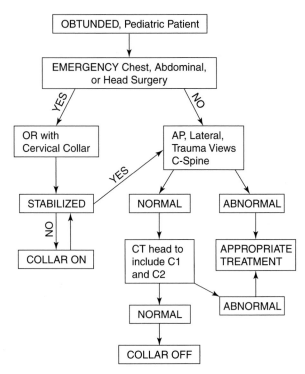

Algorithm—Pediatric Cervical Spine Trauma

**FIGURE 11–7.** Algorithm for evaluation of the cervical spine in obtunded children or those too young to cooperate with the examination. *AP,* anteroposterior. (From Mencio, G.A.; Green, N.E.. Presented at the annual meeting of the American Association of Orthopaedic Surgeons and Pediatric Orthopaedic Society of North America, 1999.)

## INCIDENCE OF SPINAL TRAUMA IN CHILDREN

Cervical spine injuries in children are relatively rare. Of 1299 cases of vertebral trauma seen at the Henry Ford Hospital, 631 were injuries to the cervical spine.[42] Only 12 of them (1.9%) were seen in individuals younger than 15 years. An additional 6 patients were added to the series for a total of 18 patients who were reviewed. Cervical spine injuries occurred more frequently in males than females, and the incidence increased with age. Injuries in the age range 0 to 2 years were rare and mainly the result of birth trauma. In those aged 3 to 5 years, the most frequent mechanisms of injury were falls from a height, automobile accidents, and child abuse. In the age range 6 to 15 years, motor vehicle accidents and sports injuries accounted for most cases. Seven of 18 patients had neurologic deficits. Only 5 of the 18 required surgery. Six of the 18 had associated major trauma to the head, chest, or abdomen.

Swimming, diving, surfing, and motor vehicle accidents are among the major causes of spinal trauma in children.[3, 27, 45] In one series,[43] four fractures of the odontoid, one dislocation of C1–C2, and six fracture-dislocations were detected. In the fracture-dislocation group, neurologic complications developed in five, and three required surgery. Vertebral compression fractures were not seen. Upper cervical spine injuries are more common in children younger than 10 years. In adolescents, the injury patterns are similar to those in adults, mainly occurring in the lower cervical spine.

In the study of Dietrich and co-workers, the average age of cervical spine trauma patients was 11 years, with a range of 2.7 to 18 years.[23] Fifty-four percent of the injuries were caused by motor vehicle accidents; sports injuries accounted for 18% and falls for 12%. Fifty-eight percent of patients had an associated head injury. A lateral radiograph was diagnostic in 98% of the patients. These authors thought that children with cervical spine injuries had two distinct patterns: lethal or intact. Other studies have confirmed similar demographic data.[29, 67]

Nitecki and Moir reviewed factors that predict the outcomes of trauma to the cervical spine in children.[72] In a review of 227 consecutively treated children aged 1 to 17 years, lower cervical spine injuries affected 73% of the patients. Of the 38 patients younger than 8 years, 87% had an injury at the C3 level or higher. Nineteen fatalities occurred, all associated with injuries at the C4 level or higher. All 11 patients with atlantoaxial fracture-dislocation died soon after the injury. All had an unstable fracture and cord transection, with subsequent cardiorespiratory collapse. Fatality rates were as follows: C1, 17%; C2, 9%; C3, 4.3%; and C4, 3.7%. No fatalities occurred in children with injuries lower than C4.

McGrory and Klassen reviewed 143 patients aged 2 months to 15 years seen at the Mayo Clinic over a 41-year period because of injury to the cervical spine.[67] Children younger than 11 years had fewer injuries as a group and were most often injured in falls; they had a predominance of ligamentous injuries to the upper cervical spine and a high rate of mortality. Children 11 through 15 years old were more often injured during sports and recreational activities, had a higher male-to-female ratio, and were more often injured in the lower cervical spine, similar to adults.

Cervical spine injuries of all types may be more common than currently recognized because of failure to diagnose these injuries. Aufdermaur[2] noted that fractures of the spine are rare in children and account for 2.5% to 3.3% of all spinal injuries. He was able to identify 12 spinal injuries at autopsy over an 8-year period. He also performed studies in three spines by stressing them in a vise to see where they would fracture. Radiographs of these spines revealed large gaping fissures and wide intervertebral joint spaces that perhaps suggested a lesion. The fracture was consistently through the endplate of the vertebral body. Of the spines seen at autopsy, seven of the injuries were in the cervical spine, four were in the thoracic spine, and one was in the lumbar spine. Ten of 12 injuries had been sustained during motor vehicle accidents, and 2 were from hyperextension at birth. Importantly, only 1 of the 12 subjects had been suspected of having a spine fracture before necropsy. These cases, then, represent a 12% incidence of spinal injury in 100 children coming to necropsy over an 8-year period. In three of the subjects, it was thought that the fracture contributed directly to death. These three had

ligament injuries as well, thus indicating that the spine was unstable. A higher incidence of spine instability occurs in patients with Down syndrome, Morquio syndrome, and rheumatoid arthritis and in those with upper airway infection.

## SPINAL INJURY IN NEONATES

Spinal column and spinal cord injuries can occur during delivery and are more common during breech delivery.[56, 73, 101] When associated with cephalic delivery, the injuries tend to occur in the upper cervical spine and are thought to result from rotation (Fig. 11–8). Injuries associated with breech delivery are usually in the lower cervical and upper thoracic spine and are thought to result from traction[101] (Fig. 11–9). At necropsy, Shulman and co-workers[93] demonstrated transection of the cord with atlanto-occipital and atlantoaxial dislocation. In a series of 600 neonatal autopsies, Tawbin[101] found a 10% incidence of brain, brain stem, or spinal injuries.

Complete C6–C7 dislocation with locked facets has also been reported in an infant.[66] This child's delivery was difficult because of a large abdominal mass, and the child was neurologically normal at birth. Complete C6–C7 dislocation with locked facets was discovered during a skeletal survey. The patient was successfully treated in traction but died at 6 months of other causes. Jones and Hensinger[50] reported a C2–C3 dislocation that occurred at birth and resulted in weakness and hypotonia. The diagnosis was made at 2 years of age. Because of hypotonia and what was considered to be ligamentous laxity, an initial diagnosis of Larsen's syndrome had been made. The patient underwent spinal fusion at 20 months. One should therefore include cervical spine injury in the differential diagnosis of a newborn with decreased tone, a nonprogressive neurologic deficit, and a negative history of familial neurologic disorders.[50]

## SPINAL CORD INJURY IN CHILDREN

Spinal cord injury (SCI) in children is unique in several ways. Depending on the age at the time of injury and the level of the lesion, spinal deformity is almost certain to develop in children with SCI. They also have a high incidence of lower extremity problems. Unique to pediatric patients is the syndrome of spinal cord injury without radiographic abnormality (SCIWORA).

## SCIWORA

This syndrome is defined as SCI in a patient with no visible fracture on plain radiographs, linear tomograms, or CT. These children can present with complete or incomplete SCI syndromes. Various theories have been put forward to explain SCIWORA. The spinal column in children is more elastic than the spinal cord in adults and can undergo considerable deformation without being

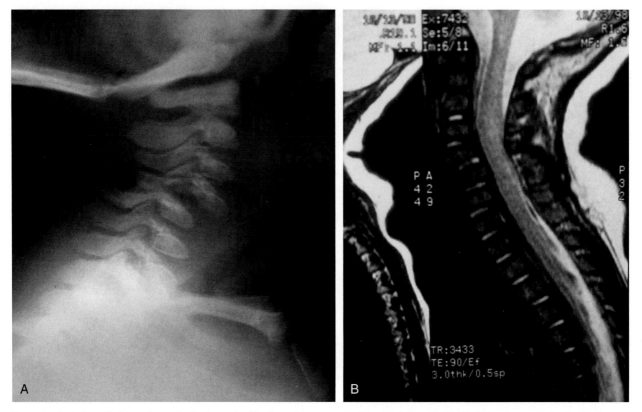

**FIGURE 11–8.** *A,* Lateral plain radiograph of a 4-month-old infant who sustained a fracture of C4 and a brachial plexus injury at birth. The fracture had healed. *B,* Magnetic resonance imaging demonstrates the absence of canal compromise.

disrupted.[14] Leventhal[56] showed that the spinal column can elongate up to 2 inches without disruption, whereas the inelastic spinal cord ruptures with only ¼ inch of elongation. A clinical example of this mechanism is the seat belt distraction injury pattern. Patients have been seen with SCIWORA and cerebrospinal fluid–mediastinal fistulas, thus demonstrating that the cord can be severely disrupted without demonstrable fracture or dislocation of the spinal column. This injury, then, involves severe flexion and distraction. Pang and colleagues[75, 76] suggested hyperextension in the thoracic and lumbar spine as a probable mechanism. They compared a series of patients with SCIWORA who were run over by cars while lying prone or while lying supine.[75] Although both groups had a variety of visceral injuries that one would expect from such a crush, only those lying prone sustained neurologic injuries, which suggests that the SCIWORA was caused by hyperextending the spine.

Other factors in SCIWORA include the relatively large head in relation to body size in children. Poor neck muscle development and head control may also be important. These speculations are supported by the fact that these injuries are more common in younger children and in the upper cervical spine.[75, 76] One must be particularly vigilant if the dire consequences of missing the diagnosis of SCIWORA syndrome are to be avoided. Although motor vehicle and pedestrian accidents are the most frequent causes, the syndrome can occur with falls or in sports. It may also have a delayed onset.

The reported incidence of SCIWORA in patients with SCI has varied from 5% to 67%.[75, 76, 113] Yngve and associates[113] reviewed a series of 71 SCI patients from

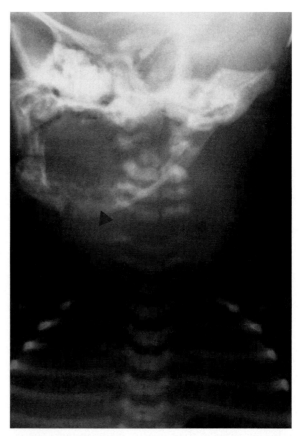

**FIGURE 11–9.** Dislocation of C4-5 (*arrowheads*) as a result of a cephalic delivery with forceps. The child had abdominal dystocia. (Courtesy of Dr. Tim Tytle.)

birth to 1 year of age. Sixteen had SCIWORA, and 55 had SCI associated with osseous injury. In another series of 55 children with SCIWORA, 22 had complete or severe SCI and 33 had incomplete or mild SCI.[75] Ten lesions were in the upper cervical spine (C1–C4), and 33 were in the lower (C5–C8); 12 were thoracic. The syndrome was more common and more likely to be severe in younger children. All but 1 of the 22 patients with complete SCI were younger than 8 years, and two thirds of the severely injured were younger than 4 years. Younger children were also more likely to have upper cervical spine injuries. Fifteen of the patients in Pang and Pollack's series[75] had a delayed onset of paralysis. Nine had transient warning signs such as paresthesias or subjective paralysis. Eight patients sustained a second episode of SCIWORA after the initial event; the second event was always more severe. In all patients with a delayed onset of the syndrome, the spine had not been immobilized after the initial trauma, and all were neurologically normal before the second event. Complete SCI developed in four, and they were left with varying degrees of residual deficit. Patients with SCIWORA have a variety of associated injuries. In one series, 18 of the patients had closed head injuries.[76] Thoracic injuries were usually the result of severe trauma, and crush injuries often had associated visceral injuries.

Pang and Pollack[75] stated that the prognosis depends on the results of the initial neurologic examination. To maximize the care of these patients, they made the following recommendations: (1) rule out occult fractures and dislocations that are unstable and require surgery, (2) identify patients who are likely to have late deterioration, and (3) prevent the recurrence of SCIWORA. After the initial examination, the patients should be evaluated by plain radiography, linear tomography, CT, and magnetic resonance imaging (MRI). None of these imaging studies has proved reliable in detecting the osseous or ligamentous injury that must be present. Myelography may be useful to localize the level of injury. In one series, a displaced end-plate was diagnosed by myelography.[113] Extravasation of myelographic dye from the spinal canal is a poor prognostic sign (Fig. 11–10). Pang and Pollack[75] found that somatosensory evoked potential (SSEP) studies were abnormal in 17 of 22 patients studied. These studies are particularly useful in patients with combined head trauma, in young children, and as a baseline for recovery.

The indications for any type of surgery in children with SCIWORA are the same as those for SCI and osseous injury. These patients usually have stable injuries and rarely require surgical stabilization. Laminectomy has not proved beneficial.[68, 75, 76, 113]

## Characteristics of Spinal Cord Injury in Children

SCI in children is rare. Most often it occurs as a result of motor vehicle accidents (38%), falls or jumps (16%), and gunshot wounds (13%).[45] Sports-related injuries are less frequent, with diving being the most common (9%). All other sports account for 1% or less of the total. Spine

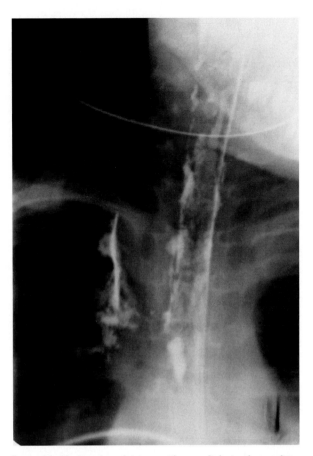

**FIGURE 11–10.** Spinal cord injury without radiologic abnormalities. This patient was struck by a car. In the emergency room, he was noted to have a T4-level complete paraplegia. The results of plain radiography and computed tomography were normal. The myelographic contrast medium extravasated into the chest at T4.

fracture without SCI is more common than fracture with SCI. Children make up a small percentage of all patients with acquired quadriplegia and paraplegia. Rang[85] reviewed the experience at Toronto Sick Children's Hospital over a 15-year period and found that paraplegia was three times more common than quadriplegia.

Hoy and Cole described the pediatric cervical seat belt syndrome over a 9-year period.[48] During that time, 541 children were admitted with injuries sustained as passengers in motor vehicle accidents. Seven (1.3%) had cervical seat belt syndrome. Five had fractures or fracture-dislocations of the proximal cervical spine, and two had injuries of the lower cervical spine. Head injury occurred in four children, and severe cervical SCI occurred in three. A fracture of the larynx and recurrent laryngeal nerve palsy occurred in one child. All these children were wearing three- or four-point restraints. Only two children recovered completely. One died, and two required continuing care for cervical cord damage. Children wearing three-point restraints were thought to be injured from flexion of the neck over the poorly fitting sash of the adult seat belt. In the four-point restraint group, the injury was thought to result from hyperflexion of the neck on a fixed torso.

Air bag deployment can also result in cranial and cervical spine injury. By 1997, automotive air bag deployment after low-speed collisions had resulted in the deaths of 49 children and serious injuries in 19 others in the United States. Marshall and associates reviewed the injury pattern in 11 cases,[63] and others have reported case studies.[40, 69] The cause of death or serious injury in every case was neurologic. Crush injuries of the skull were predominant in infants in rear-facing seats. Both skull and cervical spine trauma occurred in older children regardless of whether they were properly or improperly restrained or totally unrestrained. Morrison and colleagues reported the case of a 3½-year-old child with multiple facial, cranial, and cervical spine injuries, including atlantoaxial subluxation and fracture of the C4 body.[69] We have treated a child with complete atlanto-occipital dislocation at our institution (Fig. 11–11). These injuries result from release of the gases and the force of the deploying bag causing the head to strike the interior of the automobile. The Centers for Disease Control and Prevention recommend keeping children properly restrained, preferably in the rear seat or as far as possible from the air bags. Automobile manufacturers are currently developing air bags that sense the weight of the rider and deploy with less force.

It is of utmost importance that all children with suspected spinal injury, even though it is relatively uncommon, be properly immobilized before extraction from a vehicle or before transport. Because of the large head size relative to body size, children younger than 10 years may need a recess in the spine board for the occiput or may need to be placed on double mattresses to protect the cervical spine. In one series of 10 children younger than 10 years with cervical spine injuries, lateral radiographs revealed that the spine was improperly positioned on a standard spine board.[46]

On arrival in the emergency room, the patient's airway and cardiovascular status are checked. A careful examination is done to seek associated injuries. A child who is comatose or who has multiple organ system trauma or closed head trauma must be systematically evaluated for spinal injury. The neurologic examination must be complete and meticulous, and the sensory level and motor function must be carefully documented. After routine radiography in two planes has been performed, additional studies include supervised stress views and open-mouth odontoid views if the child is able to cooperate. Flexion-extension views in a patient with normal radiographs are of questionable value.[25] CT can be performed to demonstrate bony injury and MRI to evaluate the spinal cord. A myelogram may be necessary.

Scarrow and co-workers[90] performed a pilot study on evaluation of the cervical spine in obtunded or comatose pediatric trauma patients. Patients were evaluated with standard three-view cervical spine radiographs and CT when necessary. Those without radiographic abnormality but with altered mental status underwent flexion-extension radiographs of the cervical spine with monitoring by fluoroscopy and SSEP studies. Patients with abnormal movement by fluoroscopy or changes in SSEP underwent MRI. Fifteen patients were evaluated with this protocol. Two had movement on flexion-extension of the cervical spine, and five had SSEP changes. Three patients had MRI, with only one showing injury. Five patients had residual hemiparesis. They concluded that evaluation of the cervical spine in obtunded or comatose patients could be done safely with flexion-extension radiographs and fluoroscopic and SSEP monitoring. They thought that further studies were needed to determine the efficacy of SSEP monitoring for cervical spine clearance in this select population. D'Alise and colleagues noted that in eight patients who were obtunded or comatose and required surgery, MRI was the first test to identify the injury.[17]

SSEP studies are not readily available in the emergency room. Dr. Neil Green, one of the editors of this book, has presented a study to develop a protocol for dealing with obtunded pediatric patients. In all cases, the cervical collar was left in place until the spine was cleared or a definitive diagnosis was made. Radiographs obtained

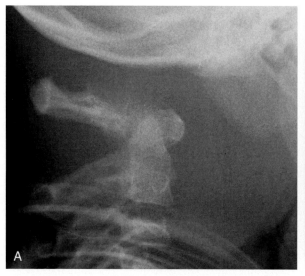 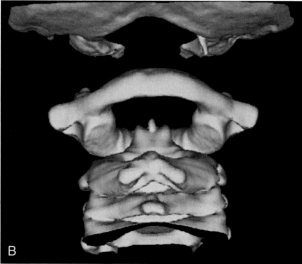

*A,* Lateral radiograph demonstrating an occipitoatlantal dislocation sustained in an air bag injury. *B,* Three-dimension computed tomography was performed before occipitoatlantal fusion.

were routine AP, lateral, and trauma oblique views. The odontoid view was obtained if the patient was cooperative. CT was performed from the occiput to C3. Flexion-extension views were not obtained acutely. In this prospective study of 116 children younger than 8 years (birth to 8 years; average, 4.7 years), 5 were lost to follow-up, leaving 111 to be studied (63 boys, 48 girls). Patients were included in the study if they had less than a grade 1 level of consciousness, neck pain or tenderness, decreased range of motion, abnormal neurologic examination, or head, neck, or face trauma. Seven injuries were identified in these 111 patients. Two were SCIWORA and five were bony abnormalities, including fractures and dislocations. No false-negative results occurred. They detected one fracture of the occipital condyles that was identified only by CT. Figure 11–7 is the algorithm that they used. These authors concluded that by using the algorithm, patients can be safely evaluated and the cervical spine either cleared or the injuries reliably detected.

Studies indicate that methylprednisolone administered in the first 8 hours after injury may improve the chances of recovery.[10–12] In a randomized, controlled study of methylprednisolone, placebo, and naloxone in the treatment of acute SCI, methylprednisolone produced improvement in motor and sensory recovery when evaluated at 6 weeks and 6 months.[12] The effect was limited to those treated within the first 8 hours of injury. Methylprednisolone was given as a bolus and for the first 23 hours after injury. The effect was observed in children with both complete and incomplete SCI. These children had a higher incidence of wound infections, but the difference was not statistically significant. No increased risk of gastrointestinal bleeding was seen. All the patients in the study were older than 13 years, so the effect on younger children is unknown.

Prospective, randomized, controlled, double-blind clinical drug studies in acute SCI have reported enhancement of neurologic recovery of motor function when both methylprednisolone and $GM_1$ ganglioside are used.[36–39] Methylprednisolone is a steroid administered at high levels, and $GM_1$ is a complex acidic glycolipid found in high levels in cell membranes in the central nervous system. The latter has neuroprotective and neurofunctional restoration potential. Patients administered both drugs had improved recovery in comparison to those given methylprednisolone alone.

Methylprednisolone is given specifically to decrease edema, as an anti-inflammatory, and to protect cell membranes by the scavenging of oxygen free radicals. It is given initially in an intravenous bolus of 30 mg/kg of body weight over a 15-minute period. An infusion of 5.4 mg/kg/hr is then administered for 23 hours to all patients who are treated less than 8 hours after the onset of blunt trauma.[10–12]

## Spinal Cord Syndromes in Children

Central cord syndrome is not common in children, but it does occur. Oller and Boone diagnosed Brown-Séquard syndrome in three victims of blunt trauma.[74] Penetrating trauma is far more likely to cause this uncommon syndrome of ipsilateral motor and proprioception loss with contralateral pain and temperature deficit. Pediatric victims frequently have no fracture.

All patients with SCI should be given prophylaxis for stress ulcers. Routine care includes a Foley catheter initially and then intermittent catheterization and a bowel program. Pressure sore prevention is of extreme importance and begins immediately.

Guidelines for the management of spinal skeletal injury are the same as those discussed for SCIWORA. Children have a better chance than adults do for some useful recovery from SCI. Hadley and co-workers[41] noted that 89% of pediatric patients with incomplete SCI improved; 20% of patients with complete SCI had evidence of significant recovery. None of the patients sustained neurologic deterioration as a result of treatment. Children with both incomplete and complete SCI showed some recovery, except for those with injuries in the thoracic area, where the prognosis was regarded as hopeless.[85] Laminectomy is not beneficial and can be harmful[68, 85, 92, 112] because it increases instability. In the cervical spine, swan neck deformity can occur after laminectomy.[92] Angular deformity at all levels is more likely after laminectomy in children.[65]

Children with acquired paraplegia require management by a variety of specialists, and treatment is best delivered by a team approach. Specialists in orthopaedics, pediatrics, urology, psychology, social services, physical and occupational therapy, orthotics, and education are crucial members of the team.

Several authors have looked at the risk of spinal deformity subsequent to SCI in children.[6, 7, 13, 65] Mayfield and associates[65] reviewed 49 patients younger than 18 years. In the 28 who sustained SCI before the teenage growth spurt, spinal deformities developed in all, and 80% of the deformities were progressive. Scoliosis developed in 93%, kyphosis in 57%, and lordosis in 18%. Sixty-one percent of these patients required spinal fusion. In most patients, orthotic management was unsuccessful, but in some, it delayed the age at which fusion was necessary. These patients experienced a high complication rate after surgery, but 93% achieved solid fusion. Thirteen had had laminectomy without benefit, and pelvic obliquity was often a problem. In patients who sustained their injuries after the teenage growth spurt, acute angular deformity at the site of the fracture developed in two thirds. Only 38% had a progressive deformity, which was not usually significant. Only one third of these patients required stabilization. Age, then, is important because younger patients are at a higher risk for the development of deformity.

In other series, additional factors were important in the development of deformity. The paralysis itself is the most important factor.[6] Children with simple fractures without SCI show good remodeling of the spine, and subsequent deformity is rare and not progressive.[48] In a series of patients with paraplegia resulting from infection, tumor, and trauma, those with paraplegia caused by infection had the highest incidence of deformity, thus indicating that it is the paraplegia itself, rather than any injury to the bony column, that is most important.[6] The level of injury is important, with higher levels carrying a higher risk of deformity.[65] Spasticity and muscle imbalance are also contributory. The development of pelvic obliquity can be catastrophic in an SCI patient with insensitive skin.[53] When pelvic obliquity develops, the pelvis follows the spine. Management of the deformity must balance the pelvis to produce a good sitting surface and a good result.[7, 53]

## Specific Cervical Spine Injuries

### OCCIPUT–C1

Injuries at this level have been infrequently demonstrated in children.[30] It may well be that these injuries are so often associated with death that they are not diagnosed, as in the studies by Aufdermaur.[2] In the study of Shulman and co-workers,[93] transection of the cord with atlanto-occipital and atlantoaxial dislocation was demonstrated at necropsy. Bohlman[9] reported a 14-year-old child with an occiput–C1 lesion that was not discovered until arteriography was performed.

A lesion is diagnosed by the demonstration of excessive mobility of the occiput on C1. No series are available with specific treatment recommendations. Because of the potential for cord injury and death, these lesions should probably be reduced and an occiput–C1 or occiput–C2 fusion performed (Fig. 11–12; see also Fig. 11–11).

Fusion of the occiput to C1–C2 is performed with the patient prone. Although a headrest can be used, I prefer a retaining fixation device that is attached to the skull and the head of the table. This device provides stable fixation, more freedom in the surgical approach, and the ability to obtain good confirmation radiographically. Before beginning the procedure, I obtain a lateral radiograph to be certain that I can adequately visualize the area to be operated and the position of C1 relative to C2. A midline incision is made from the base of the occiput to the C3 spinous process. If the occiput and C3 are not to be included in the fusion, they should be exposed as little as possible because the fusion can extend itself, and care should be taken to not enter the periosteum. If one stays in the median raphe or the ligamentum nuchae, the procedure is usually bloodless. I prefer using electrocautery down to the bone. For a C1–C2 fusion, it is carried just caudal to the C2 vertebra. I always confirm the level radiographically, before beginning the subperiosteal exposure. Lateral dissection is performed carefully with a combination of electrocautery and periosteal elevators. It continues laterally out on the lamina to the medial aspect of the facet joint. C2 is dissected first because C1 may be further anterior, and only the posterior aspect may be palpable in the midline. A small periosteal elevator is used for C1. The ring of C1 is unstable and can be pressed forward. It may also be fractured because it can be quite fragile. Care must be taken to not damage the atlanto-occipital membrane. Lateral exposure of C1 is done with care because the vertebral vein and vertebral artery are just lateral to the lateral aspect of the dissection. These vessels travel in the groove of C1, which is carefully identified.

Positioning the head in neutral alignment or slight flexion aids in exposure because such positioning helps identify the interval between the occiput and C1. After the exposure is completed, I use a small periosteal elevator or dural resector to dissect under the ring of C1. An 18-gauge wire is bent double into a loop, with the loop circumference being approximately the circumference of C1. The wire is carefully passed under C1, and the loose ends are passed through the loop of wire. The ends are pulled tight around C1, with care taken to not let the wire move anteriorly toward the dura.

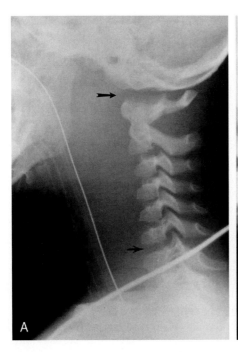 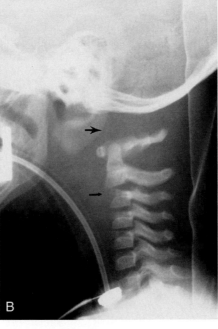

FIGURE 11–12. Atlanto-occipital dislocation. *A,* This 3-year-old girl sustained multiple trauma and was placed on a respirator. Note the massive prevertebral swelling, dislocation of the atlanto-occipital joint, and dislocation of C6-7. The patient died shortly after the study. *B,* This 3-year-old was struck by a car, resuscitated elsewhere, and transferred. Once again, note the hypopharyngeal soft tissue swelling and an additional injury at C2-3. This patient also died. (Courtesy of Dr. Tim Tytle.)

In children, C2 is usually too small to drill a hole to pass the wire through the spinous process, so I loop it under C2 and twist it with a pair of large needle holders. Before I twist the wire, an unscrubbed assistant positions the head in the fixation device, and a lateral radiograph is obtained to confirm reduction. At this point, the wire is twisted, and cortical and cancellous grafts in small bits and strips are placed from C1 to C2. C1 and C2 are decorticated carefully with a small rongeur. If the occiput is to be included, a flap of periosteum is raised over the lower aspect of the occiput. The periosteum is dissected off the inferior aspect of the occiput, and a small bur is used to drill two holes through the bone. Either two loops of wire can be passed as for C1 or a Wisconsin wire with a button can be passed through the skull, which is my preferred technique. Although I have no experience with them, twisted cables of titanium are also used in this area. These two wires can then be twisted below the spinous process of C2. Decortication of the occiput is carried out with a bur. The remainder of the fusion is similar to that of C1–C2.

Rodgers and colleagues reviewed 23 patients who had occipitocervical fusion by the technique devised by the senior author John Hall.[88] A threaded K-wire was passed through the spinous process. Occipital fixation was achieved by wiring corticocancellous bone through bur holes. The wires were wrapped around the K-wire. A halo was used in 10 patients for an average of 12.5 weeks (range, 2 to 24 weeks). Twenty-two of 23 achieved successful fusion at an average follow-up of 5.8 years. Multiple complications occurred, including pseudarthrosis (two, with persistence in one), transient quadriplegia (one), hardware failure (one), extension of the fusion, pneumonia, halo pin infection, sores under the halo vest, hydrocephalus, cerebrospinal fluid leak, and traumatic fracture of the fusion mass. The authors comment that the results are comparable with or better than the results published and the results in their patients in whom this technique was not used.

Rodgers and co-workers also reported on five children treated with occipitocervical fusion before 6 years of age in whom increased cervical lordosis developed. They recommended fusion in neutral or slight flexion in very young children to offset this predictable increase in lordosis.[89]

## SUBLUXATION OF C1 ON C2

Rotation between the occiput and C1 is minimal.[1] Fifty percent of cervical spine rotation occurs between C1 and C2. To a lesser extent, flexion, extension, and translation also occur in this joint. Roughly one third of the canal is occupied by the odontoid, one third by the cord, and one third by the SAC.[97] When rotation exceeds normal values, particularly when the ligaments are disrupted, the odontoid can cause pressure on the spinal cord. In addition, the vertebral artery is immediately anterior to the transverse foramina of C1 and C2 and can be damaged with excessive displacement. This excessive mobility can be caused by rupture of the ligaments, fracture of the odontoid, or increased ligamentous laxity.

Diagnosis of C1–C2 instability is suggested by a history of trauma to the cervical spine and is confirmed by plain or tomographic views of the cervical spine and flexion-extension views showing excursion of greater than 5 mm between the anterior cortex of the dens and the posterior cortex of the anterior ring of C1. The neurologic condition of the patient must be meticulously documented. Although these injuries may fail to heal, a trial of conservative treatment in a halo vest or Minerva cast is indicated in a child. Additional pins may be required in a small infant or child to distribute the force of the halo pins.[70]

Halo application in children can be performed under general anesthesia or with conscious sedation using ketamine or combinations of narcotic agents. If conscious sedation is chosen, the skin is infiltrated at each pin site with local anesthetic. The scalp is scrubbed with povidone-iodine (Betadine). I do not shave the hair. In children, multiple pins are used; generally, the younger the child, the more pins needed. In some patients younger than 2 to 3 years, at least 10 pins may be needed. In very young children, the torque has to be carefully controlled, and finger tightness is usually satisfactory. Two pounds is sufficient in older children. The anterior pins are placed approximately 1 cm above the eyebrows. Care must be taken that the posterior aspect is aligned so that it is inferior to the maximal prominence of the skull and just above the occiput. Placement of the pins laterally behind the hairline will perforate the temporalis and masseter muscles; the skull is quite thin in that area and poses a risk of penetration. In addition, chewing will cause motion around the pins and lead to irritation. The posterior pins are placed about 1 cm above the pinna. A ring should be selected that allows sufficient clearance for pin care and prevents impingement from edema.

The pins can be cared for by any of a variety of means. It is most important that they be cleaned daily, with removal of all dried drainage, and inspected for evidence of infection. In children, I generally tighten the pins after the first day; after that time, skull penetration is a hazard. A variety of devices can be used to position the neck and hold the halo in place before final placement.

If after 2 to 3 months of this conservative care, flexion-extension films indicate continued instability of greater than 5 mm, C1–C2 fusion should be performed. My preferred technique is the same as that described and illustrated in the later discussion on os odontoideum.

Considerable interest has been shown in the incidence of C1–C2 instability in individuals with Down syndrome.[20, 82–84, 105] In a series of 236 patients, 17% were found to have greater than 5 mm of instability.[82] Eighty-five percent were asymptomatic, and 15% had neurologic symptoms or findings. In a more recent review of 404 patients,[84] 14.6% had greater than 5 mm of displacement (59 of 404). Of these 59 patients, 53 were asymptomatic, and only 6 were symptomatic and required surgery. In follow-up, significant changes were detected clinically or radiographically.

After the early studies, the Committee on Sports Medicine of the American Academy of Pediatrics issued a policy statement.[16] The committee recommended that patients with Down syndrome who have 5 to 6 mm of instability be restricted from participating in sports that carry a risk of stress to the head and neck. Those without instability were not restricted. Follow-up was not specified. The Special Olympics organization issued a bulletin that placed even greater restrictions on particular sports.[96] The bulletin led to the belief that all individuals with Down's syndrome required examination and radiographic evaluation before participating in sports. In some instances, this examination was interpreted as an annual requirement.

In a 1988 review, Davidson[20] found little support for the hypothesis that instability predisposes to neurologic compromise or dislocation. All cases of dislocation were preceded by several weeks of readily detectable physical signs; therefore, a carefully performed physical examination (including a neurologic examination) would be more predictive. Davidson reached the following conclusions: (1) the incidence of atlantoaxial dislocation in children with Down syndrome is unknown; (2) it has not been shown that a radiograph is predictive (one patient with a normal radiograph died of the condition); and (3) atlantoaxial dislocation has not been reported in any patient with Down syndrome during participation in sports.

Instability of the cervical spine in individuals with Down syndrome is a matter of concern to those with the syndrome and their caretakers. Although instability occurs in a significant number of these individuals, the natural history of the condition is unknown. It is reasonable to obtain a baseline neurologic examination and flexion and extension films of the cervical spine. Repeat neurologic evaluation every 3 to 5 years is probably sufficient. These persons should not be unnecessarily restricted. If neurologic symptoms or signs develop, a more detailed workup is necessary. If radiographic evaluation reveals an atlantodens interval greater than 5 mm, the patient should refrain from sports that stress the cervical spine. Recognized treatment options are available for those with neurologic problems.[84] In one series, 7 of 236 patients had various neurologic deficits.[33] Early recognition and treatment led to good results; however, patients with long-standing symptoms were minimally improved by surgery.

## ATLANTOAXIAL ROTARY FIXATION

Atlantoaxial rotary fixation (AARF), which has been called by a variety of names, is a clinical condition usually characterized by pain, loss of cervical motion, and torticollis. Young patients with long-standing AARF may also have facial asymmetry. In Fielding and Herman's series of 17 cases, one of the striking features was the delay in diagnosis.[33] The condition may be difficult to diagnose with plain films, but plain tomography may be suggestive. Cineradiography or CT may be necessary to make the diagnosis.

The series of Fielding and Herman[33] included equal numbers of males and females, and the age range was 7 to 68 years (average, 20 years). Onset had been spontaneous in four patients, associated with minor trauma in three, and associated with upper respiratory infection (URI) in five; three had miscellaneous associ-

ated conditions. In another series of 16 children, 8 gave a history of minor trauma, 9 of recent URI, and 1 of juvenile rheumatoid arthritis.[81]

In Fielding and Herman's series,[33] the average delay in diagnosis was 11.6 months. Neck extension was usually decreased by as much as 50%. The characteristic position of the head was a 23° tilt to one side with a 20° rotation to the opposite side and slight flexion. Patients could actively make the deformity worse but were unable to correct it.

The diagnosis must be confirmed radiographically. An open-mouth AP view shows lateral rotation of the mass of the atlas. The lateral mass that is forward appears wider and closer to the midline, and the other lateral mass appears smaller and farther away from the midline. This arrangement creates asymmetry between the odontoid process and the lateral mass. On the side on which the atlas is rotated posteriorly, the joint between the lateral masses is obscured. On the AP view, particularly with tilt and rotation, the spinous process appears markedly deviated from the midline and on the same side as the chin. Open-mouth views with rotation of 15° and 30° to the right and left may be useful. On lateral plain films, the lateral mass of the atlas is rotated forward to the position normally held by the oval anterior arch of the atlas. Such rotation can lead to constriction of the canal. With tilting of the atlas, the two halves of the posterior arch are not superimposed. Plain tomography shows that the lateral masses are in different planes. This finding can be cause by positioning and is not diagnostic. Lateral cineradiography, when available, shows that the posterior arches of C1 and C2 move together rather than independently during neck rotation, thereby confirming the diagnosis. Recently, CT has been used for confirmation. The usual technique is to obtain 5- or 6-mm cuts from the occiput to C2. The lateral masses of C1 show rotary subluxation of 20° (Fig. 11–13).[33] Dynamic CT, in which 3-mm cuts are first taken in routine fashion and then with right and left rotation, is reported to be of benefit in making the diagnosis.[81]

Fielding and Herman[33] divided this disorder into four types, depending on the status of the atlantoaxial ligaments. Type I, the most common, is rotary fixation without any anterior displacement of the atlas. In this type, the transverse ligament is thought to be intact, thus making the condition more benign. Type II, characterized by rotary fixation and anterior displacement of less than 3 to 5 mm, is potentially dangerous. A deficient transverse ligament causes unilateral anterior displacement of one of the lateral masses. The last two types are more severe because they are associated with rupture of all the ligaments. In type III, the displacement is over 5 mm; this type is associated with deficiencies of the transverse and secondary ligaments, with both lateral masses displaced anteriorly. Type IV is an unusual type in which the atlas is posteriorly displaced because of a deficient dens.

The origin of the condition is uncertain. Inflammation, ruptured ligaments, muscle contracture, and spasm have all been suggested. Trivial trauma and URI are probably among the most common causes.[52, 81] Kawabe and co-workers[52] reviewed 17 cases and also performed

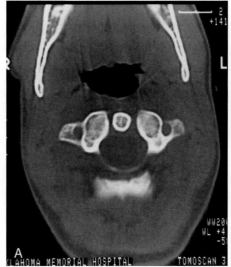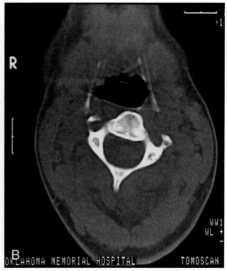

FIGURE 11–13. Computed tomographic study of atlantoaxial rotary fixation. *A,* View of C1. *B,* View of C2 obtained while the position of the head was maintained. Note the rotation of C2 relative to C1. (Courtesy of Dr. Tim Tytle.)

autopsies on 6 infant cadavers. CT studies were done on 8 patients with AARF and compared with 95 normal studies. Their article discusses a range of possible causes and notes that the facet angle of the axis is steeper in children than in adults. A meniscus-like synovial fold is also found in the occipitoatlantal and atlantoaxial joints of children that is not present in adults. These investigators concluded that inflammation or effusion from trauma could cause enfolding or rupture of these synovial folds that would result in AARF. On CT in patients with AARF, the lateral mass of C1 showed rotary subluxation of 20° anterolaterally.

The differential diagnosis of AARF includes congenital anomalies of the upper cervical spine, infection, anomalies of the dens, syringomyelia, tumor, ocular problems, and bulbar palsy. In AARF, the sternocleidomastoid is elongated, whereas in most of the other conditions it is short.

With early detection, the treatment is traction, usually with a halter, until the spasm is relieved and the deformity corrected. Maintenance of position in a collar is generally sufficient. In patients with long-standing deformity, the condition is often irreducible or only incompletely reducible. In these patients, the deformity may recur after conservative care unless fusion is carried out. In the series of Fielding and Herman,[33] which included adults and children, 11 of 13 patients were treated by skull traction followed by fusion, with good results. In the two remaining patients, one died in traction, and one had insufficient follow-up.

Marar and Balachandran[62] reviewed 12 children treated for AARF with traction and a Minerva jacket. Six of 12 had good results with this treatment. Three of 12 did not undergo reduction but were symptom free. Likewise, 3 of 12 patients did not undergo reduction but had symptoms. One of them was treated by fusion and decompression of C1 and the foramen magnum. Phillips and Hensinger[81] reviewed 23 children (average age, 7 years 6 months) treated for AARF. The key was early detection. Sixteen patients with symptoms of less than 1 month's duration responded to brief periods of halter

traction (1.3 to 2.3 kg) and were then managed in some sort of cervical immobilization. Eleven of this group had symptoms for less than 1 week. The average hospital stay was 4 days. All 7 patients who did not undergo reduction had symptoms for longer than 1 month, and these patients were treated with fusion in situ. The specific type of fusion was not mentioned, but the point was made that no reduction was attempted.

## FRACTURES OF THE ATLAS

The atlas is a diminutive structure in humans and is shielded from most forces. Most fractures of the atlas result from direct axial compression that drives the occipital condyles onto the atlas. The force is dissipated on the lateral masses (Fig. 11–14*A*). The usual fracture disrupts both the anterior and the posterior ring (Fig. 11–14*B*), and the transverse ligament can be ruptured. SCI is rare. The fracture is hard to evaluate on plain radiographs, but CT is an excellent means of demonstrating the injury (Fig. 11–13*C*). Most of these lesions heal in a halo or Minerva cast or vest. Up to 6 months of immobilization may be necessary.

## FRACTURES OF THE AXIS

Fracture of the ring of C2, called a hangman's fracture, has been reported in an infant who struck his head and sustained a central cord syndrome in a motor vehicle accident.[108] The initial films were interpreted as being normal. Later films showed a fracture of C2 immediately behind the articular surface of the lateral mass. The neural arch of C2 remained with C3 while the head and C2 moved forward. This injury was treated by skull traction through bur holes. In 18 days, neurologic function returned. By 22 days, the spine was considered to be stable, and the patient was treated with a soft collar. At 14 months, the child had residual weakness of the intrinsic muscles of the hand. This weakness was believed to be a hyperextension injury.

Sumchai and Sternbach[99] described the youngest

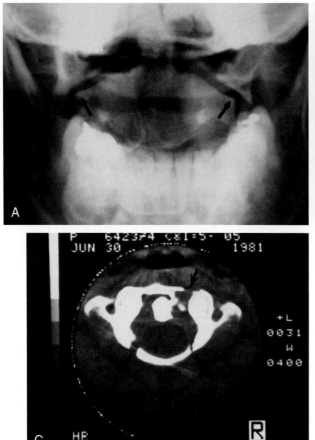

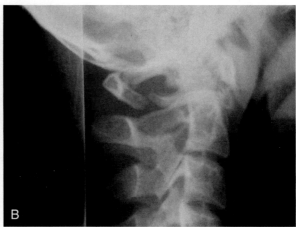

FIGURE 11–14. Fracture of C1 (Jefferson fracture). *A,* Anteroposterior view showing lateral displacement of the lateral mass and articulating facets of C1 on C2. *B,* Oblique view illustrating disruption of the posterior aspect of the ring of C1. *C,* Computed tomographic scan revealing the true extent of the injury. (Courtesy of Dr. Teresa Stacy.)

patient in the medical literature with a hangman's fracture. It occurred in a 7-week-old with bilateral avulsion of the pedicles or their synchondroses from the C2 vertebral body. Parisi and colleagues[77] reported a case in a 3-month-old infant. They warn that the subtle findings of a hangman's fracture can be confused with primary spondylolysis. Smith and associates[95] described persistent synchondrosis of the second cervical vertebra simulating a fracture in an 18-month-old child. The child had fallen from a height of approximately 2.5 m and landed headfirst. Initial radiographs were interpreted as showing an acute fracture of the posterior elements of the second cervical vertebra. CT showed a bilateral cleft of the posterior arch. The patient was immobilized in a halo vest. After 5 months of immobilization, the original tomograms were read by another physician and interpreted as a synchondrosis of the posterior arch of the second cervical vertebra. Tomograms and CT 2 years later showed no change. Five years after the fall, ossification of the synchondrosis was demonstrated. This fracture has also been reported in association with child abuse.[54] Many fractures of C2 are minimally displaced (Fig. 11–15). These injuries heal with immobilization in a cast or halo. Patients with additional injuries necessitating general anesthesia are of particular concern for the anesthesiologist.[114] Fractures of the odontoid and C1-2 dislocations are the most common pediatric cervical spine injuries.[92] Fractures of the odontoid are usually associated with head trauma from motor vehicle acci-

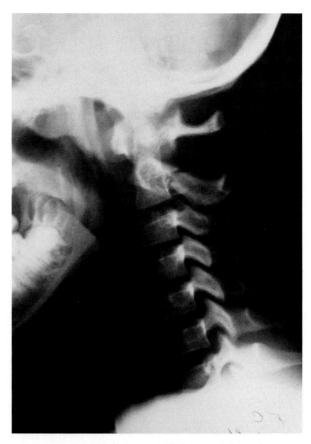

FIGURE 11–15. Fracture of C2 (hangman's fracture).

dents or falls from a height. The odontoid fracture is typically at the base, and the fragment moves with C1. The fracture can usually be reduced and held with halo traction or a halo vest or Minerva jacket for 6 to 8 weeks. Surgical reduction is rarely necessary. Results in older children are similar to those in adults. Fractures at the base and tip generally heal satisfactorily, whereas those at the level of the articular cartilage have a high failure rate when treated conservatively and usually require surgery. If unrecognized, these fractures may fail to heal.

Wang and associates reported on 16 pediatric patients (aged 3 to 15 years) with atlantoaxial instability treated by screw fixation.[107] Three had type II odontoid fractures and underwent odontoid screw fixation. The remaining 13 had posterior C1–C2 transarticular screw fixation and

Sonntag C1–C2 fusion. This second group included patients with AARF, os odontoideum, congenital atlanto-axial instability, and traumatic instability. All were treated with a Miami J-collar postoperatively. At 3 months' follow-up, all were said to have bony fusion. Complications included transient swallowing difficulty in one and extension of the fusion to C3 in another.

These acute injuries must be differentiated from os odontoideum, which typically has a remnant of the axis at the base and an apical segment separated by a wide gap (Fig. 11–16A and B). The apical segment is usually hypoplastic and may be seen with plain tomography or CT (Fig. 11–16C). In os odontoideum, instability can be demonstrated by flexion-extension plain radiography, polytomography, and flexion-extension MRI. The last is

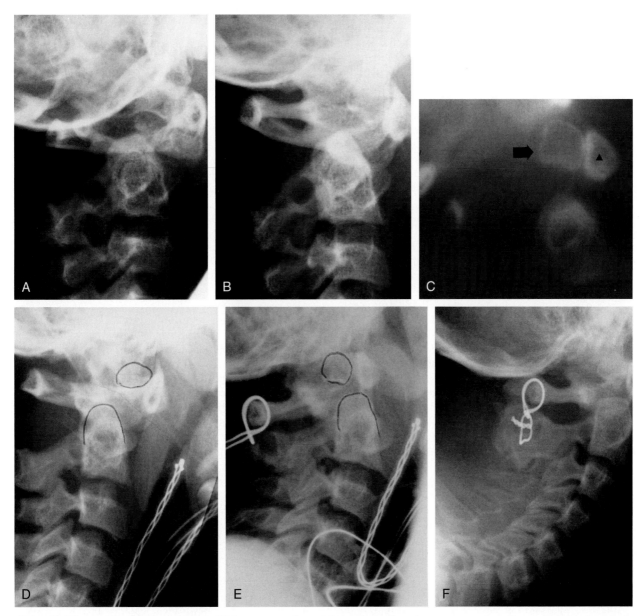

FIGURE 11–16. Os odontoideum. This patient fell from a tree and struck his neck on a branch. He was neurologically normal and had minimal findings for an acute cervical spine injury. A, His lateral cervical spine radiograph is suggestive of instability at C1-2. B, A lateral flexion view of C1-2 shows displacement of C1 on C2. C, Tomogram reveals a rounded apical segment *(thick arrow)*, a large gap above the remnant of the dens *(arrowhead)*, and movement of the apical segment with the anterior aspect of C1. D, Operative radiograph before reduction. E, Radiograph with C1 reduced on C2 and the wire placed around the ring of C1. F, Postoperative radiograph demonstrating the position of the wire.

perhaps the most valuable because it gives information about the relationship of all the components of the spinal cord and whether impingement is occurring. All patients with neurologic symptoms or findings should undergo fusion. It is a difficult decision when os odontoideum is discovered in an asymptomatic patient. I usually prefer to stabilize this area after discussing the options with the family because children are unpredictable in terms of their activity and whether they might experience trauma sufficient to displace the fragment and cause neurologic damage or death. The exact amount of instability at which stabilization should be performed has not been determined.

Wollin[110] considered os odontoideum to be a developmental anomaly of the axis in which the odontoid was divided by a transverse gap and the apical segment was left reduced without the bony support of the base of the process. Fielding and Griffin,[31] on the other hand, believed that os odontoideum was an acquired lesion. They reported three patients with radiographic evidence of a normal odontoid, in all of whom os odontoideum developed after trauma. One fell at 17 months and had a radiographically normal odontoid at 17 months; however, a lesion gradually developed by 6 years of age. Another had a normal radiograph at 18 months and os odontoideum at 8 years of age. These investigators concluded that this condition, rarely seen in young infants and seldom associated with congenital anomalies, is probably not developmental.

Os odontoideum weakens the atlantoaxial joint because it lacks a peg (see Fig. 11–16B). In the cases described, the retropharyngeal soft tissue space was wide, but the children had no history of preceding URI to explain this finding; therefore, it was thought to be swelling from the trauma. The theory was that the trauma damaged the blood supply and compromised development of the odontoid.

In Wollin's series of nine patients aged 10 to 68 years, two had severe symptoms.[110] Gwinn and Smith had seven patients aged 2 to 55 years, three of whom had severe symptoms.[40] These patients may be asymptomatic or have vague discomfort, or partial or complete quadriparesis gradually develops.

Dai and colleagues reviewed 44 patients, 5 of whom had no symptoms. Thirty-three underwent occipitocervical fusion, and all achieved solid fusion at an average follow-up of 6.5 years.[19] They concluded that this treatment is effective if atlantoaxial fusion is impossible and the patient is symptomatic.

Instability is an indication for surgical stabilization because additional trauma could be fatal. My preferred method of treatment is C1–C2 fusion (see Fig. 11–16D to F). The patient is positioned prone, and Gardner-Wells tongs are used to hold the head. Initial radiographs are obtained to be certain that the radiographic technique is sufficient and to confirm the position of C1 and C2. The exposure is facilitated if the cervical spine is in neutral flexion. One should be careful to expose only the area that is to be fused. An 18-gauge wire is passed under C1, and the free ends of the wire are passed back through the loop and tightened to grasp the ring of C1 (see Fig. 11–16D). The head is then extended and the reduction

confirmed by radiography (see Fig. 11–16E). Over-reduction must be avoided. A notch can be made in the inferior aspect of the spinous process of C2 to maintain the wire, or the wire can be passed through a hole in the spinous process if it is large enough. The wire is then twisted to maintain the position of the reduction (see Fig. 11–16F). C1 and C2 are decorticated with rongeurs, and strips of iliac bone are packed around the area to be fused. Postoperatively, the patient is placed in a SOMI (sternal-occipital-mandibular immobilization) brace for 3 months. Orthotic fixation in a young child can be difficult. In my practice, with cooperation from a competent orthotist, we have modified a commercially available Minerva jacket so that it fits young children. Lacking this customization, a fiberglass Minerva jacket or a halo can be used. Flexion-extension radiographs demonstrating stability are obtained before discontinuing use of the orthosis.

## FRACTURES AND DISLOCATIONS OF C3-7

Most of the fractures in the cervical spine in children occur at C1 and C2; fracture-dislocation in C3–C7, as seen in adults, is rare.[49–51, 80, 92] Evans and Bethem[29] reviewed 24 consecutive cases of cervical spine injury in children, which represented 1.2 cases per year in their busy hospital. Because the average age of their patients was 13 years, some could probably be regarded as adults. One must consider the mechanism of injury when choosing a treatment mode. Evans and Bethem[29] believed that flexion injuries were the culprit in 42% and hyperextension dislocations in 12%. In contrast to other series of pediatric cervical spine fractures, 29% were upper cervical spine injuries and 71% involved C3 through C7.

No definite guidelines were given regarding which patients could be treated by closed means and which ones required surgery. Treatment of most patients was nonoperative with tongs, Minerva jackets, or halo or neck orthoses. In the three patients who were treated surgically, the anterior approach was contraindicated. In flexion injuries that disrupt the anterior longitudinal ligament, this approach would increase the instability. Because most were flexion injuries, posterior spinal fusion with a wire and iliac graft was the treatment of choice. Nonoperative treatment was successful in 95% of patients. Evans and Bethem[29] concluded that surgery might be indicated for flexion injuries, which were associated with a high rate of late kyphosis. They further concluded that surgery might be indicated for burst fractures with neurologic injury in the hope that stabilization would enhance recovery. Most lower cervical spine fracture-dislocations heal when treated in closed fashion. Laminectomy is not beneficial and has been shown to cause swan neck deformity and further instability.[94]

McGrory and Klassen reviewed arthrodesis of the cervical spine for fractures and dislocations in children and adolescents.[67] Forty-two patients who had undergone arthrodesis for instability resulting from cervical spine trauma were monitored for a minimum of 7 years. The age at the time of injury ranged from 1 year 11

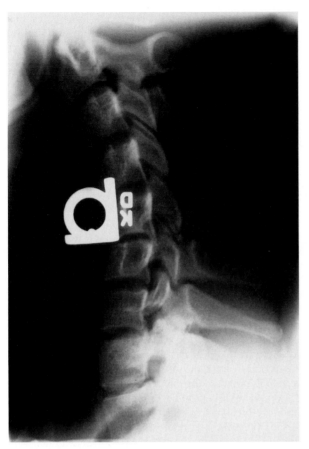

**FIGURE 11–17.** Unilateral facet dislocation. This skeletally mature patient gave a history of 3 months of pain after an automobile accident. She was neurologically normal. Note the reversal of the normal cervical lordosis and the anteriorly displaced inferior articulating facet of C6. Although it is poorly reproduced, the interspinous distance is also increased. (Courtesy of Dr. Tim Tytle.)

observed in the unfused segments. Thirty-eight percent of patients had extension of the fusion mass. These authors concluded that spinal arthrodesis for fractures and dislocations of the cervical spine in children and adolescents can be accomplished safely and with an acceptable outcome and rate of complications. A decrease in mobility was associated with an increase in osteoarthritic changes seen on radiographs.

Ligamentous instability can occur in children and adolescents, although it is less common than in adults. Pennecot and co-workers[80] described 16 cases of dislocation and ligamentous disruption, 5 at C1–C2 and 11 from C3–C7. A constant feature was the loss of a normal lordosis and a stiff neck (Fig. 11–17). This finding was confirmed on lateral radiographs in neutral and active hyperflexion. Radiographs showed a widened interspinous space, loss of parallelism of the articular facets, kyphosis in the disc space, and posterior opening. Calcification in the interspinous ligament appeared at a delayed time and was indicative of disruption and healing in the ligament. A delay in diagnosis was common. Five of eight patients were treated with posterior spinal fusion after the injury. The indications for surgery were persistent pain and radiographic evidence of worsening of the condition. These investigators cautioned that the exposure must be carefully controlled to prevent extension of the fusion mass to levels beyond the intended fusion level.

In my practice, I perform a fusion at the time of injury for patients with unstable fractures and dislocations. I believe that most purely ligamentous injuries will heal with immobilization. In those with continued instability as demonstrated by flexion-extension radiographs at 3 months, however, surgery is indicated. Some patients may elect to have surgery right away to avoid the period of immobilization in a halo or SOMI brace. With SCI, early fusion may facilitate rehabilitation by avoiding use of the halo, although rehabilitation is possible with either method.

For arthrodesis of C3–C7, exposure is accomplished through a midline incision. Dissection is by means of a subperiosteal elevator and electrocautery out to the zygapophyseal joints. Fixation may be obtained by the technique illustrated in Figure 11–18. In this method,

months to 15 years 11 months. In 76% the result was excellent, in 14% it was good, and in 10% it was fair. No patient had a poor result. No deterioration in clinical function was detected with increased duration of follow-up, and no change in stability occurred. Deformity of the fusion mass after healing was not noted with increased duration of follow-up. Osteoarthritic changes were

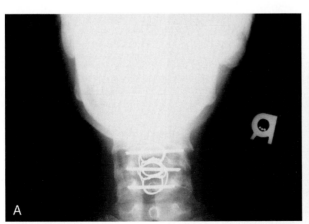
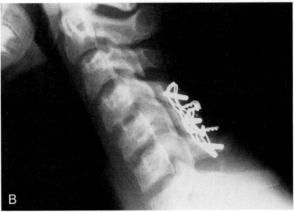

**FIGURE 11–18.** *A* and *B*, Posterior cervical fusion using pins in the spinous processes and wires.

the neck must be draped far enough laterally to allow the introduction of pins through skin punctures outside the skin incision. This approach is necessary to get the direction of the drill hole low enough so that the pin can go through the spinous process safely without penetrating the dura. Two pins may then be inserted through the spinous processes and a loop of wire passed around them. Postoperatively, the patient is immobilized in a SOMI brace.

## Thoracolumbar Spine Fractures

Thoracolumbar spine fractures in children are quite rare. As noted earlier, upper thoracic spine injuries can occur during birth. Thoracic and lumbar spine injuries in a young child can be the result of battering.[22] In the case shown in Figure 11–19, the child was noted to have a normal spine during the first year of life and a markedly deformed spine with paralysis at 2 years of age. As in many of these cases, the history was vague. Initially, a history of progressive neurologic deterioration was obtained, and a diagnosis of tuberculosis was suspected until the previous films were obtained. Child abuse was the final diagnosis.

Most thoracic and lumbar spine fractures in children result from motor vehicle accidents, pedestrian-vehicular accidents, or falls from a height.[46] Adolescents engage in a wide variety of activities that can result in spinal fractures, including sports such as tobogganing and skiing, and they can be victims of motorcycle and motor vehicle accidents.

### CLASSIFICATION

No one has yet reviewed a series of pediatric or adolescent patients to apply the three-column classification system.

These injuries are frequently described as being a result of compression, distraction, or shear. Compression injuries occur when the spine is acutely flexed forward. In some situations, particularly sporting events, the spine may be partially flexed and cause preloading.

Although it is unusual, pathologic fractures of the spine do occur. The patient in Figure 11–20 had been scheduled for evaluation of scoliosis. She was involved in a motor vehicle accident and sustained a fracture through T11. The final diagnosis was an aneurysmal bone cyst. Pathologic fractures can occur in patients with eosinophilic granuloma, leukemia, and other blood proliferative disorders. In a series from St. Jude's Hospital, 1.6% of children with acute lymphocytic leukemia had vertebral compression fractures at initial evaluation.[86] The diagnosis of leukemia was delayed in some because of the unusual symptoms, and 22 had multiple-level involvement. The symptoms abated with treatment. One must also be aware of the vertebra plana seen in patients with eosinophilic granuloma, which can be confused with a compression fracture.

Roaf[87] studied the mechanics of injury in fractures of the spine by subjecting cadaver spines of children and adults to load. With precompression and a normal disc, the annulus bulged but transmitted the load to the vertebral bodies. The blood was squeezed out of the body, and with continued pressure, the bodies cracked. After the break, the nuclear material extruded, and with further pressure, the body disintegrated. With a dehydrated disc, prolapse occurred. Compression forces were mainly absorbed by the body, and the healthy nucleus pulposus was incompressible. It was difficult to produce fractures with pure compression or pure flexion. A combination of rotation and compression could produce almost any of the commonly seen fracture patterns. Pure rotation was more likely to produce dislocation, whereas compression produced fractures.

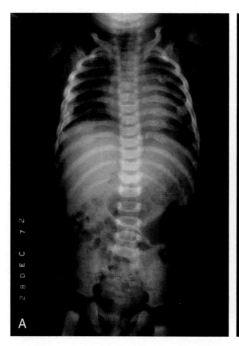
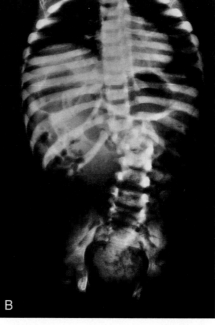

**Figure 11–19.** Child abuse. *A,* This radiograph taken during the first year of life reveals multiple rib fractures and a normal spine. *B,* A subsequent film shows a healing fracture-dislocation at the thoracolumbar junction.

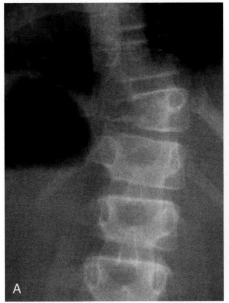
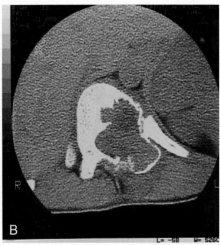

**FIGURE 11–20.** Pathologic fracture. *A,* A previous radiograph had disclosed scoliosis of 25° with the apex at T11. This exposure was made after an automobile accident. Note the absent pedicle at T11, which could also be seen on the previous film. *B,* A computed tomographic scan of T11 reveals destruction of the pedicle, erosion of the body, and extension into the soft tissues. Note the thin cortical shell over the soft tissue mass.

Distraction injuries can be produced by wearing lap seat belts.[26] American automakers have lagged in providing shoulder-type restraints for rear seat passengers. In addition, smaller children are not as effectively protected by existing shoulder harnesses. As the child is thrown forward, the lap belt, which is incorrectly positioned above the iliac crest, compresses the abdominal contents and forms a fulcrum. The more posteriorly located spine is distracted around this fulcrum, with resultant tension in the posterior aspect of the spine. If sufficient force is applied, tearing of the posterior ligaments or bony fracture plus dislocation is possible (Fig. 11–21). The classic Chance fracture is a bony injury through the vertebral body, the pedicles, and the spinous processes. Most of these injuries are stable and will heal with closed management. Variations include pure facet dislocation with disruption of the disc space and dislocation through the facet joints with fracture through the body (Fig. 11–22). One must examine carefully for intra-abdominal injury such as small bowel lacerations, renal damage, and rupture of the spleen.

A retrospective review of 365 CT studies for intra-abdominal trauma revealed five pediatric cases of lap belt injury with lumbar spine injury.[102] These injuries consisted of facet subluxation and anterior dislocation of L3 on L4. One patient had multiple compression fractures. In retrospect, the fractures were visible on the AP radiograph, but the findings were quite subtle and were best appreciated on the lateral view. Injuries to the lumbar spine occurred in less than 2% of injured children evaluated by CT. An absence of clinical symptoms may have led to failure to make the diagnosis. Children have a higher center of gravity, a large head, and an incompletely developed iliac crest, all of which may predispose to these injuries.

In another review of two cases of pediatric lumbar flexion distraction fractures associated with lap belts, the initial diagnosis was missed in both patients.[26]

Retrospectively, the injuries were visible on AP radiographs, although they were best seen on the lateral lumbar spine view. One of these patients was treated conservatively, and the other was treated surgically. At follow-up, both had maintained their reduction and had remodeling of the vertebral body. A high index of suspicion is required to make the diagnosis of such injuries. Installation of adjustable shoulder restraints might prevent these seat belt injuries. Although the injuries to the spine were serious, without the seat belt, many of these children would not have survived the accident or would have sustained other injuries such as closed head trauma.

Eighty-five cases of fracture of the vertebral limbus (a fracture between the ring apophysis and the cartilaginous rim of the vertebral end-plate) have been reported.[29, 59, 103] Twenty-four of these were in patients aged 10 to 18 years. The injury most frequently is to the superior end-plate of one of the midlumbar spines (Fig. 11–23). Mechanisms of injury have included weightlifting, shoveling, gymnastics, hyperextension, and trauma. The patients present with back and leg pain and spasm; often, they have a paucity of neurologic signs. The diagnosis is rarely made on plain radiographs, but CT with or without contrast medium is useful, although the exact diagnosis may not be apparent. Frequently, the only diagnosis that one can make is a mass in the spinal canal. This finding must be differentiated from spinal stenosis of other causes because decompression alone is of no benefit. The treatment of choice is excision of the loose fragment, which is more easily accomplished if the diagnosis is made early.

Intervertebral disc calcification occurs in children and can be confused with trauma or infection.[60, 61, 78] The patient presents with pain and neurologic signs, and a radiograph demonstrates calcification in the spinal canal. In most cases, the course is benign, and the condition resolves with conservative care.

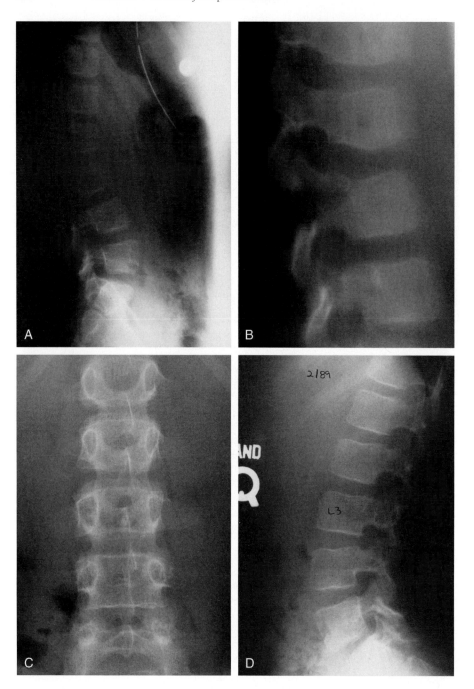

**FIGURE 11–21.** Distraction fracture-dislocation. *A,* A lateral spine film discloses loss of lumbar lordosis and an increase in the interspinous distance between L2 and L3. *B,* Tomogram confirms a fracture through the spinous process and disruption of the disc space. An extension film over a bolster showed that the fracture could be reduced by closed means. Anteroposterior (*C*) and lateral (*D*) spine radiographs 9 months later show healing of the fracture, which was treated in a plaster body jacket in extension.

## DIAGNOSIS

One must approach pediatric patients who have multiple trauma with a high index of suspicion. Those who are comatose or poorly responsive are particularly at risk. A careful search should be made for sensory level involvement and movement while ascertaining that movement is voluntary and not the result of reflexes. Rectal examination for tone and the cremasteric reflex is also important.

Radiographic evaluation in multiply traumatized patients routinely includes chest and abdominal AP and lateral radiographs and often CT studies. These images must be carefully scrutinized, with inspection of the disc spaces, the posterior aspects of the spinous processes, and the shape of the vertebral body. Children may have compression fractures at multiple levels. Small areas of avulsion may be the only subtle findings, and often these abnormalities are confused with the normal ring apophysis. As noted by Aufdermaur,[2] rupture through the growth zone and discs may be minimally visible on a radiograph.

In the absence of SCI, progression of spinal deformity is rare because children's vertebral bodies tend to remodel. In a review by Horal and associates, 53% were normal at follow-up. The patients had no significant disability, and interbody fusion was usual.[47]

## MANAGEMENT

All children with fractures of the thoracic and lumbar spine, regardless of how minimal, should be admitted to

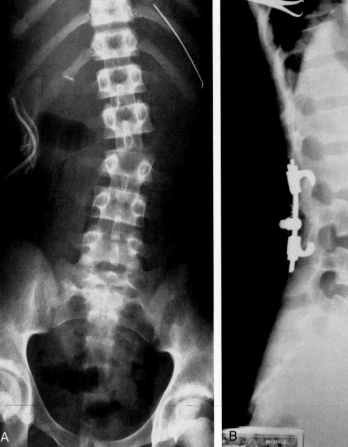

**FIGURE 11–22.** Facet dislocation. *A,* This patient sustained a distraction seat belt injury. She had an L2-3 facet dislocation. She also sustained tears in her small bowel. *B,* The spine injury was treated by open reduction, internal fixation with Harrington compression rods, and limited fusion.

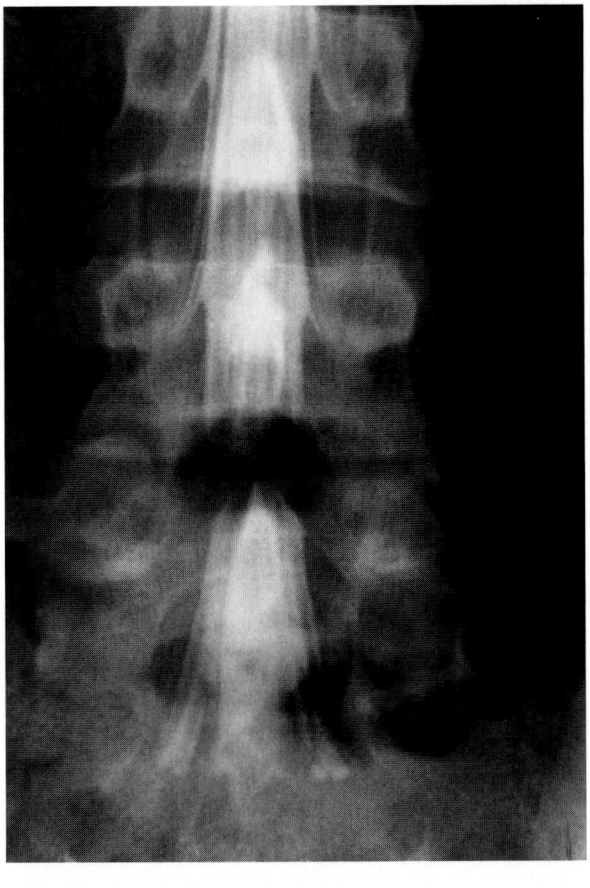

**FIGURE 11–23.** Fracture of the end-plate. This myelogram reveals a nearly complete block at L4-5. At surgery, the patient was found to have a fracture of the superior end-plate of L5.

the hospital. The risk of ileus and urinary retention is the same as in an adult. Pain must be managed, and the patient must be observed for the possibility of progressive neurologic deficit. Most children's thoracolumbar spine fractures are stable and do not require operative intervention; unstable injuries, however, may require surgery. One must determine the mechanism of injury to choose the type of instrumentation needed to restore stability. Distraction injuries should be treated with compressive forces, whereas those caused by flexion, rotation, or both are best treated by distraction. In general, the same indications exist for children as for adults. Fracture-dislocation with displacement should be reduced. The best decompression of the thoracic and lumbar spine is reduction. Laminectomy is not beneficial and can be detrimental. Instrumentation may be more difficult in children because of their smaller size. Until recently, Luque instrumentation was one of the only alternatives, but small hooks and other implants are now available for a variety of the spinal instrumentation systems.

With an incomplete neurologic injury, it is prudent to perform realignment as soon as the patient is stable. Realignment is most often obtained by posterior spinal fusion with instrumentation and iliac grafting. These injuries are not surgical emergencies unless the patient has an open wound or progressive neurologic deficit.

*Acknowledgments*

I would like to thank Drs. Teresa Stacy and Tim Tytle for supplying some of the illustrations for this chapter. These illustrations are from the superb teaching files they have developed for the Department of Radiology, University of Oklahoma, College of Medicine.

## REFERENCES

1. Anson, B.J. Morris' Human Anatomy, 12th ed. New York, McGraw-Hill, 1953.
2. Aufdermaur, M. Spinal injuries in juveniles: Necropsy findings in twelve cases. J Bone Joint Surg Br 56:513–519, 1974.
3. Babcock, J.L. Spinal injuries in children. Pediatr Clin North Am 22:487–500, 1972.
4. Bailey, D.K. The normal cervical spine in infants and children. Radiology 59:712–719, 1952.
5. Baker, C.; Kadish, H.; Schunk, J.E. Evaluation of pediatric cervical spine injuries. Am J Emerg Med 17:230–244, 1999.
6. Banniza von Bazan, U.K.; Paeslack, V. Scoliotic growth in children with acquired paraplegia. Paraplegia 15:65–73, 1977.
7. Bedbrook, G.M. Correction of scoliosis due to paraplegia sustained in pediatric age group. Paraplegia 15:90–96, 1977.
8. Boger, D.C. Cervical prevertebral soft tissues in children: An unreliable soft tissue indicator of cervical spine trauma. Contemp Orthop 5:31–34, 1982.
9. Bohlman, H.H. Acute fractures and dislocations of the cervical spine. J Bone Joint Surg Am 61:1119–1142, 1979.
10. Bracken, M.B. Treatment of acute spinal cord injury with methylprednisolone: Results of a multi-center randomized clinical trial. J Neurotrauma 8(Suppl):47–50, 1991.
11. Bracken, M.B. Pharmacological treatment of acute spinal cord injury: Current status and future projects. J Emerg Med 11:43–48, 1993.
12. Bracken, M.B.; Shepard, M.J.; Collins, W.F.; et al. A randomized, controlled trial of methylprednisolone or naloxone in the treatment of acute spinal-cord injury. Results of the Second National Acute Spinal Cord Injury Study. N Engl J Med 322:1405–1411, 1990.
13. Burke, D.C. Traumatic spinal paralysis in children. Paraplegia 9:268–276, 1971.
14. Burke, D.C. Spinal cord trauma in children. Paraplegia 9:1–14, 1971.
15. Cattell, H.S.; Filtzer, D.L. Pseudosubluxation and other normal variations in the cervical spine in children. J Bone Joint Surg Am 47:1295–1309, 1965.
16. Committee on Sports Medicine. American Academy of Pediatrics. Atlantoaxial instability in Down syndrome. Pediatrics 74:152–154, 1984.
17. D'Alise, M.D.; Benzel, E.C.; Hart, B.L. Magnetic resonance imaging evaluation of the cervical spine in the comatose or obtunded trauma patient. J Neurosurg 91(Suppl):54–59, 1999.
18. Daffner, R.H. Pseudofracture of the dens: Mach bands. AJR Am J Roentgenol 128:607–612, 1977.
19. Dai, L.; Yuan, W.; Ni, B.; Jia, L. Os odontoideum: Etiology, diagnosis, and management. Surg Neurol 53:106–108, 2000.
20. Davidson, R.G. Atlantoaxial instability in individuals with Down syndrome: A fresh look at the evidence. Pediatrics 81:857–865, 1988.
21. Davis, J.W.; Phreaner, D.L.; Hoyt, D.B.; Mackersie, R.C. The etiology of missed cervical spine injuries. J Trauma 34:342–366, 1993.
22. Dickson, R.A.; Leatherman, K.D. Spinal injuries in child abuse: A case report. J Trauma 18:811–812, 1978.
23. Dietrich, A.M.; Ginn-Pease, M.E.; Bartkowski, H.M.; King, D.R. Pediatric cervical spine fractures: Predominantly subtle presentation. J Pediatr Surg 26:995–999, 1991.
24. Dolan, K.D. Cervicobasilar relationships. Radiol Clin North Am 25:155–166, 1977.
25. Dwek, J.R.; Chung, C.B. Radiography of cervical spine injury in children: Are flexion-extension radiographs useful for acute trauma? AJR Am J Roentgenol 174:1617–1619, 2000.
26. Ebraheim, N.A.; Savolaine, E.R.; Southworth, S.R.; et al. Pediatric lumbar seat belt injuries. Orthopedics 14:1010–1033, 1991.
27. Ehara, S.; El-Khoury, G.Y.; Sato, Y. Cervical spine injury in children. AJR Am J Roentgenol 151:1175–1178, 1988.
28. Epstein, N.A.; Epstein, J.A.; Mauri, T. Treatment of fractures of the vertebral limbus and spinal stenosis in five adolescents and five adults. J Neurosurg 595–604, 1989.
29. Evans, D.L.; Bethem, D. Cervical spine injuries in children. J Pediatr Orthop 9:563–568, 1989.
30. Evarts, C.M. Traumatic occipital-atlantal dislocation. Report of a case with survival. J Bone Joint Surg Am 52:1653, 1970.
31. Fielding, J.W.; Griffin, P.P. Os odontoideum: An acquired lesion. J Bone Joint Surg Am 56:187–190, 1974.
32. Fielding, J.W.; Hensinger, R.N.; Hawkins, R.J. Os odontoideum. J Bone Joint Surg Am 62:376–383, 1980.
33. Fielding, J.W.; Herman, M.J. Atlanto-axial rotary fixation (fixed rotary subluxation of the atlanto-axial joint). J Bone Joint Surg Am 59:37–44, 1977.
34. Freiberger, R.H.; Wilson, P.H.; Nicolas, J.A. Acquired absence of the odontoid process. J Bone Joint Surg Am 47:1231, 1965.
35. Geisler, F.H.; Dorsey, F.C.; Coleman, W.P. Correction: Recovery of motor function after spinal-cord injury—a randomized, placebo-controlled trial with GM-1 ganglioside. N Engl J Med 325:1659–1660, 1991.
36. Geisler, F.H.; Dorsey, F.C.; Coleman, W.P. Recovery of motor function after spinal-cord injury—a randomized, placebo-controlled trial with GM-1 ganglioside. N Engl J Med 324:1829–1838, 1991.
37. Geisler, F.H.; Dorsey, F.C.; Coleman, W.P. GM-1 ganglioside in human spinal cord injury. J Neurotrauma 9(Suppl):407–416, 1992.
38. Geisler, F.H.; Dorsey, F.C.; Coleman, W.P. Past and current clinical studies with GM-1 ganglioside in acute spinal cord injury. Review. Ann Emerg Med 22:1041–1047, 1993.
39. Giguere, J.F.; St. Vil, D.; Turmel, A.; et al. Airbags and children: A spectrum of C-spine injuries. J Pediatr Surg 33:811–816, 1998.
40. Gwinn, J.L.; Smith, J.L. Acquired and congenital absence of the odontoid. AJR Am J Roentgenol 88:424–431, 1962.
41. Hadley, M.N.; Zabramski, J.M.; Browner, C.M.; et al. Pediatric spinal trauma. Review of 122 cases of spinal cord and vertebral column injuries. J Neurosurg 68:18–24, 1988.
42. Henrys, P.; Lyne, E.D.; Lifton, C.; Salciccioli, G. Clinical review of cervical spine injuries in children. Clin Orthop 129:172–176, 1977.

43. Hensinger, R.N.; Fielding, J.W.; Hawkins, R.J. Congenital anomalies of the odontoid process. Orthop Clin North Am 9:901–912, 1978.

44. Hensinger, R.N.; Lang, J.E.; MacEwen, G.D. Klippel-Feil syndrome: A constellation of associated anomalies. J Bone Joint Surg Am 56:1246–1252, 1974.

45. Herndon, W.A. Injuries to the head and neck. In: Sullivan, J.A.; Grana, W.A., eds. The Pediatric Athlete. Park Ridge, IL, American Academy of Orthopaedic Surgeons, 1990.

46. Herzenberg, J.E.; Hensinger, R.N.; Dedrick, D.K.; Phillips, W.A. Emergency transport and positioning of young children who have an injury of the cervical spine. The standard backboard may be hazardous. J Bone Joint Surg Am 71:15–22, 1989.

47. Horal, J.; Nachemson, A.; Scheller, S. Clinical and radiological long term follow-up of vertebral fractures in children. Acta Orthop Scand 43:491–503, 1972.

48. Hoy, G.A.; Cole, W.G. The pediatric cervical seat belt sydrome. Injury 24:297–299, 1993.

49. Jacob, B. Cervical fracture and dislocation (C3–7). Clin Orthop 109:18–32, 1975.

50. Jones, E.T.; Hensinger, R.N. C2–C3 dislocation in a child. J Pediatr Orthop 1:419–422, 1981.

51. Jones, E.T.; Hensinger, R.N. Cervical spine injuries in children. Contemp Orthop 5:17–23, 1982.

52. Kawabe, N.; Hirotani, H.; Tanaka, O. Pathomechanism of atlantoaxial rotary fixation in children. J Pediatr Orthop 9:569–574, 1989.

53. Kilfoyle, R.M.; Foley, J.J.; Norton, P.L. Spine and pelvic deformity in childhood and adolescent paraplegia. J Bone Joint Surg Am 47:659–682, 1965.

54. Kleinman, P.K.; Shelton, Y.A. Hangman's fracture in an abused infant: Imaging features. Pediatr Radiol 27:776–777, 1997.

55. Klippel, M.; Feil, A. Anomalies de la collone vertebrale par absence des vertebres cervicales; avec cage thoracique jusqu'a la bas du crane. Bull Soc Anat Paris 87:185, 1912.

56. Leventhal, H.R. Birth injuries of the spinal cord. J Pediatr Surg 56:447–453, 1960.

57. Link, T.M.; Schuierer, G.; Hufendiek, A.; et al. Substantial head trauma: Value of routine CT examination of the cervicocranium. Radiology 196:741–755, 1995.

58. Lovell, A.T.; Alexander, R.; Grundy, E.M. Silent, unstable, cervical spine injury in multiple neurofibromatosis. Anesthesia 49:453–454, 1994.

59. Lowrey, J.J. Dislocated lumbar vertebral epiphysis in adolescent children: Report of three cases. J Neurosurg 38:232–234, 1973.

60. MacCartee, C.C.J.; Griffin, P.P.; Byrd, E.B. Ruptured calcified thoracic disc in a child. J Bone Joint Surg Am 54:1272–1274, 1972.

61. Mainzer, F. Herniation of the nucleus pulposus; a rare complication of intervertebral disc calcification in children. Radiology 107:167–170, 1973.

62. Marar, B.D.; Balachandran, N. Non-traumatic atlanto-axial dislocation in children. Clin Orthop 92:220–226, 1973.

63. Marshall, K.W.; Koch, B.L.; Egelhoff, J.C. Air bag–related deaths and serious injuries in children: Injury patterns and imaging findings. AJNR Am J Neuroradiol 19:1599–1607, 1998.

64. Matar, L.D.; Doyle, A.J. Prevertebral soft-tissue measurements in cervical spine injury. Australas Radiol 41:229–237, 1997.

65. Mayfield, J.K.; Erkkila, J.C.; Winter, R.B. Spine deformities subsequent to acquired childhood spinal cord injury. Orthop Trans 3:281–282, 1979.

66. McClain, R.F.; Clark, C.R.; El-Khoury, G.Y. C6–7 dislocation in a neurologically intact neonate: A case report. Spine 14:125–126, 1989.

67. McGrory, B.J.; Klassen, R.A. Arthrodesis of the cervical spine for fractures and dislocations in children and adolescents. A long-term follow-up study. J Bone Joint Surg Am 76:1606–1616, 1994.

68. Morgan, T.H.; Wharton, G.W.; Austin, G.N. The results of laminectomy in patients with incomplete spinal cord injuries. Paraplegia 9:14–23, 1971.

69. Morrison, A.L.; Chute, D.; Radentz, S.; et al. Air bag–associated injury to a child in the front passenger seat. Am J Forensic Med Pathol 19:218–222, 1998.

70. Mubarak, S.J.; Camp, J.F.; Vuletich, W.; et al. Halo application in the infant. J Pediatr Orthop 9:612–614, 1989.

71. Murphy, M.J.; Ogden, J.A.; Bucholz, R.W. Cervical spine injury in the child. Contemp Orthop 3:615–623, 1981.

72. Nitecki, S.; Moir, C.R. Predictive factors of the outcome of traumatic cervical spine fracture in children. J Pediatr Surg 29:1409–1411, 1994.

73. Norman, M.G.; Wedderburn, L.C. Fetal spinal cord injury with cephalic delivery. Obstet Gynecol 42:355–358, 1973.

74. Oller, D.W.; Boone, S. Blunt cervical spine Brown-Séquard injury. A report of three cases. Am Surg 57:361–365, 1991.

75. Pang, D.; Pollack, I.F. Spinal cord injury without radiologic abnormality in children: The SCIWORA syndrome. J Trauma 29:654–664, 1989.

76. Pang, D.; Wilberger, J.E.J. Spinal cord injury without radiographic abnormality in children. J Neurosurg 57:114–129, 1982.

77. Parisi, M.; Lieberson, R.; Shatsky, S. Hangman's fracture or primary spondylolysis: A patient and a brief review. Pediatr Radiol 21:367–368, 1991.

78. Peck, F.C. A calcified thoracic intervertebral disc with herniation and spinal cord compression in a child. J Neurosurg 14:105–109, 1957.

79. Pennecot, G.F.; Gouraud, D.; Hardy, J.R. Roentgenographical study of the cervical spine in children. J Pediatr Orthop 4:346–352, 1984.

80. Pennecot, G.F.; Leonard, P.; Peyrot Des Gachons, S. Traumatic ligamentous instability of the cervical spine in children. J Pediatr Orthop 4:339–345, 1984.

81. Phillips, W.A.; Hensinger, R.N. The management of atlanto-axial subluxation in children. J Bone Joint Surg Am 71:664–668, 1989.

82. Pueschel, S.M. Atlanto-axial subluxation in Down syndrome. Lancet 1:980, 1983.

83. Pueschel, S.M.; Scolia, F.H. Atlantoaxial instability in individuals with Down syndrome: Epidemiologic, radiographic, and clinical studies. Pediatrics 4:555–560, 1987.

84. Pueschel, S.M.; Herndon, J.H.; Gelch, M.M.; et al. Symptomatic atlantoaxial subluxation in persons with Down syndrome. J Pediatr Orthop 4:682–688, 1984.

85. Rang, M.C. Children's Fractures. Philadelphia, J.B. Lippincott, 1983.

86. Ribeiro, R.L.; Qui, C.H.; Schell, M.J. Vertebral compression fracture as a presenting feature of acute lymphocytic leukemia in children. Cancer 61:589–592, 1988.

87. Roaf, R. A study of mechanics of spinal injuries. J Bone Joint Surg Br 42:810–823, 1960.

88. Rodgers, W.B.; Coran, D.L.; Emans, J.B.; et al. Occipitocervical fusions in children. Retrospective analysis and technical considerations. Clin Orthop 364:125–133, 1999.

89. Rodgers, W.B.; Coran, D.L.; Kharrazi, F.D.; et al. Increasing lordosis of the occipitocervical junction after arthrodesis in young children: The occipitocervical crankshaft phenomenon. J Pediatr Orthop 17:762–765, 1997.

90. Scarrow, A.M.; Levy, E.I.; Resnick, D.K.; et al. Cervical spine evaluation in obtunded or comatose patients: A pilot study. Pediatr Neurosurg 30:169–175, 1999.

91. Shaw, M.; Burnett, H.; Wilson, A.; Chan, O. Pseudosubluxation of C2 on C3 in polytraumatized children—prevalence and significance. Clin Radiol 54:377–380, 1999.

92. Sherk, H.H.; Schut, L.; Lane, J. Fractures and dislocations of the cervical spine in children. Orthop Clin North Am 7:593–604, 1976.

93. Shulman, S.T.; Madden, J.D.; Esterly, J.R.; Shanklin, D.R. Transection of spinal cord. A rare obstetrical complication of cephalic delivery. Arch Dis Child 46:291–294, 1971.

94. Sim, F.H.; Svien, H.J.; Bickel, W.H.; Janes, J.M. Swan-neck deformity following extensive cervical laminectomy. A review of twenty-one cases. J Bone Joint Surg Am 56:564–580, 1974.

95. Smith, J.T.; Skinner, S.R.; Shonnard, N.H. Persistent synchondrosis of the second cervical vertebra simulating a hangman's fracture in a child. Report of a case. J Bone Joint Surg Am 75:1228–1230, 1993.

96. Special Olympics Bulletin. Participation by individuals with DS who suffer from atlantoaxial dislocation. 1983.

97. Steel, H.H. Anatomical and mechanical consideration of the atlanto-axial articulation. J Bone Joint Surg Am 50:1481–1482, 1968.

98. Sullivan, C.R.; Bruwer, A.J.; Harris, L.E. Hypermobility of the cervical spine in children: A pitfall in the diagnosis of cervical dislocation. Am J Surg 95:636–640, 1958.

99. Sumchai, A.P.; Sternbach, G.L. Hangman's fracture in a 7-week-old infant. Ann Emerg Med 20:86–89, 1991.

100. Swischuk, L. Anterior displacement of C2 in children. Physiologic or pathologic? Radiology 122:759–763, 1977.

101. Tawbin, A. CNS damage in the human fetus and newborn infant. Am J Dis Child 119:529, 1970.

102. Taylor, J.A.; Eggli, K.D. Lap belt injuries of the lumbar spine in children: A pitfall in CT diagnosis. AJR Am J Roentgenol 150:1355–1358, 1988.

103. Techakapuch, S. Rupture of the lumbar cartilage plate into the spinal canal in an adolescent. J Bone Joint Surg Am 63:481–482, 1981.

104. Townsend, E.H.J.; Rowe, M.L. Mobility of the upper cervical spine in health and disease. Pediatrics 10:567–573, 1952.

105. VanDyke, D.C.; Gahagan, C.A. Down syndrome: Cervical spine abnormalities and problems. Clin Pediatr (Phila) 27:415–418, 1988.

106. Wagoner, C.; Pendergrass, E.P. The anterior and posterior "notch" shadows seen in lateral roentgenograms of the vertebrae of infants: An anatomic explanation. AJR Am J Roentgenol 42:663–670, 1939.

107. Wang, J.; Vokshoor, A.; Kim, S.; et al. Pediatric atlantoaxial instability: Management with screw fixation. Pediatr Neurosurg 30:70–78, 1999.

108. Weiss, M.H.; Kaufman, B. Hangman's fracture in an infant. Am J Dis Child 126:268–269, 1973.

109. Wholey, M.D.; Bruwer, A.J.; Baker, H.L. The lateral roentgenogram of the neck. Radiology 71:350–356, 1958.

110. Wollin, D.G. A separate odontoid process. J Bone Joint Surg Am 45:1459–1471, 1963.

111. Woodring, J.H.; Lee, C. The role and limitations of computed tomographic scanning in the evaluation of cervical trauma. J Trauma 33:698–708, 1992.

112. Yasuoko, F.; Peterson, H.; MacCarty, C. Incidence of spinal column deformity after multiple level laminectomy in children and adults. J Neurosurg 57:441–445, 1982.

113. Yngve, D.A.; Harris, W.P.; Herndon, W.A.; et al. Spinal cord injury without osseous spine fracture. J Pediatr Orthop 8:153–159, 1988.

114. Zanette, G.; Ori, C.; Zadra, N.; et al. Hangman's fracture in a paediatric patient: Considerations for anaesthesia. Paediatr Anaesth 7:473–475, 1997.

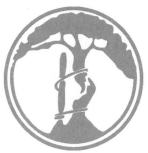

# CHAPTER 12

# *Fractures and Dislocations about the Hips and Pelvis*

Marc F. Swiontkowski, M.D.

Fractures and dislocations of the pelvis and proximal end of the femur in children are the result of high-energy trauma and are therefore rare. Because of diagnostic and treatment implications, these injuries are best grouped as pelvic fractures and dislocations (including acetabular fractures), proximal femoral fractures, and hip dislocations.

## PELVIC FRACTURES AND DISLOCATIONS

### Pathology

#### RELEVANT ANATOMY

Pelvic anatomy in children differs very little from that in adults. The pelvis consists of the ilium, ischium, and pubis, together with their apophyseal growth centers, and the sacrum (Fig. 12–1A). The acetabular cartilage complex is a unit—flat and triradiate medially and cup shaped laterally—that is interposed between the ischium, ilium, and pubis[53] (see Fig. 12–1B). The critical differences between children and adults, then, are the epiphyseal growth centers and apophyseal growth regions. This cartilaginous volume, as well as the fact that the bones are less brittle,[18] provides a greater capacity for energy absorption than that available to adults. When fractures do occur, they can arise within the cartilaginous regions and make diagnosis more difficult. Fractures in these regions can result in growth disturbances from direct trauma or result in misdirected biomechanical forces from bony malunion. The resiliency afforded by the increase in cartilage volume allows for greater displacement on impact without injury being universally apparent. In a dramatic representation of this fact, radiographically, 93% of 66 postmortem examinations of children injured by blunt trauma demonstrated bilateral posterior pelvic ring injury. Osseous vascular anatomy is also important, and it may be disturbed by direct or indirect trauma.[52, 72, 78] The major area of vulnerability is that of the femoral head.

### PREVALENCE

The true prevalence of fracture of the pelvis or acetabulum in children is difficult to determine.[27] Watts stated that 10 injuries (pelvic fractures) per year could be expected in a large children's hospital, that 97% of them would be of the stable type, and that acetabular fractures were rare.[75] Quinby identified 255 children younger than 14 years admitted to the pediatric surgery service of the Boston City Hospital for blunt trauma to the trunk over a 4-year period.[54] Twenty (7.8%) of this group, 6 girls and 14 boys with an age range of 2.5 to 13 years and a mean age of 8 years, had identifiable pelvic fractures. Of 1438 musculoskeletal injuries treated at Washington's Level I trauma center in 1 year, 5 (0.35%) were pelvic or acetabular fractures in children younger than 18 years. In a major German trauma center, 54 pelvic fractures were treated over a 19-year period; these injuries are relatively rare,[59] and associated head injuries with neurologic sequelae were found to be more common in children than in adults.[58] In a 1991 study, 2.4% of 2248 children admitted to a regional trauma center were identified as having a fracture of the pelvic ring.[7] In a 1999 review of the experience of a busy trauma center in Israel, 12.9% (15 of 116) of the pelvic fractures in children younger than 12 years were open injuries.[49]

Acetabular fractures constitute 0.8% to 15% of fractures of the pelvis in children.[11, 17, 28, 31, 32, 66]

### MECHANISM OF INJURY

Pelvic and acetabular fractures in children are generally the result of high-energy trauma for the reasons outlined earlier.[48] In Quinby's 20 cases, 19 patients were injured by impact with an automobile, truck, or train; one fell from a roof.[54] In 8 of the 19 cases of trauma produced by collisions with motor vehicles, it was suspected that the vehicle ran over or crushed the child. In an 8-year review

371

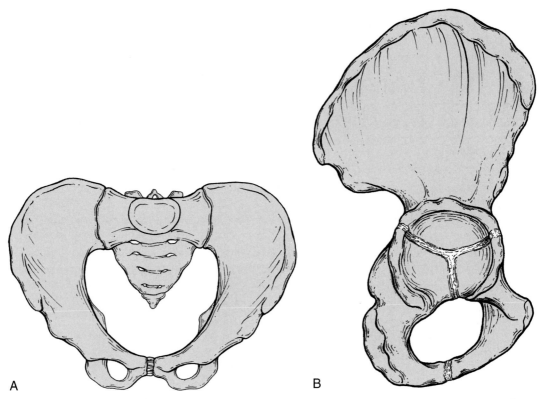

**FIGURE 12–1.** Pediatric pelvic osseous anatomy. *A,* The inlet orientation illustrates the two innominate bones, the sacrum, and the pubic symphysis. *B,* The lateral orientation reveals the triradiate cartilage as the confluence of the iliac, ischial, and pubic apophyses.

of children younger than 16 years treated at the University of Manitoba, 84 patients with pelvic fractures were identified. Of these fractures, 58% were the result of cars striking pedestrians, 17% of the patients were passengers in motor vehicles involved in accidents, 7% of the injuries were caused by impacts or falls from bicycles, and 8% were from crush injuries.[56] A 1995 report of 43 patients indicates that the mechanism of injury is related to motor vehicles in 70% of cases and to falls from significant height in 30%.[35] High-energy impact with rigid structures produces these injuries. Rarely, these injuries occur in newborns and toddlers.[39, 77]

## CONSEQUENCES OF INJURY

Because of the significant energy involved in producing fractures of the pelvis, the major consequences are from associated visceral injuries. Nineteen percent of patients in Reed's large series had associated visceral injuries,[56] most commonly involving the viscera within or just superior to the pelvic brim. Seven of the 10 associated visceral injuries involved the lower urinary tract, and 7 involved intra-abdominal structures. Three cases each of significant intrathoracic, intracranial, and soft tissue injuries occurred, again pointing to the velocity of impact involved with this blunt trauma. Of Quinby's 20 patients, 9 required laparotomy for visceral injury, and another 5 had severe hemorrhage with visceral injury requiring laparotomy in addition to the significant vascular injury.[54] Three of this latter group of five children eventually died. Forty-two percent of a series of 66

pediatric fatalities in one recent postmortem study performed in Russia expired as a result of pelvic fracture and severe hemorrhage.[35] A cohort of surviving patients was included in this report; 24 of 43 patients had at least three organ systems injured, and 62.8% of these patients were admitted with some degree of hypotension. Children who expire have higher injury severity scores and Glasgow Coma Scale scores.[50]

The major consequences of a pelvic fracture, then, are hemorrhage, shock, and death; bladder/urethral injury (particularly in males); neurologic injury (in particular, injury to the lumbosacral plexus with sacroiliac [SI] disruption or sacral fractures); and infection after open fractures that involve the perineum, rectum, or vagina.[48, 49, 58] The severity of the pelvic fracture is correlated with the risk of visceral injury. In the 1991 Children's National Medical Center series, 80% of children with multiple pelvic fractures had concomitant abdominal or genitourinary injury as compared with 33% of children with fractures of the ilium or pelvic rim and 6% of children with isolated pubic fractures.[7] In adults, the mortality from major pelvic fractures is 5% to 20%. In children, the rate has been reported to be 1.4% to 14%.[11, 50, 58] Published mortality rates for a severely traumatized group of adult patients with open pelvic fractures range from 8% to 50%; death results from hemorrhage acutely and pulmonary failure and sepsis on a delayed basis. The incidence of lower urinary tract and neurologic injury in combined large series is 12% to 15% in adults. Because of small numbers, comparable data do not exist in the literature for children. One study that compared data from the National Pediatric Trauma Registry with data from a level I trauma center documented a much lower mortality rate from hemorrhage: 5% for children and 17% for adults.[34]

Systemic consequences aside, the pelvic fracture itself results in serious sequelae. When the triradiate cartilage is involved, growth arrest can result in the "mini," shallow acetabulum described by Rodrigues[60] (Fig. 12–2). Six of 15 patients reported by McDonald[47] had injury to the triradiate acetabular cartilage; fortunately, of the 4 patients monitored long-term, the deformity described by Rodrigues[60] that results in femoral head subluxation did not develop in any. Acetabular fracture can also result in lateral subluxation of the hip, heterotopic ossification, and ankylosis.[6, 12, 29, 66] Other reported consequences of extra-acetabular pelvic fracture include delayed union, SI fusion with pelvic distortion, leg length discrepancy, and pelvic obliquity.

## COMMONLY ASSOCIATED INJURIES

As noted earlier, the injuries commonly associated with pelvic fractures are both visceral and skeletal. The visceral injuries directly related to the pelvic injury are bladder and urethral injuries, traction injury to the lumbosacral plexus, and injury to the major and minor arterial and venous systems, with resultant hemorrhage. Injuries associated with high-energy blunt trauma may involve the pulmonary, cardiac, gastrointestinal, and central nervous systems (see Chapter 4). Associated injuries occur in as many as 67% of patients with pelvic fracture.[26] Children with at least one other associated fracture had a significantly higher incidence of head and abdominal injury and an associated need for blood transfusion in a 1993 review of a 5-year experience in 79 children.[74] Chest injuries, the need for additional operative procedures, and mortality tended to be higher in the associated fracture group, but because of inadequate numbers, it did not reach statistical significance.[74] The most commonly associated fractures are those of the femur, skull, ribs, tibia and fibula, clavicle, facial bones, and humerus, in that order.[56] Identification of a pelvic injury in the primary phase of the resuscitation and injury survey should alert the physician to the possibility of these associated injuries. The associated injuries are more difficult to treat and generally affect the outcome far more than the pelvic fracture does.[59]

## CLASSIFICATION

Because of the severe nature of the associated injuries, Quinby suggested dividing pelvic fractures into those that do not require laparotomy, those that do, and those associated with severe vascular injury.[54] Although this system reflects an increasing severity of injury, complication rate, and mortality rate, it does not help the

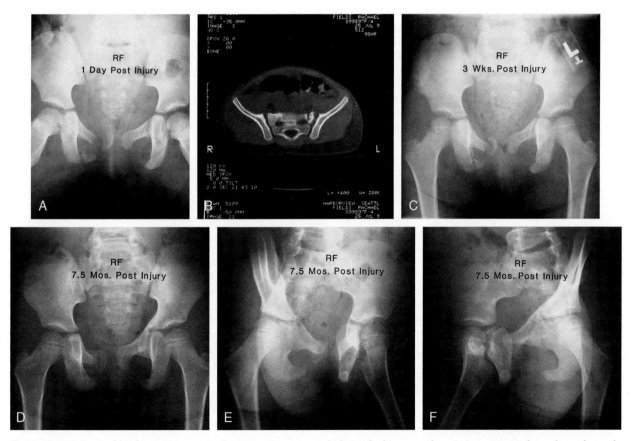

FIGURE 12–2. A 4-year-old girl was an unrestrained passenger in a motor vehicle involved in an accident. *A,* A postinjury pelvic radiograph reveals bilateral ramus fractures. *B,* Computed tomography confirms a lateral compression injury with a left-sided sacral injury. *C,* At 2 weeks, evidence of healing of all ramus fractures is seen. *D–F,* At 7.5 months, however, evidence of triradiate cartilage arrest on the left side is noted on anteroposterior, iliac, and obturator oblique radiographs.

physician with decision making or prognostic judgment. Many classification systems exist for adult pelvic fractures. The one developed by Trunkey and co-workers was applied to a series of 84 pediatric pelvic fractures.[73] This system divides pelvic fractures into stable and unstable categories. Stable injuries include pubic fractures, isolated fractures, and avulsion fractures. Unstable injuries include pubic diastasis, acetabular fractures, and diametric fractures (fractures on the sides of the pelvic ring). Watts believed that pediatric pelvic fractures are better classified according to the severity of skeletal injury, as follows[75]: (1) avulsion, such as epiphysiolysis (secondary to violent muscular activity); (2) fracture of the pelvic ring (secondary to crushing injury), stable and unstable; and (3) fracture of the acetabulum (associated with hip dislocation).

In their 1985 report on a series of 141 pelvic fractures, Torode and Zieg improved on the Watts classification and expanded it as follows[71]:

Type I—Avulsion fractures
Type II—Iliac wing fractures
Type III—Simple ring fractures, including pubic symphysis diastasis without disruption of the posterior SI joint
Type IV—Any fracture pattern that creates a free bony fragment, including bilateral pubic ramus fractures, fractures of the anterior pelvic ring with an acetabular fracture, and pubic ramus fractures or pubic symphysis disruption with a fracture through the posterior bony elements or disruption of the SI joint

In a useful addition to the literature, these authors also proposed a classification of complications based on increasing severity: type I, none; type II, occasional altered growth with subsequent remodeling; type III, occasional delayed union; and type IV, nonunion, malunion, triradiate cartilage injury, closure of the SI joint, and leg length inequality.

Tile modified Pennal's original classification of pelvic fractures in adults.[68, 69] This system, based on mechanism of injury, has the most widespread application and utility. The types are anteroposterior (AP) compression, lateral compression, and vertical shear. Burgess and colleagues recently expanded on the system in their study of 210 adults with pelvic fractures and added combined-mechanism injury as a combination of these patterns.[13] In this review, AP compression and combined mechanical disruption had the highest associated blood replacement requirement and mortality. Similarly, two retrospective reviews by McIntyre and associates[48] and Bond and co-workers[7] revealed the bilateral posterior ring fracture pattern to be associated with the greatest degree of blood loss and abdominal visceral injury. Tile's system has recently been placed into the A, B, C code system of increasing severity used by the AO/ASIF and adopted by the Orthopaedic Trauma Association[69] (Fig. 12–3, Table 12–1). This classification system is not useful for predicting patients at risk for urethral injury.[4]

Because of anticipated continued use in the literature, both the Torode-Zieg and the Pennal-Tile systems are referred to here.[69, 71] For acetabular fractures, the classification of Letournel and Judet is summarized in Figure 12–4.[38]

## Diagnosis

### HISTORY

Because of children's skeletal flexibility,[18] pelvic and acetabular fractures in the pediatric age group occur secondary to children being struck by automobiles or as a result of their being unrestrained passengers, not by minor trauma such as falls or sporting contact. A history of high-energy trauma directs the emergency medical service team to an appropriate response in the field and transfer of the patient to a regional trauma center. If shock is part of the initial findings, transportation is frequently by air ambulance. The same history of violent injury dictates a full-scale primary and secondary survey, institution of large-bore venous access, and other measures as outlined in Chapter 4. Minor apophyseal avulsion injuries, usually occurring in those 12 to 15 years of age, are generally caused by athletic injury.[40, 41, 61]

### PHYSICAL EXAMINATION

The evaluation procedure for a trauma patient is outlined in Chapter 4; the following comments are directed toward patients with a potential for pelvic or acetabular fractures. Inspection of the body surface is the initial step; the anterior surface is examined, and then the patient is logrolled so that spinal examination can be conducted at the same time. Contusions, abrasions, and areas of degloving where the subcutaneous fat has been sheared off the fascia (a Morel-Lavale lesion) are identified and recorded. Patients with acetabular fractures frequently have large peritrochanteric ecchymoses as a result of the orientation of the force that produced the fracture. Lacerations, especially anteriorly, are not uncommon in pediatric patients and are frequently associated with vascular injury.[54] In the perineum, lacerations are often the result of open fractures, with ischial fragments producing the wound.[58] Vaginal lacerations are not unusual,[33] and a digital pelvic examination should be performed in all female patients with a displaced anterior ring fracture; preferably, this examination is done with the patient under sedation or with the use of an anesthetic in prepubescent children.[51] Similarly, a digital rectal examination is done to check for gross blood, indicative of rectal perforation or sphincter injury.[48]

When the inspection is completed, pelvic stability is evaluated, preferably while the patient is still on the backboard. AP stability is assessed by the clinician placing the palms of the hands on the anterior iliac crests and applying posteriorly directed pressure (Fig. 12–5A). By placing the palms on the lateral aspect of the anterior crests and applying pressure directed toward the midline, the examiner can check for rotational instability, such as that created by an open-book fracture (Fig. 12–5B). Pain on AP or medially directed pressure in a conscious patient is carefully noted. Palpation along the posterior iliac spine, SI joint, and sacrum is performed to look for pain consistent with posterior pelvic ring injury. A final check on vertical/rotational instability can be made by assessing the relative height of the anterior superior iliac spines and relative leg lengths.

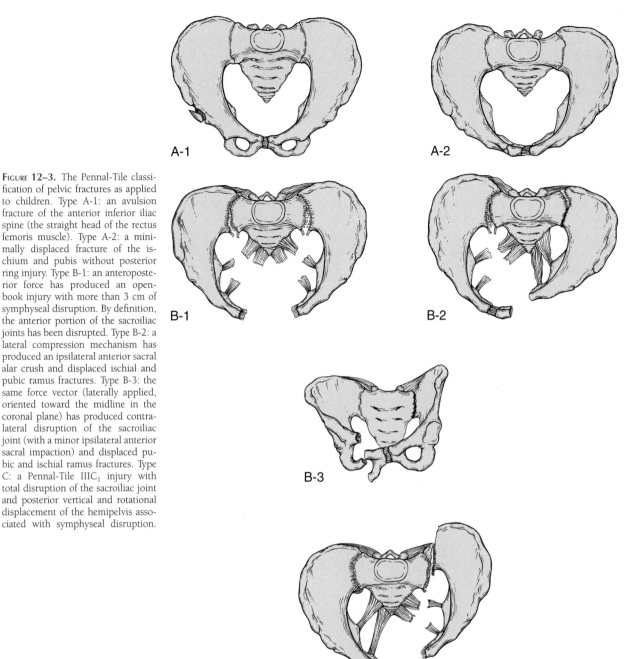

**FIGURE 12–3.** The Pennal-Tile classification of pelvic fractures as applied to children. Type A-1: an avulsion fracture of the anterior inferior iliac spine (the straight head of the rectus femoris muscle). Type A-2: a minimally displaced fracture of the ischium and pubis without posterior ring injury. Type B-1: an anteroposterior force has produced an open-book injury with more than 3 cm of symphyseal disruption. By definition, the anterior portion of the sacroiliac joints has been disrupted. Type B-2: a lateral compression mechanism has produced an ipsilateral anterior sacral alar crush and displaced ischial and pubic ramus fractures. Type B-3: the same force vector (laterally applied, oriented toward the midline in the coronal plane) has produced contralateral disruption of the sacroiliac joint (with a minor ipsilateral anterior sacral impaction) and displaced pubic and ischial ramus fractures. Type C: a Pennal-Tile $IIIC_1$ injury with total disruption of the sacroiliac joint and posterior vertical and rotational displacement of the hemipelvis associated with symphyseal disruption.

After the inspection and palpation phases are completed, a thorough evaluation of the arterial circulation is made. The femoral, popliteal, dorsalis pedis, and posterior tibial pulses are palpated; if they cannot be palpated, an ultrasound Doppler examination is done to check for biphasic pulsatile flow. Limb temperature is assessed by palpation. Finally, in an alert and cooperative patient, a gross motor examination of all major muscle groups in the lower extremity is completed bilaterally, in addition to a sensory examination to light touch and pinprick. The latter should include the perirectal area because of the frequent involvement of the sacral plexus with sacral fractures. Rectal tone should already have been assessed during the digital rectal examination.

**TABLE 12–1**

Tile's Classification of Pelvic Disruption

| Type | Characteristics |
| --- | --- |
| A | Stable |
| | $A_1$—Fracture of the pelvis not involving the ring |
| | $A_2$—Stable, minimally displaced fracture of the ring |
| B | Rotationally unstable, vertically stable |
| | $B_1$—Open-book injury |
| | $B_2$—Lateral compression, ipsilateral |
| | $B_3$—Lateral compression, contralateral (bucket-handle pattern) |
| C | Rotationally and vertically unstable |
| | $C_1$—Unilateral |
| | $C_2$—Bilateral |
| | $C_3$—Associated with an acetabular fracture |

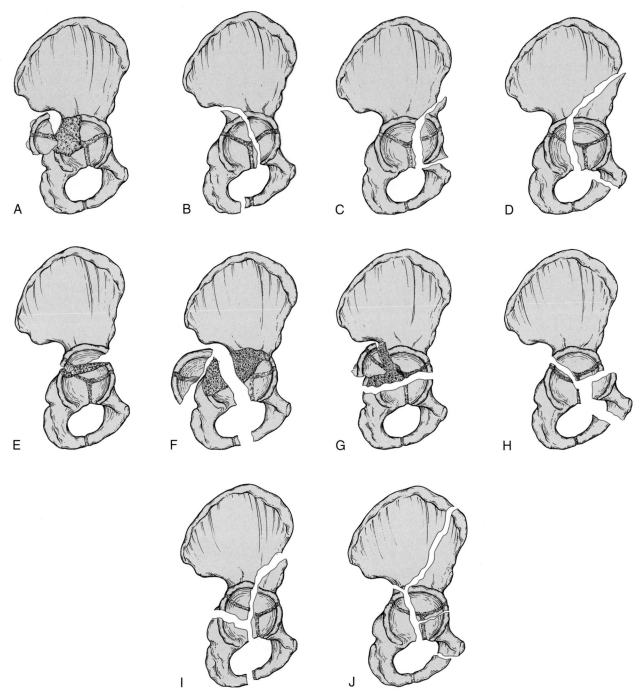

**FIGURE 12–4.** The acetabular fracture classification of Letournel and Judet. *A,* Posterior wall fracture; this fracture is often associated with impaction of the intact side of the fracture margin. *B,* Posterior column fracture. *C,* Anterior wall fracture; an atypically large fragment size is shown. *D,* Anterior column fracture; the most posterior location of the fracture line through the acetabulum is shown. *E,* Transverse fracture pattern; this location is transtectal. The fracture may cross the acetabula either higher (juxtatectal) or lower (infratectal). *F,* Associated posterior column and posterior wall fractures. *G,* Associated transverse and posterior wall fractures. *H,* T-shaped fracture. *I,* Associated anterior column and posterior hemitransverse fractures. *J,* A both-column fracture; note that no segment of the acetabulum remains attached to the intact ilium.

## RADIOGRAPHIC EVALUATION

An important part of the initial evaluation of a multiply injured child is an AP radiograph of the pelvis. Gonadal shielding should not be used because it may obscure the anterior pelvic ring.[75] Two additional views are indicated if a fracture of the AP pelvic ring is identified on the initial radiograph: a 30° to 45° (aimed distally) "inlet" view or "down shot," which demonstrates posterior pelvic ring injury more clearly, and a 40° to 45° (aimed toward the head of the patient) "tangential," "outlet," "brim shot," or "up view," which delineates the anterior pelvic ring[67, 68] (Fig. 12–6A and C). Both are helpful for delineating internal or external rotation of one of the hemipelves relative to the other. These three radiographs

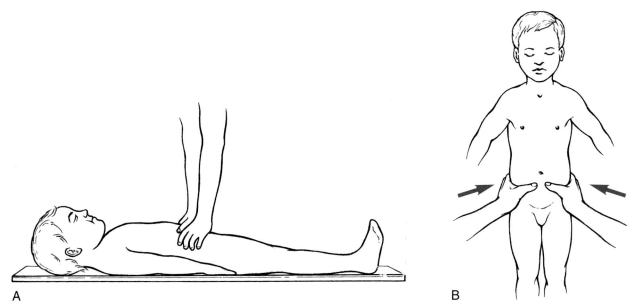

**FIGURE 12–5.** Clinical examination of pelvic stability. *A,* Examining for anteroposterior instability by applying posteriorly directed force on the anterior iliac crests. The examination is most effective when done early, while the patient is in the emergency department and still on the backboard used for transport. *B,* Examining for external rotation instability (such as that occurring in an open-book fracture, type $B_1$) by applying force on the external aspect of the pelvis and directing it toward the midline.

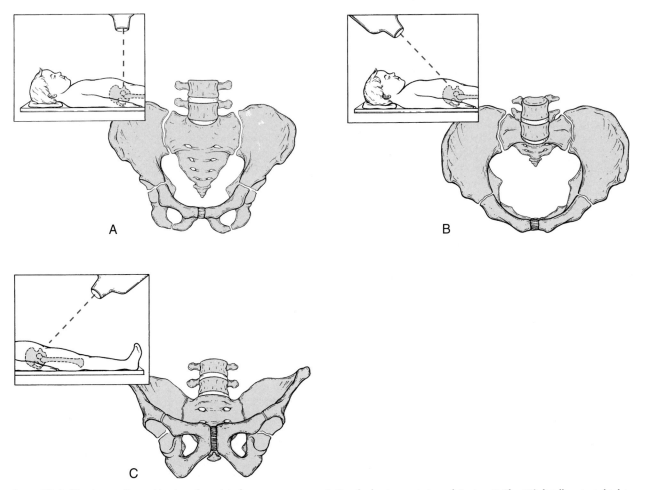

**FIGURE 12–6.** The three radiographic views for pelvic fracture assessment. *A,* Standard anteroposterior pelvis view. *B,* The 40° distally oriented inlet view demonstrates posterior ring pathology optimally. *C,* The 40° cephalically oriented tangential view demonstrates anterior ring pathology optimally.

can help determine the mechanism of injury and the form of treatment of most fractures.[79] Sacral fractures and SI joint injuries are frequently missed with standard radiographic technique. If suspicion is high because of findings on clinical examination or because of hemorrhage, shock, or radiologic abnormalities on the inlet/tangential view, computed tomography (CT) of the pelvis is indicated. CT is helpful in diagnosing pelvic hematoma, an important factor in the initial management of the patient. Cut intervals of 2.5 to 3 mm are generally sufficient to delineate the skeletal injury.[42] Images are obtained from L5 to the lower pelvic region in the axial plane by using contiguous sections with soft tissue and bone window technique.[36] Because CT is becoming more widely used to screen for abdominal injury, the images should be scrutinized by the treating orthopaedist. These images are not formatted for bone but are still useful for detecting fracture or SI joint disruption.

Because of the complex anatomy of the innominate bone, fractures of the acetabulum require a different approach for radiographic evaluation. The 45° oblique views described by Letournel and Judet are indicated when the scout AP pelvis film demonstrates involvement of the acetabulum[38] (Fig. 12–7). The iliac oblique view shows the posterior column in profile, as well as the iliac ring. The obturator oblique view places the anterior column in profile and shows the obturator foramen clearly. The two views combined with the AP pelvis view allow the physician to classify the fracture according to the scheme of Letournel and Judet[38] (see Figs. 12–4 and 12–7). CT is an important adjunct to these conventional radiographic views but is not a substitute.[42] It is especially helpful for detecting intra-articular loose fragments, which occur commonly in patients with associated hip dislocation.[2] CT also helps define fragments impacted in the acetabular margin (posterior wall), as well as occult posterior pelvic ring fractures.[42] Sacral fractures can easily be missed without CT imaging; these injuries may also be associated with disc herniation.[22] Finally, with unduly displaced, associated acetabular fracture patterns, three-dimensional reconstructions of the CT data may prove useful. Fractures with less than 2 mm of displacement may not be demonstrated with sufficient resolution on three-dimensional CT.[36]

In the case of young children (younger than 8 years) in whom fracture or dislocation of the proximal end of the femur is suspected, hip arthrography or magnetic resonance imaging (MRI) may be useful.[58] Ultrasonography is being promoted for evaluating treatment of congenital hip dislocation and may prove useful in the case of hip trauma in very young children.

## SPECIAL STUDIES

When injury to the lower urinary tract is suspected, either by blood at the penile meatus or by widely displaced anterior ring fractures, a retrograde urethrogram should be performed. By continuing the examination with larger contrast volumes once a Foley catheter has been definitely placed with appropriate urologic consultation, a cystogram can be performed to rule out bladder rupture. If renal or urethral injury is suspected from the results of physical examination or other diagnostic tests (if shown on abdominal CT scan), an intravenous pyelogram or CT scan with cystogram may be indicated to define renal and urethral anatomy and determine function.[1, 42, 58] The traditional threshold of greater than 20 red blood cells per high-power microscopic field for urine analysis cannot be used without clinical judgment as an indication for diagnostic evaluation; 28% of genitourinary tract injuries in one series would have been missed with this criterion.[1]

In the case of posterior pelvic ring injury in which sacral fracture or SI joint disruption has produced a sacral plexus injury, an electromyogram 3 to 6 weeks after injury helps define the extent and depth of the damage to neurologic function. Patients who present in shock, especially those with radiographically unimpressive pelvic fractures, may benefit from diagnostic angiography and therapeutic embolization with Gelfoam, blood clot, or coils.[5, 48, 58] This procedure may not be appropriate when open wounds are associated with major proximal (common) femoral arterial or venous injury, in which case immediate exploration and repair are indicated.[54]

## Management

### EVOLUTION OF TREATMENT

In the literature, treatment of pediatric pelvic fractures has been nearly universally conservative.[11, 58, 59] A recent retrospective study of 31 children treated with bedrest revealed that 36% had poor results, defined as continuous pain, marked disturbance in posture and gait, and loss of hip motion.[33, 35, 55, 75] Stable avulsion injuries of the anterior iliac spines, ischial hamstring origin, or iliac crests are best treated by conservative means. Open-book AP compression injuries have historically been treated by pelvic slings or spica casts. When these injuries are widely displaced or associated with severe hemorrhage or intra-abdominal injury, treatment is evolving toward external fixation or open reduction and internal fixation with small plates.[17, 35, 45, 55, 57] Stable injury to the anterior ring (isolated fractures of the pubic or ischial rami) and more severe four-ramus (or straddle) fractures have been and continue to be best treated by bedrest or spica casts (Fig. 12–8). It is for the most severe unstable pelvic fractures that treatment recommendations have changed. The standard treatment regimen for a vertical shear pelvic fracture (ipsilateral or contralateral fracture of both pubic and ischial rami or symphysis disruption anteriorly associated with a displaced fracture of the posterior iliac crest, sacrum, or SI joint) recommended in the literature has been skeletal traction with a pin through the distal end of the femur.[75] With more widespread use of external fixation, pediatric pelvic fractures of this nature have also been treated in such a fashion[35] (Fig. 12–9). Both treatments frequently result in SI joint fusion or malunion and leg length inequality; however, these outcomes are less common than when a

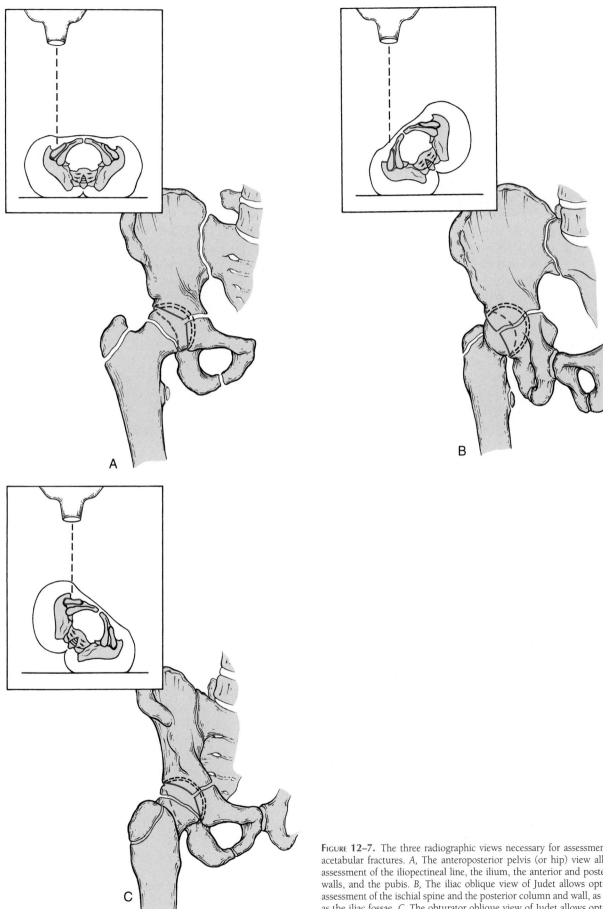

**FIGURE 12–7.** The three radiographic views necessary for assessment of acetabular fractures. *A,* The anteroposterior pelvis (or hip) view allows assessment of the iliopectineal line, the ilium, the anterior and posterior walls, and the pubis. *B,* The iliac oblique view of Judet allows optimal assessment of the ischial spine and the posterior column and wall, as well as the iliac fossae. *C,* The obturator oblique view of Judet allows optimal assessment of the iliac wing, anterior column, and anterior wall.

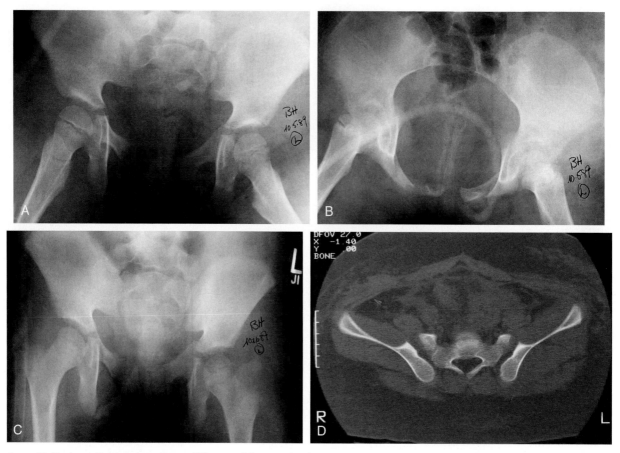

FIGURE 12–8. A type B₂ injury in an 8-year-old boy struck by a car. *A,* Admitting anteroposterior pelvis radiograph showing moderately displaced ipsilateral ischial and pubic ramus fractures. *B,* An inlet view suggests mild widening of the sacroiliac joint on that side. *C,* A tangential view confirms the anterior ring displacements. *D,* A CT scan confirms the mild widening of the right sacroiliac joint. The patient was treated with bedrest. The fractures have healed, with no residual pain or dysfunction 1 year after injury.

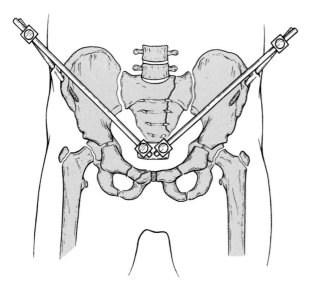

FIGURE 12–9. A simple two-pin external fixator for resuscitation of a child with hemodynamic instability from pelvic hemorrhage. The 4- or 5-mm Schanz pins are inserted through small stab wounds. Two single adjustable clamps and a tube-to-tube clamp connect two 250-mm carbon fiber rods. With the assistant compressing the pelvis externally to close the volume down, the surgeon tightens the clamps.

pelvic band or bedrest is the only treatment.[35] Optimal treatment of displaced fractures of the SI joint, posterior iliac ring, and sacrum is now considered to be reduction (closed, if possible) and internal fixation[10, 44, 45, 59, 63, 64] (Fig. 12–10).

Acetabular fractures in children have historically also been treated conservatively. Specifically, such treatment consists of bedrest or non–weight-bearing treatment for minimally displaced fractures and 4 to 6 weeks of skeletal traction for displaced fractures. Poor results have been reported, particularly for comminuted fractures, those for which traction did not improve the position of the fragments, and those that result in triradiate carti-lage injury in younger children.[6, 12, 29, 31, 32, 66, 75] In publications of clinical series when poor radiographic results have not been associated with poor clinical results, inadequate length of follow-up is generally involved.[11] Children with these injuries need to be monitored to midadulthood before one can be assured of the functional results.[31] The excellent results published for adults with displaced acetabular fractures have influenced the treatment of pediatric fractures; the current recommendation for fractures involving the major weight-bearing surface with greater than 2-mm displacement and for unstable posterior wall fracture-dislocations is open reduction and internal fixation[38, 45, 68] (Table 12–2).

## SPECIAL CONSIDERATIONS FOR POLYTRAUMA PATIENTS

Pelvic fractures associated with significant hemorrhage or concomitant intra-abdominal injury requiring laparotomy may benefit from more aggressive emergency treatment. Pelvic hemorrhage frequently responds to closing the pelvic volume down. Pneumatic antishock garments are generally effective for control of hemorrhage during patient transport.[10] The sizes appropriate for smaller children are not widely available, thus limiting the application of this technology to larger adolescents. When these garments are used, they must be removed early in the resuscitation to avoid compartment syndrome in the lower extremity and to ensure that no fractures or open wounds are missed.[2] Closing pelvic volume down is easily accomplished with simple external

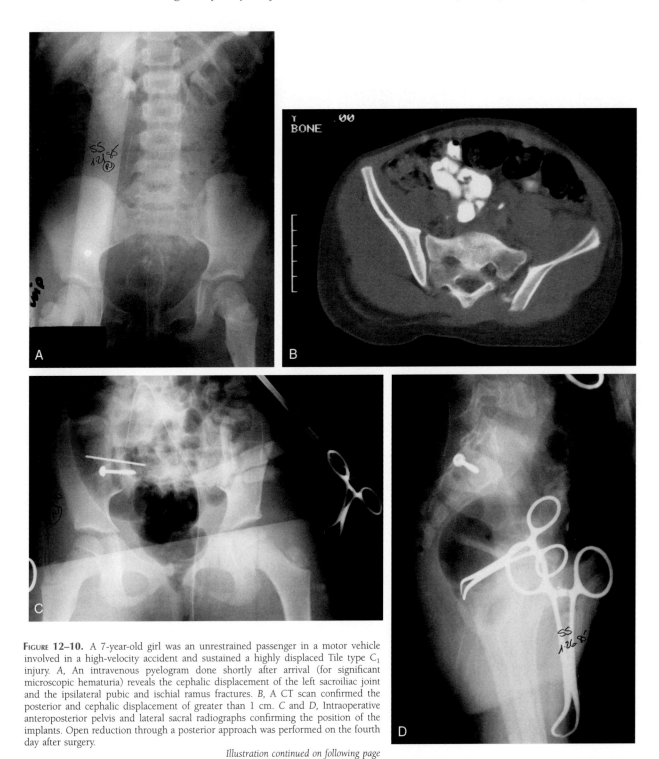

FIGURE 12–10. A 7-year-old girl was an unrestrained passenger in a motor vehicle involved in a high-velocity accident and sustained a highly displaced Tile type C₁ injury. *A,* An intravenous pyelogram done shortly after arrival (for significant microscopic hematuria) reveals the cephalic displacement of the left sacroiliac joint and the ipsilateral pubic and ischial ramus fractures. *B,* A CT scan confirmed the posterior and cephalic displacement of greater than 1 cm. *C* and *D,* Intraoperative anteroposterior pelvis and lateral sacral radiographs confirming the position of the implants. Open reduction through a posterior approach was performed on the fourth day after surgery.

*Illustration continued on following page*

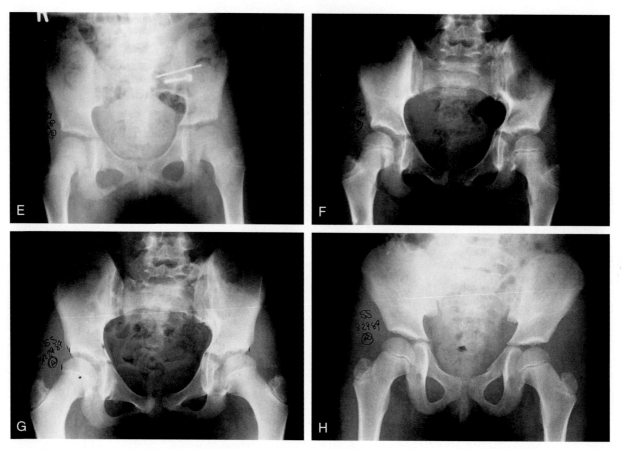

FIGURE **12–10** *Continued. E,* At 6 months after injury, the reduction was maintained, and fracture healing was apparent; the implants were removed 1 month later. *F,* At 1 year, the patient was asymptomatic; the radiograph was taken to evaluate the possibility of sacroiliac joint fusion. *G,* At 2 years, there was concern that premature acetabular triradiate cartilage closure had occurred; watchful waiting was elected. *H,* At 4 years, the patient remains asymptomatic; the sacroiliac joint and acetabular apophyses remain open.

**TABLE 12–2**

## Management of Pelvic and Acetabular Fractures

| Fracture | Description | Treatment |
|---|---|---|
| **PELVIC FRACTURES** | | |
| $A_1$, $A_2$ | Fractures not involving the pelvic ring<br>Isolated avulsions (ASIS, AIIS, ischium, ilium)<br>Isolated pubic rami fractures | Conservative management |
| $B_1$ | Open book, isolated | Conservative management<br>Exception: when associated with major hemorrhage or laparotomy or with displacement of more than 3 mm<br>External fixation vs. open reduction and internal fixation |
| $B_2$, $B_3$ | Lateral compression<br>Isolated<br>Displaced <5 mm | Conservative management<br>Exception: when associated with laparotomy, open reduction and internal fixation (if the anterior ring is amenable)<br>Exception: when widely (>1 cm) displaced, attempt closed reduction; open reduction and internal fixation if not reducible |
| $C_1$ | Vertical shear, displaced | Open reduction and internal fixation of posterior complex with or without internal or external fixation anteriorly (see Fig. 12–12) |
| **ACETABULAR FRACTURES** | | |
| | Displaced <2 mm | Conservative management |
| | Displaced ≥2 mm | Open reduction and internal fixation |

AIIS, anterior inferior iliac spine; ASIS, anterior superior iliac spine.

fixation frames with one or two pins in each iliac wing and a connecting bar (see Fig. 12–9). Generally, anterior external fixation does not optimally control displacement in the posterior pelvic ring. Posterior antishock clamps have recently been developed and have proved to be effective for SI disruption and displaced sacral fracture associated with severe hemorrhage.[25] These clamps can be difficult to apply, and their utility is limited (because of clamp size) to larger children and adolescents. They should be applied under fluoroscopic control; optimally, application of the clamps can be done in the angiography suite while the angiography team is being assembled.

In cases of open-book pelvic fractures with diastasis of 3 cm or more in which a laparotomy is being done, simple open reduction and internal fixation can be performed with a two-hole 3.5-mm dynamic compression (DC) plate and a cortical screw in each pubis (Fig. 12–11). In situations in which the patient is hemodynamically unstable and no laparotomy has been performed, a pelvic fracture of any pattern can be stabilized by a bilateral long leg spica cast with distal femoral pins incorporated.[16] In all other settings of multiple injury (not involving associated blood loss from the pelvic fracture), pelvic fracture management is best delayed 3 to 5 days and initiated after the full diagnostic evaluation is complete. Acetabular fractures should be managed similarly, with a short delay (1 or 2 days) to optimize preoperative planning.

## TREATMENT OPTIONS

For pelvic fractures, treatment options are as follows: (1) bedrest/non–weight bearing, (2) skeletal traction, (3) pelvic sling, (4) spica cast, (5) external fixation, (6) closed reduction, and (7) open reduction and internal fixation. Acetabular fractures are amenable to (1) bedrest/non–weight bearing, (2) skeletal traction, and (3) open reduction and internal fixation.

### Pelvic Fractures

#### Bedrest/Non–Weight Bearing

*Indications/Contraindications.* Bedrest treatment is indicated for all avulsion fractures of the pelvic ring and for stable pelvic fractures. These injuries include avulsion fractures of the anterior superior (sartorius origin) and anterior inferior (rectus femoris) iliac spines, the iliac apophysis (external oblique origin), and the ischial rami (hamstring origin, a common athletic injury) and isolated or bilateral pubic ramus fractures.[40, 41, 43] Probably the most severe injury that can be treated in this fashion is a straddle fracture (four rami); however, posterior ring injury must be definitively ruled out by CT and inlet/outlet radiographs. Other AP compression variants, including the minimally displaced open-book injury (<3 cm), can also be treated in this manner. Unstable pelvic injuries of the $B_1$, $B_2$, $C_1$, or $C_2$ type should not be treated in this fashion.

*Timing.* Treatment should begin as soon as all other injuries have been diagnosed and stabilized.

*Technique.* The muscle associated with an avulsion injury should be relaxed. Therefore, patients with anterior superior or anterior inferior iliac spine avulsions

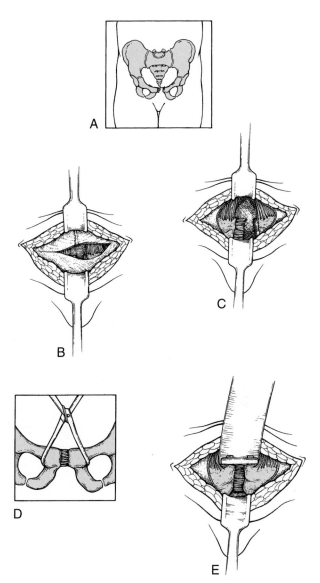

**FIGURE 12–11.** A simple two-hole plate may be used for closing an open-book deformity. *A,* If the child has (or is having) a laparotomy through a midline incision, this plate is easily applied by exposing the superior aspect of the pubis bilaterally. If not, the Pfannenstiel approach is preferred. *B,* With this approach, one side of the rectus abdominis is generally seen to be avulsed from the pubis. *C,* With a periosteal elevator, the opposite pubis is exposed. *D,* A reduction forceps is then applied to the anterior aspect of the pubis bilaterally to close the deformity. A Schanz pin 4 or 5 mm in diameter can be inserted through a percutaneous incision into the iliac crest to help with this reduction. *E,* Generally, 3.5-mm cortical screws with a four- or five-hole 3.5-mm reconstruction plate are recommended for children younger than 12 years.

or iliac apophysis avulsions and those in whom the rectus abdominis muscles are attached to pubic segments adjacent to fractures are placed in the semi-Fowler position with the hips flexed 30° to 45°.[43] Lower extremity exercises (ankle and foot) are encouraged. Patients with hamstring avulsion injuries are treated by bedrest with the hip extended and the knee flexed as much as possible. If the patient cannot be positioned in this way and made comfortable, a spica cast should be considered. The child is treated in this position for 3 to 4 weeks and then advanced to crutch ambulation (Fig. 12–12).

### Skeletal Traction

*Indications/Contraindications.* The remaining indication for distal femoral pin traction is a vertical shear injury through the iliac wing, SI joint, or sacrum that is shown to be reduced in traction.[70] This injury generally occurs in children younger than 8 to 10 years. Contraindications to skeletal traction treatment are lateral compression injuries, open-book $A_2$ injuries, and stable avulsion-type fractures.[69] Additionally, fractures that do not achieve reduction in traction should not be maintained with this form of treatment because leg length inequality will result.

*Timing.* After complete diagnosis of all injuries and institution of appropriate management, the child is

sedated or given an anesthetic. The skeletal traction pin is inserted proximal to the distal femoral physis, and the child is placed in skeletal traction. Fluoroscopic control is recommended to avoid inadvertent physeal injury. The best chance for reduction is when the traction treatment is instituted as soon as possible after injury, preferably within 24 hours.

*Technique.* A distal femoral Steinmann pin is inserted proximal to the physis by 2 to 3 cm under fluoroscopic control.[70] A Bohler traction bow is used to help prevent pin loosening with the child's increasing motion in bed. In contrast to the Kuntscher traction bow, the Bohler bow allows rotation at pin collars rather than be firmly fixed to the pin. The opposite leg is held in skin traction to prevent significant abduction; such traction is more often necessary in children younger than 8 years. Balanced

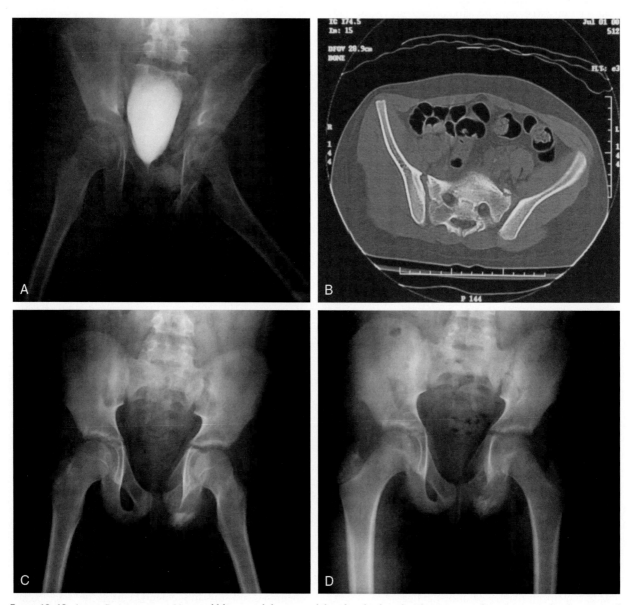

**FIGURE 12–12.** A type $B_2$ injury in an 11-year-old boy struck by a car while riding his bicycle. The trauma evaluation team ordered a retrograde urethrogram and cystogram (*A*), which reveals infolding of the left ilium and a segmental ischial fracture. *B*, a CT scan confirms the sacral compression on the left. At 6 weeks (*C*) and 20 weeks (*D*), the fracture has healed with limited weight bearing on crutches. No functional sequelae are seen 9 months after injury.

skeletal traction with a Thomas splint and Pearson attachment is helpful for toileting in older children. Inasmuch as 10 to 20 pounds may be necessary to reduce the fracture, depending on the child's age, it is helpful to elevate the foot of the bed on blocks.[75] If reduction to within 2 mm is not obtained within 5 days despite increasing weight, traction should be discontinued and consideration given to reduction and fixation. The older the child, the more frequently such is the case. Traction should continue for 4 weeks in children younger than 10 years and for 6 weeks in those aged 10 to 14 years. Strong consideration should be given to open treatment of displaced vertical shear fractures in adolescents 12 years and older. The progression is from traction for 4 to 6 weeks to several days of bedrest out of traction and, after radiographic confirmation of continued reduction, initiation of partial weight bearing with a walker or crutches.

### Pelvic Sling

*Indications.* This relatively dated form of treatment is appropriate only for $B_1$-type open-book closed pelvic injuries that are not associated with shock or hemodynamic instability.[69] Symphyseal displacement greater than 3 cm (2 cm in younger children) should be reduced, and a pelvic sling accomplishes the reduction in some instances. By definition, injuries with anterior displacement of this degree have anterior SI disruption on one or both sides and warrant reduction.[68, 69] This form of treatment is contraindicated for $B_2$ and C injuries because compression directed toward the midline will not accomplish reduction.[69]

*Timing.* Pelvic sling treatment should be instituted as soon as all other injuries have been diagnosed and stabilized. Early reduction is most likely to succeed because of less resistance to bringing the hemipelves together in the midline before the pelvic hematoma begins to organize.

*Technique.* A canvas sling 6 to 9 inches in width is placed underneath the supine patient. The ends are connected to traction rope and laterally directed pulleys with sufficient weight to suspend the patient's pelvis, generally 5 to 10 inches for most children. Greater compressive forces can be obtained by crossing the traction ropes over the patient's midline. Reduction should be confirmed by a radiograph obtained within 24 hours of initiating treatment. If the symphyseal gap is not closed down to within 1 cm or less, another form of treatment should be considered.

### Spica Cast

*Indications.* The use of a spica cast is indicated in patients who are hemodynamically unstable and internal or external fixation is not possible. Patients with severely displaced pelvic fractures and posterior ring involvement benefit from immobilization of the lower limbs in a double long leg spica cast.[16] For definitive management of pelvic injuries, the spica cast is helpful in minimally displaced pelvic fractures or avulsion injuries to allow the patient to be treated at home. Other than in the case of a $B_1$ open-book pelvic disruption, in which the spica cast is applied in the lateral position to allow reduction by gravity, these casts do not reduce displaced pelvic fractures. If the displacement is not acceptable, another form of definitive treatment should be selected.

*Timing.* Spica casts can be applied at any point during the treatment of pelvic fractures to allow mobilization of the patient. The cast should be applied emergently in the case of hemodynamic instability. If the purpose is to reduce and hold an open-book type of injury, the cast should be applied in the lateral position as soon as the patient's general status permits.

*Technique.* For general treatment purposes, the cast is applied in the supine position on a spica board for children 10 years and younger and on a fracture table equipped for casting for older children. If vertical displacement or acute hemorrhage is part of the clinical picture, it is helpful to incorporate distal femoral Steinmann pins into the cast.[16] These pins are placed under fluoroscopic control to avoid physeal injury. When applying the cast in the lateral position, a fracture table or spica box with a peroneal post that can be removed is most useful. In this instance, the reduction should be confirmed with the patient in the lateral position before the cast is completed. If reduction is not confirmed and the residual symphyseal gap is greater than 1 cm, another form of definitive treatment should be considered. These casts are left in position for a total of 6 to 8 weeks if the cast is applied after initial bedrest or traction treatment.

### External Fixation

*Indications.* The indications for this form of treatment are nearly identical to those for a spica cast. External fixation is also a useful management technique for open pelvic fractures.[57] Patients who are hemodynamically unstable will benefit from closing the intrapelvic volume down (see under Pelvic Sling). External fixation provides definitive treatment only for $B_1$-type open-book injuries. This method of treatment cannot hold reductions of displaced posterior ring injuries.[32, 48, 67]

*Timing.* Placement of the frame in circumstances of hemodynamic instability or associated open wounds must be done emergently. If an external fixator is chosen as definitive treatment of an open-book injury, the earlier it is applied, the easier it will be to achieve reduction and allow the hemipelves to be moved medially before the intrapelvic hematoma begins to organize.[70]

*Preoperative Planning.* Depending on the size of the patient, the surgeon must check on the availability of an external fixation system with pins that are appropriate for the width of the iliac crest and with connecting bars long enough for the intrailiac dimensions. The pins most commonly used are 4- and 5-mm Schanz pins, but 2.5-mm pins are available for infants and toddlers. Connecting rods 4 and 10 mm in diameter are available; the larger size is generally used, and they can be used with either the 4- or 5-mm pins.

*Anesthesia/Positioning.* General anesthesia is the technique of choice for either resuscitative application or definitive reduction. The patient is positioned supine for application of the frame.

*Technique.* In general, a modular system with a minimal number of components is prepared (see Fig. 12–11). Open wounds must be irrigated and débrided (left open) before placement of the frame.[46, 49, 62] Schanz pins or pins specific for the external system and of the appropriate diameter are selected.[57] For children older than 6 to 8 years, standard 4- to 5-mm pins are not too large. Keshishyan and co-workers determined that in children 7 years or younger, 4- to 4.5-mm pins can be used and inserted to a depth of 50 mm; in children 7 to 11 years old, 5-mm pins can be inserted to a depth of 70 mm; and in older children, it is possible to use 6-mm pins up to a depth of 110 mm. However, it is not necessary to use pins larger than 5 mm in any patient with a fractured pelvis.[35] In younger children, pins 2.5 mm in diameter may be more suitable. If the clamps are flexible enough to close down on the pin, threaded Steinmann pins of smaller diameter can be used. One or two pins in each ilium are introduced through 1-cm stab wounds (see Fig. 12–11). The pins are introduced through predrilled holes of slightly smaller diameter. The holes should just penetrate the superior iliac ring cortex, and the pins are placed by a hand chuck to minimize the chance of perforation of the inner or outer table of the ilium. Smooth K-wires can be placed on the inner and outer cortices of the iliac ring as directional guides. The bar or bars can be loosely applied, and then the assistant pushes the two sets of pins to the midline while the surgeon tightens the clamps. Reduction should be confirmed by radiograph. Adequate room should be left between the bars and the abdomen to allow the patient to sit up and to permit repeated abdominal examination.

### Closed Reduction

*Indications.* The two primary indications for attempting closed reduction by manipulation without internal fixation are a lateral compression injury with a locked symphysis and the tilt fracture described by Tile.[68] In the former, the goal is to unlock the displaced symphysis from posterior to the intact side. In the latter, the goal is to get the displaced free-floating pubic segment away from the vaginal wall in female patients. Because of the lack of stability after reduction of a vertical shear or AP compression injury, closed reduction in this setting is not indicated.

*Timing.* To optimize the chances of complete reduction, manipulation should be performed as soon as possible after injury.

*Anesthesia.* For both fracture patterns, general anesthesia is preferable with the patient in the supine position.

*Technique.* For a lateral compression injury, the displaced iliac ring is grasped on its inner aspect, and lateral traction is applied while pushing the intact ring away. If the patient's body habitus does not allow a firm grasp in the iliac ring, two Schanz screws of appropriate size (2.5, 4, or 5 mm) can be inserted to use as manipulation handles. They are removed after the reduction maneuver or incorporated into an external fixator. The reduction after manipulation of this injury is nearly always stable. The patient is kept on bedrest for 3 to 4 weeks and then mobilized with touch-down weight bearing on the injured side.

For a tilt fracture in female patients, bimanual pelvic examination is performed. If the bony fragment is palpable along the vaginal wall, reduction is indicated. With the intravaginal digit, the pubic segment is lifted anterior and superior. The external hand grasps the pubis in an attempt to coax the segment anteriorly. If reduction is obtained, it should be radiographically confirmed and

stability tested by putting lateral compression on the pelvis. If the segment is not stable, consideration should be given to placing a Steinmann pin across the medialmost fracture line through a small incision to hold the reduction. This pin is removed as soon as callus is evident on follow-up radiographs.

### Internal Fixation

*Indications.* Indications for reduction and internal fixation of pelvic fractures are an open fracture with massive displacement of the fragments and widely displaced fractures of the $A_2$, $B_1$, $B_2$, $C_1$, and $C_2$ types. Failed closed reduction and failure of an external fixator to hold a reduction are relative indications for open reduction because no other means of manipulation will be successful, especially if the injury is more than 5 days old.[49]

*Timing.* Closed or open reduction of displaced pelvic fractures is optimally done 48 to 72 hours after injury. Active hemorrhage will have ceased by then, and preoperative studies such as CT scans can be obtained and carefully reviewed. Delaying operative reduction more than 5 days increases the difficulty of obtaining anatomic reduction.

*Preoperative Planning.* Selection of the surgical approach is based on the location of the posterior ring injury. The plain radiographs and CT scans are studied to determine optimal positioning of the implants. In patients younger than 10 years, 3.5- or 4.5-mm cannulated or 3.5-mm cortical screws are the optimal implants. They must be available (special order) in lengths up to 100 mm for pediatric application. An experienced pelvic fracture surgeon should be consulted.

*Anesthesia/Positioning.* A general anesthetic is appropriate for all closed or open pelvic reductions. The patient is positioned supine for anterior ring approaches; SI joint or posterior iliac ring injuries can be addressed with the iliac fossae portion of the ilioinguinal approach.[28] For posterior approaches to the SI joint and for displaced sacral fractures, the patient is positioned supine or prone. In both instances, the patient should be on a radiolucent table; the C-arm is used to confirm placement of the hardware intraoperatively.

*Technique.* For anterior ring injuries, a Pfannenstiel approach is made to the symphysis and medial pubis. This incision is extended laterally to a formal ilioinguinal approach if more lateral displacement must be addressed. It is extended proximally to the posterior aspect of the iliac fossa for posterior iliac fractures and simple SI joint disruptions.[28] For symphysis disruptions, simple two-hole 3.5-mm DC plates or five-hole 2.7- or 3.5-mm reconstruction plates are used with 3.5-mm cortical screws (see Fig. 12–11). The longer reconstruction plates are preferred because they offer increased stability of the symphysis. The 2.7- or 3.5-mm reconstruction plates are also useful for posterior iliac fractures if long 3.5-mm cortical lag screws will not suffice. Disruptions of the SI joint may be stabilized in children with 3.5- or 4.5-mm cannulated screws placed percutaneously under fluoroscopic control and the patient in the supine position.[63, 64] Experience with this technique is required because of the high frequency of sacral anatomic variation (which may preclude the use of this technique) and the technical difficulty of this procedure; expert fluoroscopic skills are also required. This is my preferred technique. Alternatively, the joint can be stabilized in an open fashion with one or two two-hole 3.5-mm DC plates with one screw in the sacrum and one in the iliac wing. When the open posterior approach is selected for SI joint disruption, the screws are placed across the iliac wing and into the S1 body of the sacrum.[44, 45] One screw is relatively easy to place if the indirect and tangential views are observed under the fluoroscope during the procedure and if the lateral sacral view shows the screw to be inferior to the sacral slope. If adequate intraoperative visualization can be achieved, this approach is preferable to plate fixation. A technique has also been described in which CT is used as an aid to safe placement of the screw implants.[20, 21] A second screw can be placed posterior to the sacrum into the opposite intact iliac wing and capped with a washer and nut to prevent loss of compression, but a second screw is rarely necessary. This screw must not be overcompressed to prevent opening of the anterior SI joint, nor should it be overcompressed when dealing with a transforaminal sacral fracture to avoid crushing the sacral nerve roots. When dealing with comminuted sacral fractures and the percutaneous technique is used, a fully threaded screw is recommended to avoid injuring the sacral nerve roots with compression.[63, 64]

### Acetabular Fractures

**Bedrest/Non–Weight Bearing.** Bedrest or non–weight-bearing ambulation with crutches is appropriate only for nondisplaced or extremely minimally displaced (1 mm or less) fractures. Nothing specific is different about the bedrest treatment other than avoidance of pushing off with the injured limb. The patient must be closely supervised to prevent ambulation. Similarly, patients managed by touch-down weight bearing with crutches on the injured side must be carefully supervised to avoid weight-bearing forces being transmitted across the fracture surface and subsequent displacement; such treatment is appropriate only for older children who can be relied on to cooperate.

**Skeletal Traction.** Traction treatment is appropriate only for acetabular fractures that are reducible to less than 2 mm of displacement. Because of the elastic nature of skeletal tissue in children, however, such is rarely the case. A traction pin should be inserted in the distal end of the femur under fluoroscopic control and with the patient under anesthesia to avoid physeal injury. The fracture must be demonstrated to be reducible with follow-up AP and obturator and iliac oblique radiographs (with gonadal shielding) within the first 5 days. Fracture patterns that may be reducible with traction include both-column fractures and associated variants. Isolated columnar injuries or posterior wall fractures are not generally reducible with traction.

**Open Reduction and Internal Fixation.** All displaced acetabular fractures (with 2-mm or greater displacement documented on CT) should undergo operative reduction and internal fixation. The surgical approach varies according to the pattern of the fracture and the nature and direction of the displacement as

determined on preoperative AP, iliac, and obturator views and CT scans.[38, 42] All posterior wall injuries are amenable to reduction with the Kocher-Langenbeck approach. When a posterior wall fracture is combined with posterior column injuries, this surgical approach is generally effective as well. I prefer to make the Kocher-Langenbeck approach with the patient in the lateral decubitus position when it is being used for an isolated posterior wall fracture. When the approach is being performed for a fracture involving the posterior column, it should be done with the patient prone, as described by Letournel and Judet.[38] Anterior column injuries are optimally managed with the ilioinguinal approach of Letournel and Judet.[38] The associated injuries are best dealt with on an individual basis. When the posterior wall is not involved, I generally prefer the ilioinguinal approach because of the lower incidence of heterotopic ossification, better range of motion, and earlier return to function. Some transverse fractures and transverse fractures with associated posterior wall injuries may require the extended iliofemoral approach or the combined Kocher-Langenbeck incision along with the iliofemoral approach, although use of the simultaneous dual approach is rarely necessary and is associated with greater blood loss and a higher incidence of heterotopic ossification.[65] Internal fixation devices for children's fractures are generally of the 3.5-mm (small fragment) and 2.7-mm family. Extra-long screws must be specially ordered. I generally prefer 3.5- or 2.7-mm reconstruction plates for posterior wall fractures to allow early unrestricted motion of the hip (particularly unrestricted hip flexion). As a general rule, most children's associated (more complex) fractures can be treated with lag screws alone. Multiple assistants, Schanz pins with universal chucks, femoral distractors, specialized pelvic clamps, and so forth, are all useful. A surgeon well versed in acetabular fracture approaches and fixation in adults should be consulted for all operative children's fractures.[45, 68]

### Follow-up Care

**Immobilization.** The duration and type of immobilization depend on the fracture type and which treatment is selected, but the treating physician should bear in mind the following general rules: 6 to 8 weeks' healing time for pelvic and acetabular fractures, about 2 weeks less for children younger than 7 years, and 2 to 4 weeks more for adolescents older than 14 years. If the initial treatment is bedrest, traction, or a pelvic sling, the patient may be placed in a spica cast for the remaining healing time.

Beginning at about 4 to 5 weeks, cooperative children with adequate strength and coordination may be mobilized with a walker or crutches; such mobilization is possible only in those with an intact posterior pelvic ring complex on one side. The intact side is made fully weight bearing and the injured side partially weight bearing for the 3 to 4 weeks necessary for complete healing. Care must be taken when mobilizing patients who have suffered significant posterior iliac wing injuries treated by reduction in traction. Because significant leg length inequality can result from this form of treatment,[47] the patient should be taken out of bed cautiously—and only when healing has been confirmed radiographically and no clinical tenderness is present. If in doubt, the physician should err on the side of conservatism and leave the child in traction longer than strictly necessary. Patients who have been managed operatively with anterior ring open reduction and internal fixation may be treated with bedrest, bed-to-wheelchair ambulation, or a spica cast for the necessary healing time and then mobilized to full weight bearing. Children and adolescents who have been managed with anterior or posterior iliac reconstruction plating, anterior SI joint plating, or transiliac sacral screws with or without fixation to the initial posterior iliac crest can be treated with bedrest or a spica cast for the 6 to 8 weeks' healing time and then mobilized with a walker or crutches gradually, with progressive weight bearing.

Finally, patients who have been treated with external fixation may be converted to internal fixation if done within the first 7 to 10 days. Fractures older than 7 to 10 days, especially in younger children, must be considered to be malunited, and operative reduction requires removal or osteotomy of the fracture callus. If the anterior ring disruption is to be managed definitively with external fixation, it must be left in place for the required 6 to 8 weeks' healing time. The patient can generally be safely converted to a spica cast after 4 weeks of external fixation but should not be left at bedrest because external rotation forces in the pelvis may cause significant discomfort or late displacement.

Patients with acetabular fractures also require 6 to 8 weeks of healing time before weight bearing can be allowed without fear of displacement of the fracture. Younger children may be mobilized at 5 to 6 weeks; adolescents older than 12 years should be treated with partial weight bearing for 3 to 4 weeks longer (for a total of 10 to 12 weeks). Fractures that are minimally displaced and those treated with internal fixation can tolerate partial weight bearing on the injured side with a walker or crutches beginning 2 to 3 weeks after injury. Fractures reduced in traction should be held there for the full 5 to 6 weeks.

**Mobilization.** Four to 5 weeks after injury, children with radiographically documented healing pelvic fractures can be mobilized with a walker or crutches (full weight bearing on the intact side of the pelvis, partial on the injured side). Caution must be exercised in patients who have significant posterior pelvic ring displacement. Similarly, minimally displaced or operatively fixed acetabular fractures can be mobilized (partial weight bearing on the injured side) 2 to 3 weeks after injury.

**Physical Therapy.** Other than for crutch ambulation instruction, physical therapy is not generally required for children with pelvic or acetabular fractures. Swimming is excellent rehabilitative therapy for both pelvic and acetabular fractures and can be initiated 6 to 8 weeks after injury.

**Disabilities.** Barring complications, children and adolescents with pelvic fractures are fully functional by 4 to 6 months after injury. The same general time frame is valid for acetabular fractures that have been anatomically reconstructed. Patients with significant residual posterior pelvic ring displacement and those with remaining acetabular articular incongruities may have permanent disability.[31, 56, 67]

**Implant Removal.** Removal of implants is necessary only in children with significant growth remaining (see Fig. 12–10). Children younger than 10 years should have implants transfixing the SI joint or symphysis pubis removed 4 to 6 months after injury. Implants placed in the ilium, ischium, or pubis to fix anterior ring or acetabular fractures may be removed in children younger than 8 to 10 years to prevent encasement in bone and avoid the great difficulty of removing them if later reconstructive surgery is required.

## Assessment of Results

### FUNCTIONAL AND ANATOMIC PARAMETERS

Anatomic parameters, important to consider for pelvic fractures, are based on radiographic evaluation alone. For pelvic ring injury, reconstruction of normal anterior and posterior pelvic ring anatomy is the goal. The SI joint should not be fused, and the symphyseal cartilage space must be maintained. For acetabular fractures, a symmetric joint space must be maintained, with no femoral head avascular necrosis and no evidence of acetabular or femoral head osteophytes or lateral extrusion of the femoral head, as with premature closure of the triradiate cartilage.

Anatomic assessment of the results of a pelvic fracture influences the functional outcome only minimally.[8, 15] The critical result is patient function. An appropriate functional assessment for both pelvic and acetabular fractures in children includes an evaluation of pain, limping, motion of the hip, leg length inequality, activities of daily living, and sports performance, as well as an evaluation of altered activities (see Chapter 7). Females can have residual genitourinary, reproductive, and sexual problems.[15]

### RATING SCALES

Heeg and co-workers suggested that the rating scale of Harris be used to assess the functional results of acetabular fractures.[31] Until an alternative scale specific to these injuries is developed and validated, this scale is the best available. No published rating scale has been used to assess a population of children with pelvic or acetabular fractures; however, validated functional outcome scores have been used to report the results of adults with pelvic fracture.[4, 15] Physical rating scales and functional outcomes scales for children have been reviewed by Young and Wright[168] (see Chapter 7).

## Expected Results

Mortality for children with pelvic fracture ranges from 2% to 12%, not significantly different from figures published for adult pelvic fractures. Open pelvic fractures and those with significant major vascular injury carry the highest risk.[54] Patients with avulsion injuries and minor anterior pelvic disruption can be expected to have no residual disability, although nonunion can rarely result.[23] On follow-up at maturity, two thirds of patients with serious pelvic displacement have no significant functional disability, and half have normal radiographs to accompany this result. One third have residual limping and pain and have had to alter their activities.[47] Growth arrest deformities may be related to triradiate cartilage injury, but these deformities are seen much more rarely than growth arrest resulting from proximal femoral physeal injury.[14, 37]

Of the 23 patients with acetabular fractures monitored by Heeg and co-workers, 18 were treated conservatively.[31] Good to excellent functional results were achieved in 21, and radiographic results were good to excellent in 10. These investigators reported no improved results with operative management versus nonoperative treatment in patients with comminuted fractures or type V triradiate cartilage injuries.[31, 32] Excellent long-term results have been reported with widely displaced transverse fractures managed operatively.[9] As more experience is gained with the operative management of acetabular fractures in general, good to excellent functional results can be expected in 80% to 90% of children and adolescents with such fractures.

## Complications

Complications in the early phase of management of significant pelvic injury are bladder rupture, urethral injury, vaginal or rectal laceration, vascular injury, lumbosacral plexus injury, deep venous thrombosis, hemorrhage, and death. The more general complications and their prevention are covered in Chapter 4. The other associated injuries are a result of the primary trauma, and little can be done to prevent them short of preventing the initial injury.

Long-term complications of pelvic fractures include delayed union, nonunion, malunion, fusion of the SI joint, and leg length inequality. Delayed union and malunion can generally be prevented by an adequate period of immobilization. Nonunion as a complication is rare[55]; malunion is far more common.[24] Fusion of the SI joint is probably a result of the severe trauma producing the fracture, but the rate of this complication may be favorably influenced by anatomic reduction. To this extent, no less than anatomic reduction of an SI joint should be accepted in a child. These standards and an adequate period of immobilization will prevent leg length inequality. Adherence to these high standards requires a high percentage of open reductions for severe displacements in the posterior pelvic ring.

Long-term complications of acetabular fractures are premature closure of the triradiate cartilage,[12, 30, 59, 60, 78] joint space narrowing and sclerosis, femoral head subluxation, and avascular necrosis. Acceptance of no more than 1 to 2 mm of displacement in the acetabulum and careful surgical exposure minimize their incidence. The acetabular dysplasia that results from premature closure of the triradiate cartilage is distinctly different from other forms of dysplasia.[19] The marked retroversion that is produced is correctable by acetabular osteotomy, which is technically demanding.

## TREATMENT

The treatable long-term complications of pelvic fracture include leg length inequality, malunion, and nonunion. Leg length inequality in a young child is best managed by properly timed contralateral epiphysiodesis. In an older child, closed femoral shortening as developed by Winquist and colleagues is appropriate after it has been determined that the inequality is functionally significant.[76] Symptomatic nonunion is best managed by stabilization with internal fixation and bone grafting. Malunion of the anterior pelvic ring may require osteotomy and stabilization if it proves to be disabling in terms of sexual function, especially in females.

The most severe long-term complications of acetabular fractures (avascular necrosis, loss of joint space, and degenerative arthritis) are treatable only with drastic surgical measures. With these complications, temporizing with weight loss, canes, modification of activity, and anti-inflammatory medications is the wisest course. Ultimately, the choice, in most cases, is between arthrodesis and arthroplasty. The latter is best delayed as long as possible. Premature closure of the triradiate cartilage may be optimally managed by bridge resection and fat interposition, but the difficulty of surgical access and visualization makes this procedure hard to recommend except for the most experienced pelvic surgeons. The misshapen growth and lateral femoral head extrusion must be well defined and documented by CT, three-dimensional CT, or MRI before such a procedure is undertaken. The safer course may be a lateral coverage procedure, such as an acetabular osteotomy, in early adolescence.

## PROXIMAL FEMORAL FRACTURES

## Pathology

### RELEVANT ANATOMY

The relevant anatomy of the proximal end of the femur can be divided into osseous and vascular anatomy. In terms of osseous anatomy, two growth centers are of importance in the proximal part of the femur. The proximal femoral epiphysis is responsible for 13% of the overall growth in length of the femur. The greater trochanteric apophysis contributes significantly to the growth and shape of the proximal end of the femur. Damage to this apophysis before the age of 8 years produces a short greater trochanter and coxa valga.[87]

The vascular anatomy of the proximal end of the femur in a growing child plays a central role in the outcome of a proximal femoral fracture.[78] Trueta[129] and Ogden[116] investigated the proximal femoral vascular system of immature children by injection studies. The metaphyseal and epiphyseal blood supplies remain functionally separate until physeal closure at 14 to 17 years of age. Ogden, however, found some small penetrating vessels bridging the physis in the periphery of the neck.[116] These vessels may contribute to the blood supply to the femoral head until the age of 4 years.[88] The lateral circumflex system branches supply a significant anterior portion of the femoral head until 5 to 6 years of age.[116] The lateral epiphyseal branches supply most of the femoral head throughout childhood and into adult life; this vascular supply is the terminal branch of the medial femoral circumflex system.[129] The artery of the ligamentum teres generally arises from the obturator arterial system but supplies only a small amount of the femoral head.[116] This specific arrangement of the dominant medial femoral circumflex system, which Ogden identified as the posterosuperior and posteroinferior arteries,[116] as opposed to Trueta's lateral epiphyseal artery,[129] makes a child's femoral head highly susceptible to avascular necrosis after femoral neck fracture or fracture through the physis.

## INCIDENCE

Proximal femoral fractures represent less than 1% of pediatric fractures and less than 1% of all hip fractures. Most published series are compilations from orthopaedic societies or regional hospital systems or represent decades of a single institution's experience.[82, 88, 98, 103, 130] Fewer than 1000 total cases have been reported; specifically, 755 cases were reported as of 1982.[115]

## MECHANISM OF INJURY

Except when they occur through pathologic bone (usually simple bone cysts or fibrous dysplasia), proximal femoral fractures are produced by high-energy trauma.[113, 114, 120] Causes include falls from significant heights (trees), automotive accidents involving pedestrians, bicycle or motorcycle collisions, passenger injury in motor vehicle accidents, and child abuse, especially in children younger than 2 years[85, 99] (see Chapter 17).

## CONSEQUENCES OF INJURY

Proximal femoral fractures, particularly those proximal to the base of the femoral neck, carry a poor prognosis. A fracture in this region frequently results in limb shortening, deformity of the femoral head, and degenerative arthritis.[98] These problems arise from the complications of avascular necrosis and premature physeal closure,[91, 111, 119] complications that may occur more frequently in older children and adolescents (aged 8 to 16 years).[119, 130] Fortunately, such injuries are rare.

## COMMONLY ASSOCIATED INJURIES

Thirty percent of patients have significant associated injuries. Because of the high-energy nature of the trauma, chest, head, and abdominal injuries are the most common nonmusculoskeletal injuries. Fractures of the femur, tibia-fibula, and pelvis are the most commonly associated skeletal injuries.[110]

## CLASSIFICATION

Whitman was the first to report fractures of the neck of the femur in children.[132] Delbet published the standard classification of proximal femoral fractures in 1907.[90] This classification was not widely recognized until Colonna's 1929 report of 12 cases in which he used the classification.[86] Although other systems have been recommended,[112] Delbet's system remains versatile, predictive, and useful for treatment decisions.[85, 90] The Delbet classification is depicted in Figure 12–13. Some fracture patterns have been reported that transcend the standard classification.[94] A classic Salter-Harris type II fracture of the proximal epiphysis has been described; however, it may be associated with slipped capital femoral epiphysis.[128]

# Diagnosis

## HISTORY

The history of injury associated with these fractures is that of high-energy trauma in 90% of cases.* The nature of the violence directs the physical examination, as for that of a multiply injured patient (see Chapter 4).

## PHYSICAL EXAMINATION

The examination must be thorough and cover all organ systems, as established in Chapter 4. The surface of the anterior and posterior aspects of the pelvis must be inspected for contusions, abrasions, and lacerations. The affected limb is generally shortened and in external rotation. The pulses at the inguinal ligament, popliteal fossae, and dorsalis pedis and posterior tibialis locations must be assessed and compared with those of the normal limb. Finally, a screening examination for motor strength and light touch and pinprick sensation must be completed. The results of all these examinations are generally normal in these fractures.

## RADIOGRAPHIC EVALUATION

An AP pelvis radiograph is part of the screening examination for an unconscious, multiply injured patient. In a conscious patient, the complaint of groin or buttock pain generally warrants an AP pelvis radiograph, which confirms the diagnosis for each type of proximal femoral fracture. In cases of severe shortening, a traction radiograph is helpful for establishing the fracture anatomy. A cross-table lateral radiograph, with the uninjured leg flexed out of the way, is also useful for planning treatment.

---

*See references 80, 81, 89, 97, 100, 102, 105, 113, 114, 120, 125, 131, 133.

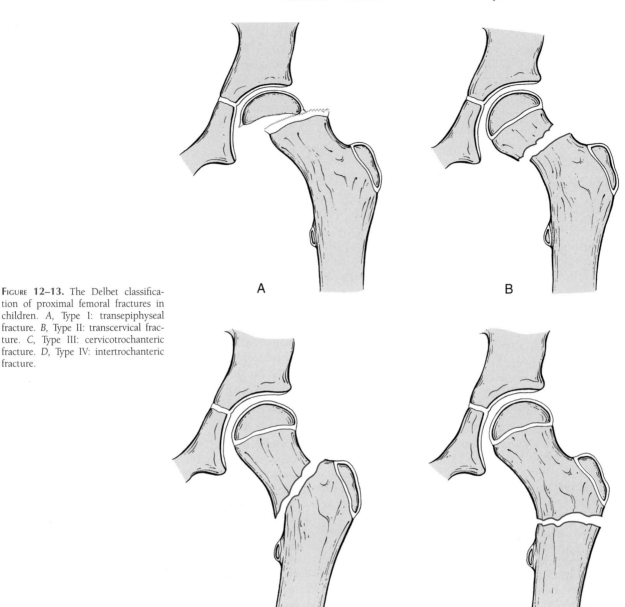

FIGURE **12–13.** The Delbet classification of proximal femoral fractures in children. *A,* Type I: transepiphyseal fracture. *B,* Type II: transcervical fracture. *C,* Type III: cervicotrochanteric fracture. *D,* Type IV: intertrochanteric fracture.

## SPECIAL STUDIES

In cases of severe trauma to the pelvis in which the pulses of the affected limb are not identified by palpation or Doppler examination, an arteriogram is indicated. Currently, no evidence has been presented that a preoperative bone scan or MRI is helpful in predicting avascular necrosis or in planning treatment.[163] In patients younger than 18 months, an arthrogram aids in diagnosing a proximal femoral epiphyseal (type I) injury.[107]

## Management

### EVOLUTION OF TREATMENT

Carrell and Carrell reviewed the recommended treatment of fractures of the proximal end of the femur before

1941.[83] The treatment to this point was primarily spica casting after closed reduction in an abducted position. In his review of 71 cases from the British Orthopaedic Association reported in 1962, Ratliff pointed out the higher incidence of nonunion when type II or type III fractures were treated conservatively.[123] Lam reviewed 75 fractures treated in Hong Kong (57 treated personally) and recommended an attempt at closed reduction and spica casting of type I to IV fractures in younger children and fixation with threaded pins in older children.[104] He advocated open reduction if closed reduction was not adequate. Canale and Bourland, in 1977, reported the Campbell Clinic experience with 61 fractures, most of which were treated with Knowles pin fixation.[82] These authors believed that the type of treatment did not affect the incidence of avascular necrosis. Heiser and

Oppenheim retrospectively reported the results in 40 cases at Children's Hospital in Los Angeles in 1980.[98] They advocated internal fixation with screws for displaced type II and III fractures and closed reduction wherever possible. They reported premature physeal closure in 23%, avascular necrosis in 17%, coxa vara in 12.5%, and nonunion in 7.5%, with fair and poor results in 35%. Pape and colleagues published similar results with the use of emergency reduction and fixation without capsulotomy in type II, III, and IV fractures.[118]

Swiontkowski and Winquist reported on 10 cases of displaced type I to III fractures treated with urgent capsulotomy and screw or pin fixation.[127] Capsulotomy was advocated and used in their series to evacuate intracapsular hematoma, which has been shown to have a detrimental effect on femoral head blood flow in adults with femoral neck fractures, as well as in animals with intact femoral necks. These results have been confirmed by Gerber and associates and Kujat and co-workers in European trauma centers.[96, 103] Although it is not completely clear that hematoma plays a major role in post-traumatic avascular necrosis in children, evacuation by means of an anterior capsulotomy produces no detrimental effect and may, in fact, help. It may play the most critical role in minimally displaced or nondisplaced fractures.[92, 96]

Currently recommended protocols are as follows:

Type I—Urgent anterior capsulotomy reduction and fixation with smooth Steinmann pins; postoperative spica cast

Type II (displaced or nondisplaced)—Urgent anterior open reduction capsulotomy and fixation with two to three lag screws short of the physis; a postoperative spica cast in children younger than 10 years

Type III (displaced or nondisplaced)—Urgent anterior open reduction capsulotomy and fixation with two to three lag screws short of the physis; a postoperative spica cast in children younger than 10 years

Type IV—Children younger than 6 years: closed reduction, pin fixation, and a spica cast. Children 6 to 12 years old: closed reduction, pin fixation, or skeletal traction for 3 to 4 weeks followed by a spica cast. Children older than 12 years and for failed closed or traction reduction: open reduction and internal fixation with a pediatric hip screw or blade plate

## SPECIAL CONSIDERATIONS FOR POLYTRAUMA PATIENTS

A displaced type I, II, or III fracture represents an orthopaedic emergency. Because of vascular compromise, which is potentially reversible, these fractures need to be reduced urgently. Therefore, this injury should be managed immediately after life-threatening injuries to the head, chest, and abdomen have been ruled out or definitively treated. Intracapsular hematoma occludes veins draining the femoral head and contributes to ischemia; it should thus be emergently evaluated. As noted earlier, such evaluation may be most critical for minimally displaced fractures.[92] Displaced femoral neck fractures may leave the critical lateral epiphyseal artery complex intact but kinked, thereby occluding flow to the femoral head.[108] An emergency reduction is therefore needed to return inflow to the femoral head. Open fractures with significant contamination should be irrigated and débrided rapidly before surgery is performed on the femoral neck fracture. All other musculoskeletal injuries take a secondary position in the hierarchy of treatment.

## INDIVIDUAL TREATMENT OPTIONS

Treatment options are given in Table 12–3.

### Type I—Closed Reduction and Spica Casting

**Indication.** The proposed indication for this treatment is a displaced type I fracture. I believe that this treatment is contraindicated, however, because of the near impossibility of obtaining anatomic reduction. Revascularization is enhanced by stable fixation.

**Timing.** To achieve the best reduction, the procedure should be done as soon as the patient's general condition allows.

**Anesthesia/Positioning.** A general anesthetic is used to provide maximal muscle relaxation.

**Technique.** The patient is positioned supine on the operating table. The limb is flexed and externally rotated, and gentle traction is instituted and a radiograph obtained. If the reduction is anatomic, a spica cast can be applied after the patient is carefully transferred to the spica board. Nothing short of anatomic reduction can be accepted. If, after a second attempt, such reduction

**TABLE 12–3**

Treatment Options for Proximal Femoral Fractures

| Type | Treatment Options | Recommended Treatment |
|---|---|---|
| I | Closed reduction and spica casting in an abducted, externally rotated position[85,93]<br>Closed reduction and smooth Steinmann pin fixation | Open reduction and smooth Steinmann pin fixation |
| II | Traction treatment in abduction and external rotation<br>Closed reduction and spica cast application<br>Closed reduction and pin or screw fixation | Open reduction and pin or screw fixation |
| III | Traction treatment in abduction and external rotation<br>Closed reduction and spica cast application<br>Closed reduction and screw fixation | Open reduction and pin or screw fixation |
| IV | Skeletal traction<br>Closed reduction and spica cast application | Closed reduction and pinning or open reduction and internal fixation |

cannot be achieved, an alternative treatment should be instituted.

### Type I—Closed Reduction and Pin Fixation

**Indication.** The indication is a displaced type I fracture.

**Timing.** The reduction should be performed as soon as feasible to optimize the reduction and minimize reversible vascular injury.

**Anesthesia/Positioning.** The patient is positioned supine on a radiolucent table, and a general anesthetic is administered. For larger children and adolescents, a fracture table is prepared.

**Technique.** After induction of anesthesia, the closed reduction is performed by simple internal rotation with gentle traction. The reduction is evaluated in the AP and lateral planes with the C-arm; if necessary, the reduction is repeated. If the reduction is anatomic, two or three smooth Steinmann pins of appropriate size are placed across the physis through a small lateral approach to the femur. If the reduction is not adequate (anatomic), an open reduction via an anterior capsulotomy should be performed.

### Type I—Open Reduction and Smooth Pin Fixation (Author's Preferred Treatment)

**Indication.** A displaced type I fracture warrants this procedure.

**Timing.** This procedure should be performed emergently.

**Anesthesia/Positioning.** See earlier.

**Technique.** After induction of anesthesia, closed reduction is performed as described earlier. If the reduction is anatomic on both views with the fluoroscope, a small linear capsulotomy is made in line with the femoral neck through a Watson-Jones approach, and the reduction is visually confirmed (see Fig. 12–17). Two or three smooth pins of appropriate size are then used to fix the fracture. If the reduction is not anatomic, the capsulotomy is extended to the acetabular labrum and then transversely along the intertrochanteric ridge. Sutures are used to retract the capsule edges, and the reduction can be performed under direct vision. A curved blunt instrument is inserted into the hip joint posterior to the femoral head, and the posterior angulation is corrected by lifting the femoral head onto the femoral neck. To facilitate this maneuver, a bone hook can be placed around the medial aspect of the femur and lateral traction applied to disimpact the fracture. Once the reduction is performed, fixation is carried out in the same manner. This approach is favored because it evacuates potential intracapsular hematoma and the reduction can be fully evaluated.[127]

### Type II—Traction in Abduction and External Rotation

**Indication.** An isolated displaced type II fracture is a possible indication for this procedure.

**Timing.** The traction should be instituted as soon as the patient's initial evaluation is completed to minimize further vascular damage to the femoral head and to provide the best chance for anatomic reduction.

**Anesthesia.** For children younger than 12 years who are awake and alert and have no contraindications, a general anesthetic should be administered.

**Technique.** The distal femoral pin is inserted under fluoroscopic control to avoid distal femoral physeal injury. The child is then placed in traction until the limb is abducted, externally rotated, and flexed. The reduction is confirmed radiographically; if nonanatomic, the weight is increased or the position altered. If the reduction in terms of the neck-shaft angle is nonanatomic, another form of treatment should be instituted. This approach is especially critical in older children. I believe that because of the increased risk of malunion and nonunion and because a potential intracapsular hematoma is not released, this treatment should not be used.

### Type II—Closed Reduction and Spica Cast Application

**Indication.** The indication is a displaced type II fracture in a child younger than 6 years.

**Timing.** Closed reduction should be done as soon as possible.

**Anesthesia/Positioning.** The patient is positioned supine, and general anesthesia with relaxation is instituted.

**Technique.** The child is placed on the spica table, and traction is applied as the limb is flexed, abducted, and externally rotated. If the intraoperative radiograph confirms an anatomic neck-shaft relationship, the cast is applied (a double long leg cast) with the limb in that position. A postcast radiograph must confirm the reduction. If perfect reduction cannot be obtained, an alternative treatment must be selected. For reasons noted earlier, this form of treatment is not recommended.

### Type II—Closed Reduction and Internal Fixation

**Indications.** A displaced type II fracture in a child older than 8 years or failure of closed reduction in a younger child warrants this treatment.

**Timing.** The operation should be done as soon as other injuries are ruled out or treated.

**Anesthesia/Positioning.** General anesthesia is required, and the patient is positioned supine on the fracture table with the C-arm available.

**Technique.** After induction of anesthesia, a closed reduction maneuver, as described earlier, is performed. If the reduction is confirmed to be anatomic, a midlateral approach to the proximal portion of the femur is made. The fracture is fixed with implants of appropriate length so that the proximal femoral physis is not violated. Cortical lag screws of 3.5 or 4.5 mm are preferred, or alternating cannulated 3.5-, 4-, or 4.5-mm cancellous screws may be used.[140] If the reduction is nonanatomic, the surgeon should proceed with open reduction. Closed reduction with internal fixation accompanied by hip joint aspiration has been documented to provide excellent results in terms of union and avoidance of avascular necrosis.[84]

### Type II—Open Reduction and Internal Fixation (Author's Preferred Treatment)

**Indications.** The indication is a type II fracture in a child (also for nondisplaced fractures) for release of intracapsular tamponade.[92, 96]

**Timing.** Same as for closed reduction.

**Anesthesia/Positioning.** Same as for closed reduction.

**Technique.** The closed reduction maneuver detailed earlier is performed. If the reduction is confirmed to be anatomic, the lateral approach is extended by detaching the vastus lateralis from the intertrochanteric ridge; the capsule is opened linearly along the femoral neck (Fig. 12–14). The reduction is confirmed by direct vision, and internal fixation is instituted as noted earlier.[84] This procedure is appropriate for nondisplaced fractures as well because of the definitive management of intracapsular tamponade. If the reduction is nonanatomic, the capsule is opened to the anterior acetabular labrum and taken off the intertrochanteric ridge 1 cm medially and laterally. With retracting sutures in place, a bone hook is placed around the medial aspect of the femur or an external fixation pin is inserted into the proximal femoral shaft, and lateral traction is initiated by the assistant. The proximal fragment is then manipulated into position with a curved, blunt instrument. The rotation of the limb must be adjusted by a nonscrubbed assistant if the procedure is done on a fracture table or by a scrubbed assistant if the leg is draped free. Once the reduction is accurate, two to three implants are placed short of the physis, as noted earlier.

### Type III—Traction Treatment

**Indications.** Indications are isolated displaced type III fractures in children aged 4 to 12 years. Contraindi-

cations include multiple injuries (especially head injury, in which case traction is poorly tolerated).

**Timing.** As with other proximal femoral fractures with the potential for vascular injury to the femoral head, these fractures should be reduced as soon as the patient can be cleared for anesthesia or sedation.

**Anesthesia/Positioning.** General anesthesia is instituted in children younger than 12 years whenever possible. The patient is positioned supine on the operating table.

**Technique.** A distal femoral pin is inserted under fluoroscopic control to avoid the distal femoral physis. The child is then placed in 5 to 10 pounds of traction in a position of abduction, flexion, and external rotation. The position of the fracture is confirmed radiographically. If the reduction is nonanatomic, more weight may be necessary, or a closed reduction maneuver should be performed. If anatomic reduction is not obtained, an alternative treatment must be selected.

### Type III—Closed Reduction and Spica Casting

**Indication.** The indication is a displaced type III fracture in a child younger than 6 years.

**Timing.** See earlier.

**Anesthesia/Positioning.** A general anesthetic is administered to a supine patient positioned on the spica board or table.

**Technique.** After induction of anesthesia, the fracture is reduced by flexing the limb while applying gentle traction and putting the limb in external rotation and abduction. The reduction is evaluated by two plain radiographs, and a double long leg spica cast is applied. The reduction is confirmed radiographically after placement of the cast. If the reduction is not acceptable, the maneuver can be repeated under fluoroscopic monitoring to evaluate limb position relative to the reduction. If anatomic reduction cannot be obtained, an open reduction should be performed.

### Type III—Closed Reduction and Screw Fixation

**Indications.** Indications include a type III fracture in a child or failure of closed treatment.

**Timing.** See earlier.

**Anesthesia/Positioning.** A general anesthetic is administered to the patient, who is positioned supine on the fracture table.

**Technique.** The technique is identical to that outlined for type II fractures. Placing the internal fixation near the physis is not as critical, however, because of the larger medial (proximal) fragment. The same implants are recommended.[140]

### Type III—Open Reduction and Screw Fixation (Author's Preferred Treatment)

**Indications.** A type III fracture in a child and failure of closed reduction are the indications. The same treatment is recommended as for release of intracapsular tamponade.[92, 96, 127]

**Timing.** See earlier.

**Anesthesia/Positioning.** General anesthesia is instituted with the child in the supine position on the fracture table or with the leg draped free on a radiolucent table.

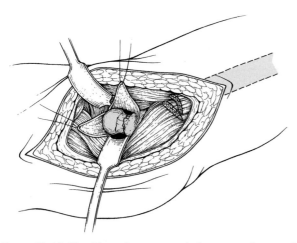

**FIGURE 12–14.** The Watson-Jones approach for open reduction of femoral neck fractures. The incision curves gently toward the interval between the tensor fasciae latae and the gluteus medius muscles from the tip of the greater trochanter and extends distally along the midlateral line of the femur. The vastus lateralis is elevated off the intertrochanteric ridge, and a T-shaped capsulotomy is performed by elevating the anterior hip capsule off the intertrochanteric ridge and extending the capsulotomy toward the center of the acetabulum to expose the femoral neck fracture. By placing sutures in the edges of the capsulotomy and inserting a Hohman retractor along the anterior aspect of the acetabulum, excellent visualization of the femoral neck fracture can be achieved.

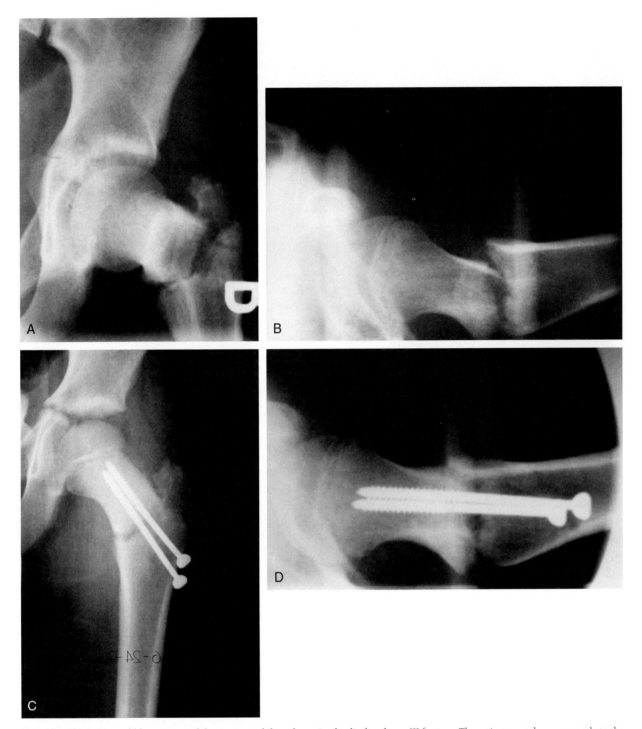

**FIGURE 12–15.** A 6-year-old boy was struck by an automobile and sustained a displaced type III fracture. The patient was taken emergently to the operating room, where capsulotomy and open reduction were performed through a Watson-Jones approach. *A* and *B,* Preoperative radiographs. *C* and *D,* Postoperative radiographs; the patient was treated for 6 weeks in a one and one-half hip spica cast.

*Illustration continued on following page*

**Technique.** The technique is identical to that outlined for type II injuries (Fig. 12–15). The same implants are used as described earlier (those able to compress the fracture site). I also recommend this treatment for nondisplaced type III fractures because intracapsular tamponade may play a role in the production of avascular necrosis.[92]

*Type IV—Skeletal Traction*

**Indication.** Displaced type IV fractures in children 6 to 12 years of age.

**Timing.** Although this distal fracture does not necessitate any vascular considerations, the best reductions are obtained when surgery is performed in the first 24 hours.

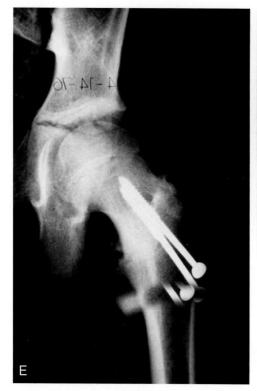

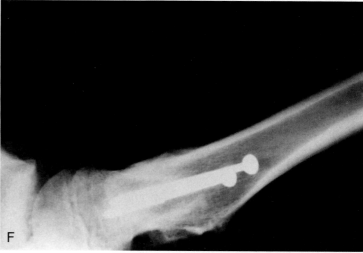

FIGURE 12–15 *Continued. E* and *F,* At 8 months, the screws were removed. The child is asymptomatic but was monitored for 3 years, the minimal length of time to definitively rule out necrosis.

**Anesthesia/Positioning.** General anesthesia is preferred, with the patient in the supine position on the standard operating table.

**Technique.** The distal femoral pin is inserted under fluoroscopic control to avoid the distal femoral physis. The limb is then placed in 10 to 15 pounds of traction (for a 60- to 80-pound child) with the limb flexed 60° to 70° in an externally rotated, flexed, and abducted position. The neck-shaft position can be controlled by increasing the weight and distal pull. This angle should be within 3° to 5° of that in the opposite normal hip. Significant varus (more than 3°) should not be accepted. If adequate reduction cannot be obtained, open reduction and fixation should be considered.

### Type IV—Closed Reduction and Spica Cast

**Indication.** A displaced type IV fracture in a child younger than 6 years is the indication.

**Timing.** See earlier.

**Anesthesia/Positioning.** General anesthesia is administered, with the child in the supine position on a spica board.

**Technique.** After induction of anesthesia, the fracture is reduced by longitudinal traction, flexion to 70°, and external rotation. The reduction is confirmed by fluoroscopic or plain film before double-leg spica casting. If a neck-shaft angle within 5° cannot be obtained and held, open reduction or closed percutaneous pinning should be considered. Frequent radiographs are necessary to confirm maintenance of reduction in the early (first 2 to 3 weeks) phase of treatment.

### Type IV—Closed Reduction and Percutaneous Pinning

**Indications.** Indications include failure to maintain reduction in a cast or in traction, multiple trauma, and an irreducible type IV fracture in a child aged 6 to 12 years.

**Timing.** See earlier.

**Anesthesia/Positioning.** General anesthesia is required. The patient is placed in the supine position on the fracture table with the **C**-arm available.

**Technique.** Closed reduction is performed, and the limb is placed in traction on the fracture table with flexion of 20° to 30° and external rotation. If the reduction is satisfactory (within 5° of the intact femoral neck-shaft angle and with good opposition on the lateral view) on fluoroscopic evaluation, the fracture can be stabilized with two to three threaded Steinmann pins inserted either percutaneously or through a small lateral approach to the lateral aspect of the proximal end of the femur. If the patient is too young to be cooperative or is large or if the stability of the fixation is in question, a one and one-half spica cast should be added.

### Type IV—Open Reduction and Internal Fixation (Author's Preferred Treatment)

**Indications.** Indications include failure to obtain adequate reduction in a child of any age by any closed technique, multiple-system trauma, and a displaced type IV fracture in a child 12 years or older.

**Timing.** If open reduction is selected as the course of treatment, the patient can be placed in skin or skeletal traction for 3 to 5 days before surgery. If the general condition of the patient allows, reduction plus fixation within the first 24 to 48 hours is preferred.

**Anesthesia/Positioning.** General anesthesia is required. The child is positioned supine on the fracture or radiolucent table, with the C-arm available.

**Technique.** After the patient is anesthetized and placed on the fracture table, traction is placed on the limb in slight external rotation. A standard lateral approach to the proximal part of the femur is made. The fragments are reduced under direct vision. In children younger than 6 years, two to three threaded pins can be used for fixation (Fig. 12–16). In children aged 6 to 12 years, limited fixation with two to three lag or cancellous screws is recommended. In both age groups, the fixation should not cross the physis and should be supplemented with a one and one-half spica cast. In patients 12 years and older, a sliding hip screw or angled blade plate should be used, with care taken to keep the fixation proximal to the physis. No supplemental casting is

indicated under normal circumstances for this type of fixation in older children.

## FOLLOW-UP CARE

**Immobilization.** The period of immobilization depends on the age of the child and the type of fracture. For type I, II, or III fractures treated with spica casting or by traction, 8 to 10 weeks is required for healing; the duration approaches 6 to 8 weeks for children 6 years and younger and 12 weeks for adolescents. If the initial treatment is by traction, the final 2 to 4 weeks can be in a spica cast. Type IV fractures have similar healing times. Type I to IV fractures managed with smooth pin or threaded Steinmann pin fixation should have supplemental one and one-half spica casts applied for the 8- to 10-week course of treatment. Children with type II or III fractures internally fixed with lag screws frequently benefit from supplemental spica casting if their ability to cooperate with non–weight-bearing regimens is suspect

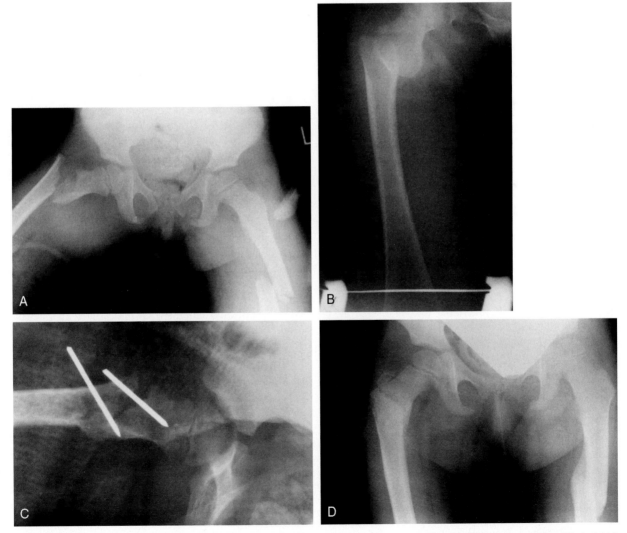

**FIGURE 12–16.** A 5-year-old girl was an unrestrained front seat passenger in a motor vehicle involved in a high-speed accident. *A* and *B*, An initial attempt was made to treat this type IV fracture by traction. The neck-shaft angle could not be adequately controlled. *C*, Through a limited open reduction, threaded Steinmann pins were inserted. The child was kept in a spica cast for 6 weeks. *D*, Radiograph taken at the time of pin removal.

(in those aged 1 to 12 years). Adolescents with rigidly fixed type IV fractures can be mobilized with crutches and partial weight bearing on the injured side beginning 10 to 14 days postoperatively.

**Mobilization.** Children from 6 years of age to adolescence benefit from a transitional period of partial weight bearing with a walker or crutches. This therapy is instituted at 8 to 10 weeks and continues for 2 to 3 weeks. Younger children can be mobilized as tolerated. Swimming pool therapy is a helpful transitional technique.

**Physical Therapy.** Formal physical therapy, other than that required for walker or crutch ambulation and possible water therapy, is not necessary for children. Adolescents (aged 15 years and older) may benefit from gait training or muscle-strengthening programs beginning 12 weeks after injury.

**Disability.** Patients with type I, II, or III injuries that heal and in which proximal physeal arrest or avascular necrosis does not develop have a 3- to 6-month period of functional disability. Those with type IV fractures that heal without coxa vara have similar periods of disability. If growth arrest develops in a child younger than 10 years, significant leg length inequality may result and lead to limping and altered gait mechanics. Avascular necrosis at any age ultimately leads to limb length inequality (and hip joint deformity in younger children), pain, and altered lifestyle in the vast majority of patients.[104, 110] In every case, the disability is progressive and permanent.[106]

**Implant Removal.** When pin fixation is selected, the pins are left long for easy retrieval and are removed 4 to 6 months after injury. Lag screws and larger implants used for type II, III, and IV fractures are removed 6 to 12 months after fracture (see Figs. 12–15 and 12–16).

## Assessment of Results

Ratliff's assessment of functional and anatomic results includes the parameters of pain, motion, activity, and radiographic findings and has been the most widely used.[123] His guidelines are presented in Table 12–4 and are recommended for continued use in the future. Currently, no long-term functional outcome data are available. Future studies will by necessity be multicenter and should involve the use of principles of outcome assessment as documented in Chapter 7.

## Expected Results

**Type I.** Avascular necrosis with poor functional results develops in well over 80% of these injuries. Urgent open reduction may affect the results positively, but a 50% minimal incidence of avascular necrosis in displaced type I fractures should be expected.[95, 111, 121, 127] The functional results are nearly always poor when this complication occurs.[118]

**Type II.** Avascular necrosis develops in 50% to 60% of displaced type II fractures, nonunion develops in 15%, and premature physeal closure after closed treatment or pin fixation develops in 50% to 60%.[82, 104, 117, 121] Urgent capsulotomy and internal fixation may favorably influence the rates of these complications[96, 103, 127] but will not reduce their incidence to zero because the initial displacement is the critical factor in producing the vascular injury. Avascular necrosis can result from nondisplaced fractures not treated with capsulotomy or aspiration of the hip capsule.[84, 92, 96]

**Type III.** Avascular necrosis develops in 30% to 40% of displaced type III fractures; these rates are favorably affected by urgent capsulotomy and fixation.[96, 103] Nonunion develops in 10% of these patients but can be minimized by optimal lag screw fixation. If the fracture is not reduced anatomically, coxa vara results in 20% of cases.[82]

**Type IV.** Coxa vara results if anatomic reduction is not obtained by whatever treatment used. It has been reported in 10% to 30% of cases and is most common with traction or cast treatment. However, carefully performed traction treatment followed by spica casting can result in preservation of normal proximal femoral anatomy.[94] Avascular necrosis and physeal closure are not anticipated in type IV injuries. Coxa vara deformity may rarely correct with time and is not by itself associated with a poor functional result.[91, 93]

In general, if avascular necrosis, premature closure, nonunion, and coxa vara can be avoided, an excellent result will be obtained. Because of the nature of these injuries, excellent results can be expected in only 40% to 50% of type I and II fractures and in 60% to 70% of type III fractures.[122] Again, urgent capsulotomy and anatomic reduction may significantly influence the rate of these complications. When these complications do develop, however, even though the results at 2 to 4 years may be functionally acceptable or rarely good, the status of the hip deteriorates with time.[104, 106, 117]

**TABLE 12–4**

Ratliff's Classification of the Results of Treatment of Fracture of the Hip

|  | Good | Fair | Poor |
|---|---|---|---|
| Pain | None or the patient ignores it | Occasional | Disabling |
| Movement | Full or only terminal restriction | >50% | <50% |
| Activity | Normal or the patient avoids games | Normal or the patient avoids games | Restricted |
| Radiograph | Normal or some deformity of the femoral neck | Severe deformity of the femoral neck and mild avascular necrosis | Severe avascular necrosis, degenerative arthritis, arthrodesis |

# Complications

The complications of avascular necrosis, premature physeal closure, nonunion, and coxa vara are generally apparent on radiographs within 6 to 9 months after injury.[81, 126] They have more severe consequences in adolescents and older children.[89, 119] Avascular necrosis of the metaphyseal region, as described by Ratliff, is not of functional significance.[123, 124] A rare associated type I fracture after fixation of a type III fracture has recently been described.[101]

## TREATMENT

**Avascular Necrosis.** No treatment of post-traumatic avascular necrosis is recognized to be effective. This complication may have the least long-term significance in children younger than 6 years because of the biologic plasticity of the bone. Acetabular and femoral osteotomies to "contain" the femoral head have been recommended by some authors, but their effect on functional outcome remains unclear.[122, 124] Seventy-eight percent of children in one long-term follow-up study required additional surgery to improve hip function.[86]

**Premature Physeal Closure.** This complication rarely results in a leg length discrepancy of greater than 1.5 cm.[97] The leg length inequality should be monitored by scanograms and distal femoral epiphysiodesis performed on the normal leg if the discrepancy is projected to be greater than 1.5 cm. This complication has very little functional impact if it occurs without avascular necrosis.[93]

**Nonunion.** If associated with varus deformity, this complication can be effectively treated by subtrochanteric valgus osteotomy and internal fixation across the nonunion. If a normal neck-shaft angle has been maintained, internal fixation with compression and bone grafting is indicated.

**Coxa Vara.** This complication is avoidable by adherence to a high standard for the initial reduction of type III and IV fractures[109] (Fig. 12–17). It can be successfully treated, when severe enough to result in effective limb shortening (less than a 130° neck-shaft angle), with a subtrochanteric or intertrochanteric valgus osteotomy and internal fixation.

# HIP DISLOCATIONS

## Pathology

### RELEVANT ANATOMY

The relevant osseous and vascular anatomy of the acetabulum and proximal end of the femur has been described previously in this chapter.

### INCIDENCE

Traumatic hip dislocation in children is rare, representing 5% or less of all pediatric dislocations.[139, 152–154, 167] The injury is not associated with any significant peak age of incidence.[139, 145] Although most hip dislocations are posterior, anterior dislocations have been reported in children.[137, 141, 149]

The ratio of boys to girls may be as high as 2:1.[157] Bilateral hip dislocation is an extremely rare injury, but the treatment principles remain the same.[161]

### MECHANISM

In contrast to other injuries presented in this chapter, hip dislocation can occur with relatively trivial injuries. The younger the child, the less the force that may be involved in dislocating the hip.[157] In a detailed report of the Pennsylvania Orthopaedic Society, four groups of mechanisms were cited[159]: (1) trivial falls (slippery surfaces or "the splits"), (2) athletic injuries (wrestling, football, or baseball), (3) falls from significant heights, and (4) being struck by a vehicle or sustaining injuries as a passenger in a motor vehicle accident. Of the 25 cases reported, 15 were in the first two groups (low energy) and 10 were in the latter two groups (high energy). The prognosis has been shown to be related to the amount of energy involved in the dislocation.

### CONSEQUENCES

Hip dislocations in children and adolescents may result in avascular necrosis or degenerative arthritis, with the resultant pain, limping, and loss of motion necessitating an adjustment in work and recreational activities.[143, 151, 159] Coxa magna of varying degree can occur in children with sufficient proximal femoral growth remaining, but it does not appear to influence patient function.[157]

### COMMONLY ASSOCIATED INJURIES

Dislocations that occur in trivial falls or with athletic activities rarely have associated injuries. Of the 67 dislocations discussed by Gartland and Benner, 9 had an associated fracture of the acetabulum, femoral head, or greater trochanter.[147] All these injuries were caused by high-energy trauma. Fracture of the ipsilateral femur is a relatively frequent association and often leads to a missed diagnosis of hip dislocation.[136, 160] In more severely injured patients, careful evaluation for head, chest, abdominal, and vascular trauma must be performed, as for any multiply injured individual (see Chapter 4). In children with significant head injury, diagnosis of a hip dislocation can be missed.[157] Associated fractures of the pelvis and upper and lower extremities in several locations have been reported.[3]

### CLASSIFICATION

Pediatric hip dislocations have traditionally been grouped according to age at injury (0 to 5 years, 5 to 10 years, 10 to 15 years), violence of the mechanism (see earlier), and direction of dislocation (anterior versus posterior). Hougaard and Thomsen[152] suggested using the Stewart-Milford[164] classification of hip dislocations to

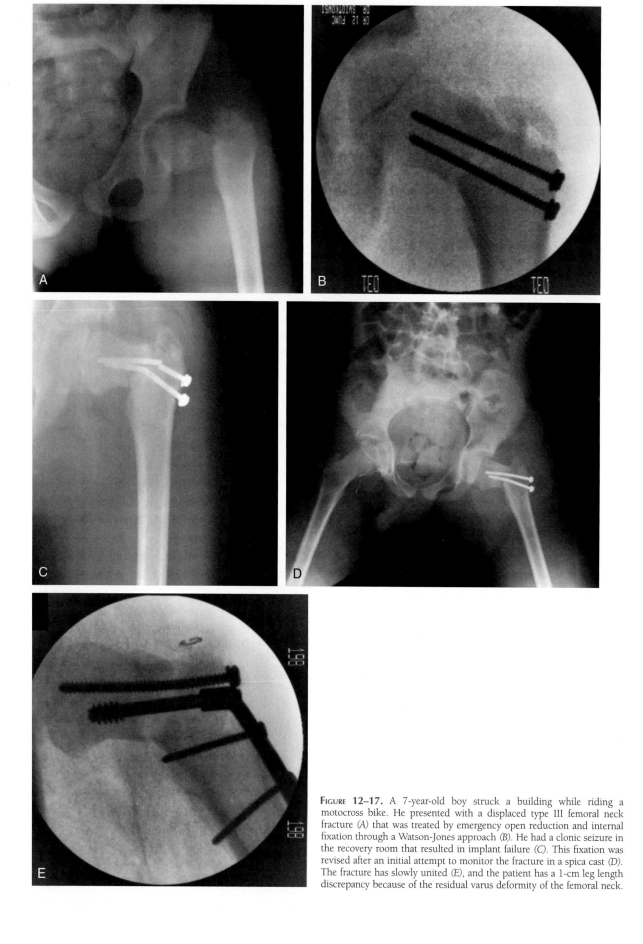

FIGURE 12–17. A 7-year-old boy struck a building while riding a motocross bike. He presented with a displaced type III femoral neck fracture (A) that was treated by emergency open reduction and internal fixation through a Watson-Jones approach (B). He had a clonic seizure in the recovery room that resulted in implant failure (C). This fixation was revised after an initial attempt to monitor the fracture in a spica cast (D). The fracture has slowly united (E), and the patient has a 1-cm leg length discrepancy because of the residual varus deformity of the femoral neck.

report associated acetabular fractures. No classification has been published specifically for hip dislocation in children.

The current classification is anterior (obturator, anteroinferior inguinal, anterosuperior) and posterior. The Stewart-Milford classification is as follows:

Grade I—No acetabular fracture or only a minor chip
Grade II—Posterior rim fracture, but stable after reduction
Grade III—Posterior rim fracture with hip instability after reduction
Grade IV—Dislocation accompanied by fracture of the femoral head and neck

When an acetabular fracture exists, the classification of Letournel and Judet[38] should be applied (see Fig. 12–14).

## Diagnosis

### HISTORY

The history associated with hip dislocation generally follows one of four lines. The accident that produces the complaint of groin and buttock pain can be a minor fall, such as on a slippery surface or doing "splits"; an athletic collision in football, wrestling, or baseball; a high-energy fall from a height; or being struck by a car or injured as a passenger. Two thirds of cases belong to the former groups of low-velocity injuries, which have the best prognosis.

### PHYSICAL EXAMINATION

Children who are the victims of high-energy trauma should be evaluated as outlined in Chapter 4. Ninety percent of hip dislocations are posterior, and the patient presents with the affected limb shortened, flexed, adducted, and internally rotated. In the more infrequent anterior dislocation, the limb is generally abducted, flexed, and externally rotated. The skin is inspected anteriorly and posteriorly for contusions, abrasions, and open wounds. The femoral, popliteal, dorsalis pedis, and posterior tibial pulses are palpated because common femoral arterial injury has been associated with hip dislocation.[137] In an alert and cooperative child, motor function is evaluated in the limb; the presence or absence (palpable contraction) of function in each major muscle group must be recorded. Finally, sensory function in response to light touch and pinprick is recorded, especially in the distal sciatic nerve distribution. This examination should be systematically repeated after attempted closed reduction.

### RADIOGRAPHIC EVALUATION

The AP pelvis examination is part of the initial evaluation in all patients who have sustained high-energy trauma with other injuries. The hip dislocation is apparent on this radiograph. A pelvis radiograph is requested for all children who present with the aforementioned physical

abnormalities. The radiograph is carefully studied for fractures of the femoral head, neck, and acetabulum. If an acetabular fracture is present, the 45° oblique views of Judet are obtained (see Fig. 12–7). After closed reduction, usually under general anesthesia, the AP pelvis radiograph is repeated to confirm a concentric reduction with symmetric joint space. A postreduction CT scan is obtained to rule out intra-articular loose bodies and fractures of the acetabulum and femoral head. In certain settings, when closed reduction has failed, it may be possible to perform CT before open reduction. This study is helpful to delineate loose bodies that need removal and acetabular fractures that may need stabilization. Reduction of the hip should never be delayed for more than an extra 45 to 60 minutes and should be done within the first 6 hours after injury, whenever possible.[144]

### SPECIAL STUDIES

A digitized technetium bone scan may be helpful for predicting avascular necrosis.[165] Although this technique has proven value in adult patients with femoral neck fractures, it has never been applied to a group of patients with hip dislocation (especially children), and its predictive value has yet to be defined. MRI has not proved to be of value in predicting avascular necrosis after femoral neck fracture in adults,[163] nor has its role in diagnosing avascular necrosis and monitoring the biologic progress of revascularization after pediatric hip dislocation been clarified. Arthrography of the hip may be useful to differentiate hip dislocation from type I proximal femoral fracture in children younger than 18 months. If an associated sciatic nerve injury is present, electromyography is helpful in defining the nature and severity of the injury a minimum of 3 weeks after injury. Arteriography is indicated when the screening physical examination with Doppler backup indicates a major proximal arterial injury.[156]

## Management

### EVOLUTION OF TREATMENT

Once sufficient experience regarding the management of hip dislocation in children was published,[141] the current standard of care was established—that is, closed reduction under general anesthesia and confirmation of concentric reduction radiographically. If reduction cannot be achieved or it is not stable or concentric, open reduction is indicated. Some evolution in the postreduction evaluation has occurred: a postreduction CT scan is now recommended to rule out loose bodies and femoral head and acetabular fracture. Developments have also occurred in reduction techniques, with some preferring skin traction to a formal closed reduction maneuver of the hip in young children. Most favor manipulative reduction for posterior dislocations and use traction with the leg in a flexed position. Great care must be taken to ensure that a nondisplaced associated femoral neck fracture is not displaced with attempted reduction.

No consensus has been reached regarding postreduction care. Bedrest, skin traction, skeletal traction, and a spica cast have all been recommended, with no clear advantage of any method. Generally, traumatic dislocations that are initially seen late should also be reduced.[138] The complication of recurrent dislocation has not been associated with any one method of postreduction treatment. For dislocations associated with displaced acetabular fractures with more than 2-mm displacement of the articular surface, most centers now recommend surgical reduction and stabilization (see under Pelvic Fractures and Dislocations).

Current treatment of pediatric hip dislocation dictates closed reduction under general anesthesia and postreduction evaluation of stability with an AP pelvis radiograph and CT scan. If reduction is not attainable, is unstable, or is associated with loose bodies, soft tissue interposition, or a displaced acetabular fracture, open reduction is recommended.

## SPECIAL CONSIDERATIONS FOR POLYTRAUMA PATIENTS

A dislocated hip, like a displaced femoral neck fracture, is a surgical emergency. Once the patient has been fully evaluated and any life-threatening head, chest, abdominal, and vascular injuries have been addressed, the hip must be reduced. Hip reduction should take precedence over all other orthopaedic problems because it can be done rapidly, especially if the child has been administered an anesthetic for any other reason. Urgency is appropriate inasmuch as it has been shown that the incidence of post-traumatic avascular necrosis is increased in hips that remain dislocated for more than 6 hours.[144]

## INDIVIDUAL TREATMENT OPTIONS

### Closed Reduction

**Indications.** An anterior or posterior dislocation noted on an AP pelvis radiograph is an indication for closed reduction. No absolute contraindications to this procedure are recognized, but if an associated displaced femoral neck fracture is noted, closed reduction will probably not succeed. In patients with a nondisplaced femoral neck fracture, the closed reduction must be gentle and done under fluoroscopic control to prevent displacing the fracture, and insertion of a percutaneous pin or screw (or two) should be considered in an effort to stabilize the fracture before closed reduction of the hip.

**Timing.** Whenever possible, the reduction should be performed within 6 hours of injury to minimize the risk of avascular necrosis.[99, 115]

**Preoperative Planning.** If an associated acetabular fracture is present, preoperative Judet views and a CT scan (if they can be done without causing significant delay) are helpful if the closed reduction is unsuccessful and open reduction is required.

**Anesthesia/Positioning.** General anesthesia with muscle relaxation is required. The patient should be positioned supine. The older or larger the patient, the

more important it is to have a surgical assistant available to stabilize the pelvis during traction.

**Technique.** If the child is older than 5 years or heavier than 50 pounds, an assistant is definitely required. The assistant provides countertraction by applying pressure with the palms of the hands on the anterior iliac crests. The surgeon flexes the hip 60° to 90° and applies traction with gentle internal and external rotation. In large adolescents, the increased force required can be provided by standing on the operating table and flexing the patient's knee between the surgeon's legs, grasping the limb just distal to the popliteal fossae with the knee bent, and using the surgeon's quadriceps and triceps surae to provide the traction necessary. The larger the patient, the more critical it is that the anesthesiologist provide excellent muscle relaxation. For posterior dislocation, the limb is in neutral position or is slightly adducted when traction is applied. The reduction maneuver differs for anterior dislocation in that traction is applied with the limb in the abducted position, and therefore the vector is somewhat lateral.

### Open Reduction

**Indications.** Indications include failed closed reduction, closed reduction that is not concentric,[140, 155, 157] dislocation with an associated displaced femoral neck fracture, and displaced acetabular fracture. (See under Pelvic Fractures and Dislocations and Proximal Femoral Fractures for details.)

**Timing.** Open reduction should be performed within 6 hours of injury or as soon as possible after the failed closed reduction.

**Preoperative Planning.** See earlier.

**Anesthesia/Positioning.** The patient is positioned on a beanbag in the lateral decubitus position with the injured hip up. General anesthesia is required.

**Technique.** A posterolateral, Kocher-Langenbeck approach is made to the hip. Great care must be taken in identifying the sciatic nerve distally and following it proximally, especially when neurologic deficits have been identified preoperatively. The nerve is carefully inspected in this setting and generally appears contused. The external rotators are evaluated and, if intact, divided 0.5 to 1 cm from their femoral insertion. Occasionally, if failure of closed reduction is the reason for the exploration, the piriformis tendon is displaced across the acetabulum and is blocking the reduction.[140, 155] The capsule is then inspected along with the labrum. Most commonly, the femoral head is buttonholed through the capsule, or the labrum is inverted. Once the soft tissue block is identified, the acetabulum must be evaluated for osteocartilaginous loose bodies. A bone hook or external fixator pin in the proximal end of the femur is helpful in laterally displacing the femoral head, and a headlamp helps with visualization. Small pituitary rongeurs make excellent grasping forceps. In older adolescents, a 5-mm Schanz screw can be inserted distal to the greater trochanteric physis and a universal chuck attached to the pin to provide lateral traction. At this point, posterior column or posterior wall fractures are reduced and internally fixed with smooth K-wires (with the ends bent to 90° to prevent migration) or small lag screws in younger children or with 2.7- or 3.5-mm lag screws and 2.7- or 3.5-mm reconstruction plates and/or one-third tubular plates as buttresses in older children (see Fig. 12–17).

## FOLLOW-UP CARE

**Immobilization.** Children younger than 6 years are immobilized in a one and one-half spica cast for 4 to 6 weeks. Older, cooperative children are placed on bedrest for 3 weeks and can then be mobilized with crutches for 3 to 4 additional weeks. Hip flexion greater than 60° should be avoided during this period, especially in the presence of posterior wall fractures.

**Mobilization.** After the 4 to 8 weeks of immobilization in a cast or with crutches, the patient can be mobilized with progressive weight bearing as tolerated. Casting is generally more appropriate for children younger than 10 years. No evidence has been presented that prolonged non–weight bearing affects the incidence or severity of avascular necrosis.[147]

**Physical Therapy.** Other than the institution of walker or crutch ambulation and hip flexion precautions, physical therapy probably does not influence the final functional result.

**Expected Duration of Disability.** Barring associated sciatic nerve injury or the complications of avascular necrosis or heterotopic ossification, one can expect the return of full function in children younger than 10 years by 3 months after injury. Adolescents, especially those who have undergone open reduction and internal fixation of an associated acetabular fracture through a posterolateral approach, may take 6 months to optimize function postoperatively.

**Timing of Implant Removal.** Though not absolutely mandatory, implants in young children should probably be removed within 6 months of surgery. In adolescents, the implants, plates, and screws can be safely left in place unless intra-articular hardware or the possibility of a later reconstructive procedure are concerns.

## Assessment of Results

**Functional and Anatomic Parameters.** Functional status assessment includes an evaluation of pain, fatigue, gait, weakness, and motion.[152] Radiographic analysis includes a direct evaluation of the hip for joint space, avascular changes in the femoral head, and osteophytes or sclerosis.[152] A suggested rating scale follows:

*Excellent*—Full motion; no pain, weakness, or fatigue; normal radiograph
*Good*—No appreciable pain in the hip (except after prolonged work or weight bearing), no greater than 25% loss of motion, slight osteoarthritic changes on radiographs, normal joint space, no avascular necrosis
*Fair*—Mild to moderate pain, moderate limping, moderate osteophytes, moderate narrowing of the joint space
*Poor*—Pain, limping, moderate to extreme limitation of motion, adduction deformity, advanced osteoarthritis,

avascular necrosis, narrowing of the joint space or sclerosis of the acetabulum

Whenever possible, validated outcome scales should be used (see Chapter 7).

## Expected Results

Few patients are reported in the literature who have been monitored for more than 5 years. Fifty of 248 children were monitored to skeletal maturity in Gartland and Benner's review.[147] Thirty-four were normal; 16 were not. Thirteen of the 16 had either a fracture about the hip or a delay in reduction of greater than 24 hours. The incidence of avascular necrosis in numerous published series is 8% to 10%. This complication is more common in older children, with delay in reduction, and with greater severity of injury.[146, 147] Twelve of 13 patients monitored for 5 to 26 years by Hougaard and Thomsen underwent reduction within 6 hours of injury and had normal hips.[152] Osteoarthritis developed in one patient with a reduction at 37 hours.

## Complications

Complications include sciatic nerve injury, avascular necrosis, osteoarthritis, and recurrent dislocation.

## TREATMENT

**Sciatic Nerve Injury.** An incidence of 24% was reported by Pearson and Mann.[158] All cases involved sensory or motor deficiency or both. All five patients had improvement in function, and in one, function returned to normal. No effective treatment has been published. Neurolysis may have a role if improvement is not forthcoming by 3 to 6 months after injury.

**Avascular Necrosis.** Avascular necrosis is the most common complication[143, 151] and is generally apparent by 3 to 6 months after injury. Patients must be examined quarterly for the first year and then annually until 4 to 5 years after injury if they are asymptomatic. Early weight bearing does not influence the rate of this complication. Younger patients with this complication fare better than older ones.[146, 147] No effective treatment is available, but acetabular or femoral osteotomy should be considered.

**Osteoarthritis.** This complication appears to be associated with a delay in reduction.[136] It is apparent only with follow-up in the 5- to 20-year range. In one retrospective review involving adolescents and adults, osteoarthritis was more prevalent in individuals who preformed manual labor; therefore, career counseling may be beneficial for individuals with hip dislocation.[166] Treatment of post-traumatic osteoarthritis is symptomatic whenever possible: weight control, modification of activity, walking aids, and anti-inflammatory medications. Surgical management should be delayed as long as possible. Options include arthrodesis, osteotomy, and arthroplasty.

**Recurrent Dislocation.** This complication has been reported in 12 children; it generally occurs in those younger than 8 years[136] and has generally been posterior in orientation.[132, 134, 135, 142, 148, 150, 162] Recurrent anterior dislocation has been reported.[142] No clear increase in incidence has been noted with more severe trauma or an inadequate period of immobilization. Although surgical exploration with repair of the posterior capsule is effective (with follow-up of less than 2 years),[148, 162] conservative care has been effective as well.[135, 150] The recommendation, therefore, is for a CT scan after the first recurrence and subsequent reduction. If the reduction is symmetric with no loose bodies, a spica cast should be applied for 6 weeks with the hip abducted 20° to 30° and flexed 45°. Patients who have a recurrence thereafter should have posterior capsular reefing.

## REFERENCES

### Pelvic Fractures and Dislocations

1. Abou-Jaoude, W.A.; Sugarman, J.M.; Fallat, M.E.; Casale, A.J. Indicators of genitourinary tract injury or anomaly in cases of pediatric blunt trauma. J Pediatr Surg 31:86–90, 1996.
2. Apprahamian, C.; Gessert, G.; Bandyk, D.F.; et al. MAST associated compartment syndrome (MACS): A review. J Trauma 29:549–555, 1989.
3. Barrett, I.R.; Goldberg, J.A. Avulsion fracture of the ligamentum teres in a child. J Bone Joint Surg Am 71:438–439, 1989.
4. Batislam, E.; Ates, Y.; Germiyangolu, C.; et al. Role of Tile classification in predicting urethral injuries in pediatric pelvic fractures. J Trauma 42:285–287, 1997.
5. Ben-Menachem, Y.; Caldwell, D.M.; Young, J.W.R.; Burgess, A.R. Hemorrhage associated with pelvic fractures: Causes, diagnosis and emergent management. Am J Radiol 157:1005–1014, 1991.
6. Blair, W.; Hanson, C. Traumatic closure of the triradiate cartilage: Report of a case. J Bone Joint Surg Am 61:144–145, 1979.
7. Bond, S.I.; Gotschall, C.S.; Eichelberger, M.R. Predictors of abdominal injury in children with pelvic fracture. J Trauma 31:1169–1173, 1991.
8. Brenneman, F.D.; Katyal, D.; Boulanger, B.R.; et al. Long-term outcomes in open pelvic fractures. J Trauma 42:773–777, 1997.
9. Brooks, E.; Rosman, M. Central fracture-dislocation of the hip in a child. J Trauma 28:1590–1592, 1988.
10. Brunette, D.D.; Fifield, G.; Ruiz, E. Use of pneumatic antishock trousers in the management of pediatric pelvic hemorrhage. Pediatr Emerg Care 3:86–90, 1987.
11. Bryan, W.J.; Tullos, H.S. Pediatric pelvic fractures: Review of 52 patients. J Trauma 19:799–805, 1979.
12. Bucholz, R.W.; Ezaki, M.; Ogden, J.A. Injury to the acetabular triradiate physeal cartilage. J Bone Joint Surg Am 64:600–609, 1982.
13. Burgess, A.R.; Eastridge, B.J.; Young, J.W.R.; et al. Pelvic ring disruptions: Effective classification system and treatment protocols. J Trauma 30:848–856, 1990.
14. Compere, E.L.; Garrison, M.; Fahey, J.J. Deformities of the femur resulting from arrestment of growth of the capital and greater trochanteric epiphyses. J Bone Joint Surg 22:909–915, 1940.
15. Copeland, C.E.; Bosse, M.J.; McCarthy, M.L.; et al. Effect of trauma and pelvic fracture on female genitourinary, sexual, and reproductive function. J Orthop Trauma 11:73–81, 1997.
16. Cotler, H.B.; LaMont, J.G.; Hansen, S.T. Immediate spica casting for pelvic fractures. J Orthop Trauma 2:222–228, 1988.
17. Craig, C.L. Hip injuries in children and adolescents. Orthop Clin North Am 11:799–805, 1979.
18. Currey, J.D.; Butler, G. The mechanical properties of bone tissue in children. J Bone Joint Surg Am 57:810–814, 1975.
19. Dora, C.; Zurbach, J.; Hersche, O.; Ganz, R. Pathomorphologic characteristics of post-traumatic acetabular dysplasia. J Orthop Trauma 14:483–489, 2000.
20. Ebraheim, N.A.; Coombs, R.; Jackson, W.T.; Rusin, J.J. Percutaneous computed tomography–guided stabilization of posterior pelvic fractures. Clin Orthop 307:222–228, 1994.
21. Ebraheim, N.A.; Coombs, R.J.; Jackson, W.T.; Holiday, B. Percutaneous computed-tomography stabilization of pelvic fractures: Preliminary report. J Orthop Trauma 1:197–204, 1987.
22. Ehrensperger, J. Fractures of the sacrum and disc herniation: Rare lesions in the pediatric surgical patient? Eur J Pediatr Surg 2:173–176, 1992.
23. Elton, R.C. Fracture-dislocation of the pelvis followed by nonunion of the posterior iliac spine. J Bone Joint Surg Am 54:648–649, 1972.
24. Ganz, R.; Gerber, C. Fehlverheilte kindliche Frakturen im Becken und Huftbereich. Orthopade 20:346–352, 1991.
25. Ganz, R.; Krushell, R.J.; Jakob, R.P.; Kuffer, J. The antishock pelvic clamp. Clin Orthop 267:71–78, 1991.
26. Garvin, K.L.; McCarthy, R.E.; Barnes, C.L.; Dodge, B.M. Pediatric pelvic ring fractures. J Pediatric Orthop 10:577–582, 1990.
27. Godfrey, J.D. Trauma in children. J Bone Joint Surg Am 46:422–447, 1964.
28. Habacker, T.A.; Heinrich, S.D.; Dehne, R. Fracture of the superior pelvic quadrant in a child. J Pediatr Orthop 15:69–72, 1995.
29. Hallel, T.; Salvati, E.A. Premature closure of the triradiate cartilage: A case report and animal experiment. Clin Orthop 124:278–281, 1977.
30. Harrison, T.J. The influence of the femoral head on pelvic growth and acetabular form in the rat. J Anat 95:12–26, 1961.
31. Heeg, M.; Klasen, H.J.; Visser, J.D. Acetabular fractures in children and adolescents. J Bone Joint Surg Br 71:418–421, 1989.
32. Heeg, M.; Viser, J.D.; Oostvogel, H.J.M. Injuries of the acetabular triradiate cartilage and sacroiliac joint. J Bone Joint Surg Br 70:34–37, 1988.
33. Heinrich, S.D.; Sharps, C.H.; Cardea, J.A.; Gervin, A.S. Open pelvic fracture with vaginal laceration and diaphragmatic rupture in a child. J Orthop Trauma 2:257–261, 1988.
34. Ismail, N.; Bellemare, J.F.; Mollitt, D.L.; et al. Death from pelvic fracture: Children are different. J Pediatr Surg 31:82–85, 1996.
35. Keshishyan, R.A.; Rozinov, V.M.; Malakhov, O.A.; et al. Pelvic polyfractures in children—radiographic diagnosis and treatment. Clin Orthop 320:28–33, 1995.
36. Kricun, M.E. Fractures of the pelvis. Orthop Clin North Am 21:573–589, 1990.
37. Laurent, L.E. Growth disturbances of the proximal end of the femur in the light of animal experiments. Acta Orthop Scand 28:255–261, 1959.
38. Letournel, E.; Judet, R. Fractures of the Acetabulum. Berlin, Springer-Verlag, 1981.
39. Lindseth, R.E.; Rosene, H.A., Jr. Traumatic separation of the upper femoral epiphysis in a newborn infant. J Bone Joint Surg Am 53:1641–1644, 1971.
40. Mader, T.J. Avulsion of the rectus femoris tendon: An unusual type of pelvic fracture. Pediatr Emerg Care 6:198–199, 1990.
41. Mader, T.J. Avulsion of the rectus femoris tendon: An unusual type of pelvic fracture [letter]. Pediatr Emerg Care 7:126, 1991.
42. Magid, D.; Fishman, E.K.; Ney, D.R.; et al. Acetabular and pelvic fractures in the pediatric patient: Value of two and three dimensional imaging. J Pediatr Orthop 12:621–625, 1992.
43. Martin, J.A.; Pipkin, G. Treatment of avulsion of the ischial tuberosity. Clin Orthop 10:108–118, 1957.
44. Matta, J.M.; Saucedo, T. Internal fixation of pelvic ring fractures. Clin Orthop 242:83–97, 1989.
45. Matta, J.M.; Mehne, O.K.; Roff, R. Fractures of the acetabulum: Early results of a prospective study. Clin Orthop 205:241–250, 1986.
46. Maull, K.I.; Sachatello, C.R.; Earnst, C.B. The deep perineal laceration—an injury frequently associated with open pelvic fractures: A need for aggressive surgical management. J Trauma 17:685–696, 1977.
47. McDonald, G.A. Pelvic disruptions in children. Clin Orthop 151:130–134, 1980.

48. McIntyre, R.C.; Bensard, D.D.; Moore, E.E.; et al. Pelvic fracture geometry predicts risk of life threatening hemorrhage in children. J Trauma 35:423–429, 1993.
49. Mosheiff, R.; Suchar, A.; Porat, S.; et al. The "crushed open pelvis" in children. Injury 30(Suppl):B14–B18, 1999.
50. Musemeche, C.A.; Fischer, R.P.; Cotler, H.B.; Andrassy, R.J. Selective management of pediatric pelvic fractures: A conservative approach. J Pediatric Surg 22:538–540, 1987.
51. Niemi, T.A.; Norton, L.W. Vaginal injuries in patients with pelvic fractures. J Trauma 25:547–551, 1985.
52. Ogden, J.A. Changing patterns of proximal femoral vascularity. J Bone Joint Surg Am 56:941–950, 1974.
53. Ponsetti, I.V. Growth and development of the acetabulum in the normal child. J Bone Joint Surg Am 60:575–585, 1978.
54. Quinby, W.C., Jr. Fractures of the pelvis and associated injuries in children. J Pediatr Surg 1:353–364, 1966.
55. Rangger, C.; Gabl, M.; Dolati, B.; et al. Kindliche Beckenfracturen. Unfallchirurg 97:649–651, 1994.
56. Reed, M.H. Pelvic fractures in children. J Can Assoc Radiol 27:255–261, 1976.
57. Reff, R.B. The use of external fixation devices in the management of severe lower-extremity trauma and pelvic injuries in children. Clin Orthop 188:21–33, 1984.
58. Reichard, S.A.; Helikson, M.A.; Shorter, N.; et al. Pelvic fractures in children: Review of 120 patients with a new look at general management. J Pediatr Surg 15:727–734, 1980.
59. Rieger, H.; Brugg, E. Fractures of the pelvis in children. Clin Orthop 336:226–239, 1997.
60. Rodrigues, K.F. Injury of the acetabular epiphysis. Injury 4:258–260, 1973.
61. Rogge, E.A.; Romano, R.L. Avulsion of the ischial apophysis. J Bone Joint Surg Am 38:442, 1956.
62. Rothenberger, D.A.; Velasco, R.; Strate, R. Open pelvic fractures: A lethal injury. J Trauma 18:184–187, 1978.
63. Routt, M.L.; Kregor, P.J.; Simonian, P.T.; Mayo, K.A. Early results of percutaneous iliosacral screws with the patient in the supine position. J Orthop Trauma 9:207–214, 1995.
64. Routt, M.L.; Meier, M.C.; Kregor, P.K.; Mayo, K.A. Percutaneous iliosacral screws with the patient supine technique. Operat Tech Orthop 3:35–45, 1993.
65. Routt, M.L., Jr.; Swiontkowski, M.F. The treatment of complex acetabular fractures using combined simultaneous anterior and posterior surgical approaches. J Bone Joint Surg Am 72:897–904, 1990.
66. Scuderi, J.G.; Bronson, M.J. Triradiate cartilage injury: Report of two cases and review of the literature. Clin Orthop 217:179–189, 1987.
67. Slatis, P.; Huittinen, V.M. Double vertical fractures of the pelvis: A report on 163 patients. Acta Chir Scand 138:799–807, 1972.
68. Tile, M. Fractures of the Pelvis and Acetabulum. Baltimore, Williams & Wilkins, 1984.
69. Tile, M. Pelvic ring fractures: Should they be fixed? J Bone Joint Surg Br 70:1–12, 1988.
70. Tolo, V.T. Orthopaedic treatment of fractures of the long bones and pelvis in children who have multiple injuries. J Bone Joint Surg Am 82:272–280, 2000.
71. Torode, I.; Zieg, D. Pelvic fractures in children. J Pediatr Orthop 5:76–84, 1985.
72. Trueta, J. The normal vascular anatomy of the femoral head during growth. J Bone Joint Surg Br 39:358–393, 1957.
73. Trunkey, D.D.; Chapman, M.W.; Lim, R.C.; et al. Management of pelvic fractures in blunt trauma injury. J Trauma 14:912–923, 1974.
74. Vazquez, D.W.; Garcia, V.F. Pediatric pelvic fractures combined with an additional skeletal injury is an indicator of significant injury. Surg Gynecol Obstet 177:468–472, 1993.
75. Watts, H.G. Fractures of the pelvis in children. Orthop Clin North Am 7:615–624, 1976.
76. Winquist, R.A.; Hansen, S.T.; Pearson, R.C. Closed intramedullary shortening of the femur. Clin Orthop 136:54–61, 1978.
77. Wojtowycz, M.; Starshak, R.J.; Sty, J.R. Neonatal proximal femoral epiphysiolysis. Radiology 136:647–648, 1980.
78. Wolcott, W.E. The evolution of the circulation in the developing femoral head and neck. Surg Gynecol Obstet 77:61–68, 1943.
79. Young, J.W.R.; Burgess, A.R.; Brumback, R.J.; Poka, A. Lateral compression fractures of the pelvis: The importance of plain radiographs in the diagnosis and surgical management. Skeletal Radiol 15:103–109, 1986.

**Proximal Femoral Fractures**

80. Allende, G.; Lezama, L.G. Fractures of the neck of the femur in children. A clinical study. J Bone Joint Surg 33:387–395, 1951.
81. Canale, S.T. Fractures of the hip in children and adolescents. Orthop Clin North Am 21:341–352, 1990.
82. Canale, S.T.; Bourland, W.I. Fracture of the neck and intertrochanteric region of the femur in children. J Bone Joint Surg Am 59:431–443, 1977.
83. Carrell, B.; Carrell, W.B. Fractures in the neck of the femur in children with particular reference to aseptic necrosis. J Bone Joint Surg 23:225–239, 1941.
84. Cheng, J.C.M.; Tang, N. Decompression and stable internal fixation of femoral neck fractures in children can affect the outcome. J Pediatr Orthop 19:338–343, 1999.
85. Chong, K.C.; Chaca, P.B.; Lee, B.T. Fractures of the neck of the femur in childhood and adolescence. Injury 7:111–119, 1975.
86. Colonna, P.C. Fracture of the neck of the femur in children. Am J Surg 6:793–797, 1929.
87. Compere, E.L.; Garrison, M.; Fahey, J.J. Deformities of the femur resulting from arrestment of growth of the capital and greater trochanteric epiphyses. J Bone Joint Surg 22:909–915, 1940.
88. Craig, C.L. Hip injuries in children and adolescents. Orthop Clin North Am 11:743–754, 1980.
89. Davison, B.L.; Weinstein, S.L. Hip fractures in children: A long-term follow-up study. J Pediatr Orthop 12:353–358, 1992.
90. Delbet, M.P. Fractures du col de femur. Bull Mem Soc Chir 35:387–389, 1907.
91. DeLuca, F.N.; Keck, C. Traumatic coxa vara. A case report of spontaneous correction in a child. Clin Orthop 116:125–128, 1976.
92. Durbin, F.C. Avascular necrosis complicating undisplaced fractures of the neck of femur in children. J Bone Joint Surg Br 41:758–762, 1959.
93. Forlin, E.; Guille, J.T.; Kumar, S.J.; Rhee, K.J. Complications associated with fracture of the neck of the femur in children. J Pediatr Orthop 12:503–509, 1992.
94. Gamble, J.G.; Lettice, J.; Smith, J.T.; Rinsky, L.A. Transverse cervicopertrochanter hip fracture. J Pediatr Orthop 11:779–782, 1991.
95. Gaudinez, R.F.; Heinrich, S.D. Transphyseal fracture of the capital femoral epiphysis. Orthopedics 12:599–602, 1989.
96. Gerber, C.; Lehmann, A.; Ganz, R. Femoral neck fractures in children: A multicenter follow-up study. Z Orthop 123:767, 1985.
97. Hamilton, C.M. Fractures of the neck of the femur in children. JAMA 178:799–801, 1961.
98. Heiser, J.M.; Oppenheimer W.L. Fractures of the hip in children: A review of forty cases. Clin Orthop 149:177–184, 1980.
99. Honton, J.L. Les fractures transcervicales recentes du femur. Rev Chir Orthop 72:3–51, 1986.
100. Ingram, A.J.; Bachynski, B. Fractures of the hip in children. Treatment and results. J Bone Joint Surg 35:867–887, 1953.
101. Joseph, B.; Mulpari, K. Delayed separation of the capital femoral epiphysis after an ipsilateral transcervical fracture of the femoral neck. J Orthop Trauma 14:446–448, 2000.
102. Kay, S.P.; Hall, J.E. Fracture of the femoral neck in children and its complications. Clin Orthop 80:53–59, 1971.
103. Kujat, R.; G-Suren, E.; Rogge, D.; Tscherne, H. Die Schenkelhalsfraktur im Wachstumsalter—Behandulungsprinzipien, Ergebnisse, Prognose. Chirurg 55:43–48, 1984.
104. Lam, S.F. Fractures of the neck in the femur in children. J Bone Joint Surg Am 53:1165–1179, 1971.
105. Lam, S.F. Fractures of the neck of the femur in children. Orthop Clin North Am 7:625–632, 1976.
106. Leung, P.C.; Lam, S.F. Long-term follow-up of children with femoral neck fractures. J Bone Joint Surg Br 68:537–540, 1986.
107. Lindseth, R.E.; Rosene, H.A., Jr. Traumatic separation of the upper femoral epiphysis in a newborn infant. J Bone Joint Surg Am 53:1641–1644, 1971.

108. Manninger, J.; Kazar, G.; Nagy, E.; Zolczer, L. Phlebography for fracture of the femoral neck in adolescence. Injury 5:244–254, 1973.
109. Marsh, H.O. Intertrochanteric and femoral-neck fractures in children. J Bone Joint Surg Am 49:1024, 1967.
110. McDougall, A. Fractures of the neck of femur in childhood. J Bone Joint Surg Br 43:16–28, 1961.
111. Milgram, J.W.; Lyne, E.D. Epiphysiolysis of the proximal femur in very young children. Clin Orthop 110:146–153, 1975.
112. Miller, W.E. Fractures of the hip in children from birth to adolescence. Clin Orthop 92:155–188, 1973.
113. Mitchell, J.I. Fracture of the neck of the femur in children. JAMA 107:1603–1606, 1936.
114. Morrissy, R. Hip fractures in children. Clin Orthop 152:202–210, 1980.
115. Niethard, F.U. Pathophysiologie und Prognose von Schenkelhalsfrakturen im Kindesalter. Unfallheilkunde 158:221–279, 1982.
116. Ogden, J.A. Changing patterns of proximal femoral vascularity. J Bone Joint Surg Am 56:941–950, 1974.
117. Ovesen, O.; Arreskov, J.; Bellstrom, T. Hip fractures in children: A long-term follow-up of 17 cases. Orthopedics 12:361–367, 1989.
118. Pape H.C.; Kretteck C.; Friedrich A.; et al. Long-term outcome in children with fractures of the proximal femur after high-energy trauma. J Trauma 46:58–84, 1999.
119. Pforringer, W.; Rosemeyer, H. Fractures of the hip in children and adolescents. Acta Orthop Scand 51:91–108, 1980.
120. Quinlan, W.R.; Brady, P.G.; Regan, B.F. Fractures of the neck of the femur in childhood. Injury 11:242–247, 1980.
121. Raju, K.K.; Tepler, M.; Dharapak, C.; Pearlman, H.S. Transepiphyseal fracture of the hips in children. Orthop Rev 13:33–45, 1984.
122. Ratliff, A.H.C. Traumatic separation of the upper femoral epiphysis in young children. J Bone Joint Surg Br 50:757–770, 1968.
123. Ratliff, A.H.C. Fractures of the neck of the femur in children. J Bone Joint Surg Br 44:528–542, 1962.
124. Ratliff, A.H.C. Fractures of the neck of the femur in children. Orthop Clin North Am 5:903–921, 1974.
125. Russell, R.H. A clinical lecture on fracture of the neck of the femur in childhood. Lancet 2:125–126, 1898.
126. Swiontkowski, M.F. Complications of hip fractures in children. Compl Orthop 4:58–64, 1989.
127. Swiontkowski, M.F.; Winquist, R.A. Displaced hip fractures in children and adolescents. J Trauma 26:384–388, 1986.
128. Thompson, G.H.; Bachner, E.J.; Ballock, R.T. Salter-Harris II fractures of the capital femoral epiphysis. J Orthop Trauma 14:510–513, 2000.
129. Trueta, J. The normal vascular anatomy of the femoral head during growth. J Bone Joint Surg Br 39:358–393, 1957.
130. Weber, U.; Rettig, H.; Brudet, J. Die Schenkelhalsfraktur im Kindesalter—Teil II: Nachuntersuchungsergebnisse. Unfallchirurg 88:512–517, 1985.
131. Weiner, D.S.; O'Dell, H.W. Fractures of the hip in children. J Trauma 9:62–76, 1969.
132. Whitman, R. Observations on fracture of the neck of the femur in children with special reference to treatment and differential diagnosis from separation of the epiphysis. Med Rec 43:227–230, 1893.
133. Wilson, J.C. Fractures of the neck of the femur in childhood. J Bone Joint Surg 22:531–546, 1940.

**Hip Dislocations**

134. Aufranc, O.E.; Jones, W.N.; Harris, H.H. Recurrent dislocation of the hip in the child. JAMA 190:291–294, 1964.
135. Barquet, A. Recurrent traumatic dislocation of the hip in childhood. J Trauma 20:1003–1006, 1980.
136. Barquet, A. Traumatic hip dislocation in childhood. A report of 26 cases and a review of the literature. Acta Orthop Scand 50:549–553, 1979.
137. Bonnemaison, M.F.E.; Henderson, E.D. Traumatic anterior dislocation of the hip with acute common femoral occlusion in a child. J Bone Joint Surg Am 50:753–755, 1968.
138. Bunnell, W.P.; Webster, D.A. Late reduction of bilateral traumatic hip dislocations in a child. Clin Orthop 147:160–163, 1980.

139. Byram, G.; Wickstrom, J. Traumatic dislocation of the hip in children. South Med J 60:805–810, 1967.
140. Canale, S.T.; Manugian, A.H. Irreducible traumatic dislocations of the hip. J Bone Joint Surg Am 61:7–14, 1979.
141. Choyce, C.C. Traumatic dislocation of the hip in childhood and relation of trauma to pseudocoxalgia: Analysis of 59 cases published up to Jan., 1924. Br J Surg 12:52–59, 1924.
142. Dall, D.; McNab, I.; Gross, A. Recurrent anterior dislocation of the hip. J Bone Joint Surg Am 52:574–576, 1970.
143. Elmslie, R.C. Traumatic dislocation of the hip in a child aged seven with subsequent development of coxa plana. Proc R Soc Med 25:1100–1102, 1932.
144. Epstein, H.C. Traumatic dislocations of the hip. Clin Orthop 92:116–142, 1973.
145. Freeman, G.E. Traumatic dislocation of the hip in children. J Bone Joint Surg Am 43:401–406, 1961.
146. Funk, F.J. Traumatic dislocation of the hip in children: Factors influencing prognosis and treatment. J Bone Joint Surg Am 44:1135–1145, 1962.
147. Gartland, J.J.; Benner, J.H. Traumatic dislocations in the lower extremity in children. Orthop Clin North Am 7:687–700, 1976.
148. Gaul, R.W. Recurrent traumatic dislocations of the hip in children. Clin Orthop 90:107–109, 1973.
149. Glass, A.; Powell, H.D.W. Traumatic dislocation of the hip in children: An analysis of 47 patients. J Bone Joint Surg Br 43:29–37, 1961.
150. Graham, B.; Lapp, R.A. Recurrent post-traumatic dislocation of the hip: A report of two cases and review of the literature. Clin Orthop 256:115–119, 1990.
151. Haliburton, R.A.; Brockenshire, F.A.; Barber, J.R. Avascular necrosis of the femoral capital epiphysis after traumatic dislocation of the hip in children. J Bone Joint Surg Br 43:43–46, 1961.
152. Hougaard, K.; Thomsen, P.B. Traumatic hip dislocation in children: Follow-up of 13 cases. Orthopedics 12:375–378, 1989.
153. MacFarlane, I.J.A. Survey of traumatic dislocation of the hip in children. J Bone Joint Surg Br 58:267, 1976.
154. Mason, M.L. Traumatic dislocation of the hip in childhood: Report of a case. J Bone Joint Surg Br 36:630–632, 1954.
155. Nelson, M.C.; Lauerman, W.C.; Brower, A.C.; Wells, J.R. Avulsion of the acetabular labrum with intraarticular displacement. Orthopedics 13:889–891, 1990.
156. Nerubay, J. Traumatic anterior dislocation of hip joint with vascular damage. Clin Orthop 116:129–132, 1976.
157. Offierski, C.M. Traumatic dislocation of the hip in children. J Bone Joint Surg Br 63:194–197, 1981.
158. Pearson, D.E.; Mann, R.J. Traumatic hip dislocation in children. Clin Orthop 92:189–194, 1973.
159. Pennsylvania Orthopaedic Society. Traumatic dislocation of the hip joint in children. J Bone Joint Surg Am 42:705–710, 1960.
160. Piggot, J. Traumatic dislocation of the hip in childhood. J Bone Joint Surg Br 43:38–42, 1961.
161. Sahin, V.; Karakas, E.S.; Turk, C.Y. Bilateral traumatic hip dislocation in a child: A case report and review of the literature. J Trauma 46:500–504, 1999.
162. Simmons, R.L.; Elder, J.D. Recurrent post-traumatic dislocation of the hip in children. South Med J 65:1463–1466, 1972.
163. Speer, K.P.; Spritzer, C.E.; Harrelson, J.M.; Nunley, J.A. Magnetic resonance imaging of the femoral head after acute intracapsular fracture of the femoral neck. J Bone Joint Surg Am 72:98–103, 1990.
164. Stewart, M.J.; Milford, L.W. Fracture dislocation of the hip. J Bone Joint Surg Am 36:315–342, 1954.
165. Strömqvist, B. Femoral head vitality after intracapsular hip fracture. 490 cases studied by intravital tetracycline labeling and Tc-MDP radionuclide imaging. Acta Orthop Scand Suppl 200:1–71, 1983.
166. Upadhyay, S.S.; Moulton, A.; Srikrishnamurthy, K. An analysis of the late effects of traumatic posterior dislocations of the hip without fractures. J Bone Joint Surg Br 65:150–152, 1983.
167. Wilson, D.W. Traumatic dislocation of the hip in children: A report of four cases. J Trauma 6:739–743, 1966.
168. Young, N.L.; Wright, L.G. Measuring pediatric physical fractures. J Pediatr Orthop 15:244–253, 1995.

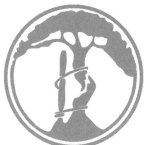

CHAPTER 13

# Fractures of the Femoral Shaft

M.L. Chip Routt, Jr., M.D.
Thomas A. Schildhauer, M.D.

Femoral shaft fractures in children continue to challenge orthopaedic surgeons. Conservative management has historically been advocated, with good results in most cases. Strategies used have included traction, splinting, and spica casting.[1, 11, 15, 24, 48, 49, 63, 65, 108] As knowledge of physiology, biomechanics, and skeletal development has expanded, the healing of pediatric femoral fractures and thus the foundation for these good results have become better understood. The orthopaedic literature is replete with reports of the outcomes of specific treatment protocols.* Other authors have noted complications of both the fracture and different treatment methods.† Skin problems, Volkmann's ischemia, pin tract infections, malunion, and other complications have been identified. Operative treatment has historically been condemned.[11, 24]

Improvements in operative technology have influenced the management of injured children. In general, children with isolated, low-energy pediatric femoral shaft fractures are treated according to accepted conservative methods, whereas polytraumatized children with femoral fractures are managed more aggressively. Operative methods must also be considered in children with numerous bony injuries to avoid prolonged immobilization.[8]

## ANATOMY AND DEVELOPMENT

Embryonic growth of the femur begins during the fourth week of gestation with the appearance of the limb bud. Rapid mesenchymal growth ensues, and endochondral ossification occurs during the eighth gestational week. Fetal development may be monitored with ultrasonography to assess femoral growth sequentially. The femoral

shaft serves as the primary ossification center, with ossification progressing circumferentially and producing trabecular bone. Ossification of the secondary centers of growth begins in the upper epiphysis at 6 months of gestational age. The distal femoral ossification center develops in the seventh month, and longitudinal and peripheral growth continues. Because of its trabecular nature and cartilage content, the femur is sufficiently malleable to accommodate passage through the birth canal. With maturation and development, the composition of the femur changes. The bone becomes more like adult bone, with less flexibility and more mineral content. The trabecular bone is remodeled along lines of stress into lamellar bone. This process increases the rigidity of the femur and its tensile strength. The greater trochanteric apophysis ossifies by 4 years of age, whereas ossification of the lesser trochanteric apophysis is usually seen radiographically by 10 years of age. Longitudinal and peripheral growth continues until skeletal maturity. The femur contributes approximately 26% of adult height.

The femoral shaft blood supply consists of endosteal (medullary) and periosteal vessels. The large muscular cuff of the thigh, together with the thick periosteum of the child's femur, provides excellent vascularity. Two nutrient arteries generally supply the femoral diaphysis, both entering posteromedially. They enter the medullary canal of the femur at the junction of the proximal and middle thirds and the distal and middle thirds of the femoral shaft. This abundant blood supply aids in both growth and healing of the skeletally immature femur. Biologically, active periosteum and osseous vascularity promote rapid formation and remodeling of callus in pediatric femoral shaft fractures.

Along with growth and vascular changes in the femur during development, architectural changes appear. Both the neck-shaft orientation and anteversion of the neck decrease with growth. In early childhood, neck-shaft angles are typically 150° and femoral anteversion begins at about 40°, with a decrease by the end of adolescence

---

*See references 1, 2, 15, 18, 24, 48, 49, 51, 63, 65, 72, 75, 76, 79, 97, 98, 106, 113, 121.
†See references 6, 16, 20, 50, 59, 89, 91, 99, 104, 107, 118.

to a neck-shaft angle of 130° ± 7° and 10° ± 4° of anteversion. The anterior curvature (mean 2.2 meter radius of curvature) of the femur is maintained during development. These unique features of the developing femur are vital to remember when planning management of pediatric femoral shaft fractures.

## INJURY

Most fractures in children are the result of accidents. Accidents are the leading cause of childhood mortality and rank second to acute infection as the cause of morbidity and visits to physicians throughout childhood.[3, 43, 44, 66, 78, 82] Almost half of all deaths in childhood are the result of accidents, as opposed to about 10% in adults, according to Gratz.[43] Between the ages of 1 and 15 years, accidents are the number one cause of death and injury to children.[41] Izant and Hubay stated that "Accidental injury is one of the poorest understood and most serious social, economic, and medical phenomenon of current times."[66] Unfortunately, minimal funding is directed to accident prevention research in children; therefore, accidents will probably continue to be responsible for high numbers of pediatric femoral shaft fractures in the future.[48] In 1990, 237,000 children younger than 15 years were treated at hospital emergency rooms for injuries related to playground equipment. Most of these injuries (58%) occurred after falls from swings or monkey bars.[3] Accidents of this type can be responsible for femoral shaft fractures, but these injuries also occur in auto-pedestrian, auto-bicycle, unrestrained auto passenger, and other high-energy mishaps. Associated injuries may complicate the management of pediatric femoral shaft fractures, and the treating physician must be aware of a 4% incidence of associated ipsilateral knee ligament injuries.[13] Incidental low-energy accidents may cause femoral shaft fractures in children with pathologic bone lesions.[27, 29] In his classic text on fractures in children, Blount stated that approximately 70% of pediatric femoral fractures are diaphyseal.[11]

The incidence of pediatric femoral shaft fractures varies according to the age and gender of the child. In a report of 851 femoral shaft fractures in children, the incidence peaked at 2 to 3 years of age, whereas the total incidence was 2.6 times higher in boys than girls.[55] The mechanisms of injury also vary according to age group. Accidental falls were the leading cause of femoral fractures in children aged 2 to 3 years, whereas traffic accidents were most common in the older age groups, with an incidence of 3.7 fractures per 10,000 population noted annually in boys 16 and 17 years of age.[55]

Femoral shaft fractures are commonly isolated injuries or are associated with minor trauma such as abrasions and contusions. High-velocity trauma in children produces unstable fracture patterns, with a constellation of other more severe and often life-threatening injuries. Blount recognized that fracture patterns and concomitant injury patterns reflect the mechanism of injury.[11] Treatment algorithms are therefore different for these two populations of children with femoral shaft fractures.

Child abuse causes a spectrum of injuries, including fractures of the femoral shaft. The incidence of child battering is estimated at 500,000 new cases annually.[90] According to Green and Haggerty, an abused child has a 50% chance of further battering and a 10% chance of death when returned home without proper therapeutic intervention.[44] Not surprisingly, the incidence of femoral fractures because of child abuse varies with age. Child abuse accounts for 67% of femoral shaft fractures in children younger than 1 year, but only 11% in those between 1 and 2 years of age.[92] One clinical study reported an overall 9% incidence of femoral shaft fractures as a result of child abuse in children younger than 4 years.[103] Direct and indirect loads applied to the pediatric femur produce fractures that are often typical of abuse. The radiographic image identifies the fracture type or pattern and may also reveal more subtle findings to alert the physician to a potential child abuse situation. These situations should be fully explored in a team approach. Ignoring these warning signs may result in more severe injury or even death of the child.[7, 37]

Stress fractures of the femur have been described in skeletally immature patients, and they result from sport activities in 50% of these children. Although more common in the tibia (47%) and fibula (21%), femoral stress fractures account for 12% of all stress fractures in children.[115]

## DIAGNOSIS

### History and Behavior

The history of the injury is important in formulating an accurate diagnosis. The parent or accompanying adult usually provides details of the traumatic event. In situations of vehicular trauma, an uninjured adult or emergency medical technician at the scene may furnish vital information to the physicians. The apparent speed of the automobile, tire skid marks, the number of people injured or dead, condition of the patient at the scene, the use of passenger restraints or car seats, and extrication times should be reported accurately. These factors are directly related to the energy of the trauma and, consequently, to the severity and type of potential injury. High-energy trauma forces the clinician to rule in or rule out associated life-threatening injuries, which are less likely in lower-velocity accidents.

Children with isolated femoral shaft fractures should be interviewed privately in a calm and quiet environment. A busy emergency room is a poor locale to obtain the history because the patient may be distracted and frightened by the surrounding activities. A private treatment room must be reserved for these instances. Such a setting allows children to tell their own story without parental involvement or active influence. Clues to potential abuse situations may be offered by the child when interviewed alone. The presence of the abuser may force the patient to alter the story in a characteristic attempt to shield the abuser for fear of retribution. The parent or accompanying adult is interviewed separately to assess discrepancies in the history. The parental history should be consistent with that of the child and the facts coincident with developmental milestones. For example, a 3-month-old infant does not "fall down while walking on the bed." Parental (or accompanying adult) behavior is likewise observed critically. Abnormal adult behavior such as excessive comforting of a stoic child or refusal to leave the child can typify abuse situations and must be further evaluated by a team approach. The patient is admitted to the hospital not only for fracture care but also for further investigation of the family situation. Potential abuse should not be forgotten in children with metabolic bone diseases, neurologic disorders, and other chronic afflictions that predispose them to fractures. Often, these patients place high demands on the caregiver that can be stressful and lead to abuse of the child.[71]

## Physical Examination

The physical examination is individualized and based on the child's developmental skills, such as the ability to communicate, as well as on the impact of the injury on the child. Infants, young children, and even older polytraumatized children are unable to provide subjective complaints to aid in localizing the physical examination. A meticulous physical examination may be the most important step in disclosing important information relevant to the injury. The patient should be reassured and informed about the details of the examination. Such an approach not only comforts an already apprehensive child but also secures trust so that the child may cooperate more fully. The examination must not be limited to the involved extremity. The patient should be disrobed carefully and examined thoroughly. Orthopaedically, a thorough examination includes palpation of each and every bone in its entirety. Deformed, painful, or swollen areas should be avoided until after all other normal-appearing regions have been evaluated. An obviously injured extremity is checked carefully for both neurologic and vascular function before manipulative reduction and splinting. The reduction should be gentle, and the splint should not be circumferential. The extremity is then retested for neurologic and vascular function to ensure that no harm was done by the manipulation. Gentle reduction and a comfortable splint should provide pain relief. A difference in the neurovascular status of the extremity after reduction or splinting mandates immediate release of all bandages and removal of the splint.

High-energy trauma changes the focus of the physical examination, which is divided into two phases: the primary resuscitative phase and the secondary definitive, injury-specific examination. Initial efforts are directed at resuscitation of the child. Airway, breathing, and circulation take priority (see Chapter 4). An unobstructed airway is secured, and the presence of breathing is established. Hemodynamic instability in a polytraumatized child may stem from numerous sources, and accordingly, all potential bleeding sources are carefully evaluated during the resuscitation phase. Hemorrhage

can occur as a result of a fractured femur, especially from high-energy trauma, and is a preventable cause of death. A team approach to the resuscitation effort, including the presence of the orthopaedist, is vital to improve survivability in these patients. All members of the team work together simultaneously rather than in a sequential or staged manner. The team approach allows evaluation, resuscitation, and initial treatment to proceed and is recommended for polytraumatized children. For example, once a patent airway is ensured and intravenous lines are placed, the orthopaedist rapidly palpates each extremity and the spine. The child must be logrolled into the lateral decubitus position to accomplish the latter examination. Crepitus, deformity, and open wounds are indicative of potential underlying bony injury. Obvious fractures can be reduced and splinted, and open wounds are covered with sterile dressings while other team members work to fully treat the child. The team leader, usually a trauma surgeon, is responsible for the resuscitation effort while prioritizing the injuries. Once stabilized, the patient is evaluated more carefully by the orthopaedist during the second phase of the examination.

Missed diagnoses may be catastrophic or produce a lifelong disability and should be preventable. Head-injured children pose a challenge and warrant repeated daily examinations, ideally by different physicians, to detect occult fractures. Femoral shaft fractures can mask an ipsilateral femoral neck fracture or hip dislocation; therefore, ecchymosis and asymmetry of the buttocks must be sought during the physical examination. Fifty percent of these injuries are late diagnoses in some reported series. Femoral head viability is affected by both missed hip dislocations and femoral neck fractures in association with ipsilateral femoral shaft fractures.[31, 57, 61, 84, 109, 114]

Because ligamentous knee instability can be associated with femoral shaft fractures, physical examination of an injured child with a femoral shaft fracture should include an examination of the knee. If possible, this examination is best performed under sedation or anesthesia and after stabilization of the femoral fracture.[13]

## Radiologic Evaluation

High-quality anteroposterior (AP) and lateral plain radiographs of the femur, including both the hip and the knee joints, generally yield the information necessary to diagnose a pediatric femoral shaft fracture. The initial films are usually obtained out of traction to assess shortening and deformity. For certain age groups, the amount of shortening noted on the initial "nontraction" radiographs determines the treatment. Traction radiographs, especially the lateral image, may underestimate the amount of soft tissue disruption. Moreover, poor-quality images must not be accepted; radiographic studies must be repeated until they are satisfactory. The physician or parent may assist in positioning and holding the extremity, as well as comforting the child during the process. These biplanar radiographs demonstrate the fracture pattern and any displacement. Unopposed muscle contractions across the fracture produce deformity and displacement. In proximal third shaft fractures, the typical deformity is flexion, external rotation, and abduction of the proximal fragment as a result of the force of the iliopsoas, gluteus medius, and gluteus maximus muscles. Shaft fractures at other levels also produce predictable deformities based on muscle attachments. Similarly, an associated ipsilateral posterior hip dislocation is heralded by adduction and internal rotation of the proximal fragment of the femoral shaft.[114] Imaging the joint both above and below the shaft fracture is mandatory so that ipsilateral associated fractures and dislocations, including physeal injuries, are not missed. Bone quality and preexisting bony abnormalities should be apparent on plain radiographs.

Computed and plain tomography may be useful in certain situations to better identify associated physeal and intra-articular fractures. Bone scans aid in diagnosing stress fractures, pathologic fractures, and other more occult problems related to the femoral shaft. Bone scans and skeletal surveys are also important in cases of child abuse to demonstrate the extent of injuries. Magnetic resonance imaging is being investigated to assess its value in trauma, but it has no routine indications at this time. Arteriography is indicated when the femoral shaft fracture is associated with absent distal pulses, knee dislocation, proximal tibial physeal fractures, or an ipsilateral tibial fracture (floating knee). Gonadal shielding for the child should be used, especially when numerous imaging studies are necessary.

## CLASSIFICATION

The classification of a femoral shaft fracture should provide specific information, guide treatment, be easy to remember, predict outcome, and allow communication among physicians. Classification of shaft fractures of the femur is usually based on skin integrity, etiology or energy, the specific fracture pattern, preexisting bony or neurologic abnormalities, and displacement.

A fracture is open when the normal skin envelope is violated. The soft tissue barrier may be disrupted by sharp bony fragments from within or by external factors. Both allow communication of the fracture with environmental pathogens, thereby increasing the potential for bone infection. Open femoral shaft fractures in children reflect high-energy trauma. The thick periosteum and muscular cuff of the thigh usually contain the bony fragments at the time of injury. Greater energy produces greater deformation of the fragments, which increases the risk for an open fracture. Contamination, comminution, and soft tissue violation determine the severity of the open fracture. Ballistic fractures are rare in young children but seem to be increasing in frequency in adolescents. Ballistic fractures are open injuries in which the severity is dependent on the missile type and energy. Rifle and shotgun blasts cause high-velocity injuries that produce extensive bony and soft tissue damage, as well as contamination because of cavitation effects. Shotgun shells contain "wadding," which is a barrier between the missiles (pellets) and the explosive charge (gunpowder).

Modern shells have pellet carriers made of plastic that are typically radiodense and therefore visible on plain radiographs. Older shotgun shell wadding was made from contaminated materials, including animal hair and fibers, and is more difficult to view on plain films. This wadding must be accounted for when treating open wounds and fractures from shotgun blasts.

The origin of most pediatric femoral shaft fractures is accidental blunt trauma. Knowledge about the energy of the injury is important to predict the behavior of the fracture. This behavior is reflected in the difficulty of obtaining and maintaining reduction and in healing times. Comminuted shaft fractures are produced by high energy and respond differently to conventional management than do low-energy fractures with minimally disrupted periosteal sleeves. High-energy trauma should alert the physician to potential associated diagnoses. Another low-energy type of femoral fracture is a "birth fracture" produced by forced traumatic vaginal delivery.[101]

The femoral shaft fracture pattern is best classified by descriptive terms. Spiral, oblique, transverse, greenstick (or unicortical), and comminuted—descriptive terms related to the direction and energy of the applied load—are familiar and easy to remember.

Femoral shaft fractures may be seen in situations of incidental, minimal trauma. These cases alert the orthopaedist to the possibility of underlying bony abnormalities. Weakened or pathologic bone may result from metabolic, inflammatory, neurologic, or other disorders. Certain pharmacologic agents interrupt normal bone calcium-phosphorus homeostasis, which may affect the strength of the diaphyseal bone. In this setting, fractures of the femoral shaft may be the result of trivial trauma, and the history must alert the physician to this possibility. The underlying cause should be treated as well as the fracture. Potential primary or metastatic tumors mandate a multidisciplinary evaluation by a pediatrician, a pediatric oncologist, and an orthopaedist with special training. Femoral shaft fractures in children with neurologic disorders may occur on a delayed basis because the fractures are not associated with the typical pain response and the clinical picture may be more suggestive of infection. Injury can result simply from rolling over in bed, with minor associated trauma being the rule.[19, 27, 29, 70]

Femoral shaft fractures are also classified according to their displacement patterns. Shortening is quantified on the nontraction lateral radiograph. Angular and rotatory deformities reflect the action of unbalanced muscle forces across the fractured shaft. Angulation is described by using the apex of the deformity as a reference. Terms such as varus and valgus usually confuse physicians other than orthopaedists. Apex angulation is more precise and more easily remembered.

## DECISION MAKING

The orthopaedic literature on pediatric femoral shaft fractures consists primarily of uncontrolled retrospective clinical series focusing on treatment alternatives.* All seem to have excellent outcomes, yet they are inadequately defined. Many factors affect the ultimate treatment plan, including considerations of the patient, physician, and institution, as well as financial concerns. Humberger and Eyring stated that "the simplest, safest, and most effective method should be the treatment of choice."[63] Dameron and Thompson outlined seven principles of pediatric femoral shaft fracture care[24]:

1. The simplest form of satisfactory treatment is the best.
2. The initial treatment should be permanent treatment whenever possible.
3. Perfect anatomic reduction is not essential for perfect function.
4. Restoration of alignment is more important than the position of the fragments with respect to one another.
5. More potential growth equals more probable restoration of normal architecture because of remodeling.
6. Overtreatment is usually worse than undertreatment.
7. The injured limb should either be immobilized in a Thomas splint or placed in skin traction before definitive therapy is begun until the patient or the limb is no longer in danger. Prolonged elevation of the limb of a child with incipient shock should be avoided because of the potential for contribution to compartment syndrome.

Most authors recommend treatment based on patient age (Table 13–1). Younger children with isolated femoral shaft fractures are managed by a variety of closed techniques, whereas older or polytraumatized children receive more aggressive intervention. The remodeling potential of the child justifies such a decision. Early (within 24 hours) versus delayed operative intervention does not affect the prevalence of pulmonary complications in children as it does in adult patients.[54] Nevertheless, pulmonary emboli as such have been described on rare occasion.[21] The family or social situation of the child affects the treatment plan. Potentially abused children require admission to the hospital while the team investigates the case, whereas children with favorable family environments may be candidates for immediate casting and discharge home. These patient-family issues can complicate management.

Physician experience and training also affect the treatment plan. Physicians with little experience may feel overwhelmed by these injuries. Pediatric femoral shaft fractures require strict attention to detail and frequent, meticulous follow-up. Parental education regarding the injury is also time consuming. These demands may overly challenge some busy practitioners, so early patient referral is advised in these situations. The hospital or institution may likewise urge transfer of the patient, especially when lack of accreditation or facilities to care for children exists. Specialized care can be cost-effective as well. Immobilization in a spica cast with early discharge home, when indicated, is less expensive.[1] External fixation of pediatric femoral shaft fractures results in decreased length of hospitalization and lower hospital cost when compared with 90-90 skeletal traction

*See references 1, 2, 11, 15, 16, 24, 39, 41, 48, 49, 51, 60, 63, 65, 72, 73, 75, 76, 79, 80, 91–98, 101, 106, 108–113, 120, 121.

**TABLE 13–1** ........................................

Recommended Treatment Options for Pediatric Femoral Shaft Fractures in Isolated and Multiple-Injury Patterns

| | Recommended Treatment Options | |
|---|---|---|
| **Age** | **Isolated Injury** | **Multiple Injuries** |
| Neonate | Splinting | Splinting |
| 1 to 6 yr | Immediate spica casting | External fixation |
| 6 to 10 yr | Immediate spica casting vs. plate osteosynthesis vs. flexible nails | External fixation vs. plate osteosynthesis vs. flexible nails |
| 10 to 15 yr | Intramedullary nail vs. plate osteosynthesis | External fixation vs. intramedullary nail vs. plate osteosynthesis |

followed by spica casting.[93] Given equivalent results, this method may be the treatment of choice when local inpatient pediatric services or familial resources are lacking.

## MANAGEMENT

Treatment alternatives include both invasive and less invasive methods (Table 13–2). Most authors use the terms *operative* and *conservative*. Some forms of conservative treatment, however, are quite aggressive both to the child and to the family, so the term *less invasive* is preferred. Some less invasive treatment methods may require hospitalization, which has social, educational, and financial implications. Spica casting, either immediately or after a period of traction, is representative of the less invasive approach. Invasive treatments include skeletal traction, pins and plaster, external fixation, medullary nailing procedures with various implants, and open and percutaneous plating for femoral shaft fractures. The invasive methods all necessitate hospitalization. Combinations of methods are occasionally indicated, as in spica casting to augment or protect internal fixation.

### Less Invasive Treatment

Less invasive techniques preserve the soft tissue envelope of the thigh. These methods are currently the predominant treatment of pediatric femoral shaft fractures in children younger than 6 years.[23, 32, 64] Uniformly reproducible good outcomes can be expected. The decision of how to treat the fracture is based on numerous factors, with patient age, mechanism of injury, initial fracture shortening, and associated injuries being the most important. Although this injury rarely occurs in utero, the youngest patient with a femoral shaft fracture is a newborn infant.[19] Birth fractures are incurred during traumatic delivery and can be difficult to diagnose. The infant may have minimal deformity and crepitus. The fractured femur may be noticed by the neonatologist or intensive care nurse as pseudoparalysis of the extremity.

**TABLE 13–2** ........................................................................................................

Advantages and Disadvantages of Various Treatment Options

| Fixation Technique | Advantages | Disadvantages |
|---|---|---|
| Spica casting | No scars, no operation | Uncomfortable, possible skin problems and loss of reduction |
| Skeletal traction | No operation, closed treatment | Possible loss of reduction, long immobilization in bed, pin tract infections |
| External fixation | Percutaneous fixation, small incisions, early mobilization | Secondary fractures and refractures, pin tract infection |
| Intramedullary nailing | Immediate stability and mobilization | Risk of avascular necrosis, implant removal necessary |
| Flexible intramedullary nails | Small incisions, immediate/early mobilization | Hardware removal necessary, possible rotational instability with necessity for temporary cast |
| Open plate osteosynthesis | Immediate stability and mobilization | Large incision and scarring, hardware removal necessary |
| Percutaneous plate osteosynthesis | Immediate stability and mobilization, small scars | Implant removal necessary |

In this setting, septic arthritis of the hip and other systemic causes must be ruled out. Plain radiographs of the femur demonstrate the fracture. Robinson in 1938 described an overhead traction apparatus for infants with femoral birth fractures, but such management is not necessary and is prone to complications.[101] Today, simple splinting is the treatment of choice to prevent excessive angular or rotational deformities. The splint is discontinued when the fracture is clinically nontender. Rapid consolidation within 3 weeks is the rule. Longitudinal growth corrects the residual minor deformities. In utero fracture or more than one birth fracture should alert the physician to a potential bone disease such as osteogenesis imperfecta.[19, 27]

## SKIN TRACTION

Skin traction requires initial hospitalization and is rarely advocated. It is generally reserved for younger children and can be used in older children as temporary immobilization before definitive treatment. Obviously, this method is not indicated in children with insensate skin regions or open wounds on the affected extremity.

**Technique.** The patient is sedated during the procedure to provide comfort, especially during transport from the stretcher to the hospital bed. The skin is cleansed and then prepared with a nonallergenic adherent dressing to prevent skin irritation. The prominences of the malleoli and heel are well protected with cast padding, and the leg is wrapped. Adhesive straps are applied to the cotton padding both medially and laterally and secured with an overwrap of elastic bandage. The straps are attached to a footplate, which is connected to the desired weights through a pulley system. The pulley system is adjusted to obtain the necessary angle of traction. Hip flexion is secured with a folded blanket posterior to the thigh or a sling about the thigh attached to a weight through a pulley system. The contralateral extremity is likewise padded, wrapped, and placed in traction. Wooden blocks or other stable items are placed beneath the bedposts. Elevation of the foot of the bed prevents the child from slipping down the bed because of the traction.

Accurate AP and lateral femoral plain radiographs are obtained to assess alignment and distraction of the fracture. Only the lateral radiograph is reliable for assessing length because the proximal fragment may be flexed by the iliopsoas muscle. Apex anterior angulation (flexion) at the fracture site may give a false impression of adequate or even excessive distraction on an AP radiograph. The amount of traction weight is adjusted after assessment of the length of the fracture on the lateral film. The patient should be comfortable in traction. Any complaint related to the lower extremities, especially the contralateral normal side, is thoroughly investigated. Frequent removal of skin wraps may be required to assess the skin because failure to recognize a skin pressure problem can be catastrophic. Skin traction is maintained until early clinical or radiographic union is noted. Early clinical union is reflected as a nontender fracture site with palpable callus. Radiographic signs of early union are callus formation and incorporation. A cast is usually applied at this point. The spica cast is maintained for a total of 6 to 8 weeks, depending on the clinical and radiographic healing response. Younger patients may require a shorter immobilization period, but each child is treated individually.

## IMMEDIATE SPICA CASTING

Casting of pediatric femoral shaft fractures should be limited to spica casting techniques. Staheli and Sheridan[107] identified five requisites for spica casting: (1) reliable parents, (2) uncomplicated femoral shaft fractures, (3) otherwise normal children younger than 8 years, (4) anesthesia possible, and (5) an initial period of traction. They believed that initial traction facilitated improved fracture reduction and consolidation before casting. Allen and co-workers[1] advocated early reduction and cast application without initial traction. They reported better results than after initial traction, lower cost, and less hospitalization with such treatment. Immediate spica casting without a period of traction is used as definitive treatment only when the initial "nontraction" plain radiographs demonstrate acceptable shortening, usually less than 1.5 cm on the lateral radiograph. Hughes and associates[62] described the effects of spica cast treatment on the families of children with femoral shaft fractures. Patient immobility was found to be the primary problem for families in this study. None of the patients were accepted back into school during casting; however, home tutoring prevented even temporary academic problems in all but two patients. Ferguson and Nicol treated children up to the age of 10 years with early spica casting and found that age older than 7 years correlated with the need for a change in treatment 7 to 10 days after injury and casting.[32]

**Technique.** The patient must be adequately sedated during cast application, and general anesthesia is frequently necessary for muscular relaxation. A pediatric fracture table affords access to the patient and simplifies the procedure (Fig. 13–1). The cast can be applied either immediately or after a period of traction. Immediate spica casting is reserved for patients with acceptable shortening based on the nontraction initial lateral radiograph. Children with unacceptable shortening are placed in casts only after an adequate amount of time in traction has allowed stable length correction and early callus formation. Recommended casting techniques vary. Both Irani and colleagues[65] and Allen and co-workers[1] advocate placement of a long leg, well-molded cast initially. Excessive padding prevents good molding and is avoided. The patient is then transferred to the fracture table, and the remainder of the spica cast is applied.

Alternatively, the patient is positioned on the table, the reduction is secured by an assistant (who should be slow to fatigue), and the spica cast is applied. Czertak and Hennrikus[23] recommended the application of a short leg cast, followed by positioning the child on the spica table. Next, the hip and knee are flexed to 90° and manual traction applied to the injured limb with the short leg cast. The spica cast is wrapped and completed with a valgus mold at the fracture site. Staheli and Sheridan[108] advocate initial placement of the patient on the fracture table followed by casting. An assistant applies fixed skin traction at the child's ankles. Before the cast is finished, radiographs are obtained to assess reduction and alignment. Distraction is evaluated on the lateral radiograph. Wedging of the cast to perfect any minor residual deformity is completed. Larger deformities may not allow cast wedging and are therefore corrected with repeat cast application. Final films confirm the reduction, and the cast is finished.

The spica cast begins at the nipple level and extends to include various portions of the extremities. A small towel temporarily placed on the chest beneath the padding permits full respiratory excursion while in the cast. The popliteal fossa as well as bony prominences are well protected with extra layers of cotton padding or thick self-adherent foam cushions applied over the cotton padding. The anterior superior iliac crest, femoral condyles, patella, malleoli, Achilles tendon, and calcaneus are the regions of concern. The groin, buttock, and

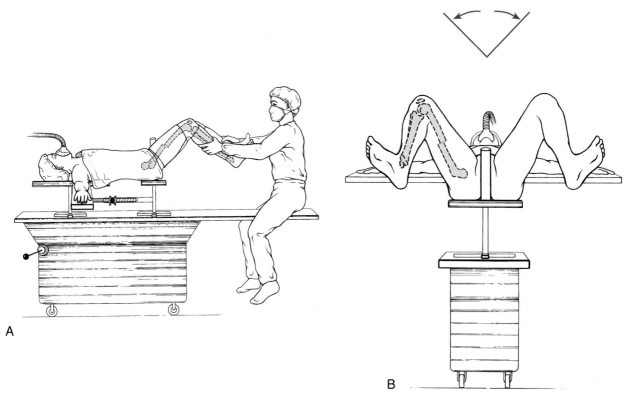

**FIGURE 13–1.** *A,* Spica casting for femoral shaft fractures. The reduction is maintained by the surgeon. Excellent condylar and buttock molding avoids the complication of shortening in the cast, but excessive padding complicates cast molding. Biplanar radiographs reveal deformities. Shortening and rotational deformities are not corrected by wedging. To correct angular deformities, wedging should be done before the crossbar is added. *B,* Hip abduction should allow perineal hygiene. Excessive abduction can injure the femoral head blood supply. The hip and knee flexions are adjusted to slightly suspend the heels from the bed.

knee areas are reinforced with splints to avoid cast breakdown. A wooden or plaster connecting bar placed anteriorly between the thighs (applied as necessary after wedging is completed) helps reinforce the construct and can also serve as a handle for patient transport. Some authors advocate inclusion of the ipsilateral foot in the cast; others advocate removal of the footplate on the affected side. Irani and colleagues reported displacement of the fracture in children whose cast included a footplate.[65] The position of the extremities in the cast provides fracture reduction and adequate perineal and toileting access for the parent. Insufficient hip abduction prevents good perineal hygiene, which is required for a child in a cast. Excessive maximal hip abduction should be avoided because of its presumed effects on blood flow to the femoral head. The hip and knee should each be flexed so that the heel is slightly suspended from the bed. Excessive knee flexion transfers pressure to the heel. Attention to detail during cast application averts many problems caused by simple positioning or plastering errors.

Immediate spica casting is a more demanding technique. Without the benefit of initial traction and early healing, the fracture remains unstable. Controlling the fracture reduction during cast application is a real challenge. The assistant works hard to maintain the proper distraction, rotation, and position of the lower extremities as the cast is applied. Even in younger, smaller children, such maintenance of position is difficult. Heavy children require more than one assistant to secure the extremities. Maintenance of distraction is critical to avoid excessive shortening or collapse of the fracture in the cast. Minor angular deformity is correctable with wedging, but excessive shortening is not. Relaxation of muscular spasm is important for achieving and maintaining reduction, and the anesthesiologist must therefore be informed. Proper padding prevents skin complications, which have been described in up to 14% of patients.[64] Nevertheless, cast molding at the femoral condyles and buttock region is critical if shortening is to be avoided. Frequent follow-up radiographs are mandatory. Both Allen and co-workers[1] and Staheli and Sheridan[108] define excessive shortening as more than 15 mm. Excessive shortening is treated with cast removal and a period of corrective traction until early fracture consolidation. Repeat casting is performed when the fracture becomes stable in length. Allen and co-workers provided guidelines to acceptable deformities: no rotational malalignment is accepted, but 10° or less of apex medial (valgus) or apex lateral (varus) angulation and less than 15° of procurvatum or recurvatum may be tolerated.[1] Irani and colleagues presented similar guidelines for acceptable deformities.[65] Most angular deformities can be prevented with precise closed reduction and can be corrected with accurate cast wedging. In a retrospective review of 47 pediatric patients with closed femoral shaft fractures, Pollack and associates identified the mechanism of injury as an important predictor of excessive shortening.[96] Twelve of 23 fractures (52%) that occurred as a result of high-energy trauma (from car vs. pedestrian or motor vehicle accidents) required repeat

reduction or additional traction. Patients with high-energy fractures demonstrating excessive shortening on the initial plain radiographs are not candidates for routine, early spica casting.

## Invasive Treatment

### SKELETAL TRACTION

Skeletal traction is generally reserved for older children with isolated fractures. It is often only a temporary measure until definitive treatment with a spica cast or internal/external fixation can be applied. The specific technique of skeletal traction varies. Distal femoral or proximal tibial sites are most frequently used for pin placement. Which bone is chosen depends on four considerations: (1) the status of the knee ligaments and local soft tissues, (2) the level of the femoral shaft fracture, (3) ipsilateral extremity trauma, and (4) the age of the patient. Proximal tibial pins are not recommended in children younger than 10 years because of the potential for proximal tibial physeal injury.[11] A distal femoral traction pin is used when the knee joint is injured or its stability is unknown. Likewise, an ipsilateral tibial fracture usually precludes placement of a proximal tibial traction pin. The femoral shaft fracture should be more easily controlled with a femoral pin.

**Technique.** The pin is placed with aseptic technique and guided by fluoroscopic imaging. The anesthetic chosen may be local, regional, or general. In younger and less cooperative patients, adequate sedation should supplement the local anesthetic. Liberal local anesthesia should include the periosteum and skin at the point of exit. Patient sedation and adequate local anesthesia improve pin insertion and accuracy. A femoral nerve block provides regional anesthesia and facilitates pin insertion. In the inguinal region, the femoral nerve is located lateral to the palpable femoral artery. The depth of the nerve depends on the amount of subcutaneous fat. In alert patients, a small-diameter, long needle is used to anesthetize the skin and subsequently the deep tissues lateral to the palpable arterial pulse. The syringe is aspirated as it is inserted to ensure proper location. The abdominal fascia is distinct when penetrated. The local anesthetic is injected beneath the fascia by using a regional infiltration technique (Fig. 13–2). Next, the local distal femoral or proximal tibial periosteum and skin of the anticipated pin site are similarly infiltrated with local anesthetic before pin insertion.

The traction pin size, location, and orientation are planned. Pin placement is critical to optimize the vector of traction pin pull and to avoid growth plate injury. The size is dependent on the type of traction bow to be used. A narrow-diameter pin tensioned adequately (Kirschner bow) is more effective than a larger pin placed in a neutral bow (Bohler bow). The pin may be smooth or threaded. Smooth pins tend to loosen within the bone over a prolonged period. The physician should consider the local anatomy carefully before pin insertion. The proximal end of the tibia has an unusual apophysis that

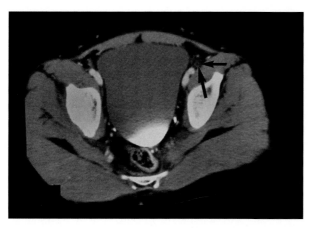

**FIGURE 13–2.** This axial image of a pelvic computed tomogram demonstrates the location of the femoral nerve *(arrow)* and its adjacent structures. The iliac vessels are enhanced by contrast. The femoral nerve is lateral to these vessels, surrounded by fat, and located on the anteromedial surface of the iliopsoas muscle.

can easily be injured by errant pin placement. Proximity to the physis is avoided during insertion, and the pin is inserted slowly with a hand drill. Heat generated during rapid pin advancement results in thermal injury to the pin tract and adjacent physis and should thus be avoided to prevent the development of a ring sequestrum or physeal bar. The orientation of the pin helps correct angular deformity if properly planned. The physician controls the point of insertion, and care is taken to avoid pin bending, especially when narrow-diameter pins are used. Bending may cause the pin to exit the bone in a potentially dangerous area. For this reason, the distal femoral pin is inserted medially and exits laterally. Medial insertion avoids popliteal vascular damage; the opposite holds true in the proximal end of the tibia. The peroneal nerve is most at risk, so the pin is inserted laterally and advanced to exit medially. Fluoroscopic imaging during pin placement provides a safe physeal margin and detects misdirection (Fig. 13–3). Alternatively, a single screw can be placed anteriorly, distal to the tibial tubercle.[53]

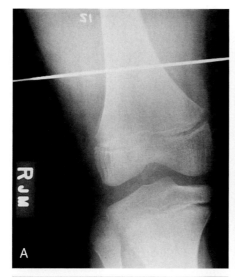

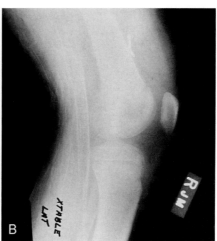

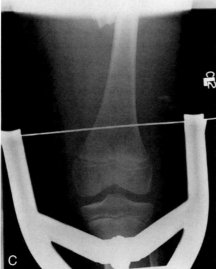

**FIGURE 13–3.** *A,* The traction pin appears to be located safely away from the physis on this anteroposterior radiograph. *B,* A lateral radiograph demonstrates the extraosseous location of the pin *(arrow).* Adequate sedation and fluoroscopic imaging during pin placement allow accurate and safe pin insertion. *C,* Smooth, narrow-diameter pins are inserted slowly and then tensioned with a Kirschner bow.

Biplanar radiographs confirm the pin's location. The skin pin sites are treated with frequent cleansing and antiseptic dressings to avoid infection. The amount of initial weight applied as traction depends on the size of the patient. An easy guide is to apply an amount of weight that slightly elevates the ipsilateral buttock from the mattress when using 90-90 traction. The amount of shortening at the fracture site is monitored with serial lateral plain radiographs. AP images are inaccurate in assessing length because of the usual anterior bowing of the femur, as well as the difficulty in obtaining a true AP image. The traction weight is adjusted according to the findings on these frequent radiographs. The frequency, determined by the fracture pattern and the difficulty in obtaining the initial reduction, is generally every third or fourth day, at a minimum, during the first 10 to 14 days of treatment. Distraction of the fracture site is painful, can cause neurovascular injury, and should thus be avoided.

## PINS AND PLASTER

Pins and plaster techniques have also been used effectively to treat femoral shaft fractures. Curtis and co-workers recommended the "pontoon" spica cast as a form of successful treatment in pediatric patients.[22] Their results were confirmed with long-term follow-up by Sahin and co-workers.[102]

**Technique.** The skeletal traction pin is placed as described earlier, and the patient is immobilized in a spica cast. The skeletal pin is incorporated into the cast and helps maintain fracture reduction. Unfortunately, the cast denies access to the skin exit sites of the pins. Systemic signs of inflammation may indicate superficial or deep pin tract infection, and pin inspection requires cast removal. Routine femoral condylar molding of the spica cast should provide similar fracture control, thereby avoiding pin site problems in most instances. Because of the inability to observe the pin sites, this method is not advocated.

## EXTERNAL FIXATION

External fixation systems have been enthusiastically recommended for pediatric femoral shaft fractures. Quintin and associates[97] advocated external fixation for children with open fractures, fractures associated with neural or vascular damage, fractures with central nervous system damage, polytrauma, and fractures that fail more traditional traction or casting treatment. Alonso and Horowitz[2] added burn patients with fractures to the list. In their series, they treated five femoral fractures with external fixation.[2] Most authors report good results with a variety of external frame constructs. The quadriceps muscle mass is minimally violated when the frame is applied laterally. Lateral half-pin frames allow control of the fracture, as well as mobilization of both the hip and knee joints. Pin placement must avoid the physes (Fig. 13–4). With external fixation treatment, a polytraumatized patient can be placed upright to restore more normal pulmonary function without jeopardizing fracture stability. Head-injured children who are combative

or have seizure activity or spasticity are more easily cared for by the nursing staff when the femoral shaft fracture has been stabilized. The frame half-pins should be capped with soft pads to prevent injury to the patient or the medical staff by the pins. External fixation systems that are simple to apply and have few parts are advantageous. These simple frame constructs can be applied rapidly (short anesthesia) and with minimal blood loss, which are important factors when dealing with severely injured or clinically unstable children. The frame can often be applied while other procedures are ongoing, such as placement of an intracranial pressure monitor and diagnostic peritoneal lavage. Fluoroscopic imaging during the application ensures accurate pin placement and fracture reduction. The reduction can subsequently be improved with minor adjustments in certain frame systems when the child is clinically more stable. However, reduction adjustments should not be delayed too long because head-injured children heal fractures rapidly. Delay in adjusting the reduction with the frame may result in malunion. When possible, the initial reduction in the frame should be optimized in all but critical situations. Serial biplanar radiographs evaluate the fracture for changes, especially in a combative or restless patient, and remanipulation is performed early. The connecting nuts should be tightened at intervals to prevent frame loosening. The half-pins are cleansed with antiseptic twice daily to avoid pin tract problems. Pin site infections and recurrent fractures at the original fracture site or at pin sites after removal of the external fixator are potential complications of external fixation.[44, 87, 105]

**Technique.** The patient is generally positioned supine for management of head, chest, or abdominal trauma or for débridement of open wounds associated with the fracture. For the latter, the skin edges must be sharply excised, all debris removed, and all nonbleeding crushed or contaminated fat and muscle débrided. The fractured bone ends are inspected and débrided through the traumatic wound and its surgical extension. This step is followed by pulsatile lavage with a minimum of 9 L of normal saline irrigant. The wound is then reinspected for the conditions noted earlier, and all nonviable (with no significant soft tissue attached) bone is removed. Irrigation may then be repeated.

Fluoroscopy directs safe and strategic pin insertion, as well as manipulative reduction. When extensive traumatic wounds are present, the reduction may be secured through the open wound. The reduction is typically achieved with manual traction in a relaxed patient, and the rotation is adjusted according to clinical and radiographic indicators. Based on study of the injury films, the initial lateral pin is placed farthest from the fracture site ("far" pin) in the longer of the two fracture fragments. The pin can be either a 5-mm standard adult pin or a 4-mm pin for smaller children. The pin is placed through a 1-cm stab wound with the use of a sleeve system that allows saline-cooled predrilling of the bone. The length of connecting bar is then selected. A carbon fiber rod is preferred for its radiolucency. Two bars are appropriate for length-unstable fracture patterns. Four pin-bar clamps are placed on each bar to be used. The clamp is attached to the "far" pin in the long fragment, and manual traction is applied. The other fragment's "far" pin is applied through the series of sleeves in the shorter of the two fracture fragments. The reduction is perfected, and the two "far" pin clamps are tightened to the connecting bars. The bar is positioned in line with the femoral shaft laterally and, to allow for thigh swelling, 5 to 10 mm from the skin. By positioning the bar directly lateral to the femoral shaft, the pins placed closest to the fracture ("near" pins) can be inserted into the femur without being inserted at an angle. Such positioning is critical when two connecting bars are stacked because an angled pin will not be captured by the most external clamp. If such is the case, a pair of bar-to-bar clamps attached to a short intermediate connecting bar can salvage the situation. This configuration also allows for adjustment of the fracture reduction after the frame has been applied. After insertion of the pins and frame assembly, the overlying soft tissues adjacent to the pin are incised enough to allow unrestricted hip and knee range of motion. Commonly, the most distal pin in the supracondylar region is poorly released from the iliotibial band, and decreased knee motion results. Early rehabilitation efforts are complicated by this decreased motion. The surgeon should ensure that the skin and deep tissues are adequately released throughout the hip and knee by applying passive range of motion. Pin site skin care is instituted the day after surgery. Sterile, saline-moistened, cotton-tipped applicators are used to débride the skin site of local crusted serous fluid and blood from around the pins two or three times daily. The parents and patient are instructed about pin site skin care and practice the technique together initially. As the patient gains confidence, skin care is performed under the parent's supervision.

After surgery, weight bearing and exercises are instituted under the direction of a licensed physical therapist. Protected "weight-of-limb" assisted ambulation using crutches or a walker allows the patient to rest the injured lower extremity on the ground during the stance phase of gait. This technique improves balance and confidence without causing pain. Active and active-assisted range-of-motion exercises target the hip, knee, and ankle joints of the injured limb. The patient is restricted to isometric strengthening exercises for 6 weeks postoperatively. After 6 weeks, findings on clinical examination of the injured limb and the radiographic signs of callus formation direct the treating physician. A fracture that is not tender to palpation along with abundant biplanar radiographic fracture callus spanning all four cortices facilitates the decision to remove the external fixation device and pins.

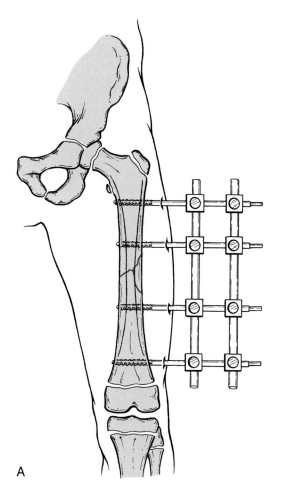

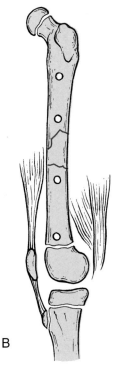

**FIGURE 13–4.** *A* and *B*, A double-bar, unilateral frame construct is shown. The pins are placed posterior to the vastus lateralis muscle.

*Illustration continued on following page*

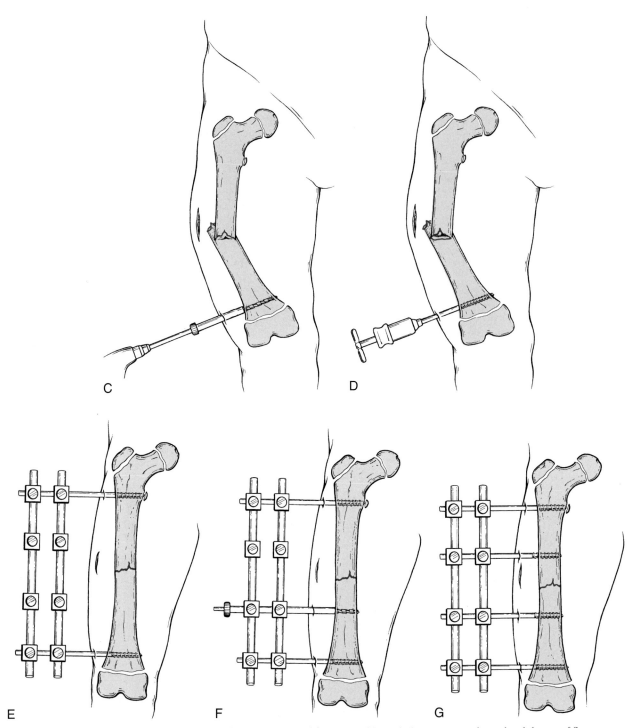

**FIGURE 13–4** *Continued. C,* Schematic representation of pin placement and frame assembly. With the patient anesthetized and the use of fluoroscopy, a saline-cooled drill is used to place the first "far" pin through a stab wound. *D,* The distal "far" pin (no. 4 pin) is seated adequately, with overpenetration avoided. *E,* The fracture is reduced and temporarily manually secured. The proximal "far" pin (no. 1 pin) is then placed after predrilling, with the desired frame construct and its clamps used as a guide. The frame must be preassembled as needed at this stage. *F,* The distal "near" pin (no. 3 pin) is placed, again using the frame and its clamps as a guide. *G,* The final frame assembly is shown after the no. 2 proximal "near" pin is inserted. The unilateral, double-bar frame provides wound access while maintaining fracture stability. Passive range of motion should be possible for the knee and hip after application of the frame. Frequently, the distal pin requires additional release to allow full knee flexion-extension. After frame application, the knee is tested for ligamentous stability. The adjacent physes are similarly reevaluated after femoral diaphyseal stability is achieved.

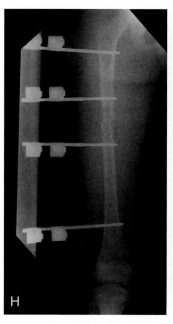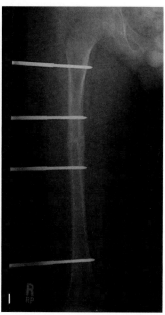

FIGURE **13–4** *Continued. H,* This patient had a diaphyseal femoral fracture treated with a unilateral, double-bar external fixation device. His reduction was positioned with cortical overlap to promote a larger callus mass at union. The pin insertions were sequenced as described earlier. Six weeks after injury, he had minimal callus formation. The peripheral external bar was removed from the frame construct in the clinic without causing pain or anxiety. His weight-bearing status was advanced progressively over the next 4 weeks. *I,* He had subsequent healing. Ten weeks after injury and under anesthesia, his knee was manipulated, the external frame and pins were then removed, and the pin sites were débrided.

Residual fracture tenderness and minimal radiographic signs of healing suggest slower fracture union. In such situations, the frame is maintained and increased weight bearing is supervised by the parent and therapist. A double-bar lateral external frame should be "destabilized" in these instances by removing the most peripheral bar. This procedure is painless, is easily performed in the clinic, and stimulates fracture healing by further loading of the femoral shaft fracture. Clinical follow-up is scheduled 4 weeks later with radiographs to ensure progressive callus formation. Eight to 10 weeks postoperatively, the pin sites typically become superficially inflamed and mandate removal. Pin removal is painful and causes anxiety in most children and their parents. Removal of the frame and pin is performed in conjunction with débridement of the pin sites under brief general anesthesia. While anesthetized, the knee is manipulated *before* frame and pin removal. Manipulation of a stiff knee after frame removal should *not* be performed because of the risk of iatrogenic refracture. Progressive, protected weight bearing on the healing femoral fracture is accomplished over the next 3 to 6 weeks. Torsional and other pivoting activities are avoided during this time. Early, unprotected weight bearing increases the risk for refracture or a new fracture at a previous pin site.

## MEDULLARY NAILING

Medullary nailing of pediatric femoral shaft fractures is an excellent treatment method. Reamed nailing in adults was popularized during World War II by Küntscher. The North American experience reported by Winquist and colleagues[119] reproduced the excellent clinical results with low rates of infection and malunion. The medullary nailing procedures in the early clinical series, however, were limited to adult patients. The medullary nailing techniques evolved, with nails placed in an antegrade fashion after reaming of the femoral canal. Reaming to the inner cortical diameter provided excellent fit and allowed the nail to function as an internal splint, thereby avoiding the need for external splinting. The traditional method of Küntscher involved placement of the medullary, antegrade nail through a greater trochanteric starting site. In children, trochanteric apophyseal arrest can occur and produce growth irregularities of the proximal end of the femur, typically a valgus femoral neck deformity. Gage has shown that after the age of 8 years, arrest of the greater trochanteric apophysis will not result in abnormal proximal femoral mechanics.[36] One must remember that the greater trochanter grows from the apophysis and from appositional growth, both of which contribute about 50% to growth of the greater trochanter. Aseptic necrosis of the femoral head is a devastating, yet rarely occurring complication after antegrade nailing. It is most likely caused by a medial starting point for the implant, which injures the vascular supply to the femoral head.[4, 14, 42, 86, 94, 95, 110] No cases of avascular necrosis of the femoral head have been reported when using a trochanteric starting point technique.[26, 39]

The lateral ascending artery from the medial femoral circumflex vessel supplies most of the blood to the developing proximal part of the femur between the ages of 3 and 10 years. This artery is located posteriorly in the cervicotrochanteric area. The ascending branches nourish the capital femoral epiphysis, and the descending metaphyseal arteries supply the apophyseal region. Interference with this vascular network about the femoral neck may produce a valgus neck deformity and aseptic necrosis of the femoral head.[42] Because of these concerns, femoral nailing in children and adolescents was historically condemned.

Kirby and co-workers[72] compared traction and casting with closed nailing in adolescents with femoral shaft fractures. In this study, the piriformis fossa (the starting point advocated by Winquist and colleagues[119]) was used without complication. Remodeling potential is less in the adolescent age group than in younger patients. These authors found that the group that received casts had stiffness of the knee, as well as rotational and angular deformities of the femur when compared with the group of adolescents treated by nailing. The nailed group had few complications, and this method was especially advocated in children 10 to 15 years old with an ipsilateral fracture of the tibia or multiple systemic injuries. Kirby and co-workers recommended that the nail be placed antegrade and left just short of the distal femoral physis to allow for the remaining longitudinal femoral growth.[72]

Momberger and colleagues[88] treated 50 femoral shaft fractures in patients aged 10 to 16 years by reamed, interlocking medullary nailing and the use of a greater trochanteric starting point. They did not observe avascular necrosis of the femoral head. Despite nail insertion through the greater trochanteric apophysis, articulotrochanteric distance measurements increased only 4.5 mm. In no patient did significant proximal femoral deformity develop. All fractures healed, and the average leg length discrepancy was 1 mm (range, −10 mm to +11 mm). They concluded that medullary nailing through a greater trochanteric starting point is a safe and effective method for treating femoral shaft fractures in the adolescent age group.[88]

Flexible or elastic medullary implants have been used to treat pediatric and adolescent femoral shaft fractures.[56, 67] Mann and associates[79] reported excellent results with Ender nailing techniques in 15 patients between the ages of 9 and 15 years. Ender nails were indicated in polytraumatized or head-injured patients. These authors also advocate Ender nailing in fractures that fail routine closed management.[79] Ligier and co-workers[76] defined elastic stable intramedullary nailing in 1988. They treated 123 pediatric femoral shaft fractures with flexible rods introduced retrogradely through two incisions in the distal metaphyseal area (see Fig. 13–9). Early patient mobilization was possible, and no delayed union occurred. Complications were minimal and consisted of skin breakdown or knee discomfort caused by the ends of the rods.[76] These results have been reproduced by Kissel and Miller[74] and by Mazda and colleagues.[83] In a small comparison series of 21 adolescent patients, Gregory and associates suggested that flexible nailing produces clinical results equivalent to those of interlocking nails, but at less cost.[46] Linhart and Roposch[77] observed rotational and axial instability and shortening of long spiral fractures, long oblique fractures, or comminuted fractures treated with elastic intramedullary nailing only. They therefore commenced to interlock modified Ender nails distally. Interlocking of screws proximally was not necessary because the proximal spongiosa is so hard that the nails anchored in a way that equals interlocking. This fixation allowed immediate mobilization and walking on crutches in their series of 17 patients aged 2.5 to 14 years. Full weight bearing was achieved at 3.5 weeks postoperatively, and the implants were removed on average after 4.1 months (range, 1 to 7 months).

Typically, flexible intramedullary nailing is performed in a retrograde fashion. Nevertheless, Carey and Galpin[17] described antegrade flexible intramedullary nailing with good results in 25 pediatric patients aged 6 to 12 years.

In 1984, Ziv and associates[120] reported their results of open Rush pinning and Küntscher medullary nailing in growing, polytraumatized children. Two incisions were used to place the implant. The lateral approach to the femoral fracture provided canal access to allow retrograde reaming. The trochanteric exit point was found by using a medullary guide. Retrograde identification of this point avoided injury to the femoral head blood supply, according to the authors. A second buttock incision was made to access the proximal fragment and enable antegrade nail passage. Open reduction was performed as the implant passed across the fracture site. These investigators stated that these methods were reliable and safe in children but stressed that single Rush pinning provided no rotational control of the fracture and thus necessitated supplemental casting. Only 10 of the 16 patients were available for direct follow-up. Because growth arrest of the proximal end of the femur is a potential problem with reamed nailing, Ziv and associates advised against reaming the proximal fragment in a growing child.[120]

This series, as well as that of Kirby and co-workers and Maruenda-Paulino and colleagues, identified no difference in femoral overgrowth with nailing versus casting techniques.[72, 81, 120] Femoral nailing has also been advocated in polytraumatized patients and in those with head injuries. This technique has advantages similar to those of external fixation, and the improved insertional guides allow percutaneous placement. Femoral nailing procedures require fluoroscopic imaging for accurate nail placement. The supine or lateral position may be used. The lateral position usually provides better access to the starting point but is contraindicated in patients with pelvic, spinal, or other unstable injuries. A fracture table simplifies the reduction and therefore the procedure, but it is not mandatory. New techniques allow medullary femoral nailing to be performed percutaneously without a fracture table.[69]

Neurologic complications occurred in 22% of 35 consecutive patients aged 10 to 17 years after femoral nailing.[100] The combination of a surgical delay of more than 48 hours allowing fracture shortening and the use of boot traction increased the incidence of all nerve palsies to 5.7 times and the incidence of peroneal palsies to 11.4 times that of patients without this combination of risk factors. Adequate traction in patients with surgical delay decreases the incidence of neurologic complications.[100]

Nail removal has been recommended at 10 to 14 months on average, and refractures have not been described.[9, 14]

### Technique

*Reamed, Locked, Antegrade Femoral Medullary Nailing.* Unstable or multiply injured patients are placed in the supine position on a radiolucent operating table with the entire abdomen, bilateral flanks, and affected lower extremity draped free, and a percutaneous nailing technique is selected.[69] A rolled blanket is placed beneath the ipsilateral flank from the sacrum to the thorax to facilitate both access to the starting point and lateral imaging of the proximal end of the femur. Similarly, the ipsilateral upper extremity is adducted across the chest and supported on a pillow or padded table attachment. If large traction forces are required, a traction pin is inserted under fluoroscopic control in the same position noted earlier. However, a traction pin is rarely necessary if the fracture is treated immediately. The fluoroscopic unit is positioned on the contralateral side of the patient with the monitor adjacent to the foot of the table. The injured limb must be adducted to allow better access to the proximal part of the femur for the trochanteric starting point. Proximal femoral shaft fractures are complicated by unopposed muscle forces causing flexion, abduction, and external rotation of the proximal fracture fragment. In these situations, a 4- or 5-mm-diameter manipulative pin can be inserted into the proximal fragment percutaneously to facilitate access to the medullary starting point and subsequent reduction. It is inserted through the lateral cortex in such a manner that the medullary cavity is not obstructed during reaming. Another reduction technique is routine preparation of the proximal fragment's medullary canal, insertion of a small-diameter cannulated nail, and manipulative reduction of the fracture with the small medullary nail used as a manipulator. A guide wire is passed through the small cannulated nail after reduction is achieved, the small nail is removed, and reaming of the distal fragment can proceed routinely. For certain proximal fractures, open fracture reduction is accomplished when these other manipulative techniques fail.

For access to the proximal fragment, a 3-mm smooth guide pin is inserted under fluoroscopic control. The pin is positioned at the lateral aspect of the greater trochanter on the AP image and in a midlateral position paralleling the medullary path on the lateral image and inserted into the medullary space of the proximal end of the femur. A 6-cm incision is made over the pin on the buttock in line with the femoral shaft. One must be certain that the guide pin enters the tip of the greater trochanter and is centered within the femoral canal on both the AP and lateral radiographic images. Once the guide pin is in perfect "center-center" position, a cannulated reamer is inserted over the 3-mm guide wire to expand the starting point, and the tip of the trochanter is reamed. The reamer then enters the femoral canal in the centered position. The cannulated reamer and 3-mm pin are removed, and a bulb-tipped guide wire of known length is inserted in the "center-center" location in the proximal fragment up to, but not across the fracture site. The fracture is then reduced as earlier, and the guide wire is passed across the fracture site into the distal end of the femur. The surgeon must be certain that the guide wire is in the distal fragment, both on the AP and lateral radiographs, and is in the center of the metaphysis of the distal part of the femur. The guide wire is positioned just proximal to the distal femoral physis. The length of the femoral canal is noted from the medullary guide wire. The femur is then reamed to 1.5 mm larger than the diameter of the nail to be used. This 1.5-mm "over-reaming" of the medullary canal facilitates uncomplicated nail insertion. Sharp reamers with deep flutes are chosen to diminish marrow element embolization. The bulb-tipped guide wire is next exchanged for a smooth guide wire through a medullary tube. The tube is removed after the smooth guide wire's medullary location is confirmed fluoroscopically for the

proximal and distal fracture fragments. The nail selected is carefully inserted. As the nail insertional device approaches the greater trochanteric entry site, the surgeon must closely monitor the nail insertion fluoroscopically and avoid "overinsertion." The insertional device is larger than the implant and may cause an iatrogenic proximal femoral fracture in certain situations. In addition, "overinsertion" of the nail distally will injure the central distal femoral physis. After the nail is placed ideally, the guide pin is removed. Next, the nail is locked. For children, pediatric femoral locking nails are produced in narrow diameters with locking options. Proximal locking is facilitated by the proximal insertional guide. Distal locking is performed with the freehand method for either position; generally, only one proximal and one distal screw is required for stable fracture patterns. For fractures located distal to the isthmus, two distal locking screws are advocated. Two locking screws are selected both proximally and distally for comminuted femoral shaft fractures. A new titanium nail is available that has been specifically designed for entry through the tip of the greater trochanter. The pediatric nail is available in an 8.5-mm diameter (Fig. 13–5).

Fracture tables can be used as well with skin or skeletal traction. Fresh fractures can generally be nailed without inserting a skeletal pin. When a fracture table is used, the foot on the injured side is stabilized with the traction boot, and gentle longitudinal distraction is applied. If large forces are required to reduce the fracture, a distal femoral traction pin should be inserted under radiographic control in the anterior 1 cm of the femur, a minimum of 1 cm proximal to the distal femoral physis. The knee can then be flexed to relax the sciatic nerve during the application of traction. The pelvis must be oblique to the surface of the fracture table so that the femoral necks do not overlie one another on the lateral fluoroscopic view. In patients with extensively comminuted femoral shaft fractures, ideal length and rotation reduction is complicated. Placing the patient in the supine position on a fracture table should improve the reduction of these difficult fractures. Clinical and fluoroscopic signs direct the reduction as well as implant insertion.

Regardless of the technique or table chosen, an accurate trochanteric starting point is mandatory. The trochanteric starting point differs from the "piriformis fossa" starting point advocated in adults. In children, the capsular blood supply to the femoral head is located peripherally relative to that in adults and therefore extends to the cervicotrochanteric area. From there, the dominant vessels ascend along the posterior aspect of the femoral neck and head. Injury to this capsular blood supply produces avascular necrosis of the femoral head in any patient with an open proximal femoral growth plate.

***Flexible Femoral Medullary Nailing.*** With the patient positioned supine on a radiolucent operating table, flexible medullary nails are inserted through two straight incisions at the distal end of the femur medially and laterally approximately 4 cm proximal to the joint line of the knee after manipulative reduction. Under image intensifier control, medial and lateral oblique cortical

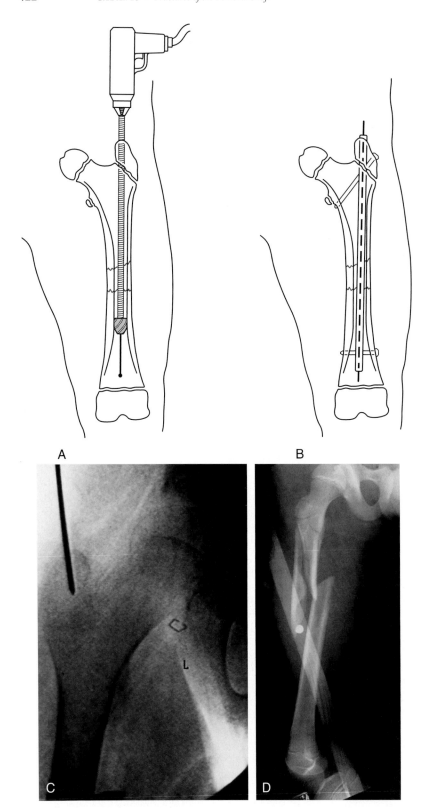

A

B

C

D

FIGURE 13–5. *A,* The starting point for the nail must enter the tip of the greater trochanter to avoid disrupting the blood supply to the femoral head. The femoral canal is reamed to within 1.5 to 2 cm of the distal femoral physis. *B,* The straight-tipped guide wire is exchanged with the bulb-tipped guide wire, and the nail is inserted over the straight-tipped guide wire after the femur has been reamed to 1.5 cm larger than the nail diameter. The guide wire is removed, and the nail is locked proximally and distally. The external guide is used for the proximal locking screw, and a freehand technique is used for the distal locking screw. Usually, only one distal locking screw is necessary unless the fracture is very comminuted or distal to the isthmus of the femur. *C,* Antero-posterior radiograph of the femur of a child who is undergoing femoral nailing. The guide wire for the 9-mm rigid reamer has been inserted through the tip of the greater trochanter before entering the femoral canal. The guide wire is inserted under fluoroscopic control to ensure accurate positioning into the tip of the greater trochanter and avoid the blood supply of the femoral head, which is at risk if one reams the femur through the pyriformis fossa. *D,* A comminuted fracture of the proximal end of the femur of a 10-year-old boy who sustained the fracture while skiing.

windows are made with an awl proximal to the distal femoral growth plate. The ideal insertion point is the proximal portion of the distal femoral metaphysis about 2 cm proximal to the distal femoral physis. The entry hole must be larger than the diameter of the chosen nail and must enter the femur in as oblique a direction as possible. One may use a drill, but curved awls (Drummond awls previously used for spinous process wiring are perfect) of various sizes are perfect for these entry holes. Two nails large enough to cover at least two thirds of the femoral canal are selected and bent into a **C** shape, with the concavity of the **C** on the same side of the nail as the bend on the leading tip of the nail. The two titanium nails must be of equal diameter. If nails of varied size are used, an angular deformity may result from the asymmetric force. The apex of the bend is located at the fracture site to provide three-point fixation and rotational stability. After adequate reduction of the fracture, the nails are directed across the fracture site one at a time. The lateral nail should be advanced so that the proximal end of the nail is just distal to the proximal extent of the greater trochanter. The medial nail is impacted into the femoral neck distal to the proximal femoral physis. The nails are then bent and cut with a nail cutter so that they are clearly positioned under the skin but are not

prominent (Fig. 13–6). A spica cast might be considered for additional stabilization in comminuted and unstable femoral shaft fractures. Normally, however, no external support is used on the extremity. The patient is quickly mobilized and ambulates with touch-down weight bearing on crutches or a walker. Patients will have increased their weight bearing within 4 weeks and will be fully weight bearing by 6 weeks after surgery. The fracture will usually be completely healed within 10 weeks postoperatively. The flexible nails may be removed by 6 months after surgery.

The risks inherent in implant removal are similar to those for implant insertion. For antegrade medullary

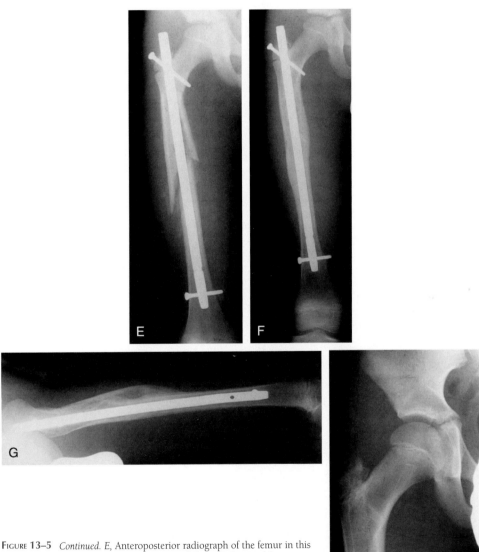

FIGURE 13–5 *Continued. E,* Anteroposterior radiograph of the femur in this child showing the nail in place. It was inserted through the tip of the greater trochanter and has been locked proximally and distally. The nail was left prominent proximal to the greater trochanter for ease of removal. *F,* Anteroposterior radiograph 5 months after the fracture was nailed. The femoral fracture has completely healed and remodeled. Again, note the starting point of the nail through the tip of the greater trochanter. *G,* Lateral radiograph of this 10-year-old child after the fracture has healed and is in the process of remodeling. *H,* Anteroposterior radiograph 1½ years after fracture and nail removal. Note the scar through the tip of the greater trochanter and across the trochanteric apophysis.

*Illustration continued on following page*

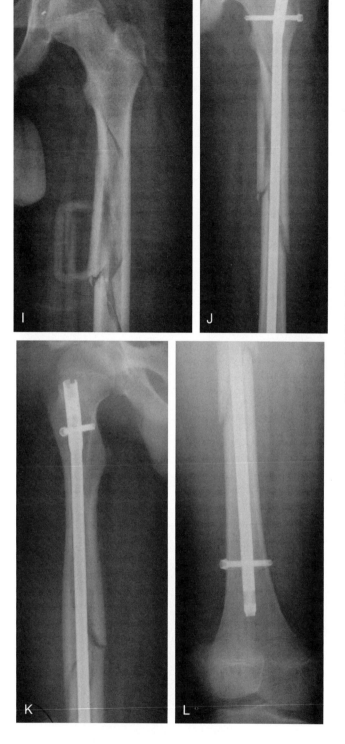

FIGURE **13–5** *Continued. I,* Another 10-year-old boy with a traumatic femoral fracture as seen on this anteroposterior radiograph. *J,* Anteroposterior radiograph after nailing of the femur with the new pediatric titanium nail designed for insertion through the tip of the greater trochanter. Note the curve in the upper end of the nail that allows trochanteric entry. *K,* Lateral radiograph of the femur after nailing of the fracture through the tip of the greater trochanter with a titanium nail. *L,* Anteroposterior radiograph of the distal end of the femur demonstrating that the nail has been locked with one distal locking screw. The distal end of the nail is well short of the distal femoral physis. (Radiographs courtesy of Dr. Neil E. Green.)

nails, risks include infection, injury to the femoral head blood supply, and sciatic nerve injury, among others. The surgeon must remember to remove all the locking screws before nail removal. Symptomatic ectopic bone in the nail insertion area should be excised at the time of implant removal.

## PLATE FIXATION

Plating techniques are rarely advocated in the orthopaedic literature for femoral shaft fractures in children. A high infection rate, extensive dissection, and the need for plate removal are concerns that accompany compression

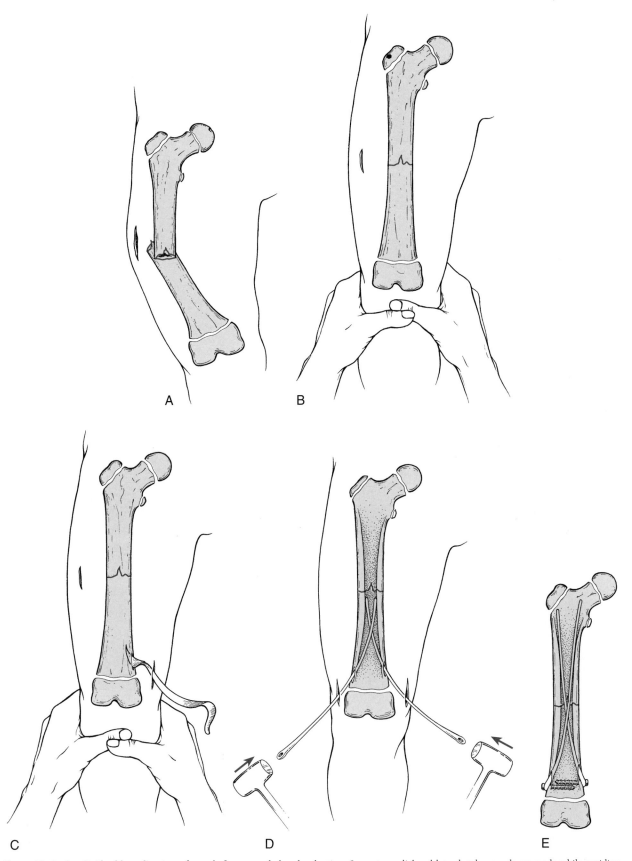

**FIGURE 13–6.** *A* to *E*, Flexible nailing is performed after manual closed reduction. Separate medial and lateral stab wounds are made while avoiding the distal femoral physis. The implants are advanced simultaneously. Additional implants are used to fill the medullary canal as needed. In this diagram, flexible and distal locked nails are illustrated.

*Illustration continued on following page*

plating.[30] Ziv and Rang[121] noted a 60% incidence of infection in four patients with five femoral shaft fractures treated with compression plates. They believed that these polytraumatized patients had a decreased resistance to infection and were more susceptible to nosocomial sepsis.[121] Three recent reports, however, found compression plating to be safe and reliable with low rates of complication.[52, 75, 98] Kregor and co-workers noted ex-

cellent results with the use of plates for femoral shaft fractures in polytraumatized children.[75] Fourteen fractures healed without infection, and overgrowth of the femur was not significant. The implant size was dependent on the size of the femur and, consequently, the age of the patient, yet all were dynamic compression plates applied with proper technique at a Level I trauma center. Postoperative spica casting was reserved for patients with

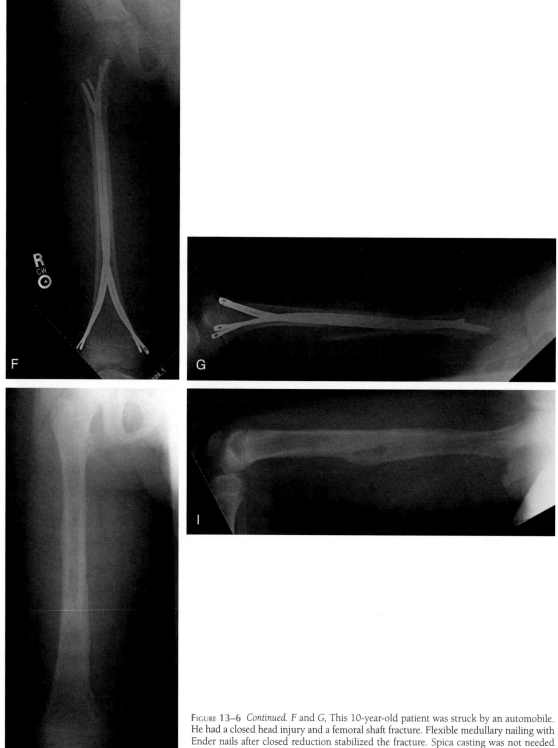

FIGURE **13–6** *Continued. F* and *G,* This 10-year-old patient was struck by an automobile. He had a closed head injury and a femoral shaft fracture. Flexible medullary nailing with Ender nails after closed reduction stabilized the fracture. Spica casting was not needed to support the implants. *H* and *I,* Uneventful healing resulted, and the implants were removed 9 months later. Note the posterior cortical union and remodeling.

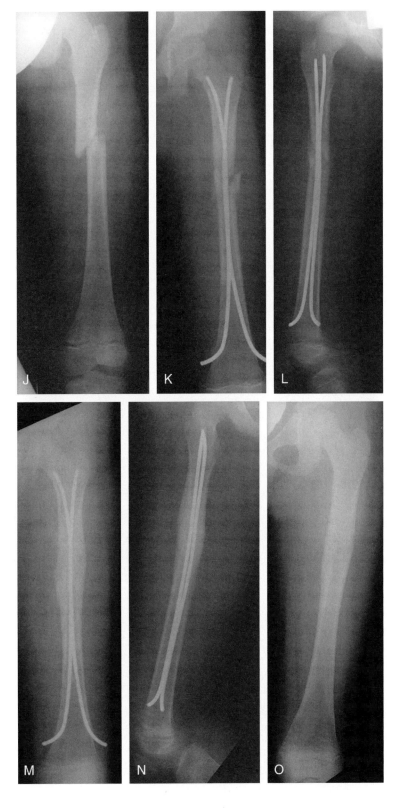

FIGURE 13–6 *Continued. J,* Nine-year-old girl who sustained a femoral fracture in a bicycle accident as demonstrated on this radiograph. *K,* Anteroposterior radiograph of the femur after internal fixation of the fracture with flexible titanium nails. The nails have been inserted distally through entry points in the femoral metaphysis medially and laterally. The nails were bent into a C shape before insertion. The nails are the same diameter, which is important because if nails of unequal diameter are used, an angular deformity is likely to result from an asymmetric force on the femoral fracture. The nails are not designed to fill the canal as with Ender nails, but use the C bend in the nail to provide three-point fixation, which provides remarkable stability of the fracture both to prevent angular deformity and to maintain rotational stability. The cephalad end of the nails has a flattened bent tip. The bend of the tip helps with passage of the nail across the fracture. The flattening of the tip, which is impacted into the compact metaphyseal bone of the proximal end of the femur, provides rotational stability of the fracture. The medial nail has been impacted into the compact metaphyseal bone of the femoral neck, and the lateral nail is inserted with the bent tip facing the greater trochanter. *L,* Lateral radiograph demonstrating flexible nailing of the fracture with excellent reduction. *M,* Anteroposterior radiograph of the femur 6 months after flexible nailing; excellent healing is evident. *N,* Lateral radiograph of the fracture 6 months after fracture demonstrating healing of the fracture. *O,* One year after fracture and 4 months after the nails were removed, the femoral fracture has fully healed. (Radiographs *J–O* courtesy of Dr. Neil E. Green.)

associated pelvic or spinal trauma requiring immobilization. In most patients, hypertrophic scarring on the lateral aspect of the thigh recurred, even after formal scar revision at the time of plate removal.[75]

Fyodorov and co-workers[35] confirmed the good results with open plate osteosynthesis in pediatric femoral shaft fractures. In 23 femoral shaft fractures in children aged 8 to 12 years, they experienced two implant failures 6 weeks postoperatively that required spica casting and revision plating, respectively. Both then healed uneventfully.

More recently, less invasive techniques for plate osteosynthesis application have evolved. Farouk and colleagues[33] in a human cadaver study showed that a minimally invasive percutaneous plating technique better preserves bone vascularity relative to the traditional open method. Additionally, Baumgaertel and co-workers[5] described faster and more effective bony bridging of a fracture gap and mineralization of callus after indirect than after open direct and anatomic reduction in an in vivo sheep study. Consequently, minimally invasive percutaneous plate osteosynthesis (MIPPO) has been performed for femoral shaft fractures[116] and is also used in children.

### Technique

*Standard Plating.* The patient is positioned supine with a soft bump under the ipsilateral flank. A straight lateral incision is made through the fascia lata. The vastus lateralis of the quadriceps is retracted anteriorly, and care is taken to identify and ligate the perforating arteries and veins. The extent of traumatic periosteal stripping adjacent to the fracture site is related to the violence of the event. Additional surgical periosteal elevation is rarely necessary for the proximal and distal fragments.

The fracture is reduced and clamped. Independent lag screws are inserted if lag screw application through the plate is not possible. The implant is selected according to the size of the femur. Either the 3.5-mm or the 4.5-mm narrow dynamic compression plating system is used. Depending on fracture comminution and orientation, plates with eight or more holes are chosen. For smaller femurs, the 3.5-mm system is used. The plate is slightly prebent for patients with transverse fracture patterns. A femoral distractor is helpful in regaining the length needed to perform the plating (Figs. 13–7 and 13–8).

*Minimally Invasive Femoral Plating.* To perform MIPPO, the patient is positioned supine on a radiolucent operating table. The skin is incised approximately 3 cm longitudinally over the greater trochanter and femoral condyles. The incisions are continued to bone. With a periosteal elevator, the interval between the vastus lateralis and periosteum is developed bluntly. A 3.5- or 4.5-mm dynamic compression plate that has been precontoured according to an AP radiograph of the

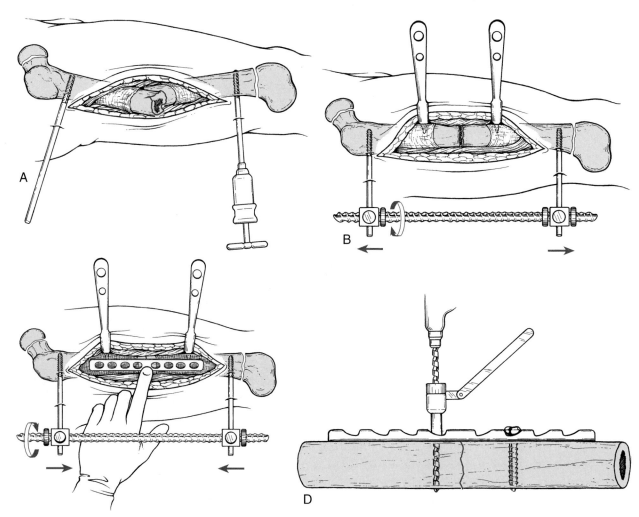

**FIGURE 13–7.** *A,* With the patient supine and the buttock elevated on a bump, a lateral surgical exposure is used. Pins are placed after predrilling. Periosteal stripping is minimized. *B,* A femoral distractor can be used to grossly align and secure the fracture. Narrow retractors are used to limit soft tissue stripping medially. The retractors should be placed in the same positions throughout the operation. Manipulation of the distractor allows perfect reduction. *C,* The distractor can then be reversed to compress the fracture. *D,* The compression plate is prebent and contoured; a template may be used. Eccentric drilling produces fracture compression when a dynamic compression plate is used.

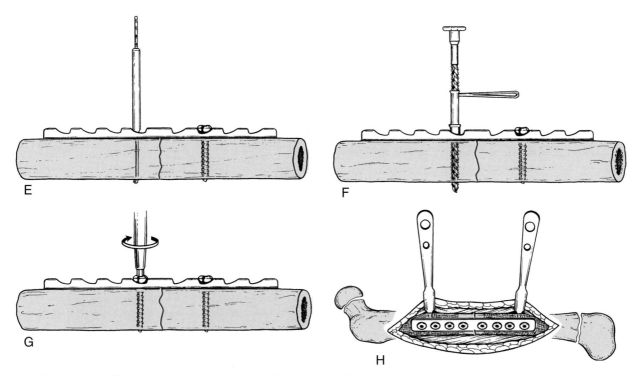

**FIGURE 13–7** *Continued. E,* A depth gauge measures length. *F,* The hole is tapped. *G,* The eccentrically placed screw is tightened. As the screw head engages the plate, the fracture is compressed. The plate must be prebent to prevent compression adjacent to the plate and distraction of the opposite cortex. *H,* Final plate appearance with the distractor removed. Notice the intact periosteum, which was preserved with careful technique.

contralateral side is then inserted into the submuscular interval under fluoroscopic control. The implant avoids both the proximal and distal physis, but it should be as long as possible for better stability of the fracture fixation. The plate is secured on one end with a percutaneously inserted screw, and the fracture is then manipulated and reduced to the plate. Femoral length and rotation at the fracture site, as well as plate positioning, are adjusted with manipulative techniques such as manual traction and rotation, percutaneously inserted pins for manipulation, and the femoral distractor, among others. The plate is stabilized to the femur with screws above and below the fracture site, similar to the concept of an external fixator using "far" screws and "near" screws (Fig. 13–9).

Patient rehabilitation after plate fixation is similar to that for both external fixation and medullary nailing. Protected weight bearing is advised for 6 weeks after surgery. Progressive loading and exercises are advanced on the basis of clinical and radiographic healing.

Plate removal from the femur is advocated for certain children. Removal is generally performed, based on the age of the patient and fracture remodeling, 6 to 18 months after the fracture.

## THE MULTIPLY INJURED CHILD

Aggressive treatment of pediatric femoral shaft fractures, especially in the polytrauma setting, has many advantages. In 1983, Marcus and co-workers[80] reported on 34 polytraumatized children with 61 total fractures, 16 of which were femoral fractures. Four patients had residual disability as a result of their femoral fractures. All four

were treated with closed reduction and spica casting. Three had limb length inequalities, and one had a flexion contracture at the knee. These authors concluded that rigid adherence to the concept of closed management in pediatric fractures may be counterproductive in polytraumatized patients and can result in increased morbidity. The residual morbidity in these conservatively managed patients was related to their orthopaedic and neural injuries. Marcus and co-workers believed that inadequate fracture alignment should not be accepted regardless of the severity of associated injuries. Because of reports of excellent function and low rates of infection with operative methods of stabilization such as external fixation, reamed nailing, flexible (Ender) nailing, and plating in multiply injured children, these approaches are being more widely advocated for isolated fractures. Ipsilateral fracture of the femur and tibia may be a relative indicator for more aggressive surgical management because of the high incidence of shortening that results.[12] This aggressive approach in polytraumatized children is in contrast to the advice of Dameron and Thompson[24] regarding isolated femoral shaft fractures. These authors asserted that "overtreatment is usually worse than undertreatment."[24] Hansen stated that although children are more tolerant of severe injury, an aggressive approach saves time, money, disability, and occasionally lives.[51]

Timmerman and Rab[112] and Reeves and associates[98] demonstrated that operative treatment decreased hospitalization. The latter investigators also estimated that conservative management of femoral fractures in children was approximately 46% more expensive than operative management. A shortened hospital stay may well have psychologic, social, educational, and economic benefit.[98]

### Conservative Management of a Multiply Injured Child

Spasticity and restlessness are the main problems in children with moderate to severe head injuries. The head-down position should be avoided because of effects on intracranial pressure. Operative fixation provides immediate stability and simplifies nursing care. Malunion occurred in 6 of 34 fractures treated nonoperatively in one study, but in none of 16 patients treated by medullary nailing. No overgrowth problems were noted in the open-treatment group.[121]

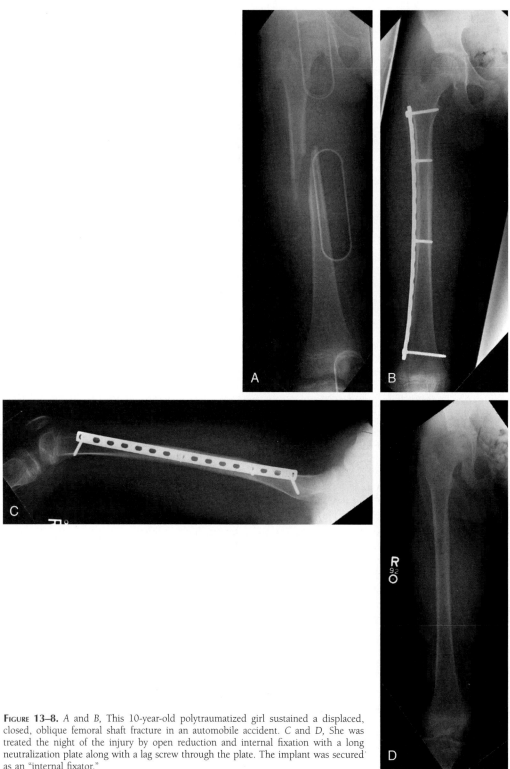

FIGURE 13–8. *A* and *B,* This 10-year-old polytraumatized girl sustained a displaced, closed, oblique femoral shaft fracture in an automobile accident. *C* and *D,* She was treated the night of the injury by open reduction and internal fixation with a long neutralization plate along with a lag screw through the plate. The implant was secured as an "internal fixator."

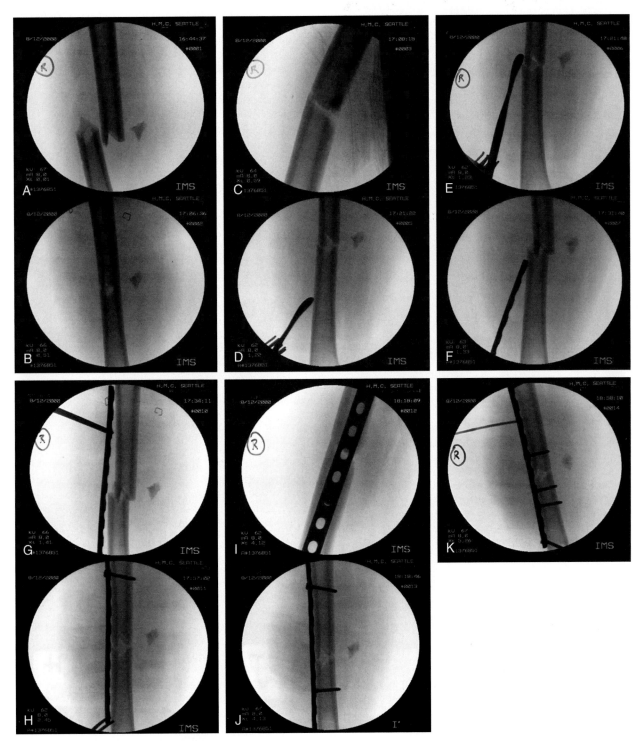

**FIGURE 13–9.** Minimally invasive plate osteosynthesis was used to treat a comminuted transverse diaphyseal femoral fracture in this 14-year-old patient. *A,* A fluoroscopic image demonstrates the displacement. *B* and *C,* These images show the alignment after closed manipulative reduction under anesthesia is accomplished. *D* and *E,* Through a small distal lateral incision, a periosteal elevator prepares the area for plate insertion. *F* and *G,* The implant is contoured according to the preoperative plan and inserted. A proximal small incision facilitates manipulation of the implant. *H,* The reduction is adjusted and the plate secured to the femur proximally with a percutaneously inserted screw after drilling and accurate depth assessment. *I,* The plate is adjusted to fit the bone on the lateral image before final screw tightening. *J,* A compression screw is inserted percutaneously in the distal fragment. *K,* Additional screws are applied percutaneously according to the preoperative plan.

*Illustration continued on following page*

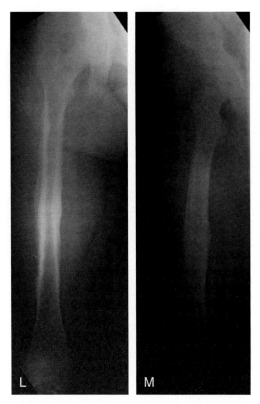

Figure 13–9 *Continued. L* and *M,* Plain radiographs demonstrate fracture union and remodeling. The implants were removed 10 months after surgery.

Of 292 children in coma with head injuries for more than 1 week, 39 had 44 femoral shaft fractures. All healed, and 32 of the 39 eventually ambulated. No complications occurred in the operatively treated group. Conservative management led to malunion, osteomyelitis, skin breakdown, excessive shortening, and rotational deformities. Open reduction and internal fixation, when feasible in a brain-injured child with a femoral shaft fracture, is an attractive solution to the overall management of this complicated injury.[34]

## Complications

### REMODELING, OVERGROWTH, GROWTH DISTURBANCE

Remodeling will never correct rotational malunion. In children older than 9 years, remodeling should not be relied on to correct angular deformity. The likelihood of correction with remodeling depends on patient age and proximity of the fracture to the physis, as well as other factors.[20] Wallace and Hoffman documented that at an average follow-up of 45 months, about 85% of the initial residual angular deformity had corrected.[116] Seventy-four percent of the correction occurred at the physes and 26% at the fracture site, and younger children remodeled only slightly better than older children.[116] These authors concluded that angular malunion of up to 25° in any place will remodel.

Overgrowth of a fractured femur seems to be most prominent in patients treated between the ages of 2 and 10 years.[92] Therefore, some shortening in the original reduction (in the range of 1.5 to 2 cm) is allowable. This phenomenon is variable in older children and adolescents, and it does not seem to be prominent with open reduction. The site of fracture, the fracture pattern, and age are not related to overgrowth, but several authors suggest that overgrowth is seen more frequently in more proximal fractures.[63] It may be related to handedness, as identified by Meals,[85] because non–dominant-side fractures overgrew more than did dominant-side fractures. Limb length inequality is the most frequent complication of femoral shaft fractures in children, and it produces limp and compensatory scoliosis. The surgeon should ensure equal leg length at injury and not accept more than 1.5 to 2 cm of shortening. Growth acceleration is probably related to the amount of osseous and soft tissue disruption, which translates to fracture hyperemia.[107] Growth disturbances of the proximal end of the femur have been reported in as many as 30% of patients younger than 13 years[41] (see Fig. 13–11).

Malunion can occur regardless of the treatment chosen. Herndon and colleagues identified seven malunions in 24 children treated nonoperatively.[60] Heinrich and co-workers reported a 9% average incidence of angular or rotational malalignment (or both) after using flexible medullary fixation.[56]

### LOSS OF REDUCTION

Loss of reduction is mainly a concern in the closed management of femoral shaft fractures, although implant failure with subsequent loss of reduction can occur as well[45] (Fig. 13–10). Illgen and co-workers[64] described a 20% incidence of loss of reduction in children younger than 6 years when treated by early sitting spica casting. They identified a spica knee flexion angle of less than 50° as predictive of eventual loss of reduction.

### EXTERNAL FIXATION PIN TRACT INFECTION/REFRACTURE

Fracture through a pin site or refracture through an incompletely united femoral shaft fracture can occur when external fixation frames are used (Fig. 13–11). In most series, pin tract infections and refracture after frame removal are the most common problems, although the rates of these complications are quite variable (Fig. 13–12). De Sanctis and co-workers[28] did not see any refractures or secondary fractures in 81 children, and Blasier and colleagues[10] described secondary fractures in only 2.1% of 139 femoral fractures. In 13 patients, one refracture and six infections of the pins were recorded in the series of Quintin and co-workers.[97] Davis and associates reported five cases of pin tract infection and one refracture in 15 pediatric patients treated with external fixation.[25] Kirschenbaum and colleagues treated 10 high-energy femoral fractures in children with a variety of lateral frames.[73] All 10 healed, with only minor deformity noted. Pin tract infections occurred in 3 of the 10 patients; all resolved with local care. One patient had spastic cerebral palsy and suffered a refracture after removal of the frame. The authors recommended brace protection after frame removal, especially in patients with spasticity.[73] Gregory and colleagues demonstrated a high rate of complications after external fixation of pediatric femoral shaft fractures. They emphasized technical problems, such as refracture secondary to a misplaced cortical pin.[47] Gregory and co-workers[45] observed pin tract infections in 52% and secondary fractures in 19% of patients, whereas Skaggs associates[105] described a 12% rate of infection in secondary fractures. The latter was statistically significantly related to the number of cortices demonstrating bridging callus (on both AP and lateral views) at the time of fixator removal. Fractures with fewer than three cortices of bridging callus had a significantly higher rate of refracture.[105] In a more recent study, Miner and Carroll[87] reported pin tract infections in 73% of 33 patients 4 to 14 years of age and a 22% rate of refracture after removal of the external fixator. The average duration in the fixator was 107 days. Children with bilateral femoral fractures had the highest risk. Such a high rate of secondary fracture and refracture might be cause for early conversion of the external fixation to internal stabilization.

Green and colleagues (personal communication, Dr. Neil E. Green) evaluated 72 children with fractures of the femur treated with an external fixation device. They found eight refractures, one of which occurred through a pin tract 26 days after removal of the fixator. The other

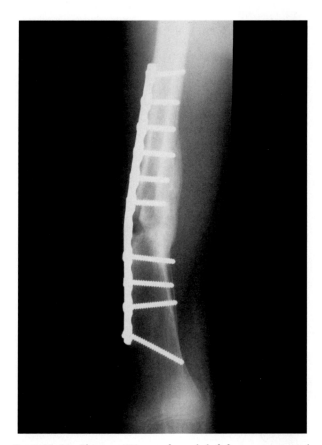

**FIGURE 13–10.** This type IIIA open femoral shaft fracture was treated with open débridement and reduction. Plate fixation was performed, but patient noncompliance resulted in plate bending.

fractures occurred within 5 days of removal of the fixation device. All the fractures in these patients were transverse. The authors found that the risk of refracture was directly proportional to the length (width) of the fracture. In other words, if the fracture was purely transverse, the length of the fracture fragment was minimal, but if the fracture was a long oblique one, the length of the fracture fragment was long. The longer the length of the fracture, the lower the risk of refracture. Therefore, a short transverse fracture had a very high risk of refracture, whereas a long oblique fracture had a very slight risk of refracture after removal of the fixator. It has been recommended that a transverse fracture not be placed in an external fixator as the best method of treatment.

Our recommendation for treatment of this fracture of the femur would be intramedullary fixation if possible as the best form of treatment. For children younger than 10 years, flexible intramedullary nails would be the device of choice, and in a child 10 years and older, a locked intramedullary nail should be chosen. Remember to insert the locked nail through a trochanteric entry point to avoid the piriformis fossa. If, on the other hand, an external fixator is used for a transverse fracture, overlapping of the fracture fragments is probably preferable to increase the volume of fracture callus and thereby reduce the risk of refracture.

## INFECTION

Infection after closed management of closed fractures is a rare, but identified phenomenon. It must be considered when pain of a different character becomes a complaint. An increase in local tissue reaction and erythema when all signs and reactions should be diminishing also brings this possibility to mind. Patients in the series of Canale and co-workers all had a primary source of infection and had a persistent febrile course.[16] Karaoglu and associates reported a deep infection after an open fracture was treated by Ender nailing.[68]

## COMPARTMENT SYNDROME

Compartment syndrome of the leg can result from prolonged elevation in Bryant's traction, even in the uninjured leg; therefore, such management is not advocated as a form of traction treatment.[67, 91] Compartment syndrome can also result from elevation of the injured limb when the patient is hypotensive.[22] When high-velocity trauma produces the fracture, compartment syndrome of the thigh must be considered a possibility (see Chapter 6). It is generally manifested as a rigid thigh, severe pain (in an alert patient), and elevated intracompartmental pressure. Fasciotomy on an emergency basis is indicated.

## REFRACTURE

Refracture after a femoral shaft fracture in children is a rare phenomenon. It is generally associated with highly comminuted fractures and extensive stripping of the bone and is related to the manipulation of stiff knees.

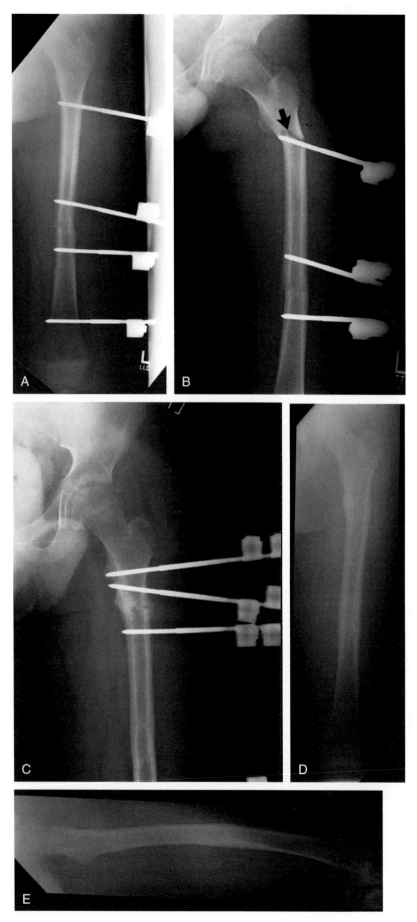

**FIGURE 13–11.** *A,* This unusual 12-year-old boy sustained forearm and femoral fractures in a motorbike accident. He smoked one pack of cigarettes per day. The femoral fracture was stabilized after closed reduction with a lateral, single-bar external fixator. Early healing was noted on this radiograph 3 weeks after injury. *B,* Five weeks after injury (while still in the frame), he fell while jumping from a trampoline against medical advice. He noted immediate pain, and radiographs revealed a displaced fracture through the proximal pin site. The diaphyseal fracture showed incomplete healing. *C,* The initial frame was removed, manipulative reduction of the acute proximal fracture was accomplished, and the subsequent external fixator was revised to span both femoral fracture sites. Two months after the initial injury, fracture healing is noted at both sites. *D* and *E,* Nine months after injury, his radiographs demonstrated remodeling of the fracture sites. He sustained an open tibial fracture in a separate motorcycle accident only 4 months later.

Refracture does not seem to correlate with treatment, deformity, or shortening because it is seen so seldom.[104] Although permanent loss of bone and density occurs with a femoral fracture, it does not predispose to refracture.[58]

## TRACTION PIN COMPLICATIONS

Traction pins may produce problems when their position is not radiographically defined. Problems include skin lacerations and disruption of the knee capsule. When a proximal tibial pin is used in an individual with an ipsilateral knee injury, the ligamentous injuries and physeal disruption can be made more severe. Finally, poor placement of a proximal tibial pin or multiple passes can result in premature tibial tubercle apophyseal closure and resultant knee recurvatum, which is a difficult problem to manage. We therefore recommend a distal femoral pin placed under radiographic control for most femoral shaft fractures in 7- to 12-year-old children.

## ECTOPIC BONE FORMATION

Symptomatic ectopic bone formation may restrict hip or knee motion and require excision. Galpin and colleagues described this complication after medullary nailing of pediatric and adolescent femoral shaft fractures.[38] Prophylaxis should be strongly considered, especially in children with associated craniocerebral trauma.

## ASEPTIC NECROSIS OF THE FEMORAL HEAD

Wide hip abduction in a spica cast allows improved perineal access but may be responsible for aseptic necrosis of the femoral head. The hips should not be overly abducted in the cast. This complication has also been reported after antegrade medullary fixation with a medial "piriformis fossa" starting point. A medially located nail insertion site, although it avoids trochanteric apophyseal damage, may injure the capsular blood supply to the femoral head.[4, 86, 110]

A trochanteric starting point avoids this complication (Fig. 13–13).

## Preferred Treatment

The following guidelines are presented according to the age of the child.

Neonate. Splinting for 2 to 3 weeks until united.
One to 5 years
 *Isolated.* Immediate spica casting if the shortening is acceptable (less than 1.5 cm), with close follow-up to limit the shortening, and wedging as indicated. If the shortening is unacceptable, external fixation or flexible nailing is indicated.
 *Multiple injuries* (especially with closed head injury). External fixation to union or, for 3 to 4

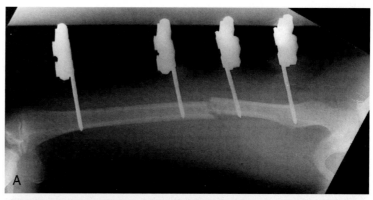

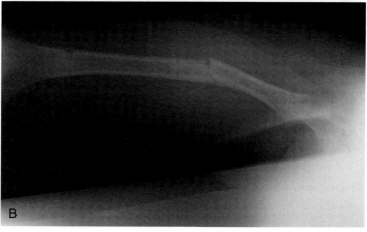

FIGURE **13–12.** *A,* This 9-year-old patient had his femoral fracture treated with an external fixator. Twelve weeks after injury, fracture healing was verified in the clinic. The pin sites were erythematous, so the frame was removed. *B,* The next day while walking, he fell and noted pain in his thigh because of a repeat fracture at the previous fracture site.

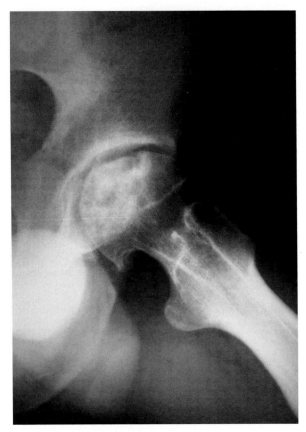

FIGURE **13-13.** Aseptic necrosis of the femoral head resulted after antegrade reamed medullary nailing. A medial starting point may have caused the necrosis.

weeks, until callus causes the length to be stable, and then conversion to a spica cast for an additional 3 to 4 weeks.

Six to 10 years

*Isolated.* Flexible nailing, external fixation, or plating.

*Multiple injuries.* Flexible nailing, external fixation, or plating.

Ten to 14 years

*Isolated.* Flexible nailing for stable fracture patterns. Antegrade, reamed, locked medullary nailing using a trochanteric starting point for larger individuals. MIPPO is also effective.

*Multiple injuries.* Hemodynamically unstable patients or those with moderate to severe head injuries are treated with external fixation, medullary nailing, or plating. Nailing is selected when all routes for stabilization of the fracture are acceptable to the anesthesia and trauma teams.

Fourteen years and older. Locked medullary nailing using the trochanteric starting point while the growth centers remain open.

### REFERENCES

1. Allen, B.L.; Kant, A.P.; Emery, F.E. Displaced fractures of the femoral diaphysis in children. J Trauma 17:8–19, 1977.
2. Alonso, J.E.; Horowitz, M. Use of the AO/ASIF external fixator in children. J Pediatr Orthop 7:594–600, 1987.
3. American Academy of Orthopaedic Surgeons. Play It Safe. Chicago, AAOS, 1991.
4. Astion, D.J.; Wilber, J.H; Scoles, P.V. Avascular necrosis of the capital femoral epiphysis after intramedullary nailing for a fracture of the femoral shaft. A case report. J Bone Joint Surg Am 77:1092–1094, 1995.
5. Baumgaertel, F.; Buhl, M.; Rahn, B.A. Fracture healing in biological plate osteosynthesis. Injury 29(Suppl 3):C3–C6, 1998.
6. Beals, R.K. Premature closure of the physis following diaphyseal fractures. J Pediatr Orthop 10:717–720, 1990.
7. Beals, R.K.; Tufts, E. Fractured femur in infancy: The role of child abuse. J Pediatr Orthop 3:583–586, 1983.
8. Beaty, J.H. Femoral shaft fractures in children and adolescents. J Am Acad Orthop Surg 3:207–217, 1995.
9. Beaty, J.H.; Austin, S.M.; Warner, W.C.; et al. Interlocking intramedullary nailing of femoral shaft fractures in adolescents: Preliminary results and complications. J Pediatr Orthop 14:178–183, 1994.
10. Blasier, R.D.; Aronson, J.; Tursky, E.A. External fixation of pediatric femur fractures. J Pediatr Orthop 17:342–346, 1997.
11. Blount, W. Fractures in Children. Baltimore, Williams & Wilkins, 1955, p. 129.
12. Bohn, W.W.; Durbin, R.A. Ipsilateral fractures of the femur and tibia in children and adolescents. J Bone Joint Surg Am 73:429–439, 1991.
13. Buckley, S.L.; Sturm, P.F.; Tosi, L.L.; et al. Ligamentous instability of the knee in children sustaining fractures of the femur: A prospective study with knee examination under anesthesia. J Pediatr Orthop 16:206–209, 1996.
14. Buford, D., Jr.; Christensen, K.; Weatherall, P. Intramedullary nailing of femoral fractures in adolescents. Clin Orthop 350:85–89, 1998.
15. Burton, V.W.; Fordyce, A.J.W. Immobilization of femoral shaft fractures in children aged 2–10 years. Injury 4:47–53, 1972.
16. Canale, S.T.; Puhl, J.; Watson, F.M.; Gillespie, R. Acute osteomyelitis following closed fractures. Report of three cases. J Bone Joint Surg Am 57:415–418, 1975.
17. Carey, T.P.; Galpin, R.D. Flexible intramedullary nail fixation of pediatric femoral fractures. Clin Orthop 332:110–118, 1996.
18. Celiker, O.; Cetin, I.; Sahlan, S.; et al. Femoral shaft fractures in children: Technique of immediate treatment with supracondylar Kirschner wires and one-and-a-half spica cast. J Pediatr Orthop 8:580–584, 1988.
19. Christensen, E.; Dietz, G. A radiographically documented intra-uterine femoral fracture. Br J Radiol 51:830–831, 1978.
20. Connolly, J.F. Fractures in children: When the growth plate is damaged. J Musculoskel Med 8:82–97, 1991.
21. Crane, S.D.; Beverley, D.W.; Williams, M.J. Massive pulmonary embolus in a 14 year old boy. J Accid Emerg Med 16:289–290, 1999.
22. Curtis, J.F.; Killian, J.T.; Alonso, J.E. Improved treatment of femoral shaft fractures in children utilizing the pontoon spica cast: A long term follow-up. J Pediatr Orthop 15:36–40, 1995.
23. Czertak, D.J.; Hennrikus, W.L. The treatment of pediatric femur fractures with early 90-90 spica casting. J Pediatr Orthop 19:229–232, 1999.
24. Dameron, T.B.; Thompson, H.A. Femoral shaft fractures in children. Treatment by closed reduction and double spica cast immobilization. J Bone Joint Surg Am 41:1201–1212, 1959.
25. Davis, T.J.; Topping, R.E.; Blanco, J.S. External fixation of pediatric femoral fractures. Clin Orthop 318:191–198, 1995.
26. Day, T.E.; Kanellopoulos, A.D.; Mendelow, M.J.; et al: Reamed, locked, intramedullary nailing of pediatric femur fractures. Paper presented at the annual meeting of the American Academy of Orthopaedic Surgeons, San Francisco, 1997, p. 266.
27. Dent, J.A.; Paterson, C.R. Fractures in early childhood: Osteogenesis imperfecta or child abuse. J Pediatr Orthop 11:184–186, 1991.
28. De Sanctis, N.; Gambardella, A.; Pempinello, C.; et al. The use of external fixators in femur fractures in children. J Pediatr Orthop 16:613–620, 1996.
29. Drennan, J.; Freehofer, A. Fractures of the lower extremity in paraplegic children. Clin Orthop 77:211–217, 1971.

30. Eikenbary, C.; Lecoq, J.F. Fracture of the femur in children. J Bone Joint Surg 14:801–804, 1932.

31. Fardon, D.F. Fracture of neck and shaft of same femur. Report of a case in a child. J Bone Joint Surg Am 52:797–799, 1970.

32. Ferguson, J.; Nicol R.O. Early spica treatment of pediatric femoral shaft fractures. J Pediatr Orthop 20:189–192, 2000.

33. Farouk, O.; Krettek, C.; Miclau, T.; et al. Minimally invasive plate osteosynthesis: Does percutaneous plating disrupt femoral blood supply less than the traditional technique? J Orthop Trauma 13:401–406, 1999.

34. Fry, K.; Hoffer, M.M.; Brink, I. Femoral shaft fractures in brain injured children. J Trauma 16:371–373, 1976.

35. Fyodorov, J.; Sturm, P.F.; Robertson, W.W., Jr. Compression-plate fixation of femoral shaft fractures in children aged 8 to 12 years. J Pediatr Orthop 19:578–581, 1999.

36. Gage, J.R.; Cary, J.M. The effects of trochanteric epiphyseodesis on growth of the proximal end of the femur following necrosis of the capital femoral epiphysis. J Bone Joint Surg Am 62(5):785–794, 1980.

37. Galleno, H.; Oppenheim, W.L. The battered child syndrome revisited. Clin Orthop 162:11–19, 1982.

38. Galpin, R.D.; Willis, R.B.; Sabano, N. Intramedullary nailing of pediatric femoral fractures. J Pediatr Orthop 14:184–189, 1994.

39. Garside, W.B.; Green, N.E.; Mencio, G. Treatment of pediatric femoral shaft fractures with reamed locked intramedullary nailing. Orthop Trans 19:156, 1995.

40. Gibson, J.M.C. Multiple injuries: The management of the patient with a fractured femur and a head injury. J Bone Joint Surg Br 42:425–431, 1960.

41. Glenn, J.; Miner, M.; Peltier, L. The treatment of fractures of the femur in patients with head injuries. J Trauma 13:958–961, 1973.

42. Gonzalzez-Herranz, P.; Burgos-Flores, J.; Lopez-Mandejar, J.A.; et al. Intramedullary nailing at the femur in children. Effects on its proximal end. J Bone Joint Surg Br 77:262–266, 1995.

43. Gratz, R.R. Accidental injury in childhood: A literature review on pediatric trauma. J Trauma 19:551–555, 1979.

44. Green, M.; Haggerty, R.J. Ambulatory Pediatrics. Philadelphia, W.B. Saunders, 1968.

45. Gregory, P.; Pevny, T.; Teague, D. Early complications with external fixation of pediatric femoral shaft fractures. J Orthop Trauma 10:191–198, 1996.

46. Gregory, P.; Sullivan, J.A.; Herndon, W.A. Adolescent femoral shaft fractures: Rigid versus flexible nails. Orthopedics 18:645–649, 1995.

47. Gregory, R.J.; Cubison, T.C.; Pinder, I.M.; Smith, S.R. External fixation of lower limb fractures in children. J Trauma 33:691–693, 1992.

48. Gross, R.H.; Davidson, R.; Sullivan, J.A.; et al. Cast brace management of femoral shaft fracture in children and young adults. J Pediatr Orthop 3:572–582, 1983.

49. Guttman, G.G.; Simon, R. Three-point fixation walking spica cast: An alternative to early or immediate casting of femoral shaft fractures in children. J Pediatr Orthop 8:699–703, 1988.

50. Haller, J. Problems in children's trauma. J Trauma 10:269–271, 1970.

51. Hansen, S.T., Jr. Internal fixation of children's fractures of the lower extremity. Orthop Clin North Am 21:353–363, 1990.

52. Hansen, T.B. Fractures of the femoral shaft in children treated with an A/O compression plate. Acta Orthop Scand 63:50–52, 1992.

53. Havranek, P.; Westfelt, J.N.; Henrikson, B. Proximal tibial skeletal traction for femoral shaft fractures in children. Treatment to discard or retain. Clin Orthop 283:270–275, 1993.

54. Hedequist, D.; Starr, A.J.; Wilson, P.; Walker, J. Early versus delayed stabilization of pediatric femur fractures: Analysis of 387 patients. J Orthop Trauma 13:490–493, 1999.

55. Hedlund, R.; Lindgren, U. The incidence of femoral shaft fractures in children and adolescents. J Pediatr Orthop 6:47–50, 1986.

56. Heinrich, S.D.; Drvaric, D.M.; Darr, K.; MacEwen, G.D. The operative stabilization of pediatric diaphyseal femur fractures with flexible intramedullary nails: A prospective analysis. J Pediatr Orthop 14:501–507, 1994.

57. Helal, B.; Skevis, X. Unrecognized dislocation of the hip in fractures of the femoral shaft. J Bone Joint Surg Br 49:293–300, 1967.

58. Henderson, R.C.; Kemp, G.J.; Campion, E.R. Residual bone-mineral density and muscle strength after fractures of the tibia in children. J Bone Joint Surg Am 74:211–218, 1992.

59. Henry, A.N. Overgrowth after femoral shaft fractures in children. J Bone Joint Surg Br 45:222, 1963.

60. Herndon, W.A.; Mahnken, R.F.; Yngve, D.A.; Sullivan, J.A. Management of femoral shaft fracture in the adolescent. J Pediatr Orthop 9:29–32, 1989.

61. Hoeksema, H.D.; Olsen, C.; Rudy, R. Fracture of femoral neck and shaft and repeat neck fracture in a child. J Bone Joint Surg Am 57:271–272, 1975.

62. Hughes, B.F.; Sponseller, P.D.; Thompson, J.D. Pediatric femur fractures: Effects of spica cast treatment on family and community. J Pediatr Orthop 15:457–460, 1995.

63. Humberger, F.W.; Eyring, E.J. Proximal tibial 90-90 traction in treatment of children with femoral shaft fractures. J Bone Joint Surg Am 51:499–503, 1969.

64. Illgen, R., 2nd; Rodgers, W.B.; Hresko M.T.; et al. Femur fractures in children: Treatment with early sitting spica casting. J Pediatr Orthop 18:481–487, 1998.

65. Irani, R.; Nicholson, J.T.; Chung, S.M.K. Long-term results in the treatment of femoral shaft fractures in young children by immediate spica immobilization. J Bone Joint Surg Am. 58:945–951, 1976.

66. Izant, R.; Hubay, M. The annual injury of 15 million children. J Trauma 6:65–74, 1966.

67. Janzing, H.; Broos, P.; Rommens, P. Compartmental syndrome as a complication of skin traction in children with femoral fractures. J Trauma 41:156–158, 1996.

68. Karaoglu, S.; Baktir, A.; Tuncel, M.; et al. Closed Ender nailing of adolescent femoral shaft fractures. Injury 28:501–506, 1994.

69. Karpos, P.A.; McFerran, M.A.; Johnson, K.D. Intramedullary nailing of acute femoral shaft fractures using manual traction without a fracture table. J Orthop Trauma 9:57–62, 1995.

70. Katz, J. Spontaneous fractures in paraplegic children. J Bone Joint Surg Am 35:220–226, 1953.

71. King, J.; Diefendorf, D.; Apthorp, J.; et al. Analysis of 429 fractures in 189 battered children. J Pediatr Orthop 8:585–589, 1988.

72. Kirby, R.M.; Winquist, R.A.; Hansen, S.T., Jr. Femoral shaft fracture in adolescents: A comparison between traction plus cast treatment and closed intramedullary nailing. J Pediatr Orthop 1:193–197, 1981.

73. Kirschenbaum, D.; Albert, M.C.; Robertson, W.W., Jr.; Davidson, R.S. Complex femur fractures in children: Treatment with external fixation. J Pediatr Orthop 10:588–591, 1990.

74. Kissel, E.U.; Miller, M.E. Closed Ender nailing of femur fractures in older children. J Trauma 29:1585–1588, 1989.

75. Kregor, P.J.; Song, K.; Routt, M.L., Jr.; et al. Plate fixation of femoral shaft fractures in multiply injured children. J Bone Joint Surg Am 75:1774–1780, 1993.

76. Ligier, J.N.; Metaizeau, J.; Prevot, J.; Lascombes, P. Elastic stable intramedullary nailing of femoral shaft fractures in children. J Bone Joint Surg Br 70:74–77, 1988.

77. Linhart, W.E.; Roposch, A. Elastic stable intramedullary nailing for unstable femoral fractures in children: Preliminary results of a new method. J Trauma 47:372–378, 1999.

78. Mann, D.C.; Rajmaira, S. Distribution of physeal and nonphyseal fractures in 2,650 long-bone fractures in children aged 0–16 years. J Pediatr Orthop 10:713–716, 1990.

79. Mann, D.C.; Weddington, J.; Davenport, K. Closed Ender nailing of femoral shaft fractures in adolescents. J Pediatr Orthop 10:651–655, 1986.

80. Marcus, R.E.; Mills, M.F.; Thompson, G.H. Multiple injury in children. J Bone Joint Surg Am 65:1290–1294, 1983.

81. Maruenda-Paulino, J.I.; Sanchis-Alfonso, V.; Gomar-Sancho, F.; et al. Küntscher nailing of femoral shaft fractures in children and adolescents. Int Orthop 17:158–161, 1993.

82. Mayer, T. Causes of morbidity and mortality in severe pediatric trauma. JAMA 245:719–721, 1981.

83. Mazda, K.; Khairouni, A.; Pennecot, G.F.; Bensahel, H. Closed flexible intramedullary nailing of the femoral shaft fractures in children. J Pediatr Orthop B 6:198–202, 1997.

84. McDougall, A. Fracture of the neck of the femur in childhood. J Bone Joint Surg Br 43:16–28, 1961.

85. Meals, R.A. Overgrowth of the femur following fractures in children: Influence of handedness. J Bone Joint Surg Am 61:381–384, 1979.

86. Mileski, R.A.; Garvin, K.L.; Crosby, L.A. Avascular necrosis of the femoral head in an adolescent following intramedullary nailing of the femur. A case report. J Bone Joint Surg Am 76:1706–1708, 1994.

87. Miner, T.; Carroll, K.L. Outcomes of external fixation of pediatric femoral shaft fractures. J Pediatr Orthop 20:405–410, 2000.

88. Momberger, N.; Stevens, P.; Smith, J.; et al. Intramedullary nailing of femoral fractures in adolescents. J Pediatr Orthop 20:482–484, 2000.

89. Mubarak, S.; Carroll, N.C. Volkmann's contracture in children: Aetiology and prevention. J Bone Joint Surg Br 61:285–293, 1979.

90. Newberger, E. The myth of the battered child syndrome. Curr Med Dialogue 40:327, 1973.

91. Nicholson, J.T.; Foster, R.M.; Heath, R.D. Bryant's traction. A provocative cause of circulatory complications. JAMA 157:415–418, 1955.

92. Nork, S.E.; Bellig, G.J.; Woll, J.P.; Hoffinger, S.A. Overgrowth and outcome after femoral shaft fracture in children younger than 2 years. Clin Orthop 357:186–191, 1998.

93. Nork, S.E.; Hoffinger, S.A. Skeletal traction versus external fixation for pediatric femoral shaft fractures: A comparison of hospital costs and charges. J Orthop Trauma 12:563–568, 1998.

94. O'Malley, D.E.; Mazur, J.M.; Cummings, R.J. Femoral head avascular necrosis associated with intramedullary nailing in an adolescent. J Pediatr Orthop 15:21–23, 1995.

95. Orler, R.; Hersche, O.; Helfet, D.L.; et al. Avascular femur head necrosis as severe complication after femoral intramedullary nailing in children and adolescents. Unfallchirurg 101:495–499, 1998.

96. Pollak, A.N.; Cooperman, D.R.; Thompson, G.H. Spica cast treatment of femoral shaft fractures in children—the prognostic value of the mechanism of injury. J Trauma 37:223–229, 1994.

97. Quintin, J.; Evrard, H.; Gouat, P.; et al. External fixation in child traumatology. Orthopedics 7:463–467, 1984.

98. Reeves, R.B.; Ballard, R.I.; Hughes, J.L. Internal fixation versus traction and casting of adolescent femoral shaft fractures. J Pediatr Orthop 10:592–595, 1990.

99. Reynolds, D.A. Growth changes in fractured long-bones. A study of 126 children. J Bone Joint Surg Br 63:83–88, 1981.

100. Riew, K.D.; Sturm, P.F.; Rosenbaum, D.; et al. Neurological complications of pediatric femoral nailing. J Pediatr Orthop 16:606–612, 1996.

101. Robinson, W. Treatment of birth fractures of the femur. J Bone Joint Surg 20:778–780, 1938.

102. Sahin, V.; Baktir, A.; Turk, C.Y.; et al. Femoral shaft fractures in children treated by closed reduction and early spica cast with incorporated supracondylar Kirschner wires: Long-term follow-up results. Injury 30:121–128, 1999.

103. Schwend, R.M.; Werth, C.; Johnston, A. Femur shaft fractures in toddlers and young children: Rarely from child abuse. J Pediatr Orthop 20:475–481, 2000.

104. Seimon, L.P. Refracture of the shaft of the femur. J Bone Joint Surg Br 46:32–39, 1964.

105. Skaggs, D.L.; Leet, A.J.; Money, M.D.; et al. Secondary fractures associated with external fixation in pediatric femur fractures. J Pediatr Orthop 19:582–586, 1999.

106. Spiegel, P.G.; Mast, J.W. Internal and external fixation of fractures in children. Orthop Clin North Am 11:405–421, 1980.

107. Staheli, L.T. Femoral and tibial overgrowth following femoral shaft fractures in childhood. Clin Orthop 55:159–163, 1967.

108. Staheli, L.T.; Sheridan, G.W. Early spica cast management of femoral shaft fractures in young children. A technique utilizing bilateral fixed skin traction. Clin Orthop 126:162–166, 1977.

109. Swiontkowski, M.F.; Hansen, S.T., Jr.; Kellam, J. Ipsilateral fractures of the femoral neck and shaft. A treatment protocol. J Bone Joint Surg Am 66:260–263, 1984.

110. Thometz, J.G.; Lamdan, R. Osteonecrosis of the femoral head after intramedullary nailing of a fracture of the femoral shaft in an adolescent. A case report. J Bone Joint Surg Am 77:1423–1426, 1995.

111. Thompson, G.H.; Wilber, J.H.; Marcus, R.E. Internal fixation of fractures in children and adolescents: A comparative analysis. Clin Orthop 188:10–20, 1984.

112. Timmerman, L.A.; Rab, G.T. Closed reamed intramedullary nail versus traction and casting in treatment of femoral shaft fractures in the 10 to 14 year old. J Pediatr Orthop 10:693, 1990.

113. Tolo, V.T. External skeletal fixation in children's fractures. J Pediatr Orthop 3:435–442, 1983.

114. Wadsworth, T.G. Traumatic dislocation of the hip with fracture of the shaft of the ipsilateral femur. J Bone Joint Surg Br 43:47–48, 1961.

115. Walker, R.N.; Green, N.E.; Spindler, K.P. Stress fractures in skeletally immature patients. J Pediatr Orthop 16:578–584, 1996.

116. Wallace, M.E.; Hoffman, E.B. Remodeling of angular deformity after femoral shaft fractures in children. J Bone Joint Surg Br 74:765–769, 1992.

117. Wenda, K.; Runkel, M.; Degreif, J.; Rudig, L. Minimally invasive plate fixation in femoral shaft fractures. Injury 28(Suppl 1): A13–A19, 1997.

118. Williamson, R.V.; Staheli, L.T. Partial physeal growth arrest: Treatment by bridge resection and fat interposition. J Pediatr Orthop 10:769–776, 1990.

119. Winquist, R.A.; Hansen, S.T., Jr.; Clawson, D.K. Closed intramedullary nailing of femur fractures. A report of five hundred and twenty cases. J Bone Joint Surg Am 66:529–539, 1984.

120. Ziv, I.; Blackburn, N.; Rang, M. Femoral intramedullary nailing in the growing child. J Trauma 24:432–434, 1984.

121. Ziv, I.; Rang, M. Treatment of femoral fracture in the child with head injury. J Bone Joint Surg Br 65:276–278, 1983.

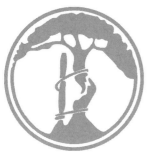

CHAPTER 14

# Fractures and Dislocations about the Knee

Lewis E. Zionts, M.D.

Traumatic forces applied to an immature knee result in fracture types that are different from those seen in adults. The presence of growing cartilage at the physes, apophyses, and articular surfaces is the key feature leading to fracture patterns that are unique to this age group. As in other anatomic regions in a growing child, the cartilaginous structures around the knee tend to be weaker and thus more vulnerable to injury than the ligaments and tendons that insert onto them.

## DISTAL FEMORAL METAPHYSEAL AND PHYSEAL FRACTURES

### Anatomy

**Bone and Soft Tissue Anatomy.** The epiphyseal ossification center of the distal part of the femur is usually present in a full-term newborn infant.

With subsequent growth, this ossification center rapidly expands to fill both condylar regions. The distal femoral physis is the largest and most rapidly growing in the body. It contributes almost 70% of the length of the femur and 40% of the length of the entire leg and averages approximately 1 cm of growth each year until maturity.[4, 95] Closure of this growth plate usually occurs between 14 and 16 years of age in girls and between 16 and 18 years in boys.[12] Any injury that partially or completely disrupts growth of the distal end of the femur may lead to significant angular deformity or shortening of the extremity. The younger the patient at the time of such injury, the greater the potential for these sequelae.

The distal epiphysis includes the entire articular surface of the lower end of the femur and serves as the origin for part of the gastrocnemius muscle.[82] Both the medial and lateral collateral ligaments originate from the distal femoral epiphysis. When a varus or valgus force is exerted on the knee, these ligaments most commonly remain uninjured because the force is transmitted to the distal femoral epiphysis and often leads to a physeal fracture.

The configuration of the distal femoral physis is unique and has been well described by Roberts.[100] The distal surface of the metaphysis consists of four gentle mounds, one in each quadrant of the cross section. These mounds fit into four shallow depressions on the proximal surface of the epiphysis. Although this undulating contour probably provides resistance to shear and torsional forces, it may also predispose regions of the epiphysis to grind against the metaphyseal projections when a separation occurs. These factors may help explain why growth disturbance after distal femoral physeal injury is so common.

**Neurovascular Anatomy.** Important neurovascular structures are positioned in close approximation to the distal end of the femur. The popliteal artery emerges from the adductor hiatus, just proximal to the distal femoral metaphysis, and enters the popliteal fossa. Within the popliteal space, the popliteal artery gives off the five geniculate arteries: paired superior and inferior and an unpaired middle artery. Although these arteries anastomose with the anterior tibial recurrent artery, they are small and too insufficient to allow continued viability of the lower part of the leg if the popliteal artery is occluded or disrupted.[39] As the popliteal artery enters the popliteal fossa, only a thin layer of fat separates the artery from the posterior surface of the femoral metaphysis. Because the artery is relatively tethered above to the femur at the adductor hiatus and below to the tibia by the fibrous arch over the soleus muscle, it is vulnerable to damage from the metaphyseal fragment of a hyperextension-type fracture of the distal femoral physis.

The posterior tibial nerve lies adjacent to the popliteal artery in the posterior part of the knee. The common peroneal nerve separates from the sciatic nerve just above the popliteal fossa and then descends along the lateral border of the fossa close to the medial border of the biceps femoris muscle. The nerve then exits the popliteal fossa between the biceps femoris muscle and the lateral head of the gastrocnemius and becomes subcutaneous just behind the head of the fibula before it wraps around the neck of the fibula deep to the peroneus longus. Because of its location, the common peroneal nerve may be prone to injury by a displaced fracture of the distal femoral physis, especially when the injury results from a hyperextension or varus stress.

## Distal Femoral Metaphyseal Fracture

### MECHANISM OF INJURY

A distal femoral metaphyseal fracture is most often caused by a direct blow to the anterior or lateral aspect of the thigh or a fall from a height. In children younger than 4 years, especially those younger than 1 year, child abuse should be considered. The lack of a reasonable explanation for the injury, an unreasonable delay in seeking medical care, or the presence of additional injuries should raise the level of suspicion of abuse.[11] A corner fracture or bucket-handle lesion at the level of the distal metaphysis makes child abuse a strong possibility.[11] In older children, nondisplaced fractures or stress fractures may occur. These patients present with local pain and tenderness, and radiographs reveal new periosteal bone. The possibility of a pathologic fracture should be considered in these patients.[31]

### DIAGNOSIS

Patients with a fracture of the distal femoral metaphysis present with local soft tissue swelling, tenderness, and deformity in the region of the distal part of the thigh and knee. The skin must be inspected for a possible open fracture. Although arterial injury here is less common than with a proximal tibial physeal fracture, careful neurovascular examination is warranted. The presence and strength of the pedal pulses and the function of the common peroneal and posterior tibial nerves should be documented. The peroneal nerve is more likely to be injured with a distal femoral fracture than is the posterior tibial nerve. The peroneal nerve may be damaged either by a direct blow to the posterolateral side of the knee (e.g., from a car bumper) or from a stretch injury to this nerve at the time of fracture angulation and displacement. Ongoing evaluation of the lower extremity is important during the first few days after the fracture so that a developing compartment syndrome may be detected promptly.

Anteroposterior and lateral radiographs of the distal end of the femur will reveal the fracture. As with any long bone fracture, radiographs of the entire bone should be taken, including the joints above and below the injury. Accordingly, radiographs of the entire femur, including the hip and knee, should be taken when the patient is initially evaluated.

### MANAGEMENT

The muscle forces on the distal fragment may present problems in obtaining and maintaining proper alignment of displaced fractures of the distal femoral metaphysis. Generally, the distal fragment will displace posteriorly, often with exaggerated flexion, because of the pull of the two heads of the gastrocnemius muscle. If the fracture line is just proximal to the distal insertion of the adductor magnus muscle, the distal fragment may also angulate into a varus position. Treatment options for this injury include traction followed by application of a hip spica cast, application of a cast brace, external fixation, percutaneous pin fixation followed by application of a hip spica cast, and open reduction and internal fixation.

**Traction and Cast Application.** In this technique, traction is applied to the lower extremity to obtain proper reduction of the fracture until enough callus has formed to allow alignment to be safely maintained in a spica cast. In a young child, skin traction can be applied to the lower part of the leg, but skeletal pin traction is preferable in children older than 3 years.

Skeletal traction may be applied through either the proximal part of the tibia or the distal end of the femur. The skeletal traction pin is either a K-wire or a Steinmann pin applied aseptically under local or general anesthesia. If a proximal tibial site is chosen, the pin should be inserted in a lateral-to-medial direction to minimize the risk of injury to the peroneal nerve. Care should also be taken to avoid the proximal tibial physis and tibial tubercle apophysis (Fig. 14–1). If a distal femoral site is chosen, the pin should be inserted medially to laterally to

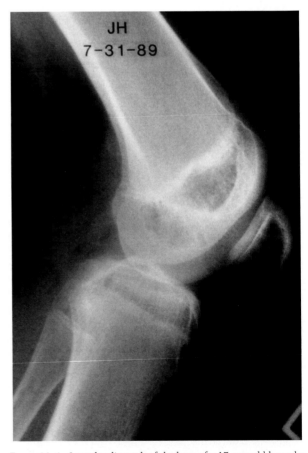

FIGURE 14–1. Lateral radiograph of the knee of a 17-year-old boy who sustained a fracture of his femur that was treated with skeletal traction. A smooth traction pin was placed through the proximal end of the tibia. Even though the pin did not penetrate the tibial tubercle, an arrest of its apophysis occurred. The resultant distal position of the tibial tubercle produced patella baja. (Courtesy of Dr. Neil E. Green.)

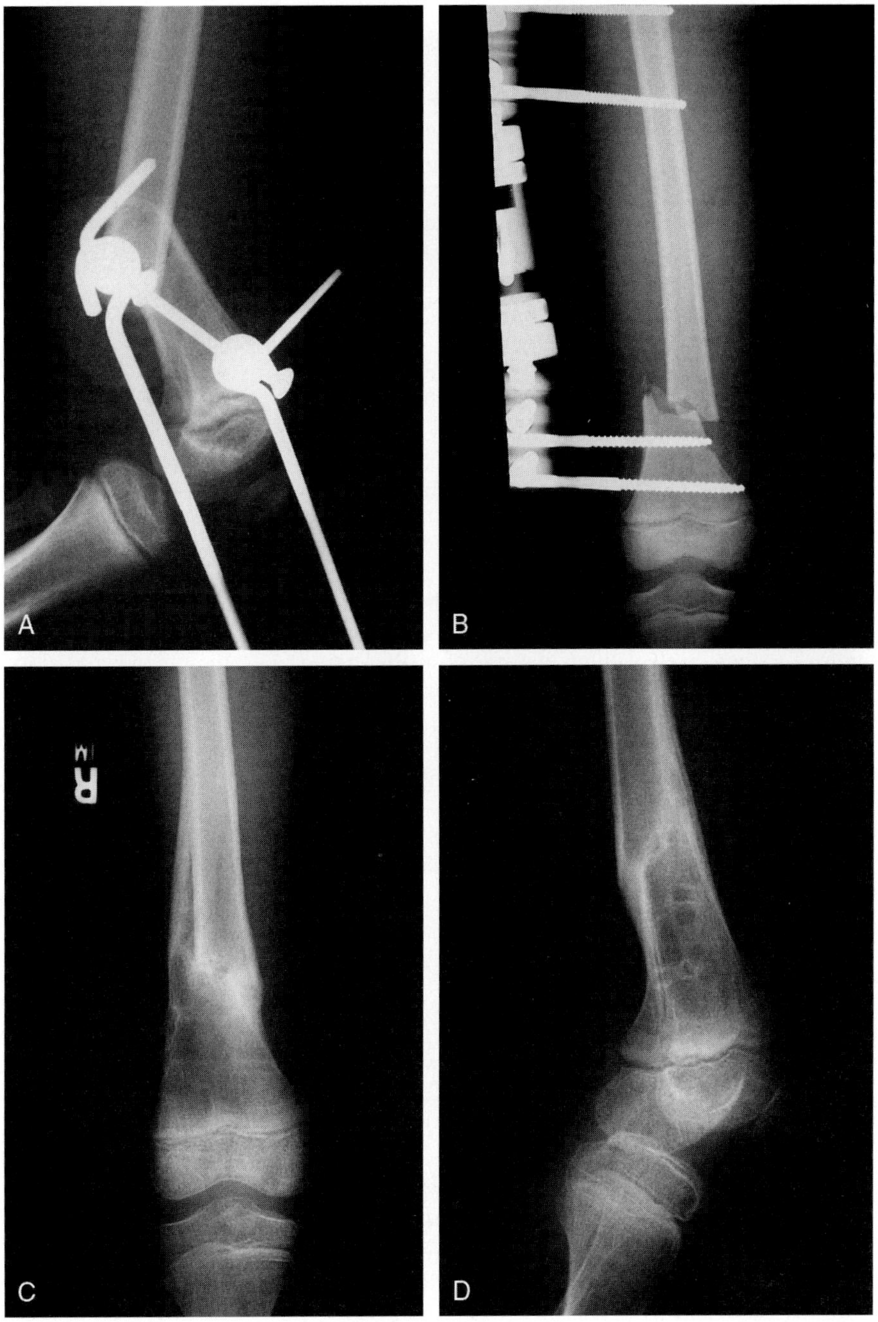

FIGURE **14–2.** Radiographs of an 8 year old who sustained a fracture of the distal end of the femur. *A,* Lateral radiograph of the distal part of the femur and knee showing a distal femoral fracture with a traction pin in the supracondylar region of the femur. The patient is in 90/90 traction, and one can see the posterior angulation of the fracture, which was difficult to control. *B,* Because of the difficulty in controlling it, the fracture was reduced in the operating room, and the reduction was held with an external fixator. *C,* Anteroposterior radiograph of the knee and distal end of the femur showing healing of the fracture 4½ months after the injury. *D,* Lateral radiograph showing good distal femoral alignment. (*A–D,* Courtesy of Dr. Neil E. Green.)

minimize the risk of injury to the femoral artery in the region of the adductor canal.

Because of the special muscle forces present, the use of a single traction pin may not maintain adequate alignment (Fig. 14–2). Double-pin traction is often needed. A proximal tibial pin will allow longitudinal traction, but it may be necessary to insert a second pin into the distal femoral fragment to provide an anteriorly directed force to achieve satisfactory position on lateral radiographs.[41] Similarly, if the distal femoral fragment is long enough, two pins may be inserted into the femoral fragment proximal to the physis. Staheli[112] described a double-pin traction technique in which one pin is placed through the metaphysis and a second pin is placed through the epiphysis. The two pins are attached to an external

fixation apparatus (such as a Roger Anderson device) through which traction is applied.

Although a two-pin traction technique may provide satisfactory sagittal plane control, the need to keep the hip and knee flexed in 90/90 traction makes it difficult to accurately determine whether a varus or valgus alignment is present. If this treatment method is selected, the child can be placed initially in 90/90 traction. Once early callus has formed and sagittal plane alignment is satisfactory, the knee can be straightened gradually; lateral radiographs are taken to ensure that the sagittal plane alignment is maintained. With the knee in a more extended position, any varus or valgus malalignment can be corrected when the hip spica cast is applied, while the callus is still relatively soft.

The duration of immobilization varies with the age of the patient: it is only a few weeks in the very young and 6 to 8 weeks in older children. After removal of the cast, rehabilitation is begun to strengthen the quadriceps and hamstring muscles. Weight bearing can be full as tolerated, but crutches are used for protection until knee motion and thigh strength are adequate to allow the patient to walk safely without assistive devices. Return to regular activities is permitted after the quadriceps has regained normal strength and full range of motion of the knee joint has been achieved.

The main complications that may result from treating a distal femoral metaphyseal fracture with traction and cast application are varus malalignment and premature closure of the anterior part of the proximal tibial physis, which leads to recurvatum deformity of the proximal end of the tibia (see Fig. 14–1). Careful traction management and cast application can prevent varus malalignment. When a proximal tibial pin is used, meticulous pin placement can avoid physeal injury to the tibial tubercle area, although some reports have noted that premature tibial tubercle growth arrest can occur in association with femur fractures, even without the use of a tibial pin.[18] Malalignment in the sagittal plane, with an apex posterior angulation at the fracture site, may result in an apparent hyperextension deformity of the knee and limited knee flexion. In a young child, this deformity largely remodels with time.

**Cast Brace Management.** A cast brace may be used after an initial period of traction in selected older children and adolescents whose fractures do not have excessive posterior angulation.

Cast brace treatment can provide an opportunity for early ambulation and avoid much of the knee stiffness and muscle atrophy that occur with spica cast immobilization.[45, 71]

In the technique described by Gross and colleagues,[45] a large (7/64 to 9/64 inch) Steinmann pin is inserted into the distal end of the femur in the operating room with the patient under general anesthesia. The pin is completely covered with cast padding, and a cylinder cast is applied with careful molding at the fracture site to prevent varus angulation. If radiographs show that satisfactory reduction has been achieved, an elliptical section of plaster is removed from the posterior part of the knee. The plaster anteriorly is transected in part, with a bridge overlying the patella left intact at this point. After hinges are applied medially and laterally, the anterior bridge of plaster is transected to allow flexion of the knee. A specially bent segment of coat hanger is incorporated over the tibia to allow traction to be applied. Postoperatively, the patient is sent to physical therapy for standing and gait training. After several days, radiographs are taken both in traction and while standing to assess alignment and shortening. Wedging of the cast is done at this stage if necessary. Weekly radiographs are mandatory to monitor length and alignment. After 4 weeks, the cast brace is changed and the pin is removed in the outpatient setting. Use of the cast brace is discontinued when clinical and radiographic union is achieved.

In general, cast braces for the treatment of femoral fractures have been used sparingly. Although other methods may be superior to a cast brace for proximal and middle-third diaphyseal femur fractures, some authors have suggested that fractures of the distal end of the femur are best suited to this technique.[71]

**External Fixation.** External fixation may be effectively used to reduce and stabilize distal femoral metaphyseal fractures (see Fig. 14–2). The best situations for the use of external fixation for this injury are in children who have sustained polytrauma, an open fracture, or a floating knee.

In cases of polytrauma with multiple fractures, abdominal injury, or head injury, stabilizing the fracture with an external fixator will allow the child to be transported for diagnostic studies or operative procedures. In persistently comatose children, external fixation will provide stability of the fracture when spasticity ensues. Tolo[120] has observed that over 90% of children in a coma for more than 48 hours will have excellent neurologic recovery. Therefore, it is important to treat all fractures in children with head injury under the assumption that full neurologic recovery will occur.

In open injuries, especially when skin loss is present, the use of external fixation to stabilize the fracture greatly facilitates care of the wound. In children who have a fractured tibia and a distal femoral metaphyseal fracture, stabilization of the distal part of the femur with an external fixator allows the tibial fracture to be treated more easily.

The use of external fixation for the management of distal femoral fractures has become more popular in response to efforts to limit the cost of prolonged hospitalization. In addition, the family may find it easier to care for a child, especially an older child, treated with an external fixator rather than a hip spica cast.

If external fixation is used to manage a distal femoral metaphyseal fracture, the surgeon should keep several technical points in mind.[120] The pins should be inserted from the lateral side under image intensifier control. It is recommended that the distal pin be placed at least 1 cm, preferably 2 cm, from the physis to avoid potential thermal injury during insertion, as well as damage from a possible pin tract infection. The external fixator pins should be applied in parallel while an assistant holds the fracture site in a reduced position. Pins should be placed into uninjured bone and through intact, uninjured skin whenever possible. In transverse fractures, an end-to-end reduction is attempted; in oblique fractures, bayonet apposition with about 5 mm of overlap should be considered in children younger than 10 years to minimize the effect of limb overgrowth. The use of an external fixation frame that allows some adjustment of varus and valgus, as well as rotation, is preferred. After placement of the frame, final adjustments are made, and radiographic confirmation of adequate reduction is obtained before the child is awakened from general anesthesia.

Pin care is taught to the child and parents while in the hospital, and this pin care is continued at home on a daily basis. If the patient is compliant, partial weight bearing with crutches can be started early. When radiographs reveal the formation of callus, weight bearing can be increased. If the fixator requires dynamization, it is done at around 4 to 6 weeks after the fracture, when callus has been present for a few weeks.

Once early fracture stability has been gained, the surgeon may choose to remove the external fixator and apply a long leg cast until healing is complete. Alternatively, the external fixator may be used for the full course of treatment. Once healing is complete, typically between 8 and 12 weeks from the time of the injury, depending on the age of the patient, the device may be removed in the outpatient setting. In most older children and all adolescents, it is best to leave the external fixator on for the full 12 weeks to minimize the risk of refracture after frame removal.

Potential complications from the use of external fixation include pin tract infection, malunion, and refracture through either a pin tract or the original fracture site. Pin tract infection can usually be avoided by good pin care. A short course of oral antibiotics may be sufficient to treat a superficial infection. The skin should be incised if tension on the skin is present. If drainage persists or if erosion around the pin is seen on radiographs, the pin should be changed or the entire device should be removed, a cast applied, and appropriate antibiotic treatment instituted.

Because the knee may be extended to assess femoraltibial alignment quite readily, varus or valgus malunion is not common if care is taken in the initial placement of the fixator. However, because of a tendency to apply the fixator with the distal fragment in slight external rotation, rotational alignment should be carefully assessed when the frame is applied.

Refracture of the femur occurs more often with fractures treated with external fixation than by other methods. A fracture may occur through the old fracture site if the frame is removed prematurely. A fracture may also occur through a pin site, particularly in young children in whom 5-mm fixator pins have been used.

Injury to the distal femoral physis is certainly a potential problem for distal femoral fractures treated with external fixation. This injury should be avoidable if the pins are kept at least 1 cm proximal to the physis when inserted. The pins should always be inserted under image intensifier control to avoid transgressing the physis.

**Closed Reduction and Percutaneous Pin Fixation.** Closed reduction and percutaneous pin fixation supplemented by the application of a single hip spica cast may be used to treat distal femoral metaphyseal fractures in selected patients. This technique is particularly useful in younger patients in whom the metaphyseal fracture is quite distal (Fig. 14–3). With the patient under general anesthesia, the fracture is reduced and smooth pins are inserted in a crossed fashion with image intensifier control. It is preferable to insert the pins through the distal metaphysis provided that sufficient metaphyseal length is available; if not, the pins may be inserted through the distal femoral epiphysis as described for distal femoral physeal fractures. The pins are bent to avoid migration. A single spica cast is applied with the knee immobilized in 20° to 30° of flexion. After 6 weeks, the cast is discontinued and the pins are removed.

**Open Reduction and Internal Fixation.** Open reduction and internal fixation may be needed for distal femoral metaphyseal fractures that cannot be reduced by other methods or if an arterial injury has occurred at the time of fracture. The most common reason for failure to obtain adequate reduction by other means is the presence of interposed muscle between the fracture fragments. If repair of an arterial injury is needed, internal fixation prevents excessive motion at the fracture site and protects the repair.

The surgical approach depends on the indication for the surgery. If interposed muscle is blocking reduction, a straight lateral approach will allow the quadriceps muscle to be reflected anteriorly and afford access to the distal end of the femur. If arterial repair is needed, the incision should be posteromedial to allow access to the femoral and popliteal arteries, as well as the saphenous vein if vein grafting is necessary.

Rigid internal fixation, as is commonly used in adults, is not usually necessary in children because casts are often applied postoperatively until fracture healing is complete. Once reduction of the fracture is obtained, crossed pins provide acceptable, provisional fixation. The pins are bent to prevent migration and are cut off just below the skin to facilitate later removal. Postoperatively, a single hip spica is applied. After the fracture has healed, use of the cast is discontinued and the pins can be removed through small skin incisions with either a local or a short-acting general anesthetic.

Compression plate fixation is rarely indicated to treat distal femoral metaphyseal fractures in a growing child, except perhaps in the polytrauma setting. In this situation, compression plating may be a useful alternative and does not cause excessive femoral overgrowth.[58] Plate removal is generally needed, followed by 4 to 6 weeks of cast immobilization to prevent fracture through the screw holes.

**Author's Preferred Method of Treatment.** In patients younger than 6 years, I base the mode of treatment on a number of factors such as the proximity of the fracture line to the physis, the presence of associated injuries, and the needs and desires of the patient's family. Traction, percutaneous pin fixation, or external fixation may be appropriate, depending on the clinical situation. In patients whose fractures are difficult to control in traction or in instances in which an extended period of hospitalization may be impractical for the family, I will use either percutaneous pin fixation or external fixation. In older children and adolescents, external fixation appears to be the best option. External fixation of these fractures may allow the patient an earlier return to school. Once the child has obtained independence in activities of daily living, the parents may be able to return to work.

## Distal Femoral Physeal Fractures

### MECHANISM OF INJURY

Fractures of the distal femoral physis account for just over 5% of all physeal injuries.[92] Most of these fractures are sustained in automobile-pedestrian accidents or

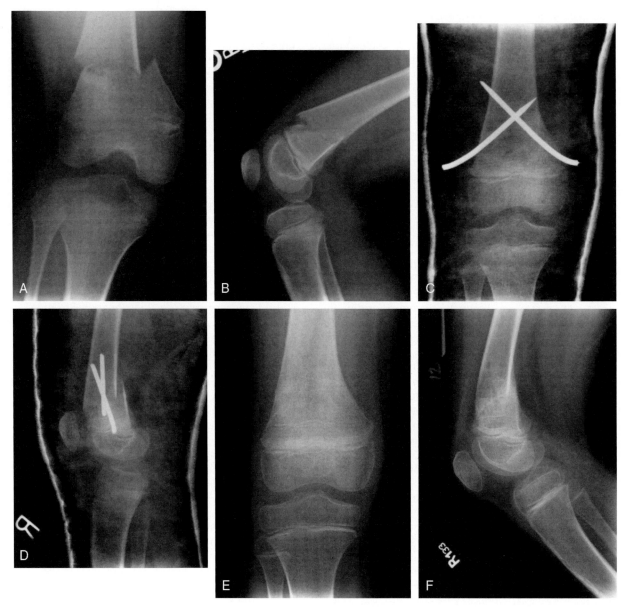

**FIGURE 14–3.** A 6-year-old girl sustained an injury to her right knee after being struck by a slowly moving automobile. *A* and *B*, Anteroposterior and lateral radiographs of the distal end of the femur show a complete supracondylar femoral fracture with medial displacement of the distal fragment. *C* and *D*, Because of the proximity of the injury to the physis, the fracture was reduced and pinned percutaneously. *E* and *F*, Anteroposterior and lateral radiographs of the left knee made after healing show excellent alignment of the fracture.

sports activities.[64, 99, 116] Riseborough and colleagues[99] observed that fractures in the juvenile group—ages 2 to 11 years—were invariably caused by severe trauma such as being struck by an automobile whereas fractures in the adolescent age group were caused by less severe trauma, most often sports related.

Because the growth plate provides less resistance to traumatic forces than the attached ligaments do, varus or valgus stress applied to an immature knee is more apt to lead to physeal separation than to a collateral ligament injury. If hyperextension of the knee occurs, the epiphysis may be displaced anteriorly.[43] This mechanism of injury is similar to the mechanism causing knee dislocation in adults. It is important to recognize this pattern of injury because of the potential for associated neurovas-

cular injury. Posterior displacement of the epiphysis is relatively uncommon and is caused by a blow to the anterior aspect of a flexed knee. Distal femoral physeal separations can also occur from birth injury, often associated with breech delivery.[99]

## CLASSIFICATION

The most commonly used classification system for distal femoral epiphyseal fractures is that of Salter and Harris.[107] Type I fractures are characterized by complete separation through the physis without any involvement of the adjacent metaphysis or epiphysis. In type II fractures, which are the most common, the fracture line traverses the physis before exiting obliquely across one corner of the metaphysis. Displacement is usually toward the side of the metaphyseal fragment. A type III injury consists of a fracture through the physis that exits through the epiphysis into the joint. A type IV injury describes a vertical, intra-articular fracture that traverses the metaphysis, physis, and epiphysis. Type V fractures are crush injuries to the physeal cartilage. These rare injuries are usually diagnosed in retrospect.

## DIAGNOSIS

A careful description of the accident should be elicited. It is particularly important to determine the direction of the force that produced the injury.

A patient with a distal femoral physeal fracture presents with effusion of the knee joint, local soft tissue swelling, and tenderness over the physis. In displaced injuries, deformity may be evident and soft or muffled crepitus can often be felt. In an anteriorly displaced, or hyperextension, injury, the patella is prominent and dimpling of the anterior skin is often evident. With posterior displacement of the epiphysis, the distal metaphyseal fragment becomes prominent just above the patella.

A careful neurovascular examination is warranted in these injuries, especially in hyperextension injuries. The presence and strength of the pedal pulses and the function of the common peroneal and posterior tibial nerves should be documented. If the clinical findings of acute ischemia are present—extremity pallor, coolness, cyanosis, or delayed capillary refill—reduction of the fracture should be attempted as soon as possible. If these findings persist after the reduction attempt, immediate vascular exploration is indicated. In the absence of an obviously ischemic limb, patients with an abnormal pulse or patients who recover pulses and perfusion after reduction of the fracture should undergo arteriography.[57, 121] As described for fractures of the distal femoral metaphysis, ongoing evaluation of the lower extremity is important during the first few days after the fracture so that a developing compartment syndrome or intimal tear with thrombosis can be detected promptly.

Anteroposterior and lateral radiographs should be obtained. Oblique radiographs may be helpful to reveal fractures that are minimally displaced. If these views show no fracture and knee instability has been noted on clinical examination, gentle stress radiographs should be obtained. Adequate analgesia is helpful to alleviate muscle spasm and protect the physis from further damage during the examination. Care should be taken to avoid excessive force that could convert a nondisplaced physeal injury to a displaced physeal separation. On occasion, magnetic resonance imaging or computed tomography may help identify fracture lines in nondisplaced injuries.[24, 78]

It is important to distinguish between a physeal fracture and a ligament injury because these two conditions are treated differently. Although ligament injuries may occur in skeletally immature individuals, physeal fractures are more common and should be the first consideration when an open physis is present.

However, it has also been shown that physeal fracture about the knee and ligament injury can both be present.[14, 20, 22, 64, 101, 116, 117] Careful evaluation of these patients, including the use of stress radiography, examination under anesthesia, and arthroscopy, will facilitate early diagnosis and appropriate management of any concomitant ligamentous insufficiency.

## MANAGEMENT

The goals of treatment are to obtain and maintain anatomic reduction and avoid further damage to the physis. The form of treatment is determined by both the fracture type and the degree of displacement.

**Salter-Harris Types I and II Fractures.** For Salter-Harris types I and II injuries, nondisplaced fractures are immobilized for 4 to 6 weeks in either a long leg cast or hip spica cast. The duration of immobilization will vary with the age of the patient. Short, obese children or patients who may be unreliable are probably better managed in a hip spica cast.[99] Displaced fractures are reduced under general anesthesia. Longitudinal traction should be used during the reduction maneuver to avoid further damage to the physis. Internal fixation makes subsequent displacement less likely, allows the use of a long leg cast with a greater margin of safety, and avoids having to place the knee in an extreme position of flexion or extension to maintain the reduction.[32, 38, 99, 119]

After the fracture is reduced under image intensifier control, smooth transphyseal pins are inserted in a crossed fashion for type I injuries and type II injuries with small metaphyseal fragments (Fig. 14–4). Type II fractures with an adequately sized metaphyseal fragment on both anteroposterior and lateral views may be stabilized with pins or screws across the metaphyseal portion of the fracture (Fig. 14–5). After fixation is achieved, the stability of the reduction is confirmed by moving the knee through a full range of motion under fluoroscopy. If smooth pins were used, they are bent to avoid migration. A long leg cast is applied with the knee immobilized in 20° to 30° of flexion. After 6 weeks, the cast is discontinued and the pins are removed in the outpatient setting.

Open reduction is indicated for fractures that cannot be reduced by closed methods or if an arterial injury has occurred at the time of fracture. If the epiphysis is displaced laterally, a medial approach will provide visualization of any obstacles to reduction and avoid disruption of the intact lateral periosteal hinge. If the epiphysis is displaced medially, a lateral approach is used. A posterior approach is necessary if arterial exploration is indicated. Once the fracture is reduced, fixation is achieved as described earlier.

**Salter-Harris Types III and IV Fractures.** Nondisplaced and stable fractures may be managed by cast immobilization. Careful follow-up of these patients at weekly intervals is needed so that any displacement may be promptly addressed. Alternatively, these injuries may be stabilized with percutaneous pins or screws to minimize the risk of late displacement.

Open reduction with internal fixation is needed for all displaced types III and IV fractures to restore congruity of the articular surface and align the physis. Because types III and IV fractures are intra-articular, a more extensive approach is needed to visualize both the articular surface and the physis or metaphysis. Type III fractures are approached through an anteromedial or anterolateral arthrotomy, depending on the location of the vertical component of the fracture through the epiphysis. After the knee joint is opened, thorough irrigation eliminates the hemarthrosis and clot from the fracture surfaces. Once accurate reduction is achieved, the fracture is stabilized with one or two AO cancellous screws placed transversely across the fracture site under image intensi-

fier control. It is preferable to not allow the threaded portion of the screw to span the fracture site in order to achieve better compression (Fig. 14–6).

For type IV fractures, the approach is made on the side of the metaphyseal portion attached to the physis. Both the joint and the metaphyseal portion of the femur are exposed. Once accurate reduction is achieved, the fracture is stabilized with one or two cancellous screws placed across the metaphysis. An epiphyseal screw is needed only if adequate stability of the fracture cannot be achieved by fixation of the metaphyseal fragment alone. Postoperatively, a long leg cast is applied. The cast is

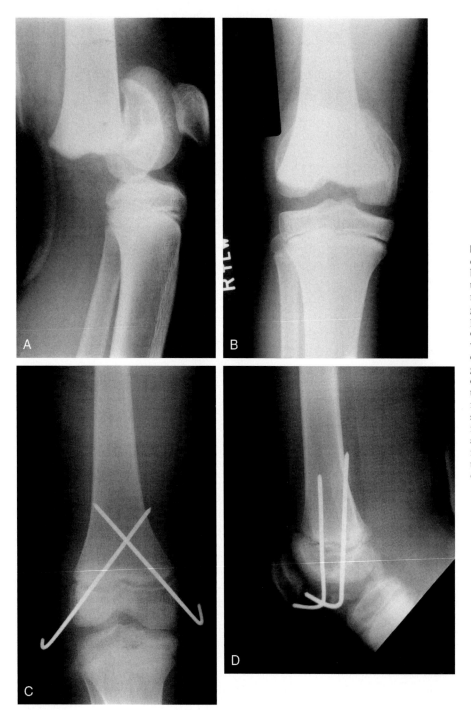

**FIGURE 14–4.** Type I fracture of the distal femoral physis of a 13-year-old boy. The patient sustained a hyperextension injury of the knee without any neurovascular injury. *A,* Lateral radiograph of the knee showing a completely displaced type I physeal injury of the distal end of the femur along with anterior displacement of the femoral condyles. *B,* Anteroposterior radiograph of the same knee demonstrating displacement of the condyles. *C,* Anteroposterior radiograph after closed reduction and percutaneous pinning showing anatomic restoration of the fracture. Note that the pins are smooth and have crossed the physis. *D,* Lateral radiograph of the knee showing anatomic reduction of the fracture. (*A–D,* Courtesy of Dr. Vernon T. Tolo).

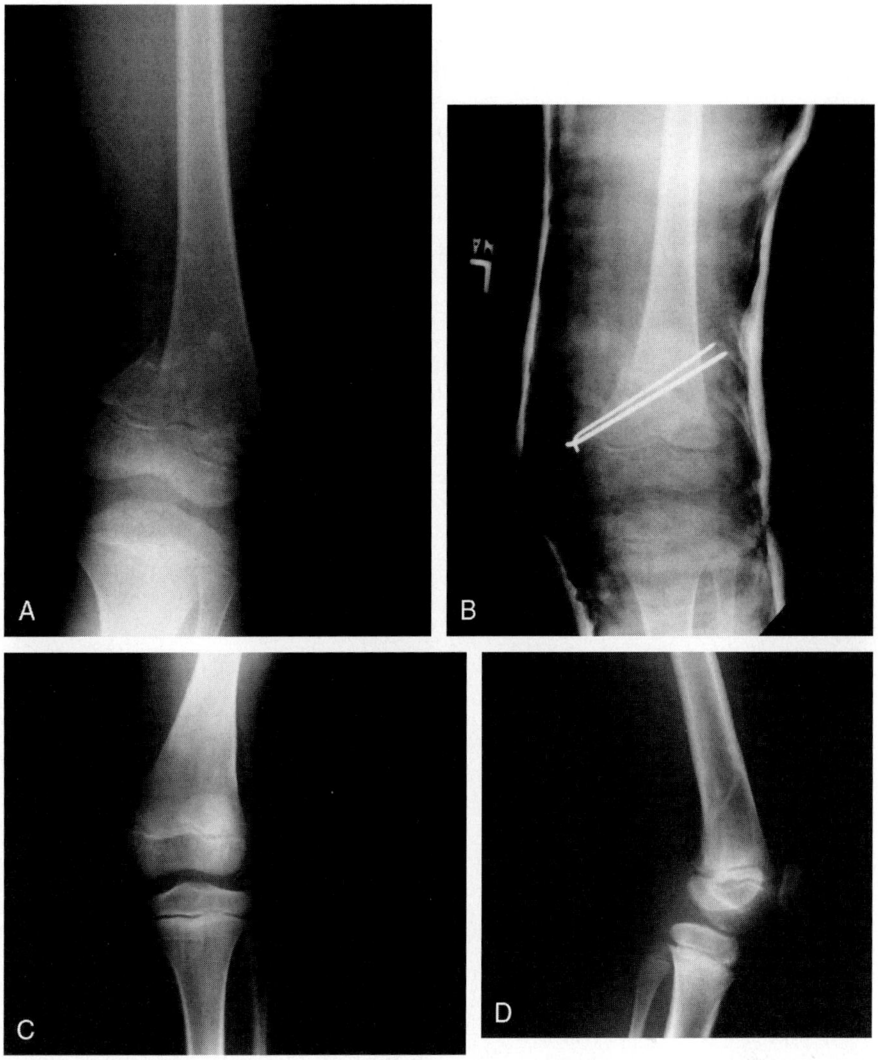

FIGURE 14–5. *A,* Anteroposterior radiograph of the left knee of a 10-year-old boy who sustained a displaced Salter type II fracture of the distal end of the left femur. *B,* Closed reduction of this fracture was attempted once but was unsuccessful. Limited open reduction with percutaneous pinning was used to obtain realignment, as shown in this postoperative anteroposterior radiograph. Pins were removed at 3 weeks, and the cast was removed 6 weeks after the fracture occurred. *C* and *D,* Anteroposterior and lateral radiographs of the left knee 18 months after the fracture. (*A–D,* Courtesy of Dr. Vernon T. Tolo.)

removed at 6 weeks and rehabilitation of the knee is begun. Because these are intra-articular fractures, weight bearing should be avoided until radiographs confirm that the fracture is fully healed.

## COMPLICATIONS

Although the prognosis for a fracture of the distal femoral physis is generally good, problems with shortening and angular deformity are more common than one might expect according to the Salter-Harris classification.[22, 64, 99, 116] The poorer than expected prognosis after distal femoral physeal injuries may be attributable to the greater force needed to cause physeal separation at this site, especially in younger patients, whose thicker periosteal and perichondral sheaths provide greater stability.[99]

Growth problems are more likely to occur after fractures that are initially displaced more than half the diameter of the shaft[64, 119] and in fractures in younger patients.[99] Riseborough and colleagues observed that fractures of the distal femoral epiphysis in juvenile

patients aged 2 to 11 years were caused by more severe trauma and were more likely to result in growth problems than similar fractures in adolescents.

Careful clinical evaluation is recommended at 6-month intervals after the injury to assess lower extremity alignment and leg length. Comparative radiographs should be taken of both lower extremities. Partial inhibition of growth, or growth deceleration, can occur after distal femoral physeal injuries.[99] Isolated instances of growth stimulation after these fractures have also been reported.[119] Therefore, it is important to monitor these patients to skeletal maturity even if radiographs show an open physis.

Leg length inequalities estimated to be less than 2 cm at skeletal maturity require no treatment. If the estimated discrepancy at maturity is between 2 and 5 cm, an appropriately timed epiphysiodesis of the contralateral extremity may be indicated. For inequalities estimated at maturity to be more than 5 cm, leg lengthening should be considered.

Angular deformities may be due to either malunion or a partial growth disturbance. Significant angular deformity caused by malunion may be managed by osteotomy or, when appropriate, by hemiepiphysiodesis. Treatment options for a progressive angular deformity caused by a partial growth disturbance include osseous bridge resection, osteotomy, or epiphysiodesis of the remaining portion of the physis. Osseous bridge resection may be considered for lesions involving less than 50% of the physis in children who have at least 2 years of growth remaining[55, 93, 100] (Fig. 14–7). Results are best if the bar is located peripherally.

The surgical incision is made either laterally or medially, depending on the location of the bar to be resected. The area of resection is determined preoperatively by the appearance of the bar on tomograms. A high-speed bur is used to excise the osseous bridge until normal physeal cartilage can be seen circumferentially within the defect. The defect is then packed with either autogenous fat (from the buttock region) or methyl methacrylate (cranioplast) to prevent re-formation of the osseous bridge. Small metal markers are placed in the metaphysis and the epiphysis to allow resumption of physeal growth to be evaluated on radiographs. If varus or valgus deformity of the distal end of the femur is greater than 20° at the time of bridge resection, a distal femoral osteotomy should also be performed to realign the knee joint.[93]

An osteotomy with epiphysiodesis of the remaining portion of the physis may be necessary when the bridge

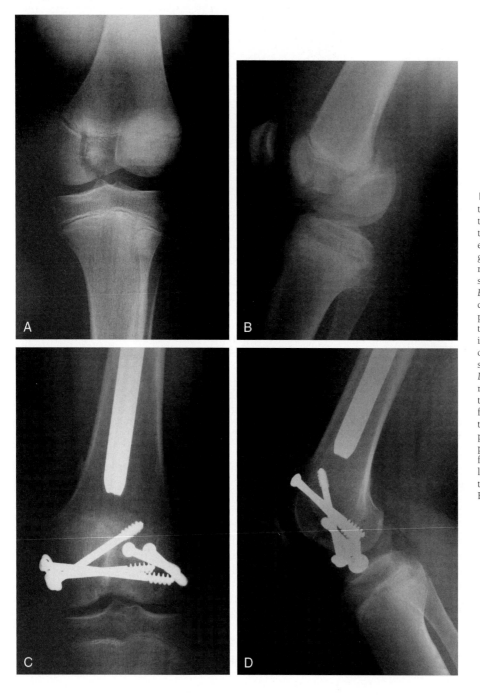

**FIGURE 14–6.** A 13-year-old boy sustained a closed midshaft fracture of the right femur and a comminuted type IV fracture of the distal femoral epiphysis. *A,* Anteroposterior radiograph of the knee showing a comminuted fracture that has split off both sides of the distal femoral epiphysis. *B,* Lateral radiograph showing the comminution of the distal femoral physeal fracture. *C,* Postoperative anteroposterior radiograph demonstrating restoration of distal femoral anatomy. The fracture was reduced and stabilized with multiple screws. *D,* Lateral radiograph demonstrating maintenance of the normal architecture of the femoral condyles. The fracture was very comminuted at the time of the injury, so screws were placed across the physis because the physis had been crushed. A distal femoral epiphysiodesis on the contralateral side was performed a short time later. (*A–D,* Courtesy of Dr. Neil E. Green.)

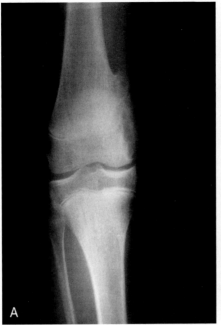

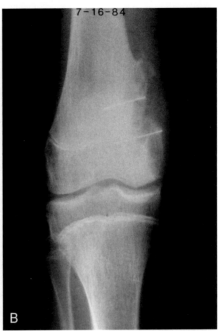

FIGURE 14–7. The knee of a 14-year-old boy who had sustained a lawn mower injury 4 years earlier. *A*, This anteroposterior radiograph demonstrates a varus deformity of the distal end of the femur, with peripheral growth arrest of the medial side of the distal femoral physis. *B*, After excision of the physeal bar, the varus deformity is corrected, with subsequent growth. (*A, B,* Courtesy of Dr. Neil E. Green.)

is too large to excise or in children who are approaching skeletal maturity.

# OSTEOCHONDRAL FRACTURES

## Mechanism of Injury

Osteochondral fractures of the knee are most often due to either a direct blow on a flexed knee or shearing forces associated with acute dislocation of the patella.[2, 46, 69, 102] These fractures occur when the dislocated patella slides back tangentially over the surface of the lateral femoral condyle.[81] Rorabeck and Bobechko[102] estimated that osteochondral fractures occur in approximately 5% of all acute patellar dislocations occurring in children. Nietosvaara and colleagues[81] found associated osteochondral fractures, either capsular avulsions or intra-articular loose bodies, in 28 of 72 (39%) children after an acute patellar dislocation. More recently, Stanitski and Paletta[115] reported arthroscopically documented articular injuries in 34 of 48 (71%) older children and adolescents after acute patellar dislocation.

These injuries occur most often in adolescents. Rosenberg[103] suggested that because adolescents have little calcified cartilage, forces tangential to the articular surface of the knee are transmitted to the subchondral region and produce a fracture that is in the horizontal plane and mostly within bone. The same forces applied to the knee in an adult often result in a chondral tear at the "tide mark" between the calcified and uncalcified zones of the articular cartilage, with sparing of subchondral bone.[49, 103]

## Classification

Rorabeck and Bobechko[102] described three patterns of osteochondral fracture that are seen in children after acute patellar dislocations: inferomedial fracture of the patella, fracture of the lateral femoral condyle, and a combination of the two (Fig. 14–8). Fractures involving the medial femoral condyle are less common and are usually caused by a direct blow to the knee.

## Diagnosis

Most patients with an osteochondral fracture will give a history of a twisting injury on a flexed knee. Usually, a painful "snap" is heard or felt. The child may report a sensation of "giving way" or that the knee "went out of joint." Hemarthrosis occurs rapidly, and the patient may experience pain on attempts to bear weight.

A child with an osteochondral fracture presents with a painful, swollen joint. Any attempt to flex or extend the knee is resisted. Tenderness may be elicited over the injured portion of the articular surface. The patient may also exhibit tenderness over the medial patellar retinaculum and a positive apprehension sign. One should ascertain the presence of hypermobility in other joints because adolescents without generalized joint laxity have a 2½-fold increased frequency of articular lesions after acute patellar dislocation.[114]

Radiographic evaluation should include anteroposterior and lateral views of the knee, as well as tunnel and patellar skyline views. Osteochondral fractures may be difficult to see on plain radiographs, especially if the ossified portion of the fragment is small.[114, 115, 124] Stanitski and Paletta[115] found that only 8 of 28 osteochondral loose bodies confirmed by arthroscopic

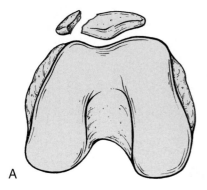

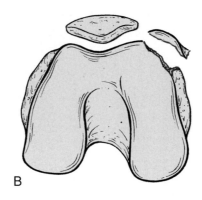

Figure **14–8.** Diagrammatic representation of an osteochondral fracture of the lateral femoral condyle *(B)* and the medial pole of the patella *(A)*, both secondary to patellar dislocation. Radiographs may appear normal, but the hemarthrosis aspirate will contain fat droplets. Arthroscopy is indicated when these chondral or osteochondral fractures are suspected.

examination could be identified on a complete four-view radiographic series.

If radiographs fail to reveal a fracture, particularly if the history suggests acute patellar dislocation, the knee joint should be aspirated under sterile conditions to confirm the presence of hemarthrosis. The presence of fat globules within a bloody aspirate is presumptive evidence of an osteochondral fracture somewhere in the knee.[103]

Although arthrography[37] or magnetic resonance imaging[76] may be useful to better visualize fragments that are largely cartilaginous, arthroscopic examination is often needed to diagnose an osteochondral or chondral fracture of the knee.[37, 81, 114, 115, 118, 123, 124]

## Management

Most authorities recommend early operative management of acute osteochondral fractures of the knee.[2, 12, 46, 69, 102, 118] Whether the fragment is excised or reattached depends on the size and origin of the fragment. However, authors do not agree on the size of

the fragment that mandates reattachment. In general, if the fragment is small and from a non–weight-bearing surface, it may be removed. Larger fragments from weight-bearing areas should be replaced.

If the osteochondral fracture is reattached, several fixation techniques have been reported. Bone pegs,[46, 54] Smillie nails,[46] countersunk AO minifragment screws,[46, 118] Herbert screws,[61, 96] small threaded Steinmann pins inserted in a retrograde fashion,[12] fibrin sealant or other adhesives,[34, 47, 118] and poly (L-lactide) pegs[68] have all been used with similar results (Fig. 14–9). Significant aseptic synovitis of the foreign body type has been reported in some patients treated with intra-articular biodegradable internal fixation.[8]

After reattachment of an osteochondral fragment, the knee is immobilized for 6 weeks in a long leg cast, during which time quadriceps muscle–strengthening exercises are started. After the cast is removed, range-of-motion exercises are added and progressive weight bearing is begun. Full weight bearing is not allowed until radiographs show that the fracture has healed.

When an acute patellar dislocation requires excision or reattachment of an osteochondral fragment, several authors have recommended additional

Figure **14–9.** *A,* Lateral radiograph of a 7-year-old child who sustained an osteochondral fracture of the medial condyle of the knee from an open injury. Note the fracture through the inferior portion of the epiphysis. *B,* Lateral radiograph of the knee after open reduction and pinning of the fracture. The smooth pins were removed after healing of the fracture. *(A, B,* Courtesy of Dr. Neil E. Green.)

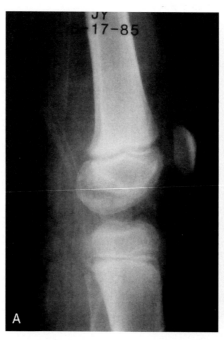

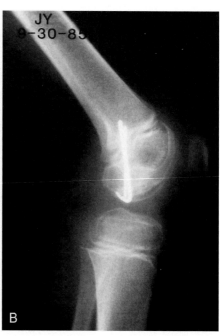

procedures to realign the extensor apparatus of the knee to prevent redislocation, especially when factors associated with patellofemoral malalignment are present.[2, 46, 69, 102, 118, 123]

## Complications

A good result may be expected after the removal of small fragments that do not involve the weight-bearing surface. The outcome is less certain after the removal of large fracture fragments from a weight-bearing surface. These defects become filled with fibrocartilage that over the long term may not be adequate to avoid late degenerative changes. Even after reattachment, a satisfactory long-term outcome is not ensured. Complications of surgical treatment include stiffness from adhesions, quadriceps atrophy, protrusion of screws or pins into the joint, and loss of knee motion.

## FRACTURES OF THE PATELLA

### Anatomy

The patella is the largest sesamoid bone in the body. It lies within the tendon of the quadriceps and functions to make the quadriceps a more efficient extensor of the knee.

The patella begins to ossify between 3 and 5 years of age. Ossification often begins as multiple foci that gradually coalesce. As the patellar ossification center expands, the peripheral margins may appear irregular and may be associated with accessory ossification centers.[83] Incomplete coalescence of a superolaterally located accessory center of ossification results in a bipartite patella (Fig. 14–10), which may be confused with a fracture. When present, a bipartite patella is

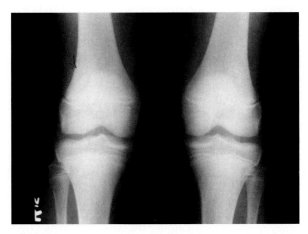

**FIGURE 14–10.** An anteroposterior radiograph of both knees demonstrates a unilateral bipartite patella. Bipartite patellas are commonly bilateral. If tenderness is present at this superolateral location, a fracture should be diagnosed. Operative treatment is rarely indicated. (Courtesy of Dr. Vernon T. Tolo.)

usually evident by 12 years of age and may persist into adult years.[84] Ossification of the patella is generally complete by late adolescence.

### Mechanism of Injury

Transverse or comminuted fractures of the main body of the patella rarely occur in children because the patella is largely cartilaginous and has greater mobility than in adults. Most of these injuries occur in adolescence when ossification is nearly complete.[65] As in adults, fractures of the patella in children may result from either direct or indirect forces.[67] An avulsion fracture of the inferior pole of the patella, the so-called sleeve fracture, is an indirect injury caused by powerful contraction of the quadriceps muscle applied to a flexed knee.

Fractures of the patella have also been attributed to repetitive stress. Hensal and colleagues[48] reported bilateral simultaneous fractures of the patella in a 17-year-old boy that resulted from indirect trauma. At surgery, sclerosis of the fracture edges was thought to be indicative of underlying areas of stress reaction. Iwaya and Takatori[52] described lateral longitudinal fractures of the patella occurring in three children aged 10 to 12 years that the authors attributed to repetitive activities. Ogden and coworkers[84] suggested that instances of painful bipartite patella may be due to a chronic stress fracture.

### Classification

Fractures of the patella in children are generally classified according to the location, pattern, and degree of displacement. One fracture unique to children is the so-called sleeve fracture that occurs through the cartilage on the inferior pole of the patella (Fig. 14–11). This fracture is most commonly seen in children 8 to 12 years of age. With this injury, a large sleeve of cartilage is pulled off the main body of the patella along with a small piece of bone from the distal pole. Grogan and colleagues[44] observed that avulsion fractures may involve any region of the periphery of the patella. They described four patterns of injury: superior, inferior, medial (which often accompanies an acute dislocation of the patella), and lateral (which they attributed to chronic stress caused by repetitive pull from the vastus lateralis muscle).

### Diagnosis

A patient with a fracture of the main body of the patella usually has local tenderness and soft tissue swelling. Hemarthrosis of the knee joint is often present. Active extension of the knee is difficult, especially against resistance. A palpable gap at the lower end of the patella indicates the presence of a sleeve fracture. A high-riding patella suggests that the extensor mechanism has been disrupted.

With marginal fractures, local tenderness and swelling over the affected region of the patella may be the only

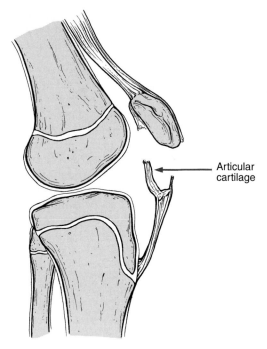

Articular cartilage

FIGURE **14–11.** Sleeve fracture of the patella. A small segment of the distal pole of the patella is avulsed with a relatively large portion of the articular surface.

findings present. In these injuries, straight leg raising may often be possible. The presence of an avulsion fracture of the medial margin suggests the diagnosis of acute patellar dislocation that may have reduced spontaneously.[44] With an associated dislocation, other findings such as medial retinacular tenderness and a positive apprehension sign may also be present.

Anteroposterior and lateral radiographs are needed to evaluate fractures of the main body of the patella. Transverse fractures are best visualized on the lateral view. A lateral radiograph taken with the knee in 30° of flexion may better define the soft tissue stability and true extent of displacement that is present.[12, 44]

Small flecks of bone adjacent to the inferior pole in a patient who has sustained an acute injury may indicate the presence of a sleeve fracture. Magnetic resonance imaging may be helpful to detect a sleeve fracture when the diagnosis is not clear from the clinical and plain radiographic findings.[9, 108] Marginal fractures that are oriented longitudinally may be best seen on a skyline view of the patella.

## Management

The treatment guidelines for transverse patellar fractures in children are generally the same as those for adults.[65, 98] Closed treatment in a cylinder cast with the knee in full extension is recommended for nondisplaced fractures, particularly if active extension of the knee is present.

Operative treatment is necessary for transverse fractures that show more than 3 mm of diastasis or step-off at the articular surface.[12, 98] Fixation may best be

achieved by using the modified tension band technique with a wire loop around two longitudinally placed K-wires.[16, 128] Other fixation options include a circumferential wire loop, interfragmentary screws, or cannulated screws in combination with a tension band wire.[13, 25] The retinaculum should be repaired at the time of osseous fixation. Similarly, sleeve fractures must be accurately reduced and stabilized by using the modified tension band technique[21, 50, 133] (Fig. 14–12). Comminuted fractures of the distal pole are best managed by partial patellectomy.[16] Total patellectomy is reserved for injuries in which the comminution is widespread.

For a small marginal fracture or a painful bipartite patella that does not respond to a period of immobilization and rehabilitation, the fragment is probably best excised.[40, 52, 84] However, screw or pin fixation should be considered for larger fragments that may involve significant portions of the articular surface.[84]

## Complications

The outcome after a fracture of the patella is generally good. Results are poorer after fractures that show greater displacement and comminution.[65] Complications that may occur after displaced fractures that are not adequately reduced include patella alta, extensor lag, and quadriceps atrophy.[12, 21]

## TIBIAL SPINE FRACTURE

### Anatomy

The anterior tibial spine, or anterior intercondylar eminence, is the distal site of attachment of the anterior cruciate ligament. Before complete ossification of the proximal end of the tibia, the surface of the anterior tibial spine is cartilaginous.[73] When excessive tensile stress is applied to the anterior cruciate ligament, the incompletely ossified tibial spine offers less resistance than the ligament, and the tensile stress thus leads to failure through the cancellous bone beneath the tibial spine.

### Mechanism of Injury

Tibial spine fractures are most likely to be caused by hyperextension of the knee in association with some rotation. Traumatic forces that would normally rupture the anterior cruciate ligament in an adult will lead to a tibial spine fracture in a child.

Fracture of the tibial spine is seen primarily in children aged 8 to 14 years. The injury almost always involves the anterior spine. Fractures of the posterior tibial spine are extremely rare in children[105] and are more likely to occur in skeletally mature individuals[79] (Fig. 14–13).

The most common event associated with fracture of

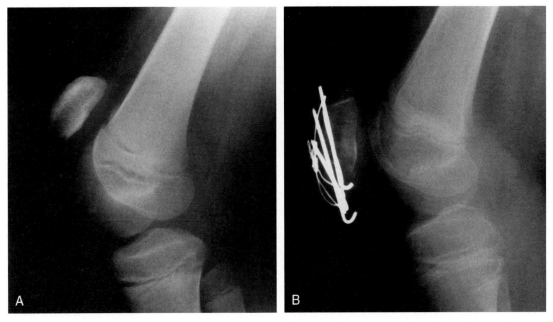

FIGURE **14–12.** Sleeve fracture of the patella. *A,* Lateral radiograph of the knee. The patella is very high riding, indicative of an injury to the patella-quadriceps mechanism. A defect noted on the inferior border of the patella represents the avulsed inferior pole of the patella. The fractured inferior portion of the patella overlies the femoral condyle and is not seen on the original radiograph. *B,* Postoperative lateral radiograph of the knee. The fractured, comminuted inferior pole of the patella was internally fixed with three smooth K-wires and a tension band. Note that the patella has been returned to its normal position. (*A, B,* Courtesy of Dr. Neil E. Green.)

the tibial spine is a fall from a bicycle. Some authors have gone as far as saying that a child who has a painful, swollen knee after falling from a bicycle must be assumed to have a tibial spine fracture until it is proved otherwise.[73, 100] These fractures have also been reported to occur in children participating in sports activities or involved in motor vehicle accidents.

## Classification

Meyers and McKeever[73, 74] classified tibial spine fractures into three main types (Fig. 14–14). In type I fractures, the fragment is minimally displaced with only slight elevation of the anterior margin. In type II fractures, the avulsed fragment has a posterior hinge with the anterior

FIGURE **14–13.** *A,* Lateral radiograph of the knee of a 15-year-old boy who sustained a fracture of the midshaft of the femur plus avulsion of the posterior cruciate ligament of the ipsilateral knee. The *arrow* points to avulsion of the posterior tibial spine. *B,* Lateral radiograph of the knee after closed femoral nailing of the femoral fracture and open reduction and internal fixation of the fracture of the posterior tibial spine through a posterior approach. (*A, B,* Courtesy of Dr. Vernon T. Tolo.)

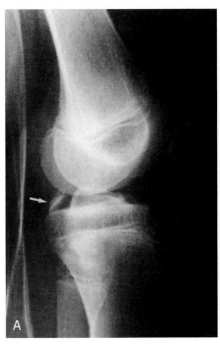
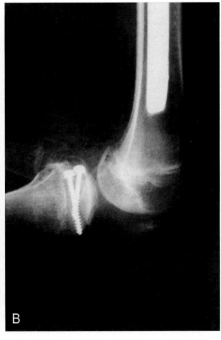

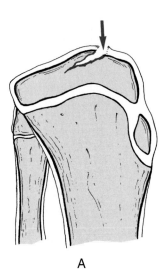
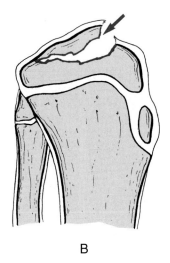
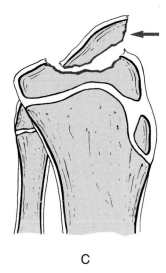

A                                                    B                                                    C

FIGURE **14–14.** Meyers and McKeever's classification of fractures of the anterior tibial spine. *A,* Type I fracture with no displacement of the fracture. *B,* Type II fracture with elevation of the anterior portion of the anterior tibial spine, but with the fracture posteriorly reduced. *C,* Type III fracture that is totally displaced.

portion being elevated from its bone bed. In type III fractures, the avulsed fragment is completely displaced and may be rotated.

## Diagnosis

A patient with a fracture of the tibial spine usually presents with pain, an effusion caused by hemarthrosis, and a reluctance to bear weight. The knee is usually held in a slightly flexed position because of hamstring spasm.

Anteroposterior and lateral radiographs will demonstrate a tibial spine fracture. The degree of displacement is best evaluated on the lateral view. The base of the tibial spine must be carefully inspected on the lateral view for discontinuity of the bony margin. When routine radiographs show only small flecks of bone in the intercondylar notch, magnetic resonance imaging may be useful to further evaluate the injury.

## Management

Treatment is based on the type of fracture present. Type I fractures and type II fractures that are minimally displaced may be treated by closed means. If a tense hemarthrosis is present, it should be aspirated under sterile conditions and a long leg cast applied. It is my preference to immobilize the knee in 10° of flexion, but not all authorities agree. Beaty and Kumar[12] recommended immobilizing the knee in 10° to 15° of flexion. Similarly, Meyers and McKeever[74] recommended immobilizing the knee in 20° of flexion. Fyfe and Jackson,[33] noting that the anterior cruciate ligament is taut in extension, recommended that the knee be immobilized in 30° to 40° of flexion to relax the ligament. One should avoid applying a cast in hyperextension to prevent excessive stretch of the popliteal artery that could result in a compartment syndrome.

After the cast is applied, radiographs should be taken to confirm reduction of the tibial spine fragment and be repeated in 1 to 2 weeks to ensure that displacement has not occurred. The cast can usually be removed in 6 weeks.

Operative reduction, either arthroscopically assisted[66, 72] or through a limited anteromedial or anterolateral arthotomy,[56, 129] is indicated for irreducible type II fractures and all type III fractures. The anterior horn of the medial meniscus, if interposed, is removed from the fracture site to facilitate accurate reduction. The fragment may be secured by passing an absorbable suture through the cartilaginous portion of the fracture fragment and either the anterior lip of the tibial epiphysis or the edge of the anterior portion of the meniscus (Fig. 14–15). Alternatively, the fragment can be secured with smooth K-wires.[134] After arthroscopic reduction, the fragment may be fixed with either absorbable sutures or a cancellous screw (Fig. 14–16). In an adolescent patient with a small fragment, fixation may be achieved by weaving a nonabsorbable pull-out suture through the anterior cruciate ligament with the ends passed through drill holes in the anterior portion of the tibia.[12]

## Complications

A good outcome may be expected for fractures of the tibial spine, at least for the short term. Nonunion of properly treated fractures is rare, but malunion of type III injuries has been reported. These patients may present with clinical instability and a mechanical block to full extension of the knee. For symptomatic patients, mobilization of the tibial spine, excision of excess bone, and reattachment of the tibial fragment in the reduced position may be used to treat the malunion.[33, 63]

Several authors have documented anterior cruciate laxity and some loss of full knee extension after tibial spine fractures, even those that have healed in an anatomic position.[5, 10, 111, 129, 130] This laxity has been attributed to the interstitial tearing of the anterior cruciate ligament that probably occurs before the fragment is avulsed.[5, 42, 53, 111, 130] Late laxity varies according to the severity of the initial injury. When compared with type I injuries, greater laxity has been noted after types II and III fractures.[10, 130] Despite the laxity, relatively few patients complain of pain or instability.[10, 130]

Few long-term outcome studies of this injury have been reported. Janarv and colleagues[53] monitored 61 children with anterior tibial spine fractures for an average of 16 years. Although most of their patients had a good clinical outcome at latest follow-up, these authors found no evidence to suggest that the anterior knee laxity that resulted from the injury diminished over time. Because of the persistent anterior knee laxity that has been docu-

mented in several reports, the long-term prognosis for this injury remains uncertain, and families of patients with this injury should be counseled accordingly.

## TIBIAL TUBERCLE FRACTURE

### Anatomy

**Bone and Soft Tissue Anatomy.** The proximal tibial physis contributes not only to longitudinal growth of the tibia but also to development of the tibial tubercle. According to Ogden,[83] the tibial tubercle, or tibial tuberosity, initially develops as an anterior extension of the proximal tibial physis at around 12 to 15 weeks of

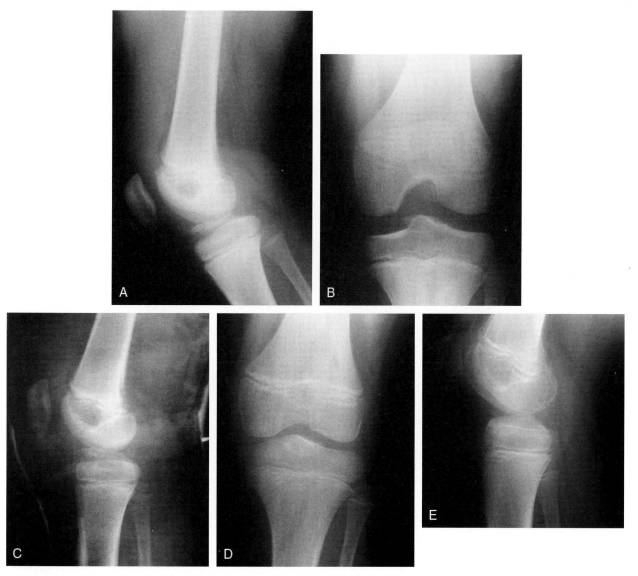

**FIGURE 14–15.** *A* and *B,* Anteroposterior and lateral radiographs of the left knee demonstrate a type II fracture of the tibial intercondylar eminence in this 9-year-old boy. *C,* A lateral radiograph after attempted closed reduction (by knee extension) demonstrates no change from the initial radiograph, which generally indicates that the meniscus is blocking fracture reduction. *D* and *E,* Anteroposterior and lateral radiographs of the left knee made 2 months postoperatively show excellent reduction and fracture healing after open reduction and suture fixation of the fracture. (*A–E,* Courtesy of Dr. Vernon T. Tolo.)

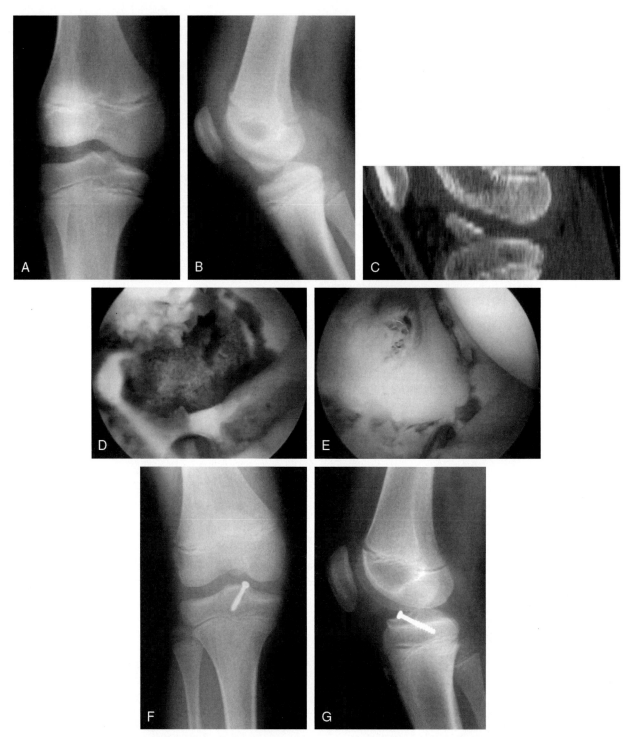

FIGURE **14–16.** Ten-year-old boy who sustained a type III fracture of the anterior tibial spine as a result of a dirt bike accident. On arrival at the emergency department, he had a large, painful effusion of his knee. *A,* Anteroposterior radiograph of the patient's knee. A displaced fracture of the anterior tibial spine is noted to be elevated from its normal position. *B,* On a lateral radiograph of the knee, the completely displaced fracture of the anterior tibial spine is seen to be displaced superiorly. *C,* A sagittal reconstruction computed tomographic scan easily demonstrates the fracture fragment displaced from its normal position. *D,* Arthroscopic view of the fracture. The bed of the fracture is seen in the middle of the photograph, and the anterior horn of the meniscus is located in the lower portion of the photograph. The fractured fragment is seen superiorly and partially overlying the superolateral portion of the fracture bed. *E,* The fragment has been replaced and internally fixed with a screw. One can see the fragment anatomically reduced into its bed. The screw has been partially countersunk into the fracture fragment. A small hook is seen retracting the anterior horn of the meniscus. *F,* Postoperative anteroposterior radiograph demonstrating that the fragment has been reinserted into its normal position and is well secured with a single cancellous screw. The screw remains entirely within the epiphysis. *G,* On this lateral radiograph, the fragment has been reduced anatomically and is internally fixed with a cancellous screw that is directed posteriorly so that the screw has adequate bone surface contact yet remains within the epiphysis and does not risk injuring the physis. (*A–G,* Courtesy of Dr. Neil E. Green.)

gestation. At birth, the tubercle is located approximately near the level of the proximal tibial epiphysis; distal migration occurs postnatally.

The epiphyseal ossification center of the proximal part of the tibia appears between the first and third months of life. The ossification center of the tibial tubercle begins in its distal region between the ages of 7 and 9 years and then gradually extends toward the proximal end of the tibia. During adolescence, these two ossification centers are separated by a small cartilaginous bridge that eventually dissipates. The physis of the tibial tubercle closes between the ages of 13 and 15 years in girls and 15 and 19 years in boys.[83]

Ogden[83] has observed that the physis underlying the tibial tubercle is initially composed almost exclusively of fibrocartilage rather than the columnar physeal cartilage that is usually present in a region of growth. He suggested that this fairly unique cytoarchitecture allowed the tubercle to better resist the normal tensile stresses applied to it by the quadriceps muscle through the patellar tendon. As the tubercle undergoes progressive ossification, the growth plate underlying the tubercle changes from fibrocartilage to columnar physeal cartilage. Because the tensile strength of columnar cartilage is less than that of fibrocartilage, these changes render the tubercle less able to resist violent tensile stresses and thus make it potentially more vulnerable to separation.

**Vascular Anatomy.** The anterior tibial recurrent artery makes a contribution to the blood supply of the tibial tubercle that has potential clinical implications. Wall[126] demonstrated by anatomic dissection numerous leashlike branches of the anterior tibial recurrent artery that terminate along the lateral border of the tibial tubercle. When these vessels were sectioned in a cadaver, he observed that they tended to retract laterally and distally under the fascia and into the muscles of the anterior compartment. The author concluded that continued bleeding from these vessels into the anterior compartment could lead to a compartment syndrome. Pape and colleagues[88] reported two adolescent boys in whom a compartment syndrome developed after an avulsion fracture of the tibial tubercle. They cited bleeding from branches of the anterior tibial recurrent artery as a predisposing factor for this complication.

## Mechanism of Injury

Tibial tubercle fractures occur most often in boys between 12 and 17 years of age. Sports activities, especially basketball and competitive jumping events, are most commonly associated with this injury.[6, 27, 28, 60, 77, 86, 131]

The mechanism of injury is either active extension of the knee with violent contraction of the quadriceps muscle, as occurs with jumping, or acute passive flexion against a contracted quadriceps muscle, as occurs when a football player is tackled.[6, 17, 60, 131]

Several authors have suggested that Osgood-Schlatter disease may predispose an individual to acute disruption of the tibial tubercle.[17, 60, 86, 131] Osgood-Schlatter dis-

ease is a common cause of knee pain in active children between the ages of 10 and 14 years. Clinically, these patients have tenderness directly over the tibial tubercle. Although this condition is self-limited and resolves when the physis of the tibial tubercle closes, affected children may require activity restriction in one form or another to allow resolution of symptoms during the early stages. Rosenberg and colleagues[104] concluded, on the basis of imaging studies, that this condition was due to inflammation of the patellar tendon at its insertion into the tubercle rather than involvement of the bone. According to Ogden and coauthors,[86] Osgood-Schlatter disease appears to involve only the anterior portion of the ossification center of the tubercle with no involvement of the physis. They postulated that this condition might somehow alter the physis of the tubercle by increasing the amount of columnar cartilage in comparison to fibrocartilage, thus predisposing the patient to acute avulsion of the entire tubercle.

## Classification

Watson-Jones classified fractures of the tibial tubercle into three types. In the first type, a small fragment of the distal portion of the tubercle is avulsed. In the second type, the entire secondary center of the tubercle is hinged upward with the apex of the angulation being at the level of the proximal tibial physis. In the third type, the fracture line propagates through the proximal tibial physis into the knee joint.

Ogden and colleagues[86] modified this classification to place greater emphasis on intra-articular extension of the fracture and comminution of the tubercle (Fig. 14–17). In type 1, only the most distal portions of the tubercle are involved. Subtype A is a fracture through the ossification center of the tubercle with little displacement. In subtype B, the fragment is separated from the metaphysis. Type 2 injuries involve separation of the entire ossification center of the tubercle. The fracture occurs through the area bridging the main tibial and tubercle ossification centers. In subtype B, the ossification center of the tubercle is comminuted and the more distal fragment may be proximally displaced. Type 3 fractures extend into the joint surface. In subtype B, the fracture fragment is comminuted.

## Diagnosis

Patients with a fracture of the tibial tubercle present with local soft tissue swelling and tenderness directly over the fracture site. Patients with a nondisplaced type 1 injury are usually able to extend the knee against gravity, and knee effusion is not generally present. In type 2 and type 3 injuries, active knee extension is not possible. Most of these patients will have hemarthrosis of the knee joint.

Accurate lateral radiographs of the tubercle are essential to evaluate this injury. Because the tubercle is just lateral to the midline of the tibia, the best profile is obtained with the tibia in slight internal rotation.

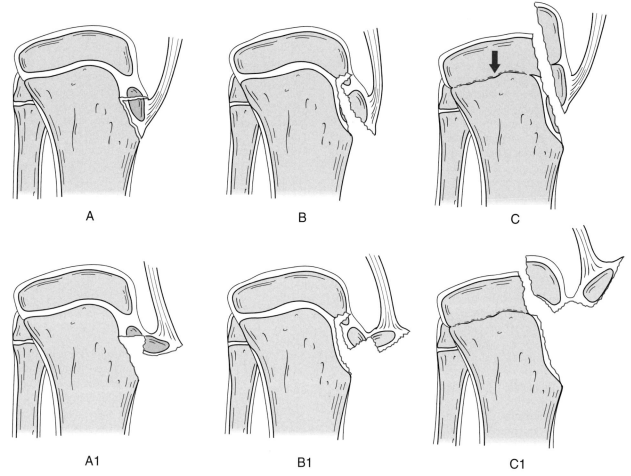

**FIGURE 14–17.** Avulsion fractures of the tibial tubercle. *A,* Type I fracture. The fracture line is through the secondary ossification center. In subtype A, the displacement is minimal. In subtype B, the fragment is hinged anteriorly and proximally. *B,* Type II fracture. The fracture occurs through the junction of the ossification centers of the proximal end of the tibia and the tuberosity. In subtype A, the fragment is not comminuted. In subtype B, the fragment is comminuted and may be more proximally displaced. *C,* A type III fracture is a true Salter-Harris type III injury that is intra-articular. In subtype A, the tubercle and anterior part of the proximal tibial epiphysis form a single unit. In subtype B, the fragment is comminuted, with the site of fragmentation being at the junction of the ossification centers of the proximal end of the tibia and the tuberosity.

Oblique radiographs of the proximal end of the tibia are helpful to fully visualize the extension of the fracture into the knee joint.[86]

## Management

Nondisplaced type 1 fractures can be treated successfully by immobilization in a cylinder or long leg cast with the knee in complete extension for 4 to 6 weeks, followed by progressive rehabilitation of the quadriceps. Type 1B, as well as nearly all type 2 and type 3 injuries, requires operative treatment. Osseous fixation may be achieved with pins or screws. My personal preference for internal fixation is one or two AO cancellous screws placed in an anterior-to-posterior direction.

The surgical approach is anterior, parallel with the patellar tendon, either medially or laterally. Hematoma and any interposed soft tissue, such as a flap of periosteum, are removed to facilitate accurate reduction. The menisci should be inspected for tears or peripheral detachments in all type 3 injuries.[131]

With the knee in full extension, the fracture is reduced and provisionally held in position with a Steinmann pin through the fracture fragment into the metaphysis. Under image intensifier control, a cancellous screw is placed in an anterior-to-posterior direction through the proximal tibial metaphysis (Fig. 14–18). Wiss and colleagues[131] recommended that 4.0-mm cancellous screws be used rather than larger implants, such as 6.5-mm screws, to lessen the incidence of bursitis that may develop over prominent screw heads. Washers may be helpful to prevent the screw head from sinking below the cortical surface. If solid fixation is not achieved with a single screw, a second screw can be added. The continuity of the patellar ligament and avulsed periosteum is also repaired. If severe comminution is present, a tension-holding suture may be necessary to secure the repair.

After operative reduction, a cylinder or long leg cast with the knee immobilized in complete extension is worn for 4 to 6 weeks, followed by progressive rehabilitation of the quadriceps. Return to regular activities is permitted after the quadriceps has regained normal strength and full range of motion of the knee joint has been achieved.

Mirbey and coworkers[77] permitted their patients to resume sports activities at an average of 3 months after injury. After type 2 and type 3 fractures, Ogden and colleagues[86] observed that patients took between 16 and 18 weeks after cast removal to return to their preinjury activity levels.

## Complications

The prognosis for a fracture of the tibial tubercle is very good. Complications are uncommon. The theoretical complication of genu recurvatum has not been reported because most of these injuries occur when the physis is nearing normal closure.

Compartment syndrome, presumably caused by tearing of nearby branches of the anterior tibial recurrent artery, has been reported after tibial tubercle fractures.[88, 131] Careful monitoring of patients treated by closed methods along with careful assessment and possible prophylactic anterior compartment fasciotomy of patients treated operatively is recommended.

Bursitis over prominent screw heads necessitates removal of the implant. Avoiding the use of larger screws may minimize the risk of this problem.[131]

## PROXIMAL TIBIAL METAPHYSEAL AND PHYSEAL FRACTURES

### Anatomy

**Bone and Soft Tissue Anatomy.** The epiphyseal ossification center of the proximal part of the tibia usually appears between the first and third months of life.[82] The proximal tibial physis contributes approximately 55% of the length of the tibia and 25% of the length of the entire leg and averages approximately 6 mm of growth each year until maturity.[4, 95] Closure of this growth plate is usually complete by 13 to 15 years in girls and 15 to 18 years in boys. Any injury that partially or completely disrupts growth of the proximal end of the tibia may lead to angular deformity or shortening of the extremity. The younger the child at the time of such injury, the greater the potential for these sequelae.

Although trauma to the region of the knee is quite common in children, fractures of the proximal tibial epiphysis are rare and account for less than 2% of all physeal injuries.[92] Several anatomic structures appear to protect the proximal tibial physis from injury.[29, 36] Laterally, the upper end of the fibula buttresses the physis. Anteriorly, the distal projection of the tibial tubercle over the metaphysis provides stability. Posteromedially, the insertion of the semimembranosus muscle spans the physis.

Several authors have suggested that the proximal tibial physis may also be protected from traumatic stress because insertion of the collateral ligaments directly into the epiphysis is limited.[3, 23, 36, 100, 109] They noted that the lateral collateral ligament inserts into the head of the fibula and has no tibial attachment whereas the medial collateral ligament has only a minor attachment to the epiphysis with most of the ligament inserting distally into the metaphysis. In contrast, Ogden[82] has described dense attachments of the collateral ligaments and joint capsule into the epiphyseal perichondrium both medially and laterally. He believes that the protection afforded to the proximal tibial physis is more likely due to anatomic factors other than the insertion of the collateral ligaments.

**Vascular Anatomy.** Of all physeal fractures, those of the proximal physis of the tibia have the greatest potential for disastrous vascular compromise.[23, 109, 132]

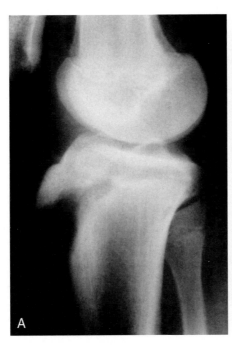 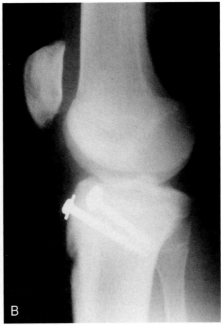

**Figure 14–18.** *A,* Lateral knee radiograph of a 14-year-old boy with a displaced fracture of the tibial tubercle. *B,* Lateral knee radiograph of the same boy after open reduction and screw fixation of the fracture. Because these fractures usually occur in adolescents whose proximal tibial physis has already partially closed, no significant growth is lost by screw fixation across the remaining physis. (*A, B,* Courtesy of Dr. Vernon T. Tolo.)

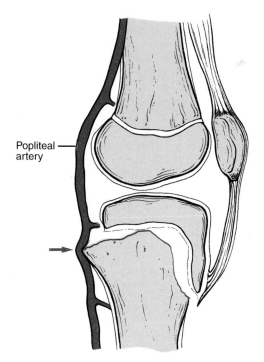

FIGURE 14–19. Lateral drawing of a knee showing a displaced proximal tibial physeal injury and demonstrating the risk of arterial injury because of the close proximity of the popliteal artery to the proximal end of the tibia.

The local vascular anatomy primarily accounts for this high risk of associated injury.

As the popliteal artery passes distally beneath the soleal arch, it divides into three branches: the anterior tibial, peroneal, and posterior tibial arteries. The vessels of this trifurcation pass distally, with the peroneal artery usually terminating in the lower part of the leg and the anterior tibial (dorsalis pedis) and posterior tibial arteries providing circulation to the foot. Just below the level of the trifurcation, the anterior tibial artery pierces the interosseous membrane as it courses into the anterior compartment of the leg and causes the arteries to be relatively tethered and immobile at this location. Because this trifurcation occurs just distal to the proximal tibial physis, any posterior displacement of the proximal end of the metaphysis may stretch or tear the popliteal artery (Fig. 14–19).

## Proximal Tibial Physeal Fractures

### MECHANISM OF INJURY

Most proximal tibial physeal fractures are due to either a hyperextension or abduction force applied to a fixed knee. The majority of these injuries occur in adolescents either during sports activities or as the result of a motor vehicle accident.[23, 109] An unusual avulsion injury involving the proximal tibial physis may occur during sports activities that involve jumping.[6, 15, 106] In this injury, the fracture begins as a tibial tubercle avulsion before propagating through the entire proximal tibial physis and exiting to include a portion of the posterior

tibial metaphysis. Lawn mower accidents, which occur most often in younger children, may result in severe open fractures of the distal tibial physis.[23]

Patients may occasionally present with physeal arrest of the anterior portion of the proximal tibial physis in association with a nonphyseal fracture of the lower extremity.[51, 87, 89] Pappas and colleagues[89] suggested that in these patients, an injury to the proximal tibial physis may have been overlooked because attention was directed to a more obvious injury. Patients who have fractures of the lower extremities that do not appear to involve the growth plate should be carefully assessed and monitored for a possible physeal injury.

### CLASSIFICATION

The most commonly used classification system for fractures of the proximal epiphysis of the tibia is that of Salter and Harris[107] as described earlier for the distal part of the femur.

### DIAGNOSIS

A careful description of the accident should be elicited to determine the direction of the force that caused the injury. A patient with a fracture of the proximal tibial physis presents with local soft tissue swelling and tenderness directly over the physis. Often, hemarthrosis is present. Deformity is evident in displaced injuries.

One must remember that because displaced fractures of the proximal tibial epiphysis may have partially or completely reduced before the patient is evaluated, an arterial injury must be considered in every patient with this injury[23] (Fig. 14–20). A careful neurovascular examination must be performed, with documentation of the presence of the dorsalis pedis and posterior tibial pulses and the function of the posterior tibial and peroneal nerves. If the clinical findings of acute ischemia are present—extremity pallor, coolness, cyanosis, or delayed capillary refill—reduction of the displacement should be performed as soon as possible. If these findings are still present after the reduction maneuver, immediate vascular exploration is indicated. In the absence of an obviously ischemic limb, patients with an abnormal pulse or those who recover pulses and perfusion after reduction of the fracture should undergo arteriography[57, 121] (Fig. 14–21). The presence or absence of pain on hyperextension of the toes should be recorded as a baseline measure to detect the possible development of an anterior compartment syndrome. As described for fractures of the distal femoral metaphysis and physis, ongoing evaluation of the lower extremity is important during the first few days after the fracture so that a developing compartment syndrome or intimal tear with thrombosis may be detected promptly.

Anteroposterior and lateral radiographs of the proximal part of the tibia and knee will usually reveal the fracture. Stress radiographs should be considered when the plain films appear normal in a patient who has tenderness localized to the physis or who has instability of the knee.[109] When performing stress radiographs, hyperextension should probably be avoided.

On occasion, computed tomography may be helpful to plan treatment of a type III or IV fracture. Magnetic resonance imaging may be useful to reveal a fracture in a patient suspected of having an occult injury to the growth plate (Fig. 14–22).

## MANAGEMENT

The goals of treatment are to obtain and maintain anatomic reduction and avoid further damage to the growth plate. The form of treatment is determined by both the fracture type and the degree of displacement.

**Salter-Harris Types I and II Fractures.** For Salter-Harris types I and II injuries, nondisplaced fractures are immobilized for 6 weeks in a long leg cast. Displaced fractures should be gently reduced under general anesthesia to minimize further damage to the growth plate. Reduction of the fracture is best done under image intensifier control. Because most of these fractures are the result of hyperextension injuries, flexion usually achieves reduction. Immobilization of the knee in marked flexion may increase the risk of vascular compromise and should be avoided. Most of these fractures tend to be unstable, so my preference is to use smooth, crossed transphyseal pins to maintain reduction.[100, 132] Type II fractures with an adequately sized metaphyseal fragment on both

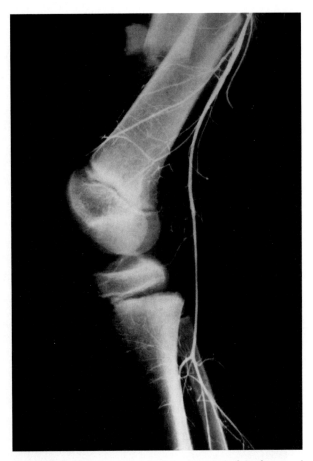

**FIGURE 14–21.** Lateral radiograph of the distal end of the femur and proximal portion of the tibia of a boy who sustained a closed femoral fracture and a displaced type I proximal tibial fracture. The arteriogram shows that the popliteal artery is narrow and under spasm, but no intimal damage to the artery is present. (Courtesy of Dr. Neil E. Green.)

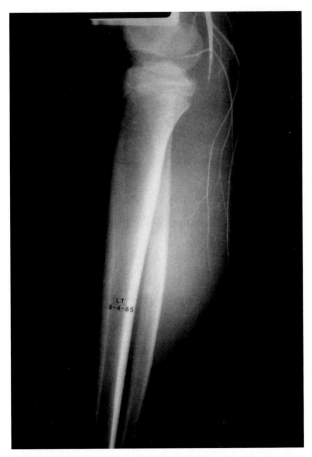

**FIGURE 14–20.** Arteriogram of the knee and proximal end of the tibia of a 13 year old who sustained a complete popliteal artery injury as a result of a displaced proximal tibial type I physeal injury that reduced spontaneously. (Courtesy of Dr. Neil E. Green.)

anteroposterior and lateral views may be stabilized by using pins or screws across the metaphyseal portion of the fracture. The use of internal fixation allows the knee to be immobilized in 20° to 30° of flexion, a position that poses less risk to the circulation and makes subsequent displacement less likely.

If satisfactory closed reduction cannot be achieved after one or at most two attempts, open reduction is required. It is more often needed in type II than type I fractures. The most common reason that closed reduction of these fractures may fail is the interposition of soft tissue in the fracture site.[29] If arterial repair is required, open reduction plus internal fixation is first performed to prevent excessive motion at the fracture site and thus afford protection to the vascular repair.

Open reduction of type I fractures may be done through an anterior approach, lateral to the tibial tubercle. In type II fractures, the incision is made over the metaphyseal fragment. Hematoma and any interposed soft tissue are removed to facilitate anatomic reduction. Smooth Steinmann pins may be used to stabilize the fracture.

Because of the proclivity to compartment syndrome with these injuries, tissue pressure in the anterior, lateral, posterior, and deep posterior compartments should be

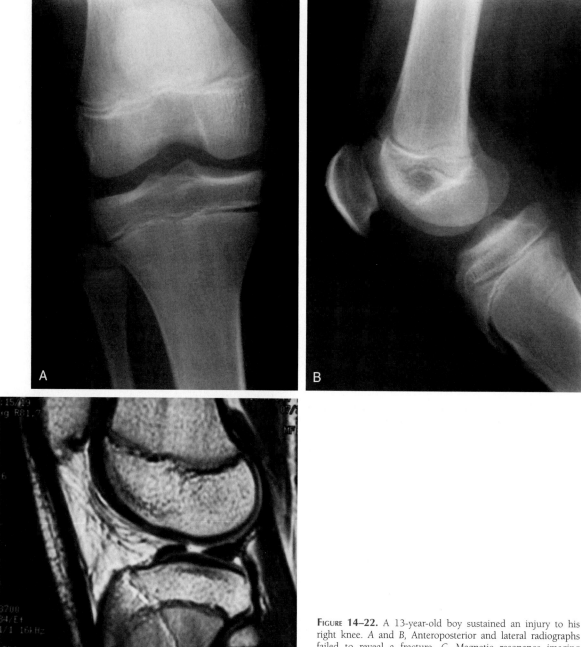

**Figure 14–22.** A 13-year-old boy sustained an injury to his right knee. *A* and *B*, Anteroposterior and lateral radiographs failed to reveal a fracture. *C*, Magnetic resonance imaging revealed a nondisplaced Salter-Harris type IV fracture of the proximal end of the tibia.

measured before leaving the operating room. If any values measure more than 40 mm Hg, appropriate fasciotomies can be performed.

**Salter-Harris Types III and IV Fractures.** Nondisplaced Salter-Harris types III and IV injuries may be placed in a long leg cast for 6 to 8 weeks. Careful follow-up of these patients at weekly intervals is needed to promptly address any displacement. Alternatively, these fractures may be stabilized with percutaneous screws.

Displaced fractures are treated by open reduction and internal fixation to restore congruity of the joint surface and align the physis. After reduction, stabilization of the

fracture may be achieved by using either smooth pins or screws inserted horizontally to avoid crossing the physis. Type III fractures may have associated tears of the medial collateral ligament.[14, 36, 94, 109] If this problem is recognized at the time of injury, primary repair of the ligament has been recommended.[14] As recommended earlier for types I and II fractures, compartment pressures should be measured before leaving the operating room.

**Postoperative Management.** After fracture reduction and stabilization have been completed and compartment pressures have been checked, a long leg splint is applied with the knee flexed at approximately 20° to 30°. Bedrest with the leg slightly elevated is maintained for 24 to 48 hours, and the child is carefully monitored for the development of compartment syndrome or an intimal tear with thrombosis. If the child is cooperative, this monitoring may be done by assessment of pedal pulses, sensation to the foot, and pain on passive movement of the toes. If the child has an associated head injury and is unconscious or otherwise uncooperative, sequential compartment measurements should be performed. If a compartment syndrome is diagnosed at any time after the fracture, emergency fasciotomy must be performed.

Once it is clear that no compartment syndrome or vascular occlusion is present or developing, a long leg cast is applied with the knee in mild flexion. After 6 weeks, use of the cast is discontinued and the pins are removed in the outpatient setting. Because these are intra-articular fractures, weight bearing after a type III or IV injury should not be begun until radiographs confirm that the fracture is fully healed.

## COMPLICATIONS

In general, the prognosis for a fracture of the proximal tibial epiphysis is good. Shortening and angular deformity are less commonly seen after these fractures than after fractures of the distal femoral physis because injuries to the proximal tibial physis tend to occur in older children and adolescents and the proximal tibial physis contributes less to overall growth of the limb than does the distal femoral physis. The younger the child at the time of a proximal tibial physeal injury, the greater the likelihood of the development of shortening and angular deformity.

Open injuries to the proximal tibial physis have a much poorer prognosis. These fractures are often due to a lawn mower mishap.[23] Angular deformities, either occurring alone or in combination with limb shortening, are frequently seen after these injuries.

Careful clinical evaluation is recommended at 6-month intervals after an injury to the proximal tibial physis to assess lower extremity alignment and leg length. Comparative radiographs of both lower extremities should be taken in both the anteroposterior and lateral planes.[35]

Angular deformities may be due to either malunion or a partial growth disturbance. Significant angular deformity resulting from malunion may be managed by osteotomy or, when appropriate, by hemiepiphysiodesis. Treatment options for progressive angular deformity caused by a partial growth disturbance include osseous bridge resection, osteotomy, or epiphysiodesis of the remaining portion of the physis. Osseous bridge resection may be considered for lesions involving less than 50% of the physis.[55, 93] Because the proximal tibial epiphysis averages approximately 6 mm of growth each year until maturity, children should have at least 3 years of growth remaining before osseous bridge resection is considered.

An osteotomy with epiphysiodesis of the remaining portion of the physis may be necessary when the bridge is too large to excise or in children who are nearing completion of growth. Lengthening may be combined with angular correction in children who have both an angular deformity and significant shortening.[87, 91]

## Proximal Tibial Metaphyseal Fractures

Fractures of the proximal metaphysis of the tibia are uncommon injuries in children. Two types of these fractures deserve special mention: a minimally displaced valgus greenstick fracture and a more displaced injury that results from higher-energy trauma.

### VALGUS GREENSTICK FRACTURE

The more common type of fracture in this region is a minimally displaced, transversely oriented greenstick fracture that usually extends two thirds of the way across the tibial metaphysis, although in some instances the fracture line may continue completely across the metaphysis. An associated fracture of the proximal end of the fibula is infrequent. Even though the fracture is relatively nondisplaced, a fracture gap on the medial side is often present. These injuries most commonly occur in children younger than 10 years and are usually the result of low-energy trauma such as playground falls or bicycle accidents.[85] Associated neurovascular problems are uncommon. Despite their innocuous appearance, a progressive valgus angulation often develops in these fractures during the period of fracture healing, as well as after union of the fracture (Fig. 14–23).

A patient with a greenstick fracture of the proximal metaphysis of the tibia presents with local pain, swelling, and tenderness at the fracture site. Anteroposterior and lateral radiographs of the proximal end of the tibia, including the knee, will reveal the fracture.

Treatment should be directed at closing the medial metaphyseal gap at the fracture site. Reduction is best accomplished by using image intensifier control with the patient under general anesthesia. The knee is straightened, and varus stress is applied across the fracture site. If reduction of the fracture has been obtained, a long leg cast is applied with the knee in nearly full extension, and varus molding is applied to the fracture site. If the fracture gap cannot be reduced by closed means, the pes anserinus or periosteum may be interposed in the fracture site.[127] In this rare instance, it may be necessary to remove the impediments to reduction through a small medial incision over the fracture site. After operative reduction, internal fixation is unnecessary. Healing of these fractures is usually complete by 4 to 6 weeks.

The most common problem associated with a greenstick fracture of the proximal tibial metaphysis is progressive valgus angulation. The angulation occurs most rapidly during the first 12 months after the injury and continues at a slower rate for as long as 18 to 24 months.[85, 136] It is important to emphasize to parents the possibility of subsequent deformity despite adequate and appropriate treatment of the fracture.

Although the exact cause of the deformity is not known, relative overgrowth of the proximal tibial physis,

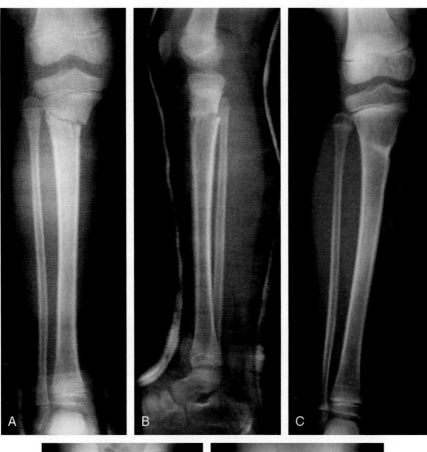

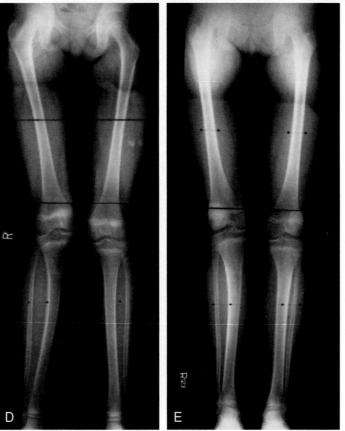

FIGURE **14–23.** A 5-year-old girl sustained a fracture of the proximal metaphysis of the tibia. *A,* An anteroposterior radiograph made after closed reduction of the fracture and application of a long leg cast shows that the fracture is properly aligned. *B,* A lateral radiograph shows excellent reduction in the sagittal plane. *C,* An anteroposterior radiograph made 1 year after the fracture shows that a valgus deformity has developed. *D,* An anteroposterior radiograph taken 2½ years after the injury reveals that the deformity is still evident. *E,* An anteroposterior radiograph taken 3 years and 2 months after the injury shows that the overall alignment of the lower extremities has improved.

presumably caused by fracture-induced hyperemia, probably plays a key role.[85, 135] Increased radionuclide activity at the proximal tibial growth plate, with proportionally greater uptake on the medial side, has been reported after a fracture of the proximal tibial metaphysis.[135] In a series of children with post-traumatic tibia valga, Ogden and colleagues[85] found both a generalized increase in longitudinal growth of the injured tibia that occurred both proximally and distally and eccentric proximal medial overgrowth in every patient.

Even though the valgus deformity resulting from the proximal tibial metaphyseal fracture is unsightly to parents, the surgeon should be in no hurry to perform a corrective valgus osteotomy. Several authors have reported spontaneous improvement of the deformity with time.[7, 70, 110, 122, 136] In addition, both recurrence of deformity and compartment syndrome have been reported after corrective tibial osteotomy for this problem.[7, 30]

McCarthy and coworkers[70] compared the results of operative versus nonoperative treatment in a series of children with post-traumatic tibia valga. These authors found no significant difference in lower extremity alignment between the operative and nonoperative groups at the time of injury, at maximal deformity, or at latest follow-up. Tuten and colleagues[122] monitored seven patients with an acquired valgus deformity after a proximal metaphyseal fracture for an average of 15 years postinjury and found that spontaneous improvement of the angulation occurred in all patients and resulted in a clinically well aligned limb in most. They concluded that patients with this deformity should be monitored through skeletal maturity and that operative intervention should be reserved for patients who have symptoms from malalignment. Because of the trend toward spontaneous improvement of the angulation with growth and because of the frequency of recurrent deformity and the risk of compartment syndrome after osteotomy in skeletally immature patients, early corrective osteotomy is not recommended.

## DISPLACED FRACTURES OF THE PROXIMAL TIBIAL METAPHYSIS

The other type of fracture of the proximal tibial metaphysis is produced by higher-energy trauma. These displaced fractures often injure the anterior tibial artery and lead to a compartment syndrome in the lower part of the leg. The fibula is generally fractured and displaced with the proximal end of the tibia and may be associated with an injury to the peroneal nerve. Because this fracture is prone to neurovascular problems, Rang[97] has labeled this injury the "arterial hazard fracture."

If adequate closed reduction can be obtained and no signs of compartment syndrome are apparent, a long leg cast may be applied with the knee immobilized in slight flexion. After reduction, the leg is slightly elevated and the patient is closely monitored for compartment syndrome over the next 24 to 48 hours. If a fasciotomy is required to treat a compartment syndrome, either external or internal fixation is needed to stabilize the fracture. An external fixator that bridges the knee allows

for fasciotomy wound care without any need to open the fracture site.[120] The fixator may be removed in a few weeks without excessive concern for residual joint stiffness. Alternatively, provisional internal fixation with smooth Steinmann pins supplemented by a splint can stabilize the fracture until wound healing is sufficient to apply a long leg cast.

## PROXIMAL FIBULAR METAPHYSEAL AND PHYSEAL FRACTURES

Most proximal fibular fractures accompany proximal tibial physeal or metaphyseal fractures. Although these fractures do not require anatomic reduction, careful evaluation of peroneal nerve function is needed whenever this injury is seen on radiographs.

Physeal fractures of the proximal portion of the fibula are among the rarest of physeal injuries.[1, 19] These fractures typically occur during adolescence, so growth disturbance is not generally a problem. If instability of the knee ligaments is not present, a long leg or cylinder cast for 3 to 4 weeks is sufficient for management. Normal function and return to athletic activities can be expected.

## OPEN FRACTURES IN THE KNEE REGION

Open fractures near the knee joint require thorough evaluation to determine whether the joint was entered at the time of injury. Sometimes, the examiner can look into the knee joint through the wound, and the diagnosis is easy. Radiographs showing air within the knee joint can be used as presumptive evidence that the wound communicates with the joint. If the diagnosis is less clear, a saline load test may be performed.[125] Under sterile conditions, 30 to 50 mL of saline or other physiologic fluid is injected into the knee through intact skin. If the wound communicates with the knee joint, the injected fluid will leak out through the wound.

Once penetration of the knee joint has been confirmed, sterile dressings are applied to the wound, tetanus prophylaxis is given if indicated, and broad-spectrum antibiotics are started intravenously. Thorough wound débridement and irrigation of the joint are performed through a formal arthrotomy.[90] If possible, the knee joint is closed over a suction drain. Similarly, the open fracture is irrigated and débrided. I prefer partial primary closure of the open fracture wound with a portion left open to close by secondary intention. As with other open fractures, antibiotics are generally continued for 3 to 5 days after the operation.

In open fractures caused by penetrating trauma such as a bullet, fracture management is somewhat different. If the bullet is a low-velocity missile causing little adjacent soft tissue injury, an open fracture of the femoral or tibial shaft does not usually require formal irrigation and débridement. However, if the bullet has lodged in the knee joint or has passed through it, arthrotomy is recommended to remove osseous and cartilaginous fragments, as well as extract the bullet. Even if a bullet is not mechanically causing a problem with knee motion, a retained bullet within the knee joint may lead to elevated serum lead levels.[62]

With gunshot wounds to the knee, vascular injury should be considered, especially when the path of the bullet is in close proximity to the popliteal vessels. Arteriography or exploration may be necessary if the bullet trajectory is in the posterior region of the knee and clinical evidence of vascular disruption is apparent. Once the wound and soft tissue injuries have been addressed, the fracture may require external fixation to allow for dressing changes; however, management has to be individualized for each open fracture in this region.

## PATELLAR DISLOCATION

### Anatomy

The patella is a sesamoid bone that lies within the tendon of the quadriceps. It allows the quadriceps muscle to be a more efficient extensor of the knee. The patella is stabilized by the trochlear groove of the distal end of the femur as it moves with flexion and extension of the knee. The alignment of the quadriceps mechanism may be estimated by the quadriceps, or Q, angle, which is defined as the angle formed by the intersection of a line extending from the anterior superior iliac spine to the center of the patella with a line extending from the center of the patella to the tibial tuberosity (Fig. 14–24). The larger the Q angle, the greater the tendency of the patella to move laterally when the quadriceps muscle is contracted.

### Mechanism of Injury

Acute dislocation of the patella occurs most often in patients between 13 and 20 years of age.[26] This injury is seen more commonly in females according to most reported series.[59, 102] The usual mechanism of injury is a twisting force applied to a flexed knee with the femur rotating internally while the foot is planted. Less commonly, the injury is caused by a direct blow to the medial edge of the patella. Most patellar dislocations are associated with falls or participation in a variety of sports activities.

### Classification

Almost all patellar dislocations are lateral (Fig. 14–25). An intra-articular patellar dislocation may occur, but it is extremely rare. Recurrent dislocations may follow an earlier dislocation. Cash and Hughston[26] found that in patients who had a patellar dislocation between 11 and 14 years of age, recurrent dislocation developed in 60%.

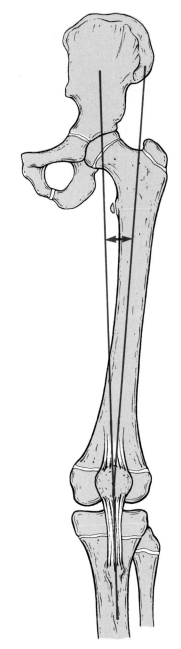

**FIGURE 14–24.** The Q angle. The quadriceps mechanism has a normal valgus alignment. This angle is measured by drawing a line from the anterior superior iliac spine to the center of the patella. The angle that this line makes with a line drawn along the center of the longitudinal axis of the patella and then from the center of the patella to the center of the tibial tubercle is called the Q angle.

The incidence of recurrent dislocation dropped to 33% in patients who had a patellar dislocation between 15 and 18 years of age. These authors also found that the incidence of recurrent dislocation was greater in patients who demonstrated a predisposition for dislocation as determined by evaluation of the unaffected knee. Predisposing signs included passive lateral hypermobility of the patella, a dysplastic distal third of the vastus medialis obliquus muscle, and a high or lateral position of the patella.

## Diagnosis

An acute dislocation of the patella will often reduce spontaneously before the patient is evaluated in the emergency department. Therefore, this diagnosis should be considered in any child or adolescent who presents with an acutely painful and swollen knee.[75]

A patient with acute dislocation of the patella may give a history of a twisting injury on a flexed knee. A painful "snap" is heard or felt. A sensation of "giving way" or that the knee "went out of joint" may also be described.

On physical examination, the child generally has diffuse tenderness in the parapatellar region. Pain and apprehension may be elicited with any attempt to laterally displace the patella. A defect in the medial patellar retinaculum may be palpated if the patient is examined before significant knee effusion has formed. On occasion, a defect may be palpated in the region of attachment of the vastus medialis obliquus to the patella if this muscle has been avulsed.

When hemarthrosis is present, the possibility of an osteochondral fracture should be considered. If the history or clinical findings suggest patellar dislocation, the knee joint may be aspirated under sterile conditions to relieve the hemarthrosis. The presence of fat globules within a bloody aspirate is presumptive evidence of an osteochondral fracture somewhere in the knee.[103] These fractures usually originate from the medial facet of the patella or from the lateral femoral condyle and have been described in an earlier section (see Osteochondral Fractures).

Anteroposterior and lateral views of the knee, as well as tunnel and patellar skyline views, should be taken to determine the presence of an osteochondral fracture. Radiographs may fail to demonstrate these lesions, especially if the ossified portion of the fragment is small.[114, 115, 124] Because of the difficulty in detecting osteochondral fractures on plain radiographs, diagnostic arthroscopy has been recommended in most cases of acute hemarthrosis of the knee in children and teenagers.[37, 81, 114, 115, 118, 124]

## Management

Because most patellar dislocations reduce spontaneously, reduction in the emergency department is rarely necessary. If the patella has not reduced, reduction is obtained by manipulation. Under appropriate sedation with the hip flexed to relax the quadriceps femoris muscle, reduction is achieved by slowly extending the knee while gently pushing the patella medially.

Surgery is rarely necessary for acute patellar dislocations in children.[26, 59] It may be needed to repair a completely avulsed vastus medialis obliquus insertion. If an osteochondral fracture has occurred, arthroscopy may be necessary to remove the fragment. If the fracture is large and involves the weight-bearing surface, open reduction and internal fixation may be indicated.

Once the presence of an osteochondral fracture has been ruled out, immobilization in a cylinder cast for approximately 4 weeks is recommended. When the cast is removed, the patient begins rehabilitative exercises with emphasis on strengthening the quadriceps muscles.

## Complications

The outcome after acute patellar dislocation is generally good. Cash and Hughston[26] noted a 75% rate of satisfactory results after nonoperative treatment in pa-

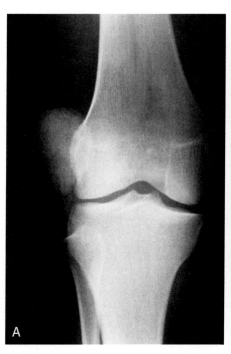
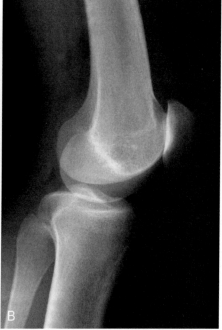

FIGURE 14–25. *A*, Anteroposterior radiograph of the knee of an adolescent girl who sustained a patellar dislocation. Note that the patella is laterally displaced. *B*, Lateral radiograph demonstrating that the patella overlies the distal femoral condyle, a finding indicative of patellar dislocation. (*A, B*, Courtesy of Dr. Neil E. Green.)

tients who showed no signs of a predisposition to subluxation or dislocation in the unaffected knee. In patients who showed evidence of a congenital abnormality of the extensor mechanism in the unaffected knee, the rate of satisfactory results after nonoperative treatment was only 52%.

Recurrent subluxation or dislocation of the patella is more common in patients whose first dislocation occurs in the early teenage years.[26, 59] Other predisposing factors to recurrent dislocation include passive lateral hypermobility of the patella, dysplasia or atrophy of the vastus medialis obliquus muscle, a high or lateral position of the patella, an increased Q angle, and radiographic evidence of dysplasia of the patella or lateral femoral condyle.

Imaging studies that may be used to detect patellar subluxation include plain radiography, computed tomography, and ultrasonography. The lateral radiograph reveals whether a high position of the patella, also referred to as patella alta, is present. A tangential view, also known as a sunrise view, taken with the knee in 30° of flexion can show lateral displacement or tilt of the patella. Stanciu and colleagues[113] found that a computed tomographic scan taken with the knee in 15° of flexion was more sensitive than standard radiographs for the detection of patellar subluxation. Ultrasonography has been used to evaluate patellar tracking and detect the presence of a proximally or laterally positioned patella.[80]

In patients who continue to have recurrent episodes of patellar subluxation despite aggressive physical therapy to strengthen the quadriceps muscle, one should consider surgical correction. The mainstay of surgical correction is release of the lateral retinaculum combined with imbrication of the medial retinaculum (Fig. 14–26A). If dysplasia of the vastus medialis obliquus muscle is present, it may be advanced at the time of the lateral retinacular release.

In patients with a significantly increased Q angle, distal realignment procedures may be indicated. In children with open physes, transfer of the tibial tubercle is contraindicated because of the possibility of causing a growth disturbance resulting in genu recurvatum. The Roux-Goldthwait procedure involves medial transfer of the lateral half of the patellar tendon (Fig. 14–26B and C). In this procedure, the lateral half of the divided patellar tendon is transposed medially, underneath the medial half of the patellar tendon, and sutured to the periosteum.

Transfer of the semitendinosus tendon may also be used in skeletally immature patients (Fig 14–26D). This procedure may be indicated in patients who have problems with continued instability after proximal realignment, or it may be combined with proximal realignment in children who have severe ligamentous laxity, such as in Down's syndrome. In this procedure, the semitendinosus tendon is detached from the muscle, with the distal attachment onto the tibia left intact. The tendon is then routed through a drill hole in the patella from the inferomedial to the superolateral margin and sutured back onto itself.

Postoperatively, these patients are maintained in a cylinder cast with the knee immobilized in extension for approximately 4 to 6 weeks. After that time, rehabilitative exercises are begun to strengthen the quadriceps muscle.

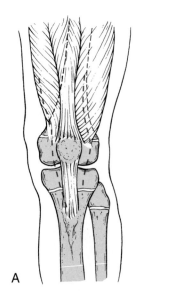
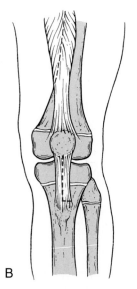
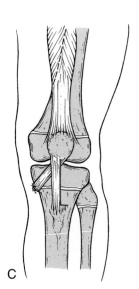
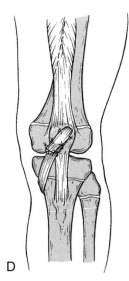

A          B          C          D

**FIGURE 14–26.** Surgical technique for the treatment of patellar subluxation or dislocation. *A,* Lateral retinacular release. The lateral retinaculum has been released well up into the vastus lateralis, and the vastus medialis plus the medial retinaculum has been plicated. *B,* Roux-Goldthwait reconstruction. A lateral retinacular release is performed, plus plication of the medial retinaculum and advancement of the medialis obliquus. In addition, the lateral half of the patellar ligament is split off from the medial half and detached from the tibial tubercle extraperiosteally. *C,* The lateral half is then transferred medially underneath the medial half of the patellar ligament and sutured to the periosteum of the proximal end of the tibia. *D,* Semitendinosus tenodesis. The semitendinosus has been released at its musculotendinous junction and pulled distally. It is passed through a drill hole in the patella and then sutured back onto itself.

# DISLOCATION OF THE KNEE

## Mechanism of Injury

Complete dislocation of the knee is rare in children. This injury is more commonly seen in older adolescents and adults because the forces needed to produce a dislocated knee are more likely to cause a fracture of the distal femoral or proximal tibial physis in a child. Complete dislocation of the knee is usually associated with violent accidents, such as a motor vehicle accident or a fall from a significant height.[39]

## Diagnosis

A patient with complete dislocation of the knee will generally have an obvious deformity. Arterial injury must be considered in every patient with this injury. Green and Allen[39] found that a popliteal artery injury was present in 32% of patients with acute dislocation of the knee. They also reported that vascular injury resulted in amputation if it was not repaired within 6 to 8 hours of injury.

A careful neurovascular examination must be performed to document the presence of the dorsalis pedis and posterior tibial pulses and the function of the posterior tibial and peroneal nerves. If clinical signs of ischemia are present, the knee dislocation is reduced as soon as possible and the vascular status of the limb is reassessed. If signs of ischemia are still present after the reduction maneuver, immediate vascular exploration is indicated. In the absence of an obviously ischemic limb, patients with abnormal pedal pulses or those who recover pulses after reduction of the knee should undergo arteriography.[57, 121] Ongoing evaluation of the lower extremity is important during the first few days after the dislocation so that a developing compartment syndrome or an intimal tear with thrombosis may be detected promptly.

Anteroposterior and lateral radiographs of the knee will confirm the direction of the dislocation. The films should be carefully examined for any occult fractures of the distal femoral physis, proximal tibial physis, or the tibial spines. Stress radiographs may be needed to help differentiate a physeal injury from a collateral ligament injury.

## Management

No series of knee dislocations in children are available on which to base recommendations for treatment. Older adolescents approaching skeletal maturity can be managed by repair or reconstruction of the ligaments as described in reports of knee dislocations in adults. The most important element of the initial management of a child with a dislocation of the knee is the early detection of injury to the popliteal artery.

## REFERENCES

1. Abrams, J.; Bennett, E.; Kumar, S.J.; Pizzutillo, P.D. Salter-Harris type III fracture of the proximal fibula: A case report. Am J Sports Med 14:514–516, 1986.
2. Ahstrom, J.P. Osteochondral fracture in the knee joint associated with hypermobility and dislocation of the patella: Report of eighteen cases. J Bone Joint Surg Am 47:1491–1502, 1965.
3. Aitken, A.P. Fractures of the proximal tibial epiphyseal cartilage. Clin Orthop 41:92–97, 1965.
4. Anderson, M.; Green, W.T.; Messner, M.B. Growth and predictions of growth in the lower extremities. J Bone Joint Surg Am 45:1–14, 1963.
5. Bachelin, P.; Bugmann, P. Active subluxation in extension; Radiological control in intercondylar eminence fractures in childhood. Z Kinderchir 43:180–182, 1988.
6. Balmant, P.; Vichard, P.; Pem, R. The treatment of avulsion fractures of the tibial tuberosity in adolescent athletes. Sports Med 9:311–316, 1990.
7. Balthazar, D.A.; Pappas, A.M. Acquired valgus deformity of the tibia in children. J Pediatr Orthop 4:538–541, 1984.
8. Barfod, G.; Svendsen, R.N. Synovitis of the knee after intraarticular fracture fixation with Biofix. Report of two cases. Acta Orthop Scand 63:680–681, 1992.
9. Bates, D.G.; Hresko, M.T.; Jaramillo, D. Patellar sleeve fracture: Demonstration with MR imaging. Radiology 193:825–827, 1994.
10. Baxter, M.P.; Wiley, J.J. Fractures of the tibial spine in children: An evaluation of knee stability. J Bone Joint Surg Br 70:228–230, 1988.
11. Beals, R.K.; Tufts, E. Fractured femur in infancy: The role of child abuse. J Pediatr Orthop 3:583–586, 1983.
12. Beaty, J.H.; Kumar, A. Fractures about the knee in children. J Bone Joint Surg Am 76:1870–1880, 1994.
13. Berg, E.E. Open reduction internal fixation of displaced transverse patella fractures with figure-eight wiring through parallel cannulated compression screws. J Orthop Trauma 11:573–576, 1997.
14. Bertin, K.C.; Goble, E.M. Ligament injuries associated with physeal fractures about the knee. Clin Orthop 177:188–195, 1983.
15. Blanks, R.H.; Lester, D.K.; Shaw, B.A. Flexion-type Salter II fracture of the proximal tibia. Proposed mechanism of injury and two case studies. Clin Orthop 301:256–259, 1994.
16. Bostman, O.; Kiviluoto, O.; Santavirta, S.; et al. Fractures of the patella treated by operation. Arch Orthop Trauma Surg 102:78–81, 1983.
17. Bowers, K.D. Patellar tendon avulsion as a complication of Osgood-Schlatter's disease. Am J Sports Med 9:356–359, 1981.
18. Bowler, J.R.; Mubarak, S.J.; Wenger, D.R. Tibial physeal closure and genu recurvatum after femoral fracture: Occurrence without a tibial traction pin. J Pediatr Orthop 10:653–657, 1990.
19. Brenkel, I.J.; Prosser, A.J.; Pearse, M. Salter type 2 fracture separation of the proximal epiphysis of the fibula. Injury 18:421–422, 1987.
20. Brone, L.A.; Wroble, R.R. Salter-Harris type III fracture of the medial femoral condyle associated with an anterior cruciate ligament tear: Report of three cases and review of the literature. Am J Sports Med 26:581–586, 1998.
21. Bruijn, J.D.; Sanders, R.J.; Jansen, B.R. Ossification in the patella tendon and patella alta following sports injuries in children. Arch Orthop Trauma Surg 112:157–158, 1993.
22. Buess-Watson, E.; Exner, G.U.; Illi, O.E. Fractures about the knee: Growth disturbances and problems of stability at long-term follow-up. Eur J Pediatr Surg 4:218–224, 1994.
23. Burkhart, S.S.; Peterson, H.A. Fractures of the proximal tibial epiphysis. J Bone Joint Surg Am 61:996–1002, 1979.
24. Carey, J.; Spence, L.; Blickman, H.; Eustace, S. MRI of pediatric growth plate injury: Correlation with plain film radiographs and clinical outcome. Skeletal Radiol 27:250–255, 1998.
25. Carpenter, J.E.; Kasman, R.A.; Patel, N.; et al. Biomechanical evaluation of current patella fracture fixation techniques. J Orthop Trauma 11:351–356, 1997.
26. Cash, J.D.; Hughston, J.C. Treatment of acute patellar dislocation. Am J Sports Med 16:244–249, 1988.

27. Chow, S.P.; Lam, J.J.; Leong, J.C. Fracture of the tibial tubercle in the adolescent. J Bone Joint Surg Br 72:231–234, 1990.

28. Christie, M.J.; Dvonch, V.M. Tibial tuberosity avulsion fracture in adolescents. J Pediatr Orthop 1:391–394, 1981.

29. Ciszewski, W.A.; Buschmann, W.R.; Rudolph, C.N. Irreducible fracture of the proximal tibial physis in an adolescent. Orthop Rev 18:891–893, 1989.

30. Dal Monte, A.; Manes, E.; Cammrota, V. Post-traumatic genu valgum in children. Ital J Orthop Traumatol 9:5–11, 1983.

31. Davies, A.M.; Carter, S.R.; Grimer, R.J.; Sneath, R.S. Fatigue fractures of the femoral diaphysis in the skeletally immature simulating malignancy. Br J Radiol 62:893–896, 1989.

32. Edmunds, I.; Nade, S. Injuries of the distal femoral growth plate and epiphysis: Should open reduction be performed? Aust N Z J Surg 63:195–199, 1993.

33. Fyfe, I.S.; Jackson, J.P. Tibial intercondylar fractures in children: A review of the classification and the treatment of malunion. Injury 13:165–169, 1981.

34. Gaudernak, T.; Zifko, B.; Skorpik, G. Osteochondral fractures of the knee and the ankle joint: Clinical experiences using fibrin sealant. Acta Orthop Belg 52:465–478, 1986.

35. Gautier, E.; Ziran, B.H.; Egger, B.; et al. Growth disturbances after injuries of the proximal tibial epiphysis. Arch Orthop Trauma Surg 118:37–41, 1998.

36. Gill, J.G.; Chakrabarti, H.P.; Becker, S.J. Fractures of the proximal tibial epiphysis. Injury 14:324–331, 1984.

37. Gilley, J.S.; Gelman, M.I.; Edson, D.M.; Metcalf, R.W. Chondral fractures of the knee: Arthrographic, arthroscopic and clinical manifestations. Radiology 138:51–54, 1981.

38. Graham, J.M.; Gross, R.H. Distal femoral physeal problem fractures. Clin Orthop 255:51–53, 1990.

39. Green, N.E.; Allen, B.L. Vascular injuries associated with dislocation of the knee. J Bone Joint Surg Am 59:236–239, 1977.

40. Green, W.T. Painful bipartite patellae: A report of three cases. Clin Orthop 110:197–200, 1975.

41. Griffin, P.P. Fractures of the femoral diaphysis in children. Orthop Clin North Am 7:633–638, 1976.

42. Groenkvist, H.; Hirsch, G.; Johansson, L. Fracture of the anterior tibial spine in children. J Pediatr Orthop 4:465–468, 1984.

43. Grogan, D.P.; Bobechko, W.P. Pathogenesis of a fracture of the distal femoral epiphysis. J Bone Joint Surg Am 66:621–622, 1984.

44. Grogan, D.P.; Carey, T.P.; Leffers, D.; Ogden, J.A. Avulsion fractures of the patella. J Pediatr Orthop 10:721–730, 1990.

45. Gross, R.H.; Davidson, R.S.; Sullivan, J.A.; et al. Cast brace management of femoral shaft fracture in children and adults. J Pediatr Orthop 3:572–582, 1983.

46. Hammerle, C.P.; Jacob, R.P. Chondral and osteochondral fractures after luxation of the patella and their treatment. Arch Orthop Trauma Surg 97:207–211, 1980.

47. Harper, M.C.; Ralston, M. Isobutyl 2-cyanoacrylate as an osseous adhesive in the repair of osteochondral fractures. J Biomed Mater Res 17:167–177, 1983.

48. Hensal, F.; Nelson, T.; Pavlov, H.; Torg, J.S. Bilateral patellar fractures from indirect trauma: A case report. Clin Orthop 178:207–209, 1983.

49. Hopkinson, W.J.; Mitchell, W.A.; Curl, W.W. Chondral fractures of the knee: Cause for confusion. Am J Sports Med 13:309–312, 1985.

50. Houghton, G.R.; Ackroyd, C.E. Sleeve fractures of the patella in children: A report of three cases. J Bone Joint Surg Br 61:165–168, 1979.

51. Hresko, M.T.; Kasser, J.R. Physeal arrest about the knee associated with non-physeal fractures in the lower extremity. J Bone Joint Surg Am 71:698–703, 1989.

52. Iwaya, T.; Takatori, Y. Lateral longitudinal stress fracture of the patella: Report of three cases. J Pediatr Orthop 5:73–75, 1985.

53. Janarv, P.M.; Westblad, P.; Johansson, C.; Hirsch, G. Long-term follow-up of anterior tibial spine fractures in children. J Pediatr Orthop 15:63–68, 1995.

54. Johnson, E.W.; McLeod, T.L. Osteochondral fragments of the distal end of the femur fixed with bone pegs. J Bone Joint Surg Am 59:677–678, 1977.

55. Kasser, J.R. Physeal bar resections after growth arrest about the knee. Clin Orthop 255:68–74, 1990.

56. Kendall, N.S.; Hsu, S.Y.; Chan, K.M. Fracture of the tibial spine in adults and children. A review of 31 cases. J Bone Joint Surg Br 74:848–852, 1992.

57. Kendall, R.W.; Taylor, D.C.; Salvian, A.J.; O'Brien, P.J. The role of arteriography in assessing vascular injuries associated with dislocations of the knee. J Trauma 35:875–878, 1993.

58. Kregor, P.J.; Song, K.M.; Routt, M.L.; et al. Plate fixation of femoral shaft fractures in multiply injured children. J Bone Joint Surg Am 75:1774–1780, 1993.

59. Larsen, E.; Lauridsen, F. Conservative treatment of patellar dislocations: Influence of evident factors on the tendency to redislocation and the therapeutic result. Clin Orthop 171:131–136, 1982.

60. Levi, J.H.; Coleman, C.R. Fracture of the tibial tubercle. Am J Sports Med 4:254–263, 1976.

61. Lewis, P.L.; Foster, B.K. Herbert screw fixation of osteochondral fractures about the knee. Aust N Z J Surg 60:511–513, 1990.

62. Linden, M.A.; Manton, W.I.; Stewart, R.M.; et al. Lead poisoning from retained bullets: Pathogenesis, diagnosis, management. Ann Surg 195:305–313, 1982.

63. Lipscomb, A.B.; Anderson, A.F. Open reduction of a malunited tibial spine fracture in a 12-year-old male. Am J Sports Med 13:419–422, 1985.

64. Lombardo, S.J.; Harvey, J.P. Fractures of the distal femoral epiphysis. J Bone Joint Surg Am 59:742–751, 1977.

65. Maguire, J.K.; Canale, S.T. Fractures of the patella in children and adolescents. J Pediatr Orthop 13:567–571, 1993.

66. Mah, J.Y.; Adili, A.; Otsuka, N.Y.; Ogilvie, R. Follow-up study of arthroscopic reduction and fixation of type III tibial-eminence fractures. J Pediatr Orthop 18:475–477, 1998.

67. Makhdoomi, K.R.; Doyle, J.; Maloney, M. Transverse fracture of the patella in children. Arch Orthop Trauma Surg 112:302–303, 1993.

68. Matsusue, Y.; Nakamura, T.; Suzuki, S.; Iwaski, R. Biodegradable pin fixation of osteochondral fragments of the knee. Clin Orthop 322:166–173, 1996.

69. Mayer, G.; Seidlein, H. Chondral and osteochondral fractures of the knee joint—treatment and results. Arch Orthop Trauma Surg 107:154–157, 1988.

70. McCarthy, J.J.; Kim, D.H.; Eilert, R.E. Posttraumatic genu valgum: Operative versus nonoperative treatment. J Pediatr Orthop 18:518–521, 1998.

71. McCollough, N.C.; Vinsant, J.E.; Sarmiento, A. Functional fracture-bracing of long-bone fractures of the lower extremity in children. J Bone Joint Surg Am 60:314–319, 1978.

72. Medler, R.G.; Jasson, K.A. Arthroscopic treatment of fractures of the tibial spine. Arthroscopy 10:292–295, 1994.

73. Meyers, M.H.; McKeever, F.M. Fracture of the intercondylar eminence of the tibia. J Bone Joint Surg Am 41:209–222, 1959.

74. Meyers, M.H.; McKeever, F.M. Fracture of the intercondylar eminence of the tibia. J Bone Joint Surg Am 52:1677–1684, 1970.

75. Micheli, L.J.; Foster, T.E. Acute knee injuries in the immature athlete. Instr Course Lect 42:473–481, 1993.

76. Mink, J.H.; Deutsch, A.L. Occult cartilage and bone injuries of the knee: Detection, classification, and assessment with MR imaging. Radiology 170:823–829, 1989.

77. Mirbey, J.; Besancenot, J.; Chambers, R.T.; et al. Avulsion fractures of the tibial tuberosity in the adolescent athlete: Risk factors, mechanism of injury, and treatment. Am J Sports Med 16:336–340, 1988.

78. Naranja, R.J.; Gregg, J.R.; Dormans, J.P.; et al. Pediatric fracture without radiographic abnormality: Description and significance. Clin Orthop 342:141–146, 1997.

79. Nichols, J.N.; Tehranzadeh, J. A review of tibial spine fractures in bicycle injury. Am J Sports Med 15:172–174, 1987.

80. Nietosvaara, A.Y.; Aalto, K.A. Ultrasonographic evaluation of patellar tracking in children. Clin Orthop 297:62–64, 1993.

81. Nietosvaara, Y.; Aalto, K.; Kallio, P.E. Acute patellar dislocation in children: Incidence and associated osteochondral fractures. J Pediatr Orthop 14:513–515, 1994.

82. Ogden, J. Tibia and fibula. In: Skeletal Injury in the Child. Philadelphia, Lea & Febiger, 1990, pp. 787–863.

83. Ogden, J.A. Radiology of postnatal skeletal development. X. Patella and tibial tuberosity. Skeletal Radiol 11:246–257, 1984.

84. Ogden, J.A.; McCarthy, S.M.; Jokl, P. The painful bipartite patella. J Pediatr Orthop 2:263–269, 1982.
85. Ogden, J.A.; Ogden, D.A.; Pugh, L.; et al. Tibia valga after proximal metaphyseal fractures in childhood: A normal biologic response. J Pediatr Orthop 15:489–494, 1995.
86. Ogden, J.A.; Tross, R.B.; Murphy, M.J. Fractures of the tibial tuberosity in adolescents. J Bone Joint Surg Am 62:205–215, 1980.
87. Olerud, C.; Danckwardt-Lilliestrom, G.; Olerud, S. Genu recurvatum caused by partial growth arrest of the proximal tibial physis: Simultaneous correction and lengthening with physeal distraction. Arch Orthop Trauma Surg 106:64–68, 1986.
88. Pape, J.M.; Goulet, J.A.; Hensinger, R.N. Compartment syndrome complicating tibial tubercle avulsion. Clin Orthop 295:201–204, 1993.
89. Pappas, A.M.; Anas, P.; Toczylowski, H.M. Asymmetrical arrest of the proximal tibial physis and genu recurvatum deformity. J Bone Joint Surg Am 66:575–581, 1984.
90. Patzakis, M.J.; Dorr, L.D.; Ivler, D.; et al. The early management of open joint injuries. J Bone Joint Surg Am 57:1065–1071, 1975.
91. Pennig, D.; Baranowski, D. Genu recurvatum due to partial growth arrest of the proximal tibial physis: Correction by callus distraction. Arch Orthop Trauma Surg 108:119–121, 1989.
92. Peterson, C.A.; Peterson, H.A. Analysis of the incidence of injuries to the epiphyseal growth plate. J Trauma 12:275–281, 1972.
93. Peterson, H.A. Partial growth plate arrest and its treatment. J Pediatr Orthop 4:246–258, 1984.
94. Poulsen, T.D.; Skak, S.V.; Toftgarrd Jensen, T. Epiphyseal fractures of the proximal tibia. Injury 20:111–113, 1989.
95. Pritchett, J.W. Longitudinal growth and growth-plate activity in the lower extremity. Clin Orthop 275:274–279, 1992.
96. Rae, P.S.; Khasawneh, Z.M. Herbert screw fixation of osteochondral fractures of the patella. Injury 19:116–119, 1988.
97. Rang, M. Children's Fractures. Philadelphia, J.B. Lippincott, 1983, pp. 297–307.
98. Ray, J.M.; Hendrix, J. Incidence, mechanism of injury and treatment of fractures of the patella in children. J Trauma 32:464–467, 1992.
99. Riseborough, E.J.; Barrett, I.R.; Shapiro, F. Growth disturbances following distal femoral physeal fracture-separations. J Bone Joint Surg Am 65:885–893, 1983.
100. Roberts, J.M. Operative treatment of fractures about the knee. Orthop Clin North Am 21:365–379, 1990.
101. Robinson, S.C.; Driscoll, S.E. Simultaneous osteochondral avulsion of the femoral and tibial insertions of the anterior cruciate ligament. J Bone Joint Surg Am 63:1342–1343, 1981.
102. Rorabeck, C.H.; Bobechko, W.P. Acute dislocation of the patella with osteochondral fracture: A review of eighteen cases. J Bone Joint Surg Br 58:237–240, 1976.
103. Rosenberg, N.J. Osteochondral fractures of the lateral femoral condyle. J Bone Joint Surg Am 46:1013–1026, 1964.
104. Rosenberg, Z.S.; Kawerblum, M.; Cheung, Y.Y. Osgood-Schlatter lesion: Fracture or tendinitis? Scintigraphic, CT, and MR imaging features. Radiology 185:853–858, 1992.
105. Ross, A.C.; Chesterman, P.J. Isolated avulsion of the tibial attachment of the posterior cruciate ligament in childhood. J Bone Joint Surg Br 68:747, 1986.
106. Ryu, R.K.N.; Debenham, J.O. An unusual avulsion fracture of the proximal tibial epiphysis. Case report and proposed addition to the Watson-Jones classification. Clin Orthop 194:181–184, 1985.
107. Salter, R.B.; Harris, R. Injuries involving the epiphyseal plate. J Bone Joint Surg Am 45:587–622, 1963.
108. Shands, P.A.; McQueen, D.A. Demonstration of avulsion fracture of the inferior pole of the patella by magnetic resonance imaging: A case report. J Bone Joint Surg Am 77:1721–1723, 1995.
109. Shelton, W.R.; Canale, S.T. Fractures of the tibia through the proximal tibial epiphyseal cartilage. J Bone Joint Surg Am 61:167–173, 1979.
110. Skak, S.V. Valgus deformity following proximal tibial metaphyseal fracture in children. Acta Orthop Scand 53:141–147, 1982.
111. Smith, J.B. Knee instability after fractures of the intercondylar eminence of the tibia. J Pediatr Orthop 4:462–464, 1984.
112. Staheli, L.T. Fractures of the shaft of the femur. In: Rockwood, C.A.; Wilkins, K.E.; King, R E., eds. Fractures in Children. Philadelphia, J.B. Lippincott, 1991, pp. 1121–1163.
113. Stanciu, C.; Labelle, H.B.; Morin, B.; et al. The value of computed tomography for the diagnosis of recurrent patellar subluxation in adolescents. Can J Surg 37:319–323, 1994.
114. Stanitski, C.L. Articular hypermobility and chondral injury in patients with acute patella dislocation. Am J Sports Med 23:146–150, 1995.
115. Stanitski, C.L.; Paletta, G.A. Articular cartilage injury with acute patellar dislocation in adolescents: Arthroscopic and radiographic correlation. Am J Sports Med 26:52–55, 1998.
116. Stephens, D.C.; Louis, E.; Louis, D.S. Traumatic separation of the distal femoral epiphyseal plate. J Bone Joint Surg Am 56:1383–1390, 1974.
117. Sullivan, A.J. Ligamentous injuries of the knee in children. Clin Orthop 255:44–50, 1990.
118. Ten Thue, J.H.; Frima, A.J. Patellar dislocation and osteochondral fractures. Neth J Surg 35(5):150–154, 1986.
119. Thomson, J.D.; Stricker, S.J.; Williams, M.M. Fractures of the distal femoral epiphyseal plate. J Pediatr Orthop 15:474–478, 1995.
120. Tolo, V.T. External fixation in multiply injured children. Orthop Clin North Am 21:393–400, 1990.
121. Treiman, G.S.; Yellin, A.E.; Weaver, F.A.; et al. Examination of the patient with a knee dislocation: The case for selective arteriography. Arch Surg 127:1056–1063, 1992.
122. Tuten, H.R.; Keeler, K.A.; Gabos, P.G.; et al. Posttraumatic tibia valga in children: A long-term follow-up note. J Bone Joint Surg Am 81:799–810, 1999.
123. Ure, B.M.; Tiling, T.; Roddecker, K. Arthroscopy of the knee in children and adolescents. Eur J Pediatr Surg 2:102–105, 1992.
124. Vaheasarja, V.; Kinnuen, P.; Serlo, W. Arthroscopy of the acute traumatic knee in children. Acta Orthop Scand 64:580–582, 1993.
125. Voit, G.A.; Irvine, G.; Beals, R.K. Saline load test for penetration of periarticular lacerations. J Bone Joint Surg Br 75:732–733, 1996.
126. Wall, J.J. Compartment syndrome as a complication of the Hauser procedure. J Bone Joint Surg Am 61:185–191, 1979.
127. Weber, B.G. Fibrous interposition causing valgus deformity after fracture of the upper tibial metaphysis in children. J Bone Joint Surg Br 59:290–292, 1977.
128. Weber, M.J.; Janecki, C.J.; McLeod, P.; et al. Efficacy of various forms of fixation of transverse fractures of the patella. J Bone Joint Surg Am 62:215–220, 1980.
129. Wiley, J.J.; Baxter, M.P. Tibial spine fractures in children. Clin Orthop 255:54–60, 1990.
130. Willis, R.B.; Blokker, C.; Stoll, T.M.; et al. Long-term follow-up of anterior tibial eminence fractures. J Pediatr Orthop 13:361–364, 1993.
131. Wiss, D.A.; Schilz, J.L.; Zionts, L. Type III fractures of the tibial tubercle in adolescents. J Orthop Trauma 5:475–479, 1991.
132. Wozasek, G.E.; Moser, K.D.; Haller, H.; Capousek, M. Trauma involving the proximal tibial epiphysis. Arch Orthop Trauma Surg 110:301–306, 1991.
133. Wu, C.D.; Huang, S.C.; Liu, T.K. Sleeve fractures of the patella in children. A report of five cases. Am J Sports Med 19:525–528, 1991.
134. Zaricznyj, B. Avulsion fracture of the tibial eminence: Treatment by open reduction and pinning. J Bone Joint Surg Am 59:1111–1114, 1977.
135. Zionts, L.E.; Harcke, H.T.; Brooks, K.M.; MacEwen, G.D. Posttraumatic tibia valga: A case demonstrating asymmetric activity at the proximal growth plate on technetium bone scan. J Pediatr Orthop 7:458–462, 1987.
136. Zionts, L.E.; MacEwen, G.D. Spontaneous improvement of post-traumatic tibia valga. J Bone Joint Surg Am 68:680–687, 1986.

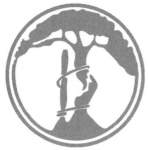

# CHAPTER 15

# Fractures of the Tibia and Fibula

George H. Thompson, M.D.
Fred F. Behrens, M.D.

Nonphyseal fractures of the tibia and fibula are among the most common injuries involving the lower extremities in children and adolescents.[41, 130, 191, 222, 232] The fracture patterns, mechanisms of injury, and anatomic locations of these fractures vary according to the age of the child. Most can be treated nonoperatively with satisfactory long-term results and minimal complications. However, certain tibia fractures pose unique problems that must be carefully evaluated and treated to avoid complications.

## PATHOLOGY

**Relevant Anatomy.** The shafts of the tibia and fibula each consist of a proximal metaphysis, central diaphysis, and distal metaphysis. This chapter is not concerned with fractures involving the proximal or distal epiphyses and their physes, which are discussed elsewhere (see Chapter 2). The blood supply to the tibia consists of (1) a nutrient artery, which is a branch of the posterior tibial artery that enters at the junction of the distal and middle thirds of the tibia and is responsible for the endosteal or medullary blood supply; (2) periosteal vessels, which are segmented and enter from surrounding tissues; and (3) epiphyseal vessels. The inner two thirds of the cortex is supplied by the endosteal vessels, and the outer third is supplied by the periosteal vessels. Proximally, the epiphyseal and periosteal vessels are branches of the medial and lateral inferior geniculate arteries from the popliteal artery. The collateral circulation is rich proximally, especially on the medial aspect.[182] Tibia fractures distal to the nutrient artery may deprive the distal fragment of its medullary blood supply, and in such cases, the distal end of the tibia must rely on its periosteal and metaphyseal blood supply for healing. This supply is limited because of a lack of muscle attachment, and a slower rate of healing generally results. Periosteal and soft tissue stripping of the distal fracture from the injury or

surgical intervention will further slow the healing process.

The blood supply to the fibula is from the peroneal artery, which gives off a nutrient artery that enters the diaphysis just proximal to its midpoint. The rest of the artery supplies multiple segmental musculoperiosteal vessels that pass circumferentially around the fibula and supply both the fibula and the adjacent muscles.

From a surgical perspective, it must be remembered that the popliteal artery descends between the posterior aspects of the medial and lateral femoral condyles. It passes between the medial and lateral heads of the gastrocnemius muscle and along the distal border of the popliteus muscle before dividing into the anterior and posterior tibial arteries. The anterior tibial artery passes anteriorly between the two heads of the tibialis posterior muscle and enters the anterior compartment of the leg by passing through the proximal aspect of the interosseous membrane at the flare of the proximal tibial and fibular metaphyses.[182] Displaced fractures in this region may damage the anterior tibial artery.[46, 76, 201] Fortunately, such fractures rarely occur. The foramen in the interosseous membrane is long and narrow; it affords some protection inasmuch as the anterior tibial artery is allowed to move both proximally and distally. Corrective varus or valgus osteotomies of the proximal portion of the tibia can also damage the anterior tibial artery.[231] Subperiosteal dissection in the region below the tibial tubercle allows protection of this vessel.

**Fracture Patterns.** Nonphyseal fracture patterns involving the tibia and fibula include compression (torus), incomplete tension-compression (greenstick), and complete fractures. Plastic deformities can also occur but predominantly involve the fibula.[139, 155, 238] Complete fractures can be further classified according to the direction of the fracture (spiral, oblique, or transverse) and as comminuted or segmental. Tibia and fibula fractures may also be open or closed, depending on the integrity of the overlying skin and soft tissues.

472

**Prevalence.** Fractures of the tibial and fibular shafts are the most common long bone fractures of the lower extremity[130, 191, 222, 232] and represent approximately 15% of all pediatric fractures[41, 232]; they occur more frequently in boys than girls. Parrini and co-workers[191] reported on 1027 long bone fractures in children between 1 and 11 years of age, including 326 tibia fractures (32%). One hundred fifty-seven isolated fractures of the tibia and 169 fractures of both the tibia and fibula were noted, as well as 151 femur fractures. The remaining fractures involved the upper extremity. In a more recent study, Cheng and Shen[41] studied 3350 children with 3413 limb fractures in Hong Kong and also found tibial shaft fractures to be the most common lower extremity fracture, with a relatively static prevalence of 9% to 12% throughout various pediatric age groups. Only fractures of the upper extremity, including the distal ends of the radius and humerus (supracondylar) and the forearm, were more common overall.

An epidemiologic study by Karrholm and associates[130] in Lund, Sweden, in 1981 showed an annual incidence of 190 tibia fractures per 10,000 boys between infancy and 18 years of age and 110 tibia fractures per 10,000 girls in the same age range. In boys, the incidence peaked between 3 and 4 years of age and again between 15 and 16 years of age. The first peak involved predominantly spiral or oblique fractures, and the second peak involved primarily transverse fractures. In girls, the incidence was relatively even up to 11 to 12 years of age, with a tendency toward a declining incidence with advancing age.

**Mechanisms of Injury.** Fractures of the tibia and fibula may be the result of direct as well as indirect forces. Direct trauma frequently produces a transverse fracture or segmental fracture pattern, whereas indirect forces are typically rotational and produce an oblique or spiral fracture.

Steinert and Bennek[232] in 1966 analyzed 263 tibia fractures in children and found that falls were the most common mechanism of injury. Falls accounted for 45% of the fractures, and approximately half of them involved falls from a height. Motor vehicle accidents were the most common cause of complete fractures, which occurred in 43% of cases. Drewes and Schulte[64] analyzed 212 fractures in children younger than 14 years. The frequency and mechanism of injury varied according to the age of the child. In 51 children younger than 4 years, 17 fractures (35%) were caused by bicycle spoke accidents. In 160 children between 4 and 14 years of age, sports and motor vehicle accidents were the major mechanisms of injury.

In the study by Karrholm and associates,[130] motor vehicle accidents involving children as passengers, as bicycle riders, or as pedestrians were the most common mechanism of tibia fractures. The age range of children in motor vehicle accidents was 8 to 14 years. It was interesting that winter sports activities had almost the same incidence as motor vehicle accidents in girls. Similar results regarding winter sports were reported in England, where the risk for tibia fracture in children involved in skiing accidents was 10 times higher than that for adults.[103] Falls were the most common mechanism of injury in young children.

In a 1988 study by Shannak[222] of 142 tibial shaft fractures, motor vehicle accidents caused 63% of the fractures; falls, 18%; direct violence, 15%; and sports, only 4%. Cheng and Shen[41] did not analyze the mechanisms of injury in their study.

**Consequences of Injury.** Despite the frequency of pediatric tibia and fibula fractures, the consequences for most children are minimal. These fractures heal readily with minimal complications. Children typically have a rapid return to normal activities, including sports, and minimal disability. However, in a small percentage of cases, especially those involving open fractures or severe soft tissue injury, residual disability may occur.

**Associated Injuries.** It is not uncommon for children who sustain tibia and fibula fractures to have associated injuries, especially children who are victims of high-energy trauma, such as motor vehicle–related accidents. In the study by Karrholm and associates,[130] 27 of 480 children (6%) with tibia and fibula fractures sustained associated injuries, the most common being head injuries, fracture of the femur, and injury to an upper extremity. Other body areas (face and neck, chest, and abdomen) may also be injured, depending on the severity of the trauma. Children with open tibia fractures have the highest incidence of associated injuries[39, 49, 106, 115, 140, 266] (see later in this chapter).

**Classification.** A classification of nonphyseal fractures of the tibia and fibula is presented in Table 15–1. A modification of the classification of Dias,[60] this classification divides the tibial and fibular shafts into their three major anatomic areas: proximal metaphysis, diaphyses, and distal metaphysis. Fractures of the tibial and fibular diaphyses are subdivided according to the location (proximal third, middle third, and distal third) and the combination of bones fractured. Each of these subgroups may be further divided according to the fracture pattern: compression (torus), incomplete tension-compression (greenstick), or complete. This classification is useful for determining treatment methods and understanding the potential long-term results and possible complications.

## DIAGNOSIS

**History.** The typical symptom of a tibia or fibula fracture is pain. However, the severity of the pain varies

---

**TABLE 15–1** . . . . . . . . . . . . . . . . . . . . . . . . . . . . . .

Classification of Tibia and Fibula Fractures

. . . . . . . . . . . . . . . . . . . . . . . . . . . . . . . . . . . . . . . . . . .

Fractures of the proximal tibial metaphysis
Fractures of the tibial and fibular shafts
Isolated fractures of the tibial shaft
Isolated fractures of the fibular shaft
Fractures of the distal tibial metaphysis

. . . . . . . . . . . . . . . . . . . . . . . . . . . . . . . . . . . . . . . . . . .

Adapted from Dias, L.S. Fractures of the tibia and fibula. In: Rockwood, C.A., Jr.; Wilkens, K.E.; King, R.E., eds. Fractures in Children. Philadelphia, J.B. Lippincott, 1984, pp. 983–1041.

with the magnitude of injury, the mechanism, and the age of the child. Frequently, a history is unavailable because the injury was not observed and the child is unable to verbalize symptoms or the mechanism of injury. In these cases, child abuse or battered child syndrome must also be considered[187] (see Chapter 17). In young children, an inability to walk may be the only sign or symptom. If the child is able to speak, it is important to ascertain the mechanism of injury, if possible.

**Physical Examination.** Because pain is the major symptom in a tibial or fibular shaft fracture, it is important to have the child point to the most painful area. Palpation in this area may reproduce or increase the child's discomfort. Deformity is not a common finding in young children because many tibia fractures are nondisplaced. Swelling or edema of the lower part of the leg also varies according to the mechanism of injury, the extent of soft tissue injury, and the presence of displacement. Usually, the soft tissue swelling is maximal at the fracture site. Stress examination may reveal instability or crepitation but invariably increases pain. A stress examination is usually unnecessary when a fracture is suspected. Injured extremities with a suspected tibia fracture are best splinted before radiographic evaluation, usually with a long leg posterior plaster splint, which relieves pain, prevents additional injury to the soft tissues, and allows more accurate positioning of the extremity for radiographs.

Nerve damage in association with closed tibia and fibula fractures is very uncommon (see under Neurologic Injury). However, in all fractures it is important to check dorsiflexion and plantar flexion of the foot and toes, as well as sensation, especially to touch. Nerve damage, if present, is most likely the result of a direct injury to the peroneal nerve at the proximal fibular metaphysis.

Arterial injuries associated with a closed tibial shaft fracture are also very uncommon (see under Vascular Injury). The peripheral pulses of the dorsalis pedis and posterior tibial arteries must be evaluated and recorded at the initial physical examination. Unfortunately, the presence of pulses does not completely eliminate the possibility of an associated arterial injury (see under Vascular Injury). Arterial injuries are most likely to be associated with a displaced proximal tibial metaphyseal fracture or an open fracture. Capillary circulation, sensation to the toes, pain on passive stretch, and pain out of proportion to the injury must be monitored carefully because compartment syndromes can occur in children after tibia fractures (see under Compartment Syndrome).

The soft tissues of the lower part of the leg must also be evaluated. It is important to assess the integrity of the skin at the fracture site. Fractures in association with bicycle spoke injuries may ultimately result in full-thickness skin loss requiring delayed skin grafting. Any evidence of skin penetration at the fracture site is an indication that the fracture is open and contaminated (see under Open Tibia and Fibula Fractures).

**Radiographic Evaluation.** When a tibial or fibular shaft fracture is suspected, radiographs must be taken. After splinting of the injured extremity, anteroposterior (AP) and lateral radiographs are obtained. They must include the knee and ankle joints to rule out an associated epiphyseal fracture. Comparison radiographs may be indicated in complicated injuries, but this situation is unusual. Occasionally, incomplete fractures, such as a torus fracture, may be difficult to visualize. A spiral fracture of the tibial shaft with an intact fibula may be visible on only one view. It is therefore imperative that orthogonal radiographs always be obtained. Oblique radiographs may be beneficial if the initial radiographic appearance is normal but a fracture is suspected.

**Special Diagnostic Studies.** Special diagnostic imaging studies of the tibia and fibula may include technetium bone scans, computed tomography (CT), and magnetic resonance imaging (MRI).

Technetium bone scans may be useful in identifying occult fractures, especially in infants.[160, 190] Park and colleagues[190] found that bone scans could be used to differentiate occult fractures of the femur or tibia from early acute osteomyelitis in infants. Images obtained early (1 to 4 days after the onset of symptoms) demonstrated a subtle increase in uptake along the entire length of the injured bone when an occult fracture was present. The distribution of uptake was similar regardless of the fracture pattern. In early acute osteomyelitis, focal uptake was observed at the site of infection.

A CT scan of the tibia can be used to assess torsional alignment after complex unilateral fractures.[119] It can also be used in the assessment of pathologic fractures of the tibia to determine the presence, size, and intralesional contours of the lesion.[126]

MRI has been demonstrated to detect early stress fractures accurately. This procedure, though expensive, avoids the high doses of radiation incurred with bone scans and CT.

## MANAGEMENT

### Fractures of the Proximal Tibial Metaphysis

Proximal tibial metaphyseal fractures are relatively uncommon injuries that generally occur in children between 3 and 6 years of age (range, 1 to 12 years).[1, 52, 114, 125, 182, 184, 208, 216, 225] The male-to-female ratio of approximately 3:1 closely parallels the incidence of tibia fractures by gender in children. Skak and co-workers[225] in 1987 reported an incidence of approximately 6 proximal tibial metaphyseal fractures per 100,000 children per year. These fractures are typically the result of a direct injury to the lateral aspect of the extended knee. The fracture patterns are the same as for other tibia fractures—compression (torus), incomplete tension-compression (greenstick), and complete. Most of these fractures have minimal or no displacement and appear benign radiographically, but they may, in fact, be followed by a post-traumatic valgus deformity. Greenstick and complete fractures are most commonly associated with a valgus deformity,[204, 225] but such deformities are unusual after a torus fracture. In a greenstick fracture, the medial cortex (tension side) fractures while the lateral cortex (compression side) remains intact or hinges slightly. If the lateral cortex hinges, a valgus deformity occurs. However, displacement is not usually seen, and apposition remains normal. The fibula is typically intact but may occasionally sustain either a fracture or plastic deformation. Radiographically, the degree of angulation can be difficult to ascertain unless radiographs are obtained of both lower extremities symmetrically positioned on a long cassette and the true angulation measured. Oblique views and occasionally fluoroscopy may be beneficial in defining the fracture and any angulation.

The most important, as well as the most common, sequela of a fracture of the proximal tibial metaphysis is the development of a transient, progressive valgus deformity and overgrowth of the tibia. Cozen[47] in 1953 reported four cases of valgus deformity after nondisplaced or minimally angulated fractures of the proximal tibial metaphysis. Since then, numerous other reports have been published regarding this complication.* Interestingly, similar valgus deformities have been reported in association with other conditions affecting the proximal metaphysis of the pediatric tibia, including acute and chronic osteomyelitis,[10, 237] harvesting of a bone graft,[133] excision of an osteochondroma,[184, 251] and osteotomy.[237]

The incidence of valgus deformity after proximal tibial metaphyseal fractures is variable. Salter and Best[216] reported 21 cases of proximal tibial metaphyseal fracture in which 13 (62%) showed a valgus deformity between 11° and 22° at the time of cast removal. At follow-up, this angle had increased to 18° to 25°. Ten of their patients required surgical correction of the valgus deformity. Robert and associates[204] studied 25 patients with fractures of the proximal tibial metaphysis, in 12 (48%) of whom a genu valgum deformity later developed. In a review of 40 consecutive patients by Skak and co-workers,[225] valgus deformities developed in 4 (10%). These deformities occurred only after greenstick fractures. Boyer and colleagues[34] reported no valgus deformities in seven children aged 2 to 5 years who sustained fractures while jumping on trampolines with heavier children or adults.

Theories regarding the etiology of valgus deformity have included injury to the lateral aspect of the proximal tibial physis, inadequate reduction, premature weight bearing, hypertrophic callus formation, dynamic muscle action, soft tissue interposition, tethering from an intact fibula, and asymmetric growth stimulation. Blount[28] initially thought that the lateral aspect of the proximal tibial physis was damaged by the original injury. Goff[80] and Ben-Itzhak and associates[21] supported this concept, but it has not been substantiated in subsequent reports.

Best[23] and Salter and Best[216] believed that inadequate reduction of the fracture was the major cause of the initial valgus deformity. Others concurred.[9, 201] Pollen[196] believed that early weight bearing in a cast contributed to

the valgus angulation as a result of asymmetric compression in the preexisting valgus position. However, the valgus deformity has also occurred in nonambulatory children with myelodysplasia who sustained nondisplaced bilateral proximal tibial metaphyseal fractures.[127] One of the major reasons for the difficulty in obtaining anatomic reduction has been the interposition of soft tissues such as periosteum, pes anserinus, or the medial collateral ligament in the medial fracture gap. Weber[258] explored four acute fractures of the proximal tibial metaphysis and found that the periosteum and the insertion of the pes anserinus were stripped from the medial surface of the tibia and were interposed into the fracture gap. When these soft tissues were removed from the fracture gap, anatomic alignment could be achieved. These fractures then healed uneventfully and without a subsequent valgus deformity. Visser and Veldhuizen[255] reported a similar case. Weber[258] believed that with soft tissue interposition, biomechanical equilibrium was lost between the medial and lateral soft tissues. Traction on the medial metaphyseal portion from the pes anserinus was lost, but traction on the lateral side remained intact, thereby producing a bending moment on the tibia that resulted in a progressive valgus deformity.

Bassey[14] repaired the pes anserinus at the time of corrective osteotomy for a recurrent valgus deformity after proximal tibial osteotomy. He claimed that loss of the pes anserinus medial tether led to medial overgrowth as a result of hemichondrodiastasis (physeal lengthening). The deformity did not recur. Similar observations were made by Potthoff.[197] Brougham and Nicol,[37] however, reported a case in which the pes anserinus was repaired in a 2-year-old child in whom an acquired valgus deformity nonetheless developed. Coates[43] also reported two cases in which the superficial portion of the medial collateral ligament was interposed in the fracture gap and prevented anatomic alignment. After removal, anatomic alignment was achieved and the fractures healed without valgus deformity. Others have theorized that an intact fibula tethers the tibia and, as mild overgrowth occurs, a progressive valgus deformity is produced.[47, 118, 139] However, valgus deformity has been reported after complete fractures of the proximal ends of the tibia and fibula.[10, 204]

Currently, most authors attribute valgus deformity to asymmetric growth of the proximal part of the tibia.† Cozen[47] and Jackson and Cozen[118] thought that hypertrophic callus formation resulted in asymmetric growth from the medial aspect of the proximal tibial epiphysis. Bahnson and Lovell[9] studied five children with unilateral genu valgum after a fracture of the proximal tibial metaphysis. A mean of 6.7° of valgus deformity was observed in the initial cast. The deformity increased during the next 12 to 14 months to 10.8° and then improved to a mean of 8.7° over the next 2 years. These investigators concluded that weight bearing caused compression forces laterally and distraction medially, with subsequent asymmetric growth. Houghton and

---

*See references 1, 9, 10, 14, 21, 23, 37, 43, 48, 51, 52, 80, 82, 101, 114, 118, 125, 127, 156, 157, 166, 184, 197, 204, 208, 209, 216, 225, 237, 249, 255, 258, 268, 269.

†See references 5, 9, 10, 47, 51, 97, 108, 109, 118, 127, 166, 182, 184, 249, 269.

associates,[108, 109] in experimental studies with immature rabbits, found that medial hemicircumferential division of the periosteum resulted in valgus overgrowth. They believed that if the medial periosteum is torn during a proximal tibial metaphyseal fracture, asymmetric overgrowth occurs and produces a valgus deformity. Balthazar and Pappas[10] studied nine patients with acquired valgus deformity of the tibia in childhood—seven secondary to acute fracture and two from osteomyelitis of the proximal end of the tibia. In the children with osteomyelitis, one had undergone surgical drainage through the medial metaphysis, and the other had a pathologic metaphyseal fracture. In all nine children, the valgus angulation was associated with longitudinal overgrowth of the tibia. These investigators believed that both the valgus deformity and the overgrowth were caused by asymmetric growth stimulation. The maximum deformity (17° to 30°) was attained approximately 18 months after injury. Green[82] demonstrated an asymmetric growth arrest line in the proximal end of the tibia 1 year after a nondisplaced metaphyseal fracture in association with a valgus deformity. This line indicated increased growth on the medial aspect of the physeal plate. Bohn and Durbin[29] observed asymmetric, proximal tibial growth arrest lines in three boys after ipsilateral fractures of the femoral shaft and proximal tibial metaphysis. Herring and Moseley[101] observed similar asymmetry in the proximal end of the tibia in a 2-year-old child after corrective osteotomy for an acquired valgus deformity. The deformity recurred after the osteotomy and then underwent spontaneous correction. Spontaneous correction with growth has subsequently been observed by other authors.[156, 166, 184, 249, 268]

Aronson and co-workers[5] in 1990 reported on an experimental model with immature rabbits that confirmed asymmetric growth as the cause of post-traumatic valgus deformity. Twenty-two 8-week-old rabbits were divided into two equal groups. In one group, the periosteum on the medial aspect of the proximal tibial metaphysis was excised and a partial osteotomy involving the medial half of the metaphysis was performed. In the other group, the same procedure was performed on the lateral side. Parallel K-wires were inserted above and below the partial osteotomy. A valgus deformity (mean of 12°) occurred in the first group, and a varus deformity (mean of 10°) developed in the second. In each animal, the K-wires remained parallel, thus indicating that the deformity occurred at the physis. Despite the asymmetric growth, the light microscopic appearance of the physes was normal. The deformities were therefore attributed to asymmetric physeal growth, which was not demonstrable histologically. Ogden[182] reported that the normal circulation to the knee has a more extensive medial geniculate blood supply, especially in the proximal tibial region, than a lateral geniculate supply, which may be responsible for transient eccentric growth. Jordan and associates[127] also concluded that asymmetric growth stimulation was secondary to an increased vascular response. Harcke and co-workers[97] and Zionts and colleagues[269] supported the concept of eccentric growth in quantitative scintigraphic studies by demonstrating proportionally greater uptake on the medial side than the lateral side

and overall increased uptake on the injured as compared with the uninjured side. In 1995, Ogden and colleagues[184] performed detailed measurements of the metaphyseal-diaphyseal-metaphyseal distances medially and laterally of the injured and noninjured tibias of 17 children with 19 proximal tibial metaphyseal fractures (2 children had bilateral fractures) monitored for a mean of 3.7 years (range, 2 to 7 years). The difference between the medial and lateral sides of the injured tibias was 7.4 mm, an indication of eccentric medial growth. Interestingly, the 3.3-mm difference noted between the injured and uninjured lateral sides was a reflection of overall growth stimulation on the injured side. These observations occurred with or without an intact fibula.

It is clear from these publications that a valgus deformity is not usually a complication of the initial reduction but, instead, is secondary to differential growth between the medial and lateral aspects of the proximal tibial epiphysis.

## EVOLUTION OF TREATMENT

It is important to understand the current concepts regarding the natural history of a valgus deformity before beginning a discussion of current treatment. It is now accepted that a valgus deformity will stabilize and then improve with growth and development. The deformity usually develops within 5 months of injury, reaches its maximum within 18 to 24 months, stabilizes, and then begins to improve by a combination of longitudinal growth and physeal (proximal and distal) realignment.[156, 166, 184, 249, 268] Unfortunately, no data indicate how much improvement can be anticipated. Salter and Best[216] found no improvement in 13 cases, and 10 later required proximal tibia varus osteotomy. Visser and Veldhuizen[255] reported no spontaneous improvement in the valgus deformity from the proximal tibial epiphysis but did observe some correction in alignment from the distal tibial epiphysis. Taylor[237] noted improvement in some patients, but not in all. Of the 12 children with valgus deformities reported by Jordan and associates,[127] 11 had documented improvement, although 4 subsequently underwent corrective osteotomy. Two children had their deformities recur, and two had postoperative compartment syndromes. Six of the children who were observed had complete correction of their deformities.

Jackson and Cozen[118] and later Ippolito and Pentimalli[114] observed that deformities of 15° or less usually remodeled completely, especially in young children. More severe deformities did not completely correct. Bahnson and Lovell[9] found some improvement in the valgus deformity of five children whom they monitored for a minimum of 3 years after injury. Balthazar and Pappas[10] reported that two of nine patients who were treated nonoperatively resolved their valgus deformities over a period of 1 to 3 years. Skak and co-workers[225] reported that valgus deformities tended to increase during the first year after injury, remain constant for 1 to 2 years, and then improve. Only one of their six patients had a significant residual deformity at final follow-up.

MacEwen and Zionts[156] and Zionts and MacEwen[268] monitored seven children with post-traumatic tibia valga for a mean of 39 months after injury. These children ranged in age from 11 months to 6 years. It was found that the valgus deformity progressed most rapidly during the first year after injury and then continued at a slower rate for as long as 17 months; overgrowth of the tibia accompanied the valgus deformity. The mean overgrowth was 1 cm, with a range of 0.2 to 1.7 cm. Clinical correction with subsequent growth occurred in six of the seven patients. These authors recommended a conservative approach to management of both the acute fracture and the subsequent valgus deformity. If the valgus deformity fails to correct satisfactorily by early adolescence, a tibial osteotomy can be performed. They also recommended that the mechanical tibiofemoral angle, as described by Visser and Veldhuizen,[255] be used to measure the alignment of the lower extremity rather than the metaphyseal-diaphyseal angle of Levine and Drennan.[149] The latter measures only the alignment of the proximal end of the tibia. This angle is useful in the immediate postinjury stage but not in the follow-up period because considerable correction of the deformity is a result of distal realignment.[156, 184, 225, 255, 268] The distal tibial epiphysis tends to reorient itself perpendicular to the pressure forces, thereby resulting in eccentric growth and an S-shaped appearance of the tibia radiographically.[75, 193]

In an experimental study in dogs, Karaharju and associates[128] observed that the tibial physes changed their direction of growth after an osteotomy and residual valgus angulation. In the study by Ogden and colleagues,[184] no true correction of the proximal tibia valga was observed, but eccentric growth was present distally and led to realignment of the ankle joint toward its normal parallel alignment with the floor and knee.

Tuten and associates[249] reevaluated the seven children of Zionts and MacEwen[268] at a mean follow-up of 15.3 years (range, 10.4 to 19.9 years). Every patient had spontaneous improvement of the metaphyseal-diaphyseal and mechanical tibiofemoral angles. However, most of the correction was thought to have occurred in the proximal end of the tibia. The mechanical axis of the limb remained lateral to the center of the knee joint in every patient with a mean deviation of 15 mm (range, 3 to 24 mm). The affected tibia was slightly longer. The affected knee score was excellent in five patients and fair in two. One patient required a tibial osteotomy because of knee pain secondary to malalignment. The authors concluded that post-traumatic tibia valga should be observed throughout growth and that operative intervention should be reserved for patients with symptoms from malalignment.

McCarthy and associates[166] made similar recommendations after their study of 15 children with post-traumatic genu valgum, 10 of whom were managed nonoperatively and 5 operatively. At approximately 4 years of follow-up, they found essentially no difference in the complementary physeal shaft and tibiofemoral angles and maximal valgus deformity of the two groups. They recommended nonoperative treatment and observation, especially for children 4 years or younger when injured.

## CURRENT ALGORITHM

Most proximal tibial metaphyseal fractures can be treated nonoperatively with closed reduction techniques. Treatment consists of correction of any valgus angulation of greenstick fractures and immobilization in a long leg cast with the knee in extension for 4 to 6 weeks or until the fracture is well united. Slight overcorrection, if possible, may be desirable.[182] Displaced fractures require reduction as well as correction of any residual valgus angulation. However, normal apposition is not always necessary. Currently, indications for operative management of these fractures are limited. An inability to correct a significant valgus deformity under general anesthesia rather than failure to close the medial fracture gap is probably the major indication. The latter is usually indicative of soft tissue entrapment, but this complication does not contribute to subsequent overgrowth.

After satisfactory fracture reduction and cast application, fracture alignment should be assessed radiographically at least weekly for the first 3 weeks after injury. Any loss of alignment should be corrected. During this initial period, the child must avoid weight bearing to minimize compression forces and the possibility of valgus angulation at the fracture site in the cast.

## SPECIAL CONSIDERATIONS FOR MULTIPLE TRAUMA

Children who are victims of multiple trauma may sustain an unrecognized proximal tibial metaphyseal fracture, especially if an ipsilateral femoral shaft fracture is present. Bohn and Durbin[29] reported three males with proximal tibial metaphyseal fractures and ipsilateral femoral fractures in whom post-traumatic genu valgum and lower extremity overgrowth of 1.8 to 2.2 cm developed. In one, a 20° deformity resolved over a 5-year period. It is important that during the secondary survey the lower part of the legs be carefully evaluated for occult injuries and that radiographs be obtained in suspicious cases. The presence of a proximal tibial metaphyseal fracture may necessitate a change in treatment plan for the other musculoskeletal injuries. If an associated femoral shaft fracture is present, stabilization by either internal or external fixation may be necessary so that adequate closed reduction of the proximal tibial metaphyseal fracture can be achieved and maintained.

## TREATMENT OPTIONS

Proximal tibial metaphyseal fractures may be treated by either nonoperative or surgical techniques.

**Nonoperative Management.** The vast majority of angulated or displaced proximal tibial metaphyseal fractures are amenable to closed reduction and immobilization in a long leg plaster cast. Such management is almost always performed under general anesthesia to ensure adequate relaxation and pain relief. In some instances, the intact lateral cortex of a greenstick fracture must be fractured to achieve correct alignment. Once satisfactory alignment is obtained, the leg must be immobilized in a long leg cast with the knee in extension.

An AP radiograph of both lower extremities on a long cassette should document correction of the valgus deformity and symmetric alignment with the opposite uninvolved extremity. Slight overcorrection (5°, if possible) is desirable to counter any valgus overgrowth. A lateral radiograph of the fractured tibia is also obtained.

After a satisfactory closed reduction, repeat radiographs are obtained weekly for the first 3 weeks to assess maintenance of alignment. These radiographs usually consist of a non–weight-bearing AP view of both lower extremities on a long cassette and a lateral view of the fractured extremity. Subtle changes in alignment may not be appreciated unless both extremities are included on the radiograph. Any loss of alignment should be corrected by cast wedging techniques or repeat closed reduction. Repeat closed reduction may require general anesthesia, depending on the age of the child, the amount of correction necessary, and the degree of healing. Immobilization is continued until the fracture is well healed radiographically.

**Surgical Management.** Surgery is rarely indicated. Usually, the best alignment by closed reduction is accepted. Only if significant residual valgus deformity is present, with or without closure of the medial fracture gap (entrapped soft tissue), is open reduction considered. At surgery, after any entrapped soft tissue has been removed, the fracture can typically be reduced anatomically and the periosteum repaired. Internal fixation is not generally necessary, and fracture alignment is maintained by a long leg plaster cast with the knee in extension. The child is then monitored as described for nonoperative management.

Open proximal tibial metaphyseal fractures are rare but can occur in children who are victims of polytrauma. They are managed in the same manner as other open tibial shaft fractures (see under Open Tibia and Fibula Fractures). An external fixator may be necessary for stabilization, especially in children with segmental bone loss, instability, or other significant fractures or body area injuries. Alonso and Horowitz[3] and Behrens[17] reported on open proximal tibial metaphyseal fractures treated with an external fixator. Epiphyseal pins may be necessary in these fractures to achieve adequate stability.

The final step in either management method is to advise the family that even though satisfactory or anatomic alignment of the fracture has been obtained, valgus deformity and tibial overgrowth are possible as a natural consequence of this fracture. Such counseling prepares the family for this complication, should it occur. The necessity of long-term follow-up must be emphasized.

**Treatment of Valgus Deformities.** Treatment of valgus deformities after proximal tibial metaphyseal fractures is controversial. Conservative management with an orthosis has been suggested, but no evidence is available to substantiate the efficacy of this method.[60, 101, 114] Surgical correction was initially believed to be necessary. Salter and Best[216] reported that 10 of 13 patients with valgus deformity required tibial osteotomy for correction. Balthazar and Pappas[10] pointed out that even with osteotomies, the valgus deformity can recur. Such recurrence has been attributed to the same asymmetric overgrowth phenomenon that led to the valgus deformity initially. In their six patients who had osteotomies, the valgus deformity recurred, though to a lesser degree. Similar results were reported by DalMonte and co-workers,[52] who observed recurrent valgus deformities in 7 of 16 patients (44%) after proximal tibial osteotomies. No significant difference was seen in the prevalence of recurrence in children younger than 5 years (60%) and those between 5 and 10 years old (36%), except that the younger children experienced a greater recurrent deformity. These authors concluded that the osteotomy is essentially a second fracture and therefore has the same pathologic factors. Recurrent valgus deformity after corrective osteotomy has been documented by others.[14, 37, 127, 204]

Zionts and MacEwen[268] and Tuten and associates[249] recommend that most valgus deformities be observed until early adolescence. If spontaneous improvement fails to provide sufficient clinical correction or if the malalignment is causing pain, a proximal tibial varus shortening osteotomy and fibular diaphyseal osteotomy may be necessary. Zionts and MacEwen[268] also suggested medial epiphysiodesis as another method for simultaneous correction of both the angular deformity and any remaining lower extremity length inequality. Medial epiphysiodesis has also been recommended by Robert and associates.[204] Although tibial overgrowth is not usually excessive, it may be important for both the valgus and the overgrowth to be corrected simultaneously if surgery is performed.

## FOLLOW-UP CARE AND REHABILITATION

Once fracture healing is complete, the long leg cast can be removed. Initially, the child is allowed full weight bearing, and knee range-of-motion exercises are encouraged. Failure to achieve satisfactory knee motion within 2 weeks of cast removal is an indication for supervised physical therapy, but such therapy is rarely necessary. Radiographic follow-up at 3-month intervals is usually performed during the first year and should consist of a standing AP view of both lower extremities on a long cassette to assess alignment. Orthogonal radiographs or scanograms may be necessary if significant tibial overgrowth has occurred. It is important that all children be monitored for at least 2 years after a fracture. Longer follow-up is necessary if a valgus deformity or significant lower extremity length inequality occurs.

## RESULTS

It appears that in approximately 50% of children who sustain proximal tibial metaphyseal fractures, a clinically apparent valgus deformity, tibial overgrowth, or both will develop. Zionts and MacEwen[268] showed that the maximal deformity induced by overgrowth is present by approximately 18 months after injury. Improvement begins thereafter, and maximal improvement has usually been achieved by 4 years after injury. Minor residual deformities may continue to correct with subsequent growth and physeal alignment. Significant deformities persisting after 12 years of age may require surgical correction.

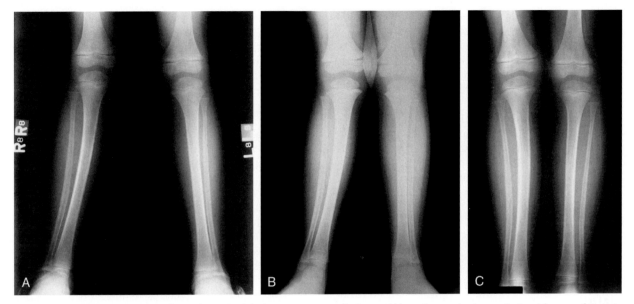

**FIGURE 15–1.** *A,* Anteroposterior standing radiograph of the lower extremities of a 5-year-old boy who sustained a nondisplaced fracture of the right proximal tibial metaphysis 15 months previously. The fracture healed uneventfully. The valgus deformity occurred shortly after cast removal. In terms of the mechanical axis, the right knee has a 22° valgus alignment versus 5° on the left. *B,* A repeat radiograph 1 year later demonstrates improvement in the right genu valgum to approximately 18°. Overgrowth of the tibia is also occurring. Observe the increased width between the distal tibial physis and the physeal growth arrest line on the right as compared with the left. *C,* Repeat radiograph 40 months after injury showing further improvement in alignment of the right tibia. Although the tibia is longer, the genu valgum measures only 12°. A significant proportion of the realignment has occurred in the distal end of the tibia. The articular surface of the right ankle joint is now parallel to the ground and perpendicular to the weight-bearing axis.

## AUTHORS' PREFERRED METHOD OF TREATMENT

In the initial management of an acute fracture, any angular or valgus deformity may be corrected, or even slightly overcorrected, by nonoperative closed reduction techniques under general anesthesia, and the parents must be warned of possible valgus deformity and tibial overgrowth. To evaluate alignment after closed reduction, adequate radiographs must be obtained. Alignment of the lower extremities should be assessed on an AP view of both lower extremities symmetrically positioned on a long cassette. With this method, the true alignment of the tibia can be measured directly and compared with the opposite side. If correction of a valgus deformity cannot be achieved by closing the medial fracture gap or fracturing the lateral cortex, open reduction is indicated. Failure to close the medial fracture site is typically indicative of soft tissue interposition from the periosteum, pes anserinus, medial collateral ligament, or a combination thereof. After satisfactory reduction is achieved, a long leg cast is applied with the knee in extension. Only by having the knee in extension is it possible to radiographically assess alignment of the tibia. The child is reevaluated radiographically at weekly intervals for the first 3 weeks after injury. Any change in position of the alignment in the cast is an indication for cast wedging or repeat closed reduction.

Treatment of valgus deformities is not usually considered for 2 to 3 years after injury, depending on the age of the patient and the degree of valgus. We do not believe that the use of orthoses or night splints will correct or alter the growth abnormality. Families are advised that

approximately 50% correction of any valgus deformity will occur during the first 3 to 4 years after injury (Fig. 15–1). Only after this time is it possible to determine whether further treatment will be necessary. If the maximal valgus deformity exceeds 20°, the residual deformity may be too severe to accept, and a proximal tibia vara and shortening osteotomy with a fibular diaphyseal osteotomy may be necessary. Valgus deformities are not generally clinically significant until they are 5% to 10% greater than on the normal side.[101]

If a corrective osteotomy is performed, it is usually a closing wedge proximal tibial and oblique diaphyseal fibular osteotomy. It is important that a fasciotomy of the anterior compartment be performed to minimize the risk of compartment syndrome. The deformity should be slightly overcorrected at the time of surgery because of the tendency for recurrence. Internal fixation with staples or crossed Steinmann pins can be used. Compression plates can also be considered, but they require a second, more extensive operative procedure for removal. We recommend stabilization after the osteotomy to maintain alignment, and we prefer percutaneous crossed Steinmann pins or a simple external fixation system consisting of a single threaded Steinmann pin placed above and below the osteotomy and secured with an external fixation clamp. This simple technique maintains apposition and prevents rotation and angulation. The leg is then immobilized in a long leg cast with the knee in extension. The child is closely monitored radiographically to assess alignment and healing. Once the osteotomy site has healed (usually in 6 weeks), the Steinmann pins are removed, typically in an outpatient clinic.

Temporary stapling of the medial aspect of the proximal tibial epiphysis is also an attractive treatment option because it allows correction with growth and does not provide the same magnitude of stimulation as a corrective osteotomy, which can contribute to recurrence. The authors have no experience with this procedure for this condition.

After satisfactory healing, the child is allowed full weight bearing, and knee range-of-motion exercises are encouraged. If satisfactory motion of the knee has not been obtained after 2 weeks, supervised physical therapy is instituted. The child should be monitored for at least 2 years to observe for recurrent valgus deformity, tibial overgrowth, or both. Standing radiographs are obtained at 3- to 6-month intervals, and scanograms are obtained annually.

## Fractures of the Tibial and Fibular Shafts

Fractures involving both the tibial and the fibular diaphyses are more common than isolated fractures of the tibia.[175, 204] In a 1988 review by Shannak[222] of 117 children with tibial shaft fractures, 85 (73%) had an associated fracture of the fibula. The mean age at fracture was 8 years (range, 1 to 15 years). Boys were involved three times more frequently than girls. These children had 104 fractures (90%) that involved the middle or lower third of the tibial shaft. Oblique (35%) and comminuted (32%) were the most common fracture patterns. Only four fractures (3%) were open. Parrini and co-workers[191] also found that tibia and fibula fractures were more common than isolated tibial shaft fractures in children between 1 and 11 years of age. Typically, fractures of both the tibia and the fibula require greater energy than an isolated tibial shaft fracture does. They generally result from direct injury rather than from rotation, as occurs in the latter. This mechanism accounts for the increased incidence of oblique, transverse, and comminuted fracture patterns.

### EVOLUTION OF TREATMENT

The major problems with fractures of the tibial and fibular shafts are shortening, angulation, and malrotation. Valgus deformities are common because of the action of the long flexor muscles of the lower part of the leg. However, these problems are not usually severe, and almost all fractures are amenable to nonoperative or closed methods of treatment. In the study by Shannak[222] in which 117 pediatric tibial shaft fractures were monitored for a mean of 3.9 years (range, 3 to 10 years), it was determined that satisfactory results can almost always be expected with conservative treatment and that surgery is usually not indicated or justified. Similar results have been reported by others.[95, 104, 232] Shortening of 5 mm or less is compensated by growth acceleration, and mild varus angulations undergo spontaneous correction; however, valgus malalignment and rotational deformities persist and must be corrected.[222, 234] For these reasons,

the conservative methods of treatment of tibial and fibular shaft fractures have changed little in this century. However, in certain situations, surgical management with either internal or external fixation may be advantageous. These selected indications are presented in Table 15–2.

### CURRENT ALGORITHM

Nearly all closed tibial and fibular shaft fractures in children can be managed by nonoperative techniques. Nondisplaced fractures are immobilized in a long leg cast with the knee flexed 20° to 60°.[28, 84, 196, 201, 222] Depending on the fracture pattern, the child is kept from weight bearing for 3 to 4 weeks or until early radiographic healing is evident. A long leg cast with the knee extended may then be applied, and full weight bearing is allowed until complete healing has occurred. In diaphyseal fractures of the distal third, a patellar tendon–bearing (PTB) or short leg cast may be applied instead.

Displaced closed fractures require closed reduction, with strict attention to maintenance of tibial length and correct angulation and rotation alignment. This procedure can usually be accomplished with manipulation and application of a long leg cast with the knee flexed 20° to 60°. If the tibia fracture is oblique or comminuted, maintenance of length may be difficult, and surgical treatment may need to be considered. After application of the long leg cast, the patient must be monitored closely, usually weekly, to assess maintenance of fracture alignment. Minor alterations in angulation can be corrected by cast wedging techniques. When the fracture is stable both clinically and radiographically, usually 4 to 6 weeks after injury, a long leg weight-bearing cast with the knee in extension or possibly a PTB or short leg cast, depending on the fracture type and location, may be applied for an additional 2 to 3 weeks until the fracture is well healed.

Unstable closed fractures (oblique or comminuted) in a child who is a victim of polytrauma may benefit from the more aggressive operative methods of management, especially external fixation.

**TABLE 15–2** ......................................

Indications for Internal or External Fixation of Pediatric Tibia and Fibula Fractures

Open fractures
   Type III and some type II[79, 80]
   Segmental bone loss
Unstable closed fractures
   Segmental
Neurovascular injuries
Multiple trauma
   Severe body area injuries
   Head injuries with spasticity or combativeness
   Ipsilateral femoral fractures
   Multiple fractures
Soft tissue abnormalities
   Burns
   Skin loss
   Compartment syndromes (fasciotomies)

.........................................

Modified from Thompson, G.H., et al. Clin Orthop 188:10–20, 1984.

## SPECIAL CONSIDERATIONS FOR MULTIPLE TRAUMA

Children who are victims of multiple trauma and have additional long bone fractures or significant injuries to other body areas may benefit from having their fractures stabilized surgically (see Table 15–2). Surgical stabilization enhances their overall care by improving both stability and mobility. The child is more easily cared for, and other diagnostic studies such as CT and MRI are facilitated by allowing the child to be transported and properly positioned in the gantry. The most common method of surgical stabilization of pediatric tibia and fibula fractures is external fixation. A variety of half-pin cantilever systems and small-pin transfixation rings have been used for external fixation of tibia fractures in children.[3, 17, 55, 69, 83, 132, 202, 242, 243] The former is usually the preferred method because of the ease and speed of application and the decreased risk of neurovascular injury; in addition, this system does not block surgical exposure to any associated wounds. Wires, pins, and screws are occasionally used as surgical adjuncts. Compression plates are not generally recommended because of the extensive dissection necessary for application, the increased risk of infection, and the need for a second extensive procedure for hardware removal. Intramedullary rods, commonly used in adults, are rarely used because of the risk of damaging the proximal tibial physes.

## TREATMENT OPTIONS

Closed fractures of the tibial and fibular diaphyses in children are usually uncomplicated, and their healing is typically rapid in comparison to similar fractures in adults. Current treatment methods consist of nonoperative and surgical management; the latter includes both internal and external fixation techniques.

**Nonoperative Management.** Most closed fractures of the tibial and fibular shafts can be managed by closed reduction and immobilization in a long leg cast.[28, 84, 196, 201, 222]

Displaced fractures usually require reduction under general anesthesia, whereas nondisplaced fractures can frequently be managed with a cast after sedation. This first cast usually has the knee flexed 20° to 60° to discourage weight bearing. Once satisfactory alignment has been achieved, the fracture is assessed radiographically at weekly intervals for the first 3 weeks. Minor changes in alignment can be corrected with cast wedging techniques. Significant loss of alignment may require repeat closed reduction under general anesthesia. After 1 to 4 weeks, depending on the type of fracture and degree of radiographic healing, a weight-bearing long leg cast with the knee in extension may be applied.[222] The cast is worn until fracture healing is complete. In patients with fractures in the lower third of the tibia and fibula, a PTB cast or possibly a short leg cast may be used instead. A functional brace, as described by Sarmiento and colleagues,[217] should also be considered for older adolescents. Sarmiento's group applied the functional brace approximately 2 weeks after the injury and initial treatment with a long leg plaster cast. They reported minimal problems with shortening, angulation, malrotation, and delayed union or nonunion.

The major problem when both the tibial and the fibular shafts are fractured is shortening.[95, 222] Angulation can also develop inasmuch as the long flexor muscles tend to produce a valgus rather than a varus deformity at the fracture. Recurvatum may occur as well, especially in children with considerable soft tissue swelling at the time of initial reduction and cast application. Wedging of the cast may be required to correct the angulation.[222] Often, it is best to wait 1 to 2 weeks for the soft tissue swelling to resolve and for the fracture to develop some stability. If considerable swelling is observed initially, it may be better to apply a posterior splint and then perform the definitive manipulative reduction 4 to 7 days later when the swelling has subsided, the risk of compartment syndrome has passed, and a more appropriate, well-fitting cast can be applied.

For unstable fractures of the tibial and fibular diaphyses, especially those that are displaced, comminuted, and with appreciable shortening, other methods of closed management have been proposed. Steinert and Bennek[232] recommended an unpadded long leg cast with the foot in mild plantar flexion. After 3 weeks, the cast is changed and the foot is brought to the neutral position. Weber and associates[259] and Shannak[222] recommended skeletal traction with a Steinmann pin through the os calcis of the heel. After 10 to 14 days, sufficient healing has usually occurred to allow application of a long leg cast with the knee in extension. These methods are rarely used today. Most authors prefer surgical stabilization with some type of external fixation.

**Surgical Management.** The principles of surgical management of pediatric fractures are distinctly different from those used in skeletally mature adults. When surgical management of pediatric fractures is indicated, the general principles of Spiegal and Mast[229] must be considered. These principles are applicable both in polytrauma patients and in specific tibia fractures (see Table 15–2). The principles applicable to tibial shaft fractures include the following: (1) satisfactory, possibly anatomic alignment should be achieved, with particular attention to rotation and angular orientation; (2) internal fixation devices, if used, should be easy to remove; (3) rigid fixation to maintain fracture alignment rather than allow immediate mobilization of the lower part of the leg is usually the goal, and therefore a supplemental plaster cast may be required; and (4) external fixators, when used, should be removed as soon as any soft tissue wounds have healed or the fracture is stable and will not become displaced. Cast immobilization is continued until complete healing has occurred. The three basic surgical techniques of open reduction and internal fixation, closed reduction and percutaneous internal fixation, and external fixation may be considered for pediatric tibial shaft fractures.[240] The last is the most commonly used method. Hansen[96] stated that the choice of surgical treatment of pediatric fractures should be guided by analyzing the extent of soft tissue injury, the location of the fracture, the fracture pattern, and the extent of other associated injuries.

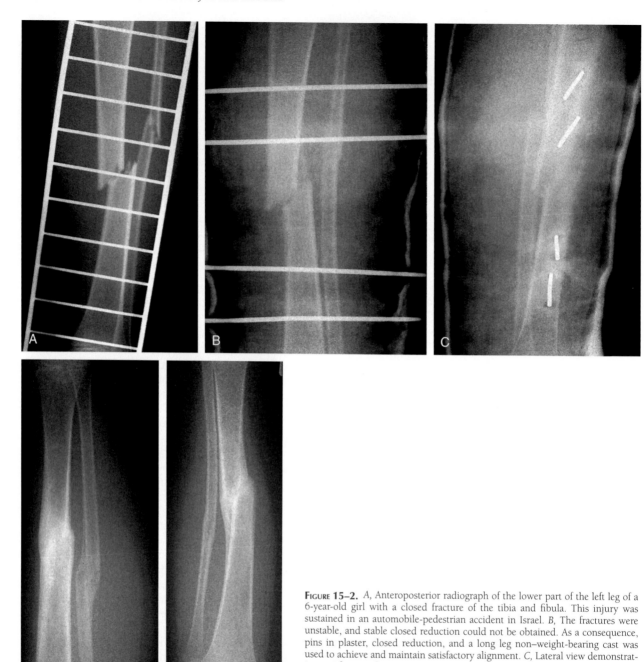

**Figure 15–2.** *A,* Anteroposterior radiograph of the lower part of the left leg of a 6-year-old girl with a closed fracture of the tibia and fibula. This injury was sustained in an automobile-pedestrian accident in Israel. *B,* The fractures were unstable, and stable closed reduction could not be obtained. As a consequence, pins in plaster, closed reduction, and a long leg non–weight-bearing cast was used to achieve and maintain satisfactory alignment. *C,* Lateral view demonstrating satisfactory alignment. *D,* Anteroposterior radiograph 4 months postinjury and after returning to the United States. Good healing and satisfactory alignment are evident. *E,* Lateral view.

*External Fixation.* External skeletal fixation is the surgical procedure of choice for most pediatric tibia and fibula fractures.* It is particularly useful in open tibia fractures but may be beneficial in closed, but unstable or other specific fractures (see Table 15–2). Techniques include pins above and below the fractures that are incorporated into a plaster cast[13] (Fig. 15–2) or a variety of commercial half-pin and ring fixator systems.[3, 17, 69, 83, 132, 202, 240, 243] Methyl methacrylate in a

tube has been used as an external fixator in selected cases.[55] External fixation is usually maintained until adequate callus formation has been achieved and the fracture is stable. At that time, the fixator is removed and replaced by a long leg cast with the knee in extension. Tolo[242] reported that the use of external fixators increased the healing time and was associated with a significant prevalence (50%) of superficial pin tract infections and a high rate of refracture. Three of 13 tibia fractures (23%) refractured 5 to 10 months after injury. Whether the refractures were caused by stress shielding, premature frame removal, or relative ischemia from the

---

*See references 3, 13, 17, 55, 69, 83, 132, 202, 240, 242, 243.

local trauma was unknown. All three refractures healed with immobilization in long leg casts. As experience with external fixators in pediatric tibia fractures has been gained, the incidence of these complications has significantly decreased.[69, 83]

The advantages of external fixation of pediatric tibial shaft fractures include rigid immobilization, direct surveillance of the lower part of the leg and any associated wounds, facilitation of wound dressing and management, patient mobilization for other diagnostic studies and management of other body area injuries, and possible application under local anesthesia in severely injured children.

***Internal Fixation.*** Closed or open reduction with internal fixation of pediatric tibial and fibular diaphyseal fractures is not commonly performed. Operative techniques include limited internal fixation with K-wires, Steinmann pins, and cortical lag screws; compression plates and screws[179] (Fig. 15–3); and intramedullary rods. Although Thompson and associates[241] reported that the latter are the most common devices for achieving stable fixation in pediatric fractures, intramedullary rods are not commonly used in tibial shaft fractures. One possible indication would be an unstable segmental fracture that could not be satisfactorily aligned by closed methods or with an external fixator. Compression plates and screws may be considered in similar situations, but these devices require extensive dissection and periosteal stripping, which can increase the risk of infection or delayed union or nonunion because of further disruption of the blood supply to the bone. Highland and LaMont[102] reported six cases of deep, late infection after

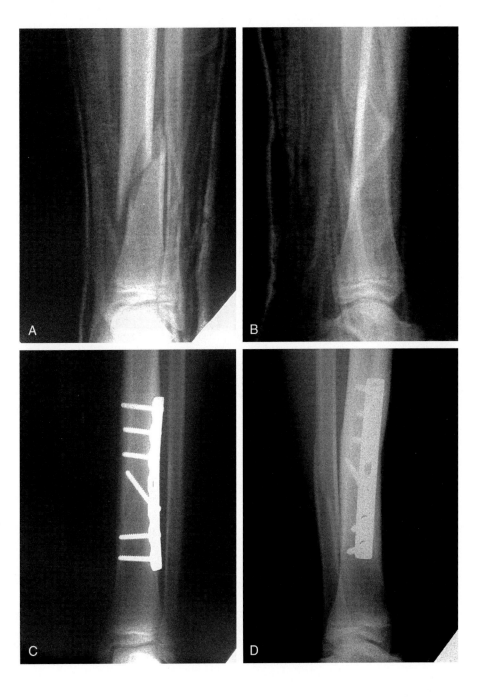

FIGURE 15–3. *A*, Anteroposterior radiograph of the lower part of the left leg of a 13-year-old boy with an unstable oblique fracture of distal ends of the tibia and fibula. *B*, A lateral radiograph more clearly demonstrates the fibular fracture. *C*, Anteroposterior radiograph 18 months after open reduction and internal fixation of the fibular fracture. The fractures are well healed. *D*, Lateral view.

internal fixation of proximal femoral osteotomies. They recommended routine removal of internal fixation devices in children, which is a second relatively extensive procedure and an additional disadvantage to the use of plates and screws.

Intramedullary rodding of a pediatric tibia fracture has not been indicated until recently because of possible injury to the proximal tibial epiphysis, physis, and tibial tubercle, which are near the usual entry points. In 1985, Ligier and co-workers[151] from France reported on the results of using two flexible intramedullary rods in 19 pediatric tibia fractures. Such treatment produced elastic stability at the fracture site, which enhanced the formation of bridging external callus by eliminating shear forces and allowing compression forces across the fracture site. One rod was inserted through the medial and the other through the lateral proximal tibial metaphysis, distal to the physis and posterior to the apophysis of the tibial tubercle, and then passed distally across the fracture site to terminate proximal to the distal tibial physis. These workers reported that no cast immobilization was necessary and all fractures healed within 3 months. The major indications for intramedullary fixation were predominantly for unstable fractures that failed nonoperative management. In 1988, Verstreken and associates[252] from Belgium also used the technique of elastic stable rodding in children. They recommended its use for tibia fractures with contralateral lower limb injuries in children 6 years and older, especially those who are victims of multiple trauma. In 2001, Qidwai[199] from Saudi Arabia reported on 84 tibial fractures, including 30 open fractures treated with a similar technique of intramedullary K-wires (2.5 to 3.5 mm in diameter). The mean age at fracture was 10.2 years (range, 4 to 15 years), and 54 had an associated fibular fracture. The fractures healed at a mean of 9.5 weeks (range, 8 to 14 weeks), and the implants were removed at a mean of 5.6 months postoperatively. The mean follow-up was 18 months (range, 13 to 16 months). No delayed unions, nonunions, or lower extremity length discrepancies greater than 1.0 cm were observed. One child had a 10° varus malunion that remodeled with growth. No postoperative infections occurred in the 54 closed fractures. However, in the 30 open fractures, 5 postoperative infections (4 superficial and 1 deep) were reported. They concluded that their technique was simple and produced good clinical, radiographic, and functional results.

## FOLLOW-UP CARE AND REHABILITATION

Most children with tibia and fibula fractures do not require physical therapy for rehabilitation. They usually regain full knee and ankle motion within the expected time and wish to return to full activities much sooner than their parents and orthopaedic surgeons would like. An inability to regain full knee and ankle motion within 2 to 3 weeks after the cast is removed is a common indication for physical therapy. Once motion is regained, muscle strength returns to normal, and radiographs show solid union, normal activities, including sports, can be allowed, usually 4 to 6 weeks after the last cast is removed. The child is then monitored at 3- to 6-month intervals for approximately 2 years to assess function, leg length, and resolution of any residual problems such as mild angulation.

## RESULTS

The results after nonoperative management of uncomplicated closed tibial and fibular shaft fractures are uniformly satisfactory. The fractures heal rapidly, depending on age, and minor discrepancies in length and angulation may correct spontaneously with subsequent growth.[95, 104, 222, 232] Shannak[222] reported union in a mean of 37 days, with or without preliminary traction, in children with a mean age of 8 years (range, 1 to 15 years). Hansen and colleagues[95] reported healing in 2 to 18 weeks in children in the same age group. Young children healed quickly, and adolescents took the longest.

Approximately 25% of children with tibial and fibular shaft fractures have minor tibial length inequalities and angulatory changes at initial healing.[95, 222] Significant rotational problems are fortunately uncommon. Because the amount of overgrowth of the tibia and fibula secondary to fracture stimulation is small, it is important to maintain adequate length during healing. In tibia fractures in boys older than 12 years and in girls older than 10 years, an attempt must be made to achieve full length. Excessive shortening must be avoided if equal leg length is to be reached by maturity. The amount of shortening that can be accepted after closed reduction of these fractures is 5 to 10 mm in girls 3 to 10 years of age and boys 3 to 12 years of age.[84, 203, 222, 234] Older children and adolescents require alignment that is as close to anatomic as possible. Younger children may have overgrowth in both the tibia and femur, whereas older children and young adolescents may actually experience growth retardation. The type of fracture and the presence of residual angulation do not appear to affect the amount of overgrowth. The growth stimulation process is usually complete 2 years after injury.[234] Reynolds[203] demonstrated that within 3 months of injury, the rate of growth was at its maximum and was 38% in excess of normal. The growth rate then decreased but remained significantly elevated for 2 years; it returned to normal in the tibia approximately 40 months after injury.

It is also important to correct any coexistent angular or rotational deformity. Angular deformities may improve with growth, but rotational malalignment does not.[84, 222] Varus deformities of up to 15° in young children can undergo spontaneous correction.[222] However, valgus and posterior angulation tend to persist, as do rotational deformities, particularly medial or internal rotation. In uncomplicated fractures, function can be expected to return to normal.

## AUTHORS' PREFERRED METHOD OF TREATMENT

Because closed tibia and fibula fractures in children usually heal rapidly and with satisfactory long-term results, we recommend closed reduction and immobilization in a long leg cast for the vast majority of cases.

Only a small percentage of closed fractures require operative management with either external or internal fixation.

Most nondisplaced fractures are managed by a long leg cast applied with the knee in 20° to 60° of flexion. Weight bearing is avoided for 2 to 3 weeks; a long leg cast is then applied with the knee in extension, and toe-touch weight bearing is allowed. Once callus formation is visible, the cast may be changed to either a PTB or a short leg cast, depending on fracture location and the degree of radiographic healing. A long leg cast is always used initially because a PTB or short leg cast will fail to control motion at the fracture site, thus causing pain and possible displacement of the fracture.

Displaced fractures of the tibia and fibula are reduced under general anesthesia. When displacement is present, extensive injury to the surrounding soft tissues has usually occurred. These children have an increased risk for compartment syndrome and are admitted to the hospital for observation after reduction and immobilization in either a posterior splint or a long leg cast, depending on the degree of soft tissue swelling. If a splint is used initially, the long leg cast should be applied 4 to 7 days later to allow resolution of the soft tissue swelling; the procedure is usually performed under general anesthesia. After immobilization, the patient is evaluated radiographically at weekly intervals for the first 3 weeks. If alignment is lost, the need for cast wedging or repeat closed reduction must be considered. In most cases, the displacement is minor and can be managed by cast wedging.

For an unstable fracture with unacceptable alignment after closed reduction, an external fixator may be necessary. We prefer half-pin systems. They are easy to apply, but care must be taken to avoid injury to the proximal and distal tibial physes. The use of fluoroscopy ensures safe application of these devices. These systems control length, angulation, and rotation. They are typically supplemented with a posterior splint for the first several weeks to immobilize both the knee and the ankle for comfort. Depending on the age and reliability of the child, partial weight bearing may be allowed 2 to 4 weeks after injury. Transverse fractures that heal with small areas of callus may require longer periods with the frame in place to prevent recurrent deformity. Once callus is confirmed radiographically and any associated wounds have healed, the external fixation device is removed and replaced with a long leg or PTB cast until fracture healing is complete.

We have had limited experience with intramedullary fixation with flexible nails but believe that such fixation is also becoming an acceptable method of treatment. Care must be taken to avoid injury to the tibial tubercle during rod insertion.

## Isolated Fractures of the Tibial Diaphysis

Fractures of the tibial shaft with an intact fibula are common in children.[36, 191, 222, 232, 238, 265] They can be either incomplete tension-compression (greenstick) or complete fractures. Steinert and Bennek[232] reported that 70% of 263 fractures were isolated tibia fractures and 30% were complete fractures of both the tibia and the fibula. However, as discussed previously, Shannak[222] and Parrini and co-workers[191] found fractures involving both the tibia and fibula to be more common. Shannak observed that only 32 (27%) of 117 children with tibia fractures had isolated tibial diaphyseal fractures. Briggs and associates[36] reported a similar incidence, with 25 of 65 children (38%) having isolated tibia fractures.

Teitz and colleagues[238] reported on 45 patients younger than 20 years (range, 3 to 19 years) with isolated tibial shaft fractures. In this group, falls were the most common mechanism of injury, followed by skiing and motor vehicle accidents. Most fractures were spiral and involved the middle or distal third of the shaft. Briggs and associates[36] reported that low-velocity trauma or an indirect twisting injury caused all 25 isolated tibia fractures in their study. The mean age of their patients was 6.1 years (range, 1 to 12.4 years). Most of the fractures in their study also occurred at the junction of the middle and distal thirds of the tibial shaft. Similar findings were reported by Yang and Letts[265] in a study of 95 patients in 1997. The mean age at injury was 8.1 years (range, 0.3 to 17 years); 77 (81%) were due to indirect trauma, and 69 (73%) occurred in the distal third of the tibia. It therefore appears that fractures involving both the tibia and the fibula are more commonly the result of severe, high-energy accidents, such as motor vehicle accidents, whereas isolated tibial shaft fractures result from less severe types of trauma, such as falls or sporting accidents.

Isolated tibial fractures are caused predominantly by torsional forces, and most will be localized in the distal third or at the junction of the middle and distal thirds of the tibia.[232, 265] The most common mechanism of torsion was lateral rotation of the body while the foot was in a fixed position on the ground. The fracture line began distally on the anteromedial surface of the tibia and progressed proximally to the posterolateral aspect. The intact fibula and periosteum prevent significant displacement or shortening. However, angulation can occur, especially varus angulation. When the fibula is intact, the tendency toward shortening is converted to a torsional deformity at the fracture site, and a varus deformity is produced. This abnormality is caused predominantly by the effect of the long flexor muscles across the fracture site inducing a rotational force. Briggs and colleagues[36] and Yang and Letts[265] found that secondary varus angulation was most likely to develop in oblique and spiral fractures. Transverse fractures tended not to angulate. Occasionally, plastic deformation of the fibula may also be present.[139, 155, 238] The degree of deformation is usually minimal, which may present difficulties when realigning the tibia unless the plastic deformation of the fibula is corrected simultaneously.

Teitz and colleagues[238] corroborated clinical observations with biomechanical studies on tibia fractures with an intact fibula. They found that when the fibula remains intact, a tibiofibular length discrepancy develops and causes altered strain patterns in the tibia and fibula. These strain patterns may lead to delayed union, nonunion, or malunion of the tibia. They found a lower incidence of these complications in children and adolescents and attributed it to greater compliance of their fibulas and soft tissues.

Treatment of an isolated tibial shaft fracture is predominantly nonoperative, with immobilization in a long leg cast alone[36, 191, 222, 232, 238, 265] (Fig. 15–4). Closed reduction may be necessary, especially if a varus deformity greater than 15° is present along with coexistent plastic deformation of the fibula. Flexing the knee 30° to 90° and placing the foot in some degree of plantar flexion during the first 2 or 3 weeks may negate some of the deforming force from the long toe flexors.[36] Children should be monitored radiographically at weekly intervals for the first 3 weeks because secondary varus angulation can occur, especially in those with oblique and spiral fractures. A repeat closed reduction may be necessary if the angulation exceeds 15°. After fracture stability is achieved, a long leg weight-bearing cast with the knee in extension is applied. The cast is usually

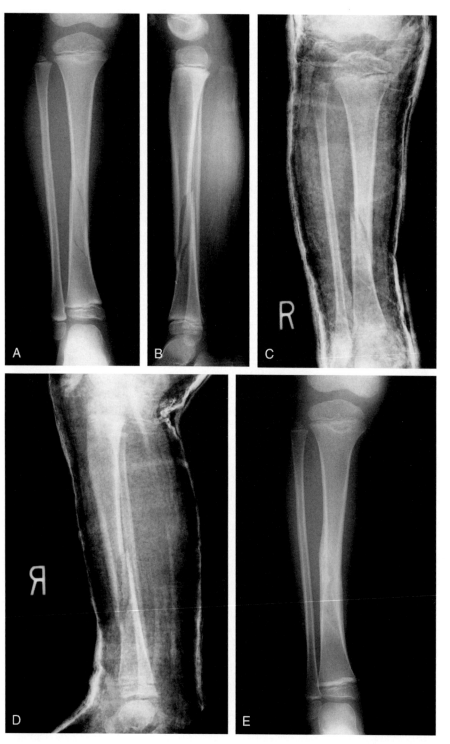

**Figure 15–4.** *A,* Anteroposterior radiograph of the lower part of the right leg of a 4-year-old boy who fell through a boat hatch. An isolated spiral fracture of the distal third of the tibia is apparent. The fibula is intact. *B,* A lateral radiograph demonstrates that the spiral fracture is minimally displaced. *C,* Slight varus angulation of 5° occurred during immobilization in a long leg plaster cast. Shortening at the fracture site was minimal. *D,* A lateral radiograph shows no change in alignment from the initial radiographs. *E,* Three months after injury, the fracture is well healed. Despite the slight varus angulation, the articular surface of the ankle is parallel to the floor and perpendicular to the weight-bearing axis.

maintained until healing is complete. A PTB cast, fracture brace, or short leg cast can be used for distal fractures. Indications for surgical intervention in children with isolated tibial shaft fractures are limited. Even in children with multiple trauma, these fractures can be treated by simple immobilization with a long leg cast. Severe soft tissue damage, such as with burns or open fractures, or a diaphyseal fracture with significant residual angulation may be better managed by open reduction and internal fixation or an external fixator. Qidwai[199] recently reported on 30 isolated tibial shaft fractures treated by intramedullary fixation with 2.5- to 3.5-mm K-wires. The fractures healed quickly, and no postoperative infections occurred in the closed fractures.

Isolated tibia fractures usually heal uneventfully, and the child quickly returns to normal activities. Briggs and associates[36] reported that the mean time to healing in their 25 patients was 46 days (range, 18 to 73 days) and that time to healing increased with advancing age. Similar results were reported by Yang and Letts[265] and by Qidwai.[199] Tibial length inequality is not a problem, and any associated varus deformity is usually not appreciable clinically. Varus deformities up to 15° usually remodel sufficiently, but the outcome is less true for diaphyseal, more proximal fractures.

## Special Tibial Shaft Fractures

### TODDLER'S FRACTURE

In children between 9 months and perhaps 6 years of age, torsion of the foot may produce an oblique fracture of the distal aspect of the tibial shaft without a fibula fracture.[65, 94, 169, 170, 187, 223, 239] The term *toddler's fracture* was first used by Dunbar and co-workers[65] in 1964. These fractures are usually the result of a trivial or seemingly innocuous event, such as tripping while walking or running, stepping on a ball or toy, or falling from a modest height. It is most common in younger children, hence the name toddler's fracture. Dunbar and co-workers[65] reported 76 cases, with 63 occurring in children younger than 2.5 years. Tenenbien and colleagues[239] in 1990 reported 37 cases in children between 1 and 4 years of age.

The physical findings and radiographic appearance are often subtle. These children are typically seen because of failure to bear weight, a limp, or pain when forced to stand on the involved extremity. Usually, the child does not have any soft tissue swelling, ecchymoses, or deformity. Localized tenderness is the most common physical finding. Local warmth may be noted during palpation at the fracture site.[239] The traumatic episode may not be witnessed.[187]

AP and lateral radiographs of the entire tibia and fibula are necessary for diagnosis and may demonstrate a spiral fracture of the distal end of the tibia. However, the radiographs may also be normal.[65, 94, 223, 239] The characteristic finding is a faint oblique fracture line crossing the distal tibial diaphysis and terminating medially. When routine radiographs are normal but a fracture is suspected, an internal rotation oblique view may be

beneficial.[65] Occasionally, a series of oblique films in various degrees of rotation are of value, with two being made in external rotation and two in internal rotation.[60] The fracture line may be visualized on only one film. If a fracture is suspected but not visualized, immobilization is still indicated. A technetium bone scan may reveal increased uptake, thereby confirming the fracture.[6, 53, 68, 124, 173] However, such scanning is rarely indicated unless the child is febrile and osteomyelitis is a concern.[6, 173] Repeat radiographs 7 to 10 days after injury usually demonstrate subperiosteal new bone formation, thereby substantiating the fracture. Halsey and associates[94] recently reported that of 39 children with a suspected toddler's fracture and negative initial radiographs, 16 (41%) had a toddler's fracture confirmed on follow-up radiographs.

The periosteal reaction can vary from slight to abundant. Treatment of this fracture is immobilization in a long leg cast for 2 to 4 weeks, depending on the age of the child (Fig. 15–5). When the fracture is discovered 2 weeks or more after injury, immobilization may not be necessary, provided that callus formation is adequate and the child has no tenderness on stress examination.

Tenenbien and colleagues[239] differentiated the radiographic features of a typical toddler's fracture from those of child abuse or the battered child syndrome. In the latter, the fracture is usually midshaft and less oblique. It is important to distinguish between these two entities. In a review by Oudjhane and associates[187] of 500 consecutive radiographic evaluations of children younger than 5 years with an acute limp, excluding cases of child abuse, occult fracture of the tibia or fibula was the most common cause (56 cases). These fractures occurred predominantly in the distal metaphysis, occasionally in the proximal metaphysis, and only rarely in the diaphysis. Similar findings regarding occult tibia fractures in young children have been reported by others.[169, 224]

### BATTERED CHILD SYNDROME

Fractures are second only to soft tissue injuries as the most common finding in battered child syndrome.[77] Approximately 25% to 50% of abused children have fractures.[2, 77, 135] The humerus, femur, and tibia are the most commonly fractured long bones in published series, in various order.[2, 77, 135, 138, 146, 153, 186] In some series, the metaphyseal bucket-handle or corner fracture pattern is the most frequent type, but in recent publications, the transverse pattern was more common. In 1986, Kleinman and co-workers,[136] in a combined histologic and radiographic study, demonstrated that a corner fracture is not an avulsion of the metaphyses at the site of attachment of the periosteum or ligaments but, instead, is a subepiphyseal fracture through the most immature portion of the metaphysis. Depending on the size of the injury, the degree of involvement of the metaphysis, and the radiographic projection, the lesion may appear as a bucket-handle fracture, a corner fracture, or metaphyseal radiolucency. Thus, these fractures are complete rather than avulsion types.

King and colleagues,[135] in a review of 750 children seen at the Children's Hospital of Los Angeles between

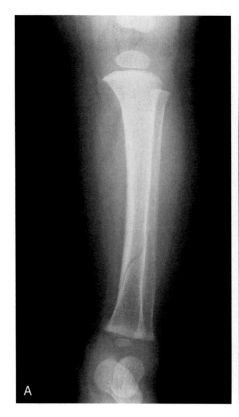
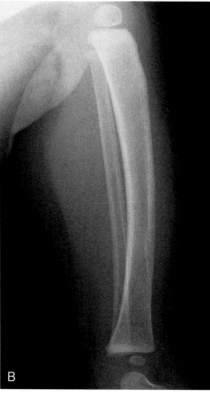

FIGURE 15–5. *A,* Toddler's fracture in a 9-month-old girl. She fell while taking her first independent steps. A faint oblique fracture is seen crossing the distal tibial diaphysis and terminating medially and distally. This fracture healed with 2 weeks of immobilization in a long leg plaster cast. *B,* A lateral radiograph shows that the fracture is barely visible with no displacement.

1971 and 1981 who were considered to be victims of battered child syndrome, found that 189 children (25%) sustained 429 total fractures. The median age was 7 months, with the range being 1 month to 13 years. Most were 2 years or younger. In this series, the most commonly fractured bones were the humerus, tibia, and femur. However, the most commonly fractured bones per patient were the humerus, femur, and tibia. Of all the long bone fractures, 48% were transverse, 26% were spiral, 16% were avulsion, 10% were oblique, and only 1.5% were comminuted fractures. When fracture combinations were analyzed, avulsion or metaphyseal corner fractures were the fourth most common pattern involving the proximal third of the tibia. A similar fracture pattern involving the distal third was the sixth most common pattern. Twenty-eight percent of the patients had a history of previous fractures. Ultimately, 10 of the children (5%) died.

The findings of King and colleagues[135] are similar to those in other studies. O'Neill and associates[186] demonstrated that 29 of 110 abused children (26%) had fractures. In this study, the humerus, femur, and tibia were the most commonly involved long bones. In a 1974 study by Akbarnia and co-workers[2] of 74 abused children with fractures, the ribs were the most commonly fractured bones, but the humerus, femur, and tibia were the most common long bones fractured. Also in 1974, Kogutt and colleagues[138] reported that tibia fractures were second only to femoral shaft fractures. In 1982, Galleno and Oppenheim[77] reported that metaphyseal corner fractures were the most common fracture pattern and occurred in 29 of 36 children with fractures. Of their 24 diaphyseal fractures, 17 were transverse and only 5

were spiral or oblique. Their study included 89 fractures in 36 children. Fifteen fractures involved the tibia, the second most common bone fractured. In 1983, Leonidas[146] emphasized that diaphyseal fractures were more common than epiphyseal-metaphyseal fractures. In 1991, Loder and Bookout,[153] in a study of 75 battered children with fractures, found that the skull was the most common bone fractured but that the tibia was the most common long bone fractured. Transverse fracture patterns occurred in 40% of the long bone fractures, and metaphyseal corner fractures occurred in 28%.

The diagnosis of battered child syndrome requires a high index of suspicion. Typically, the injuries are unobserved, and the parents' descriptions are vague. Physical examination may reveal soft tissue injuries in various stages of healing, failure to thrive, and emotional abnormalities resulting from deprivation and fear. Another potential problem in the evaluation of a child with battered child syndrome is distinguishing between nonaccidental injuries and osteogenesis imperfecta. Usually, diagnosis of the latter is not difficult because of the existence of a family history and the presence of fractures at birth, blue scleras, dentogenesis imperfecta, and other characteristic findings. However, these factors may not always be present. In a comparison of fracture patterns in these two disorders, Dent and Paterson[56] found that in osteogenesis imperfecta, the peak incidence for fractures was between 2 and 4 years of age; lower limb fractures, especially the distal portion of the femur and the tibial diaphysis, were more frequent than upper extremity fractures, and severe displacement of the fracture fragments was more common. Metaphyseal, spiral, and transverse fractures were common, whereas greenstick and torus fractures were not. However, even when the diagnosis of osteogenesis imperfecta is clear, the possibility of nonaccidental injury must be considered. Knight and Bennet[137] in 1990 reported the case of a 2-year-old boy with osteogenesis imperfecta who was the victim of child abuse. They noted that most children with osteogenesis imperfecta and fractures do not have associated bruising or soft tissue injuries. When soft tissue injuries are present, the possibility of child abuse must be considered.

Care must also be taken in distinguishing a toddler's fracture from fracture in an abused child. Mellick and Reesor[169] recognized another accidental spiral tibia fracture that occurs in children between 2 and 6 years of age. It is similar to a toddler's fracture and overlaps the same age range, although it requires more energy and is more visible radiographically. The fracture begins more proximally at the middle rather than the distal third of the tibia. The fibula is not involved. This fracture is usually the result of a fall with a torque or rotational component. Most tibia fractures in abused children are diaphyseal and transverse rather than distal and spiral. Also, a concomitant fracture of the fibular shaft is suggestive of an abused child because the energy necessary to fracture both bones is much greater than that causing a toddler's fracture or an isolated spiral fracture in an older child. Skeletal surveys are necessary in suspected cases to assess for previous healing fractures and evidence of subperiosteal new bone formation

secondary to blunt trauma. If a truly accidental origin cannot be confirmed immediately, the child requires admission to the hospital and evaluation by the child abuse team.

Management of tibia fractures in battered children is similar to that described for isolated tibia and combined tibial and fibular shaft fractures. Closed reduction with simple cast immobilization is usually sufficient in these young children. The most important aspect is the diagnosis and appropriate intervention to prevent further injuries and possible death.

## BICYCLE SPOKE INJURIES

Bicycle spoke injuries of the lower extremity, especially over the medial malleoli, are relatively common in children. They may be caused by the lower part of the leg becoming trapped between the spokes of the wheel and the frame of the bicycle when the child is being transported as a passenger. They may also result from bicycling accidents. These injuries can produce severe compression or crushing of the soft tissues over the foot and ankle. A fracture may also result[71] (Fig. 15–6). Karrholm and associates[130] reported that 39 of 462 pediatric tibial and fibular shaft fractures (8%) were caused by spoke injuries. Izant and co-workers[117] reviewed 60 cases of bicycle spoke injuries and found that most of the children were between 2 and 8 years old, with a mean of 5 years. In almost every instance the

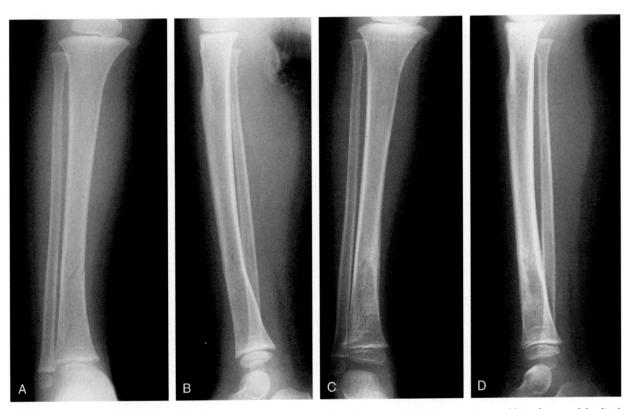

FIGURE 15–6. *A*, Anteroposterior radiograph of the lower portion of the right leg of a 3-year-old girl demonstrating an oblique fracture of the distal end of the right tibia and an intact fibula. This injury occurred when her leg was trapped between bicycle spokes and a rear fender support while sitting in an unprotected rear passenger seat. The skin and subcutaneous tissues were contused and abraded, but no lacerations occurred. *B*, A lateral radiograph demonstrates mild anterior angulation of the fracture. *C*, Two months after the injury, the fracture is well healed. *D*, Lateral radiograph demonstrating no change in alignment.

injury occurred while two children were on a bicycle built for one.

The initial appearance of the extremity can be deceiving. The skin may appear to only be abraded, but over the next 2 to 3 days an area of full-thickness skin loss may develop. These injuries bear a striking similarity to wringer injuries of the upper extremity. Izant and colleagues[117] recognized three aspects of this injury: (1) laceration of the tissues from the knifelike action of the spokes, (2) crushing from impingement between the wheel and the bicycle frame, and (3) shearing injuries from the coefficient of these two forces. Lacerations usually involve the area over the medial malleoli or the Achilles tendon. Simple suture closure may result in dehiscence of the wound, which may prolong secondary healing. The decision to perform a skin graft must await adequate demarcation of the area of necrosis and wide débridement. The most common site of skin necrosis is over the malleoli, where the skin and subcutaneous tissues are thin. All children with spoke injuries should be admitted to the hospital for observation. Treatment recommendations after fracture management, if necessary, include well-padded splints over dressings, mild elevation, and frequent wound inspection. Débridement is performed as necrosis becomes apparent, followed by early split-thickness skin grafting. Closure of initial lacerations is done only after careful débridement, with special attention to defatting the thick skin flaps when the laceration involves the heel.

## STRESS FRACTURES

Pediatric stress fractures are uncommon and frequently lead to misdiagnosis, especially in young children. The pattern of stress fractures in children is different from that in adults. The tibia and fibula are the most common pediatric bones to sustain stress fractures,[172] and boys are affected more frequently than girls. Stress fractures are more common in adolescents and are similar to those in adults. A stress fracture incurred by a young child may resemble osteomyelitis or a malignant process. Roberts and Vogt[205] in 1939 were the first to describe stress fractures of the tibia in children. They found 12 children who had stress fractures, or "pseudofractures," involving the proximal third of the tibia. Since their report, numerous authors have described stress fractures involving the tibia in children.*

Children typically present with mild pain and a limp that was gradual in onset. Although no history of a specific injury may be elicited, frequently, an older child has participated in vigorous physical activities, such as sports, to which the child is unaccustomed or not properly conditioned.[27, 113, 172, 236] In a review of pediatric stress fractures, Devas[57] confirmed that the proximal end of the tibia is the most common site, with the peak incidence between 10 and 15 years of age. The pain is typically relieved by rest and exacerbated by returning to activities. The most common positive physical finding is local tenderness to palpation or percussion over the

fracture site. Typically, no soft tissue swelling, erythema, or ecchymoses are present.

The radiographic diagnosis of a stress fracture of the tibia and fibula is frequently difficult, especially in young children.[67, 145, 171, 198, 213, 218] Radiographic changes may even be absent. Pediatric tibial stress fractures most commonly involve the posteromedial or posterolateral aspect of the proximal third of the tibia. They do not occur in the anterior aspect. Engh and colleagues[67] recognized that the typical radiographic changes occur in three phases. Initially, a small area of radiolucency is seen in the cortex in the posterior wall of the tibia. This abnormality is associated with some metaphyseal and endosteal increase in bone density and a fine haze of periosteal reaction. These findings are usually present 2 to 3 weeks after the onset of symptoms, but this phase is often missed in children. No linear fracture is seen radiographically, and follow-up radiographs show a gradual increase in periosteal and endosteal new bone formation. The second phase is sometimes associated with the appearance of a definite incomplete defect in the posterior cortex. If a complete fracture does not occur, the third phase involves maturation and partial resorption of the periosteal and endosteal new bone formation. If a fracture line becomes apparent, it is typically that of a nondisplaced fracture, and the characteristic radiographic sequence then follows.

In difficult cases, technetium bone scans may be of benefit. In 1977, Prather and associates[198] reported on 42 patients suspected of having stress fractures. Of the 21 in whom stress fractures were ultimately diagnosed, radiographs were normal in 15, but bone scans were positive in each case, including eight stress fractures of the tibia and one involving the fibula. These investigators found that bone scans were a highly sensitive technique for the early diagnosis of stress fractures and that the findings on bone scans can be identified long before radiographic changes. Roub and co-workers[213] reported that the typical bone scan appearance of a stress fracture of the tibia consists of a sharply marginated oval or fusiform area of increased radiodensity located posteromedially. It occasionally extends the width of the bone at the area of involvement. The medial aspect of the tibial cortex is more commonly involved. Meurman and Elfving[171] found that the mean delay between positive bone scans and positive radiographs in stress fractures in adults was 10.5 days. Currently, MRI may also be beneficial in recognizing stress fractures while avoiding the use of ionizing radiation. Lee and Yao[145] described characteristic MRI features of stress fractures that are useful in distinguishing between occult fractures and other subtle abnormalities. These changes include intraosseous bands of very low signal intensity that are continuous with the cortex, as well as juxtacortical or periosteal findings of high signal intensity.

Stress fractures of the fibula can also occur.[40, 58, 85, 113, 172] Devas and Sweetnam[58] stated that the fibula may sustain a stress fracture at a younger age than any other bone. Griffiths[85] reported eight children between 2 and 8 years of age who had stress fractures in the distal third of the fibula. Ingersoll[113] reported three patients with stress fractures of the lower part of the

---

*See references 22, 27, 57, 67, 98, 113, 145, 172, 219, 236.

fibula. All three were ice skaters, but the process may also occur in other children who participate in vigorous physical activities.

Clinical examination usually shows an area of tenderness proximal to the lateral malleolus. The involved area is generally tender to palpation, and mild soft tissue swelling may be present. Plain radiographs may be diagnostic, but in difficult cases, a technetium bone scan may be indicated.

Treatment of tibial or fibular stress fractures is usually conservative. In most cases, restriction of physical activities relieves the discomfort and allows healing of the fracture. Occasionally, immobilization in a long or short leg plaster cast, depending on the involved bone, may be necessary for 2 to 4 weeks in children with significant discomfort. A stress fracture of the distal end of the fibula may also be treated with a removable air stirrup splint.

## IPSILATERAL TIBIA AND FEMUR FRACTURES

Ipsilateral tibial and femoral shaft fractures in children are severe injuries, usually the result of high-velocity accidents such as motor vehicle collisions.[26, 29, 147, 267] As a consequence, these fractures are commonly open, and the victims often sustain other body area injuries. These fractures produce the so-called "floating" knee. In 1975, Blake and McBryde[26] reported on nonoperative treatment in eight children (eight extremities) with ipsilateral tibia and femur fractures. Four patients (50%) had significant lower extremity length discrepancy or angular malunion. Letts and colleagues[147] in 1986 in a study of 15 children with this combined injury found the treatment difficult. Results were poor when both fractures were treated nonoperatively, and it was recommended that at least one of the fractures be rigidly stabilized by either internal or external fixation techniques. Stabilization maintains alignment of the knee and minimizes problems with angulation and malrotation.

Bohn and Durbin[29] reviewed 44 consecutive ipsilateral femur and tibia fractures in 42 children and skeletally immature adolescents. Thirty patients (32 limbs) had a mean follow-up of 5.1 years (range, 1 to 14 years), and 19 were available for personal examination and radiographs. The 24 boys and 6 girls had a mean age of 10.5 years (range, 3.6 to 16.6 years). Twenty-seven of the children sustained their fractures in automobile-related accidents, including 17 automobile-pedestrian accidents. Three injury patterns were identified: double-shaft fractures (femur and tibia both fractured in the diaphysis), juxta-articular fractures, and epiphyseal fractures. Twelve of the 30 children had one or both fractures open, 17 children had at least one additional fracture, and 15 had another body area injury, especially cranial. Closed methods of treatment of both fractures were used in 18 patients. Ten patients had operative stabilization of one fracture, and 10 had operative stabilization of both fractures. Eight patients had operative fixation of their femur fractures (closed intramedullary rod, open intramedullary rod, or compression plate and screws), including one of the three open fractures. Twenty-three patients (24 limbs) had

their tibia fractures treated by closed reduction and cast immobilization. External fixation was used in five open fractures, and pins in plaster were used in four unstable fractures. One fracture was treated by open reduction and internal fixation.

These authors found age to be the most important variable related to the clinical course. Of the 15 patients who were younger than 10 years, the mean time to unsupported weight bearing was 13 weeks and the mean combined femoral and tibial overgrowth was 1.8 cm. Three children had early complications. Of the 15 patients who were older than 10 years, 8 had early complications, the mean time to unsupported weight bearing was 20 weeks, and femoral and tibial growth was variable. The younger children were treated successfully with closed techniques for both fractures, whereas the older children were more successfully treated with reduction and surgical stabilization of the femur fracture. The older group had the highest incidence of complications, including four with unrecognized ipsilateral knee ligament injuries. These injuries included four anterior cruciate ligament tears and two medial collateral ligament injuries. Careful examination of the knee was recommended at the time of initial evaluation. The juxta-articular injury patterns in the older children had the highest incidence of early and late complications. Of the 19 patients who were personally evaluated by the authors, only 7 had normal function. The remainder had compromised results consisting of lower extremity length inequality, angular deformity, or knee instability.

In 2000, Yue and associates[267] studied 29 children (30 extremities) with ipsilateral femur and tibia fractures treated nonoperatively (group 1) and operatively with rigid stabilization of one or both fractures (group 2). The mean follow-up was 8.6 years (range, 1.1 to 18.6 years). The nonoperative group consisted of 16 patients (16 extremities) treated by skeletal traction of the femoral fracture, closed reduction and splinting or casting of the tibia fracture, and an eventual hip spica cast. The operative group of 13 patients (14 extremities) had one or both fractures treated by open reduction and internal fixation (Fig. 15–7). The same criteria of Bohn and Durbin[29] were used in the evaluation of these patients to make the studies comparable. Despite higher modified injury scores and skeletal injury scores, the children and adolescents treated operatively had significantly reduced hospital stays, 20.1 versus 34.9 days, respectively; decreased time to unsupported weight bearing, 16.8 versus 22.3 weeks; and fewer complications. Operative stabilization of the femur had a significant effect on decreasing the length of hospital stay and the time to unassisted weight bearing. The patients were also analyzed according to their age at injury: 9 years or younger and 10 years and older. The younger children treated nonoperatively had an increased rate of lower leg length discrepancy, angular malunion, and need for a secondary surgical procedure when compared with younger children treated operatively with rigid fixation. Based on the results of this study, the authors recommended operative stabilization of at least the femur and preferably both fractures in a child with a "floating" knee, even for younger children.

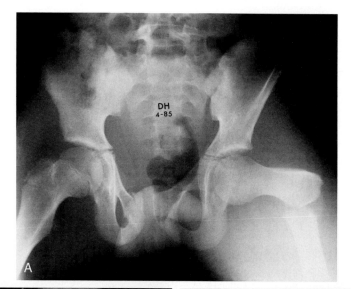

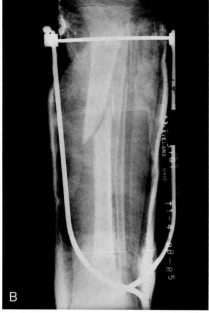

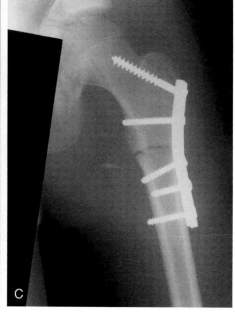

FIGURE 15–7. *A,* Anteroposterior radiograph of the pelvis of an 11-year-old boy who was struck by an automobile. A closed, displaced left subtrochanteric femur fracture can be seen. Minimally displaced fractures of the right superior and inferior pubic rami have occurred. This child also sustained an ipsilateral closed, displaced tibial and fibular shaft fracture. The subtrochanteric fracture was initially treated with skeletal traction via a threaded Steinmann pin through the proximal part of the tibia. *B,* The tibia fracture was reduced and immobilized in a long leg plaster cast incorporating the proximal tibial traction pin. Unfortunately, alignment of both the femoral and tibial fractures was unsatisfactory. *C,* The left subtrochanteric femoral fracture was subsequently managed by open reduction and internal fixation with a compression plate and screws.

## TIBIA FRACTURES IN CHILDREN WITH NEUROMUSCULAR DISORDERS

Children with neuromuscular disorders such as myelo-meningocele,* paraplegia from spinal cord injury or tumor,[63, 73, 159, 207] head injury,[264] spinal muscular atrophy,[159] muscular dystrophy,[159] cerebral palsy,[159, 167] and arthrogryposis multiplex congenita, especially those who are nonambulatory, are at risk for fractures and epiphyseal displacement of the tibia and fibula. These fractures must be treated in accordance with the underlying diagnosis and the degree of functional impairment. Although comprehensive care programs, including aggressive orthotic management and appropriately timed surgery, may prevent fractures by increasing the exposure of bone to weight bearing, maximal

*See references 35, 74, 79, 81, 92, 120, 152, 159, 192, 200, 228, 233, 244.

function may expose the patient to an increased risk of fractures.

The major pathophysiologic change in the bones of children with neuromuscular disorders is osteopenia. Abnormal mechanical properties secondary to lack of weight bearing and normal joint motion result in osteoporosis and inherent fragility and predispose to fracture with minimal trauma. Osteoporotic bone has been demonstrated to be physically soft and therefore has less strength and less stiffness than normal bone does.[61] Developing bone deprived of neuromuscular activity has diminished cross-sectional area, cortical thickness, and bone circumference, and qualitatively and quantitatively inferior bone results.[200] Walton and Warrick[257] correlated the severity of change with the age at onset of the neuromuscular disease and emphasized the importance of muscle activity in normal growth and development of bone. Although decreased bone mass may result from loss of motor function, when sensory loss is also present, the bone effects are increased.[154] In these cases, epiphyseal separation can occur. Stern and co-workers[233] reported separation of the distal tibial and fibular epiphyses in a child with myelodysplasia. Other cases of unilateral slippage of the proximal and distal tibial epiphyses have been reported.[81, 228] These abnormalities occurred with minimal or no injury and resembled osteomyelitis both clinically and radiographically.

Neuromuscular disorders in children disturb the normal pattern of bone growth and development in a variety of ways and result in bone with thin cortices and decreased mass. Loss of muscle and weight-bearing forces produces abnormal bone and joint shape. Associated soft tissue contractures resulting from muscle imbalance and weakness may also predispose to fracture by placing excessive stress on the adjacent metaphyseal

regions, especially about the knee. Makin[158] demonstrated that shortening of the lower portion of the leg in children secondary to acute poliomyelitis in infancy was asymmetric and that the fibula was shorter than the tibia. This length discrepancy may contribute to deformity of the ankle, tibia, and knee. In addition, an association with abnormal stresses and fracture may be seen. Similar observations regarding shortening of the fibula were made by Dias in an analysis of 86 children with myelomeningocele.[59]

The clinical features of fractures of the tibia and fibula in a child with a neuromuscular disease are commonly modified. Fractures may occur with no history of trauma or after a trivial injury. Even gentle physical therapy and passive exercise may unintentionally cause a fracture. Boytim and colleagues[35] recognized that myelodysplastic

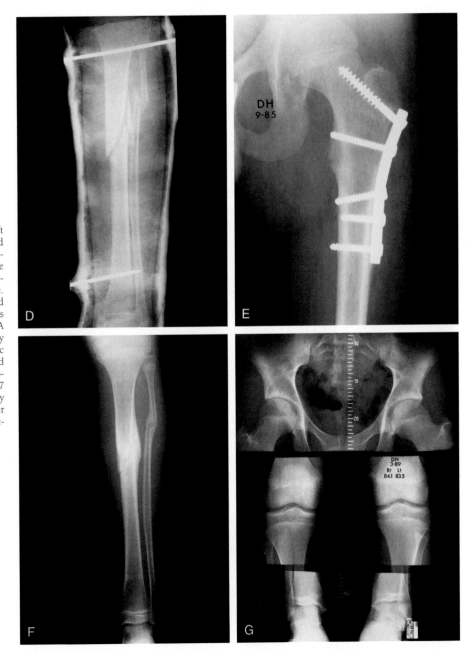

FIGURE 15–7 *Continued. D,* The left tibia and fibula fractures were treated by repeat closed reduction and immobilization in a long leg cast after the addition of a second threaded Steinmann pin distal to the tibia fracture. Satisfactory alignment was achieved and maintained. This radiograph was obtained 2 months after injury. *E,* A radiograph taken 5 months after injury demonstrates that the subtrochanteric fracture is well healed. *F,* The tibia and fibula fractures also healed satisfactorily. *G,* A scanogram obtained 47 months after injury demonstrates only 6 mm of shortening in the left lower extremity. The patient is almost skeletally mature and is asymptomatic.

infants with thoracic and upper lumbar neurologic levels and soft tissue contractures were prone to fractures during physical therapy. Common physical signs include warmth, erythema, and swelling. If sensation is normal, pain is obviously present. However, in the absence of sensation, as occurs in myelomeningocele and spinal cord injury, fever may also be present. Townsend and associates[244] reviewed a series of myelomeningocele patients with fractures who had elevated temperatures averaging 38.2°C and whose white blood cell counts were over 11,000 cells/mm.[3] The erythrocyte sedimentation rate may also be elevated, but calcium phosphorus and alkaline phosphatase values are usually normal.[63] An occasional patient may become toxic and extremely ill, as noted by Freehafer and co-workers.[74]

Whatever the underlying neuromuscular disorder, the goals of treatment are to achieve satisfactory alignment of the extremity and return the patient to the preinjury level of function. The major principle is to provide minimal immobilization of the patient and the limb compatible with union in a satisfactory position. What constitutes an acceptable position is based on the ambulatory abilities of the individual. Functional alignment, including rotation, must be achieved so that standing, walking, use of an orthosis, or wheelchair sitting will not be compromised. In displaced fractures in nonambulators, less than perfect alignment may be adequate. The specific method of treatment is individualized for the child, the underlying diagnosis, and the functional level.

Fractures of the tibia and fibula in children with neuromuscular diseases are characterized by rapid healing and absence of serious displacement. As a consequence, nonoperative methods are usually sufficient, as well as desirable. In nonambulatory children, bulky cotton roll dressings or pillow splints may be all that is necessary to maintain satisfactory alignment of the fractured tibia. Plaster or thermoplastic splints may also be used. Once the acute swelling subsides, the patient's orthosis may be used to support the fracture. If a child is able to stand, standing should be allowed as soon as possible after injury. If the fracture displacement, angulation, or rotation is too severe, a short or long leg plaster cast may be required.

Matejczyk and Rang[159] reviewed the distribution of fractures in children with neuromuscular disorders at the Hospital for Sick Children in Toronto. They found that most fractures occurred in the region of the knee joint. The femur, followed by the tibia, was most commonly fractured, especially the distal femoral and proximal tibial metaphyses. In children with myelodysplasia, fractures tended to occur predominantly in areas with no functioning muscles. Fractures occurred most often after falls and removal of postoperative hip spica casts or after immobilization for other reasons. Freehafer and co-workers[74] demonstrated that the occurrence of fractures after immobilization can be minimized by allowing the child to stand in the postoperative spica cast as soon as possible after surgery.

The major problem with fractures in children with muscular dystrophy is decreased ambulatory ability. Even short periods of immobilization without weight bearing may result in premature loss of walking ability. Falls are the most common cause of fracture, and fractures occur in children who are walking with orthoses or fall from a wheelchair. Fractures of the tibial shaft and proximal and distal metaphyses are most frequent in children who are still ambulatory.

McIvor and Samilson,[167] as well as Matejczyk and Rang,[159] found that only severely involved institutionalized patients with cerebral palsy have an increased risk for fracture of the extremity. McIvor and Samilson[167] reported a 7% prevalence of fractured extremities in more than 1000 patients confined to a state hospital. Severe preexisting disuse osteoporosis was associated with fractures and was similar to that seen in other neuromuscular disorders. Internal fixation was successful if nonoperative treatment was precluded because of spasticity.

## PATHOLOGIC FRACTURES

Fractures through preexisting osseous tumors, benign or malignant, may be the first indication of a pathologic process (see Chapter 3). These fractures are usually realigned and temporarily immobilized in a long leg posterior splint while a thorough evaluation of the pathologic lesion is performed. Pathologic fractures in the proximal metaphysis may result in an acquired valgus deformity. Jordan and associates[127] reported a 14° valgus deformity over a 2-year period in a 4-year-old boy after fracture through a large simple bone cyst in the proximal end of the tibia. The deformity spontaneously corrected to 4° over the next 7 years. Pathologic fractures of the proximal tibial metaphysis resulting in acquired valgus deformities have also been reported after osteomyelitis.[9] Definitive management is based on the diagnosis and natural history of the lesion.

## Isolated Fractures of the Fibular Diaphysis

Isolated fracture of the fibular shaft is rare and usually the result of a direct blow to the lateral aspect of the leg. These fractures may be compression (torus), incomplete tension-compression (greenstick), complete, or plastic deformation (bend) fractures. Such fractures typically heal with only simple immobilization (Fig. 15–8). A peroneal nerve palsy may accompany a proximal fibula fracture in direct injuries to the nerve itself. Complications in healing and subsequent growth are rare; however, it is important to rule out the presence of an associated physeal injury of the distal end of the tibia because a high fracture of the fibula can be seen in pronation-eversion–external rotation injuries to the ankle.[60]

## Fractures of the Distal Tibial Metaphysis

The distal tibial metaphysis may sustain fractures similar to those in the proximal end of the tibia. These injuries are predominantly compression (torus) or incomplete

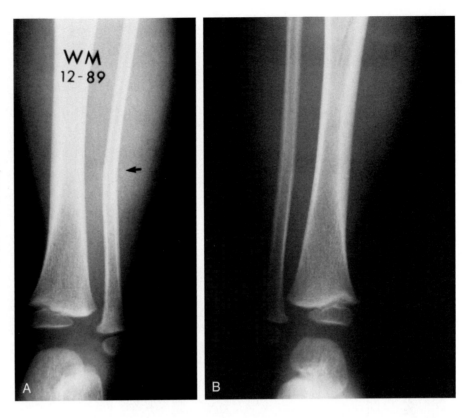

**FIGURE 15–8.** *A,* Anteroposterior radiograph of the lower part of the left leg of a 2-year-old child who was observed to be limping. No history of injury was elicited. Plastic deformation of the distal third of the fibula has produced a slight valgus deformity *(arrow). B,* Comparison view of the lower portion of the right leg. The fibula is normal.

tension-compression (greenstick) fractures. Complete fractures may occur, but the thick tibial periosteum and the tendency for the fibula to remain intact or to plastically deform limit major displacement.[182] The most common fracture is a greenstick fracture, in which the posterior cortex is fractured and the anterior cortex impacted and angulated. This mechanism results in a radiographic and occasionally a clinical recurvatum deformity.

Metaphyseal fractures of the distal end of the tibia are typically visible on standard AP and lateral radiographs. Toddler's fractures may occasionally not be visible on the initial radiographs but should be treated symptomatically if a fracture is suspected. Special radiographic studies such as technetium bone scans are not usually indicated.

Treatment of distal tibial metaphyseal fractures depends on the displacement or angulation of the fracture. Nondisplaced fractures require only simple immobilization in a long leg cast. A short leg cast may be appropriate in certain cases, depending on the fracture pattern and the child's age and reliability. Any angular deformity should be corrected, especially varus or valgus angulation. If significant recurvatum is present, closed reduction should be performed. This technique is usually difficult because of impaction and requires general anesthesia. Immobilization in a long leg cast with the foot in plantar flexion for 3 to 4 weeks, followed by a short leg walking cast until healing is complete, will maintain alignment.

Fractures of the distal tibial metaphysis generally heal quickly and without significant deformity (Fig. 15–9). They are not associated with the problems of asymmetric overgrowth and progressive angular deformity, which occur in fractures of the proximal metaphysis.

## Open Tibia and Fibula Fractures

Open fractures of the tibia and fibula in children are serious injuries with a high complication rate.* They are invariably the result of high-velocity trauma. Motor vehicle–related accidents account for over 80% of open fractures, and most occur in children older than 2 years. Even in adolescents, athletic activities account for less than 5% of open fractures. Although some open tibia fractures may involve the proximal or distal tibial metaphyses, most occur in the diaphyses or shafts.

The prevalence of open tibial and fibular shaft fractures in children varies between 2% and 14%.[95, 115, 142, 222, 230, 253, 254, 266] Hansen and colleagues[95] in 1976 reported that 14 of 102 pediatric tibia fractures treated in 1971 (14%) were open. In larger, more recent studies, the incidence is less. Yasko and Wilber[266] in 1989 reported that 53 of 1049 consecutive tibia fractures (5%) in skeletally immature patients seen between 1972 and 1988 were open. Irwin and associates[115] in 1995 found that 58 of 1400 consecutive tibial fractures (4%) were open. It has been estimated that 1% of open tibia fractures occur before the age of 2 years, 15% to 20% from 2 to 6 years of age, and about 40% each in those aged 6 to 10 years and 10 to 14 years.[253, 254] The rarity of open fractures in children

---

*See references 12, 25, 38, 39, 49, 50, 86, 106, 115, 140, 142, 199, 206, 227, 253, 254, 266.

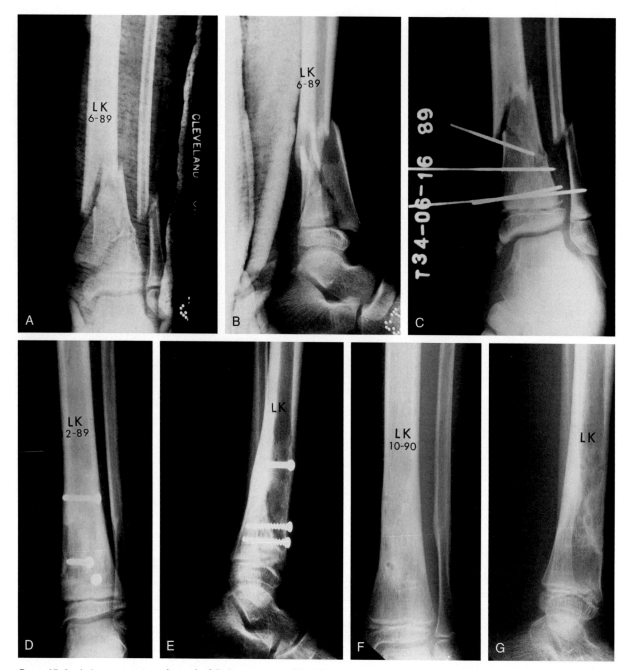

**FIGURE 15–9.** *A,* Anteroposterior radiograph of the lower portion of the left leg of a 9-year-old girl who was struck by an automobile while riding her bicycle. A very comminuted fracture involving the left distal tibial metaphysis is evident. In addition, she has a Salter-Harris type II distal tibial epiphyseal fracture. *B,* A lateral radiograph demonstrates displacement of the anteromedial portion of the metaphysis of the Salter-Harris type II epiphyseal fracture. *C,* Limited internal fixation was performed because the fracture was unstable, and satisfactory alignment could not be achieved by closed reduction. Initial alignment was obtained with multiple K-wires followed by cortical screws. *D,* Nine months after surgery, the fractures have healed and the distal tibial physis remains open. *E,* Lateral radiograph confirming no evidence of premature physeal closure. *F,* Fourteen months after surgery, the screws have been removed. The distal tibial physis is open, and normal growth and development are occurring. *G,* Lateral radiograph 14 months after surgery.

younger than school age is related to their small body mass and large amount of protective subcutaneous fat. In addition, young children are rarely exposed to high-velocity injuries, which threaten life rather than limb in this age group.

Because most open tibia and fibula fractures are caused by severe trauma, the incidence of other body area injuries is high. These injuries include other

fractures, closed head injuries, and blunt abdominal and chest trauma* (see Chapter 4). The prevalence of associated injuries in children with open tibia fractures has varied between 15% and 74% in recent studies.[39, 49, 106, 115, 140, 206, 266] In closed fractures, both the

---

*See references 12, 25, 38, 39, 49, 50, 86, 95, 106, 115, 140, 142, 206, 222, 227, 253, 254, 266.

tibia and the fibula are fractured in about 33% of cases, whereas in open fractures, both bones are fractured approximately 85% of the time.[115] Comminution is also more common in open fractures. It occurs in approximately 33% of open fractures as opposed to only 5% to 10% of closed fractures.

## ASSESSMENT AND INJURY CLASSIFICATION

In the past, open tibia and fibula fractures were managed as closed fractures, with the exception of local wound care. Recent studies indicate that these fractures must be managed similar to open fractures in adults, with the possible exception of fracture stabilization. The type and incidence of complications are similar, but children appear to have better long-term results.[25, 206] The classification system of open fractures by Gustilo and associates,[88, 89] which was based on adult injuries, is also used to classify pediatric open tibia and fibula fractures and to guide subsequent management.

Despite advances in prehospital resuscitation and the development of free flaps and microvascular reconstruction,[107, 116, 148, 168] many limbs with severe open fractures, including those with vascular compromise[54, 152] or partial amputation, cannot be salvaged. Some of the most severe open tibia fractures may be better managed with a below-knee amputation than with extensive reconstructive procedures that may leave the patient with a poor cosmetic result and only marginal function. A number of investigators have developed severity indices to provide some guidance when the decision is between limb salvage and amputation.[30, 123] Johansen and co-workers[123] in 1990 developed the Mangled Extremity Severity Score, which is a rating scale for lower extremity trauma based on skeletal and soft tissue damage, limb ischemia, shock, and age of the patient. Although reproducibility of the score has been questioned, scores of seven and higher have, in a number of studies, been a good indicator for the need to amputate.[100] To what extent this score is useful for the assessment of pediatric lower extremity injury is not known at this time. Minimal requirements for a functional restorable limb include (1) an intact or restorable blood supply and (2) a sufficient sleeve of viable muscle to provide for stable soft tissue coverage and limb function that is superior to a below-knee amputation. When amputation is inevitable, early intervention enhances patient survival, reduces pain and disability, and shortens the length of hospitalization.[30]

It has also become apparent that some closed fractures caused by violent force may result in extensive soft tissue destruction without resulting in an open lesion.[246, 247] Typically, these injuries are characterized by skin contusions, deep abrasions, burns, or frank separation of the cutis from the subcuticular tissue. Even in children, these lesions can result in delayed partial or full skin and subcutaneous loss and secondary infection of the fracture site. To avoid such catastrophes, these lesions must be treated as open fractures. Tscherne and Oestern[247] developed a classification system that describes four severity grades of these injuries. This system can be useful in choosing among different treatment options.

## TREATMENT

The goals of treatment of open tibia fractures in children are the same as for adults: (1) preventing wound sepsis, (2) ensuring healing of soft tissues, (3) achieving bone union, and (4) returning the patient to optimal function.[87, 90] Measures to achieve these goals include emergency resuscitation and a thorough initial evaluation focusing in sequence on vital functions, limb-threatening injuries, and then the extremity fracture that is compromising the soft tissues. Other important measures include appropriate antimicrobial therapy, extensive and possibly repeated wound débridement, fracture stabilization, measures that facilitate wound closure, early autogenous cancellous bone grafting, and vigorous rehabilitation[88–91] (Fig. 15–10). These measures are discussed in more detail in Chapter 19.

After initial resuscitation and careful assessment of the whole patient, priorities and plans for the treatment of all injuries are established with participation of the key medical services while the patient is still in the emergency room. There, the patient will also receive tetanus prophylaxis and the appropriate antibiotic or antibiotics.

More extensive evaluation of the wound, the initial débridement, and stabilization of the principal fracture fragments occur in the operating room. Fracture stabilization reduces pain, prevents additional injuries to surrounding soft tissues, decreases the spread of bacteria, and allows for early soft tissue and bone repair. For fractures with more extensive soft tissue injury, the method of stabilization must allow for free limb access to assess limb viability and to carry out repeated débridement. It must also be sufficiently rigid to permit early range-of-motion exercises of adjacent joints and possibly partial weight bearing.

**Splints and Casts.** Plaster splints and plaster-reinforced cotton-wool dressings (Robert Jones dressings) can be used for the early care of some stable type I and type II open fractures.[142, 222] Once the soft tissue swelling has subsided and the wounds are closed, better fracture stabilization is needed. In many children, such stabilization can be achieved with a well-padded long leg cast with the knee in approximately 10° of flexion.[95, 104, 115, 206, 230] Younger children, up to 8 years of age, can be immobilized in a long leg cast until their fractures are healed, usually 6 to 10 weeks after injury. In older children, the long leg cast is exchanged for a well-molded short leg cast after 4 to 5 weeks, when early callus formation is evident radiographically. The short leg cast remains in place for another 1 to 2 months, when most open tibia fractures have healed.

**External Fixation.** Splints and casts cannot prevent shortening of unstable fractures. Such lesions and most type II and type III open fractures, which may require prolonged observation, repeated débridement, secondary flap procedures, or bone grafts, are best managed with external fixators.[16, 19, 141, 206] When properly applied, external fixators allow free access to the wound for repeated débridement. The fixator frames should be of sufficient rigidity to prevent further injuries to the soft tissues, preserve length, and allow progressive weight bearing with dynamization.[3, 15, 17–19, 95, 115, 132, 202]

In older children and adolescents, external fixators designed for adults are ideal. However, for smaller children, fixators used for adult wrist fractures or a combination of smaller pins with adult clamps and connecting rods is more appropriate.[52] The diameter of the fixator pins should not exceed a quarter of the diameter of the tibia; thus, pins with diameters ranging from 2.5 to 4 mm are most appropriate for children younger than 12 years.[17]

To construct fixator frames of sufficient rigidity, many surgeons use such optimizing methods as a wide pin spread, dual longitudinal bars, and two-plane unilateral or two-plane bilateral designs.[20, 243] Nevertheless, with

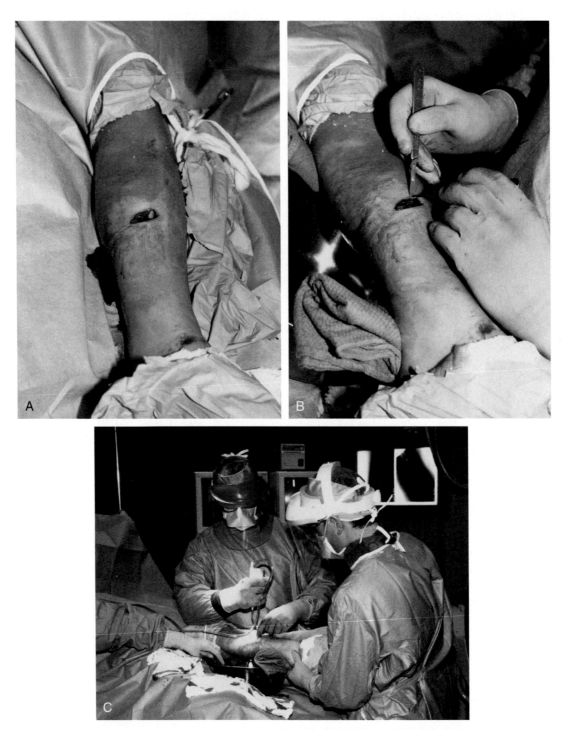

FIGURE 15–10. *A*, Intraoperative clinical photograph of a type IIIB open tibia and fibula shaft fracture in an 11-year-old girl who was struck by an automobile. *B*, Débridement of the skin margins, subcutaneous tissues, and muscle and direct visualization of the fracture and inspection of the bone ends. *C*, Pulsed irrigation with 7 to 10 L of normal saline.

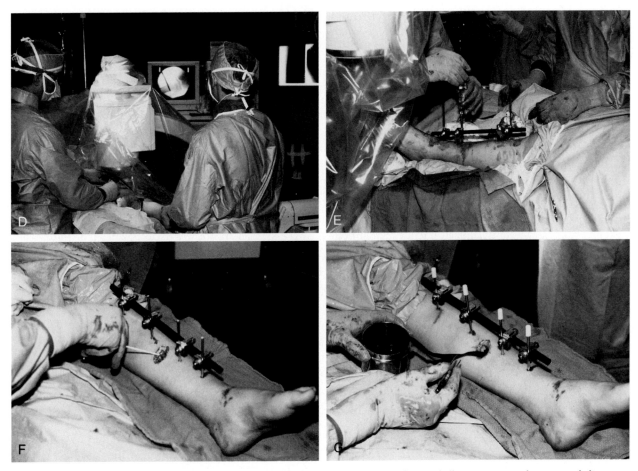

FIGURE 15–10 *Continued. D,* Application of an external fixator under fluoroscopic control. Such control allows proper pin placement and alignment, avoids possible physeal injury, and facilitates final reduction. *E,* Final adjustments of the half-frame external fixator. *F,* Tissue for culture is obtained intraoperatively after débridement, irrigation, and application of the external fixator. *G,* Packing of the wound. In this case, povidone-iodine (Betadine)-soaked gauze was used, followed by the application of sterile dressings and a long leg posterior plaster splint.

the exception of athletic or obese teenagers, simple one-plane unilateral frames routinely achieve sufficient rigidity for early weight bearing. Ring fixators using wires under tension are useful to treat tibial fractures with extensive comminution and fractures extending close to the epiphyseal plates. These devices, which are generally more versatile than unilateral frames, are also preferred for correction of length discrepancy, malalignment, and soft tissue contracture. Ring fixators, however, tend to obstruct the wound.

To provide optimal stabilization with minimal complications, three basic criteria are used when external fixators are applied: (1) they should not damage vital anatomy, (2) they should provide sufficient wound access for débridement and secondary procedures, and (3) the frame should be appropriate to the mechanical demands of the patient.[19]

As a limb segment in which the principal long bone lies eccentrically, the tibia is ideally suited for the application of an external frame. The anteromedial aspect of the tibia is a safe corridor where pins can be inserted without the risk of impaling neurovascular structures or myotendinous units. Occasionally, pins may be inserted into the epiphysis. Great care must be taken when pins are placed periarticularly because the undulating shape

of the physis creates an unsafe zone that varies in width from 1 to 2 cm.[3] Pins injuring the physis can cause growth disturbances. Epiphyseal pins also demand meticulous pin care to prevent osteomyelitis and septic arthritis. With careful technique and the use of an image intensifier, epiphyseal pins can be placed safely and can be highly effective in the management of fractures, especially those with a comminuted metaphyseal component.

External fixators are applied in the operating room under general anesthesia and sterile conditions. The leg is draped so that the knee and ankle joint are within the operating field to aid in clinical limb alignment. The most proximal and distal pins are inserted first under image intensification to avoid injuries to the physes. The remaining pins are then inserted, including those for a segmental fragment. An image intensifier is used routinely to check pin location, depth of penetration, and overall limb alignment.[3, 17] Holes for the pins are predrilled with a sharp drill bit through a trocar sleeve that helps protect the soft tissues and facilitates accurate pin placement. Universal articulations that allow for easy alignment are routinely used. If the AO/ASIF fixator is used, care must be taken to avoid malrotation, which is difficult to correct after the insertion of all four pins.[3]

Once the frame is applied, final fracture alignment is documented by long orthogonal radiographs. For pin care, we have found that cleaning the leg and the pin sites once a day with warm water and soap is most effective. This regimen in conjunction with the use of titanium pins has rendered major pin tract complications a rarity. Unless bone loss is a factor, many children and adolescents can bear full weight with minimal external support within 3 to 4 weeks.

**Internal Fixation.** Although the use of screws, plates, and intramedullary nails has revolutionized the treatment of open tibial fractures in adults, they have had less influence on the care of these injuries in children. Screws alone may have a place in the fixation of simple metaphyseal fractures but lack the axial and bending stability needed to hold tibial shaft fractures.[141] In both adults and children, plating of tibial fractures has been accompanied by a higher infection rate.[8, 227] As long as the proximal tibial physis is open, standard intramedullary nails are contraindicated. Flexible intramedullary nails can be an alternative to external fixation.[8, 102, 199, 206, 230] In 2001, Qidwai reported intramedullary fixation in 30 open tibia fractures, including 9 type I, 10 type II, and 11 type III (8 type IIIA and 3 type IIIB) fractures. Eighteen patients underwent primary wound closure, whereas 12 had delayed wound closure. Five patients (17%) had a postoperative infection—four superficial and one deep. The latter occurred in a type IIIB fracture that underwent delayed wound closure. All infections were successfully treated by débridement and intravenous antibiotics. All fractures healed rapidly with good functional outcomes.

## FOLLOW-UP CARE AND REHABILITATION

Once the soft tissues have healed and bone union progresses, rehabilitation is accelerated. Typically, range-of-motion exercises of the knee and ankle are followed by muscle strengthening and gait training. It is important that children undergo long-term follow-up to assess ultimate outcome with respect to function, alignment, and lower extremity length equality.

## RESULTS

The initial results of treatment of open tibia fractures in children were primarily speculative and were included with the results of closed tibia fractures in children.[95, 104, 222, 230] In 1966, Stanford and co-workers[230] studied 94 pediatric tibia fractures, 19 of which were open. They reported on the results of treatment of 18 children, 16 of whom were treated by closed techniques and healed at a mean of 3.1 months. Infection developed in the two fractures treated by open reduction. Healing occurred at 11 and 24 months. Hoaglund and States[104] in 1967 reported on 43 pediatric tibia fractures. Five fractures were open and were treated by closed techniques without complications, with a union time of 3 months. Hansen and colleagues[95] in 1976 reported 14 open fractures treated by cast immobilization that healed without complications. Shannak[222] in 1988 reported on

117 pediatric tibia fractures, 4 of which were open. Three fractures were treated with os calcis traction and one with pin fixation. No complications related to these fractures occurred.

As external fixation of fractures gained popularity in adults, it began to be used in children, especially those with open tibia fractures. The initial results were controversial because of a high incidence of infection and refracture after removal of the device. Alonso and Horowitz[3] reported on use of the AO/ASIF external fixator in children, including 10 of 20 children with tibia fractures (most were open). In one patient with an open proximal metaphyseal fracture, a 12° progressive valgus deformity and 2.5 cm of overgrowth developed, and another patient had a refracture 6 months after injury. The external fixator was used for a mean of 7 weeks, and then a cast was applied. Union was achieved at a mean of 16 weeks. Tolo[242] reported on 13 open tibia fractures treated by external fixation. He reported that half had superficial pin tract infection, although osteomyelitis did not develop in any of the children. Three patients had refracture 5 to 10 months after injury. Two children had mild angular deformities, and three had overgrowth of 1 to 1.4 cm. The fixator was used for a mean of 11 weeks before being removed. Union was achieved at a mean of 21 weeks. This author believed that fracture healing was slightly delayed by use of the external fixator. Bohn and Durbin[29] reported that 8 of 30 children with ipsilateral femur and tibia fractures had open tibia fractures, 5 of whom were treated by external fixation. Two patients had refractures 2 and 14 weeks after they resumed walking. One superficial pin tract infection developed along with two cases of pin tract osteomyelitis that required sequestrectomy.

Between 1989 and 1995, numerous large, relatively standardized studies investigating open tibia fractures in children were conducted.[39, 49, 106, 140, 266] The studies used the classification of Gustilo and associates[88, 89] and followed their treatment recommendations.[88, 90, 91] These studies have demonstrated the true spectrum of pediatric open tibia fractures.

In 1989, Yasko and Wilber[266] presented the results of 53 open tibia fractures in children with a mean age at injury of 10 years (range, 2 to 15 years) and found similar results. These children had 24 type I, 17 type II, and 12 type III (3 type IIIA, 4 type IIIB, and 5 type IIIC) fractures that were monitored for a mean of 5.5 years (range, 6 months to 16 years). In this series, the most common mechanism of injury was motor vehicle accidents (82%). Thirteen children (25%) had other body area injuries, including 9 children with other fractures. External fixation was used in 12 fractures, including 3 type I, 4 type II, and 5 type III injuries (Fig. 15–11). Uncomplicated healing occurred in all type I fractures, whereas delayed union or nonunion occurred in 12% and 50% of the type II and type III fractures, respectively (Fig. 15–12). The overall sepsis rate was 8%, with 6% and 30% of the type II and type III fractures becoming infected, respectively. Two delayed amputations were necessary in type III fractures because of severe sepsis. Four children had delayed union (8%), including one

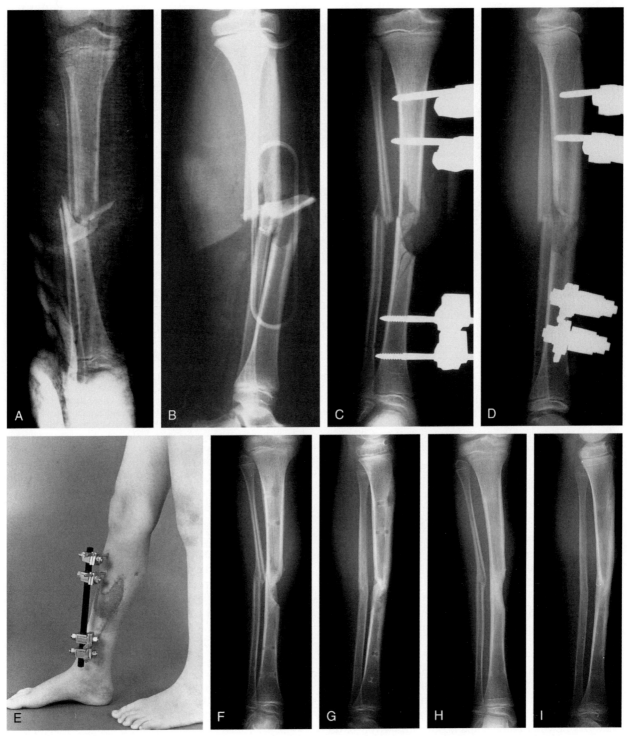

FIGURE 15–11. *A,* Anteroposterior radiograph of the lower part of the right leg of a 6-year-old girl with a comminuted, displaced type IIIB open fracture of the tibial and fibular diaphyses. These fractures were sustained when she was struck by an automobile. *B,* A lateral radiograph demonstrates malrotation and a large, transversely oriented tibial fracture segment. *C,* Radiograph obtained 1 month after débridement, removal of the devascularized tibial fracture fragment, irrigation, stabilization with an external fixator, and a soleus muscle rotation flap covered with a meshed, split-thickness skin graft. A large residual defect is present in the tibia. Leg length was maintained because of reduction of the lateral cortices of the tibia. *D,* Lateral radiograph demonstrating satisfactory alignment. *E,* Clinical photograph 2 months after injury. The wounds are well healed, and the patient is allowed partial weight bearing with crutches. Cancellous bone grafting of the tibial defect was performed at this time. *F,* Anteroposterior radiograph 3 months after injury and 1 month after cancellous bone grafting and removal of the external fixator. The tibial defect is healing satisfactorily. The patient then had 2 months of additional immobilization in a short leg weight-bearing fiberglass cast. *G,* Lateral radiograph showing maintenance of satisfactory alignment. *H,* Six months after injury, excellent reconstitution of the tibial defect has occurred. At this time, the patient was allowed unprotected weight bearing. *I,* Lateral radiograph demonstrating excellent healing and alignment.

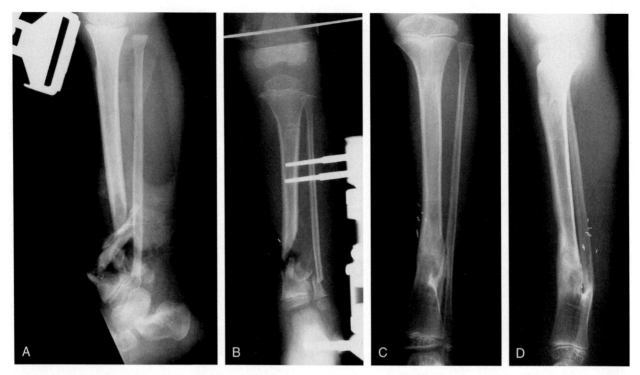

**FIGURE 15–12.** *A,* Anteroposterior radiograph of the lower portion of the left leg of a 3-year-old boy who sustained an open, comminuted, type IIIC fracture of the distal ends of the tibia and fibula when he was struck by an automobile. The closed ipsilateral femoral shaft fracture compromised circulation to the left foot. An arteriogram demonstrated occlusion of both the anterior tibial and the peroneal arteries. Blood flow through the posterior tibial artery was intact. *B,* Radiograph 1 month after extensive débridement, irrigation, application of an external fixator, vascular repair, wound coverage with a rotational skin flap, and cancellous bone grafting. The femoral shaft fracture was treated with skeletal traction through the distal part of the femur. *C,* Radiograph 28 months after injury. The child experienced delayed union and required two additional bone grafts. He ultimately underwent a free microvascular muscle transfer and split-thickness skin grafting to obtain vascularized soft tissue coverage over the fracture. Union ultimately occurred. The patient has equal leg length and normal function. *D,* Lateral radiograph confirming satisfactory alignment, although slight posterior angulation is present.

type II and three type III fractures. One nonunion (2%) occurred in a type IIIC fracture that required bone grafting procedures before union was obtained at 1 year. This study revealed a significant morbidity rate associated with open tibia fractures in children.

In 1990, Buckley and co-workers[39] reported the results of 41 children with 42 open tibia fractures who were monitored at least to fracture healing. The mean age at injury was 9 years 9 months (range, 3 to 16 years), and the mean follow-up period was 15 months (range, 3 to 96 months). This series consisted of 32 boys and 9 girls, for an almost 4:1 ratio. The mechanism of injury was predominantly automobile-pedestrian accidents, which occurred in 29 patients (71%). Twenty-one fractures (50%) were comminuted, and 33 fractures involved the tibial diaphysis. The fibula was fractured in 38 (90%) of the 42 extremities. Twelve type I, 18 type II, and 12 type III (6 type IIIA, 4 type IIIB, and 2 type IIIC) fractures were noted. Nineteen children (46%) had other associated injuries—14 had other fractures, 9 had closed head injuries, 2 had abdominal injuries, and 1 had a pulmonary contusion. Twenty-two of the fractures were immobilized in long leg plaster casts, and 20 had external fixators applied. The indications for external fixation included severe soft tissue injury, the need for a fasciotomy, and an unstable fracture pattern with tibial shortening. Two patients had elevated compartment

pressures that required a four-compartment fasciotomy. All fractures were immobilized until evidence of healing both clinically and radiographically. Wound infection developed in three patients, one of whom progressed to osteomyelitis. Pin tract infections developed in 4 of the 20 patients who were treated with external fixation. All pin tract infections resolved with appropriate treatment. At the time of healing, four fractures had 10° or more of angulation. Spontaneous correction secondary to growth and remodeling occurred in three patients. Corrective osteotomy was necessary in one patient for a 25° diaphyseal angulation—the same patient in whom osteomyelitis and delayed union developed. Four patients had lower extremity length discrepancies greater than 1 cm (range, 1.3 to 2.5 cm). The involved tibia was longer in all four patients, but shortening of more than 1 cm did not occur in any of the children. The average time to union of the fractures was 4.8 months (range, 2 to 22 months); six patients (15%) had delayed union. Most of the delayed unions were directly related to the severity of the soft tissue injury and the fracture pattern. Delayed union occurred in two type II fractures, three type IIIB fractures, and one type IIIC fracture. The patients with segmental bone loss took the longest time to heal. In no children did nonunion occur. The authors thought that their data demonstrated that children with open fractures of the tibia have an incidence of vascular injury,

compartment syndrome, infection, and delayed union similar to that reported for adults. Type I fractures, however, were not associated with these complications and tended to heal relatively quickly in a manner similar to closed fractures. The factor that was unique to open fractures of the tibia in children was tibial overgrowth associated with severe open fractures.

Cramer and colleagues[49] in 1992 studied 40 open diaphyseal fractures, including 22 open tibia fractures, in 35 children with a mean age at injury of 11 years (range, 3 to 16 years). Twenty-six children (74%) had associated injuries, and 30 (86%) were injured in motor vehicle–related accidents. One type I, 10 type II, and 11 type III open tibia fractures occurred, including 4 type IIIC fractures that required arterial repair. Four children needed fasciotomies because of impending compartment syndrome. External fixation was used in 15, casts in 5, and limited internal fixation in 2 fractures. Four patients required amputation—two immediately because of incomplete amputations and 2 because of delayed infection. All amputations occurred in children with type IIIC injuries. Delayed union developed in eight fractures (36%) and nonunion in three (14%). These complications tended to occur in older children with severely comminuted or segmental fractures that were managed by external fixation. They were treated with bone grafting, a change in instrumentation, or prolonged use of external fixation before union was obtained at a mean of 53 weeks (range, 26 to 155 weeks). Infection developed in 10 of the 40 fractures (25%), including 4 children with pin tract infection, 4 with deep soft tissue infection, and 2 with osteomyelitis. Other complications included fat embolism and deep venous thrombosis in one child each. No patient had growth arrest, and less than 1 cm of leg length discrepancy was observed in 34 extremities. These authors concluded that open fractures in children, especially type II and III injuries, have a high rate of complications, including infection, delayed union, and nonunion. However, the incidence was still less than that seen in adults with similar injuries.

Hope and Cole,[106] also in 1992, reported their results of treatment of 92 children between 3.1 and 16 years of age with open tibia fractures. Their series consisted of 22 type I, 51 type II, and 19 type III injuries (5 type IIIA, 13 type IIIB, and 1 type IIIC). Half the children had multiple injuries, and three died of head injuries within 24 hours of injury. Fifty-one wounds with minimal soft tissue injury were closed primarily, and 41 were left open and allowed to heal secondarily (18) or with delayed split-thickness skin grafts or free flaps (23). Sixty-five fractures (71%) were treated by closed reduction and immobilization in long leg casts. External fixation was used for unstable fractures (3), for those with extensive soft tissue injury (17), and in children with multiple injuries (6). Short-term complications included compartment syndrome (4), superficial infection (7), deep infection (3), delayed union (15), nonunion (7), and malunion (6). The authors believed that these short-term complications were similar to those reported in adults. At late follow-up ranging from 1.5 to 9.8 years, 29 patients had continuing morbidity, usually those with type III injuries. The morbidity included pain at the fracture site,

restriction of sporting activities, joint stiffness, cosmetic defects, and minor leg length discrepancies. They concluded that open tibia fractures in children are associated with a high incidence of early and late complications and that these complications are more frequent in older children and those with type III injuries.

In 1995, Kreder and Armstrong[140] reviewed 56 open tibia fractures in 55 children. The mean age at injury was 10 years (range, 3 to 17 years), and most injuries occurred in boys and were related to motor vehicle accidents. These children had 14 type I, 16 type II, and 26 type III injuries (12 type IIIA, 8 type IIIB, and 6 type IIIC). Most of their patients had other body area injuries. Four patients died in the first 48 hours after injury. Four patients with five injured extremities (7%) required amputation, including four of the six type IIIC injuries. Infections occurred in eight patients and eight extremities (four superficial and four deep infections), for a prevalence of 14%. Twenty-three fractures were treated by external fixation. Fourteen children experienced delayed union (10) or nonunion (4). The 10 children with delayed union required prolonged immobilization and subsequently healed. The four patients with nonunion each underwent bone grafting and internal fixation before union was obtained. At follow-up, two extremities required treatment for leg length discrepancy and three for malunion. Important factors leading to complications were older age, severity of the injury, neurovascular injury, and delay in getting the patient to the operating room. These authors also documented that open tibia fractures have a high incidence of complications and require careful evaluation and treatment.

Since 1995, most studies have focused on specific fixation methods,[50] more severe injuries,[12, 38] and the factors that most clearly affect prognosis.[25, 100, 206, 227]

In 1996, Cullen and colleagues[50] reported the results of treatment of 40 of 83 open tibial fractures with percutaneous Steinmann pins and casts. Malunion of 14° to 17° developed in four patients (10%) treated with this technique, whereas five patients (13%) had tibial overgrowth in excess of 1 cm. In the final analysis, percutaneous pinning and casts carried a higher overall complication rate than did external fixation alone. Nevertheless, the authors thought that this treatment technique led to good anatomic and functional results.

Buckley and co-workers[38] reviewed 20 children with type III open tibial fractures. There were 7 type IIIA, 10 type IIIB, and 3 type IIIC fractures. Ninety percent of these patients required repeated débridement, and most were initially stabilized with an external fixator. To cover the wounds, 25% required split-thickness skin grafts, 15% needed local muscle flaps, and 30% underwent free muscle transfers. Three patients with segmental bone loss were treated with autologous bone grafts after the soft tissue injuries had healed. The limbs in three patients who had interpositional vein grafts for injuries to one or both tibial arteries survived, although the grafts failed. In one of these patients, a deep infection and delayed union with 3.5 cm of shortening developed. Osteomyelitis developed in three patients (30%) with type IIIB fractures. The average healing time was 29 weeks (range,

8 to 104 weeks) for all type III tibial fractures, 16 weeks for type IIIA fractures, 35 weeks for type IIIB fractures, and 36 weeks for type IIIC fractures. Simple fractures healed in 16 weeks and comminuted fractures in 33 weeks. Fractures without bone loss healed in 24 weeks, and those with a segmental bone defect healed at an average of 59 weeks. The average healing time for uninfected fractures was 29 weeks, whereas those with osteomyelitis required 33 weeks for union. Only two patients had leg length discrepancy in excess of 1 cm. All patients with osteomyelitis were successfully treated, with no amputations. The authors concluded that with proactive wound care and fracture management, children with severe open fractures of the tibia have a good prognosis for limb salvage.

Blaiser and Barnes[25] reviewed 33 consecutive open fractures of the tibia prospectively and focused, in particular, on the relationship of age to various treatment parameters. They separated their patient population into children younger than 12 years (group A) and those 12 years and older (group B). Both groups were similar regarding mechanism, severity of soft tissue injury, and method of immobilization. The authors found that patients in group A had significantly fewer complications, a lower rate of osteomyelitis, a diminished need for bone grafts, and faster healing times. These results confirmed the previous observations of Cramer and associates,[49] who reported average healing times of 3 months for type I fractures, 4.6 months for type II fractures, 6.8 months for type IIIA fractures, 17.8 months for type IIIB fractures, and 11.6 months in the only type IIIC fracture in the study. Similar observations regarding age at injury, complications, and results were published in 1996 by Grimard and associates[86] in a study of 90 children with open tibia fractures from Quebec and by Song and colleagues[227] in 38 children from Seattle.

**Summary of Recent Studies.** In reviewing the key articles published during the last quarter of the century, it appears that between 5% and 15% of all fractures of the tibia and fibula are open. The vast majority of these fractures are caused by collisions of motor vehicles with pedestrians or bicycles and falls from heights. About 30% of these injuries are type I, 40% are type II, and another 30% are type III in severity.[227] The severity of the soft tissue injury directly correlates with the number and severity of associated injuries, which occur in about 25% of those with type I, 50% with type II, and 80% with type III open fractures. About 3% of patients sustain a compartment syndrome. Amputation rates are difficult to estimate because primary amputations are not usually reported. Many open tibial fractures, particularly those of lesser severity, are managed with primary wound closure and immobilization in a long leg cast, whereas repeated débridement and external fixation have become the accepted standard of care for the most severe injuries. Expected complication rates are 30% for infection, 40% for delayed union, 5% for nonunion, 6% for malunion, and about 2% for leg length discrepancy in excess of 1 cm. According to recent studies, children younger than 12 years fair significantly better than those who are older.[50, 86, 206, 227] They have fewer complications and healing times are faster than in older children and

adolescents. This difference may relate to the energy of the trauma involved in older children. These studies show that expert care of even type IIIB and type IIIC fractures may still result in overall outcomes superior to below-knee amputation.[38, 199, 227]

## AUTHORS' PREFERRED METHOD OF TREATMENT

Tetanus prophylaxis, parental antibiotics, and thorough wound débridement remain key for the optimal care of open tibial fractures. Good evidence can now be found in the literature that primary loose wound closure is well tolerated in lower-grade injuries[50, 106] but, in most type III lesions, repeated débridement is usually required.[227] Stable fractures with minimal soft tissue injury can be successfully managed with a long leg cast. However, most children with multiple injuries, those with second- and third-degree burns or other skin conditions, those with unstable fracture patterns, and children with higher-grade open wounds are best managed with external fixation.[38, 227] Simple unilateral frames are ideal for most diaphyseal fractures, but ring fixators are more effective in highly comminuted lesions, in some metaphyseal fractures close to the growth plate, and in fractures with bone loss that may eventually require bone transport. We do not normally use plates and screws because of their high complication rates[38] but will occasionally use elastic nails in older children with stable fracture patterns.

## Delayed Union

Delayed union (6 months or longer) in closed pediatric tibia fractures is uncommon. The total time to satisfactory healing depends on the child's age and the type of fracture. In the series of Steinert and Bennek,[232] the duration of immobilization was 8 to 10 weeks. In Hoaglund and States' report of 43 tibia fractures in children younger than 16 years,[104] the mean healing time for 38 closed fractures was 10 weeks (range, 6 to 25 weeks).

Typically, younger children heal faster than older children. In addition, comminuted, displaced fractures take longer to heal than simple nondisplaced fractures in which the periosteum is intact. Delay in healing usually represents inadequate vascularization of the fracture site. This problem may be caused by an injury to the nutrient artery, the overlying musculature or periosteum, or a combination thereof. Additional time for revascularization and healing is therefore necessary. Moreover, inadequate immobilization that allows motion at the fracture site may contribute to delayed union or possibly to nonunion.

Delayed union after closed tibia fractures is usually managed by autogenous bone grafting from the iliac crest and proper immobilization until healing occurs. Internal or external fixation is not usually necessary but may be beneficial, especially in children with instability or malalignment.

In open fractures, delayed union is more common. The reported prevalence has been between 5% and

36%.* This increase is predominantly the result of compromised vascularity, as discussed previously. Delayed union is also more likely to occur with open fractures in older children and adolescents.

## Nonunion

Nonunion of closed pediatric tibia fractures is very uncommon.[95, 150] Hansen and colleagues[95] reported no nonunions in 85 tibia fractures in children 1 to 15 years of age. Lewallen and Peterson,[150] in a study of 30 nonunions of long bone fractures, including 15 tibia fractures, found that they tend to occur in older children and adolescents, in high-energy fractures, and in open fractures (13 cases), especially in children with soft tissue loss and infection. The association of nonunion with open fracture is clearly evident in recent publications on this subject, although Buckley and co-workers[38] reported two nonunions (20%) in their series of type III fractures. Recent studies involving open tibia fractures have shown a low occurrence of nonunion, usually 10% or less.[50, 86, 140, 227] Again, nonunions tend to occur more commonly in open fractures in older children and adolescents. In addition, when nonunion is associated with an open fracture, infection should be considered a possible etiology.

Autogenous bone graft from the iliac crest and appropriate fracture stabilization form the basis of treatment of pediatric tibial nonunion. In patients with inadequate vascularization of the fracture site, a delayed muscle or myocutaneous flap using microvascular techniques as well as cancellous bone grafting may be beneficial in achieving union. Immobilization can be accomplished with either external fixation frame compression or flexible intramedullary rods, plate, and screws. Ring fixators (Ilizarov) and callotasis have been used successfully for tibial nonunion associated with bone loss.[188] We prefer external fixation because it does not require a second procedure for metal removal and the soft tissue damage at the time of the initial bone grafting is less severe. Flexible intramedullary rods can be considered for nonunion. This technique was used successfully in two cases by Cramer and colleagues.[49]

## Angular Deformity

Angular deformities after closed or open tibia fractures are primarily caused by inadequate alignment before union and occasionally by transient asymmetric overgrowth. The latter is typically associated with a proximal tibial metaphyseal fracture, which has already been discussed.

Fractures of long bones, including the tibia, in children with angular deformities may undergo spontaneous correction with subsequent skeletal growth.[39, 75, 95, 206, 222] Certain generalities can be stated

regarding remodeling[75]: (1) the younger the child, the greater the capacity for correction; (2) the closer the fracture to the physis, the more the remodeling potential; (3) the smaller the remaining angulation, the more complete the correction should be; and (4) residual angulation in the same plane as the movement of the adjacent joints has a greater capacity for correction. Correction of residual angular deformities results from a combination of asymmetric epiphyseal growth, both proximally and distally, and remodeling of the fracture site according to Wolff's law. However, the amount of correction is not predictable and varies with each long bone.

Shannak[222] identified several factors associated with spontaneous correction of angulated tibial malunions. These factors included varus and anterior angulation, spiral fractures, and younger age at injury (more remaining skeletal growth). Hansen and colleagues[95] reported angular deformities in 25 of 85 children (29%) who were monitored clinically and radiographically for a mean of 2 years. These deformities were mild and varied between 4° and 19°. They found only a 14% correction of angular deformities of the tibia in children. Correction ceased 18 months after injury and was independent of the child's age. Shannak[222] reported that 43 (37%) of 117 children had residual varus or valgus angulation. In 25 children it was mild and varied from 1° to 10°, and in 18 children it was moderate, being greater than 10° but less than 22°. At a mean follow-up of 3.9 years (range, 1 to 10 years), 91 children had no residual angulation, 20 had 1° to 10°, and only 6 had more than 10°. Thus, one third of the children with greater than 10° of angulation had persistent deformity, which was typically valgus or anterior angulation, or both. Even when remodeling is incomplete at the diaphyseal level, epiphyseal realignment, both proximally and distally, compensates for some of the residual deformity.[193, 259] Such compensation occurs with varus more than with valgus deformities and with posterior more than with anterior deformities.

Management of angular deformities is prevention. It is important that tibia fractures be monitored closely radiographically and that any residual angulation in the frontal and sagittal planes be corrected before fracture healing. Angulations of 10° can be accepted because many will improve with growth. Deformities greater than 10° need to be corrected before healing, especially in older children and adolescents, because corrective osteotomy may be required at a later time. Hope and Cole[106] reported that two of six malunions after open tibia fractures were corrected by hemiepiphysiodesis. Unfortunately, these two cases were not discussed in detail.

## Malrotation

Pediatric tibia fractures that are allowed to heal in a malrotated position will not correct or remodel with subsequent skeletal growth. External rotation of the distal fracture fragment results in an out-toed gait, as well as increased stress along the medial aspect of the knee and pronation of the ankle and foot. Internal rotation of

---

*See references 38, 39, 49, 50, 86, 106, 115, 140, 199, 206, 227, 266.

the distal fracture fragment results in an in-toed gait. It may also produce internal rotation at the knee joint level and supination of the foot.

Fortunately, the incidence of functionally significant rotational malunion is low. Hansen and colleagues[95] reported that only 5 of 85 patients (6%) seen in follow-up had rotational deformities between 10° and 20°. In Shannak's series,[222] 3 of 117 children (3%) had rotational deformities—two internal and one external. These deformities persisted after 3.9 years of follow-up. All three children were 12 years or older at injury. Bohn and Durbin[29] reported no rotational malalignment in 30 children (32 limbs) with ipsilateral femur and tibia fractures monitored for a mean of 5.1 years. Yue and associates[267] reported one malrotation in 16 patients with ipsilateral femur and tibia fractures treated nonoperatively and none in the 13 patients (14 extremities) treated by operative stabilization.

It is important that accurate rotational alignment be achieved during reduction of a tibia fracture and application of a long leg cast or an external fixator. Any degree of malrotation should be avoided. If adequate radiographic assessment cannot be made by matching cortical widths of the proximal and distal fragments, a CT scan, including views of the opposite intact tibia, can be helpful.[119] If the fracture is allowed to heal in excessive rotational malalignment, surgical correction may be necessary. The location of surgery depends on the level of the deformity. Surgery is usually performed either proximally but inferior to the tibial tubercle or in the supramalleolar area. Concomitant osteotomy of the fibula may be necessary, depending on the severity of the malrotation. The risk of compartment syndrome is lower if the osteotomy is performed distally below the origin of the calf musculature. If performed proximally, an anterior compartment fasciotomy should be performed concomitantly.

## Proximal Tibial Physeal Closure

Asymmetric closure of the proximal tibial physis with subsequent genu recurvatum is a rare complication after a nonphyseal tibial fracture.[110, 174] It has also been described after femoral shaft fractures,[33] Osgood-Schlatter disease,[121] avulsion fractures of the tibial tubercle,[183] tibial tubercle transfer,[72] prolonged immobilization for congenital (developmental) dislocation of the hip,[31] excessive pressure on the tibial tubercle from a cast or brace,[185] skeletal traction,[189, 250] and minor trauma.[235]

Kestler[134] in 1947 reported on premature cessation of epiphyseal growth about the knee joint. He recognized infectious and noninfectious causes involving the hip but also noted an idiopathic group without a pathologic process. Morton and Starr[174] in 1964 reported this complication after a nonphyseal tibia fracture in two children. Both patients sustained comminuted fractures of the tibial diaphysis with no apparent injury to the knee. The fractures were reduced, and K-wires were used in the proximal fracture segment but were 4 cm distal to the tibial tubercle. A genu recurvatum deformity second-

ary to anterior closure of the proximal tibial physis later developed in both patients. Subsequently, similar cases have been described after both tibial and femoral shaft fractures.[29, 60, 110, 189, 226] The mean age at injury for children who seem to be at increased risk for this complication is between 10 and 12 years.[110, 189] The clinical deformity is usually noticed 1 to 3 years later.

The cause of closure of the anterior aspect of the proximal tibial physis is unknown. Hresko and Kasser[110] speculated on two possible mechanisms: (1) direct blunt trauma to the subcutaneous tibial tubercle resulting in anterior growth arrest and recurvatum and (2) compression injury to the anterior part of the proximal tibial physis generated by hyperextension of the knee. These mechanisms may damage the perichondrial ring of the tibial tubercle or the periosteum at the edge of the tubercle which, during healing, results in the formation of an osseous bridge. The initial injury is not recognizable radiographically.[110, 174, 189] This mechanism may explain the case report of Takai and associates,[235] who described this complication after minor trauma to the knee in a 14-year-old boy.

Genu recurvatum deformities are best managed by an opening wedge osteotomy of the proximal end of the tibia with triangular iliac crest bone grafts. Epiphysiodesis of the remainder of the proximal tibial physis is necessary in adolescents to prevent recurrence. It is important that the osteotomy restore the normal posterior slope of the articular surface of the proximal part of the tibia. Care must be taken to not excessively stretch the skin anteriorly because such stretching may predispose to wound dehiscence and skin necrosis. Osteotomy followed by lengthening (callotasis) can also be used.[194] Fasciotomy of the anterior compartment and closed suction drainage should be performed to minimize the risk of compartment syndrome. Epiphysiodesis of either or both the distal femoral and proximal tibial epiphysis of the contralateral extremity may be required in children with significant tibial shortening to achieve equal leg length at skeletal maturity.

In a young child with an angular deformity less than 20°, resection of the osseous bridge and interposition with fat or other inert material may restore growth and allow spontaneous correction.[143, 195] When the deformity exceeds 20°, a corrective osteotomy combined with osseous bridge resection is recommended.[195]

Recently, Navascues and associates[181] reported on seven patients with premature central physeal closure of the distal femoral or proximal tibial physis or both after tibial diaphyseal fractures. All patients were 12 to 15 years of age at injury, and mild lower extremity length discrepancies (8 to 30 mm) subsequently developed. No children had angular deformities. The exact etiology of the premature closure was unknown, but a vascular etiology was suspected.

## Lower Extremity Length Inequality

As with other long bone fractures in children, the periosteal stripping, callus formation, and increased blood flow to the involved bone result in stimulation of the adjacent physes and a transient acceleration in growth. However, it does not occur with the same magnitude as in femoral shaft fractures, with the possible exception of children with open tibia fractures. Greiff and Bergmann[84] and Swaan and Oppers[234] reported tibial overgrowth of approximately 5 mm in girls 3 to 10 years of age and boys 3 to 12 years of age. Older children and young adolescents may actually have growth retardation induced by the fracture. Additional overgrowth of 1 to 3 mm can occur in the ipsilateral femur. The overgrowth is not usually affected by the fracture pattern or any residual angulation and lasts for 1 to 2 years after injury. Shannak,[222] however, found that comminuted fractures, proximal and distal fractures, and fractures with significant shortening had the greatest overgrowth. Similar results were reported in the Italian literature in 1985.[42, 62, 191] In their study of 121 tibia fractures, DiLeo and co-workers[62] reported that the greatest incidence of overgrowth occurred in children 3 to 8 years of age with proximal metaphyseal fractures in which the fracture line encroached on the physis.

Open fractures, especially those treated by external fixation, also seem to have a greater propensity for overgrowth than would normally be anticipated.[3, 29, 39, 232, 242] Tolo[242] reported overgrowth of 1 to 1.4 cm in 3 of 13 open tibia fractures. He recommended slight overriding of the fracture fragments in children between 2 and 12 years of age to compensate for this expected overgrowth.

Overgrowth and the resultant length inequality of the lower extremities appear to be a problem in younger children whose fractures are reduced end-on or anatomically.[38, 39, 50]

Open reduction and the use of intramedullary rods in open and closed fractures may cause overgrowth, assuming that the proximal physis is not injured. Steinert and Bennek[232] reported three cases of overgrowth of 2 to 3 cm with this technique. However, Qidwai[199] reported no cases of overgrowth of 1.0 cm or greater in 84 tibia fractures, including 30 open fractures treated by intramedullary fixation.

Trotter and Gleser[245] and others[4, 11, 93, 248] demonstrated that a mean of 5 mm (range, 5 to 12 mm) of length discrepancy may be seen in the lower extremities of normal children. Therefore, some degree of luck is involved in obtaining equal leg lengths, especially if the fractured extremity was originally the larger one.

Based on these data, it is important that accurate restoration of length be achieved in the management of pediatric tibial shaft fractures. Fortunately, most instances of shortening are not clinically significant. Discrepancies of 2 cm or less as an adult do not usually produce a limp or predispose to other problems. If overgrowth or shortening should occur, the child must be monitored with periodic radiographic measurements (scanograms) and bone age determinations to assess the behavior of the discrepancy and determine whether epiphysiodesis will be necessary to achieve relatively equal leg lengths at skeletal maturity.

## Vascular Injury

Vascular injuries in association with closed tibial shaft fractures are very uncommon in children.[29, 46, 76, 221, 256] Shaker and colleagues[221] reported that only 8 of 118 children (7%) younger than 15 years with upper and lower extremity fractures seen between 1965 and 1975 had vascular injuries and that most were from supracondylar fractures of the distal end of the humerus. No vascular injuries were reported in association with tibia fractures. When vascular injuries secondary to tibia fractures are present, they are usually the result of high-velocity injuries and open fractures, such as occur in motor vehicle accidents.[29, 39, 46, 70, 106, 180, 266] Males are more commonly involved than females. Between 1% and 18% of open tibia fractures in the most recent studies had associated vascular injuries (type IIIC).[38, 39, 49, 86, 106, 115, 140, 227, 266] These injuries frequently lead to amputation.

Vascular injuries in association with closed tibia fractures are most often seen with displaced fractures of the proximal metaphysis or diaphysis.[29, 44, 76, 93, 105, 180, 201] Fractures in the proximal tibial metaphysis may damage the anterior tibial artery as it passes in a posterior-to-anterior direction through the interosseous membrane. Proximal tibial diaphyseal fractures may also damage the popliteal artery or its trifurcation of the anterior tibial, posterior tibial, and peroneal arteries.[29, 105] Another fracture that may involve the anterior tibial artery occurs in the lower aspect of the tibia when the distal fragment is displaced posteriorly. Isolated injuries to the posterior tibial artery as a consequence of a tibial shaft fracture are very rare.

Prompt recognition, evaluation, and vascular reconstruction are critical for initial limb salvage and avoidance of late complications. The cardinal signs of an arterial injury are known as the five P's: pulselessness, pain, pallor, paresthesias, and paralysis.[180, 256] However, the presence of palpable pulses on Doppler flowmetry does not rule out an arterial injury. If such an injury is suspected, an arteriogram should be obtained. Compartment syndromes can have many of the same features as an arterial injury and may also occur after vascular repair (see under Compartment Syndrome).[211, 214] Fasciotomies at the time of vascular repair have been recommended.[29, 46] If a fasciotomy is not performed, sequential or continuous compartment pressure measurements need to be taken.

Friedman and Jupiter[76] reported the results of seven children with vascular injuries associated with closed extremity fractures, including three with tibia fractures that were not diagnosed initially and underwent delayed repair. Early complications included wound infection, below-knee amputation, deep vein thrombosis, and motor and sensory deficits. Late follow-up revealed two cases of limb overgrowth and one of limb undergrowth. Minor motor and sensory deficits persisted, but the overall function was good. These authors recommended arteriography in all children with a suspected vascular injury after fracture. If the arteriogram reveals a major vascular lesion, it should be repaired immediately, usually after fracture stabilization with internal or external fixation. This strategy is applicable even with adequate collateral circulation to keep the limb viable. This study indicated that as the child grows and places greater functional demands on the extremity, the collateral circulation may be inadequate to meet the increased demands, and altered growth or intermittent ischemia-like symptoms related to activity may result. However, it is important to remember that arteriography is not without complications and should be used only in children in whom the index of suspicion for an associated vascular injury is high. Thrombosis is a recognized complication after angiography in children.[221] As a consequence, Friedman and Jupiter[76] recommended the use of digital subtraction angiography to evaluate long-term vascular patency in children.

Another potential vascular complication after tibia fractures is traumatic arterial spasm. Diffuse arterial spasm without a specific arterial injury can occur and result in gangrene. Children appear to be more susceptible to this condition than adults are. Russo[215] reported a 9-year-old boy who sustained a type IIIC open tibia, fibula, and calcaneus fracture; traumatic arterial spasm developed and resulted in gangrene of the lower part of the leg and foot that required below-knee amputation. Arteriography showed only diffuse arterial spasm. The spasm was not relieved by vasodilating agents. Treatment options for this rare condition, as discussed by Russo,[215] include intra-arterial injection of vasodilating agents such as papaverine, sodium nitroprusside, reserpine, tolazoline, and prostaglandin E. Surgical measures may include external irrigation with warm lactated Ringer's solution, application of local anesthetics or 32% papaverine, and adventitial stripping. If these measures fail, dilatation of the artery with mechanical dilators or catheters may be beneficial.

Treatment of fractures associated with arterial injury in children is controversial. Generally, the fracture is stabilized by an external fixator before arterial repair. However, Wolma and co-workers,[263] as well as Friedman and Jupiter,[76] demonstrated satisfactory results with conservative management. Each case must be individualized and the vascularity to the lower portion of the leg restored as rapidly as possible. Some fracture patterns may prevent initial vascular repair and necessitate reduction and stabilization before repair. If limb viability is in question, the arterial repair should be performed first or an intraluminal shunt used.[122] When limb viability is not in question, the fracture should be stabilized first to allow for more normal anatomic restoration of the bone and soft tissue.

## Neurologic Injury

Neurologic injuries associated with pediatric tibia fractures are uncommon, even in open fractures. The most common neurologic injury involves the peroneal nerve as it passes around the lateral aspect of the proximal end of the fibula. The nerve is more likely to be damaged by a direct blow than by a fracture fragment. It is important when fractures occur in this area that the function of the muscles innervated by the peroneal nerve be well documented. Bohn and Durbin[29] reported two transient, partial peroneal nerve palsies in children with ipsilateral femur and tibia fractures. One occurred during skeletal traction and the other at the time of injury or during fracture reduction and application of a hip spica cast. In studies on open tibia fractures in children, the prevalence has been quite variable. Some studies have reported no neurologic injuries,[49, 106, 226, 266] whereas others have reported a prevalence between 2% and 14%.[38, 39, 50, 86, 106, 140] The peroneal and posterior tibial nerves are the most frequently injured nerves.

Perhaps the most common mechanism for a neurologic injury with a pediatric tibia fracture is the post-traumatic compartment syndrome.

## Compartment Syndrome

A compartment syndrome caused by bleeding and extravasation of tissue fluid into one or more of the four compartments of the lower part of the leg can and does occur in children, as well as in adults, after fracture of the tibial shaft.[66, 176] It can also be a complication of proximal tibial corrective osteotomies, tibial lengthening procedures, and use of the tibia for bone graft donor sites in children.[163, 176, 220, 231] Increased tissue pressure results in an increased net force per unit area exerted on the vessels within one or more compartments. This force increases local venous pressure, which decreases the local arteriovenous gradient and reduces local blood flow and oxygenation; as a consequence, local tissue function (muscle and nerve) and viability are compromised.[7] The tolerance for increased compartment pressure varies with the local arterial pressure, the duration of the pressure, and possibly the local metabolic needs of the tissues.[161] Prompt diagnosis and surgical decompression are essential to preserve the viability and function of tissues within the compartment. Failure to diagnose and treat either an incipient or an established compartment syndrome may result in irreversible ischemia of the extrinsic muscles of the lower part of the leg and possibly amputation.[144, 176, 212] Mubarak and Carroll[176] in 1979 presented a review of 55 children with Volkmann's ischemic contracture seen between 1955 and 1975 at the Hospital for Sick Children in Toronto. This series included 11 children with lower leg compartment syndromes, 5 of which were complications of tibial shaft fractures. All but one patient had a delay in diagnosis of greater than 3 days. As a result, 1 below-knee amputation and 10 cases of residual functional deficit (5 severe, 4 moderate, and 1 mild) occurred.

Although most compartment syndromes occur in closed fractures, the presence of an open fracture with supposed compartment disruption does not preclude the possibility.[39, 49, 50, 106, 115] It is more likely to occur in type I or type II injuries, in which compartment disruption may be limited. Buckley and co-workers[39] reported 2 compartment syndromes in 42 open pediatric tibia fractures (5%). Both were type II injuries. Cramer and colleagues[49] reported compartment syndromes in 4 of 22 open tibia fractures (18%), including 3 type II and

1 type III injury. Hope and Cole[106] treated 4 compartment syndromes in 92 open tibia fractures (4%), including 2 type I, 1 type II, and 1 type III injury. Irwin and associates[115] reported 1 compartment syndrome (a type II injury) in 58 open tibia fractures (2%). Other authors have reported no cases of compartment syndrome in their studies on open tibia fractures.[38, 86, 140, 227, 266]

The clinical findings of compartment syndrome are subjective, and detection depends heavily on patient cooperation. In children, such cooperation can be difficult because of pain, fear, and anxiety. The physician must therefore have a high index of suspicion during evaluation. Intracompartment pressure measurements by a variety of techniques allow a more objective method of evaluating and monitoring compartment pressure (see Chapter 4 for more detail). The first and most important symptom of an impending acute compartment syndrome is pain out of proportion to that expected from the fracture.[165, 175–178, 210, 211] Other symptoms may include a feeling of tenseness in the involved compartments and paresthesias of the nerves that traverse those compartments.

The earliest clinical finding is a swollen and tense compartment caused by the increased intracompartment pressure. Pain with passive stretch of the muscles in the involved compartment is a common finding but is subjective.[175, 211] Unfortunately, children with sensory deficits resulting from a proximal nerve injury may not exhibit stretch pain, even in the presence of elevated intracompartment pressure.

The most reliable physical finding of a compartment syndrome is sensory deficit.[175] Most compartments of the lower part of the leg are traversed by nerves with distal sensory distribution. Decreased sensation to light touch, pinprick, or two-point discrimination in the distal sensory distribution is an important finding. However, differentiating between paresthesias from a proximal nerve injury and a compartment syndrome can be difficult.

Except in the presence of major arterial injury, peripheral pulses and capillary filling are usually intact in children with compartment syndrome.[175] As a consequence, the presence of palpable distal pulses and good capillary filling is no assurance that a compartment syndrome does not exist.[261]

The most complex problem after a tibial shaft fracture is distinguishing among compartment syndrome, arterial occlusion, and proximal nerve injury (neurapraxia).[175, 177, 220] Similar problems can also occur after a proximal tibial osteotomy.[163, 231] These conditions frequently coexist, and their clinical findings can overlap. Mubarak and Hargens[177] developed an algorithm to assist in differentiating them and in choosing appropriate treatment. Arterial injuries normally have absent peripheral pulses but no increased compartment pressure. Children with neurapraxia have no pain with passive stretch of muscles within a given compartment, no increased compartment pressure, and normal peripheral pulses. These characteristics are generalities, and each child must be carefully evaluated for these possibilities.

Mubarak and co-workers[178] identified three groups of patients in whom it is difficult to elicit and interpret the physical findings of compartment syndrome and in whom measurement of intracompartment pressure may be extremely helpful: (1) patients who are unresponsive; (2) those who are uncooperative or unreliable, as commonly occurs in young children; and (3) those with peripheral nerve deficits attributable to other causes, such as peroneal nerve palsy. Several methods have been developed for the measurement of compartment pressure, including needle, continuous infusion, Wick catheter, and slit catheter techniques. The last technique appears to be the most popular and affords an accurate method for continuous monitoring of intracompartment pressure.[175] The pressure threshold for diagnosis of compartment syndrome varies for each of these techniques. The orthopaedic surgeon must be familiar with the advantages, disadvantages, and pressure thresholds for each technique. Whitesides and associates,[260] using the needle technique, recommended decompression when compartment pressures rise to within 10 to 30 mm Hg of diastolic blood pressure. Matsen and colleagues,[165] using the infusion technique, suggested that fasciotomies be performed in patients with clinical findings of compartment syndrome and pressure greater than 45 mm Hg. Using the Wick and slit catheter techniques, Mubarak,[175] Mubarak and co-workers,[178] Rorabeck,[210, 211] Rorabeck and MacNab,[212] and Russell and associates[214] recommended decompression when intracompartment pressure exceeds 30 to 35 mm Hg and the appropriate clinical findings are present. It is important that pressure measurements be taken at the level of the fracture because pressure declines at increasing distances proximal and distal to the fracture.[45] Incorrect technique could result in a serious underestimation of maximal compartment pressure.

The anterior compartment syndrome occurs most often after a fracture of the tibial shaft and is characterized by pain referred to the anterior compartment on passive flexion of the toes and mild weakness of the extensor hallucis longus followed by the extensor digitorum longus. The last sign to appear is hypoesthesia in the first web space.[32, 212] Although the anterior compartment syndrome is the most common, other compartments may be involved concomitantly or individually. A deep posterior compartment syndrome can occur in children. It was initially described in 1975 by Matsen and Clawson[162] and characterized by pain, plantar hyperesthesia, weakness of toe flexion, pain on passive toe extension, and tenseness of the fascia between the tibia and the triceps surae in the distal medial part of the leg. Decompression of the deep posterior compartment within 12 hours of onset of the syndrome prevented permanent sequelae. Karlstrom and colleagues,[129] as well as Bohn and Durbin,[29] reported on the sequelae of unrecognized deep posterior compartment syndrome. Karlstrom and colleagues[129] found 23 cases, 2 of which occurred in adolescents younger than 15 years. These patients presented with a clawed foot and limited ankle and subtalar motion secondary to fibrous contractures of the muscles of the deep posterior compartment. The muscle changes were attributed to vascular damage, soft tissue swelling, or severe muscle laceration.

Because involvement of multiple compartments is common, it is now recommended that during the initial evaluation, pressure measurements be made in all four compartments and, if a fasciotomy is required, all compartments be released simultaneously.[212]

Incipient compartment syndromes can also exist and should be suspected in children who complain of inordinate pain under the cast but in whom no frank signs of compartment syndrome are present. The first step in the management of incipient compartment syndrome involves bivalving the cast and splitting the underlying padding. Garfin and associates[78] demonstrated that univalving and spreading a cast on the hind limb of an experimental animal reduced compartment pressure by a mean of 65% and that cutting the underlying padding further reduced the pressure by an additional 10% to 20%. Thus, by splitting a cast and cutting the soft dressings, it is possible to decrease compartment pressure by as much as 85%. Rorabeck[211] stated that bivalving a long leg cast in a patient with a fracture of the tibial shaft and cutting the underlying padding may reduce compartment pressure by as much as 50%. Bingold,[24] in an experimental model, made similar observations. Elevation of an extremity with incipient compartment syndrome is not recommended. It was noted both experimentally and clinically that elevation of the limb reduced the mean arterial pressure and therefore reduced blood flow to the compartment.[7, 164, 176] In addition, elevation reduces the arteriovenous gradient and hence increases the susceptibility of the limb to compartment syndrome by reducing oxygen perfusion to the muscles. An extremity with an incipient compartment syndrome should be positioned to be level with the heart to promote arterial inflow.

In an established compartment syndrome, the patient has the clinical signs and symptoms of a compartment syndrome along with elevation of intracompartment pressure. Rorabeck[210, 211] identified the indications for surgical decompression in patients with established compartment syndrome. These indications include (1) clinical signs of an acute compartment syndrome with demonstrable motor or sensory loss, (2) elevated compartment pressure above 35 mm Hg when using either the slit or the Wick catheter technique or above 40 mm Hg with the needle technique in a conscious or unconscious patient, and (3) interrupted arterial circulation to an extremity for more than 4 hours. Mubarak and Carroll[176] also recommended prophylactic fasciotomies, especially of the anterior compartment, for all elective tibial operations in children. The most common methods for decompression of all four compartments of the lower part of the leg in an established compartment syndrome include fibulectomy, perifibular fasciotomy, and double-incision fasciotomy.

Fibulectomy as a method of decompression has been popularized by Kelly and Whitesides.[131] It is particularly useful for a deep posterior compartment syndrome. However, it is usually contraindicated in children because of the risk of residual pseudarthrosis of the

fibula, which may result in fibular shortening from asymmetric growth and a valgus deformity of the ankle, as well as external tibial torsion.[111, 112, 262] This risk is especially high when fibulectomy is performed in children 10 years or younger. Friedman and Jupiter[76] used either a fibulectomy, which leaves the periosteum intact, or multiple-incision fasciotomies for their pediatric patients who had fractures associated with vascular injuries. The former allowed re-formation of the fibula. Hsu and co-workers[112] and Wiltse[262] recommended bone grafting for fibular pseudarthrosis after partial fibulectomy. Perifibular fasciotomy, which was recommended by Matsen and colleagues,[165] has the advantage of allowing access to all four compartments through a single lateral incision. This technique is useful, provided that the anatomy of the extremity has not been distorted. The double-incision technique has been used by Mubarak and co-workers[178] and was studied extensively by Bourne and Rorabeck[32] and by Rorabeck.[210, 211] The procedure is easy to perform, and no structures are likely to be damaged, with the exception of the saphenous vein medially. This technique allows easy access to all four compartments. It is important to perform generous skin incisions because the skin envelope can also contribute to increased compartment pressure.[45]

Once the diagnosis of compartment syndrome has been made, it is imperative that decompression be performed immediately. Rorabeck and MacNab[212] reported complete recovery when fasciotomies were performed for anterior compartment syndrome within 6 hours of the onset of symptoms. In 18 patients who underwent fasciotomies after 6 hours or more (mean, 18 hours), 14 had persistent weakness of dorsiflexion, complete footdrop was seen in 3, and below-knee amputation was required in 1. However, in a follow-up study of 18 patients with various acute compartment syndromes, Rorabeck[211] demonstrated that acceptable results could still be obtained up to 24 hours after the onset of symptoms.

Fracture management after fasciotomies in children is controversial. In adults, Rorabeck[210] recommended stabilization with an external fixator, intramedullary nail, or compression plate. Mubarak and Carroll[176] recommended either internal or external fixation of pediatric tibia fractures associated with compartment syndrome to allow for easier management of the fasciotomy wounds. One of the major reasons for stabilization is that fasciotomies convert a closed fracture into an open fracture that, in most cases, must be left open and later closed secondarily. In a child, such stabilization may not always be necessary. The decision regarding fracture stabilization must be made on the basis of associated injuries and fracture stability. If rigid stabilization is necessary, it usually involves the use of an external fixator. In certain cases, however, young children may be managed conservatively with a long leg posterior splint followed by a long leg plaster cast.

## REFERENCES

1. Aadalen, R.J. Proximal tibial metaphyseal fractures in children. Minn Med 62:785–788, 1979.

2. Akbarnia, B.; Torg, J.S.; Kirkpatrick, J.; Sussman, S. Manifestations of the battered child syndrome. J Bone Joint Surg Am 56:1159–1166, 1974.

3. Alonso, J.E.; Horowitz, M. Use of the AO/ASIF external fixator in children. J Pediatr Orthop 7:594–600, 1987.

4. Anderson, M.; Messner, M.B.; Green, W.T. Distribution of lengths of the normal femur and tibia in children from one to eighteen years of age. J Bone Joint Surg Am 46:1197–1202, 1964.

5. Aronson, D.D.; Stewart, M.C.; Crissman, J.D. Experimental tibial fractures in rabbits simulating proximal tibial metaphyseal fractures in children. Clin Orthop 255:61–67, 1990.

6. Aronson, J.; Garvin, K.; Seibert, J.; et al. Efficiency of the bone scan for occult limping toddlers. J Pediatr Orthop 12:38–44, 1992.

7. Ashton, H. The effect of increased tissue pressure on blood flow. Clin Orthop 113:15–26, 1975.

8. Bach, A.W.; Hansen, S.T., Jr. Plates versus external fixation in severe open tibial fractures. Clin Orthop 241:89–94, 1989.

9. Bahnson, D.H.; Lovell, W.W. Genu valgum following fractures of the proximal tibial metaphysis in children. Orthop Trans 4:306, 1980.

10. Balthazar, D.A.; Pappas, A.M. Acquired valgus deformity of the tibia in children. J Pediatr Orthop 4:538–541, 1984.

11. Barfod, B.; Christensen, F. Fractures of the femoral shaft in children with special reference to subsequent over-growth. Acta Chir Scand 116:235–250, 1959.

12. Bartlett, C.S., III; Weiner, L.S.; Yang, E.C. Treatment of type II and type III open tibia fractures in children. J Orthop Trauma 11:357–362, 1997.

13. Bassey, L.O. The use of P.O.P. integrated pins as an improvisation on the Hoffmann's apparatus: Contribution to open fracture management in the tropics. J Trauma 29:59–64, 1989.

14. Bassey, L.O. Valgus deformity following proximal metaphyseal fractures in children: Experiences in the African tropics. J Trauma 30:102–107, 1990.

15. Behrens, F. A primer of fixator devices and configurations. Clin Orthop 241:5–14, 1989.

16. Behrens, F. General theory and principles of external fixation. Clin Orthop 241:15–23, 1989.

17. Behrens, F. External fixation in children: Lower extremity. Instr Course Lect 39:205–208, 1990.

18. Behrens, F. Fractures with soft tissue injuries. In: Browner, B.D.; Jupiter, J.B.; Levine, A.M.; Trafton, P.G., eds. Skeletal Trauma. Philadelphia, W.B. Saunders, 1991.

19. Behrens, F.; Searls, K. External fixation of the tibia. Basic concepts and prospective evaluation. J Bone Joint Surg Br 68:246–254, 1986.

20. Behrens, F.; Johnson, W. Unilateral external fixation: Methods to increase and reduce frame stiffness. Clin Orthop 241:48–56, 1989.

21. Ben-Itzhak, I.; Erken, E.H.W.; Malkin, C. Progressive valgus deformity after juxta-epiphyseal fractures of the upper tibia in children. Injury 18:169–173, 1987.

22. Berkebile, R.D. Stress fracture of the tibia in children. AJR Am J Roentgenol 91:588–596, 1964.

23. Best, T.N. Valgus deformity after fracture of the upper tibia in children. J Bone Joint Surg Br 55:222, 1973.

24. Bingold, A.C. On splitting plasters. A useful analogy. J Bone Joint Surg Br 61:294–295, 1979.

25. Blake, R.; McBryde, A. The floating knee: Ipsilateral fractures of the tibia and femur. South Med J 68:13–16, 1975.

26. Blaiser, R.D.; Barnes, C.L. Age as a prognostic factor in open tibial fractures in children. Clin Orthop 331:261–264, 1996.

27. Blatz, D. Bilateral femoral and tibial shaft fractures in a runner. Am J Sports Med 9:322–325, 1981.

28. Blount, W.P. Fractures in Children. Baltimore, Williams & Wilkins, 1955, pp. 183–194.

29. Bohn, W.W.; Durbin, R.A. Ipsilateral fractures of the femur and tibia in children and adolescents. J Bone Joint Surg Am 73:429–439, 1991.

30. Bondurant, F.J.; Cotler, H.B.; Buckle, R.; et al. The medical and economic impact of severely injured lower extremities. J Trauma 28:1270–1273, 1988.

31. Botting, S.; Scrase, W.H. Premature epiphyseal fusion of the knee complicating prolonged immobilization for congenital dislocation of the hip. J Bone Joint Surg Br 47:280–282, 1965.

32. Bourne, R.B.; Rorabeck, C.H. Compartment syndromes of the lower leg. Clin Orthop 240:97–104, 1988.

33. Bowler, J.R.; Mubarak, S.J.; Wenger, D.R. Tibial physeal closure and genu recurvatum after femoral fracture: Occurrence without a tibial traction pin. J Pediatr Orthop 10:653–657, 1990.

34. Boyer, R.S.; Jaffe, R.B.; Nixon, G.W.; Condon, V.R. Trampoline fractures of the proximal tibia in children. AJR Am J Roentgenol 146:83–85, 1986.

35. Boytim, M.J.; Davidson, R.S.; Charney, E.; Melchionni, J.B. Neonatal fractures in myelomeningocele patients. J Pediatr Orthop 11:28–30, 1991.

36. Briggs, T.W.R.; Orr, M.M.; Lightowler, C.D.R. Isolated tibia fractures in children. Injury 23:308–310, 1992.

37. Brougham, D.I.; Nicol, R.O. Valgus deformity after proximal tibial fractures in children. J Bone Joint Surg Br 69:482, 1987.

38. Buckley, S.L.; Smith, G.R.; Sponseller, P.D.; et al. Severe (type III) open fractures of the tibia in children. J Pediatr Orthop 16:627–634, 1996.

39. Buckley, S.L.; Smith, G.; Sponseller, P.D.; et al. Open fractures of the tibia in children. J Bone Joint Surg Am 72:1462–1469, 1990.

40. Burrows, H.J. Fatigue fractures of the fibula. J Bone Joint Surg Br 30:266–279, 1948.

41. Cheng, J.C.Y.; Shen, W.Y. Limb fracture pattern in different pediatric age groups: A study of 3,350 children. J Orthop Trauma 7:15–22, 1993.

42. Cigola, F.; Rega, A.N.; Lotito, F.M. Growth disturbances following fractures of the femur and tibia in children. Ital J Orthop Traumatol 11:121–125, 1985.

43. Coates, R. Knock-knee deformity following upper tibial "greenstick" fractures. J Bone Joint Surg Br 59:516, 1977.

44. Cofer, J.B.; Burns, R.P.; Clements, J.B. Popliteal artery injury associated with tibial fracture in a five year old. J Tenn Med Assoc 79:430–432, 1986.

45. Cohen, M.S.; Garfin, S.R.; Hargens, A.R.; Mubarak, S.J. Acute compartment syndrome. Effect of dermotomy on fascial decompression in the leg. J Bone Joint Surg Br 73:287–290, 1991.

46. Cole, W.G. Arterial injuries associated with fractures of the lower limbs in childhood. Injury 12:460–463, 1981.

47. Cozen, L. Fracture of the proximal portion of the tibia in children followed by valgus deformity. Surg Gynecol Obstet 97:183–188, 1953.

48. Cozen, L. Knock knee deformity after fracture of the proximal tibia in children. Orthopedics 1:230, 1959.

49. Cramer, K.A.; Limbird, T.J.; Green, N.E. Open fractures of the diaphysis of the lower extremity in children. Treatment, results, and complications. J Bone Joint Surg Am 74:218–232, 1992.

50. Cullen, M.C.; Roy, D.R.; Crawford, A.H.; et al. Open fracture of the tibia in children. J Bone Joint Surg Am 78:1039–1046, 1996.

51. Currarino, G.; Pickney, L.E. Genu valgum after proximal tibial fractures in children. AJR Am J Roentgenol 136:915–918, 1981.

52. DalMonte, A.; Manes, E.; Cammarota, V. Posttraumatic genu valgum in children. Ital J Orthop Traumatol 11:5–11, 1985.

53. DeBoeck, K.; VanEldere, S.; DeVos, P.; et al. Radionuclide bone scan imaging in toddler's fracture. Eur J Pediatr 150:166–169, 1991.

54. Dellinger, E.P.; Miller, S.D.; Wertz, M.J.; et al. Risk of infection after open fracture of the arm or leg. Arch Surg 123:1320–1327, 1987.

55. Demetriades, D.; Nikolaides, N.; Filiopoulos, K.; Hager, J. The use of methylmethacrylate as an external fixator in children and adolescents. J Pediatr Orthop 15:499–503, 1995.

56. Dent, J.A.; Paterson, C.R. Fractures in early childhood: Osteogenesis imperfecta or child abuse? J Pediatr Orthop 10:542–544, 1990.

57. Devas, M.B. Stress fractures in children. J Bone Joint Surg Br 45:528–541, 1963.

58. Devas, M.B.; Sweetnam, R. Stress fractures of the fibula. J Bone Joint Surg Br 38:818–829, 1956.

59. Dias, L.S. Ankle valgus in children with myelomeningocele. Dev Med Child Neurol 20:627–633, 1978.

60. Dias, L.S. Fractures of the tibia and fibula. In: Rockwood, C.A., Jr.; Wilkens, K.E.; King, R.E., eds. Fractures in Children. Philadelphia, J.B. Lippincott, 1984, pp. 983–1041.

61. Dickenson, R.P.; Hutton, W.C.; Stott, J.R.R. The mechanical properties of bone in osteoporosis. J Bone Joint Surg Br 63:233–238, 1981.

62. DiLeo, P.; Lispi, A.; Marciano, R. Growth disturbances following fractures of the femur and tibia in children. Ital J Orthop Traumatol 11:127–131, 1985.

63. Drennan, J.C.; Freehafer, A.A. Fractures of the lower extremities in paraplegic children. Clin Orthop 77:211–217, 1971.

64. Drewes, J.; Schulte, H.D. Bruche im Bereich des Unterschenkels bei Kindern infolge von Fahrradspeichenverletzungen. Chirurg 36:464–468, 1965.

65. Dunbar, J.S.; Owen, H.F.; Nogrady, M.D.; McLesse, R. Obscure tibial fracture of infants—the toddler's fracture. J Can Assoc Radiol 25:136–144, 1964.

66. Ellis, H. Disabilities after tibial shaft fractures with special reference to Volkmann's ischemic contracture. J Bone Joint Surg Br 40:190–197, 1956.

67. Engh, C.A.; Robinson, R.A.; Milgram, J. Stress fractures in children. J Trauma 10:532–541, 1970.

68. Englaro, F.E.; Gelfand, M.J.; Paltiel, H.J. Bone scintigraphy in preschoolers with lower extremity pain of unknown origin. J Nucl Med 33:351–354, 1992.

69. Evanoff, M.; Strong, M.L.; MacIntosh, R. External fixation maintained until fracture consolidation in the skeletally immature. J Pediatr Orthop 13:98–101, 1993.

70. Fabian, T.C.; Turkleson, M.L.; Connelly, T.L.; Stone, H.H. Injury to the popliteal artery. Am J Surg 143:225–228, 1982.

71. Felman, A.H. Bicycle spoke fractures. J Pediatr 82:302–303, 1973.

72. Fielding, J.W.; Liebler, W.A.; Tambakis, A. The effect of a tibial-tubercle transplant in children on the growth of the upper tibial epiphysis. J Bone Joint Surg Am 42:1426–1434, 1960.

73. Freehafer, A.A.; Mast, W.A. Lower extremity fractures in patients with spinal-cord injury. J Bone Joint Surg Am 47:683–694, 1965.

74. Freehafer, A.A.; Anscheutz, R.H.; Shaffer, J.W. Fractures of the lower limbs in patients with myelomeningocele. Interclin Information Bull 18:11–12, 1982.

75. Friberg, S. Remodeling after fractures healed with residual angulation. In: Houghton, G.R.; Thompson, G.H., eds. Problematic Musculoskeletal Injuries in Children. London, Butterworths, 1983, pp. 77–100.

76. Friedman, R.J.; Jupiter, J.B. Vascular injuries and closed extremity fractures in children. Clin Orthop 188:112–119, 1984.

77. Galleno, H.; Oppenheim, W.L. The battered child syndrome revisited. Clin Orthop 162:11–19, 1982.

78. Garfin, S.R.; Mubarak, S.J.; Evans, K.L.; et al. Quantification of intracompartmental pressures and volume under plaster casts. J Bone Joint Surg Am 63:449–453, 1981.

79. Gillies, C.L.; Hartung, W. Fracture of the tibia in spinal bifida vera. Radiology 31:621–623, 1938.

80. Goff, C.W. Surgical Treatment of Unequal Extremities. Springfield, IL, Charles C Thomas, 1960.

81. Golding, C. Museum pages. III: Spina bifida and epiphyseal displacement. J Bone Joint Surg Br 42:387–389, 1960.

82. Green, N.E. Tibia valga caused by asymmetrical overgrowth following a nondisplaced fracture of the proximal tibial metaphysis. J Pediatr Orthop 3:235–237, 1983.

83. Gregory, R.J.H.; Cubison, T.C.S.; Pinder, I.M.; Smith, S.R. External fixation of lower limb fractures of children. J Trauma 33:691–693, 1992.

84. Greiff, J.; Bergmann, F. Growth disturbance following fracture of the tibia in children. Acta Orthop Scand 51:315–320, 1980.

85. Griffiths, A.L. Fatigue fracture of the fibula in childhood. Arch Dis Child 27:552–557, 1952.

86. Grimard, G.; Naudie, D.; Laberge, L.C.; Hamdy, R.C. Open fractures of the tibia in children. Clin Orthop 332:62–70, 1996.

87. Gustilo, R.B. Principles of the management of open fractures. In: Gustilo, R.B., ed. Management of Open Fractures and Their Complications. Philadelphia, W.B. Saunders, 1982.

88. Gustilo, R.B.; Anderson, J.T. Prevention of infection in the treatment of one thousand and twenty-one fractures of long bones: Retrospective and prospective analyses. J Bone Joint Surg Am 58:453–458, 1976.

89. Gustilo, R.B.; Mendoza, R.M.; Williams, D.N. Problems in the management of type III (severe) open fractures: A new classification of type III open fractures. J Trauma 24:742–746, 1984.

90. Gustilo, R.B.; Merkow, R.L.; Templeman, D. Current concepts review. The management of open fractures. J Bone Joint Surg Am 72:299–304, 1990.

91. Gustilo, R.B.; Granninger, R.P.; Davis, T. Classification of type III (severe) open fractures relative to treatment and results. Orthopaedics 10:1781–1788, 1987.

92. Gyepes, M.T.; Newbern, D.H.; Neuhauser, E.B.D. Metaphyseal and physeal injuries in children with spina bifida and meningomyeloceles. AJR Am J Roentgenol 95:168–177, 1965.

93. Haas, L.M.; Staple, T.W. Arterial injuries associated with fractures of the proximal tibia following blunt trauma. South Med J 62:1439–1448, 1969.

94. Halsey, M.F.; Finzel, K.C.; Carrion, W.V.; et al. Toddler's fracture: Presumptive diagnosis and treatment. J Pediatr Orthop 21:152–156, 2001.

95. Hansen, B.A.; Greiff, J.; Bergmann, F. Fractures of the tibia in children. Acta Orthop Scand 47:448–453, 1976.

96. Hansen, S.T. Internal fixation of children's fractures of the lower extremities. Orthop Clin North Am 21:353–363, 1990.

97. Harcke, H.T.; Zapf, S.E.; Mandell, G.A.; et al. Quantitative bone scintigraphy in the evaluation of angular deformity of the lower extremity. Radiology 164:437–440, 1987.

98. Hartley, J.B. Fatigue fracture of the tibia. Br J Surg 30:9–14, 1942.

99. Heckman, M.M.; Whitesides, T.H., Jr.; Grewe, S.R.; Rooks, M.D. Compartment pressure in association with closed tibial fractures. The relationship between tissue pressure, compartment, and the distance from the site of the fracture. J Bone Joint Surg Am 76:1285–1292, 1994.

100. Helfet, D.L.; Howey, T.; Sanders, R.; Johansen, K. Limb salvage versus amputation: Preliminary results of the mangled extremity severity score. Clin Orthop 256:80–86, 1990.

101. Herring, J.A.; Moseley, C. Post-traumatic valgus deformity of the tibia. Instructional case. J Pediatr Orthop 1:435–439, 1981.

102. Highland, T.R.; LaMont, R.L. Deep, late infections associated with internal fixation in children. J Pediatr Orthop 5:59–64, 1985.

103. Hill, S.A. Incidence of tibial fractures in child skiers. Br J Sports Med 23:169–170, 1989.

104. Hoaglund, F.T.; States, J.D. Factors influencing the rate of healing in tibial shaft fractures. Surg Gynecol Obstet 124:71–76, 1967.

105. Hoover, N.W. Injuries of the popliteal artery associated with fractures and dislocation. Surg Clin North Am 41:1099–1112, 1961.

106. Hope, P.G.; Cole, W.G. Open fractures of the tibia in children. J Bone Joint Surg Br 74:546–553, 1992.

107. Horowitz, J.H.; Nichter, L.S.; Kenney, J.G.; Morgan, R.F. Lawnmower injuries in children: Lower extremity reconstruction. J Trauma 25:1138–1146, 1985.

108. Houghton, G.R.; Dekel, S. The periosteal control of long bone growth. Acta Orthop Scand 50:635–637, 1979.

109. Houghton, G.R.; Rooker, G.D. The role of the periosteum in the growth of long bones: An experimental study in the rabbit. J Bone Joint Surg Br 61:218–220, 1979.

110. Hresko, M.T.; Kasser, J.R. Physeal arrest about the knee associated with non-physeal fractures in the lower extremity. J Bone Joint Surg Am 71:698–703, 1989.

111. Hsu, L.C.S.; O'Brien, J.P.; Yau, A.C.M.C.; Hodgson, O.B.E. Valgus deformity of the ankle resulting from fibular resection for a graft in subtalar fusion in children. J Bone Joint Surg Am 54:585–594, 1972.

112. Hsu, L.C.S.; O'Brien, J.P.; Yau, A.C.M.C.; Hodgson, A.R. Valgus deformity of the ankle in children with fibular pseudarthrosis. J Bone Joint Surg Am 56:503–510, 1974.

113. Ingersoll, C.F. Ice skater's fracture. A form of fatigue fracture. AJR Am J Roentgenol 50:469–479, 1943.

114. Ippolito, E.; Pentimalli, S. Post-traumatic valgus deformity of the knee in proximal tibial metaphyseal fractures in children. Ital J Orthop Traumatol 10:103–108, 1984.

115. Irwin, A.; Gibson, P.; Ashcroft, P. Open fractures of the tibia in children. Injury 26:21–24, 1995.

116. Iwaya, T.; Kiyonori, H.; Yamada, A. Microvascular free flaps for the treatment of avulsion injuries of the feet in children. J Trauma 22:15–19, 1982.

117. Izant, R.J.; Rothman, B.F.; Frankel, V. Bicycle spoke injuries of the foot and ankle in children: An underestimated "minor" injury. J Pediatr Surg 4:654–656, 1969.

118. Jackson, D.W.; Cozen, L. Genu valgum as a complication of proximal tibial metaphyseal fractures in children. J Bone Joint Surg Am 53:1571–1578, 1971.

119. Jakob, R.P.; Haertel, M.; Stussi, E. Tibial torsion calculated by computerized tomography and compared to other methods of measurements. J Bone Joint Surg Br 62:238–242, 1980.

120. James, C.C.M. Fractures of the lower limbs in spina bifida cystica: A survey of 44 fractures in 122 children. Dev Med Child Neurol Suppl 22:88–93, 1970.

121. Jeffreys, T.E. Genu recurvatum after Osgood-Schlatter's disease. A case report. J Bone Joint Surg Br 47:298–299, 1965.

122. Johansen, K.; Bandyk, D.; Thiele, B.; et al. Temporary intraluminal shunts: Resolution of a management dilemma in complex vascular injuries. J Trauma 22:395–401, 1982.

123. Johansen, K.; Daines, M.; Howey, T.; et al. Objective criteria accurately predict amputation following lower extremity trauma. J Trauma 30:568–573, 1990.

124. John, S.D.; Moorthy, C.S.; Swischuk, L.E. Expanding the concept of the toddler's fracture. Radiographics 17:367–376, 1997.

125. Johnson, P.H. Beware: Greenstick fractures of the proximal tibial metaphysis. J Ark Med Soc 80:215–218, 1983.

126. Jones, E.T. Use of computed axial tomography in pediatric orthopaedics. J Pediatr Orthop 1:329–338, 1981.

127. Jordan, S.E.; Alonso, J.E.; Cook, F.F. The etiology of valgus angulation after metaphyseal fractures of the tibia in children. J Pediatr Orthop 7:450–457, 1987.

128. Karaharju, E.O.; Ryoppy, S.A.; Makinen, R.J. Remodeling by asymmetrical epiphyseal growth. J Bone Joint Surg Br 58:122–126, 1976.

129. Karlstrom, G.; Lonnerholm, T.; Olerud, S. Cavus deformity of the foot after fracture of the tibial shaft. J Bone Joint Surg Am 57:893–900, 1975.

130. Karrholm, J.; Hansson, L.I.; Svensonn, K. Incidence of tibiofibular shaft and ankle fractures in children. J Pediatr Orthop 2:386–396, 1982.

131. Kelly, R.P.; Whitesides, T.E., Jr. Transfibular route for fasciotomy of the leg. J Bone Joint Surg Am 49:1022–1023, 1967.

132. Kendra, J.C.; Price, C.T.; Songer, J.E.; Scott, D.S. Pediatric applications of dynamic axial external fixation. Contemp Orthop 19:477–486, 1989.

133. Kessel, L. Annotations on the etiology and treatment of tibia vara. J Bone Joint Surg Br 52:93–99, 1970.

134. Kestler, D.C. Unclassified premature cessation of epiphyseal growth about the knee joint. J Bone Joint Surg Am 29:788–797, 1947.

135. King, J.; Diefendorf, D.; Apthorp, J.; et al. Analysis of 429 fractures in 189 battered children. J Pediatr Orthop 8:585–589, 1988.

136. Kleinman, P.K.; Marks, S.C.; Blackbourne, B. The metaphyseal lesion in abused infants: A radiologic-histopathologic study. AJR Am J Roentgenol 146:895–905, 1986.

137. Knight, D.J.; Bennet, G.C. Nonaccidental injury in osteogenesis imperfecta. A case report. J Pediatr Orthop 10:542–544, 1990.

138. Kogutt, M.S.; Swischuk, L.E.; Fagan, C.J. Patterns of injury and significance of uncommon fractures in the battered child syndrome. Radiology 121:143–149, 1974.

139. Komara, J.S.; Kottamasu, L.; Kottamasu, S.R. Acute plastic bowing fractures in children. Ann Emerg Med 15:585–588, 1986.

140. Kreder, H.J.; Armstrong, P. A review of open tibia fractures in children. J Pediatr Orthop 15:482–488, 1995.

141. Krettek, C.; Haas, N.P.; Tscherne, H. External fixation of ninety-nine open tibial shaft fractures: Advantages with supplemental lag screws? Orthop Trans 15:807, 1991.

142. Kurz, W.; Vinz, H. Zur Epidemiologie und Klinik der geschlossenen diaphysaren Unterschenkelfraktur im Kindesalter. Zentralbl Chir 104:1402–1409, 1979.

143. Langenskiold, A. Surgical treatment of partial closures of the growth plate. J Pediatr Orthop 1:3–11, 1981.

144. Leach, R.E.; Hammond, G.; Stryker, W.S. Anterior tibial compartment syndrome. J Bone Joint Surg Am 49:451–462, 1967.

145. Lee, J.D.; Yao, L. Stress fractures: MR imaging. Radiology 169:217–220, 1988.

146. Leonidas, J.C. Skeletal trauma in the child abuse syndrome. Pediatr Ann 12:875–882, 1983.

147. Letts, M.; Vincent, N.; Gouw, G. The "floating knee" in children. J Bone Joint Surg Br 68:442–446, 1986.

148. Letts, R.M. Degloving injuries in children. J Pediatr Orthop 6:193–197, 1987.

149. Levine, A.M.; Drennan, J.C. Physiological bowing and tibia vara. The metaphyseal-diaphyseal angle in the measurement of bowleg deformities. J Bone Joint Surg Am 64:1158–1163, 1982.

150. Lewallen, R.P.; Peterson, H.A. Nonunion of long bone fractures in children: A review of 30 cases. J Pediatr Orthop 5:135–142, 1985.

151. Ligier, J.N.; Metaizeau, J.P.; Prevot, J.; Lascombes, P. Elastic stable intramedullary pinning of long bone shaft fractures in children. Z Kinderchir 40:209–212, 1985.

152. Lock, T.R.; Aronson, D.D. Fractures in patients who have myelomeningocele. J Bone Joint Surg Am 71:1153–1157, 1989.

153. Loder, R.T.; Bookout, C. Fracture patterns in battered children. J Pediatr Orthop 5:428–433, 1991.

154. Lodge, T. Bone, joint, and soft tissue changes following paraplegia. Acta Radiol 46:435–445, 1956.

155. Mabrey, J.D.; Fitch, R.D. Plastic deformation in pediatric fractures: Mechanism and treatment. J Pediatr Orthop 9:310–314, 1989.

156. MacEwen, G.D.; Zionts, L.E. Proximal tibial fracture in children. In: Uhthoff, H.K.; Wiley, J.J., eds. Behavior of the Growth Plate. New York, Raven, 1988, pp. 141–152.

157. Mahnken, R.F.; Yngve, D.A. Valgus deformity following fracture of the tibial metaphysis. Orthopaedics 11:1320–1322, 1988.

158. Makin, M. Tibio-fibular relationship in paralysed limbs. J Bone Joint Surg Br 47:500–506, 1965.

159. Matejczyk, M.B.; Rang, M. Fractures in children with neuromuscular disorders. In: Houghton, G.R.; Thompson, G.H., eds. Problematic Musculoskeletal Injuries in Children. London, Butterworths, 1983, pp. 178–192.

160. Matin, P. The appearance of bone scans following fractures, including immediate and long-term studies. J Nucl Med 20:1227–1231, 1979.

161. Matsen, F.A., III. A practical approach to compartment syndromes. Part I. Definition, theory, and pathogenesis. Instr Course Lect 32:88–91, 1983.

162. Matsen, F.A., III; Clawson, D.K. The deep posterior compartmental syndrome of the leg. J Bone Joint Surg Am 57:34–39, 1975.

163. Matsen, F.A., III; Staheli, L.T. Neurovascular complications following tibial osteotomy in children. Clin Orthop 110:210–214, 1975.

164. Matsen, F.A., III; Krugmire, R.B., Jr.; King, R.V. Increased tissue pressure and its effects on muscle oxygenation in level and elevated human limbs. Clin Orthop 144:311–320, 1979.

165. Matsen, F.A., III; Winquist, R.A.; Krugmire, R.B. Diagnosis and management of compartmental syndromes. J Bone Joint Surg Am 62:286–291, 1980.

166. McCarthy, J.J.; Kim, D.H.; Eilert, R.E. Posttraumatic genu valgum: Operative versus nonoperative treatment. J Pediatr Orthop 18:518–521, 1998.

167. McIvor, W.C.; Samilson, R.L. Fractures in patients with cerebral palsy. J Bone Joint Surg Am 48:858–866, 1966.

168. Meland, N.B.; Fisher, J.; Irons, G.B.; et al. Experience with 80 rectus abdominis free-tissue transfers. Plast Reconstr Surg 83:481–487, 1989.

169. Mellick, L.B.; Reesor, K. Spiral tibial fractures of children: A commonly accidental spiral long bone fracture. Am J Emerg Med 8:234–237, 1990.

170. Mellick, L.B.; Reesor, K.; Demers, D.; Reinker, K.D. Tibial fractures in young children. Pediatr Emerg Care 4:97–101, 1988.

171. Meurman, K.O.A.; Elfving, S. Stress fracture in soldiers: A multifocal bone disorder. Radiology 134:483–487, 1980.

172. Micheli, L.J.; Gerbino, P.G. Etiologic assessment of stress fractures of the lower extremity in young athletes. Orthop Trans 4:51, 1980.

173. Miller, J.H.; Sanderson, R.A. Scintigraphy of toddler's fracture. J Nucl Med 29:2001–2003, 1988.

174. Morton, K.S.; Starr, D.E. Closure of the anterior portion of the upper tibial epiphysis as a complication of tibial-shaft fracture. J Bone Joint Surg Am 46:570–574, 1964.

175. Mubarak, S.J. A practical approach to compartment syndromes. Part II. Diagnosis. Instr Course Lect 32:92–102, 1983.

176. Mubarak, S.J.; Carroll, N.C. Volkmann's contracture in children. Aetiology and prevention. J Bone Joint Surg Br 61:285–293, 1979.

177. Mubarak, S.J.; Hargens, A.R. Diagnosis and management of compartmental syndromes. In: American Academy of Orthopaedic Surgeons: Symposium on Trauma to the Leg and Its Sequelae. St. Louis, C.V. Mosby, 1981.

178. Mubarak, S.J.; Owens, C.A.; Hargens, A.R.; et al. Acute compartment syndromes: Diagnosis and treatment with the aid of the Wick catheter. J Bone Joint Surg Am 60:1091–1095, 1978.

179. Mueller, M.E.; Allgower, M.; Schneider, R.; Willenegger, H. Manual of Internal Fixation, 2nd ed. New York, Springer-Verlag, 1979.

180. Navascues, J.A.; Gonzalez-Lopez, J.L.; Lopez-Valverde, S.; et al. Premature physeal closure after tibial diaphyseal fractures in adolescents. J Pediatr Orthop 20:193–196, 2000.

181. Navarre, J.R.; Cardillo, P.J.; Gorman, J.F.; et al. Vascular trauma in children and adolescents. Am J Surg 143:229–231, 1982.

182. Ogden, J.A. Tibia and fibula. In: Ogden, J.A., ed. Skeletal Injury in the Child, 2nd ed. Philadelphia, W.B. Saunders, 1991, pp. 587–591.

183. Ogden, J.A.; Tross, R.B.; Murphy, M.J. Fractures of the tibial tuberosity in adolescents. J Bone Joint Surg Am 62:205–215, 1980.

184. Ogden, J.A.; Ogden, D.A.; Pugh, L.; et al. Tibia valga after proximal metaphyseal fractures in childhood: A normal biologic process. J Pediatr Orthop 15:489–494, 1995.

185. Olerad, C.; Danckworth-Kiliestrom, G.; Oternd, S. Genu recurvatum caused by partial growth arrest of the proximal tibial physis: Simultaneous correction and lengthening with physeal distraction. Arch Orthop Trauma Surg 106:64–68, 1986.

186. O'Neill, J.A., Jr.; Meachan, W.F.; Griffin, P.P.; Sawyer, J.C. Patterns of injury in the battered child syndrome. J Trauma 13:332–339, 1973.

187. Oudjhane, K.; Newman, B.; Oh, K.S.; et al. Occult fractures in preschool children. J Trauma 28:858–860, 1988.

188. Paley, D.; Catagni, M.A.; Argnani, F.; et al. Ilizarov treatment of tibial nonunions with bone loss. Clin Orthop 241:146–165, 1989.

189. Pappas, A.M.; Anas, P.; Toczylowski, H.M., Jr. Asymmetrical arrest of the proximal tibial physis and genu recurvatum deformity. J Bone Joint Surg Am 66:575–581, 1984.

190. Park, H.-M.; Kernek, C.B.; Robb, J.A. Early scintigraphic findings of occult femoral and tibia fractures in infants. Clin Nucl Med 13:271–275, 1988.

191. Parrini, L.; Paleari, M.; Biggi, F. Growth disturbances following fractures of the femur and tibia in children. Ital J Orthop Traumatol 11:139–145, 1985.

192. Parsch, K.; Rossak, K. Die pathologischen Frakturen bei Spina bifida. Arch Orthop Unfallchir 68:165–178, 1970.

193. Pauwels, F. Grundriss einer Biomechanik der Fraktur Heilung. Verh Dtsch Orthop Ges 34:62–108, 1940.

194. Pennig, D.; Baranowski, D. Genu recurvatum due to partial growth arrest of the proximal tibial physis: Correction by callus distraction. Arch Orthop Trauma Surg 108:199–211, 1989.

195. Peterson, H.A. Partial growth plate arrests and its treatment. J Pediatr Orthop 4:246–258, 1984.

196. Pollen, A.G. Fractures and Dislocations in Children. Baltimore, Williams & Wilkins, 1973.

197. Potthoff, H. Ein Beitrag zur Behandlung der Proximalen metaphysaren Tibiafraktur in Kindesalter. Aktuelle Traumatol 12:127–128, 1982.

198. Prather, J.L.; Nusynowitz, M.L.; Snowdy, H.A.; et al. Scintigraphic findings in stress fractures. J Bone Joint Surg Am 59:869–874, 1977.

199. Qidwai, S.A. Intramedullary Kirschner wiring for tibia fractures in children. J Pediatr Orthop 21:294–297, 2001.

200. Ralis, Z.A.; Ralis, H.M.; Randall, M.; et al. Changes in shape, ossification, and quality of bone in children with spina bifida. Dev Med Child Neurol 18(Suppl 37):29–41, 1976.

201. Rang, M. Children's Fractures, 2nd ed. Philadelphia, J.B. Lippincott, 1983.

202. Reff, R.B. The use of external fixation devices in the management of severe lower extremity and pelvic injuries in children. Clin Orthop 188:21–33, 1984.

203. Reynolds, D.A. Growth changes in fractured long-bones. A study of 126 children. J Bone Joint Surg Br 63:83–88, 1981.

204. Robert, M.; Khouri, N.; Carlioz, H.; Alain, J.L. Fractures of the proximal tibial metaphysis in children: Review of a series of 25 cases. J Pediatr Orthop 7:444–449, 1987.

205. Roberts, S.M.; Vogt, E.C. Pseudofracture of the tibia. J Bone Joint Surg 21:891–901, 1939.

206. Robertson, P.; Karol, L.A.; Rab, G.T. Open fractures of the tibia and femur in children. J Pediatr Orthop 16:621–626, 1996.

207. Robin, G. Fracture in childhood paraplegia. Paraplegia 3:165–170, 1966.

208. Rooker, G.D.; Coates, R.L. Deformity after greenstick fractures of the upper tibial metaphysis. In: Houghton, G.R.; Thompson, G.H., eds. Problematic Musculoskeletal Injuries in Children. London, Butterworths, 1983, pp. 1–13.

209. Rooker, G.; Salter, R. Prevention of valgus deformity following fracture of the proximal metaphysis of the tibia in children. J Bone Joint Surg Br 62:527, 1980.

210. Rorabeck, C.H. A practical approach to compartment syndromes. Part III. Treatment. Instr Course Lect 32:102–113, 1983.

211. Rorabeck, C.H. The treatment of compartment syndromes of the leg. J Bone Joint Surg Br 66:93–97, 1984.

212. Rorabeck, C.H.; MacNab, I. Anterior tibial compartment syndrome complicating fractures of the shaft of the tibia. J Bone Joint Surg Am 58:549–550, 1976.

213. Roub, L.W.; Gumerman, L.W.; Hanley, E.N.; et al. Bone stress: A radionuclide imaging perspective. Radiology 132:431–438, 1979.

214. Russell, W.L.; Apyan, P.M.; Burns, R.P. Utilization and wide clinical implementation using the Wick catheter for compartment pressure measurement. Surg Gynecol Obstet 160:207–210, 1985.

215. Russo, V.J. Traumatic arterial spasm resulting in gangrene. J Pediatr Orthop 5:486–488, 1985.

216. Salter, R.B.; Best, T. The pathogenesis and prevention of valgus deformity following fractures of the proximal metaphyseal region of the tibia in children. J Bone Joint Surg Am 55:1324, 1973.

217. Sarmiento, A.; Gersten, L.M.; Sobol, P.A.; et al. Tibial shaft fractures treated with functional braces. J Bone Joint Surg Br 71:602–609, 1989.

218. Savoca, C.J. Stress fractures. A classification of the earliest radiographic signs. Radiology 100:519–524, 1971.

219. Sawmiller, S.; Michener, W.M.; Hartman, J.T. Stress fracture in childhood. Cleve Clin Q 32:119–123, 1965.

220. Schrock, R.D. Peroneal nerve palsy following derotation osteomies for tibial torsion. Clin Orthop 62:172–177, 1969.

221. Shaker, I.J.; White, J.J.; Signer, R.D.; et al. Special problems of vascular injuries in children. J Trauma 16:863–867, 1976.

222. Shannak, A.O. Tibial fractures in children: Follow-up study. J Pediatr Orthop 8:306–310, 1988.

223. Shravat, B.P.; Harrop, S.N.; Kane, T.P. Toddler's fracture. J Accid Emerg Med 13:59–61, 1996.

224. Singer, J.; Towbin, R. Occult fractures in the production of gait disturbance in childhood. Pediatrics 64:192–196, 1979.

225. Skak, S.V.; Toftgard, T.; Torben, D.P. Fractures of the proximal metaphysis of the tibia in children. Injury 18:149–156, 1987.

226. Smillie, I.S. Injuries of the Knee Joint, 2nd ed. Baltimore, Williams & Wilkins, 1951.

227. Song, K.M.; Sangeorzan, B.; Benirschke, S.; Browne, R. Open fractures of the tibia in children. J Pediatr Orthop 16:635–639, 1996.

228. Soutter, F.E. Spina bifida and epiphyseal displacement. J Bone Joint Surg Br 44:106–109, 1962.

229. Spiegal, P.G.; Mast, J.W. Internal and external fixation of fractures in children. Orthop Clin North Am 11:405–421, 1980.

230. Stanford, T.C.; Rodriguez, R.P.; Hayes, J.T. Tibial-shaft fractures in adults and children. JAMA 195:1111–1114, 1966.

231. Steel, H.H.; Sandrow, R.E.; Sullivan, P.D. Complications of tibial osteotomy in children for genu varum or valgum. J Bone Joint Surg Am 53:1629–1635, 1971.

232. Steinert, V.V.; Bennek, J. Unterschenkelfrakturen im Kindesalter. Zentralbl Chir 91:1387–1392, 1966.

233. Stern, M.B.; Grant, S.S.; Isaacson, A.S. Bilateral distal tibial and fibular epiphyseal separation associated with spina bifida. Clin Orthop 50:191–196, 1967.

234. Swaan, J.W.; Oppers, V.M. Crural fractures in children. Arch Chir Neerl 23:259–272, 1971.
235. Takai, R.; Grant, A.D.; Atar, D.; Lehman, W.B. Minor knee trauma as a possible cause of asymmetrical proximal tibial physis closure. A case report. Clin Orthop 307:142–145, 1994.
236. Tauton, J.E.; Clement, D.B.; Webber, D. Lower extremity stress fractures in athletes. Physician Sports Med 9:77–86, 1981.
237. Taylor, S.L. Tibial overgrowth: A cause of genu valgum. J Bone Joint Surg Am 45:659, 1963.
238. Teitz, C.C.; Carter, D.R.; Frankel, V.H. The problems associated with tibial fractures with intact fibulae. J Bone Joint Surg Am 62:770–776, 1980.
239. Tenenbien, M.; Reed, M.H.; Black, G.B. The toddler's fracture revisited. Am J Emerg Med 8:208–211, 1990.
240. Thompson, G.H.; Wilber, J.H. Fracture management in the multiply injured child. In: Marcus, R.E., ed. Trauma in Children. Rockville, MD, Aspen, 1986, pp. 99–146.
241. Thompson, G.H.; Wilber, J.H.; Marcus, R.E. Internal fixation of fractures in children and adolescents. A comparative analysis. Clin Orthop 188:10–20, 1984.
242. Tolo, V.T. External skeletal fixation in children's fractures. J Pediatr Orthop 3:435–442, 1983.
243. Tolo, V.T. External fixation in multiply injured children. Orthop Clin North Am 21:393–400, 1990.
244. Townsend, P.F.; Cowell, H.R.; Steg, N.L. Lower extremity fractures in children simulating infection in myelomeningocele. Clin Orthop 144:255–259, 1979.
245. Trotter, M.; Gleser, G.C. Estimation of stature from long bones of American whites and Negroes. Am J Phys Anthropol 10:463–514, 1952.
246. Tscherne, H.; Gotzen, L. Fractures with Soft Tissue Injuries. Berlin, Springer-Verlag, 1984.
247. Tscherne, H.; Oestern, H.J. Die Klassifizierung des Weichteilschadens bei offenen und geschlossenen Frakturen. Unfallheilkunde 85:111–115, 1982.
248. Tupman, G.S. A study of bone growth in normal children and its relationship to skeletal maturation. J Bone Joint Surg Br 44:42–67, 1962.
249. Tuten, H.R.; Keeler, K.A.; Gabos, P.G.; et al. Posttraumatic tibia valga in children: A long-term follow-up note. J Bone Joint Surg Am 81:799–810, 1999.
250. Van Meter, J.W.; Branick, R.I. Bilateral genu recurvatum after skeletal traction. A case report. J Bone Joint Surg Am 62:837–839, 1980.
251. Verhelst, M.P.; Spaas, F.M.; Fabry, G. Progressive valgus deformity of the knee after resection of an exostosis at the proximal medial tibial metaphysis. A case report. Acta Orthop Belg 41:689–694, 1975.
252. Verstreken, L.; Delronge, G.; Lamoureux, J. Orthopaedic treatment of paediatric multiple trauma patients. Int Surg 73:177–179, 1988.
253. Vinz, H. Die Behandlung offener Frakturen bei Kindern. Zentralbl Chir 105:1483–1493, 1980.
254. Vinz, H.; Kurz, W. Die offene diaphysare Unterschenkefraktur im Kindesalter. Zentralbl Chir 105:32–38, 1980.
255. Visser, J.D.; Veldhuizen, A.G. Valgus deformity after fracture of the proximal tibial metaphysis in childhood. Acta Orthop Scand 53:663–667, 1982.
256. Voto, S.J.; Pigott, J.; Riley, P.; Donovan, D. Arterial injuries associated with lower extremity fractures. Orthopaedics 11:357–360, 1988.
257. Walton, J.N.; Warrick, C.K. Osseous changes in myopathy. Br J Radiol 27:1–15, 1954.
258. Weber, B.G. Fibrous interposition causing valgus deformity after fracture of the upper tibial metaphysis in children. J Bone Joint Surg Br 59:290–292, 1977.
259. Weber, B.G.; Brunner, C.; Freuler, F., eds. Treatment of Fractures in Children and Adolescents. Berlin, Springer-Verlag, 1980.
260. Whitesides, T.E., Jr.; Haney, T.C.; Morimoto, K.; Harada, H. Tissue pressure measurements as a determinant for the need of fasciotomy. Clin Orthop 113:43–51, 1975.
261. Willhoite, D.R.; Moll, J.H. Early recognition and treatment of impending Volkmann's ischemia in the lower extremity. Arch Surg 100:11–16, 1970.
262. Wiltse, L.L. Valgus deformity of the ankle: A sequel to acquired or congenital abnormalities of the fibula. J Bone Joint Surg Am 54:595–606, 1972.
263. Wolma, F.J.; Larrieu, A.J.; Alsop, G.C. Arterial injuries of the legs associated with fractures and dislocations. Am J Surg 140:806–809, 1980.
264. Wood, D.; Hoffer, M.M. Tibial fractures in head-injured children. J Trauma 27:65–68, 1987.
265. Yang, J-P; Letts, R.M. Isolated fractures of the tibia with intact fibula in children: A review of 95 patients. J Pediatr Orthop 17:347–351, 1997.
266. Yasko, A.; Wilber, J.H. Open tibial fractures in children. Orthop Trans 13:547–548, 1989.
267. Yue, J.J.; Churchill, R.S.; Cooperman, D.R.; et al. The floating knee in the pediatric patient. Nonoperative versus operative stabilization. Clin Orthop 376:124–136, 2000.
268. Zionts, L.E.; MacEwen, G.D. Spontaneous improvement of posttraumatic tibia valga. J Bone Joint Surg Am 68:680–687, 1986.
269. Zionts, L.; Harcke, T.H.; Brooks, K.M.; MacEwen, G.D. Posttraumatic tibia valga: A case demonstrating asymmetric activity of the proximal growth plate on technetium bone scan. J Pediatr Orthop 7:458–462, 1987.

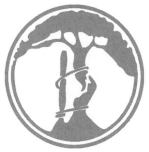

# CHAPTER 16

## Fractures and Dislocations of the Foot and Ankle

Alvin H. Crawford, M.D., F.R.C.S.
Mohammed J. Al-Sayyad, M.D., F.R.C.S.(C.)

Fractures and injuries about the foot and ankle in children are important. A pain-free and deformity-free foot and ankle after injury allow a child the freedom to run, play, explore the environment, and satisfy unlimited personal curiosities. If a residual deformity lingers after injury, the child limps, which causes agony for the parents, who may feel that they did not do enough to prevent their child's angular deformity. The child is teased and taunted by peers or has an arthritic problem that causes pain and leads to unfulfilled wishes—whether they be simply to walk through a meadow and smell the flowers or to be a great athlete like Michael Jordan. Our collected thoughts and those of our referenced colleagues are intended to guide the reader to a safe resolution of foot and ankle injuries in children.

## THE ANKLE

### Relevant Anatomy

The ankle joint is a true mortise joint, or a modified hinge joint, that consists of three bones: the tibia, fibula, and talus. The joint essentially moves in only one plane, from plantar flexion to dorsiflexion. The lateral malleolus allows minimal rotation to accommodate the changing width of the talar dome. The talar dome is broader anteriorly than posteriorly and, as a result, allows less rotation when the foot is in dorsiflexion than when it is in plantar flexion. The anatomic relationships and limited joint motion render the distal fibular epiphysis particularly vulnerable to crushing and twisting injuries (Fig. 16–1).

The ligaments about the ankle are attached to the epiphyses (Fig. 16–2). The deltoid ligament arises from the tip of the medial malleolus distal to the growth plate; it consists of two sets of fibers—superficial and deep. The superficial fibers are attached to the navicular bone (tibionavicular fibers), talus (posterior tibiotalaris), and

sustentaculum tali (tibiocalcanean). The deep portion inserts into the medial surface of the talus (anterior tibiotalar). On the lateral aspect of the ankle, support is provided by three separate ligaments. Their tension and spatial orientation change according to the position of the ankle joint: plantar flexion, neutral, or dorsiflexion. These ligaments have their origin on the fibula distal to the physis. The anterior talofibular ligament runs anteriorly and medially from the anterior margin of the lateral malleolus to the talus anteriorly. The posterior talofibular ligament runs horizontally from the sulcus on the back of the lateral malleolus to the posterior aspect of the talus. The calcaneofibular ligament extends downward and slightly posterior from the tip of the lateral malleolus to a tubercle on the lateral aspect of the calcaneus; it is in close relationship to the peroneal tendons and their sheath. The growth plate is more likely than the ligaments to fail during the years of skeletal development. The tibiofibular syndesmosis consists of four ligaments—the anterior and posterior inferior tibiofibular ligaments, the interosseous ligament, and the anterior transverse ligament—in addition to the interosseous membrane. The anterior tibiofibular ligament runs downward between the anterior margin of the tibia and fibula; its origin in the fibula is also distal to the growth plate. The tibiofibular syndesmosis is rarely injured in children because the ligament is stronger than the growth plates, which tend to give more easily. In an adolescent in whom the growth plate has closed, disruption of the tibiofibular syndesmosis can occur. In 1995, Xenos and co-workers determined that to evaluate disruption of the syndesmosis, a stress lateral radiograph has a much higher correlation with anatomic diastasis than does a stress mortise radiograph.[162] Historically, orthopaedists have evaluated this injury on an external rotation stress mortise view to determine whether diastasis has occurred. On a true lateral view under external rotation stress, cadaveric studies have shown that posterior displacement of the fibula is a more accurate observation when release of the tibiofibular syndesmosis has been

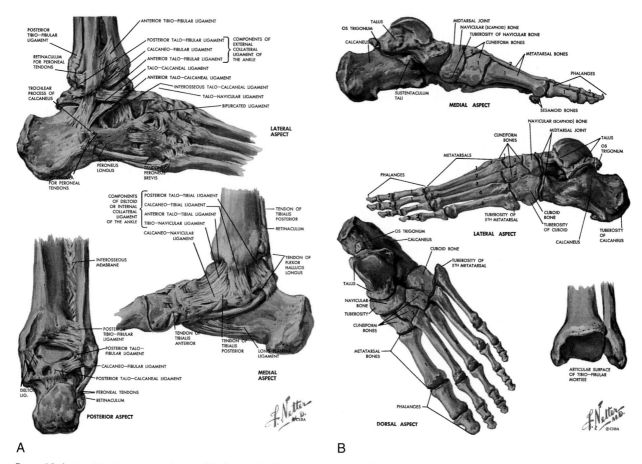

A                                                          B

FIGURE 16–1. *A* and *B,* The anatomic bones of the foot and ankle; anteroposterior and lateral views, including ligaments. (From Netter, F. Ciba-Geigy Corp. Clin Symp 17:1, 1965.)

carried out. Furthermore, both intraobserver and interobserver data suggest that stress lateral radiographs are more reliable. It is possible that the prevalence of this injury is higher than previously reported because of the difficulty of diagnosing it with the stress mortise view.[162]

The distal tibial physis begins to close about 18 months before complete cessation of tibial growth, first closing in its midportion, then medially, and finally laterally.[98] Longitudinal growth of the distal tibial epiphysis ceases at about 12 years of age in girls and 13 years in boys.[80] The fusion process does not occur uniformly but is instead asymmetric (Fig. 16–3). Fusion begins in the area of the tibial "hump," which is located centrally and is seen on the anteroposterior (AP) view as a small bump over the area of the medial edge of the talus. As fusion progresses, the medial part of the plate closes and then progresses posteriorly; finally, the anterolateral part of the plate fuses. The average time to fusion is 18 months. The fused part of the epiphyseal plate is no longer weak and prone to fracture but becomes an area of relative strength.[80] The irregular fusion pattern and the resulting areas of relative strength and weakness are responsible for the unusual transitional fracture patterns, specifically, juvenile Tillaux and triplane fractures.

Accessory ossicles of the malleoli are common in skeletally immature individuals. They usually appear

between the ages of 7 and 10 years and eventually fuse with the secondary ossification center of the malleolus at skeletal maturity.[112] The lateral ossicle has been termed the os subfibulare. Most of these ossification variations are identified only fortuitously, when radiographs are taken to evaluate an injury to the ankle or foot. They may be confused with a sleeve fracture-avulsion of the medial or lateral malleolus. If the patient is symptomatic and presence of a lesion is uncertain, a positive technetium bone scan may support a diagnosis of injury.[28]

## Incidence and Mechanism of Injury

Injuries are commonly caused by indirect violence, with the fixed foot being forced into eversion-inversion, plantar flexion, external rotation, or dorsiflexion. Fractures may also be sustained by direct violence, the usual history being an automobile accident, a fall from a height, or participation in contact sports. Injuries to the lower part of the leg and foot are more common in boys and usually occur between the ages of 10 and 15 years.[37, 77, 115, 141] Those about the ankle constitute 10% to 25% of all physeal injuries.[97] Distal tibial and fibular epiphyseal and physeal injuries account for 4% of all ankle injuries. Fractures of the distal end of the tibia

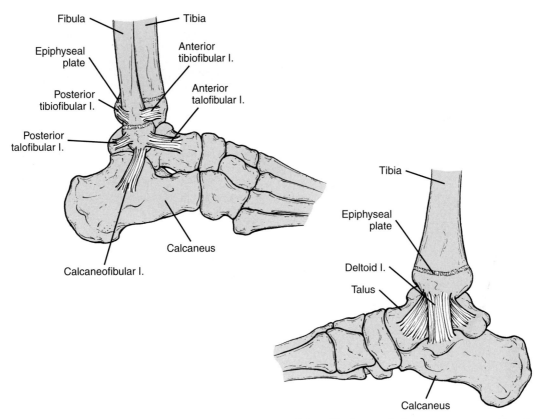

**Figure 16–2.** The ligaments of the foot. Medial and lateral views of the ankle showing the ligamentous anatomy. Note the relationship of the physes to the ligaments. (From McNealy, G.A.; et al. AJR Am J Roentgenol 138:683, 1982. Copyright 1982, American Roentgen Ray Society.)

often involve the articular surface and the physis (growth plate). If left unreduced, these injuries can predispose to articular and growth deformities and eventually arthritis. The distal tibial epiphysis is the second most common site of epiphyseal fracture in children, after the distal end of the radius.[115] The bone of a child is more capable of elastic and plastic deformation than adult bone is.[126] Ligamentous injuries are rare because the ligaments are stronger than the physes. Adduction injuries are most common (15%) and also account for the highest rate of complications. The patterns of separation of the epiphyseal plate, when it is subjected to indirect trauma, usually result from avulsive or rotational forces applied to the fixed foot and leg, with subsequent transmission of the shearing and sliding forces to the epiphyseal plate. These forces are transmitted to the medial part of the tibia by the ligamentous pull of the deltoid ligaments. Laterally, forces are transmitted by the anterior and posterior tibiofibular ligaments, the anterior and posterior talofibular ligaments, and the calcaneofibular ligaments.[73] The tendency for physeal compression during adduction injury is also greater. With an adduction injury, medial migration of the talus is usually blocked by the medial malleolus, and the medial malleolus is subsequently fractured. Pronation injuries involve eversion and external rotation and are caused by an abduction force in 40% of cases.[71] External rotation injuries are seen in 25% of leg and foot injuries.

## Consequences of Injury

The prognosis for injuries to the foot and ankle involves several criteria. The skeletal maturity of the patient determines the resulting bone, ligament, or growth plate injury. At different skeletal ages, the same mechanical twisting, torsional force, or related trauma to the foot and leg causes different injuries. Children are more prone to epiphyseal injuries, which of course are subject to more complications than shaft or metaphyseal injuries are. The more severe the injury (e.g., compound, grossly contaminated, comminuted with or without soft tissue crushing), the greater the possibility of secondary devitalization with consequent delayed union, nonunion, pseudarthrosis, or osteomyelitis. The adequacy of reduction directly influences the rate of union; the more bony contact, the less healing time required. All things considered, anatomic reduction is especially important for epiphyseal fractures because anatomic alignment reduces the incidence of angular deformity and shortening secondary to growth arrest, as well as degenerative arthritis secondary to persistent joint incongruity (step-off) and instability. The prognosis after fractures involving the distal end of the tibia in children depends on the skeletal maturity of the patient, the severity of the injury, the fracture type, the degrees of comminution and displacement of the fracture, and the adequacy of reduction.[141]

Epiphyseal plate

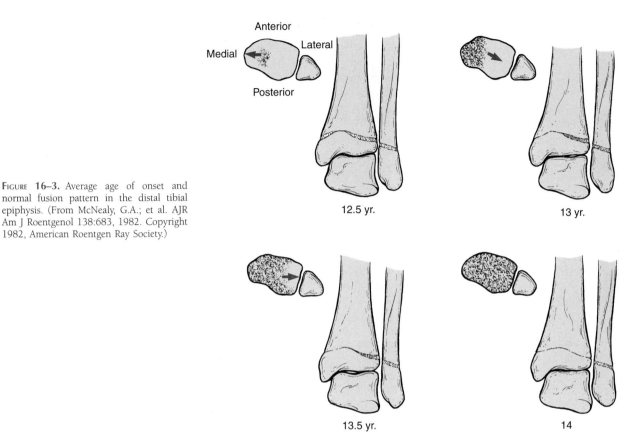

**FIGURE 16–3.** Average age of onset and normal fusion pattern in the distal tibial epiphysis. (From McNealy, G.A.; et al. AJR Am J Roentgenol 138:683, 1982. Copyright 1982, American Roentgen Ray Society.)

Anterior

Medial ← Lateral

Posterior

12.5 yr.          13 yr.

13.5 yr.          14

## Radiologic Evaluation

AP and lateral views of the injured area should always be taken. If swelling is present and no injury can be seen, an oblique view is recommended. One should assess the soft tissue very carefully.[129] The normal fat stripe surrounding a bone may be thickened after a nondisplaced fracture. In addition, joint effusion after nondisplaced articular fractures may result in a positive fat pad, or synovial, sign, especially in the anterior of the ankle over the talar neck or the posterior of the ankle with displacement of the Achilles tendon fat stripe (Fig. 16–4). Computed tomography (CT) is recommended for imaging articular fractures when plain radiographs show displacement of greater than 2 mm. Polycycloidal tomography is still preferred for mapping a physeal bar after premature growth arrest. Even though the C-arm image intensifier is excellent for achieving reduction in

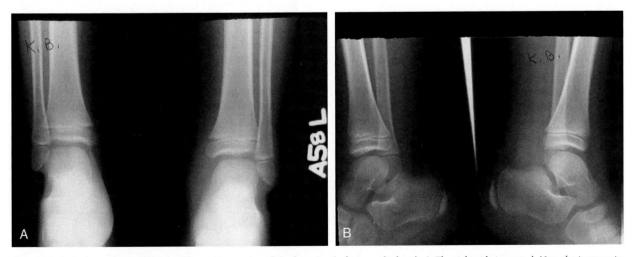

**FIGURE 16–4.** Radiographic evaluation of foot with notation of the fat stripe (soft tissue shadows). *A,* The right side is normal. Note the increase in soft tissue density adjacent to and below the medial malleolus on the left side. *B,* The left lateral ankle view (right side) shows an increase in the soft tissue posterior to the ankle joint. The soft tissue density is limited by the fat stripe just anterior to the Achilles tendon shadow.

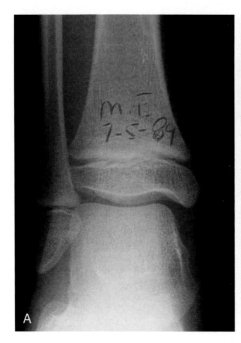
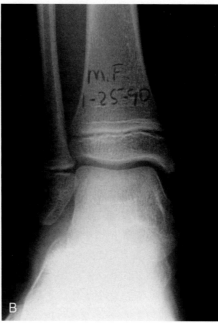

FIGURE **16–5.** "Sprain" injury to the ankle, with the subsequent development of Park-Harris lines. *A,* A radiograph taken at the time of injury demonstrates soft tissue swelling below the malleoli. *B,* Six months later, a horizontal line is seen just superior to the physis of both the tibia and fibula—the Park-Harris growth arrest line. The line should always be horizontal and parallel to the physis when growth is normal.

the operating room, we recommend permanent plain radiographs after reduction and before waking the patient. This is our hard copy "report card." The worst time to discover failure of anatomic reduction and stabilization is when examining radiographs taken in the recovery room or while the patient is being transferred to the floor. After treatment, if the patient has any stiffness or fails to achieve adequate range of motion, a contrast CT scan or magnetic resonance imaging (MRI) is indicated to rule out any intra-articular cartilaginous (silent) fragments.

When monitoring fractures about the ankle in children, it is extremely important to observe the Park-Harris growth arrest lines. These lines represent transient calcification of physeal cartilage during injury repair and are an excellent marker for observing growth after injury. The lines are parallel to the physis if growth is occurring normally (Fig. 16–5). In children with physeal damage, the line may be tented or angular. Special attention to this phenomenon is indicated in Salter-Harris types III and IV injuries to the medial malleolus (Fig. 16–6).

## Classification (Historical Data)

In 1898, Poland, based on an anatomic study of amputation specimens, showed that pure separation of the epiphysis at the physis was rarer than separation of the epiphysis with a fracture of the metaphysis.[122] Ashhurst and Bromer in 1922 presented a classification of the mechanisms of fracture of the leg bones involving the ankle.[4]

In 1932, Bishop differentiated physeal injuries of the ankle based on the Ashhurst-Bromer classification according to the direction of the force that produced the fracture: external rotation, abduction, adduction, axial compression, and direct injury.[9] Each mechanism was subdivided into first-, second-, and third-degree external rotation, abduction, and adduction. This classification

was confusing and often inaccurate; as a result, it is rarely used today.

Aitken in 1936 classified fractures of the physeal cartilage into three distinct types according to the relationship of the fracture line to the various zones of the physis.[1]

Lauge-Hansen in 1950, through a series of experimental studies and clinical observations, proposed a new classification of ankle fractures in adults.[82] According to his study, three elements are important in ankle injury: axial load, position of the foot at the moment of trauma, and direction of the abnormal forces.

In 1955, Carothers and Crenshaw added the plantar flexion mechanism to the classification of Bishop.[21] This

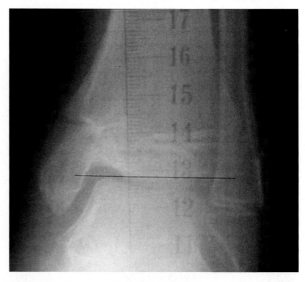

FIGURE **16–6.** Scanogram of the left ankle illustrating a physeal bar; the image was taken 1 year after a Salter-Harris type IV fracture of the medial malleolus. The physis is obliterated just above the medial corner of the mortise, and trabeculae can be seen connecting the epiphysis to the metaphysis. The Park-Harris growth arrest line can be seen lateral to the bony bar and is angulated, indicative of arrest on the medial side.

system describes five mechanisms of injury: plantar flexion, external rotation, abduction, adduction, and direct injury/axial compression. They described six cases in which no fracture of the fibula accompanied posterior displacement of the entire tibial epiphysis.

Salter and Harris in 1963 classified physeal injuries into five types.[131] Ogden classified physeal injuries into seven types with subgroupings.[111] Although more anatomically inclusive, the Ogden classification has not gained widespread use; the Salter-Harris classification is the most generally accepted and widely used.

In 1978, Dias and Tachdjian introduced a new classification of children's fractures that incorporated the concepts of Lauge-Hansen.[37] To classify the fracture properly, radiographs are necessary; AP, lateral, and oblique views must be taken, and tomograms may also be necessary. In their classification (Table 16–1), the first part of the type name describes the position of the foot at the moment of trauma, and the second notes the abnormal force applied to the ankle joint: supination-inversion, pronation-eversion–external rotation, supination–plantar flexion, or supination–external rotation (Fig. 16–7).

**TABLE 16–1**

Classification of Physeal Injuries of the Ankle in Children (Modified from Lauge-Hansen)

| Type | Grade | Position of Foot | Injuring Force | Pattern of Fracture | Comment |
|---|---|---|---|---|---|
| Supination-inversion | 1 | Supinated | Inversion | Usually Salter-Harris I or II fracture-separation of distal fibular physis<br>Occasionally rupture of lateral ligament or fracture of tip of lateral malleolus | Displacement minimal and almost always medial |
| | 2 | Supinated | Inversion | Usually Salter-Harris III or IV fracture of medial part of tibial epiphysis<br>Rarely Salter-Harris I or II fracture with medial displacement of entire tibial epiphysis | Caution: asymmetric growth arrest causes varus ankle |
| Supination–plantar flexion | 1 | Supinated | Plantar flexion | Commonly Salter-Harris II fracture of tibial epiphysis<br>Rarely Salter-Harris I fracture of tibial physis<br>No associated fracture of fibula<br>Metaphyseal fragment and displacement posterior<br>Fracture line best seen on lateral radiograph | Prognosis good<br>Caution: do not damage growth plate by forced manipulation<br>Posterior displacement will remodel |
| Supination–lateral rotation | 1 | Supinated | Lateral rotation | Salter-Harris II fracture of distal tibial epiphysis with long spiral fracture of distal tibia starting laterally at distal tibial growth plate | Distinguishing feature is direction of fracture line starting laterally and running medially and proximally |
| | 2 | Supinated | Lateral rotation | Grade 1 plus spiral fracture of distal fibular shaft | |
| Pronation-eversion–lateral rotation | 1 | Pronated | Eversion–lateral rotation | Salter-Harris II fracture of distal tibial epiphysis<br>Metaphyseal fragment lateral or posterolateral<br>Displacement lateral or posterolateral<br>Fibular fracture short, oblique, 4–7 cm from tip of lateral malleolus | |
| **MISCELLANEOUS** | | | | | |
| Adolescent Tillaux | — | Neutral? | Lateral rotation | Salter-Harris III fracture of lateral part of distal tibial epiphysis<br>Should not be any metaphyseal fragment<br>Displacement anterolateral | Medial part of distal tibial physis closed |
| Triplane, three fragments | — | ? | Lateral rotation | Fracture in three planes—coronal, sagittal, and transverse<br>Combination of Salter-Harris II and III<br>Fracture produces three fragments | Medial part of distal tibial physis open |
| Triplane, two fragments | — | ? | Lateral rotation | Fracture in three planes—coronal, sagittal, and transverse<br>Combination of Salter-Harris II and III<br>Fracture creates two fragments | Medial part of distal tibial physis usually closed |
| Comminuted fracture of distal end of tibia | — | ? | Crushing injuries<br>Direct violence | Comminuted fracture involving distal tibial epiphysis<br>Physis often damaged<br>Fibula fracture at various levels | Poor prognosis |

*Source:* Tachdjian, M.O. Pediatric Orthopedics, 2nd ed. Philadelphia, W.B. Saunders, 1990.

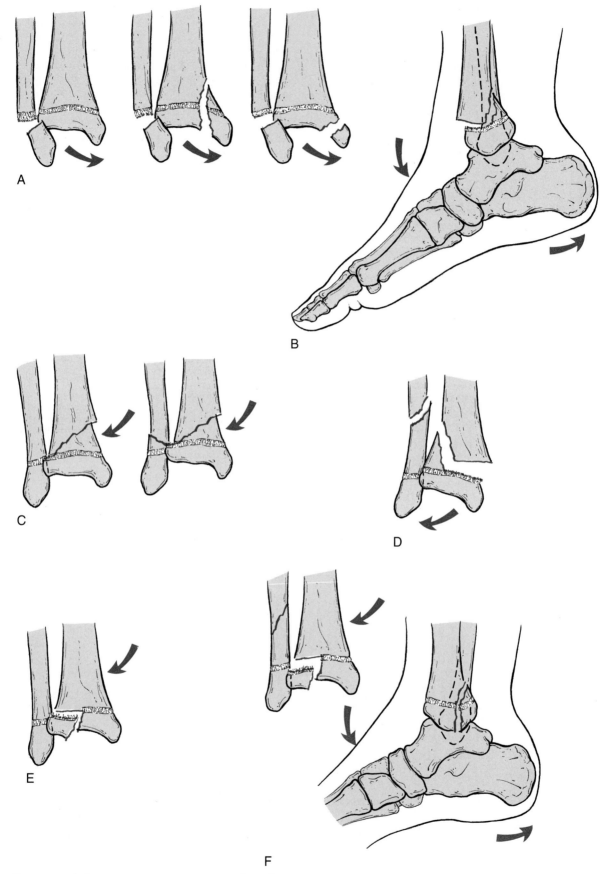

FIGURE **16–7.** *A,* Supination-inversion. *B,* Supination–plantar flexion. *C,* Supination–external rotation. *D,* Pronation-eversion. *E,* Salter-Harris III fracture, distal tibial epiphysis. *F,* Triplane fracture. (From Dias, L.S.; Tachdjian, M.O. Clin Orthop 136:230, 1978.)

Spiegel and co-workers (Fig. 16–8) monitored 184 of a series of 237 fractures of the distal end of the tibia, fibula, or both for an average of 28 months after injury.[141] Using the Salter-Harris classification, they differentiated three groups according to their risk for shortening of the leg, angular deformity of the bone, or incongruity of the joint. The low-risk group consisted of 89 patients, 6.7% of whom had complications; this group included all type I and type II fibula fractures, all type I tibia fractures, type III and type IV tibia fractures with less than 2 mm of displacement, and epiphyseal avulsion injuries. The high-risk group consisted of 28 patients, 32% of whom had complications; this group included type III and type IV tibia fractures with 2 mm or more of displacement, juvenile Tillaux fractures, triplane fractures, and comminuted tibial epiphyseal fractures (type V). The unpredictable group was made up of 66 patients, 16.7% of whom had complications; only type II tibia fractures were included. The incidence and types of complications were correlated with the type of fracture (Carothers and Crenshaw classification), the severity of displacement or comminution, and the adequacy of reduction.[141]

de Sanctis and co-workers monitored 113 of a series of 158 fractures of the distal end of the tibia, fibula, or both for an average of 6 years after injury. Using the Salter-Harris classification and the Carothers and Crenshaw traumatic mechanism classification, they reported that fractures more likely to result in permanent damage to the physis are those caused by a traumatic adduction-supination mechanism that can produce Salter-Harris type III, IV, and V fractures of the distal part of the tibia; they also reported that the combination of compression and adduction may cause a Salter-Harris type V injury

with type III and IV fractures. However, type V lesions are often diagnosed late. In 11 of their 12 poor results, 6 were caused by adduction-supination injuries and 5 were compressive injuries.[35]

In spite of their complexity, ankle fractures in children can be roughly divided into avulsion and epiphyseal fractures.[155] Adequately reduced avulsion fractures can be expected to heal well; epiphyseal fractures, however, may give rise to late complications. Vahvanen and Alto proposed that classification of ankle fractures in children be based on radiographic findings, primarily with respect to epiphyseal lesions, as well as on a simple grouping with regard to risk for clinical purposes: group I, low-risk avulsion fractures and epiphyseal separations; and group II, high-risk fractures through the epiphyseal plate. We agree completely with this simplistic concept. Most avulsion fractures in children heal very well and have few complications; those that involve the epiphyseal plate tend to lead to either failure of continued growth because of damage to the endochondral ossification sequence or the potential for arthritis from interfragmentary gaps or step-offs of greater than 3 mm.[155]

In this chapter, the Salter-Harris classification is used to describe injuries to the growth plates. Radiographs must be studied carefully to determine the type of Salter-Harris physeal injury and the direction of displacement of the epiphyseal-metaphyseal fracture fragments in relation to localized swelling and tenderness. Various published studies noting the importance of the mechanism of injury are cited. Unfortunately, our clinical experience is that children are seldom able to recall the exact position of the foot and leg at the time of injury (Fig. 16–9).

## Indications for Surgical Treatment

Primary indications for surgical treatment include open fractures, inability to obtain or maintain an adequate closed reduction, displaced articular fractures, displaced physeal fractures, or any evidence of massive soft tissue injury.

## Surgical Technique

Every effort should be made to reduce the fracture anatomically and attain formal alignment of the physis and articular surface. If one is able to achieve anatomic reduction by closed manipulation, strong consideration should be given to stabilizing the fracture with percutaneous Steinmann pins/K-wires or a cannulated screw. Indirect reduction as an adjunct to closed manipulation is extremely effective in treating children's ankle fractures. It is most effective when the fracture is fresh or before an interfragmentary clot has formed. We have performed indirect reduction of medial malleolar and Tillaux fractures by using a Steinmann pin through the distal fragment as a levering device or "joystick" to anatomically align the fragment; direct manual compression is then applied, and the pin is continued across the fracture site. Once anatomic reduction and alignment are

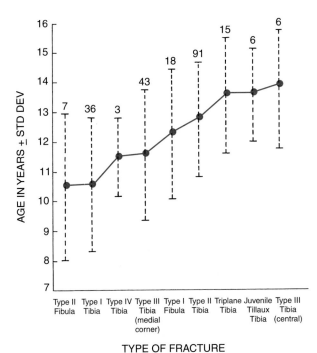

**FIGURE 16–8.** Type of fracture based on age (age versus type of fracture). (From Spiegel, P.G.; et al. J Bone Joint Surg Am 60:8, 1978.)

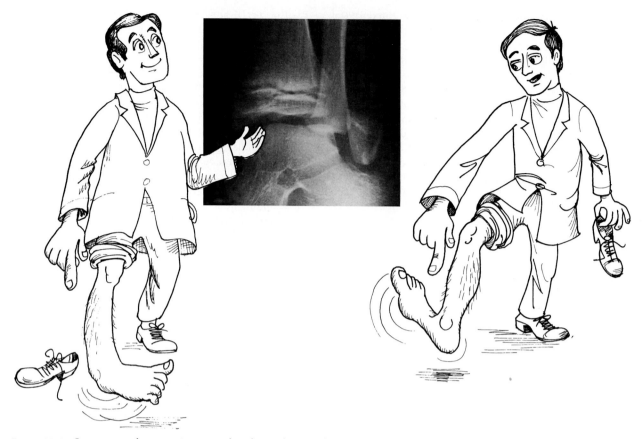

FIGURE 16–9. One surgeon demonstrating to another the mechanism of an ankle injury. (From Rang, M. *Children's Fractures*. Philadelphia, J.B. Lippincott, 1974.)

achieved, one can either use a plaster-of-Paris cast or place a cannulated screw over the pin to maintain stability. Over the past 10 years, the senior author (A.H.C.) has preferred this indirect reduction technique over open reduction whenever possible.

If one has to perform open reduction, adequate exposure of the physis, articular surfaces, or both is mandatory. Every effort should be made to diminish the amount of soft tissue dissection by placing the incision over the area of the fracture gap. One can usually see elevation of the periosteum at the level of the fracture, and little additional dissection is necessary. By irrigating the wound, removing any clots, and extracting any bony debris by curettage, it is usually possible to realign the fracture anatomically. If anatomic reduction is prevented by a distal metaphyseal fragment, such as that found with a Salter-Harris type IV fracture, it is possible to remove the metaphyseal fragment and obtain anatomic alignment of the epiphysis without damaging the physeal line. On occasion, a periosteal flap may prevent anatomic reduction. Once anatomic alignment has been achieved, one should pin the epiphysis to the epiphysis and, if it was not necessary to remove the metaphyseal fragment, the metaphysis to the metaphysis. We strongly recommend *against* placing a pin obliquely across the physis in a growing child. Unless evidence of closure of the middle of the physis is seen, we would not place an oblique pin across the fracture site, similar to the technique used in adults for medial malleolar fractures.

Epiphyseal injuries about the ankle are very common and are probably second only to epiphyseal injuries of the distal end of the radius. The classifications help identify the injury pattern, suggest a treatment, and imply a prognosis. We strongly recommend treating most displaced injuries under general anesthesia so that the child is completely relaxed and adequate reduction can be achieved. Percutaneous Steinmann pin fixation with cast immobilization or cannulated screw fixation followed by splinting and padding is strongly recommended if closed reduction results in anatomic alignment. Because of projectional distortion, the image intensifier film may fail to show the same degree of clarity as plain films. We therefore firmly recommend three-view plain radiographs for all displaced physeal and articular fractures before applying the cast in the operating room.

## Salter-Harris Distal Tibial Fractures

### TYPE I FRACTURE

A type I injury is rare and is most often noted in neurologically impaired children or those subjected to child abuse. Most type I injuries are diagnosed as ankle sprains or strains on initial radiographs because no definite fracture can be identified.

**Physical Examination.** Because the patient has pain and swelling around the ankle, little deformity, if any, can be seen. Adequate range of motion of the ankle is usually possible but may be limited by pain.

**Radiographic Examination.** Radiographs may show some displacement of the tibial epiphysis on the metaphysis or may show only mild widening of the tibial physis (Fig. 16–10). No special studies are required for this injury because the diagnosis is generally fairly straightforward.

**Management.** Often, the child has been treated initially with an elastic bandage for a sprain but returns in 2 or 3 days with complaints of continued pain and swelling. Radiographs then reveal widening of the growth plate and an increase in density of the metaphyseal border. The child is treated for 4 weeks with a below-knee walking cast. The pain is relieved and the growth plate is restored to its normal thickness, but significant complications may rarely occur.[12] The fibula may also be involved. We recommend follow-up in 6 months to rule out growth arrest of the distal end of the tibia.

Three cases of rotational displacement of the lower tibial epiphysis secondary to trauma have been reported. The injury is a Salter-Harris type I distal tibial fracture. In this rare injury to the distal tibial growth plate, the distal tibial epiphysis undergoes true rotational displacement with posterior displacement of the fibula, but without fracture of the fibula.[13, 88, 109] The fibula in these cases appears to be plastic enough to twist without breaking.

Reduction is achieved with an audible click, probably caused by the fibula snapping back into the metaphyseal portion of the incisura fibularis and having retained its normal relationship and attachments to the displaced tibial epiphysis. No permanent damage to the growth plate was noted with these injuries.

## TYPE II FRACTURE

Type II injuries are the most common and are usually caused by a fixed supination and external rotation force. The fibula is often fractured with it. The ankle is swollen and painful, and the deformity is obvious. The circulation and motor-sensory nerve function are documented, and radiographs are obtained.

**Radiographic Evaluation.** A metaphyseal spike, or the Thurston-Holland sign, is usually seen on the distal medial part of the tibia; however, the metaphyseal fragment may pull off the lateral aspect (Fig. 16–11). The fibula may or may not be injured.

**Management.** Closed reduction is usually easily performed if relaxation is achieved; in most cases, fentanyl analgesia and a muscle relaxant produce sufficient relaxation. The distal fragment may be rotated, and the rotatory displacement is not appreciated radiographically. An oblique view generally identifies any displacement of the distal fragment. Unlike the shoulder or hip joint, the ankle is a single-action hinge joint. Malalignment in the plane of motion of the ankle joint corrects spontaneously in the young. Most important is the fact

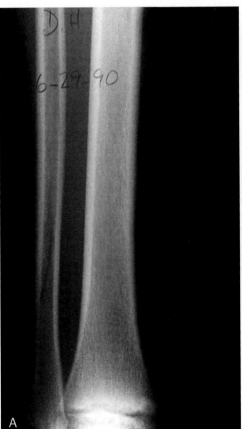
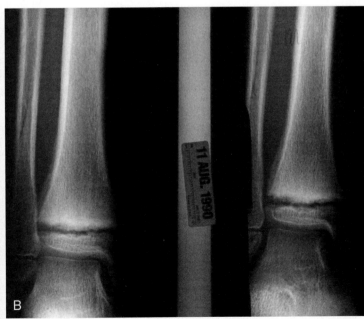

**FIGURE 16–10.** Salter-Harris type I fracture of the distal ends of the tibia and fibula. *A,* The initial radiograph shows only soft tissue injury, with no evidence of fracture. *B,* A follow-up radiograph 2 months later shows widening of the physis, as well as some deposition of bone or early callus in the interosseous space. The ankle was asymptomatic.

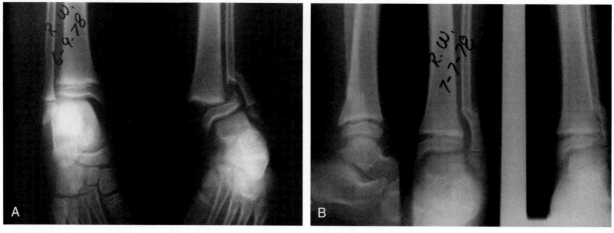

**FIGURE 16–11.** Salter-Harris type II fracture of the distal end of the tibia with a fibular shaft fracture. *A,* This Salter-Harris type II fracture is an abduction injury. The Thurston-Holland fragment sign on the distal end of the tibia is on the lateral aspect. *B,* After the reduction, the injury healed with no difficulty.

that neither rotation nor varus or valgus malalignment corrects spontaneously. Reduction can usually be achieved by closed methods; however, it may be necessary to perform an open reduction in some cases. An above-knee cast with 30° of knee flexion is indicated for immobilization. The cast is changed at 2 weeks, and a below-knee walking cast is applied. Because malalignment in the plane of motion will correct spontaneously, it is far better to accept a less than perfect reduction than to risk physeal damage by delayed or repeated manipulation.

## TYPE III FRACTURE

Salter-Harris types III and IV injuries of the medial malleolus are somewhat unusual.[42] These injuries are usually the result of a supination-inversion force on the ankle. After separation of the distal fibular epiphysis, the inversion-adduction force of the talus striking the medial malleolus produces either of these two fracture patterns. The child presents with complaints of pain and swelling over the medial aspect of the ankle. The fibula may be involved and may also be painful. The injury occurs most often in children younger than 10 years or before the growth plate begins to close.

**Radiographic Evaluation.** Type III injuries to the medial malleolus are less common, but radiographs do show the fracture to involve less than one third of the medial-lateral distance across the epiphysis. The fracture line extends vertically to the physis and exits medially through the physis (Fig. 16–12).

**Management.** Closed reduction can usually be achieved with fentanyl analgesia and good muscle relaxation. Failure to reduce the interfragmentary gap to less than 2 mm has been associated with growth arrest and angular deformity.[77] Anatomic reduction is required,

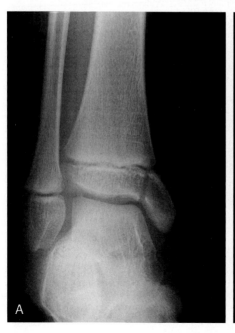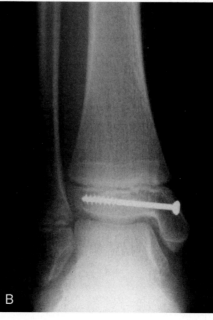

**FIGURE 16–12.** Salter-Harris type III fracture treated by a percutaneous interfragmentary screw. *A,* In this adduction injury, the fracture occurred just above the superomedial aspect of the talar dome. The fracture line of the epiphysis ends at the physis. *B,* The injury was treated by closed reduction and a percutaneous interfragmentary screw. Note the horizontal Park-Harris line, indicative of normal growth after treatment. The screw should never cross an open growth plate obliquely.

followed by application of an above-knee cast with 30° to 40° of knee flexion. We recommend reduction under general anesthesia if displacement of the subchondral surface is greater than 3 mm. The greater degree of muscle relaxation obtained under general anesthesia should enable a more anatomic reduction. Determining the precise extent of displacement in these fractures is crucial, for a significant gap may lead to growth arrest. As the fracture unites, the ossification process above and below the physis may span the growth plate and form a bony bridge anchored in the metaphyseal and epiphyseal calluses. The width and, in turn, the strength of that bridge depend on the size of the residual interfragmentary gap. A thin, weak bridge may have no adverse effect on growth, disruption of which requires substantial force.[42]

Open reduction under general anesthesia is performed if the displacement is greater than 2 mm after reduction. A medial Kocher, **J**, or "hockey-stick" incision may be used. The fracture site is obvious by virtue of the hematoma. The fragment is rotated outward on the deltoid ligament, and interfragmentary debris is removed. Anatomic reduction is performed under image intensification. A guide wire is placed across the fracture site, and a cannulated screw is inserted. Because of the potential instability after reduction, internal fixation is advisable. We recommend a cannulated 4.0-mm interfragmentary screw or percutaneous threaded Steinmann pins.

The interfragmentary screw, which can be inserted quite neatly when cannulated, allows excellent control and can be inserted percutaneously if closed reduction to within 2 mm is achieved. The problem with an interfragmentary screw is that when one attempts to remove the screw, it may be overgrown with healing callus. We believe that it is acceptable to leave the screw in. Percutaneous pinning is less traumatic; operative exposure, with potential vascular compromise and infec-

tion, is avoided; and the reduction is adequately stabilized. Another advantage of the percutaneous Steinmann pin technique is that the pin can be removed in 3 to 4 weeks at the time of cast change.

## TYPE IV FRACTURE

With the patient under general anesthesia and the use of image intensification control, open reduction of type IV fractures is performed in the operating room. The previously described medial incision and reduction techniques are carried out. One should try to insert the transfixion implant from the epiphysis to the epiphysis or from the metaphysis to the metaphysis. Every effort should be made to avoid placing the screw from the epiphysis across the physis into the metaphysis unless the physis is closing. Physeal arrest may occur after oblique cross-physeal pinning, as performed for adult fractures. After anatomic reduction of type IV injuries (Fig. 16–13), one should place transverse epiphysis-to-epiphysis or metaphysis-to-metaphysis Steinmann pins or cannulated 4-mm screws. Because the metaphyseal fragment is often warped or fragmented, it may be necessary to discard it to ensure anatomic reduction of the epiphysis. Removing the fragment also prevents the formation of a bony bridge (Fig. 16–14). After reduction, an above-knee nonwalking cast is applied for 3 weeks, followed by an above-knee walking cast for 3 weeks. If a percutaneous Steinmann pin is used, it should be removed when the cast is changed. If interfragmentary screw fixation is used, the screw may be removed about 1 year after treatment. If the screw is not removed within 1 to 1.5 years, exuberant callus may overgrow it. Removing it then would subject the extremity to more trauma than simply leaving the pin in place. We have no experience with the use of bioabsorbable implants for the management of these fractures. Closed reduction of this injury may be successful when the fracture is not

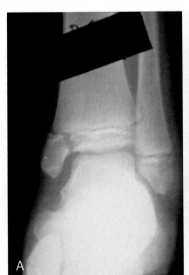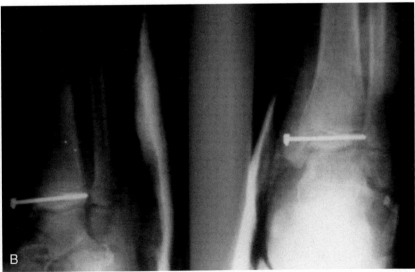

**FIGURE 16–13.** Salter-Harris type IV fracture treated by open reduction and interfragmentary screw fixation. *A,* The initial radiograph shows a vertical fracture through the epiphysis with a small metaphyseal fragment. Soft tissue density is increased. *B,* Radiograph of the leg through plaster showing anatomic reduction and screw placement.

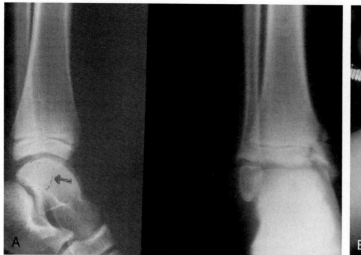
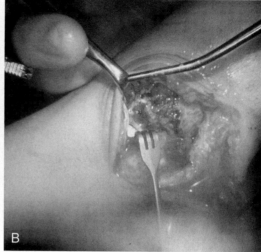

**FIGURE 16–14.** This Salter-Harris type IV fracture required open reduction and anatomic repair. *A,* Type IV fracture of the tibia, with the vertical component extending through the epiphysis and obliquely through the metaphysis. A Salter-Harris type I fracture of the lateral malleolus is also present. *B,* Note the articular surface of the talus, the bony epiphysis, and the physeal line on the operative photograph. The metaphyseal fragment should be discarded if it prevents anatomic reduction.

displaced and anatomic reduction is achieved and maintained (Fig. 16–15). It is almost always necessary to stabilize this injury by internal fixation (Fig. 16–16). Rarely can one obtain and maintain satisfactory closed reduction without internal fixation if the fracture is displaced.

## TYPE V FRACTURE

Type V injuries are extremely rare and appear to result from axial compression. The Salter-Harris type V injury supposedly causes partial or complete physeal arrest by virtue of a crush injury to the germinal cells of all or a portion of the physis. In such an injury, no obvious fracture of the epiphysis or metaphysis can be found, and the initial radiograph may show no evidence of injury. The diagnosis of a type V injury is therefore a retrospective one made only after premature closure has

been established in a growth plate that was previously considered uninjured. It is believed that this injury causes unrecognized damage to physeal cells either directly or secondary to injury to the blood supply of the germinal cell layer of the physis. Controversy surrounds the contribution of premature closure of the growth plate to crush injury of the germinal cell layers alone.

Two cases of tibia fracture have been reported in which symmetric premature closure of the entire proximal tibial physis caused a leg length discrepancy without any angular deformity.[117] A compression injury to the entire physis would be unlikely unless a uniform longitudinal force were the mechanism of injury, as in a fall from a height. However, the clinical history and the configuration of the associated fractures were not consistent with a purely longitudinal force in their cases. Peterson and Burkhart[118] considered the proposition that premature closure of the growth plate results from

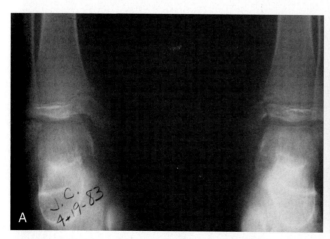
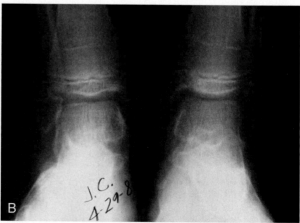

**FIGURE 16–15.** Salter-Harris type III fracture of the right ankle and Salter-Harris type IV fracture of the left ankle treated by closed reduction and monitored for 1 year. *A,* The initial radiograph shows less than 2-mm displacement of either fracture. The positions were accepted, and bilateral fiberglass casts were applied. *B,* A radiograph 1 year later shows both fractures to be healed. The horizontal Park-Harris lines show that no physeal bar developed.

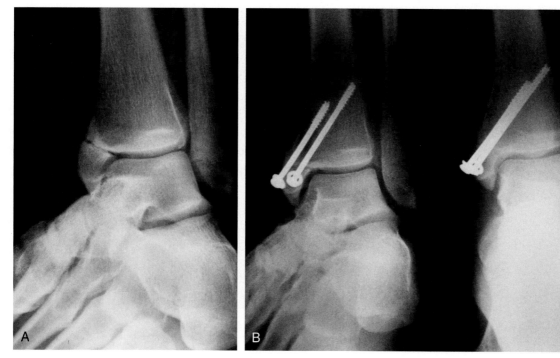

**FIGURE 16–16.** Nonunion of a medial malleolar fracture after closed reduction without internal fixation. *A,* Mortise view of the ankle revealing nonunion of the medial malleolar fragment. *B,* Anteroposterior and mortise views of ankle 6 months later showing closure of the fracture line after compression from percutaneous cannulated screws.

compression at the time of the accident to be speculative. Because the two cases cited by Salter and Harris[131] did not have a normal radiographic appearance at the time of injury, another type could have been present. These investigators further concluded that all type V injuries reported in the literature involved the knee.[118] On review of the literature, they concluded that the common factor in all these conditions, including the trauma cases, seemed to be prolonged immobilization. Thus, an intriguing possibility is that post-traumatic physeal fusion is not always caused by direct damage to the growth plate at the time of injury, but rather by factors associated with immobilization.

Peterson and Burkhart studied symmetric premature closure of the physis after trauma and found that when treated by immobilization, premature closure is more likely to be the result of ischemia secondary to immobilization rather than physeal compression.[118] Furthermore, the type V classification may unwittingly be stifling investigation into equally plausible mechanisms of premature growth arrest. Bone scan at the time of injury has been proposed as an investigative measure to aid and confirm a crush injury.[158] We have not encountered this injury. The most severe compression injury in our experience resulted in an angular deformity (Fig. 16–17).

### TYPE VI FRACTURE

Ablation of the perichondrial ring has been categorized as a type VI injury. Avulsion or compression injury to the periphery of the physis is rarely seen. Lawn mower injuries and degloving injuries, which occur when the leg is dragged across concrete or pavement, may remove the perichondrial ring. The ensuing callus may cause the development of a bridge between the metaphysis and epiphysis as described by Rang.[126] We have not encountered this fracture about the ankle.

## Transition Fractures

The juvenile fracture of Tillaux and triplane fractures are considered to be transition fractures. These fractures occur in and about the early part of the second decade during the pubescent transition to skeletal maturity. They occur as a result of an external rotational force. The pattern of closure of the distal tibial physis (i.e., middle, medial, lateral) is responsible for propagation of the fracture after injury.

### JUVENILE FRACTURE OF TILLAUX

The juvenile fracture of Tillaux is an isolated fracture of the lateral portion of the distal tibial epiphysis. It is a transition fracture and usually occurs early in the second decade, when the medial half of the distal growth plate is closed and the lateral portion remains open. This fracture is generally the result of an external rotational force. With external rotation, the anterior tibiofibular ligament holds firmly to the tibial epiphysis, which separates through the junction of the middle and lateral open physis. When displacement of the fragment is minimal, the vertical and horizontal fracture lines may be difficult to visualize. It is a Salter-Harris type III epiphyseal fracture, and mild or moderate displacement of the fragment may be present.

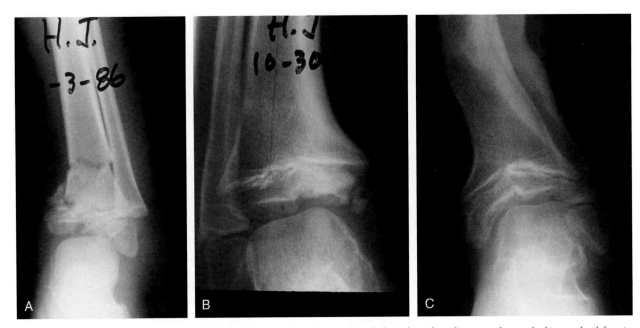

**FIGURE 16–17.** Axial compression injury with multiple fractures around the metaphyseal-physeal-epiphyseal juncture that resulted in angular deformity treated by osteotomy. *A,* The initial radiograph shows soft tissue swelling and a markedly comminuted tibial epiphyseal fracture. The fibular epiphysis is medially displaced. *B,* Nine months later, a dense bone scar is located over the medial physis, with angulation of the lateral Park-Harris line; the ankle is in varus. Note the horizontal Park-Harris line of the fibula. *C,* A valgus overcorrection osteotomy was performed and resulted in good clinical alignment. Note the medial bone scar and the multiple Park-Harris lines over the lateral tibial metaphysis. The deformity subsequently recurred.

The pattern of the injury is thought to result from the closure sequence of the distal tibial physis.[75]

The distal physis of the tibia closes first on its medial half at the age of 13 or 14 years; the lateral part closes at 14½ to 16 years. Closure of the distal tibial physis occurs first in the middle, then in the medial, and finally in the lateral physis. Because the lateral physis is still open, the fracture crosses through it. The fracture line extends from the articular surface proximally; it traverses the epiphysis and then continues along the physis laterally. It is equivalent to the Tillaux lesion in adults. Local tenderness and swelling may be seen over the anterolateral aspect of the distal tibial epiphysis.

A variably sized portion of the anterolateral bony epiphysis is pulled off by the anterior tibiofibular ligament when the foot is forcibly externally rotated, a variation of a supination–external rotation mechanism. If the fragment is large enough, a residual deformity in the joint surface may lead to an increased risk of osteoarthritis. The importance of preventing this problem in adolescents cannot be overstated.[27]

**Management.** Closed reduction may be performed with analgesia and a muscle relaxant if it is done within the first 24 hours. Reduction is usually achieved by gentle internal rotation of the foot, and anatomic reduction should be attained in every case. If closed reduction is successful, we recommend percutaneous fixation with a threaded Steinmann pin or cannulated screw.[30] An above-knee cast is applied for 3 weeks, followed by a below-knee walking cast for 3 weeks (Fig. 16–18). If the gap after reduction appears to be less than satisfactory (>3 mm), further radiographic studies are indicated (Fig. 16–19). CT scanning provides accurate assessment of the reduction; three-dimensional re-formation produces a readily interpretable image that does not require mental reconstruction of two-

dimensional films and provides a permanent record of the reduction[83] (Fig. 16–20). If closed reduction is not satisfactory, open reduction with transfixion may be required. The screw or percutaneous Steinmann pin can

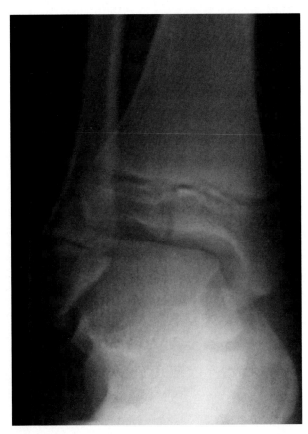

**FIGURE 16–18.** This nondisplaced Salter-Harris type III fracture was treated by cast immobilization with an uneventful outcome.

cross the physis in this particular situation because the middle and medial sections of the growth plate are usually closed. If the growth plate is not closed or closing, the implant should not cross the physis. Growth discrepancy is an unusual sequela of this injury because most of the physis has closed. The more significant complication is arthritis resulting from either a step-off of the articular surface or a residual interfragmentary gap greater than 3 mm.

## TRIPLANE FRACTURE

A triplane fracture is an injury unique to the closing distal tibial growth plate. The fracture line crosses the articular surface through the epiphysis, the physis, and finally the posterior tibial metaphysis in the sagittal, transverse, and coronal planes, respectively. The multi-planar Salter-Harris type IV injury created is thought to be caused by external rotation of a supinated foot.

**Radiographic Evaluation.** Triplane fractures of the distal end of the tibia are sometimes quite difficult to identify on plain radiographs. AP, lateral, and mortise views should be taken. The fracture appears to be a Salter-Harris type III injury on the AP view and a Salter-Harris type II injury on the lateral projection. In the AP projection, the fracture can be seen as a vertical line crossing the central area of the epiphysis, with widening of the mortise. The appearance in this projection is remarkably similar to that of a juvenile Tillaux fracture, and care must be taken to not confuse the two. Mortise views may show more displacement than the AP ones.[45] The apparent Salter-Harris type II fracture seen on the lateral view may be minimally displaced and occasionally obscured. This radiographic fracture pattern in a growing child should always suggest a triplane fracture. CT studies have simplified identification of all facets of this injury. The fracture may consist of two or three fragments, depending on closure of the distal tibial physis. The fracture generally involves three or four parts in children younger than 10 years and two parts in children older than 10 years.

In 1957, Johnson and Fahl presented a figure illustrating a triplane injury.[67] The nature of this unusual fracture was not appreciated until Marmor's publication in 1970. Marmor noted widening of the ankle mortise after closed reduction of what appeared to be a Salter-Harris type II fracture.[93] After reduction, he observed that the fracture extended in three planes—

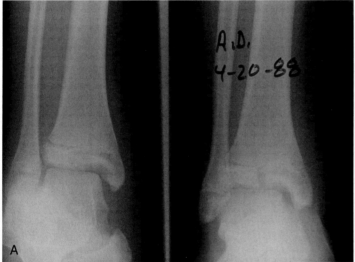

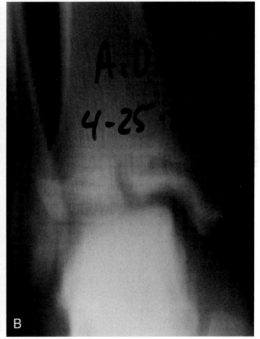

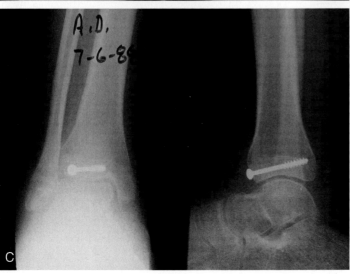

FIGURE 16–19. This child sustained a Salter-Harris type III fracture of the lateral tibial epiphysis that required open reduction and internal fixation. *A,* Mortise and anteroposterior views of a juvenile Tillaux fracture. *B,* A polytomogram after closed reduction shows that the fracture-separation at the subchondral surface was greater than 3 mm; therefore, open reduction was performed. *C,* Complete closure of the physis occurred within 3 months after open reduction.

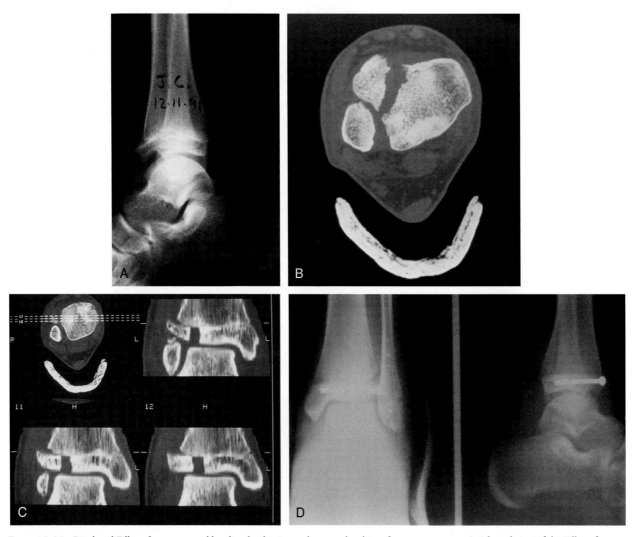

**FIGURE 16–20.** Displaced Tillaux fracture treated by closed reduction and a cannulated interfragmentary screw. *A,* A lateral view of the Tillaux fracture shows anterior displacement. *B,* Computed tomography (CT) taken with the leg in a splint just above the ankle joint shows displacement of the anterior lateral fragment. *C,* CT with a three-dimensional reconstructed cranial view confirms the amount of displacement. *D,* After indirect reduction and percutaneous fixation with a cannulated interfragmentary screw, the fracture was anatomically reduced and aligned. (From Crawford, A.H. AAOS Instr Course Lect 44:320, 1995.)

sagittal, transverse, and coronal—and involved three parts of the distal end of the tibia: the shaft, an anterolateral epiphyseal fragment, and an unattached fragment consisting of the remainder of the epiphysis with a metaphyseal spike.

The triplane fracture was named by Lynn, who reported two fractures with a three-dimensional configuration that required open reduction and internal fixation.[90] Torg and Ruggiero also noted that the fracture was intrinsically unstable and needed internal fixation.[152] Cooperman and colleagues thought that most triplane fractures had no free anterolateral epiphyseal fragment and were therefore two-part fractures in three planes[25] (Fig. 16–21). Dias and Giegerich postulated that the same mechanism—external rotation of the foot on the leg—causes both triplane fractures and juvenile Tillaux fractures and believed that the resulting injury is solely determined by the patient's age.[36] The triplane fracture occurs earlier in adolescence than the juvenile Tillaux fracture does because the epiphyseal plate is still

completely open in early adolescence, thus allowing the horizontal fracture to run through its entire anterior portion. In the older group, the growth plate's medial area has already closed, so the horizontal break extends only through its anterolateral portion and is met by the vertical fracture near the closed medial epiphyseal line.[45] If growth plate closure is more advanced, no anterolateral epiphyseal fragment is produced, and the result is a two-part fracture. Denton and Fischer described a medial triplane fracture caused by adduction and axial loading.[33] Karrholm stated that such a fracture type occurs at a low peak age, is associated with complications such as medial growth retardation or arrest, and stressed that it should not be confused with other types of triplane fracture.[70] Intramalleolar triplane fractures have been reported.[49,137] Shin and associates published a classification of intramalleolar triplane fractures and pointed out that three-dimensional CT has great advantage over plain radiographs and two-dimensional CT for evaluation of this injury. They described three classes: intramalleolar, intra-articular fracture at the junction of the tibial plafond and medial malleolus (type 1); intra-articular fracture of the medial malleolus (type 2); and extra-articular intramalleolar fracture (type 3), which is the most prevalent. Operative reduction is required when intra-articular incongruity exists.[137] None of the patterns fit into a Salter-Harris type.[43, 45, 46] Ertl and associates completed a long-term (3 to 13 years) follow-up of this intra-articular fracture and found that it leads to significant arthritis in adults when less than anatomic reduction was achieved.[45] Although symptoms were absent on early follow-up, about half their patients were symptomatic at long-term evaluation. Karrholm published the results of 21 of his cases with a 4-year follow-up and a review of the literature (209 cases); in total, about 80% displayed excellent results, 16% had minor symptoms, and 4% had more pronounced symptoms combined with degenerative changes.[70] When the epiphyseal fracture extended into the weight-bearing arch of the ankle, residual displacement of greater than 2 mm was associated with suboptimal results. In Rapariz and associates' series, of the 35 patients treated for triplane fractures, the only two patients in whom degenerative changes were seen in their ankle radiographs were those with residual intra-articular displacement of 3 mm.[127] Anatomic reduction by either closed or open means is mandatory in the treatment of triplane fractures.

The choice between open and closed reduction depends on the amount of residual displacement after reduction. Impending growth arrest is not usually a consideration because the growth plate is approaching closure. Even though this fracture seems to be intrinsically unstable, it is only at the articular surface, where permanent disruption definitely predisposes to degenerative joint disease, that loss of reduction is crucial.

Anatomic reduction of the articular surface is mandatory. Ertl and associates found that none of their patients with initial displacement of greater than 3 mm on AP or mortise radiographs had successful closed reduction.[45] Interposition of soft tissue at the fracture site was responsible for the failure of closed reduction in six of eight open operations. The soft tissue was identified as periosteum in five patients and was found to be the extensor hallucis longus tendon in one.[45] A diastasis or step-off of more than 3 mm in any plane at the articular surface requires anatomic reduction.

**Management.** General anesthesia is required for complete relaxation. The knee is flexed to 90°, and the foot is plantar-flexed and internally rotated. If anatomic reduction is achieved, we prefer percutaneous threaded Steinmann pin fixation (Fig. 16–22). A cannulated interfragmentary screw may be placed over the pin with the same result. The extremity is placed in an above-knee, non–weight-bearing cast for 4 weeks, at which time the pin is removed, followed by a below-knee cast for 2 to 3 weeks.[30]

If the interfragmentary gap after reduction is greater than 3 mm, open reduction is necessary. Open reduction is not easy and may require anterolateral and posteromedial approaches to reduce the fractures under direct vision. Only after the posteromedial fragment is reduced can the anterolateral (Tillaux) fragment be reduced. Through an anterolateral approach, the anterolateral fragment is identified and displaced. The posteromedial fragment, if displaced, is first reduced under direct vision by internal rotation and dorsiflexion of the foot. When reduced, the posteromedial fragment is fixed with a Steinmann pin or cancellous screw. If the posteromedial fragment cannot be reduced by manipulation, it should be reduced under direct vision through a posteromedial incision. If displaced, the fibula fracture is reduced next.

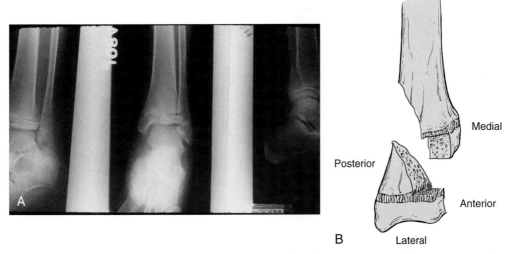

FIGURE 16–21. Radiograph and artist's drawing of a two-part triplane fracture. A, On an ankle composite view, the mortise view shows little evidence of bony injury. The anteroposterior view reveals a Salter-Harris type III fracture of the distal tibial epiphysis and an anterior view of the medial tibial metaphyseal triangular fragment. On the lateral view, the Salter-Harris type II fragment of the distal end of the tibia is seen. B, Artist's rendition of a two-fragment triplane fracture. (B, From McNealy, G.A.; et al. AJR Am J Roentgenol 138:688, 1982. Copyright 1982, American Roentgen Ray Society.)

Finally, the displaced anterolateral fragment (Tillaux) is reduced and fixed with a Steinmann pin or screw.[76] A non–weight-bearing, above-knee cast is applied for 3 weeks, followed by a below-knee walking cast for 4 weeks. If percutaneous Steinmann pins are used, they are removed at the time of cast change.

Distal tibial growth is nearly complete when this injury occurs, so shortening from growth arrest is rarely a problem. Ertl and associates' long-term reevaluation showed marked deterioration with time in ankles in which reduction of the articular surface was not accomplished. At an average of more than 6 years after injury, the result was that 15 patients had declined at least one grade.[45] None of these patients improved during

follow-up after injury to the articular cartilage. Even in individuals with anatomic reduction, delayed long-term symptoms still occurred. The symptomatic patients monitored for 20 years were only in their third decade and could experience continued deterioration. Residual 2- to 3-mm displacement of the articular cartilage in the weight-bearing area may result in late-onset degenerative arthritis.[45]

## Distal Fibular Fractures

Isolated distal fibular shaft injuries are somewhat uncommon and are more often associated with tibia fractures.

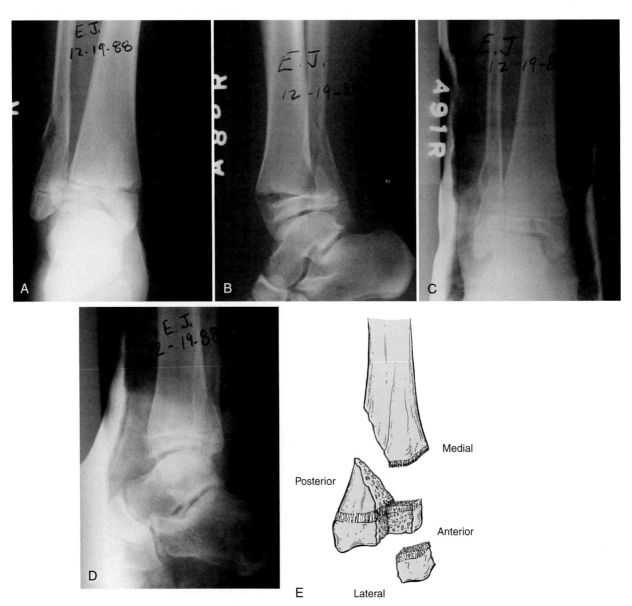

FIGURE 16–22. Triplane fracture treated by closed reduction and percutaneous Steinmann pinning. *A,* An anteroposterior radiograph shows a Salter-Harris type III fracture of the distal end of the tibia and a nondisplaced distal fibular fracture. *B,* Lateral radiograph showing an apparent Salter-Harris type II fracture of the distal part of the tibia. *C,* An anteroposterior radiograph after closed reduction reveals less than anatomic reduction of the Salter-Harris type III distal tibial fracture. *D,* Lateral radiograph after closed reduction, with the Salter-Harris II component slightly posterior and the Salter-Harris III component slightly anterior. This position was not considered acceptable. *E,* Artist's rendition of three fracture fragments and three planes of fracture.

*Illustration continued on following page*

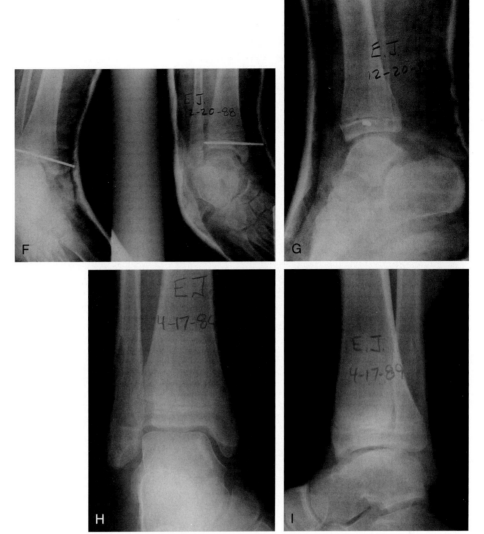

FIGURE 16–22 *Continued. F,* Anteroposterior and mortise views after closed reduction and percutaneous Steinmann pin fixation. *G,* Lateral view after closed reduction and percutaneous Steinmann pin fixation. The reduction is anatomic. *H,* Anteroposterior radiograph 3 months after pin removal. The subchondral surface is anatomic. *I,* Lateral radiograph 3 months after pin removal. (*E,* From McNealy, G.A.; et al. AJR Am J Roentgenol 138:689, 1982. Copyright 1982, American Roentgen Ray Society.)

The Salter-Harris type I distal fibula injury is the most common type of ankle fracture in children.[141] If the injury occurs through the physis, the diagnosis may be difficult to make because the displacement is usually minimal. Pain and swelling ("goose egg") are generally observed over the lateral malleolus.

**Radiographic Evaluation.** Fragment displacement is usually minimal. The soft tissue ("goose egg") appearance over the lateral malleolus is generally diagnostic (Fig. 16–23).

**Management.** A compression dressing of three layers of Webril and an elastic bandage is used for 1 week to diminish the swelling. A below-knee walking cast is then applied for 3 weeks. Many of these injuries are misdiagnosed as sprains or strains and are thus treated initially with a compression bandage. When the patient is reevaluated at 10 days to 2 weeks, ecchymosis may be seen extending down the lateral aspect of the lower third of the leg into the foot. These patients tend to do well. Fractures that are displaced, unstable, and not treated may undergo chronic nonunion that gives rise to epiphysiolysis. This problem is extremely rare, except for patients with neurologic disorders.

Isolated distal fibular shaft fractures above the tibiofibular syndesmosis are uncommon in children. They are most often associated with injuries to the deltoid ligament (pronation injuries) if no fracture of the tibia is seen. Failure to recognize the medial ligamentous instability associated with distal-third isolated fibula fractures has been responsible for the development of chronic instability and early degenerative joint disease. We recommend open reduction and compression plate fixation for these injuries. An above-knee, non–weight-bearing cast is applied initially for 3 weeks, followed by a below-knee walking cast; the plate is removed at 1 year.

A small chip fracture of the inferior tip of the epiphysis may be caused by the initial ankle injury and not be diagnosed, especially if the fracture occurs through the cartilaginous epiphysis. The history given is that the patient sustained an ankle sprain and, although the radiographs were negative, the patient continues to experience pain and instability. A repeat radiograph shows a small rounded ossicle just inferior to the epiphysis. This ossicle, the os subfibulare, is thought to be a post-traumatic development and not a normal variant. A below-knee walking cast or Aircast may relieve

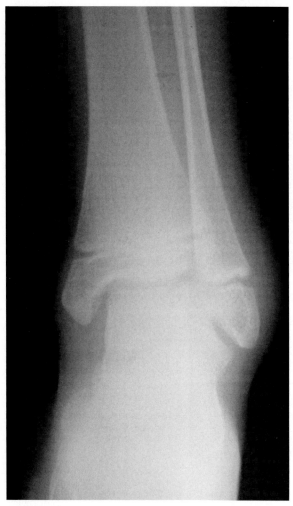

**FIGURE 16–23.** Anteroposterior radiograph of an ankle with a soft tissue "goose egg" swelling over a nondisplaced fibular Salter-Harris type I fracture.

the symptoms, but rarely does the ossicle unite to the fibula. Occasionally, the problem progresses to chronic pain and instability. Removal of the ossicle and ligamentous repair followed by a below-knee walking cast for 4 weeks are recommended (Fig. 16–24).

## Dislocation of the Ankle Joint

Ankle dislocation without fracture is a rare event that has prompted isolated case reports in the literature.[102] Most dislocations are posteromedial and manifested as open injuries on the anterolateral side of the joint, with gross disruption of the lateral capsular ligamentous complex (Fig. 16–25). The majority of patients are young adults; few ankle dislocations have been reported in children.[102, 110] Nusem and associates reported a closed posterior ankle dislocation in a 12-year-old girl that was successfully treated with closed reduction and a short leg cast.[110] Most posterior or medial dislocations are stable in neutral or slight dorsiflexion. In this position, the torn lateral ligamentous complex is approximated. Although the dislocation is invariably posteromedial, rarely is repair of the deltoid ligament necessary, and stability usually occurs.

The mechanism of injury is generally marked plantar flexion with inversion. Local distraction occurs anterolaterally, with rapid rupture of the lateral ligamentous complex from front to back or through the fibular physis in children. This injury is akin to a flexion-distraction injury in the spine. In addition to separation of the lateral ligamentous complex, the physis, or both, the skin, extensor tendons, and neurovascular structures frequently rupture in an open dislocation. As the plantar-flexed foot is carried into inversion, varus tilting and rotation of the talus occur, followed by dislocation, usually in the posteromedial position. The deltoid

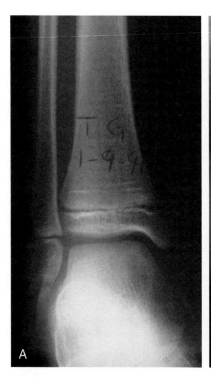

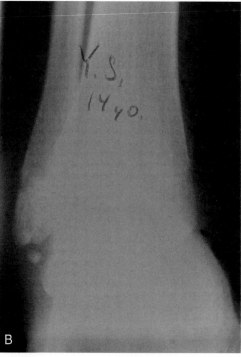

**FIGURE 16–24.** *A,* An anteroposterior radiograph of the ankle 2 months after injury shows delayed union of the distal end of the fibula and horizontal Park-Harris lines of the tibial metaphysis. The ankle was asymptomatic. *B,* Anteroposterior radiograph of this 14-year-old boy's ankle after a sprain. Soft tissue swelling is apparent, and an ossicle is seen beneath the fibula. The child is an avid soccer player with a history of repeated sprains. The ossicle is round and smooth and probably represents an old nonunited fracture.

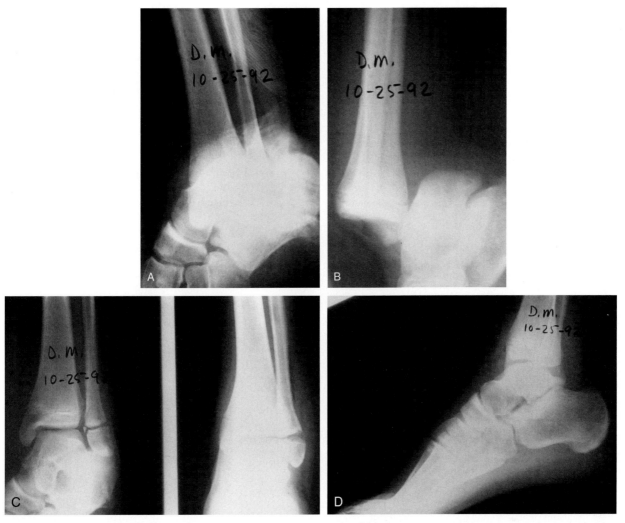

**FIGURE 16–25.** This 15-year-old boy injured his right ankle while playing basketball. He apparently came down on an opposing player's foot and severely inverted and twisted his ankle. The boy complained of severe pain and deformity but no numbness or tingling. The injury was open. He underwent reduction with open inspection and irrigation of the joint. The fracture-dislocation extended through the fibular physis, and the distal fibular malleolar fragment remained with the foot component. The anterior, posterior, and inferior talofibular ligaments were intact. Anatomic reduction was achieved by transfixion of the fibular malleolus with Steinmann pins. The wound was closed over a drain. The extremity was placed in a bulky dressing for 10 days, followed by a below-knee cast. When seen 2 years later, the ankle was stable. *A,* Oblique view of the ankle revealing superimposition of the medial malleolus over the talus in the dislocated position. *B,* True lateral view showing posterior dislocation of the foot on the ankle (note the subcutaneous air). *C,* Anteroposterior and mortise views after closed reduction. *D,* True lateral view of the ankle joint after closed reduction.

*Illustration continued on following page*

ligament is always injured, but except in cases of gross displacement, it usually retains a significant amount of integrity and provides a posteromedial hinge that affords stability when the ankle is reduced and held in dorsiflexion.

Most of these injuries are open, and débridement and irrigation of the joint are required. In an adult, the lateral ligamentous structures are repaired; however, in a child, where the injury is transphyseal through the fibula, the anterior posterior and lateral talofibular ligaments appear to be intact, and anatomic reduction and fixation of the fibular physis are normally all that is necessary. The wound may be closed over a drain if the soft tissues will allow it; otherwise, delayed primary closure and possibly skin grafting are required. The ankle is placed in a compressive protective dressing for 7 to 10 days, after which a non–weight-bearing cast in the neutral planti-

grade position is worn for 4 to 6 weeks. After cast removal, progressive weight bearing is permitted after rehabilitation restores ankle motion, strength, and proprioception.

## THE FOOT

### Anatomy

The foot has 26 bones and a variable number of sesamoids and accessory ossicles (Fig. 16–26). All are held together by interconnecting ligaments. The five rays of the foot each contain a metatarsal and its phalanges—two for the first toe and three for the others. The epiphysis of the first metatarsal is located at its proximal end, similar to a phalanx, rather than at the distal end, as it is for the other metatarsals.

The first three rays have a cuneiform bone at the base; the fourth and fifth share the cuboid bone at the base. The tarsal navicular is interposed between the head of the talus and the cuneiform, and the talus sits "sidesaddle" on the calcaneus. Thus, the talus lies roughly in the axis of the first ray, and the calcaneus lies in the axis of the fourth ray.

The foot is customarily divided into the forefoot, midfoot, and hindfoot (metatarsus, midtarsus, and tarsus). The forefoot contains the 5 metatarsals and 14 phalanges; it is separated from the midfoot by the tarsometatarsal joint (of Lisfranc). The midfoot contains the three cuneiforms, the navicular, and the cuboid, and it is separated from the hindfoot by the transverse midtarsal joint of Chopart. The hindfoot contains two bones, the talus and the calcaneus. The reader is referred to comprehensive articles by Mann[91] and Morris[104] for a thorough description and discussion of foot and ankle biomechanics.

The foot presents myriad interesting anatomic features. It is not well ossified at birth, and of the tarsal bones present at birth, only the calcaneus and talus are fully ossified; however, the cuboid ossifies shortly after birth. The calcaneus may be bifid in certain syndromes (e.g., Larsen, Williams) (Fig. 16–27), and this variation may be interpreted as a fracture. The cartilaginous model is retained for an extended period.

Reduction of foot deformities after fractures in children is important because remodeling cannot always be predicted with growth. Fifty percent of the mature length has been achieved in 1-year-old girls and 1.5-year-old boys. In contrast, the femur and tibia do not reach 50% of their length until 3 years before comparable physeal closure in the long bones.[144] Severe malalignment after foot fractures does not usually have enough time to correct spontaneously.

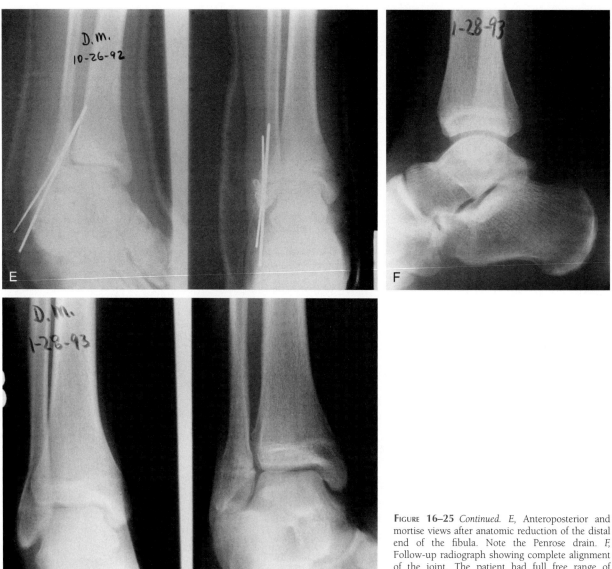

FIGURE 16–25 *Continued. E,* Anteroposterior and mortise views after anatomic reduction of the distal end of the fibula. Note the Penrose drain. *F,* Follow-up radiograph showing complete alignment of the joint. The patient had full free range of motion. *G,* Anteroposterior and mortise views showing complete healing of the fractured fibula.

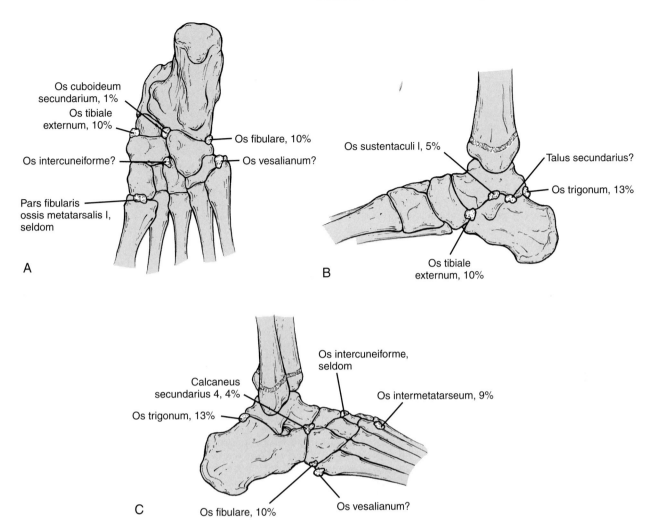

**FIGURE 16–26.** The normal bones of the foot and the accessory ossicles. (From Tachdjian, M.O. Pediatric Orthopedics, 2nd ed. Philadelphia, W.B. Saunders, 1990.)

## Osteochondroses and Variants

Several osteochondroses occur that may or may not be anatomic variants. Sever's disease has been thought to be epiphyseal ischemic necrosis of the calcaneal apophysis; this area may be the site of trauma, as well as developmental problems. The clinical condition usually occurs in very active youngsters and is manifested as heel pain. Radiographs show fragmentation of the calcaneal

apophysis. We have found identical fragmentation of the calcaneal apophysis in asymptomatic feet of children in whom radiographs are taken for other reasons (Fig. 16–28); therefore, this finding is not diagnostic. The clinical condition most likely results from an overuse syndrome or traction apophysitis of the calcaneus similar to the tibial apophysitis of Osgood-Schlatter disease. Symptomatic treatment and an explanation to the child and parents are usually successful. Treatment ranges

**FIGURE 16–27.** The presence of multiple calcaneal centers usually implies a malformation syndrome. This patient with four calcaneal centers, which eventually fused, had Williams' (Beuran's) elfin facies syndrome. (From Oestrich, A.O.; Crawford, A.H. Atlas of Pediatric Orthopaedic Radiology. New York, Thieme, 1985.)

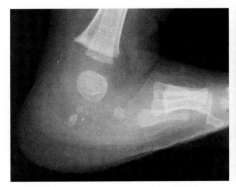
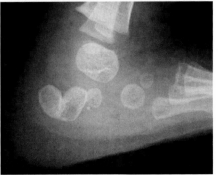

from rest to a ¼-inch heel lift to a sponge cushion heel insert.

A pseudoepiphysis may occur at the distal end of the first metatarsal and may be interpreted as a fracture. The epiphysis of the first metatarsal is proximal; in the other metatarsals (second through fifth), secondary ossification centers develop distally (Fig. 16–29). The base of the fifth metatarsal may have an ossification center just lateral to it, commonly called the os vesalianum or os peroneum; it is frequently mistaken for an avulsion fracture (Fig. 16–30). The middle phalanges may occasionally lack secondary ossification centers.

Variation in the sequence of ossification of the epiphyseal structures is common. Ossification of the lateral cuneiforms usually occurs by the end of the first year. The navicular ossification center appears between 3 and 5 years of age and is the last of the ossification centers of the foot to appear. The secondary ossification centers of the metatarsals and phalanges appear by 5 years of age. The calcaneal apophysis is present by 6 to 10 years of age and tends to unite with the body of the calcaneus at 15 to 18 years of age. An accessory navicula is found on radiographs in 10% of feet[111] and may come to clinical attention because of either trauma or repetitive overuse syndrome (Fig. 16–31). The os trigonum is a posterolateral process of the talus found at the same level as the groove for the flexor hallucis longus; it may occasionally become separated

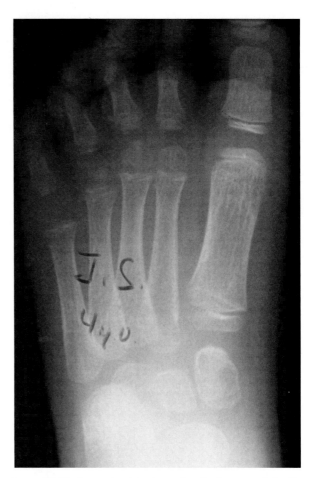

**FIGURE 16–29.** A pseudoepiphysis on the distal aspect of the first metatarsal. The normal epiphysis is located at the proximal end of the first metatarsal.

and be interpreted as a fracture on radiographs (Fig. 16–32). Structural variations in ossification patterns are the rule rather than the exception and may occur in 22% of children. The orientation of the trabecular patterns in the os calcis may mimic a unicameral bone cyst (Fig. 16–33).

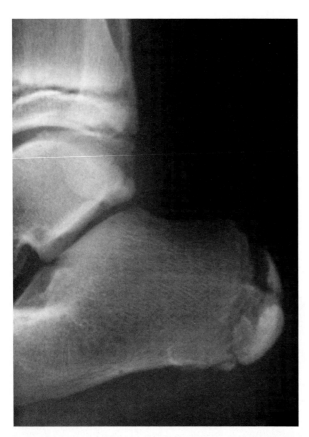

**FIGURE 16–28.** Sever's disease. Note the fragmentation of the calcaneal apophysis. Heel pain diagnosed as Sever's disease is probably an overuse syndrome.

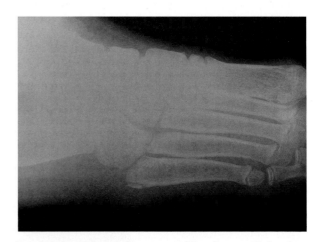

**FIGURE 16–30.** The os vesalianum is an oblique bony ossicle found just lateral to the base of the fifth metatarsal ray. It is normal.

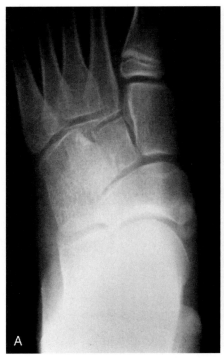
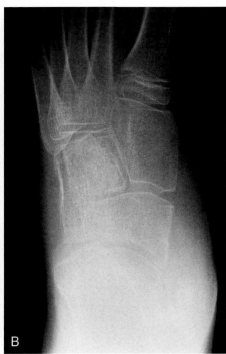

Figure 16–31. Preoperative and postoperative radiographs of a child with an accessory tarsal navicula. An accessory navicular ossicle is seen on the proximal medial aspect of the navicular bone; this one has round, smooth edges. *A,* An accessory navicula may be either separate from the bone and found in the posterior tibialis tendon or partially attached to the navicular bone itself. In those that are partially attached, injury to the attachment is thought to occur as a result of overuse and pull from the posterior tibialis tendon, which causes the patient to be symptomatic. *B,* After excision of the ossicle and medial tuberosity of the navicula.

## Types of Injuries

The senior author (A.H.C.) undertook a review of foot injuries managed by the resident service at the Children's Hospital Medical Center, Cincinnati, Ohio, in December 1990 (Table 16–2).[29] Two hundred fifteen patients were identified, and their charts and radiographs were examined; 175 patients with definitive fractures and follow-up to completion of treatment were identified and reviewed. Metatarsal fractures accounted for 90% of the fractures, with 66% occurring in the lesser second through fifth metatarsals, 25% in the isolated base of the fifth metatarsal, and 9% at the base of the first metatarsal, with or without other injuries. Phalangeal fractures (18%) were the next most common group, including proximal (64%), distal (29%), and middle (7%) phalangeal fractures. The navicular (5.1%) was the most common tarsal bone fracture, followed by the talus (2.3%) and cuboid (1.1%). Coexistent unrecognized fractures of the distal ends of the tibia and fibula occurred in 8% of all fractures studied. Dislocation of the phalanges occurred in 2.3%, and conditions initially mistaken as fractures were talofibular ligament tear, tarsal coalition, foreign body, and sesamoid fracture, each occurring once. Sixty-two percent of the children in this study were boys and 38% were girls. The left side was involved in 64% of cases and the right side in 36%.[29] This study is referred to throughout the discussion of foot fractures.

Few firm guidelines are available for the treatment of foot injuries in children. Fractures of the metatarsals, phalanges, and proximal fifth metatarsal occur most commonly. Injury to the chondro-osseous components of a child's foot is uncommon.

Most foot fractures result from direct violence, such as being crushed by a falling object, being run over by the wheel of an automobile, falling, or jumping from a height. The foot is so flexible and resilient that force applied to it is usually transmitted higher up and causes ankle and leg injuries. The soft tissue component of a foot injury is most important, and if the area is swollen and tense, elevation and decompression should be instituted early. Preservation of soft tissues, particularly the ligaments essential to long-term function of the longitudinal and transverse arches, is just as important as actual fracture reduction in restoring complete function to an injured foot. Fractures involving a joint surface carry a worse prognosis than do nonarticular fractures, especially when the tarsal bones are involved. Articular fractures in mobile joints require anatomic reduction to prevent early degenerative arthritis.

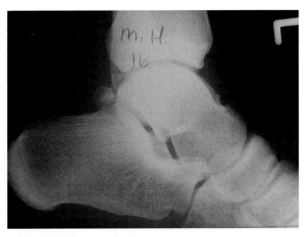

Figure 16–32. Note the round os trigonum just posterior to the talus. The os trigonum is considered to be a normal component of the posterior lateral process of the talus. A bone scan determines whether current injury or a fracture is present.

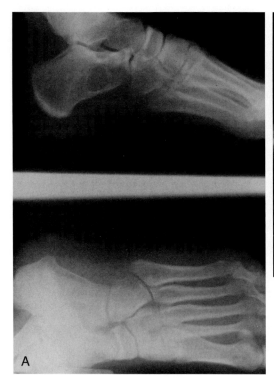

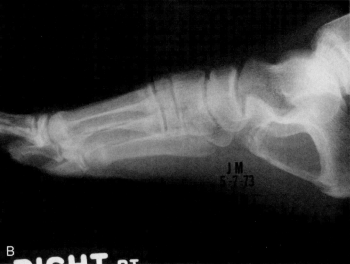

**FIGURE 16-33.** Calcaneal radiographs showing cystic lesions. *A,* The appearance of a simple bone cyst of the calcaneus. The oblique view is not as convincing. This finding may be normal and related to convergence of the trabecular patterns. *B,* An example of a true unicameral bone cyst of the calcaneus. Note the pathologic fracture on the proximal inferior cortex.

## Talus

In a recent study by Thermann and co-workers, the prevalence of talus fractures was found to be 0.008% of all childhood fractures.[148] This infrequent injury in children is a potential problem injury because of the precarious blood supply.[106] The posterior tibial artery gives off small branches that enter the region of the posterior tubercle to supply a portion of the body of the talus. The anterior tibial artery creates small branches that enter the superior surface of the head and neck of the talus. Formation of the primary talar ossification center depends on a functioning vascular supply (Fig. 16–34). When compared with adults, children appear to have less dominance of a single system with retrograde flow from the neck into the body, and avascular (ischemic) necrosis is a rare complication after talus fracture. Much of its surface is covered by articular cartilage, with only the constricted neck left to accept the majority of nutrient vessels. Unfortunately, the neck is the area where most injuries occur. A displaced fracture of the neck of the talus is consistent with impending avascular necrosis.[18] Talar neck fractures can be overlooked in children and may become apparent only after the onset of osteonecrosis (Fig. 16–35). Avascular necrosis may not be appreciated for up to 6 months after injury.

## TYPES OF FRACTURES

**Talar Neck Fractures.** The most common talus fracture occurs through the neck and is slightly angulated, usually with minimal displacement. Ankle pain, swelling, and decreased joint motion may be noted. Weight bearing is not tolerated. Radiographs reveal the injury in most cases (Fig. 16–36). Angulation of up to 30° can usually be accepted. The apex of the angulation is in a plantar direction. Gentle, maximal plantar flexion with image intensification control under general anesthesia should be carried out if the angulation is greater than 30°. One has to weigh the risk of further displacement

**TABLE 16–2** •••••••••••••••••••••••••••••••••••••••

Distribution of 175 Foot Injuries* from Cincinnati Children's Hospital Resident Fracture Service, 1990

| Area of Injury | Number | Percentage |
|---|---|---|
| Metatarsals | | |
|   Lesser (2–4) | 104 (66.24) | 59.42 |
|   Buckle base | 14 (8.91) | 8 |
|   Base of 5th | 39 (24.84) | 22.2857 |
| Navicular | 9 | 5.14 |
| Talus | 4 | 2.285 |
| Calcaneus | 4 | 2.285 |
| Cuboid | 2 | 1.142 |
| Cuneiform | 1 | 0.571 |
| Phalanges | 31 | 17.71 |
|   Proximal | 20 (64.51) | 11.4285 |
|   Distal | 9 (29.0) | 5.14285 |
|   Middle | 2 (6.45) | 1.14285 |
| Talofibular ligament | 1 | 0.571 |
| Fibula | 8 | 4.57 |
| Sesamoid | 1 | 0.571 |
| Tarsal coalition | 1 | 0.571 |
| Foreign body | 1 | 0.571 |
| Medial malleolus | 3 | 1.71 |
| Distal tibial articular surface | 2 | 1.142 |
| Dislocation (MP/IP) | 4 | 2.285 |

•••••••••••••••••••••••••••••••••••••••••••••••••••••••••••••

*Sixty-two percent of the injuries occurred in boys, 38% in girls, and the left foot was involved 64% of the time, with the right foot injured in 36%. IP, interphalangeal; MP, metaphalangeal.
*Source:* Crawford, A.H. Fractures about the foot in children. A radiographic analysis. Cincinnati, OH, The Children's Hospital Medical Center, 1991 (unpublished data).

and vascular compromise against acceptance of the angulation. Rarely does the angulation inhibit ankle motion. If plantar flexion is required to maintain reduction, a non–weight-bearing, above-knee cast is worn for 3 to 4 weeks, followed by an Aircast. Treatment otherwise consists of a below-knee, non–weight-bearing cast for 3 to 4 weeks. Radiographs should be monitored for evidence of subchondral osteopenia of the proximal fragment. The vascular resorption Hawkins sign is an indication that the blood supply is intact.[59]

Displaced talar neck fractures tend to occur in older children (Fig. 16–37). They require open anatomic reduction. Early reduction by open or closed means enhances fracture healing but may not influence the occurrence of avascular necrosis. Because the distal tibial growth plates are closing, a medial malleolar osteotomy may be performed to allow direct visualization of the fracture. The reduction is stabilized with interfragmentary screws, and the osteotomy is repaired. An above-knee cast is applied with the knee flexed 30° and the

ankle plantar-flexed 20° for 4 to 6 weeks, followed by a below-knee, weight-bearing cast. The parents should be strongly advised of the possibility of avascular necrosis. Radiographs of the talus should be monitored for evidence of subchondral osteopenia of the proximal fragment. If no Hawkins' sign is apparent and the proximal fragment becomes sclerotic, we recommend a patellar tendon–bearing (PTB) brace to prevent talus collapse.

In a computerized search (1990–1997) performed at Children's Medical Center in Cincinnati to detect patients with talar neck fractures, 16 fractures were identified in 15 patients with an average age of 5.5 years (range, 1.6 to 17.5 years) and an average clinical follow-up for the group of 3.2 years, with all fractures monitored to beyond the point of clinical healing. In 12 instances, the talar neck fracture occurred in conjunction with other ipsilateral lower extremity fractures, with tibial fractures being most common. Four of the talar neck fractures were discernible, but not recognized on the initial

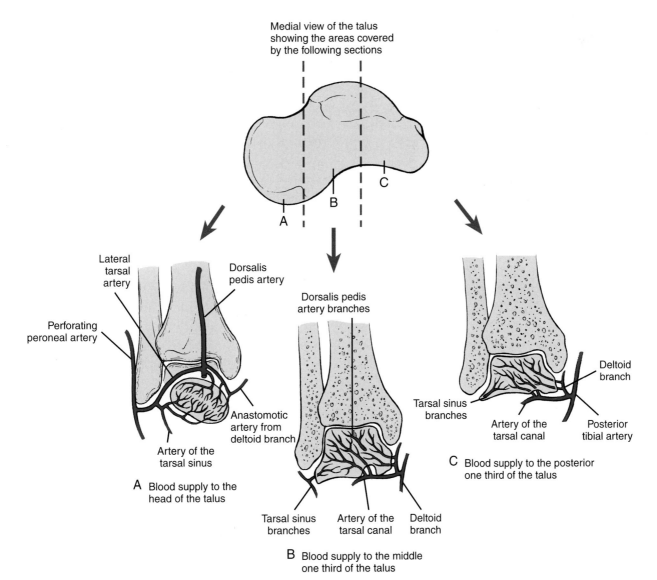

**FIGURE 16–34.** Diagram showing the blood supply to the talus in coronal sections. (From Mulfinger, G.L.; Trueta, J. J Bone Joint Surg Br 52:160, 1970.)

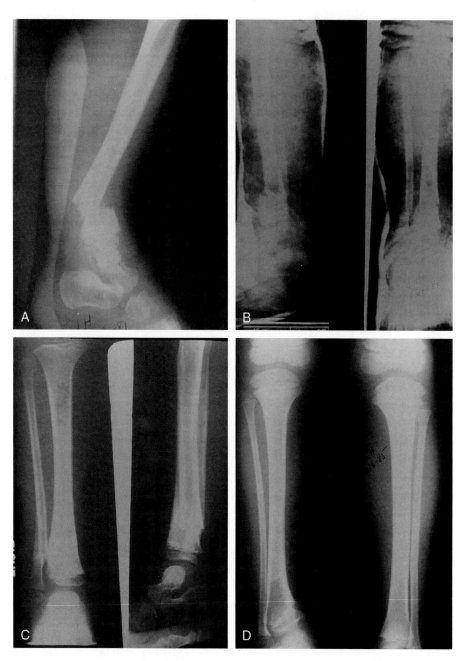

**Figure 16–35.** An example of unrecognized injury to the talus resulting in osteonecrosis. This child sustained a tibial fracture that was reduced and healed uneventfully. He was subsequently noted to have avascular necrosis of the talus over the dome. Another unrecognized injury was a Salter-Harris type IV injury to the medial malleolus. The injury resulted in a severe varus deformity that finally caused his return to the hospital. *A,* Lateral radiograph of the leg showing a displaced, posteriorly angulated distal tibial fracture. The talar fracture was not recognized. *B,* Anteroposterior and lateral radiographs of the leg showing adequate reduction. *C,* Anteroposterior and lateral radiographs 2 months later showing avascular necrosis of the talar dome that had not been recognized. *D,* The patient was seen in consultation 3½ years after the injury because of an ankle varus deformity secondary to growth arrest of the medial malleolar fracture. The talus was collapsed, and the ankle or subtalar joint had very little motion.

radiographs. All fractures were minimally displaced. The nonoperative protocol outlined earlier was carried out. No cases of avascular necrosis were found. Clinical outcomes analysis revealed no trouble with shoe wear, mild limp or stiffness in 2 patients, mild pain in 2 patients, and 12 patients participating in unrestricted sports. A high index of suspicion is appropriate when an ipsilateral tibial fracture is present because one may be dealing with a "floating ankle."[99]

**Compression Fracture of the Dome of the Talus.** This injury is rare in children. The cartilage-to-bone ratio tends to cushion the impact of the tibial and subtalar joints, and the bone is well protected in the mortise. These compression fractures are most common in older adolescents and young adults; thus, they are not discussed here.

**Lateral or Medial Process Fractures.** These fractures may occur after a twisting injury to the ankle. The patient complains of pain beneath the malleolus. Rarely does displacement occur, and treatment of nondisplaced fractures consists of non–weight bearing in a below-knee cast for 4 weeks and then 2 weeks of progressive weight bearing as tolerated in a walking cast.

Kirkpatrick and co-workers showed that lateral process fractures represented 15% of all the ankle injuries related to snowboarding in their study.[74] A common mechanism for this fracture is dorsiflexion of the ankle and inversion of the hindfoot. The physician should be very suspicious of anterolateral ankle pain in a snowboarder. Many of these fractures are not visible on plain radiographs and require CT for diagnosis. If small displaced fragments or significant comminution is found,

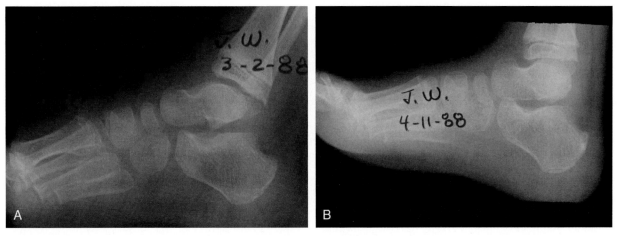

FIGURE 16–36. Minimally angulated talar neck fracture in a 6-year-old after a dorsiflexion injury to his foot. *A,* Lateral radiograph at the time of injury. Minimal plantar angulation is seen. *B,* Lateral radiograph at the time of healing. The neck remains slightly angulated.

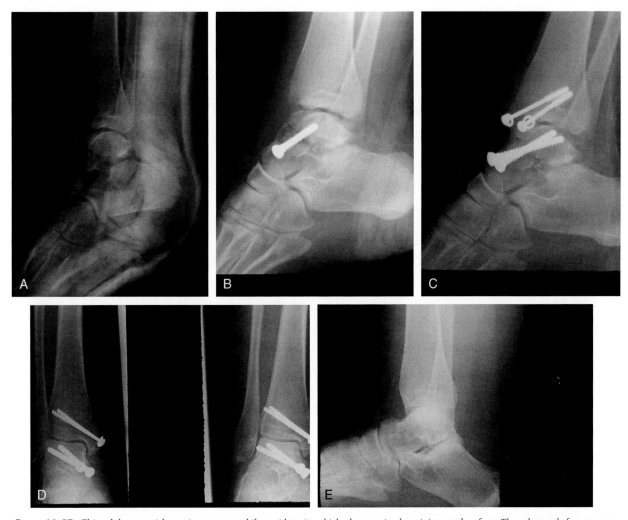

FIGURE 16–37. This adolescent girl was in an automobile accident in which she sustained an injury to her foot. The talar neck fracture was displaced. As a result, she underwent open reduction through a medial malleolar osteotomy and internal fixation. Because of avascular necrosis, the child was maintained in a brace for 1½ years; she healed uneventfully. *A,* Original lateral radiograph of the foot in a posterior plaster splint showing a displaced talar neck fracture. *B,* Intraoperative radiograph showing anatomic reduction of the talar neck fracture with cortical screw fixation. *C,* Final postoperative radiograph showing fixation of the talar neck fracture, as well as the medial malleolar osteotomy. *D,* Anteroposterior and mortise views 3 months after injury. Note the absence of subchondral osteopenia (Hawkins' sign). The talus had undergone avascular necrosis. *E,* Lateral view of the ankle 3 years later. The ankle was protected with a patellar tendon–bearing brace for 2 years. Some ankle joint space has been lost.

most authors favor early excision with weight bearing as tolerated.[74, 105] If CT demonstrates a large displaced fracture, open reduction plus internal fixation is the recommended treatment.[74]

**Transcondylar Fractures (Osteochondritis Dissecans).** This entity is discussed separately under Osteochondral Fractures.

## COMPLICATIONS

Complications of talus fractures depend on the location of the fracture line and the amount of displacement. Commonly, after reduction of fractures with significant displacement, the complication is avascular necrosis.

### Avascular Necrosis

The talus is the anatomic keystone for the ankle joint; it is the linchpin between the anatomic foot and ankle. Collapse of the talar dome may occur after avascular necrosis of the talus, but this condition is extremely rare in children younger than 10 years. Talkhani and co-workers reported a case of avascular necrosis of the talus after a minimally displaced talar neck fracture in a 6-year-old child.[146] We had a similar case in a 5-year-old child (presented in Fig. 16–35). The anatomy and function of the talus are usually stable until the collapse occurs. The subsequent alteration in its shape leads to ankle joint incongruity, instability, and later, degenerative joint disease. A bone scan is indicated after the treatment of all displaced talus fractures to rule out avascular necrosis. It has been questioned whether the avoidance of weight bearing has an effect on the outcome of talar avascular necrosis. Management is usually similar to that for Legg-Perthes disease, with no weight bearing and active motion in a PTB articulated ankle brace until evidence of revascularization.

Avascular necrosis developed in 5 of 17 children with nondisplaced fractures of the talus, as reported by Canale and Kelly[18] and by Letts and Gibeault.[84] Consequently, Gross[55] suggested that children may be as much at risk as adults for the development of avascular necrosis after nondisplaced fractures. These reports contradict the prevailing philosophy that pediatric avascular necrosis is unusual because displacement is uncommon in children (see Fig. 16–35).

Hawkins in 1970 detailed his experience with a series of 57 fractures of the talus in adults and outlined a useful classification.[59] Type I fractures were nondisplaced, and in his series, avascular necrosis did not appear. Type II fractures were displaced, with subtalar dislocation or subluxation. All united, but the rate of avascular necrosis was 42%. Type III fractures were accompanied by subluxation or dislocation at the subtalar and ankle joints, and a 91% rate of avascular necrosis was found in this group.[59] After injury and reduction, the Hawkins sign, a radiolucent subchondral line, is usually an indication that the blood supply is intact, even though avascular necrosis may have occurred. Because this sign accompanies disuse atrophy, it may be absent in children immobilized for only brief periods. A bone scan can demonstrate whether avascular necrosis has occurred and has been used by Canale and Kelly to determine

when weight bearing can be resumed.[18] We have treated talar avascular necrosis by PTB bracing in an effort to prevent collapse. This method has not been completely successful; in one child, the talus underwent flattening, with stiffness of the ankle and shortening of the extremity. Pain has not been a consistent complaint, but 5 years after the injury the child is only 10 years old, and symptoms may occur as maturity progresses.

## OS TRIGONUM

The lateral tubercle, also called the os trigonum, sometimes separates, usually at the attachment of the talocalcaneal ligament. The os trigonum may be considered a developmental analogue of a secondary ossification center, similar to the posterior calcaneal apophysis.[54] The normal ossification process within the body of the talus is characterized by progressive posterior extension toward the posterior tubercle. Radiographic studies suggest that the prevalence may be as high as 14% to 25% and that the condition is usually bilateral.[68]

Hindfoot pain can have a myriad of causes and may be acute or chronic; radiographs show evidence of chondroosseous separation (see Fig. 16–32). When the clinical findings are difficult to differentiate from other causes of posterior ankle pain, a positive response to a fluoroscopically guided injection of local anesthetic into the region of the synchondrosis between the os trigonum and the posterior aspect of the talus can help confirm the diagnosis.[69] A bone scan can be used to determine whether the lesion should be treated as an undisplaced fracture with probable microscopic delayed union or nonunion. A below-knee weight-bearing cast is indicated for symptomatic treatment; although the radiographs may not change, the patient becomes asymptomatic. On rare occasion, excision may be indicated.

## OSTEOCHONDRAL FRACTURES

In 1888, Konig first used the term *osteochondritis dissecans* to describe loose bones in the knee joint.[79] It was not until 1932 that Rendu reported an intra-articular fracture of the talus that appeared to be similar in nature to that described by Konig.[128] The condition occurs most frequently in the second decade; however, it has been seen in a 3-year-old (Fig. 16–38). Osteochondral fractures of the talus usually result from eversion-inversion injuries.[6, 17] The initial complaint is usually ankle pain and an associated limp. A history of trauma was reported in 64% to 92% of patients.[6, 113, 142] The condition has been described in siblings and has also been associated with dwarfism[2, 121, 132, 160, 163] and with endocrine abnormalities.[153] Medial osteochondritis dissecans is usually a deeper lesion, and the clinician is not always able to elicit a history of injury. Lateral osteochondritis dissecans is generally caused by a more significant injury; however, it is also more shallow. In addition, the lateral fragment has a greater tendency to become displaced into the joint.

Berndt and Harty coined the term *torsional impaction,* which is useful in understanding the mechanism of injury in these lesions.[6] They classified the lesion into

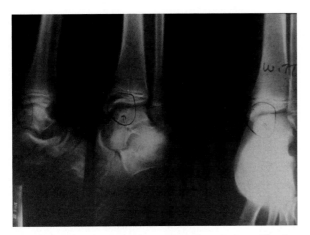

**FIGURE 16–38.** These composite radiographs of the ankle show medial talar osteochondritis dissecans in a 3-year-old child. The child was treated with a below-knee walking cast, and the lesion healed.

four stages: (1) a small area of compression of subchondral bone, (2) a partially detached osteochondral fragment, (3) a completely detached osteochondral fragment remaining in the crater, and (4) a displaced osteochondral fragment (Fig. 16–39). They suggested that the lesion may represent nonunion of an osteochondral fracture or separation of articular cartilage and underlying subchondral bone by means of a localized vascular insult. They produced the posteromedial lesion by inversion and plantar flexion of the foot combined with external rotation of the tibia. Traumatic inversion and ankle dorsiflexion and compression of the talus against the lateral malleolus produce the anterolateral lesion, which may be accompanied by rupture of the fibular collateral ligaments (Fig. 16–40). The

posteromedial lesion is slightly more common. The osteochondrotic fragment consists of viable hyaline cartilage with underlying necrotic bone. The radiolucent line between the dead bone and the remainder of the talus is formed by a dense layer of fibrous connective tissue that acts as a barrier to capillary ingrowth. The primary objective of any treatment is to obtain bony union between the osteochondrotic fragment and the remainder of the talus. MRI is superior to CT arthrography if detachment or displacement of the fragment cannot be identified on plain radiographs (Fig. 16–41). MRI findings that have been reported in osteochondral lesions are a low-intensity area on T1-weighted images and signal rims observed between the talar bed and the osteochondral fragment on T2-weighted images; the first suggests the presence of the lesion and the second evaluates the stability of the lesion. Postoperative MRI of these lesions is useful in assessing healing of osteochondral lesions. MRI findings that suggest healing are a decreasing size of the low-intensity area on T1-weighted images and disappearance of the signal rims behind the osteochondral fragment on T2-weighted images.[60]

Taranow and co-workers suggested a new classification for talar osteochondral lesions. The classification uses findings from preoperative MRI and arthroscopic findings. The condition of the cartilage and bone together determines the type of surgical treatment. Cartilage is classified as viable and intact (grade A) or breached and nonviable (grade B). The bone component is described as follows: stage 1 is subchondral compression or a bone bruise, which appears as high signal on T2-weighted images; stage 2 lesions are subchondral cysts and are not seen acutely; stage 3 lesions are partially separated or detached fragments in situ; and stage 4 represents displaced fragments.[147] When drilling was indicated,

| Stage I | Stage II | Stage III | Stage IV |
|---|---|---|---|

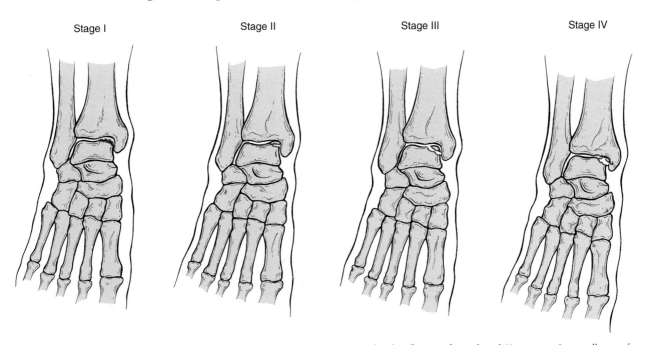

**FIGURE 16–39.** The four stages of an osteochondral lesion of the talus according to the classification of Berndt and Harty: stage I, a small area of subchondral compression; stage II, a partially detached fragment; stage III, a completely detached fragment remaining in the crater; and stage IV, a fragment that is loose in the joint. (From Canale, S.T.; Belding, R.M. J Bone Joint Surg Am 62:97, 1980.)

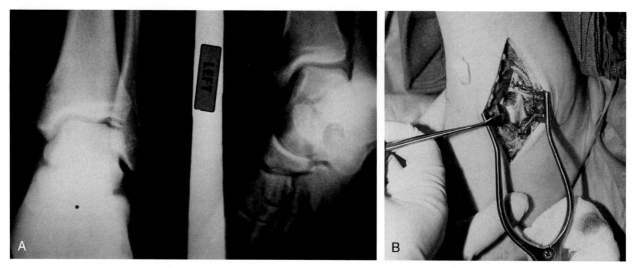

**FIGURE 16–40.** Acute injury to the ankle resulting in an anterolateral talar osteochondral fracture. *A*, Anteroposterior and mortise views of the ankle showing the loose body (osteochondral fragment) lying on the skin over the anterior lateral junction of the ankle joint. *B*, Operative view showing the defect in the anterior lateral dome of the talus. The osteochondral fragment is shown lying across the ankle. It was not large enough to be replaced. After removal of the fragment, bone wax was placed over its bed. The patient was immobilized for 10 days, followed by active range-of-motion and ankle-strengthening exercises in a bivalved cast.

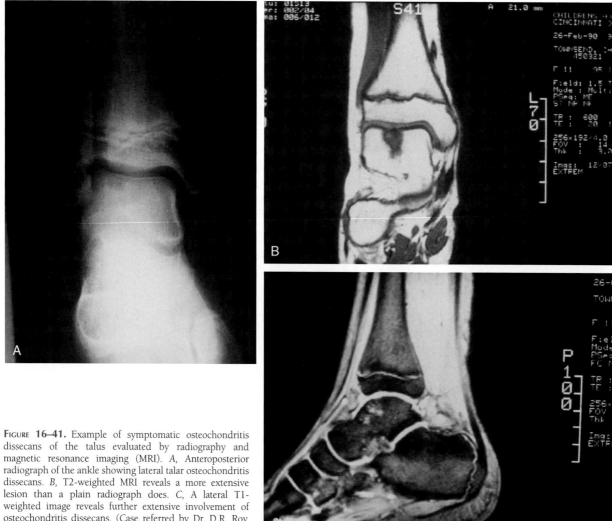

**FIGURE 16–41.** Example of symptomatic osteochondritis dissecans of the talus evaluated by radiography and magnetic resonance imaging (MRI). *A*, Anteroposterior radiograph of the ankle showing lateral talar osteochondritis dissecans. *B*, T2-weighted MRI reveals a more extensive lesion than a plain radiograph does. *C*, A lateral T1-weighted image reveals further extensive involvement of osteochondritis dissecans. (Case referred by Dr. D.R. Roy, Cincinnati, OH.)

retrograde drilling was suggested in patients with grade A cartilage.

Canale and Belding recommended that undisplaced lesions be treated conservatively with casts and that displaced lesions be treated with excision and curettage.[17] The literature is pessimistic about the use of a cast and no weight bearing to obtain healing of lateral osteochondritis.[6, 17] We have been successful in the treatment of nondisplaced lesions in children younger than 10 years with the application of an above-knee, non–weight-bearing cast for 3 months. Displaced lesions and those that do not respond to non–weight bearing warrant surgical intervention. Because arthroscopic treatment of these lesions has yielded outcomes as good as or better than arthrotomy, we advocate this method. Advantages of arthroscopic surgery include minimal iatrogenic trauma during surgery and rapid mobilization of patients after surgery. We recommend arthroscopically assisted transtalar retrograde drilling in patients in whom continuity of the cartilaginous surface and stability of the lesion have been confirmed, possibly allowing easier access to posteromedial lesions (Fig. 16–42). For larger lesions, open reduction plus fixation of unstable osteochondral fragment is recommended, and transmalleolar osteotomy may be required. We perform arthroscopic excision and drilling of the base of the lesion if the osteochondral fragment is small and completely detached. If the fragment is completely detached and the bed of the defect is forming granulation tissue, excision of only the fragment may be indicated. The current authors have no experience with the treatment of these lesions by autologous osteochondral grafting.[58]

In a recent literature review, Tol and associates showed the average success rate of nonoperative treatment in a mixed group of patients to be 45%; the highest success rate (85%) was achieved with excision, curettage, and drilling, but the great diversity in the articles included in the review does not allow any definite conclusions to be made.[150]

In summary, surgery is to be recommended infrequently in the younger age group because children through the age of adolescence usually do well after a period of activity modification, immobilization, or both.

Two case reports discussed patients with osteochondritis dissecans of the talar head. Both patients were 16 years old, and one of these patients had a history of trauma. One patient did well after nonoperative symptomatic treatment and the other required surgical excision and drilling because of persistent symptoms and was doing well at the 2-year follow-up provided in the case report.[39, 123]

## Calcaneus

Schofield reviewed 2025 fractures of the calcaneus; his youngest patient was an 18-year-old male.[134] Essex-LoPresti reported only 12 patients between the ages of 9 and 20 years among 241 with fractures of the calcaneus.[46] Thomas in 1969 reported five boys aged 6 to 12 years who had sustained fractures of the calcaneus.[149]

Matteri and Frymoyer reported three fractures of the calcaneus in children.[95] Schmidt and Weiner detected 59 fractures of the calcaneus in patients younger than 20 years, 46 of which were in skeletally immature children.[133] One third of their patients had associated injuries; three sustained lumbar vertebral fractures. Ten percent of adults with calcaneal fractures have spinal injuries, whereas only 5% of children have such injuries. This lower prevalence, however, does not mean that spinal injury should not be looked for in children. Calcaneal fractures were initially unrecognized in 16 of the 59 fractures reviewed. Most of these fractures were minimal, which led to the conclusion that the injury has a benign prognosis. More recently, Inokuchi and co-workers reported on 20 fractures of the calcaneus in children 14 years and younger, and Brunet reported on 19 fractures in 17 patients 13 years and younger.[14, 64]

### CLASSIFICATION

The patterns of fracture modified from Rowe by Ogden include type 1, fracture of the tuberosity, sustentaculum tali, or anterior process; type 2, a beak fracture or avulsion fracture of the tendo Achillis insertion; type 3, an oblique fracture in the posterior portion of the bone not involving the subtalar joint and similar to a metaphyseal fracture of a longitudinal bone; type 4, involvement of the subtalar region, with or without actual articular involvement; type 5, a central depression fracture with varying degrees of comminution; and type 6, involvement of the secondary ossification center[111] (Table 16–3). Schmidt and Weiner[133] developed a composite classification to include the compound fractures that are so common with lawn mower injuries in children. The soft tissue injury is usually serious and includes significant bone loss and loss of insertion of the Achilles tendon (Fig. 16–43).

### CONSEQUENCES OF INJURY

The calcaneus is largely cartilaginous in children. Fracture of the calcaneus is a common, disabling injury in adults, yet it is rarely reported in infancy or in early childhood.[95, 151] However, it is probably the most frequent tarsal injury seen in children.[133] Fracture of the calcaneus was recognized in 4 of 175 patients seen in the pediatric foot fracture study from the Children's Hospital Medical Center in Cincinnati.

Stress or occult fractures may occur, and clinicians should beware of a young child who refuses to bear weight or who limps, especially when no radiographic evidence of a fracture can be found.[132] Schindler and colleagues reported on five children 14 to 33 months of age treated for calcaneal fractures who had a history of trauma followed by limping or refusal to walk.[132] Their initial radiographs were negative. Four patients were treated with above-knee casts with the presumptive diagnosis of fracture, and one was treated with a bandage. All fractures healed without complications, and although no bone scans were performed, radiographs taken 2 to 4 weeks after treatment confirmed the diagnosis. These authors recommended a bone scan only

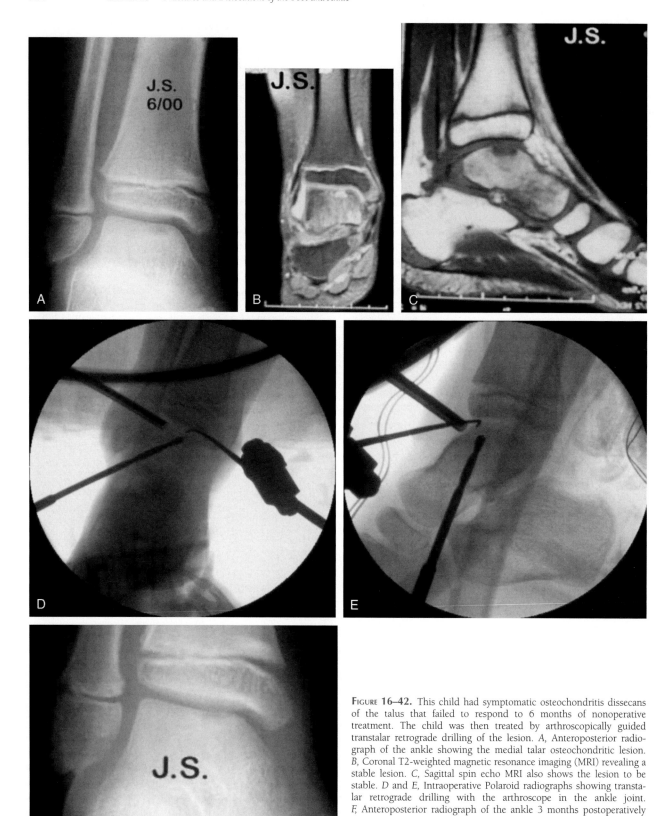

**Figure 16–42.** This child had symptomatic osteochondritis dissecans of the talus that failed to respond to 6 months of nonoperative treatment. The child was then treated by arthroscopically guided transtalar retrograde drilling of the lesion. *A,* Anteroposterior radiograph of the ankle showing the medial talar osteochondritic lesion. *B,* Coronal T2-weighted magnetic resonance imaging (MRI) revealing a stable lesion. *C,* Sagittal spin echo MRI also shows the lesion to be stable. *D* and *E,* Intraoperative Polaroid radiographs showing transtalar retrograde drilling with the arthroscope in the ankle joint. *F,* Anteroposterior radiograph of the ankle 3 months postoperatively showing no evidence of extension of the lesion. (Case referred by Dr. Eric Wall, Cincinnati, OH.)

if the follow-up radiographs showed no evidence of a healing fracture or if the symptoms persisted after treatment. Depending on the degree of primary ossification, stress fracture is extremely difficult to diagnose early. Later, a sclerotic oblique line may be seen over the trabecular pattern, an indication of the reparative process. It is possible that a bone scan would identify the problem early. A below-knee, weight-bearing cast for 3 to 4 weeks is usually sufficient treatment.

Heel pain may be a result of overuse or a symptom of

····································

Calcaneal Fracture Patterns

| Type | Description |
|------|-------------|
| 1 | Fracture of the tuberosity |
| | Fracture of the sustentaculum tali |
| | Fracture of the anterior process |
| 2 | "Beak" fracture |
| | Avulsion fracture of the tendo Achillis insertion |
| 3 | Oblique fracture in the posterior portion not involving the subtalar joint; corresponds to a metaphyseal fracture of a longitudinal bone |
| 4 | Fracture involving the subtalar region with or without actual articular involvement |
| 5 | Central depression with varying degrees of comminution |
| 6 | Involvement of the secondary ossification center |

····································

*Source:* Rowe, C.R., at al. JAMA 184:920, 1963. Copyright 1963, American Medical Association.

systemic disease such as osteomyelitis or leukemia. The appearance of the secondary ossification center of the calcaneus is often fragmented on radiographs and leads to the assumption that an injury is present. This pattern of fragmentation of the apophysis in young children is more the rule than the exception. The clinical condition of pain about the heel with this radiographic finding carries the diagnosis of Sever's disease. We consider Sever's disease to be an overuse syndrome or the result of repetitive microtrauma (see Fig. 16–28).

Most calcaneal fractures result from a significant fall. Parmar and co-workers reported a fracture of the calcaneus and an anterior column injury of L4 after a water tubing (pulling of an inner tube behind a power boat) injury when a 17-year-old patient went feet first into the dock.[114] Radiographs are usually taken in the AP, lateral, and axial planes, although internal and external oblique views of the foot, as well as a CT scan, may be necessary. If the patient sustained a significant fall from a height, AP and lateral views of the thoracolumbar spine should be taken to rule out vertebral fracture (Fig. 16–44). Calcaneal injuries may also result from vehicular and lawn mower accidents (Fig. 16–45) or from a heavy object falling onto the foot (Fig. 16–46).

Intra-articular injuries affect the subtalar joint and are most often caused by the inferior protruding lateral process of the talus (Fig. 16–47). The process jams superiorly into the calcaneus during impact, with

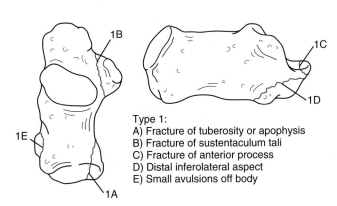

Type 1:
A) Fracture of tuberosity or apophysis
B) Fracture of sustentaculum tali
C) Fracture of anterior process
D) Distal inferolateral aspect
E) Small avulsions off body

A

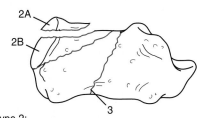

Type 2:
A) Beak fracture
B) Avulsion fracture of insertion of Achilles tendon

Type 3:
A) Linear fracture not involving subtalar joint

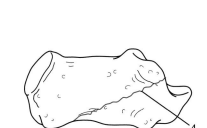

Type 4:
Linear fracture involving subtalar joint

B

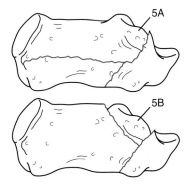

Type 5:
Linear fracture involving subtalar joint
A) Tongue type
B) Joint-depression type

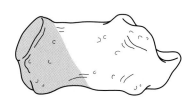

Type 6:
Significant bone loss of posterior aspect with loss of Achilles tendon insertion

C

FIGURE 16–43. Classification used to evaluate calcaneal fracture patterns in children. *A*, Extra-articular fractures. *B*, Intra-articular fractures. *C*, Type 6 injury, with significant soft tissue injury, bone loss, and loss of insertion of the Achilles tendon. (From Schmidt, T.L.; Weiner, D.S. Clin Orthop 171:151, 1982.)

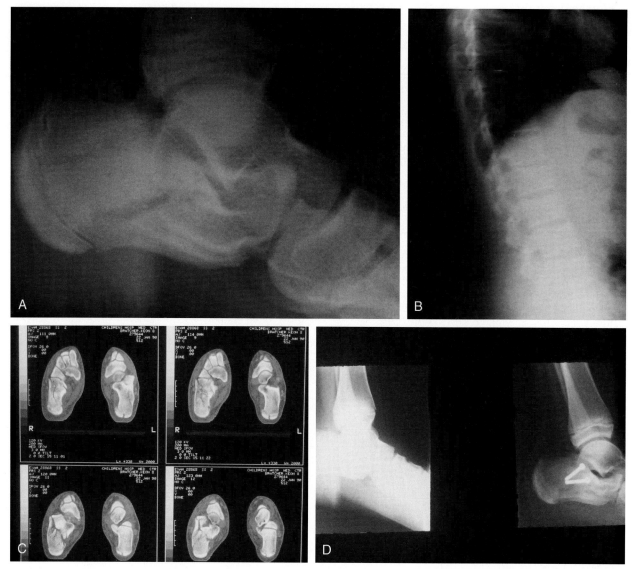

FIGURE 16–44.  Comminuted calcaneal fracture in association with a thoracolumbar spine injury. This child jumped from a height and sustained a calcaneal fracture; he also had back pain. The lateral thoracolumbar spine film shows a compression injury at the T12–L1 junction. The calcaneal fracture was treated by open reduction and internal fixation. *A,* Lateral view of the foot showing a comminuted, dorsally displaced calcaneal fracture. *B,* Lateral thoracolumbar spine radiograph showing mild compression fractures of T12, L1, and L2. *C,* Multiple coronal-view computed tomographic scans of both feet revealing a comminuted right calcaneal fracture and nondisplaced fractures of the left calcaneus. *D,* Preoperative and postoperative lateral views of the right foot show reduction and fixation with two cortical screws.

cracking of the calcaneus in a dorsal-to-plantar direction. Most young children with fractures of the calcaneus are assumed to have ankle sprains. The initial radiographs may not show the fracture, and in suspected cases, a bone scan is indicated. A nondisplaced fracture of the calcaneus is treated by immobilization. This injury in children produces minimal disability in comparison to fractures of the calcaneus in adults.[96] For a displaced calcaneal fracture, initial treatment should be directed toward the soft tissue swelling, which may be extensive. One should make every effort to achieve anatomic reduction of all articular surfaces to prevent subsequent degenerative joint disease. After reduction, the foot and ankle should be immobilized in a well-padded compression dressing and the leg elevated for 2 to 3 days. A cast should not be applied until the bulk of the swelling has

subsided. A below-knee walking cast is sufficient for immobilization of most calcaneal fractures not requiring open reduction. After open reduction, a well-padded above-knee cast is indicated for 3 to 4 weeks, followed by a below-knee walking cast for 3 to 4 weeks.

Cole and co-workers[24] reported on avulsion fractures of the tuberosity of the calcaneus in children and reviewed the literature. In contrast to the usual recommendation to treat skeletally immature patients with calcaneal fractures by immobilization, they recommend open reduction and internal fixation. Of the four patients in their series (all of whom were older than 12 years), open reduction and internal fixation gave the best results. None of their patients had displaced intra-articular injuries, and the purpose of the open reduction was to prevent any functional loss from a shortened heel cord.

The recommendation is to first attempt closed reduction under general anesthesia and to place the child in an above-knee cast with the knee in flexion and the ankle in 30° to 45° of plantar flexion. If closed reduction fails and if the degree of displacement is such that functional disability, nonunion, or breakdown of soft tissue is likely, the fracture should be treated by open reduction and internal stabilization plus avoidance of fixation across the immature calcaneal apophysis.

Intra-articular fractures prevail in adult series (56% to 75%).[133] In the present series, 37% of children sustained intra-articular fractures and 63%, extra-articular fractures. A review of the association between fracture type and age further illustrated that extra-articular fractures were more characteristic of younger children. In children through the age of 7 years, 92% of the fractures were extra-articular. From ages 8 through 14 years, 61% of the fractures were extra-articular. In children 15 years and older, the adult pattern was present, with 38% of the fractures extra-articular and 62% intra-articular. The predominance of extra-articular fractures in younger children seems predictable in view of the fact that the mechanism of vertical compressive load (e.g., a fall) is responsible for most intra-articular fractures and occurs twice as frequently in adults as in children. In addition, the resiliency of the cartilage and adjacent soft tissues tends to act as a resorbing factor in children who sustain vertical compressive loads. It is probable that the ability to absorb the stress from vertical loading results in fewer displaced intra-articular fractures in children than in adults. On the contrary, two series in the literature reported a predominance of intra-articular fractures in children; the first is by de Beer and associates, who reported on nine fractures in eight patients aged 18 months to 12 years (mean, 6 years), and six of the nine fractures (66%) were intra-articular.[32] The second report is by Brunet, who reported on 19 fractures in 17 patients aged 1.6 to 13 years (mean, 6.2 years); 14 of the 19 fractures (74%) were intra-articular.[14]

Inokuchi and associates reported on 20 calcaneal fractures, with ages at the time of injury ranging from 1 to 14 years (mean, 8.2 years). The fractures were extra-articular in 12 and intra-articular in 8. Four of the intra-articular fractures were associated with displacement. Only two cases required surgical intervention: one was a displaced avulsion fracture of the Achilles tendon insertion and the other was a displaced intra-articular fracture of the joint depression type. The results were favorable in all patients except one who suffered an associated neurologic injury after an L5 burst fracture. Inokuchi and colleagues concluded that surgical therapy should be performed on displaced avulsion fractures of the portion of the calcaneus where the Achillis tendon inserts and on intra-articular fractures in which displacement is present.[64]

Brunet reported on the long-term results of the treatment of 19 calcaneal fractures in 17 children. Their age at the time of injury ranged from 1.6 to 13 years (mean, 6.2 years). Follow-up ranged from 13.2 to 22.7 years with an average of 16.8 years. Extra-articular fractures occurred in 6 and intra-articular fractures in 14. The fracture pattern of these 14 intra-articular fractures consisted of 2 tongue type, 2 centrolateral, 1 involving the sustentaculum tali, 6 grossly comminuted, and 3 minimally displaced. All fractures were managed in a cast without manipulative reduction, with the exception of

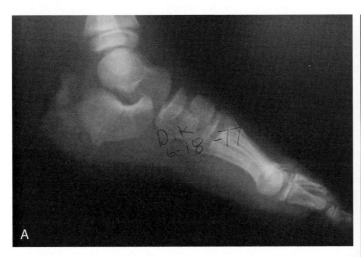

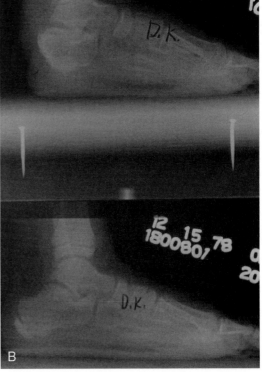

**FIGURE 16–45.** This child sustained a lawn mower injury that clipped away the posterior half of the calcaneus. After injury, the bone had minimal posterior growth. *A,* Lateral radiograph of the foot showing extensive soft tissue and bony injury to the posterior of the calcaneus. The wound was débrided and the Achilles tendon sutured to bone. Unfortunately, the apophysis was crushed and had to be discarded. *B,* Comparison lateral views of both feet 1½ years later showing loss of the calcaneal apophysis and failure of continued posterior growth of the bone.

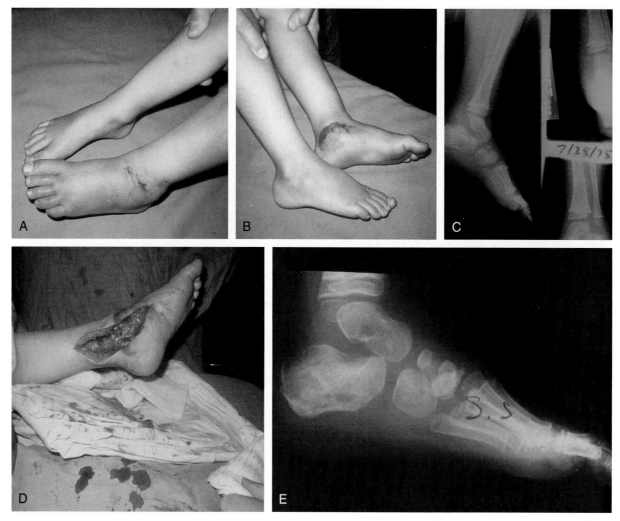

**FIGURE 16–46.** This child was watching her father erect a wall of concrete blocks when one of the blocks fell on her left foot and caused tremendous swelling of the foot and toes. A clinical diagnosis of impending compartment syndrome was made. Immediate decompression was carried out to save the foot. The fracture healed uneventfully. Swelling and congestion of the foot and toes constitute a surgical emergency. *A,* Anterior clinical photograph of both feet showing the tension edema of the foot and toes. *B,* Side view showing swelling of the medial aspect of the left foot with focal blanching "ischemia" on the plantar portion. *C,* Anteroposterior, lateral, and mortise views. *D,* Operative photograph at the time of decompression. *E,* Follow-up lateral radiograph of the foot. The calcaneus is healed, and the wounds were approximated by delayed primary closure.

one that required open treatment for wound débridement. At follow-up, a few children complained of cramps in the foot with abrupt barometric pressure changes and sensitivity to cold weather. All but two patients had full or slightly reduced range of motion of the subtalar joint, and these two patints sustained an ipsilateral fracture of the neck of the talus. All patients were unaware of any functional restriction resulting from their injury. They could all walk comfortably on uneven ground. Mild to moderately severe osteoarthritic changes were seen in two patients on radiographic assessment: one involved the subtalar joint and the other involved the calcaneocuboid joint. Many who suffered joint depression and comminution had been and were still involved in high-performance sports such as long-distance running. It was suggested that children younger than 10 years have sufficient remodeling potential at the damaged articular surfaces of the calcaneum that when the immature talus grows into the defect produced by the depressed calcaneus, the final result is relative anatomic congruity of the subtalar joint.[14]

## COMPLICATIONS

Subtalar arthritis may occur with persistent displacement and instability of osteochondral fractures in the subtalar joint. Late surgery to reduce and align the joint surfaces is rarely successful, and subtalar or triple arthrodesis may be required. In Brunet's long-term study, subtalar joint osteoarthritis developed in only 1 of 14 intra-articular fractures. This patient was 11.8 years old at the time of the injury and suffered a severely comminuted fracture of his calcaneus. The patient had minimal symptoms and scored 90 out of 100 on the American Orthopaedic Foot and Ankle Society rating score.[14] Injury to the growth plate has been noted after open fracture secondary to a lawn mower injury (see Fig. 16–45); otherwise, growth plate injury to the calcaneus is extremely rare.

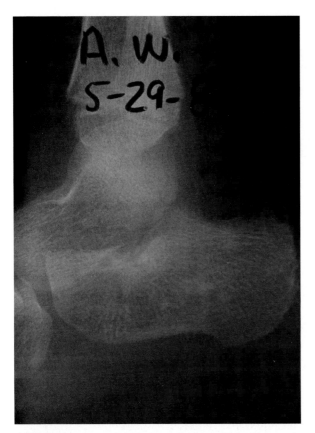

**FIGURE 16–47.** Fracture through the medial facet of the calcaneus. This fracture is thought to be caused by the lateral process of the talus impacting between the posterior and medial facets. The injury healed uneventfully.

## Navicular Bone

The tarsal navicular bone is injured only occasionally in children, and the fracture is rarely displaced. Nine navicular fractures were seen in 175 fractures reviewed from the Cincinnati Children's Hospital.

Because of the variability in ossification, a fracture may be confused with Köhler's disease. The radiographic picture of a sclerotic, thin, fragmented tarsal navicular bone, commonly called Köhler's disease, may represent repetitive microtrauma, an abnormal ossification pattern, or an overuse syndrome (Fig. 16–48). In Waugh's study of 52 boys and 52 girls, on radiographs taken at 6-month intervals from 2 to 5 years, 10 boys and 16 girls showed abnormal ossification.[159] Radiographs of the foot taken for other reasons often show irregularity of tarsal navicular ossification. It is still questioned whether Köhler's disease is a normal variant or represents overuse. Treatment of this injury is usually uncomplicated because the bone is minimally displaced, if at all.

Borges and colleagues found that patients treated without casting had symptoms lasting an average of 10 months. Patients treated with casting were completely asymptomatic within an average of 3 months. Treatment with a below-knee walking cast for about 8 weeks rendered the individual pain free in the shortest period. The average time required for complete restoration of normal bone structure was 1 year 4 months, with a minimum of 4 months and a maximum of 4 years.[10]

The most frequent navicular fracture in children is a dorsal proximal chip fracture, which is best seen on a lateral radiograph of the foot (Fig. 16–49). This injury

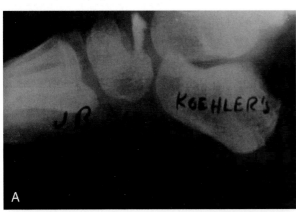

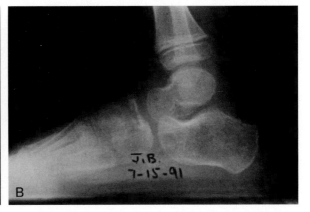

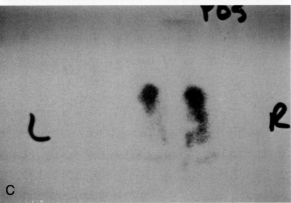

**FIGURE 16–48.** *A,* Köhler's disease of the navicular bone in a 6-year-old. This disease is believed to be an inflammatory condition; however, asymptomatic feet may have similar radiographic findings. *B,* Lateral radiograph illustrating osteopenia of the tarsal navicular bone. *C,* Bone scan of the patient's foot showing a photopenic tarsal navicular bone. Bone scanning is not recommended to investigate this condition.

may represent an avulsion pull-off of an apophyseal fragment from the dorsal tarsal ligament. Treatment of this injury is usually uncomplicated because of the minimal, if any displacement. A below-knee walking cast is applied for 3 to 4 weeks. Even though the small chip may not unite to the navicular body, the symptoms subside.

Displaced fractures of the tarsal navicular bone in children are usually associated with severe trauma and possible dislocation. We recommend anatomic reduction and percutaneous pinning with a threaded Steinmann pin. If closed anatomic reduction cannot be achieved, open reduction and internal fixation are indicated. If soft tissue injury has occurred, compression and elevation are required until the problem is resolved. A below-knee, non–weight-bearing cast is then applied.

## Cuboid Fractures

Fractures of the cuboid in children are very uncommon. Cuboid fractures accounted for 1.1% of the fractures in our series.[61] Simonian and associates described eight fractures of the cuboid in children younger than 4 years. All fractures were first diagnosed with a bone scan because the early radiographs were read as normal.[140] For these nondisplaced fractures, a short-leg walking cast is the treatment of choice, primarily for comfort. Cuboid

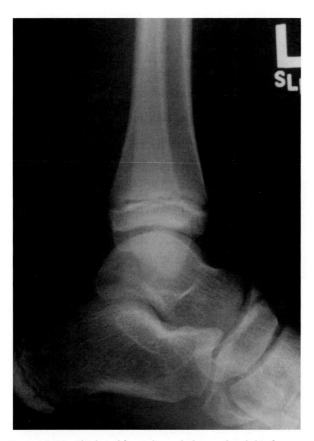

FIGURE 16–49. This lateral foot radiograph shows a dorsal chip fracture of the navicular bone, which is the most common navicular fracture in children.

fractures should be considered in the differential diagnosis of a limping toddler, and a bone scan is helpful in making the diagnosis.

## Tarsometatarsal Fractures

These injuries are rare[161] and may result from indirect injury, such as the violent plantar flexion and dorsiflexion found in toe walking or trying to break speed while sledding or tobogganing, or from direct injury, which is more common, secondary to an object falling onto the foot. The unique pattern of tarsometatarsal joint injuries described by numerous authors is related to the anatomic features of this joint complex and the mechanism of injury. The most relevant anatomic features are the fixed, mortised position of the base of the second metatarsal and the ligamentous attachments to its base. A detailed review of the anatomy was provided in a recent review by de Palma.[34] A fracture of the base of this metatarsal is a sentinel feature of a tarsometatarsal joint injury.[161] Trillat and associates reviewed 81 fracture-dislocations of the tarsometatarsal joint and concluded that "the lesion is not seen in children."[154] Wiley reported 18 tarsometatarsal injuries in children younger than 16 years.[161]

### MECHANISM OF INJURY

Wiley[161] described three basic mechanisms of injury (Fig. 16–50):

1. Traumatic impact while in the tiptoe position. An example would be jumping from a height to the ground and landing on the toes. This mechanism usually causes metatarsal joint dislocation plus fracture of the base of the second metatarsal.
2. Heel-to-toe compression. In this instance, the victim is in a kneeling position when the impact load strikes the heel. The second, third, fourth, and fifth metatarsals may be laterally dislocated, and the second metatarsal base may be fractured.
3. The fixed forefoot. In this situation, the patient falls backward while the forefoot is fixed to the ground by a heavy weight. The patient's heel resting on the ground becomes the fulcrum for the forefoot injury.

No specific injury pattern is typical; the pattern depends on the character of the impact and the distance. The soft tissue injury is the most important.

Lisfranc's joint is rarely injured, but when injury does occur, it usually involves the second metatarsal. Swelling is noted, with a serious potential for further damage. Decompression of soft tissue may be necessary. Extensive soft tissue injury, particularly injury involving disruption of major vessels, may require amputation, although this complication is extremely rare in children.

### MANAGEMENT

One should always obtain AP, lateral, and oblique radiographs. Small displaced osteochondral fractures with joint displacement may be missed on the AP and

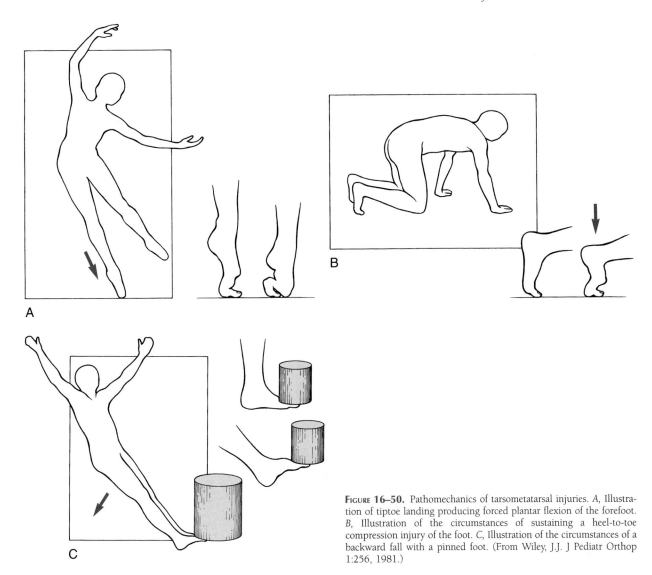

**Figure 16–50.** Pathomechanics of tarsometatarsal injuries. *A,* Illustration of tiptoe landing producing forced plantar flexion of the forefoot. *B,* Illustration of the circumstances of sustaining a heel-to-toe compression injury of the foot. *C,* Illustration of the circumstances of a backward fall with a pinned foot. (From Wiley, J.J. J Pediatr Orthop 1:256, 1981.)

lateral views, however. A fracture of the base of the second metatarsal implies a more severe injury. The combination of a fracture at the base of the second metatarsal and fracture of the cuboid bone usually results from tarsometatarsal dislocation. Recent advances in MRI have allowed the detection of disruption of Lisfranc's ligament and may be a valuable technique in assessing patients who have normal plain films after tarsometatarsal joint injury.[124]

Treatment consists of not only reduction of the fracture, if it is displaced, but also elevation of the extremity and compression. A below-knee walking cast is then applied when the swelling is down and the patient is comfortable. Closed reduction should be performed for displacement. The key to reduction involves aligning the base of the second metatarsal anatomically. Percutaneous pinning may be used to obtain stability of the reduction, especially when swelling is present. Failure to obtain anatomic reduction can cause persistent pain and swelling. A compression dressing is applied until the swelling subsides, followed by a short-leg walking cast.

## Metatarsal Fractures

Metatarsal fractures accounted for 90% of the fractures of the foot seen in the study from the Cincinnati Children's Hospital.[29] The injury usually occurs as a result of direct trauma from a falling object; indirect trauma after torsional stress may result in oblique fractures. An avulsion fracture of the base of the fifth metatarsal is the most common isolated metatarsal injury in children. Stress fractures can occur in a foot subjected to repetitive trauma, such as jogging and track-and-field activities. The injury occurs most commonly in the second metatarsal, although other metatarsals may be involved.

The necks of the metatarsals are rarely injured. The fracture pattern may be oblique, transverse, or linear. If the articular surface or condylar epiphysis is not injured, the injury usually resolves readily. Treatment consists of a below-knee walking cast for 3 weeks.

Metatarsal shaft fractures usually occur from a direct crushing blow, and solitary fractures are generally nondisplaced. Reduction of shaft injuries requires particular attention. Lateral displacement of metatarsal fractures is acceptable, but dorsal or plantar angulation is not. Residual dorsal or plantar angulation may give rise to subsequent problems because of abnormal weight distribution. Malunion and nonunion are rare but may occur.

Usually, the base of the metatarsal is injured only in patients with other associated injuries, except for the bases of the first and fifth metatarsals. Isolated fracture of the first metatarsal base is not uncommon, and this injury may predispose to growth plate injury. The child's symptoms are usually swelling, pain, or ecchymosis across the forefoot. Evidence of fracture may or may not be seen on initial radiographs. Fractures of the base of the fifth metatarsal are more common in adolescent athletes involved in jumping sports.

Displaced fractures of the bases of the metatarsals are usually caused by strong, avulsive forces. It is important to appreciate the fibrous compartment of the interossei and short plantar muscles in patients with foot injuries, especially those with significant swelling. One should consider early fasciotomies, similar to those performed in the hand, in patients who have marked swelling with the skin stretched and taut or in those with significant venous congestion of the toes. One should be especially wary if multiple fractures are present and should not hesitate to perform fasciotomies.

Growth plate injuries to the metatarsals are rare but do occur under certain conditions: (1) the chondroepiphysis may be avulsed, (2) a fracture may extend into the epiphysis, or (3) the condylar surface of the secondary ossification center may be avulsed. Treatment of these injuries is usually a below-knee walking cast for 3 to 4 weeks. Growth inhibition is unusual; overgrowth is more common. Condylar fractures rarely require open reduction. Growth rates may be affected differently, depending on the type of injury.

## TREATMENT

Significant displacement is rare. If swelling is present, one should refrain from the immediate use of a circular cast around the ankle, which would lead to dorsal pressure and a tourniquet effect. One should consider using only a bulky dressing initially in all cases, even those with minimal displacement. After reduction of swelling, a below-knee cast is applied. Skeletal traction can be used for a severely swollen foot with multiple displaced fractures to achieve alignment and decrease swelling (Fig. 16–51). Open reduction plus internal fixation is indicated in only the most unstable displaced fractures.

## MANAGEMENT OF SPECIFIC INJURIES

### First Metatarsal

The first metatarsal is often fractured. The injury occurs most frequently in the first decade, and as a result, the mechanism of injury is elusive. The child presents with a limp, and the parents may simply state that the child "fell on the foot." The radiograph shows a buckle at the base of the metatarsal just distal to the physis, which the senior author (A.H.C.) has termed *buckle base* (Fig. 16–52), similar to the torus radial forearm fracture. One should look carefully at the physis for evidence of injury. In contrast to the other metatarsals, the physis is located on the proximal end of the first metatarsal. A pseudo-epiphysis may occur at the distal end. If the physis is injured, shortening may result and produce a deficiency on the longitudinal arch with further growth of the other bones. A buckle base injury may appear to be isolated on the initial radiograph; however, on follow-up, callus may be noted over other metatarsals, which is indicative of healing of nondisplaced fractures. A below-knee walking cast is all that is needed once the swelling is down.

Osteochondritis of the first metatarsal has been reported but is extremely rare.[47] Four cases of painful

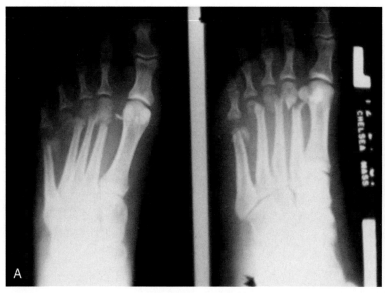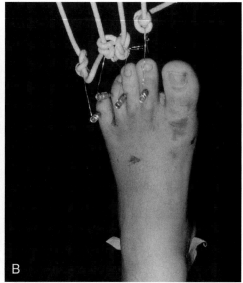

**FIGURE 16–51.** Skeletal traction for the management of severe injuries to the foot. This child presented with a tremendously swollen foot and multiple metatarsal neck fractures. Pins were placed through the phalanges, and the foot was hung in traction. The swelling receded, and adequate alignment was obtained. *A,* Anteroposterior radiographs of the foot showing multiple metatarsal neck fractures. *B,* Clinical photograph of the foot in traction; 18-gauge needles were placed through the phalanges, and 22-gauge wires were attached to traction.

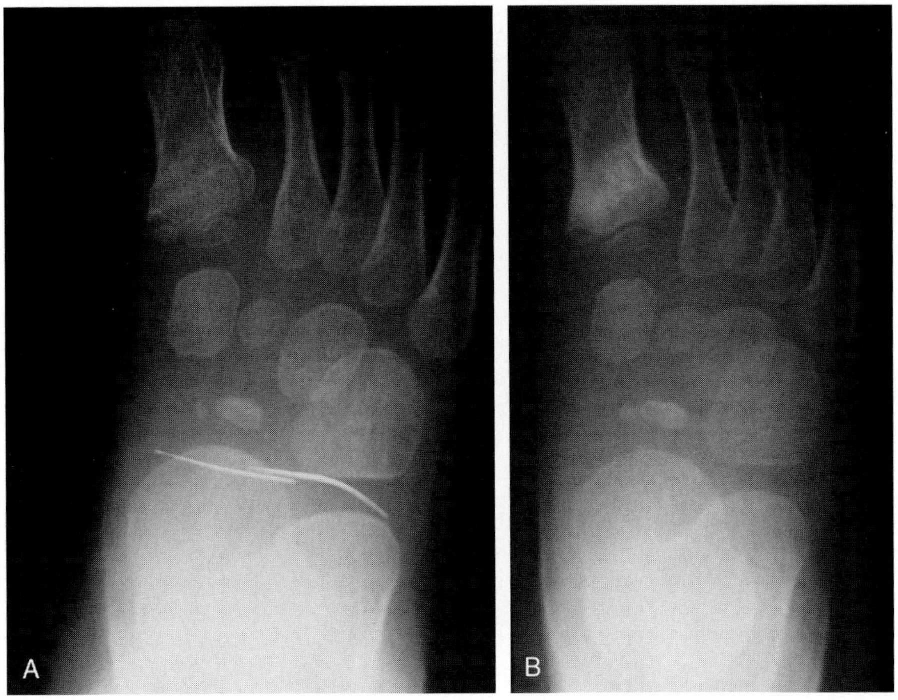

**FIGURE 16–52.** Fractures of the base of the first metatarsal tend to buckle and have been termed the "buckle base" injury; these injuries heal uneventfully. *A,* Initial anteroposterior radiograph showing a buckle fracture of the base of the first metatarsal. *B,* Follow-up anteroposterior radiograph 3 weeks later; the fracture has healed, and remodeling is taking place.

osteochondritis of the basal epiphysis of the first metatarsal have been described; the children are usually active in running sports. Radiographic findings are usually noted at the initial evaluation, and a bone scan, if necessary, confirms the diagnosis. Treatment is symptomatic, with immobilization in plaster and arch supports providing adequate management. When subtle radiographic changes consisting of slight irregularities of the subchondral surface of the first metatarsal are seen in a child with transitory foot pain, osteochondritis should be suspected. A technetium 99m bone scan is diagnostic.

### Second Metatarsal

Isolated fractures of the second metatarsal are rare. Fracture of this bone was associated with fractures of other metatarsals in 30 of 51 fractures of the lesser second through fifth metatarsals in the study from the Cincinnati Children's Hospital.[29] The most common mechanism of injury was indirect, such as jumping from a height of less than 5 feet. Other direct mechanisms included objects such as a rock, table, or chair falling on the foot. The fractures were rarely displaced, except with severe trauma (e.g., foot run over by a car or a lawn mower). Most of these fractures can be treated with below-knee walking casts once the swelling is down.

The second metatarsal is more often subject to stress fracture. The injury occurs early in the second decade, is commonly called a march fracture, and usually occurs in runners. We have seen the injury in sedentary children who suddenly increase their walking or running activity (Fig. 16–53). The child complains of persistent pain under the metatarsal arch. The initial radiographs may be negative, but a bone scan is positive. Periosteal cortical hypertrophy or new bone is generally present within 2 weeks after complaints of pain (Fig. 16–54). Treatment

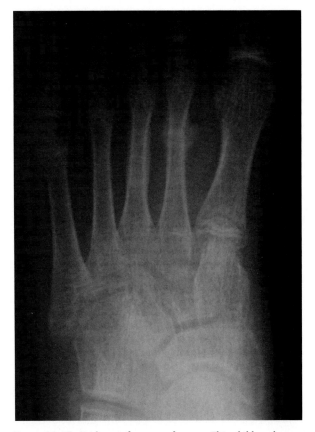

**FIGURE 16–53.** Evidence of a stress fracture. This child underwent excision of a calcaneonavicular bar and was required to be immobile for 6 weeks and not participate in sports. She was an avid soccer player and on return to soccer noted foot pain and swelling. An anteroposterior radiograph of the foot shows a stress fracture with exuberant callus of the second metatarsal and healing callus over the shaft of the third metatarsal.

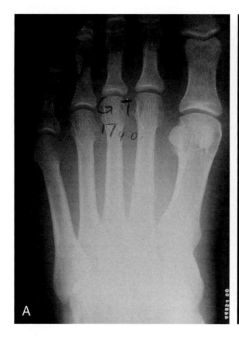
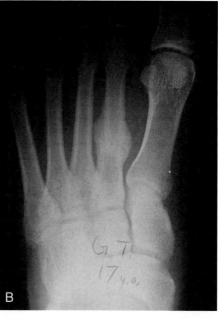

FIGURE 16–54. Stress fracture of the second metatarsal. *A,* The initial radiograph reveals a nondisplaced proximal second metatarsal fracture. *B,* On follow-up, bulbous callus is noted around the fracture line at the base of the second metatarsal.

most often consists of wearing a hard-soled shoe; rarely is a cast indicated. Displacement of the fragments is hardly ever seen.

Freiberg's infraction is an uncommon disorder, and no estimate of its incidence is available. The diagnosis is not difficult, although initial radiographs may be negative. Athletic adolescent girls predominate. Freiberg first described infraction of the second metatarsal head in 1914.[52] The first patient in whom the lesion was recognized was a 16-year-old girl who stubbed her foot in a tennis game. His original article included six patients, four of whom sustained trauma. In 1915, Köhler, independent of Freiberg's report, also described the disorder.[78] In Europe, the disorder is commonly known as Köhler's second disease, the first being avascular necrosis of the tarsal navicula.

Freiberg's disease, or osteochondrosis of the second metatarsal head, may be confused with a fracture.[52] The second metatarsal is the longest and most rigidly fixed metatarsal (Fig. 16–55). Repetitive trauma to the articular surface of the distal end of the second metatarsal may cause this injury. The injury usually occurs after intensive training for running sports and has been seen in avid young soccer players. Conservative treatment by rest or wearing a below-knee walking cast is recommended. Small osteochondral fragments may be left in the second metatarsophalangeal joint. Open débridement may be necessary to prevent degenerative joint disease. Prevention can be accomplished only if the débridement is performed very early; otherwise, in patients with multiple fragments in various stages of union, open débridement is not indicated. We recommend rest as early treatment if an acute injury is present, but afterward, a hard toeplate should be inserted in the shoe to allow the child to participate in sports activities, if desired. We have had no experience with shortening of the metatarsal for this condition.

Other authors have recommended resection of the entire metatarsal head, bone grafting, dorsiflexion osteotomy, or a combination of these procedures. Recently,

el-Tayeby described interpositional arthroplasty with the tendon of the extensor digitorum longus used for resurfacing and also to act as a spacer; 11 adolescent patients were treated with this technique, and excellent/good results were obtained in 85% of the cases.[44] Early

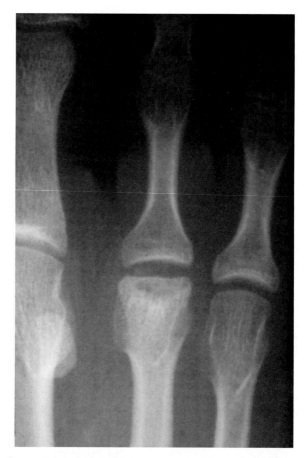

FIGURE 16–55. This example of Freiberg's disease was noted in an avid soccer player; the head of the second metatarsal of the right foot is flattened. A hard toeplate was inserted in the soccer shoe, and the patient continued playing with minimal difficulty.

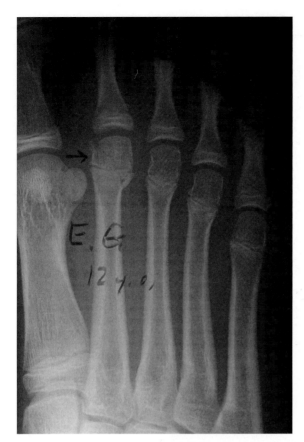

**FIGURE 16–56.** Salter-Harris type IV condylar fracture of the metatarsal head. It healed uneventfully.

débridement for symptomatic lesions is our choice of treatment.

Fractures of the chondroepiphysis of the second metatarsal occur most frequently as Salter-Harris type II fractures of the neck. The injury is rarely displaced. Even fractures with plantar flexion tend to remodel. The condylar fractures are usually oblique Salter-Harris type IV fractures and rarely result in growth injuries (Fig. 16–56). All these injuries have been treated by below-knee casts, with good results.

### Third and Fourth Metatarsals

The third and fourth metatarsals are usually injured as a result of indirect trauma; these injuries may occur anywhere along the shaft. More often than not, these fractures are nondisplaced and may not even be seen on initial radiographs (Fig. 16–57). Exceptions are cases involving severe trauma such as vehicular or lawn mower accidents. Persistence of plantar displacement or angulation after reduction is to be avoided because of the prominence over the weight-bearing surface and the development of painful calluses. Nonunion of these metatarsals has been noted after severely displaced fractures but tends to be asymptomatic (Fig. 16–58).

### Fifth Metatarsal

The fifth metatarsal is a relatively common area of fracture. This bone was injured in 39 of 104 children and adolescents with metatarsal fractures; their average age was 12 years. The most common mechanism of injury was jumping during an athletic activity, such as basketball or volleyball.[29] The patient may complain of acute pain over the base of the lateral aspect of the foot and cease the activity immediately, or the child may present with a painful limp several days later. Initial radiographs may be negative and show only soft tissue swelling over the lateral aspect of the foot. The presence of the os vesalianum in this age group may cause it to be confused with a fracture. The os vesalianum has an oblique distribution, or a sagittal line between it and the metatarsal (Fig. 16–59). A true fracture through the metatarsal

**FIGURE 16–57.** Nondisplaced fractures of the base of the metatarsals. The child presented with pain across the base of the forefoot, but no fractures were observed. After being placed in a below-knee walking cast, the child was noted 3 weeks later to have fracture healing lines of the second, third, and fourth metatarsals. *A,* Anteroposterior radiograph of the foot showing soft tissue swelling but little evidence of fracture. *B,* Anteroposterior radiograph 1 month later showing healing bone scars at the base of the inner metatarsals.

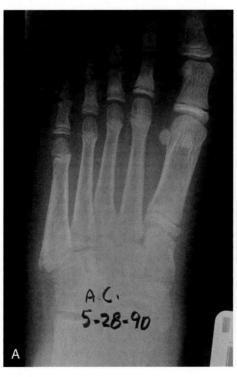

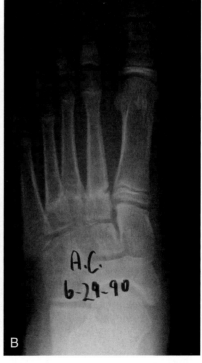

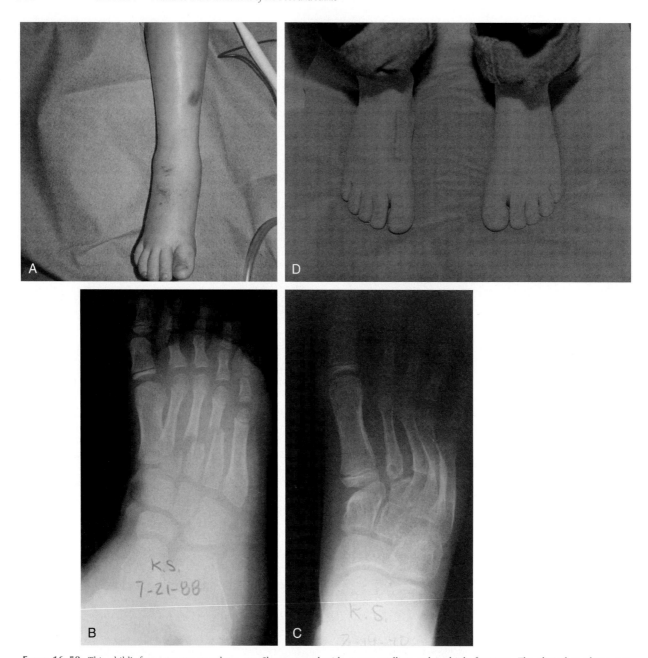

**FIGURE 16–58.** This child's foot was run over by a car. She presented with severe swelling and multiple fractures. The clinical condition was consistent with compartment syndrome. Immediate decompression was achieved with two longitudinal incisions over the lateral aspect of the first ray and the medial aspect of the fifth ray. The wounds were closed with delayed primary closure. The patient has some tendency to varus positioning of her metatarsals and nonunion of the base of the second metatarsal, but she is asymptomatic. *A,* Clinical photograph at the time of injury. The forefoot was tense. *B,* Initial radiograph showing soft tissue swelling and displaced metatarsal fractures. *C,* Radiograph 18 months later showing union of the third and fourth metatarsals and tenuous union of the second metatarsal. *D,* Clinical photograph at last follow-up; the patient was asymptomatic.

usually has a transverse orientation (Fig. 16–60). Avulsion of the base of the fifth metatarsal by the action of the peroneus brevis at its insertion might be considered, but it usually applies to a Jones fracture, which is a proximal diaphyseal fracture that occurs in 15- to 20-year-olds; it is not an avulsion fracture.

Kavanaugh and colleagues emphasized that a Jones fracture is a fracture of the proximal part of the diaphysis of the fifth metatarsal and not an avulsive fracture of the base (despite the incorrect common use of the term).[72] A Jones fracture appears to result from a combination of

vertical loading and medial lateral forces, with the patient bearing weight on the metatarsal heads and concentrating force at the proximal fifth metatarsal (Fig. 16–61).

It is possible that the avulsion fracture that occurs in children is a result of the tendinous portion of the abductor digiti minimi and the tough lateral cord of the plantar aponeurosis inserting into the base. Most of these fractures can be treated by below-knee walking casts. Nonunion is rare, although it occasionally takes longer than 4 to 6 weeks for radiographic bony union. Patients not showing union are immobilized only until they are

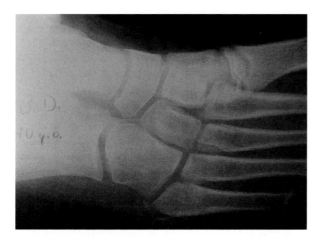

FIGURE 16–59. Fracture of the os vesalianum, an unusual fracture through the accessory apophysis.

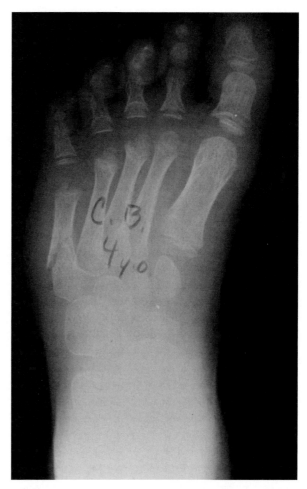

FIGURE 16–61. Jones fracture through the proximal portion of the fifth metatarsal. A true Jones fracture is quite rare in children, who most often sustain an avulsion fracture of the fifth metatarsal base.

pain free and are then allowed to return to their athletic activity.

Traction apophysitis of the tuberosity of the fifth metatarsal (Iselin's disease) has been reported rarely in the literature.[19, 65, 125] Canale and Williams reported on four cases.[19] The condition occurs in older children and young adolescents at about the time of appearance of the tuberosity of the fifth metatarsal. A history of significant trauma is generally absent, although symptoms begin after an inversion injury. Children who are involved in

sports that cause inversion stress on the forefoot appear to be especially prone. Examination shows the tuberosity to be larger than on the opposite side, with local soft tissue swelling and tenderness at the area of insertion of the peroneus brevis. Radiographs show enlargement of the apophysis and often fragmentation; in addition, the chondro-osseous junction may be widened (Fig. 16–62).

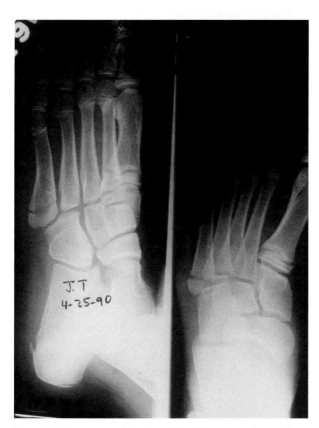

FIGURE 16–60. Fracture of the base of the fifth metatarsal. An oblique radiograph shows anatomic alignment. The anteroposterior view shows minimal displacement.

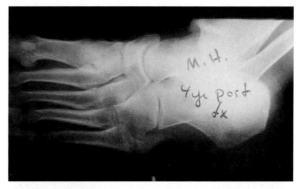

FIGURE 16–62. Example of Iselin's disease of the base of the fifth metatarsal. This condition is treated only until it is asymptomatic. The child was asymptomatic when seen for another problem approximately 4 years after his initial treatment.

Immobilization appears to help with the acute pain, and when the tenderness is completely resolved, physical therapy will increase strength and coordination. Bony union will occur in most patients. If conservative treatment fails, Iselin's disease can develop into nonunion and surgical excision is recommended.[125] Early recognition and treatment may prevent long-term complications.

## Phalangeal Fractures

Phalangeal fractures occurred in 31 of 175 children with fractures about the foot. Twenty fractures (64%) occurred in the proximal phalanges, 9 (29%) in the middle, and 2 (6.4%) in the distal phalanges. Indirect trauma, such as stubbing a toe, or direct trauma from a falling object was the usual mechanism of injury. Rarely is operative reduction of a phalangeal fracture necessary; usually, traction, manipulative reduction, and buddy-taping (i.e., taping the toe to an adjacent toe) after reduction is all that is needed (Fig. 16–63). If the swelling allows, wearing a hard-soled shoe is the only measure necessary; if not, a below-knee walking cast will suffice.

Fracture of the growth plate of the proximal phalanx of the great toe may involve the articular surface (Fig. 16–64). The percentage of articular surface involved and its displacement determine the need for anatomic reduction. Open reduction and internal fixation of the fragment are indicated when more than 30% of the articular surface is involved or displacement is greater

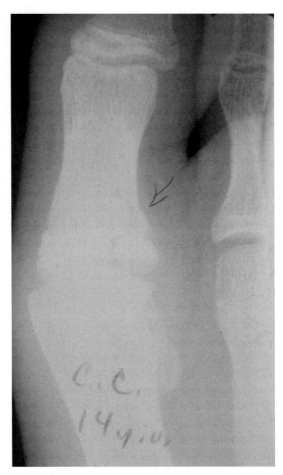

**FIGURE 16–64.** Salter-Harris type III fracture through the articular surface of the proximal phalanx. Reduction and fixation are indicated if the fracture involves more than one third of the articular surface and shows more than 2 mm of separation after reduction.

than 3 mm. After anatomic reduction, the fragment should be pinned to prevent displacement. If pinning is not performed, instability may occur and cause a step-off of the fragments. Degenerative arthritis and hallux rigidus may occur. Rarely does incomplete reduction result in the formation of a bony bridge.

A distal phalangeal epiphyseal fracture of the great toe may be open because of its proximity to the nail matrix (Fig. 16–65). The crushing nature of the injury leaves cracks or breaks in the skin that allow bacterial contamination. The possibility of osteomyelitis should be recognized, and prophylactic antibiotics are recommended for 10 days after this injury. Other management may include irrigation and débridement; reduction, which is rarely necessary if the fracture is not particularly displaced; buddy-taping; a hard-soled shoe; or a below-knee walking cast.

Fractures of the proximal phalanges of the lateral four toes rarely require more than symptomatic treatment. They are seldom displaced enough to require operative treatment, and buddy-taping tends to work well for these fractures. They occasionally become malaligned, and the angulation does not always correct. Fortunately, these disturbances hardly ever cause clinical problems.

Open fractures of the phalanges require débridement and irrigation. The patient should be given parenteral

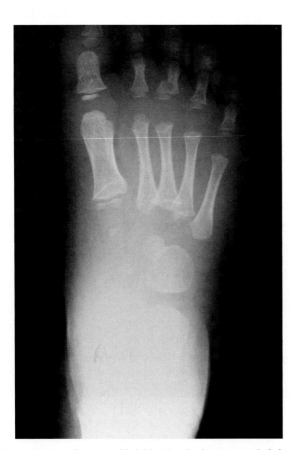

**FIGURE 16–63.** Three-year-old child with a third-ray proximal phalangeal fracture. These injuries may be buddy-taped and tend to do well.

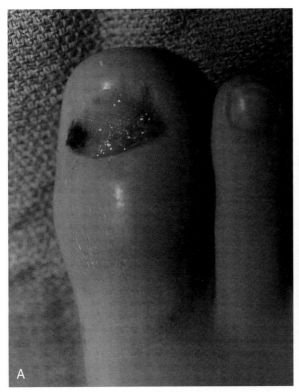

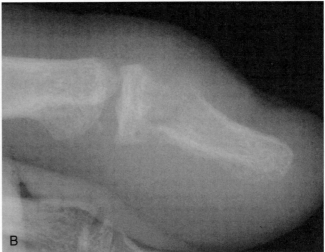

A

B

**FIGURE 16–65.** "Stubbed-toe" osteomyelitis should be assumed in patients with a great toe distal phalangeal injury that extends through the nail matrix. Prophylactic antibiotics are indicated. This child was thought to have an ingrown toenail and the toenail was removed, at which time the treating health care professional noted pus draining from the base and referred the child to a children's hospital. *A,* Clinical photograph of the great toe after removal of the nail. *B,* Lateral radiograph of the great toe showing changes consistent with osteomyelitis at the fracture site.

broad-spectrum antibiotics, a tetanus booster, adequate aggressive and thorough débridement, and wound dressing changes. It is better to return to the operating room for delayed primary closure than to perform immediate closure of these injuries. Internal fixation is indicated only if the neurovascular bundles are torqued or under tension and are not adequately perfused at the time of surgery. It is better to have malunion or growth plate injury in these patients than osteomyelitis.

## Dislocations

Dislocations of the joints of the foot are extremely rare. Only 4 patients with dislocation of the bones of the foot were seen in 175 children with fractures and other injuries about the foot[29]; 3 of the 4 were older than 10 years. All except one sustained proximal interphalangeal joint dislocations of the second and third digits (Fig. 16–66). One child dislocated the metatarsophalangeal joint of the fifth ray (Fig. 16–67). Reductions of all the dislocations were uneventful; treatment consisted of buddy-taping and a hard-soled shoe.

## Compartment Syndrome

Silas and co-workers reviewed compartment syndrome of the foot in children in 1995.[139] They found that the cause of compartment syndrome was a crush injury in six patients and a motor vehicle accident in one. All patients

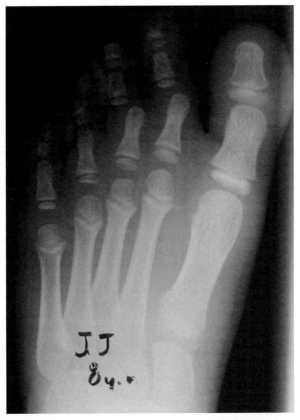

**FIGURE 16–66.** Interphalangeal joint dislocations of the second and third toes. Reduction was easily accomplished by longitudinal traction and maintained by buddy-taping.

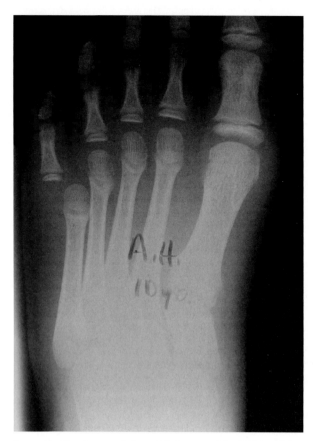

**FIGURE 16–67.** Metatarsophalangeal dislocation of the fifth toe. Reduction and stabilization were achieved by traction and buddy-taping.

had swelling and pain with passive motion, but none had neurovascular deficits. Only the two oldest children had osseous injuries that necessitated open reduction and internal fixation, but all had elevated compartment pressure ranging from 38 to 55 mm Hg (5.07 to 7.33 kPa). An unusual case report discussed a toddler whose leg and foot were hanging on the side of his bed for hours and who went to the emergency department with compartment syndrome of his leg and foot. Complete fasciotomies of the leg and foot were performed, followed by secondary closure and skin grafting; at 1 year the child had a normally functioning lower extremity.[56]

Orthopaedists managing children who have traumatic injuries to the foot, especially crush injuries, should have a high index of suspicion for compartment syndrome, even in the absence of severe fracture. Neurovascular symptoms do not occur until much later; however, some children experience so much pain and tenderness that the weight of the bed sheet on the foot may be more than they can tolerate. If compartment syndrome is suspected, pressure measurements should be obtained in the central and interosseous compartments because they are more sensitive indicators of occult compartment syndrome of the foot.[89, 92, 107, 139]

Severe soft tissue injury may occur with injury to the interossei and short plantar flexor muscles contained in the tightly closed fascial compartments of the foot. Fasciotomy is indicated if the swelling is severe. Similar to injuries to the hand, the clinical indications for

fasciotomy are marked swelling, taut skin, and decreased sensation. The incisions should be generous and extend down to the bone. Medial and lateral longitudinal incisions are made over the second and fourth metatarsals; they are packed open, and the foot is elevated. K-wire fixation can be used to stabilize the bones but is rarely necessary. Delayed primary closure is carried out in 5 to 7 days.

## Lawn Mower Injuries

Lawn mowers remain a common source of serious injury and morbidity for children. An estimated 75,000 lawn mower–related injuries occur annually in the United States.[97] The estimated annual cost for these injuries is $253 million, not including monetary damage for pain and suffering. It is estimated that 7 million new lawn mowers are purchased annually and that more than 30 million are used in the United States.[87]

Lawn mower injuries in children differ from comparable injuries in adults in several ways. First, a child's growth potential may be altered by direct injury to the physis, indirect stimulation of growth by the repair process, or inhibition of growth from neurovascular injury to that part. Second, vessel size may influence the choice of free tissue transplant,[62] the ability to repair a vessel, or both. Third, children in general tolerate prolonged immobilization better than adults do, and children tend to have better rehabilitative potential.[40]

These injuries represent some of the more contaminated injuries that one sees in pediatric orthopaedics.[85] Dormans and colleagues recommend that all patients be treated with fluid replacement, blood replacement (when appropriate), and intravenous triple antibiotics (penicillin, cefazolin, and an aminoglycoside).[40] Tetanus status should be evaluated and appropriate coverage implemented. They further recommend that all wounds be débrided no fewer than two times and that early closure be avoided. In patients who do not respond readily to standard empirical broad-spectrum antibiotics, infection caused by *Stenotrophomonas* (formerly *Xanthomonas*) *maltophilia* should be considered, and cotrimoxazole is the best initial antibiotic of choice.[31] Two types of lawn mower injuries have been identified: a shredding injury, which is most common and usually intercalary or distal (Fig. 16–68), and a paucilaceration type of injury (Fig. 16–69). The shredding injuries had the worst results. As a matter of fact, the only factors that appeared to correlate with outcome were the severity of the initial injury and the presence or absence of injury to vital structures, such as arteries, nerves, physeal plates, and articular cartilage (i.e., shredding-type injuries versus single laceration–type injuries).[40]

Farley and associates reported on 24 children who suffered lawn mower injuries. Eight injuries were fractures, 10 were amputations, and 6 were combined fractures with amputations. The average age at injury was 4.7 years, and the average clinical follow-up was 36 months. All 18 children were injured by riding mowers, and 16 of the 18 were injured in their own yard. The initial average hospital stay was 2 weeks. The children had an average of three irrigation and débridement procedures, and completion of amputation was necessary in 16. Five children required readmission, and three were admitted for a third time. Three of the children had significant psychologic distress, half the children had altered their goals and plans for the future despite reporting normal athletic ability, and most of the children reported moderate regular pain.[48]

Vosburgh and associates found that ride-on mower injuries were more severe and resulted in a poorer functional outcome and more surgical procedures than did walk-behind mower injuries.[156] All their cases of below-knee amputation, ankle disarticulation, and free vascularized grafting resulted from ride-on mower injuries. No patient sustaining an injury from a walk-behind mower required blood transfusion. They identified two

areas that are somewhat controversial and in which their series differed from other reported series. The first was the conclusion that great toe amputation did not lead to severe disability in children. This statement is in contrast to Myerson and co-workers,[108] who concluded that amputation of the hallux proximal to the insertion of the flexor mechanism leads to instability of the first ray, loss of intrinsic strength, and lateral shift of forefoot pressure to the lesser toes. Because Vosburgh and colleagues' series showed no significant problems, those authors found that heroic surgical measures to preserve the great toe were not required to ensure a satisfactory functional outcome for this particular foot injury.

The second area involves lacerations of the Achilles tendon. Vosburgh and associates determined that it was more important to obtain a clean wound for closure than

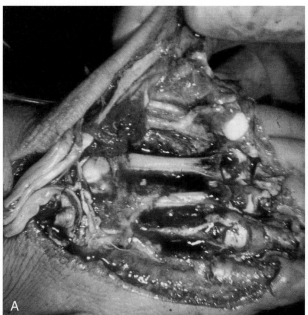

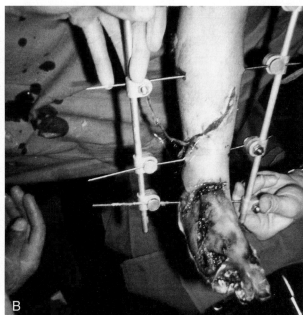

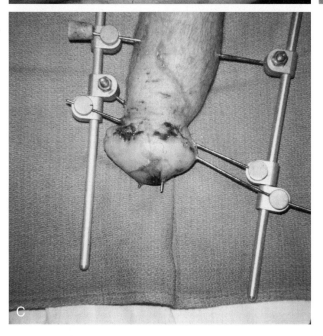

**FIGURE 16–68.** Shredding injury. A severe contaminated lawn mower injury with comminuted tibial and fibular fractures was treated by external fixation and closure of the dorsal foot wound. The wound was closed, possibly injudiciously, but the parents refused to accept immediate amputation. After referral, the severe foot injury was treated definitively by Boyd-Syme amputation. *A,* Initial clinical photograph showing complete destruction of soft tissue over the dorsal lateral aspect of the foot. The wound was extensively débrided and closed. *B,* At the time of referral, the dorsal soft tissue was completely necrotic. Because of the extensive loss of tendons and bone, a Boyd-Syme amputation was performed, with the plantar skin and heel pad maintained to allow weight bearing. Delayed primary closure was performed in 5 to 6 days. *C,* Two threaded Steinmann pins were used to secure the weight-bearing skin to the calcaneus. The fracture united uneventfully, and the child was able to fully ambulate on the stump.

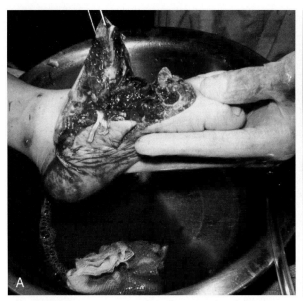
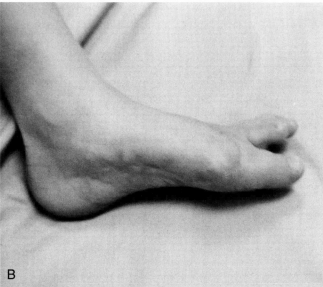

FIGURE 16–69. Paucilaceration injury. A lawn mower injury to the medial portion of the forefoot severed the extensor hallucis longus, the extensor digitorum longus, and the brevis tendons and fractured the first metatarsal. It was treated by vigorous débridement and delayed primary closure. *A*, At initial débridement, the extensor hallucis longus and extensor digitorum longus and brevis were all lacerated, and the first metatarsal bone was filleted. Aggressive débridement was performed, with a "second look" carried out in 3 days, at which time the long and short extensors were repaired, the fracture was pinned, and the wound was closed over a drain. *B*, Six months after the injury, the wound is completely healed and the child has excellent function, except for extension of the great toe. This type of result can be expected only in young children.

to consider repair and transfer early after Achilles tendon lacerations. They found that three of four patients with complete disruption and segmental loss of the Achilles tendon were able to ambulate independently without orthoses or special shoes when a "physiologic tendon" was permitted to develop by scar formation after irreparable laceration of the triceps surae.[156]

Because of the severe injuries related to ride-on mowers, certain recommendations for injury prevention have been advocated by Vosburgh and associates: (1) blade safety devices for ride-on mowers that disconnect the blade from the power source when the operator leaves the operating position, (2) automatic blade disengagement when the mower is placed in reverse gear, and (3) labels on the mower housing warning against pediatric passengers.[156] These measures might decrease the rate of accidents in the future. No passengers should be permitted on ride-on mowers, and children younger than 12 to 13 years should not be permitted to operate these machines. These measures alone would have eliminated half the accidents in all published series to date. Chopra and co-workers made more stringent recommendations for prevention of lawn mower injuries after studying such injuries in Canadian children from 1990 through 1998: (1) children younger than 15 years should not operate lawn mowers, (2) children younger than 15 years should not be in the yard when the lawn is being mowed, (3) no passengers should be carried on ride-on mowers, and (4) wearing hard closed-toe shoes should be mandatory.[23]

In a multicenter study, Loder and colleagues reported on gas-powered lawn mower injuries in 144 children with an average age at injury of 7 years. The child was the machine operator in 36 cases, a bystander in 84, and a passenger in 21. Amputations occurred in 67 children; the most common level was the toes (63%). Children injured by a riding lawn mower were typically younger, had a longer hospital stay, and required more surgery. Blood transfusions were given to 35 children. Fifty-six procedures were performed after initial hospital discharge. They reported that if children younger than 14 years had not been permitted around the lawn mowers, approximately 85% of the injuries in their report would have been prevented.[86]

Lawn mower and threshing machine injuries are quite common in children in rural communities. Considerable judgment is required when managing these injuries. Most often, the child is riding on the mower with one of the parents rather than with a sibling. The usual history is that the child leaves to take a break, such as to go to the bathroom. Because of the noise from the mower, the parent is unaware that the child has returned until hearing a crunching sound in the rotor blades. The force of injury causes soft tissue contamination by grass, shoe leather, socks, and various other debris. One should never make an early decision concerning the sterility or the ultimate viability of the tissue. The force may cross the physis at multiple levels, possibly even excising the growth center. The injury may include loss of the articular surfaces and the collateral ligaments. Vigorous débridement and irrigation are carried out immediately. Avulsed tissue is usually less vital than it appears when first seen. This severe trauma may involve degloving of the bone and detachment of the perichondrial rings, with the subsequent development of a callus bridge between the epiphysis and metaphysis resulting in bar formation across the physes.[126] Vigorous débridement, delayed primary closure, and split-thickness skin grafting (initially with mesh) followed by a cast, brace, or splint are indicated (Fig. 16–70). We urge resistance against early aggressive closure (e.g., cross-leg pedicle) until the issue of wound viability and sterility is resolved.

## Free Tissue Transfer

The distal portion of the lower extremity is occasionally injured to the extent that either severe loss of soft tissue occurs or the injury results in nonviable tissue. In this case, coverage is extremely important, and free tissue transfer may be required. Such transfer is especially necessary when extensive exposure of the fracture site has occurred, the periosteum is exposed or, worse, stripped, and devitalized bone is exposed. Indications for free tissue transfer include open joints, soft tissue destruction (usually to the extent that the adjacent soft tissue is avascular, necrotic, or nonvital), facilitation of future reconstruction (i.e., avulsion of a major tendon such as the anterior tibial or Achilles tendon), or intercalary avulsion of the soft tissue envelope from bone such as the midshaft of the tibia.

The preferred donor sources for free tissue transfer in children include the latissimus dorsi, the rectus abdominis, and the gracilis. The attraction and advantages of the latissimus dorsi are its large size, its ability to drape well into any configuration, and the fact that the donor site has minimal morbidity. The gracilis is used most frequently in adults for small wound areas, but in children, a wound small enough to require gracilis transfer is usually one that would respond to dressing changes, granulation, and possibly split-thickness skin grafts. To a lesser extent, groin flaps have been also used as a donor site. The advantages of a groin flap are that it is large, primary closure of the donor site is possible, iliac crest bone grafts can be taken simultaneously, and no hair is incorporated in the flap.[57]

The distal extremity in children often accepts split-thickness skin grafting. We have on occasion allowed skin defects as well as adjacent bone to granulate, at which time split-thickness skin grafts are acceptable. The split-thickness graft may be meshed or vented to allow for drainage if necessary. The use of cross-extremity flaps with linkage of a bilateral lower extremity external fixator in place of traditional casting has also been described with good success.[103]

Most often, in children with severe soft tissue destruction plus bone and joint involvement, a free tissue transfer is indicated. It is important that stability of the extremity be achieved, especially if fractures are present or if the stabilizing tendons (i.e., anterior tibial tendon, Achilles tendon, or both) have been destroyed (Fig. 16–71). We recommend achieving stability of the joint and the fracture with the use of a small external fixator; our preference ranges from the Roger-Anderson universal external fixator to the AO Synthes or Orthofix. The polyaxial universal joints of these fixators allow for multiple configurations and constructs, and they are extremely adaptable. Although the Orthofix is the most stable, the Synthes appears to be more adaptable for smaller children. The wound is usually radically débrided of all necrotic and nonviable tissue, followed by application of the external fixator. The wound is acutely packed with a saline-, povidone-iodine (Betadine)-, or antibiotic-soaked dressing, and the child is returned to the operating room within 48 hours, where débridement is performed again. If the necrotic tissue has been completely resected with good tissue margins, a free tissue transfer or flap is considered. Most often, the latissimus dorsi is used and placed over the affected area, and a split-thickness skin graft is placed over the muscle. The graft is usually vented, and compression dressings are applied. The wound is observed in the hospital until adequate "take" of the graft and the transfer is

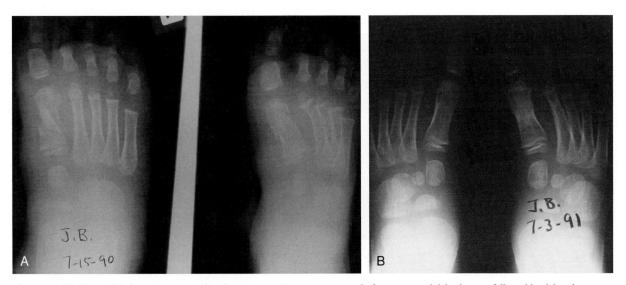

**FIGURE 16–70.** This child's foot was run over by a lawn mower. Treatment consisted of irrigation and débridement, followed by delayed primary closure. *A,* Initial anteroposterior and oblique radiographs showing a markedly comminuted fracture of the first metatarsal and Salter-Harris type II fractures of the third and fourth metatarsal necks, with marked soft tissue swelling. A pseudoepiphysis can be seen at the distal end of the first metatarsal. *B,* Anteroposterior radiograph 1 year later showing healing of all fractures.

apparent. A strategy is then planned to allow for further reconstruction or rehabilitation (or both) of the extremity.

Byrd and colleagues advocate the following 12-step approach to open tibia fractures with associated tissue loss[16]:

1. Emergency department care is as follows: tetanus prophylaxis, prophylactic cephalosporin antibiotics, moist sterile Betadine dressings over the wound, immobilization of the fracture with a splint, and wound culture.
2. Surgery is initiated within 6 to 8 hours of the injury, with copious water jet irrigation of the soft tissue and fracture.
3. Extensive radical soft tissue débridement is performed. All nonviable tissues can be removed from the wound with the assurance that a well-vascularized soft tissue envelope can be provided. The skin is excised according to the pattern of fluorescence or until bleeding dermis is encountered. All exposed subcutaneous tissue and fascia are removed. The surrounding muscle is excised if any

question remains about its viability, as evaluated by the parameters of color, turgor, bleeding, and contractibility. Fluorescein is not relied on to assess muscle viability. Any small chips of bone not attached to soft tissue are removed. Large fragments of bone, whether attached or unattached, are retained in the wound. Every effort is made to clean embedded foreign material from these fragments of bone. All fragments, regardless of size, that have maintained viable soft tissue attachments are left in the wound. Nerves, vessels, and important tendons are preserved.

4. Compartment fasciotomy is performed whenever the muscles are bulging from edema or when arterial repair is required.
5. Percutaneous pin fixation or external fixation is the preferred method of stabilizing the fracture.
6. Detached, but viable muscles are draped over the fracture and any exposed bone. In patients with minimal devascularization of the muscles, formal myoplasty is undertaken to effect coverage of the wound. When the injury is more extensive, the wound and any exposed bone or fracture are

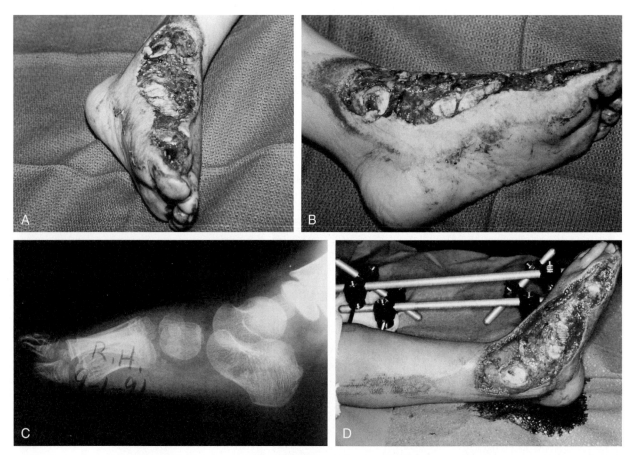

**Figure 16–71.** This 4-year-old boy was in an auto accident in which the medial aspect of his left foot was dragged across a concrete surface and all the soft tissues overlying the medial malleolus, tarsals, metatarsal, and phalanges of the great toe were abraded off. He underwent débridement and external fixation followed by free tissue transfer, skin grafting, and subsequent peroneus longus tendon transfer. *A,* Soft tissue loss over the medial malleolus, tarsals, metatarsal, and phalanges of the great toe, with exposure of the underlying joints. The tibialis anterior and extensor hallucis longus tendons were abraded off. *B,* Medial view. *C,* Radiograph of the foot at the time of injury. No evidence of bony injury was noted. An external fixator was applied to allow for management of the wound while immobilizing the ankle to prevent deformity from asymmetric muscle forces. *D,* After placement of an external fixator and initial débridement before reconstruction of the defect.

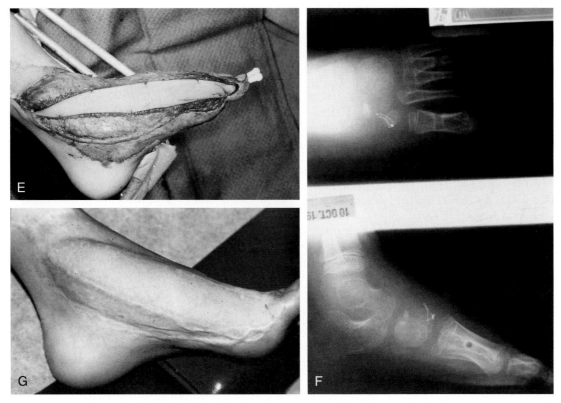

FIGURE **16–71** *Continued. E,* Closure of the defect with a free latissimus dorsi microvascular flap and split-thickness skin grafting. End-to-side reanastomosis was performed on the posterior tibial artery, high above the zone of injury. *F,* Radiographs after peroneal tendon transfer for the anterior tibialis. *G,* Four-year follow-up. (Courtesy of Dr. David Billmire, Director of Plastic Surgery, Children's Hospital Medical Center, Cincinnati, OH.)

covered with a Betadine-soaked gauze dressing to avoid desiccation.

7. A second-look operation under anesthesia is undertaken 48 to 72 hours after the injury to assess for progression of devitalized tissue. All flaps are released to allow thorough inspection of the wound bed. Débridement is repeated, and a definitive muscle, myocutaneous flap, or free flap transfer is provided if minimal devitalized tissue is present. When devitalized tissue is found, a moist dressing is applied and a third débridement is scheduled in 48 hours, at which time definitive flap coverage is anticipated.

8. Definitive wound coverage is provided within the first 5 days of injury. The preferred methods are local muscle flaps, local myocutaneous flaps, or distant microvascular myocutaneous free flap coverage. Skin grafts to exposed muscle are applied primarily or secondarily.

9. The extremity is elevated to 30° to 45° postoperatively.

10. Ambulation with weight bearing is begun in the first 3 weeks after injury.

11. Fixation is changed to a PTB below-knee plaster brace when the soft tissues and fractures are stable.

12. The extremity is fitted with Jobst support hose when the plaster is removed.

## Amputation

On occasion, the severity of an injury to an extremity is such that neither free tissue transfer, skin grafting, nor reimplantation can be achieved (see Fig. 16–68). In that case, amputation must be carried out. Amputations in children are occasionally performed at unconventional sites, as opposed to the ankle, Lisfranc, or Chopart joint. More often than not, every effort is made to maintain length. For foot amputations, we prefer a Boyd-Syme type of amputation. If the child has a shredding laceration that includes all of the dorsum of the foot, it is important to make an effort to preserve the plantar skin of the foot, which is good for weight bearing. The level of amputation is sometimes determined by the most viable proximal segment of tissue and bone. Tibial injuries above the ankle joint may require transdiaphyseal amputation. The parents and child are informed of the strong possibility of stump overgrowth and the need for revisions until skeletal maturity. Transmetatarsal amputations are not necessarily as good as through-the-joint amputations (e.g., Chopart's or Lisfranc's joint) because of the possibility of stump overgrowth of the metatarsal segments, which may necessitate additional operations in the future. Prosthetic fitting is easier with a Boyd-Syme amputation. Even Boyd-Syme amputations can present problems over the long term because of the attachment of the tendo calcaneus to the os calcis. If a Boyd-Syme amputation or ankle disarticulation amputation is to be performed, we strongly recommend that a segment of no less than 1 inch of tendo calcaneus be excised. The tenotomized Achilles tendon will reattach itself and apply constant pressure on the calcaneus that pulls it or the weight-bearing heel pad into the midcalf area. In a young child (younger than 10 years), when a midfoot amputation through Chopart's joint is a possibility, we recommend excising the talus, débriding the cartilage from the mortise as well as the dorsum of the calcaneus, and fusing the calcaneus to the mortise. The malleoli will shrink down over the years and will not present a problem for prosthetic fitting at the heel or with a SACH (solid ankle–cushion heel) Seattle type of foot in the future. If one is to preserve the plantar weight-bearing heel pad skin over the calcaneus, it is most important to affix it with pins and suture it to the anterior distal flap of skin with interrupted sutures. We do not believe that it is as important to use an immediate-fit prosthesis in a child as it is in an adult, but we have used this concept with varying degrees of success. Some children readily take to their unfinished prostheses in the recovery room, whereas others have considerable psychologic problems associated with it. If one prefers to perform a Chopart-level amputation in a young child, it is important that balance of the anterior tibial or peroneal tendons be preserved; otherwise, it is possible that persistent plantar flexion contractures will develop secondary to overpull of the tendo Achillis.

The problem seen most frequently with amputations in children is that of stump overgrowth. One should make an effort to inform the parents of this possibility, especially with a transbone or metaphyseal type of amputation. Several methods of preventing stump overgrowth have been used in the past, such as Silastic plugs and periosteal flaps. Unfortunately, none of them have had any degree of success and thus they are rarely used.

## Laceration Injuries of the Foot

Laceration of soft tissue structures may occur in association with open fractures in the foot. One should carefully examine the limb for injury to nerves, vessels, or tendons. Laceration injuries of the foot may result in deformity, especially if the heel cord, the anterior tibial tendon, or the posterior tibial tendon is involved. These tendons are the only ones requiring immediate or delayed repair. Little indication exists for direct repair of the extensor hallucis longus, the long-toe flexor, or the long-toe extensors because little disability occurs.

## Puncture Wounds

Puncture wounds require adequate débridement, tetanus toxoid, and a broad-spectrum antibiotic. A small puncture wound may be all that is evident on clinical inspection (Fig. 16–72A). In children who have stepped on a nail, the diagnosis is clear; in the absence of such a history, a radiograph to rule out a radiopaque foreign body is indicated. Careful exploration of the wound, open Wick catheter drainage, and antibiotics usually resolve the problem. If pain and swelling persist, osteomyelitis is a possibility (Fig. 16–72B and C). If the presence of osteomyelitis is uncertain, one should perform a bone scan with either technetium or gallium. *Pseudomonas* is the most common organism cultured from children who have stepped on nails.[100] The age-old question of tennis sneaker glue harboring *Pseudomonas* has not been answered. With osteomyelitis, local pain and swelling usually last for 2 or 3 days after the puncture, and it takes about 5 to 10 days before the local reaction becomes more apparent. One should make a surgical incision and drain the wound along with aggressive débridement to remove any contaminated tissue. Carbenicillin and gentamicin are the antibiotics of choice. The wound should be left open with a drain inserted. Two cases of *Mycobacterium fortuitum* osteomyelitis secondary to a nail puncture wound in the foot have been described; one affected the cuboid and the other affected the calcaneus. Treatment of *M. fortuitum* osteomyelitis requires surgical drainage in addition to antibiotic therapy with a combination of two or more of the following: amikacin, imipenem, ciprofloxacin, and clarithromycin.[101] One should be aware of the possibility of premature physeal arrest or avascular necrosis at the epiphysis. If the metatarsophalangeal joint is involved, early chondrolysis of the articular surfaces with fibrosis and subsequent arthritis may occur (Fig. 16–73). The family should be informed of the possibility of growth plate involvement and be advised to continue follow-up examination. Several times each year, older children present with short third or fourth toes and vague histories of stepping on nails or with occult foot injuries incurred at an earlier age. It appears in retrospect that osteomyelitis, avascular necrosis, and growth arrest occurred (Fig. 16–74).

## Foreign Body

If a child complains of pain and has a persistent limp with no clear history of injury, one has to consider the possibility of a retained foreign body. The object may or may not be visible on radiographs. Although CT and MRI have been used in the past to localize objects, we now use ultrasonography. Ultrasonography picks up both radiodense and radiolucent lesions. The object may be localized and removed under ultrasonic control (Fig. 16–75). Occasionally, a foreign body such as a needle is seen in the foot of an asymptomatic patient who receives a radiograph for other reasons (Fig. 16–76). We do not recommend removal of these asymptomatic objects.

Shells from gunshot wounds are a notorious type of foreign body (Fig. 16–77). Most often, the wound is accidental, self-inflicted, and located in the forefoot. Depending on the size and caliber of the bullet, a large amount of soft tissue injury and debris such as shoe leather and socks may be seen. Segmental loss of bone may also occur. The wound should be vigorously

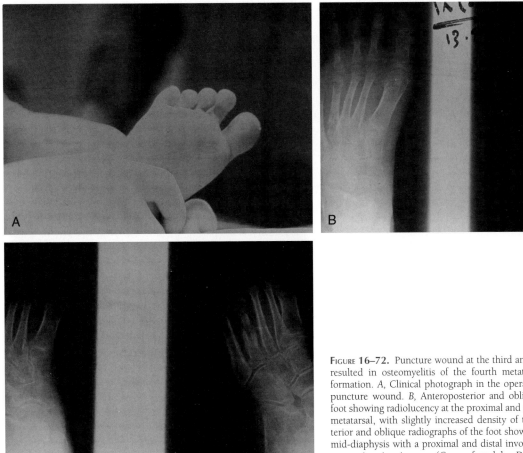

FIGURE 16–72. Puncture wound at the third and fourth interspace that resulted in osteomyelitis of the fourth metatarsal, with sequestrum formation. *A,* Clinical photograph in the operating room showing the puncture wound. *B,* Anteroposterior and oblique radiographs of the foot showing radiolucency at the proximal and distal poles of the fourth metatarsal, with slightly increased density of the shaft. *C,* Anteroposterior and oblique radiographs of the foot showing a sequestrum of the mid-diaphysis with a proximal and distal involucrum; the sequestrum was swimming in pus. (Case referred by Dr. Fouad Hussan, King Hussein Medical Center, Amman, Jordan.)

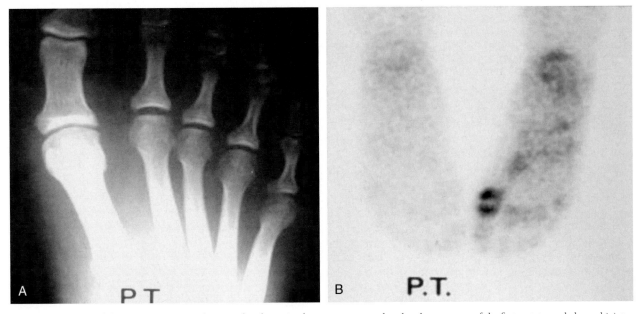

FIGURE 16–73. This adolescent patient stepped on a nail and sustained a puncture wound at the plantar aspect of the first metatarsophalangeal joint. Inadequate superficial débridement was initially performed elsewhere and the patient started on oral antibiotics. The child subsequently was referred 3 weeks later with forefoot pain and swelling in addition to a low-grade fever. A diagnosis of septic arthritis was made and an incision and drainage carried out. *A,* An anteroposterior radiograph of the foot shows joint space narrowing of the first metatarsophalangeal joint and soft tissue swelling. *B,* A nuclear bone scan revealed increased uptake at the level of the first metatarsophalangeal joint with a concomitant increase in the first metatarsal head, as well as the base of the proximal phalanx, suggestive of both septic arthritis and osteomyelitis. *Pseudomonas aeruginosa* was isolated from the intraoperative cultures; however, aspiration of both the metatarsal head and the proximal phalanx failed to reveal a positive culture. (Case referred by Dr. Charles Mehlman, Cincinnati, OH.)

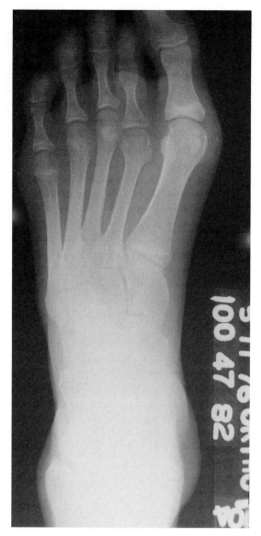

FIGURE 16–74. This child was seen because a short second toe was developing. The history revealed that a nail had penetrated the child's foot when he was younger and the toe became infected. We believe the retrospective history to be that of osteomyelitis involving the physis, with subsequent growth arrest of the metatarsal.

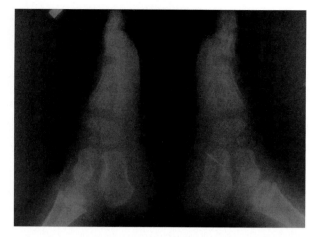

FIGURE 16–76. A needle in the foot. This child was seen for another problem; the needle had apparently lodged in the foot several years earlier. Removal of an incidentally seen asymptomatic foreign body is contraindicated and is to be condemned.

irrigated and débrided but not closed. Multiple dressing changes are carried out, followed by mesh skin graft coverage. Reconstructive procedures should be considered only after all wounds are cleaned and closed, which might take 6 to 8 months.[143]

## Miscellaneous Causes of Foot Pain

Foot pain and reluctance to bear weight with no direct history of trauma should lead one to consider other conditions, including tarsal coalitions, stress fractures, tumors, and early inflammatory arthritis. The cause of the pain is usually age related. If plain radiographs are normal, a bone scan is indicated. Pediatric orthopaedists are often faced with vague, nondescript pain known by the six Ps: puzzling and perplexing pain problems in

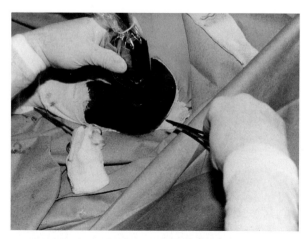

FIGURE 16–75. The use of ultrasonography to remove foreign bodies allows the visualization of nonradiopaque as well as radiopaque objects. We strongly recommend its use to prevent the extensive dissection occasionally required to remove nonopaque foreign bodies.

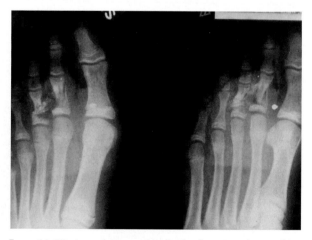

FIGURE 16–77. A gunshot wound to the forefoot. Note the significant soft tissue swelling, phalangeal fractures, and metallic fragments. Most such injuries are self-inflicted through accident. They require extensive débridement, with the possibility of later skin grafting. Amputation is indicated for vascular compromise distal to the metatarsophalangeal joint.

pediatric patients. Bone scans have been of tremendous benefit in these situations.

## STRESS FRACTURES

Stress fractures usually occur after a sudden increase in activity in a skeletally maturing adolescent who is starting to participate in intensive or repetitive sports training. The condition may be seen as early as 8 to 12 years of age. The most frequent sites are the proximal part of the tibia in 10- to 15-year-olds, the distal end of the fibula in 2- to 5-year-olds, and the second metatarsal in older adolescents (see Figs. 16–54 and 16–55). Navicular stress fractures have also been reported in older adolescents and occur mainly in basketball players.[3] If the fracture is nondisplaced, we recommend 6 weeks of a short leg cast that is non–weight bearing, and healing is then assessed with a CT scan. If displacement, delayed union beyond 12 weeks, or frank nonunion has occurred, bone grafting and internal fixation are indicated.[64]

## PATHOLOGIC FRACTURES

Metabolic disease such as end-stage renal osteodystrophy may cause weakening of the bone at the metaphyseal-epiphyseal junction, with subsequent fractures after trivial trauma. In these same patients, brown tumors may also develop after secondary hyperparathyroidism, with resultant bone weakening. In addition, the bone may be undermined by constitutional disorders such as idiopathic juvenile osteoporosis, osteogenesis imperfecta, and congenital insensitivity to pain (Fig. 16–78) and by therapeutic procedures such as chemotherapy for leukemia or anticonvulsant medication such as phenytoin (Dilantin) for seizure disorders (Fig. 16–79).

## BICYCLE SPOKE INJURIES

These injuries occur in early walkers, usually between 2 and 8 years of age. A fracture, if present, is often not as important as the soft tissue injury. Initially, the foot may appear to be normal, with no significant injury, because none of the bones are broken.[66] The foot subsequently tends to swell and exhibit soft tissue problems. This pathobiologic picture is similar to that seen in a crush injury caused by a washing machine wringer. We recommend that soft tissue decompression be performed early, if necessary, followed by delayed primary closure or a skin graft. It is more important to resolve the issue of crush injury to the tissue than to manage the fracture in this situation. Bicycle spoke injuries can be prevented if the bicycle is equipped with already fitted spoke guards and a child carrier with adjustable pedals and foot straps.[135] A meshed disk that covers the spokes would prevent further injuries without increasing wind resistance.[41]

## REFLEX SYMPATHETIC DYSTROPHY (COMPLEX REGIONAL PAIN SYNDROME)

Reflex sympathetic dystrophy (RSD) is a syndrome characterized by severe regional pain with swelling, dysesthesia to light touch, and vasomotor instability that can lead to chronic trophic soft tissue changes, joint contractures, and osteoporosis. Recently, in an attempt to classify patients by clinical signs and symptoms rather than pathophysiology, newer terminology has been proposed to replace the term RSD. The new term is complex regional pain syndrome (CRPS), which is divided into two types: CRPS type I to replace RSD and CRPS type II to replace causalgia.[53] The role of the sympathetic nervous system in many aspects of the illness is not clear, and dystrophy may not occur in all patients. Childhood RSD (CRPS type I) is much more common in girls, and a history of trauma is present in a minority of cases. Lower extremity involvement is much more common than upper extremity involvement in children, with a significant number of patients having knee involvement. Knee involvement is often misdiagnosed as chondromalacia patellae, especially in the preadolescent and adolescent girls who constitute a large proportion of the patient population. Radiographic studies are not usually helpful in diagnosing CRPS type I

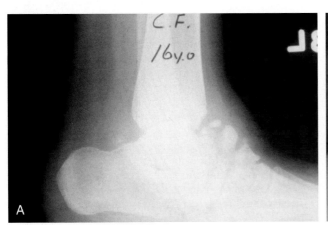
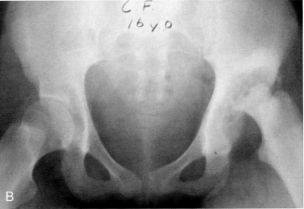

**FIGURE 16–78.** This child has familial dysautonomia (congenital insensitivity to pain). *A,* This lateral radiograph of the foot and ankle shows Charcot-like joints at the talonavicular cuneiform joints. *B,* An anteroposterior view of the pelvis shows very similar Charcot-like changes in the hip with complete dissolution of the femoral head and marked distortion of the acetabulum.

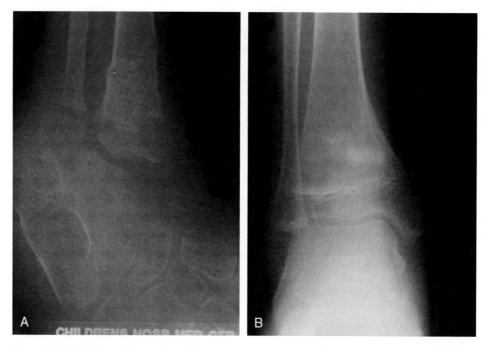

**FIGURE 16–79.** Pathologic fractures through osteopenic bone. *A,* Pathologic fracture in a child with phenytoin (Dilantin)-induced rickets and abnormal bone. Note the widened fibular and tibial physis. *B,* An anteroposterior radiograph shows horizontal trabecular densities and osteopenia in a young girl in whom juvenile osteoporosis was diagnosed.

in children. The spotty or patchy osteopenia typical of adults with RSD is rare in children.[38] RSD accounts for 11% of pediatric pain of uncertain etiology.[43] Because the syndrome is relatively uncommon in children, diagnosis and treatment are often delayed. The delay in diagnosis prolongs the painful period and results in unnecessary and potentially morbid diagnostic procedures.

CRPS type I in childhood most commonly affects the lower extremities. Dysesthesia, vasomotor instability, and swelling of the affected area are found in most reported cases. Vasomotor instability (most commonly discoloration, temperature difference, and tache cérébrale) is present in almost all cases, and the diagnosis of RSD should not be considered in its absence. Tache cérébrale is elicited by stroking the skin in the affected area with a blunt object, such as the head of a safety pin, with the contralateral limb used as a control. Autonomic dysfunction is demonstrated by the appearance of an erythematous line 15 to 30 seconds after the stimulus; the line may persist as long as 15 minutes. This sign may be present before other signs of autonomic dysfunction appear.[38] The child may have a trivial injury to the lower extremity, followed by the full manifestations of CRPS type I. Dietz and colleagues[38] reported signs of vasomotor instability in 83% of cases, including color changes (60%), decreased temperature (58%), altered sweating (14%), and decreased pulses (16%). Local swelling was noted in 70% of their cases. The regional distribution was the foot and ankle (52%), arm (21%), knee (14%), hand (8%), and shoulder (5%). Limb length discrepancy can develop in children secondary to altered blood flow and trophic changes.[53]

The psychogenic aspects of this syndrome in children are important and have been noted by several authors.

Situations involving family dysfunction, including loss of a parent, alcohol and substance abuse, a psychiatric illness in the family, physical or sexual abuse of the patient, and divorce and remarriage, must be considered as precipitating factors for this disorder.[7, 22, 50, 94]

When children present with pain of the upper or lower extremity, CRPS type I does not usually head the list of possible diagnoses. Most recently, bone scanning has been used to assist in the elucidation of pain disorders in the extremities of children, but it lacks sensitivity and specificity for RSD in children. Of 35 bone scans reported in the literature on childhood RSD, 31% were normal, 31% showed diffuse increased uptake, and 37% showed diffuse decreased uptake.[38]

Bryan and associates[15] described a technique for the early diagnosis of RSD.[15] The authors measured pressure pain thresholds with an instrument called a dolorimeter that was developed by Atkins and Kanis.[5]

A technique of modified differential spinal blockade has been described to determine whether the pain is sympathetic, somatic, or central in origin. Saline is used as a placebo, and 5% procaine is used to induce pharmacologic spinal blockade. If the patient's pain is relieved by saline, the pain is possibly psychogenic in origin because no pharmacologic blockade has been administered. However, 5% procaine effectively blocks all somatic and sympathetic fibers. If its introduction does not provide pain relief, the pain may be considered to be central (malingering, psychogenic, or encephalized because of the extended duration of pain). If patients obtain relief with procaine, they are monitored for return of pinprick sensation and motor function, skin temperature, and changes in blood pressure. If the pain returns simultaneously with the return of pinprick sensation, it can be assumed to be somatic in origin because the larger somatic neural fibers recover from the anesthesia faster than the smaller sympathetic fibers do. If the pain relief persists after the return of motor function and pinprick sensation but while sympathetic function remains blocked, the pain is sympathetic in origin.

Early recognition and treatment of this disorder provide the most optimism for a good outcome. Some of these patients have undergone extensive diagnostic testing, as well as diagnostic arthroscopy in the case of adolescent girls with knee pain. Most authors believe that physical therapy and mobilization are the best methods of treatment of this disorder; unfortunately, when most children complain of pain, immobilization is the first step in treatment, a measure that may exacerbate CRPS type I.

Nonpharmacologic therapy has been successful in most cases reported in children. Physical therapy and mobilization alone or with transcutaneous nerve stimulation have been used in over 70% of patients.[38]

Sherry and colleagues reported on 103 children with type I CRPS. Forty-nine of their patients were monitored for more than 2 years (mean, 5 years). These patients were treated with an intense exercise therapy program (most received a daily program of 4 hours of aerobic and functionally directed exercise and 1 to 2 hours of hydrotherapy and desensitization). Seventy-seven percent were referred for psychologic counseling. The mean duration of exercise therapy was 14 days. Ninety-two percent of these patients initially recovered from all symptoms and regained full function. The long-term outcome of the 49 children studied was excellent, with 88% being fully functional without pain after a mean of more than 5 years. Recurrent episodes were seen in 31% and developed in most within the first 6 months; the majority resolved with self-initiation of their exercise program.[136]

Other treatments used successfully in small numbers of patients include systemic corticosteroids, regional blocks with reserpine or guanethidine, sympathetic blockade, propranolol, and neuroprobing.[38]

It is most important to evaluate the family situation before embarking on treatment. A dysfunctional family may or may not predispose to the disorder, and family counseling may be necessary to assist with or speed up management of the disorder. Although surgical sympathectomy is considered in adults if the patient responds to sympathetic blocks, its use in children is discouraged because CRPS type I appears to be self-limited. The chronic trophic changes and contractures characteristic of adults are not commonly seen in children. Treatment of children includes massage, primarily the application of lanolin skin cream three times a day, and mobilization with encouragement of weight bearing and range-of-motion exercises in spite of the discomfort. A careful explanation of the disorder is necessary to reassure the patient and the parents that no damage will be done in spite of the pain. These exercises should be performed at least three times a day for 5 to 10 minutes each.[38]

A team approach to patients with chronic pain is important. The team should include a leader—an orthopaedist, anesthesiologist, or rehabilitation medicine specialist—as well as physical and occupational therapy support. A psychologist can also provide the necessary emotional and mental support.

Early recognition of this disorder may prevent a prolonged diagnostic encounter in these children with significant morbidity. Practitioners who manage children should be familiar with this disorder and consider it when a child (usually female) presents with considerable pain and a positive tache cérébrale test of the lower extremity after trivial trauma, especially when one is aware of potential psychologic disturbances or a dysfunctional family.

## COMPLICATIONS OF INJURIES TO THE DISTAL TIBIAL AND FIBULAR GROWTH PLATES

### Angular Deformity Secondary to Asymmetric Arrest of the Distal Tibial Growth Plate

The deformity is usually varus and is most frequently seen after Salter-Harris type III and IV medial malleolar injuries. An adduction injury most commonly results in a varus deformity. After an adduction injury, a direct compressive force applied to the epiphyseal plate by the talus results in premature closure of that part of the plate and subsequent angular deformity (Fig. 16–80). Anatomic reduction by open or closed means is necessary when the fracture involves the medial malleolus (Salter-Harris type III or IV) because incomplete anatomic reduction will result in later deformity.[77] Anatomic reduction and fixation usually prevent this problem. Creative opening or closing wedge osteotomies have been used successfully to lessen minimal leg length discrepancy caused by partial growth arrest. Epiphysiodesis of the distal ends of the tibia and fibula may be performed to prevent an angular deformity if the child has less than 2 years of growth remaining. Correction by epiphysiolysis may be successful if less than 50% of the cross-sectional area of the physis is involved.[112] Epiphysiolysis is an adequate, if not excellent procedure when partial growth arrest of the distal part of the tibia has occurred. The child should have more than 3 years of growth remaining. MRI is an excellent modality for imaging physeal bars. The amount of involvement of the growth plate can be well documented graphically by the use of anterior and lateral polycycloidal tomography to map out the physeal bar.[20] Imaging data can be processed to yield both three-dimensional rendered and projection physeal maps that are particularly useful in preoperative planning. The projection technique is superior because it provides a more reliable and anatomically detailed depiction of the physis; it also uses software that is already available on many MRI systems, and it requires less operator input and is therefore less time consuming[11, 26] (Fig. 16–81).

Even though the attending physician has made the family aware of the potential for physeal arrest or has discussed the radiographs demonstrating angulation of the Park-Harris growth arrest line, if the child does not complain of pain, that child may not be returned for follow-up. Most often, the child presents sometime later because of the development of a varus deformity. The technique of placing a proximal window in the metaphysis and approaching the bar from above for central bars and directly for peripheral ones has worked out satisfactorily.[116] It is most important that the bar be completely excised and that after excision, normal-appearing physeal cartilage be identified circumferentially. An interposition substance is necessary to prevent rebridging, and subcutaneous fat[81] or cranioplasty has been used most often. Cranioplasty appears to be more attractive because it allows immediate weight bearing. However, if indicated, removal of the interpositional substance may be difficult. Compromised host immunity has been associated with release of the methyl methacrylate monomer.[119, 120] If the angular deformity of the ankle exceeds 20°, a corrective osteotomy is indicated. Nearly normal longitudinal growth and correction of moderate angular deformities can be expected with bridges that occupy less than 25% of the physis. It is important to place metallic markers (a small Steinmann pin or vascular clip) into the epiphysis and metaphysis to determine whether growth results from the epiphysiolysis. Berson and colleagues suggested a decision-making process that they used to divide their 24 patients into three groups: group 1 consisted of children with less than 2 years of growth remaining, less than 9° of predicted angulation, and less than 2 cm of predicted discrepancy. This group was treated by observation. Group 2 consisted of children with less than 9° of existing angulation, more than 2 cm of predicted leg length discrepancy, or more than 9° of predicted angulation. This group was treated with bilateral distal tibial and fibular epiphysiod-esis. Group 3 consisted of children with more than 9° of existing angulation and greater than 2 cm of predicted leg length discrepancy. This group was treated by osteotomy to correct the angulation and either lengthening or epiphysiodesis to correct the leg length discrepancy. They did not include physeal bar excision because they did not have great success with it. This approach resulted in satisfactory correction in 22 of 24 patients.[8]

Takakura and colleagues reported their results after opening wedge osteotomy for the treatment of post-traumatic varus deformity of the ankle. A corrective osteotomy was indicated for children only when they had ankle pain after walking for long distances, had difficulty participating in sports, and had a progressive deformity as well as uneven wear of the sole of the shoe, with more rapid wear on the lateral part. In four of the nine cases discussed, the initial injury was an epiphyseal fracture of the distal end of the tibia. The average age of these patients was 14 years, and the average follow-up was 9 years. The tibial shaft and the tibial joint surface angle (TAS angle) on the AP radiograph was an average of 73° in this group (this angle is 88° in normal Japanese). The ankle joint radiographs also showed evidence of subchondral sclerosis and osteophyte formation. The osteotomy was performed 2 to 3 cm proximal to the epiphyseal plate, and an oblique osteotomy of the fibula was performed first (Fig. 16–82). The space created anteromedially was filled with iliac crest bone graft. The average time for osseous union was 6.5 weeks, and the average postoperative TAS angle was 89°. Improvement in leg length discrepancy was also reported. On latest follow-up, these patients were able to participate in physical education classes at school, and two of them were able to participate in competitive basketball and athletic activities.[145]

Foster and colleagues published a report on the use of

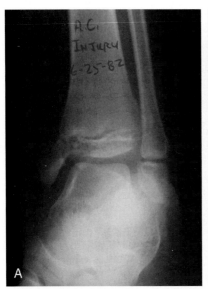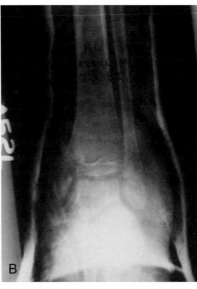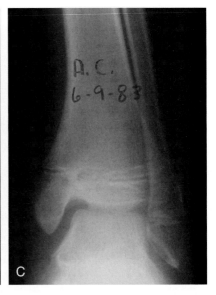

**FIGURE 16–80.** This child sustained a Salter-Harris type IV medial malleolar fracture of the distal end of the tibia that resulted in a growth plate injury. The growth plate injury in turn resulted in a physeal bar that caused a varus deformity. The bar was removed, fat was interposed, and growth was reestablished. *A,* Initial radiograph of the ankle showing minimal displacement. *B,* Radiograph through a plaster cast, consistent with anatomic reduction. *C,* Radiograph 1 year later showing a bony bar. Note the Park-Harris line angulated from the bar.

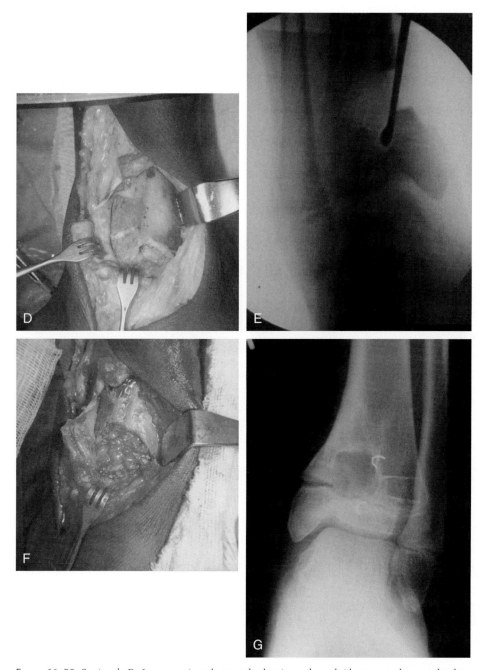

Figure 16–80 *Continued. D,* Intraoperative photograph showing a bone bridge across the growth plate. *E,* Intraoperative Polaroid radiograph showing a curette across the resected physeal bar. *F,* Operative photograph showing fat through the bone window. *G,* Anteroposterior radiograph after excision of the bar and resumption of growth. The metallic clips are used as markers to monitor future growth.

free fat interpositional grafts acutely in severe physeal injuries of the distal end of the tibia, particularly in injuries with complete peripheral detachment of the zone of Ranvier. The physeal, cancellous epiphyseal, and metaphyseal debris was removed, fractures were stabilized, and fat grafting was performed. After an average follow-up of 4 years (for distal tibial injuries), no angular deformity of the leg was present, and the distal tibial growth plate remained open.[51]

## Angular Deformity Secondary to Growth Arrest of the Distal Fibular Growth Plate

Growth arrest of the distal fibular physis is a rare complication of distal fibular growth plate fractures. This complication may result in valgus malalignment of the ankle joint. When detected early, screw epiphysiodesis of the distal tibial physis may suffice (Fig. 16–83).

## Angular Deformity Secondary to Malunion

This unusual complication is seen more frequently in older adolescents. Angulation of less than 20° can be expected to remodel in children younger than 10 years. We tend to give injuries with less than 20° of angulation approximately 2 years to remodel to within 10°, or to within limits acceptable to the parents, before considering an osteotomy. Angulation of less than 15° rarely causes functional disability. Residual valgus deformities are generally more acceptable than varus deformities. Angular deformities in the plane of motion tend to remodel more readily. A supramalleolar osteotomy is usually considered when the child is too old for epiphysiolysis, as a complement to bar excision in an older child, or when residual varus or valgus angulation is greater than 20°.

## Leg Length Discrepancy

Direct bone lengthening is another option in the management of growth problems after fractures. Ten percent to 30% of lengthening procedures on the lower extremity are carried out for correction of discrepancies after injury to the growth plates. One-stage step-cut procedures or opening or closing wedge osteotomies may

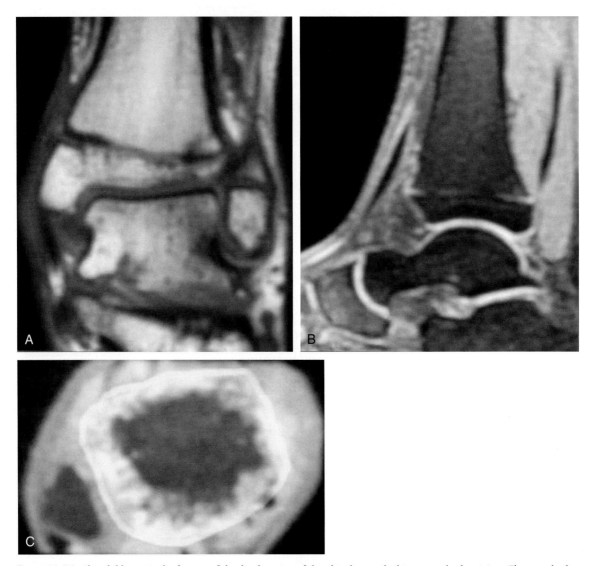

**Figure 16–81.** This child sustained a fracture of the distal portion of the tibia that resulted in a growth plate injury. The growth plate injury in turn resulted in a large physeal bar. Rarely is there documentation of the circumferential diameter of a physeal bar as illustrated in this figure. *A,* Coronal T1-weighted magnetic resonance image (MRI) of the ankle showing obliteration of the physis in its middle segment (high signal intensity); the peripheral linear low signal intensity represents the open physis. *B,* Sagittal gradient-recalled-echo MRI of the ankle showing a large bony bar (low signal intensity); the line of high signal intensity represents the open physis. *C,* A gradient-recalled-echo maximal intensity projection (MIP) image in the axial plane outlining the perimeter of the distal tibial physis and showing a large centrally located physeal bar (represented by the central area of low signal intensity). (Case referred by Dr. Tal Laor, Cincinnati, OH.)

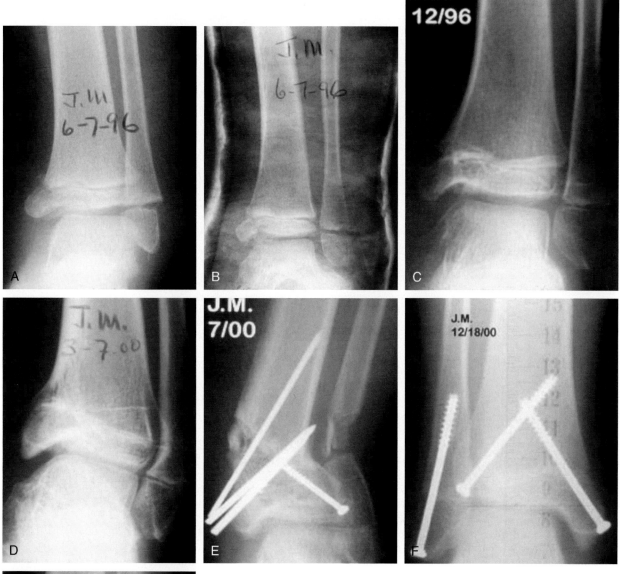

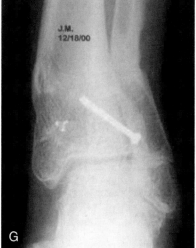

**FIGURE 16–82.** This child sustained a Salter-Harris type IV medial malleolar fracture of the distal end of the tibia that resulted in a growth plate injury, as well as a Salter-Harris type I distal fibular fracture that went on to normal healing. The tibial growth plate injury in turn resulted in a physeal bar involving greater than 50% of the physis that produced a significant varus deformity. *A,* Initial anteroposterior (AP) radiograph of the ankle showing displacement of the medial malleolar fracture, as well as the fibular physeal fracture. *B,* AP radiograph through a plaster cast consistent with anatomic reduction. *C,* Radiograph 6 months later illustrating the Park-Harris growth lines of both the fibula and the tibia. Note on the fibula that the Park-Harris growth line is horizontal and shows consistent growth from the physis. The Park-Harris line of the tibia ends in the medial aspect of the tibial metaphysis immediately lateral to Poland's hump (most often associated with physeal injuries). Failure of continuous parallel growth of the Park-Harris line of the tibia in addition to angulation of it into the area of the previous fracture site (Poland's hump) is highly indicative of an early physeal bar. Unfortunately, the patient was not referred at that time. *D,* An AP radiograph of the ankle at our institution revealed the continued obliquity of the Park-Harris line into the area of physeal arrest. Note that the ankle has gone into significant varus and that the lateral physis is still open. *E,* An opening wedge supramalleolar osteotomy was performed in addition to lateral tibial physeal screw epiphysiodesis and fibular osteotomy. *F,* Postoperative radiograph showing screw epiphysiodesis performed on the distal ends of the contralateral tibia and fibula to minimize future leg length discrepancy. *G,* Final correction obtained after removal of the hardware except for the lateral tibial epiphysiodesis screw.

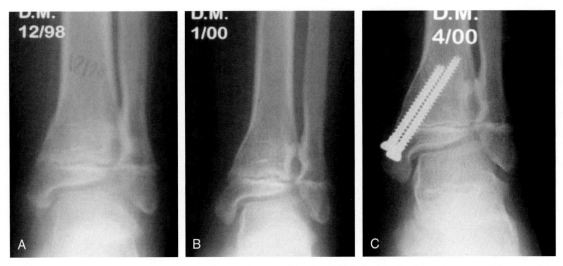

**FIGURE 16–83.** This child sustained a Salter-Harris type I fracture of the distal tibial physis and a Salter-Harris type V fracture of the distal end of the fibula at the age of 8 years. The fractures were treated by closed reduction and casting. The fibular growth plate injury in turn resulted in a physeal bar that caused a mild valgus deformity of the ankle joint. The deformity appeared to be progressive and thus warranted treatment. *A,* Radiograph of the ankle 1 year after injury showing distal fibular arrest with the fibular physis at the same level as the tibial physis. In normal growth of children without neurologic conditions, the fibular physis should never be above the level of the joint line. Note in this child the symmetric Park-Harris line of the distal end of the tibia. The child did not have any incremental Park-Harris line of the distal fibular physis inferring physeal arrest. *B,* Radiographs 1 year after injury showing worsening of the valgus malalignment of the ankle as the distal tibial epiphysis increases in size and incorporates its secondary ossification center. *C,* Radiographs 2 months after screw epiphysiodesis of the medial aspect of the distal tibial physis was carried out to prevent further progression of the ankle valgus deformity.

be performed for the correction of discrepancies within 1 inch. Greater discrepancies can be addressed by contralateral open or closed epiphysiodesis or by ipsilateral leg lengthening. The most frequently used lengthening procedures include the Wagner gradual distraction procedure, followed by osteosynthesis,[157] and the callotasis techniques of Renzi-Brivio[130] or Ilizarov.[63] The axial distraction osteogenesis and callotasis methods used for lengthening the leg by means of periosteally stimulated regenerate bone are most popular at the time of this writing. All have been found to be quite satisfactory in the management of limb length inequality. The most popular techniques use the monoaxial fixator or the circular frame. The monoaxial fixator frame is less bulky than the circular frame lengthener. It is an excellent method to use for the femur. The monoaxial fixator may cause the tibia to go into valgus unless it is applied in an AP direction instead of laterally. The circular frame is preferred when angular and rotational deformity is associated with tibial shortening and length discrepancy.

## Osteoarthritis

Osteoarthritis may occur secondary to persistent residual joint incongruity. The condition usually follows failure to achieve anatomic reduction of interfragmentary gaps greater than 3 mm. The use of current radiographic imaging technology may increase our awareness of this problem and prevent its occurrence. Prevention may be achieved by open or closed anatomic reduction and stabilization.

Another cause of osteoarthritis may be unappreciated

damage to articular cartilage. The impact of the trauma may damage the subchondral plate. Irreversible damage to these cartilage cells causes localized failure of the articular weight-bearing surface, which leads to shearing down to subchondral bone and chondrolysis. In addition, damage may occur to the articular component of the tibia or the talar dome or both.

## Rotational Deformities

This complication is unusual and, if significant, can be easily corrected by supramalleolar osteotomy. Both bones should be osteotomized; however, it may not be necessary to transfix the fibula.

## Nonunion or Delayed Union

These complications are extremely rare but may occur. Operative management of nonunion or delayed union is rarely required for fractures below the distal third of the tibia. Nonunion of the metacarpals may be asymptomatic and thus not require treatment. The senior author (A.H.C.) has treated segmental loss of a metatarsal after a lawn mower injury by autologous fibular interposition grafting, with good results.

## Avascular Necrosis of the Distal Tibial Physis

This extremely rare condition has been reported only once in the English language literature.[138]

# APHORISMS FOR ANKLE AND FOOT INJURIES

Parents should be made aware of the possibility of a growth injury any time that an epiphysis is fractured. If the child is seen in the emergency department, the attending physician should impress on the parents how serious this issue is. The parents must be informed and made aware of the injury's potential to cause growth-related problems. The worst scenario occurs when growth arrest occurs and the parent did not even know about the possibility.

Closed reduction is usually possible for most injuries around the foot and ankle. If the patient is under general anesthesia and anatomic reduction is accomplished, we strongly recommend percutaneous Steinmann pinning or percutaneous use of an interfragmentary screw. The new cannulated cancellous screws are optimal for this technique. The need for open reduction is minimal if the injuries are treated within 48 hours.

Soft tissue "goose egg" swelling over the distal end of the fibula usually represents a Salter-Harris type I growth plate injury. A fibular physeal fracture may or may not accompany a distal tibial physeal injury. After several weeks of treating an ankle sprain, the appearance of calcification around the distal fibular metaphysis or in the interosseous ligament is indicative of a previously unrecognized fracture.

Epiphyseal injuries should be reduced within the first 24 to 48 hours; repeat manipulation after 5 or 6 days may be difficult and can cause epiphyseal damage. We would rather accept the malreduction after 1 week than risk injury to the growth plate.

The distal tibial and fibular ossification centers can vary, and sometimes these variants make the diagnosis of a fracture difficult. In most of these instances, the fracture is minor, with minimal displacement, and is adequately treated by simple immobilization. A bone scan can differentiate an anomalous ossification pattern from a fracture.

Close attention must be paid to the direction of growth plate displacement after injury, especially the metaphyseal fragment. The direction of displacement of the metaphyseal fragment determines the mechanism of injury in most circumstances.

Epiphyseal articular fragment displacement of greater than 2 mm requires reduction. CT can be used not only to diagnose these injuries but also to assess the reduction. It is more important that the articular cartilage rather than the metaphyseal-epiphyseal junction be anatomically reduced. The latter tends to remodel unless angulation is excessive or growth plate arrest has occurred. If the metaphyseal fragment of a medial malleolar Salter-Harris type IV fracture cannot be reduced, it can usually be discarded as long as the epiphyseal fracture is anatomically reduced.

An eccentric bony bridge is more likely to cause angular deformity than to significantly slow growth in a distal tibial injury because the central growth plate is too strong.

After injury, one should look closely at the growth arrest lines (Park-Harris) for evidence of bony bridging. These lines should be horizontal, and any tendency toward angulation into the fracture site indicates bony bridge formation.

A residual deformity with greater than 2-mm displacement of the weight-bearing articular surface after reduction is not compatible with a good result. An interfragmentary gap greater than 3 mm on the initial radiograph is not consistent with successful closed reduction. Open reduction should be considered if manipulation under general anesthesia does not enable better apposition of the fragments. After having achieved anatomic reduction, one should be alert for possible instability; consequently, we strongly recommend a percutaneous pin or percutaneous interfragmentary screw to maintain stability. Following apparent anatomic reduction confirmed by the image intensifier, a hard copy anteroposterior and lateral radiograph are mandatory as a "report card."

Unrecognized damage to the articular cartilage at the time of injury may lead to chondrolysis and long-term symptoms in spite of adequate reduction and normal-appearing radiographs. The articular cartilage has poor remodeling potential, and injury tends to lead to arthritic changes.

Growth arrest is rare in triplane fractures. The child is usually an adolescent without much longitudinal growth remaining. The major residual problem is joint incongruity or an interfragmentary gap greater than 3 mm resulting in degenerative arthritis. All radiographs of the ankle should be made in no fewer than three planes; if necessary, a polytomogram or a limited CT scan can be used to determine the direction and reduction of the fracture fragments.

Mandatory follow-up of growth plate injuries for 1 year in children younger than 12 years is necessary. Managed health care plans are becoming more prevalent, with patients constantly switching physicians as the plan dictates. This movement makes it extremely difficult to monitor patients who may or may not have a current problem but have suffered a growth plate injury with a predictable future disability. One must be aware of "disappearing patients."

Angular deformity and shortening are usually asymptomatic. The patient returns because of deformity and not pain. Joint incongruity and articular cartilage injury leading to degenerative joint disease are more significant long-term problems that do cause pain.

The compartments of the foot are tight. Decompression is indicated for any persistent swelling, venous congestion, or taut skin or when multiple bones are involved. Compartment syndrome should be considered regardless of whether fractures are seen.

Displacement of metatarsal fractures is rare, but nonunion is not uncommon. Lateral displacement of the middle metatarsal (second through fourth) fracture fragments with varus or valgus angulation is acceptable, tends to remodel, and does not cause problems. Dorsal or plantar displacement is not acceptable because the resulting angular deformity will alter the weight-bearing pattern and lead to painful calluses.

One should avoid a primary circular cast for most ankle injuries because of the possibility of a tourniquet effect. We recommend the use of a bulky dressing for initial management of these injuries. After several days, when the swelling is decreased, a well-molded cast is satisfactory.

Open reduction plus internal fixation of foot fractures is rarely indicated and should be avoided, if possible. Growth inhibition in and around the foot is unusual; overgrowth is more common. Usually, the only indications for open reduction of foot fractures are open injuries and significant soft tissue injury.

## REFERENCES

1. Aitken, A.P. The end results of the fractured distal tibial epiphysis. J Bone Joint Surg 18:685–691, 1936.
2. Anderson, D.V.; Lyne, E.D. Osteochondritis dissecans of the talus: Case report on two family members. J Pediatr Orthop 4:356–357, 1984.
3. Arendt, E.A. Orthopaedic Knowledge Update, Sports Medicine 2. Rosemont, IL, American Academy of Orthopaedic Surgeons, 1999.
4. Ashhurst, A.P.; Bromer, R.S. Classification and mechanism of fractures of the leg bones involving the ankle. Arch Surg 4:51–129, 1922.
5. Atkins, R.M.; Kanis, J.A. The use of dolorimetry in the assessment of post-traumatic algodystrophy of the hand. Br J Rheumatol 28:404–409, 1989.
6. Berndt, A.L.; Harty, M. Transchondral fractures (osteochondritis dissecans). J Bone Joint Surg Am 41:988–1020, 1959.
7. Bernstein, B.H.; Singsen, B.H.; Kent, J.T.; et al. Reflex neurovascular dystrophy in childhood. J Pediatr 93:211–215, 1978.
8. Berson, L.; Davidson, R.S.; Dormans, J.P.; et al. Growth disturbances after distal tibial physeal fractures. Foot Ankle 21:54–58, 2000.
9. Bishop, P.A. Fractures and epiphyseal separation fractures of the ankle: Classification of 332 cases according to mechanism of their production. AJR Am J Roentgenol 28:49–67, 1932.
10. Borges, J.L.; Guille, J.T.; Bowen, J.R. Kohlers bone disease of the tarsal navicular. J Pediatr Orthop 15:596–598, 1995.
11. Borsa, J.J.; Peterson, H.A.; Ehman, R.L. MR imaging of physeal bars. Radiology 199:683–687, 1996.
12. Brogle, P.J.; Gaffney, J.T.; Denton, J.R. Acute compartment syndrome complicating a distal tibial physeal fracture in a neonate. Am J Orthop 28:587–589, 1999.
13. Broock, G.J.; Greer, R.B. Traumatic rotational displacements of the distal tibial growth plate. J Bone Joint Surg Am 52:1666–1668, 1970.
14. Brunet, J.A. Calcaneal fractures in children. Long-term results of treatment. J Bone Joint Surg Br 82:211–216, 2000.
15. Bryan, A.S.; Klenerman, L.; Bowsher, D. The diagnosis of reflex sympathetic dystrophy using an algometer. J Bone Joint Surg Br 73:644–646, 1991.
16. Byrd, H.S.; Cierny, G., III; Tebbetts, J.B. The management of open tibial fractures with associated soft-tissue loss: External pin fixation with early flap coverage. Plast Reconstr Surg 68:73–79, 1981.
17. Canale, S.T.; Belding, R.H. Osteochondral lesions of the talus. J Bone Joint Surg Am 62:97–102, 1980.
18. Canale, S.T.; Kelly, F.B., Jr. Fractures of the neck of the talus. Long-term evaluation of 71 cases. J Bone Joint Surg Am 60:143–156, 1978.
19. Canale, S.T.; Williams, K.D. Iselin's disease. J Pediatr Orthop 12:90–93, 1992.
20. Carlson, W.O.; Wenger, D.R. A mapping method to prepare for surgical excision of a partial arrest. J Pediatr Orthop 4:232–238, 1984.
21. Carothers, C.O.; Crenshaw, A.H. Clinical significance of a classification of epiphyseal injuries at the ankle. Am J Surg 89:879–887, 1955.
22. Casten, D.F.; Betcher, A.M. Reflex sympathetic dystrophy. Surg Gynecol Obstet 100:97–101, 1955.
23. Chopra, P.; Soucy, P.; Laberge, J.M.; et al. Know before you mow: A review of lawn mower injuries in children, 1990–1998. J Pediatr Surg 35:665–668, 2000.
24. Cole, J.R.; Brown, H.P.; Stein, R.E.; Pearce, R.G. Avulsion fracture of the tuberosity of calcaneus in children. J Bone Joint Surg Am 77:1568–1571, 1995.
25. Cooperman, D.R.; Spiegel, P.G.; Laros, G.S. Tibial fractures involving the ankle in children: The so-called triplane epiphyseal fracture. J Bone Joint Surg Am 60:1040–1046, 1978.
26. Craig, J.G.; Cramer, K.E.; Cody, D.D.; et al. Premature partial closure and other deformities of the growth plate: MR imaging and three-dimensional modeling. Radiology 210:835–843, 1999.
27. Lichtman, D.M.; Crawford, A.H. Pediatric Orthopaedic Surgery. Burbank, CA, Science Image Communications, 1988.
28. London, W.D.; Crawford, A.H. Triplane fracture. Orthop Consult 4:8–12, 1983.
29. Crawford, A.H. Fractures about the foot in children: A radiographic analysis. Cincinnati, OH, The Children's Hospital Medical Center, 1991 (unpublished data).
30. Crawford, A.H. Ankle fractures in children. Instr Course Lect 44:317–324, 1995.
31. Daley, A.J.; McIntyre, P.B. *Stenotrophomonas maltophilia* and lawn mower injuries in children. J Trauma 48:536–537, 2000.
32. de Beer, J.D.; Maloon, S.; Hudson, D.A. Calcaneal fractures in children. S Afr Med J 76:53–54, 1989.
33. Denton, J.R.; Fischer S.J. The medial triplane fracture: Report of an unusual injury. J Trauma 21:991–995, 1981.
34. de Palma, L.; Santucci, A.; Sabetta, S.P.; Rapali, S. Anatomy of the Lisfranc joint complex. Foot Ankle 18:356–364, 1997.
35. de Sanctis, N.; Della Corte, S.; Pempinello, C. Distal tibial and fibular epiphyseal fractures in children: Prognostic criteria and long-term results in 158 patients. J Pediatr Orthop B 9:40–44, 2000.
36. Dias, L.S.; Giegerich, C.R. Fractures of the distal tibial epiphysis in adolescence. J Bone Joint Surg Am 65:438–444, 1983.
37. Dias, L.S.; Tachdjian, M.O. Physeal injuries of the ankle in children: Classification. Clin Orthop 136:230–233, 1978.
38. Dietz, F.R.; Matthews, K.D.; Montgomery, W.J. Reflex sympathetic dystrophy in children. Clin Orthop 258:225–231, 1990.
39. Dolan, A.M.; Mulcahy, D.M.; Stephens, M.M. Osteochondritis dissecans of the head of the talus. Foot Ankle 18:365–368, 1997.
40. Dormans, J.P.; Azzoni, M.; Davidson, R.S.; et al. Major lower extremity lawn mower injuries in children. J Pediatr Orthop 15:78–82, 1995.
41. D'Souza, M.S.; Hynes, D.E.; McManus, F.; et al. The bicycle spoke injury: An avoidable accident. Foot Ankle 17:170–173, 1996.
42. Ehrlich, M.G. The problem: Distal tibial fracture in a child. Orthop Consult 7:1–10, 1986.
43. Ehrlich, M.G.; Zaleske, D.J. Pediatric orthopaedic pain of unknown origin. J Pediatr Orthop 6:460–468, 1986.
44. el-Tayeby, H.M. Freiberg's infraction: A new surgical procedure. J Foot Ankle Surg 37:23–27, 1998.
45. Ertl, J.P.; Barrack, R.L.; Alexander, A.H.; Van Buecken, K. Triplane fracture of the distal tibial epiphysis: Long-term follow-up. J Bone Joint Surg Am 70:967–976, 1988.
46. Essex-LoPresti, P. The mechanism, reduction technique, and results in fractures of the os calcis. Br J Surg 39:395–419, 1952.
47. Falkenberg, M.P.; Dickens, D.R.; Menelaus, M.B. Osteochondritis of the first metatarsal epiphysis. J Pediatr Orthop 10:797–799, 1990.
48. Farley, F.A.; Senunas, L.; Greenfield, M.L.; et al. Lower extremity lawn-mower injuries in children. J Pediatr Orthop 16:669–672, 1996.
49. Feldman, D.S.; Otsuka, N.Y.; Hedden, D.M. Extra-articular triplane fracture of the distal tibial epiphysis. J Pediatr Orthop 15:479–481, 1995.
50. Fermaglich, D.R. Reflex sympathetic dystrophy in children. Pediatrics 60:881–883, 1977.
51. Foster, B.K.; John, B.; Hasler, C. Free fat interpositional graft in acute physeal injuries: The anticipatory Langenskiöld procedure. J Pediatr Orthop 20:282–285, 2000.
52. Freiberg, A.H. Infraction of the second metatarsal bone, a typical injury. Surg Gynecol Obstet 19:191–193, 1914.
53. Gellman, H. Reflex sympathetic dystrophy: Alternative modalities for pain management. Instr Course Lect 49:549–557, 2000.

54. Grogan, D.P.; Walling, A.K.; Ogden, J.A. Anatomy of the os trigonum. J Pediatr Orthop 10:618–622, 1990.

55. Gross, R. Fractures and dislocations of the foot. In: Rockwood, C.A.; Green, D.P., eds. Fractures. Philadelphia, J.B. Lippincott, 1975.

56. Haasbeek, J.F. Lower extremity compartment syndrome resulting from a toddler's bed. Pediatrics 102:1474–1475, 1998.

57. Hahn, S.B.; Lee, J.W.; Jeong, J.H. Tendon transfer with a microvascular free flap for injured feet in children. J Bone Joint Surg Br 80:86–90, 1998.

58. Hangody, L.; Kish, G.; Karpati, Z.; et al. Treatment of osteochondritis dissecans of the talus: Use of the mosaicplasty technique—a preliminary report. Foot Ankle 18:628–634, 1997.

59. Hawkins, L.G. Fractures of the neck of the talus. J Bone Joint Surg Am 52:991–1002, 1970.

60. Higashiyama, I.; Kumai, T.; Takakura, Y.; Tamail, S. Follow-up study of MRI for osteochondral lesion of the talus. Foot Ankle 21:127–133, 2000.

61. Holbein, O.; Bauer, G.; Kinzl, L. Fracture of the cuboid in children: Case report and review of the literature. J Pediatr Orthop 18:466–468, 1998.

62. Horowitz, J.H.; Nichter, L.S.; Kenney, J.G.; Morgan, R.F. Lawn mower injuries in children: Lower extremity reconstruction. J Trauma 25:138–146, 1985.

63. Ilizarov, G.A.; Devitav, A.A. Operative elongation of the leg with simultaneous correction of deformities. Ortop Travmatol Protez 30:32–37, 1969.

64. Inokuchi, S.; Usami, N.; Hiraishi, E.; Hashimoto, T. Calcaneal fractures in children. J Pediatr Orthop 18:469–474, 1998.

65. Iselin, H. Wachstumbeschwerden zur Zeit dur Knochernen Entwicklung der Tuberositas metatarsi quinti. Dtsch Z Chir 117:529–535, 1912.

66. Izant, R.J., Jr.; Rothmann, B.F.; Frankel, V.H. Bicycle spoke injuries of the foot and ankle in children: An underestimated "minor" injury. J Pediatr Surg 4:654–656, 1969.

67. Johnson, E.W., Jr.; Fahl, J.C. Fractures involving the distal epiphysis of the tibia and fibula in children. Am J Surg 93:778–781, 1957.

68. Johnson, R.P.; Collier, B.D.; Carrera, G.F. Os trigonum syndrome:Use of bone scan in the diagnosis. J Trauma 24:761–764, 1984.

69. Jones, D.M.; Saltzman, C.L.; El-Khoury, G. The diagnosis of the os trigonum syndrome with a fluoroscopically controlled injection of local anesthetic. Iowa Orthop J 19:122–126, 1999.

70. Karrholm, J. The triplane fracture: Four years of follow-up of 21 cases and review of the literature. J Pediatr Orthop B 6:91–102, 1997.

71. Karrholm, J.; Hansson, L.I.; Laurin, S. Pronation injuries of the ankle in children: Retrospective study of radiographical classification and treatment. Acta Orthop Scand 54:1–17, 1983.

72. Kavanaugh, J.H.; Brower, T.D.; Mann, R.V. The Jones fracture revisited. J Bone Joint Surg Am 60:776–782, 1978.

73. Kaye, J.J.; Bohne, W.H. A radiographic study of the ligamentous anatomy of the ankle. Radiology 125:659–667, 1977.

74. Kirkpatrick, D.P.; Hunter, R.E.; Janes, P.C.; et al. The snowboarder's foot and ankle. Am J Sports Med 26:271–277, 1998.

75. Kleiger, B.; Mankin, H.J. Fracture of the lateral portion of the distal tibial epiphysis. J Bone Joint Surg Am 46:25–32, 1964.

76. Kling, T.F., Jr. Operative treatment of ankle fractures in children. Orthop Clin North Am 21:381–392, 1990.

77. Kling, T.F., Jr.; Bright, R.W.; Hensinger, R.N. Distal tibial physeal fractures in children that may require open reduction. J Bone Joint Surg Am 66:647–657, 1984.

78. Köhler, A. Typical disease of the second metatarsophalangeal joint. AJR Am J Roentgenol 10:705–710, 1915.

79. Konig, F. Ueber freie Korper in den Gelenken. Dtsch Z Chir 27:90–109, 1888.

80. Kump, W.L. Vertical fractures of the distal tibial epiphysis. Clin Orthop 73:132–135, 1970.

81. Langenskiöld, A. Surgical treatment or partial closure of the growth plate. J Pediatr Orthop 1:3–11, 1981.

82. Lauge-Hansen, N. Fractures of the ankle. Combined experimental-surgical and experimental-roentgenological investigations. Arch Surg 60:957–985, 1950.

83. Leitch, J.M.; Cundy, P.J.; Paterson, D.C. Case report: Three-dimensional imaging of a juvenile Tillaux fracture. J Pediatr Orthop 9:602–603, 1989.

84. Letts, R.M.; Gibeault, D. Fractures of the neck of the talus in children. Foot Ankle 1:74–77, 1980.

85. Letts, R.M.; Mardirshah, A. Lawn-mower injuries in children. Can Med Assoc J 116:1151–1153, 1977.

86. Loder, R.T.; Brown, K.L.; Zaleske, D.J.; Jones, E.T. Extremity lawn-mower injuries in children: Report by the Research Committee of the Pediatric Orthopaedic Society of North America. J Pediatr Orthop 17:360–369, 1997.

87. Love, S.M.; Grogan, D.P.; Ogden, J.A. Lawn mower injuries in children. J Orthop Trauma 2:94–101, 1988.

88. Lovell, E.S. An unusual rotatory injury to the ankle. J Bone Joint Surg Am 50:163–165, 1968.

89. Lower, R.F.; Kenzora, A.J.E. The diabetic neuropathic foot: A triple crush syndrome—measurement of compartmental pressures of normal and diabetic feet. Orthopaedics 17:241–248, 1994.

90. Lynn, M.D. The triplane distal tibial epiphyseal fracture. Clin Orthop 86:187–190, 1972.

91. Mann, R.A. Biomechanics of the foot. In: American Academy of Orthopedic Surgeons. Atlas of Orthotics. Biomechanical Principles and Applications. St. Louis, C.V. Mosby, 1975, pp. 257–266.

92. Manoli, A., II; Weber, T.G. Fasciotomy of the foot: An anatomical study with special reference to release of the calcaneal compartment. Foot Ankle 10:267–275, 1990.

93. Marmor, L. An unusual fracture of the tibial epiphysis. Clin Orthop 73:132–135, 1970.

94. Matles, A.I. Reflex sympathetic dystrophy in a child: A case report. Bull Hosp Jt Dis 32:193–197, 1971.

95. Matteri, R.E.; Frymoyer, J.W. Fracture of the calcaneus in young children: Report of 3 cases. J Bone Joint Surg Am 55:1091–1094, 1973.

96. McFarland, B. Industrial aspect of fractures of os calcis. BMJ 1:607–610, 1937.

97. McIntire, M.S. Injury Control for Youth and Children. Elk Grove Village, IL, Committee on Accident and Poison Prevention, American Academy of Pediatrics, 1987.

98. McNealy, G.A.; Rogers, L.F.; Hernandez, R.; Pozananski, A.K. Injuries of the distal tibial epiphysis: Systematic radiographic evaluation. AJR Am J Roentgenol 138:683–689, 1982.

99. Mehlman, C.T.; Strub W.M.; Todd, L.T. Talar fractures in children. J Am Osteo Acad Orthop 37:38–41, 2000.

100. Miller, E.H.; Semian, D.W. Gram-negative osteomyelitis following puncture wounds of the foot. J Bone Joint Surg Am 57:535–537, 1975.

101. Miron, D.; El, A.L.; Zuker, M.; et al. *Mycobacterium fortuitum* osteomyelitis of the cuboid after nail puncture wound. Pediatr Infect Dis J 19:483–485, 2000.

102. Moehring, H.; Tan, R.T.; Marder, R.A.; et al. Ankle dislocation. J Orthop Trauma 8:67–172, 1994.

103. Mooney, J.F., 3rd; DeFranzo, A.; Marks, M.W. Use of cross-extremity flaps stabilized with external fixation in severe pediatric foot and ankle trauma: An alternative to free tissue transfer. J Pediatr Orthop 18:26–30, 1998.

104. Morris, J.M. Biomechanics of the foot and ankle. Clin Orthop 122:10–17, 1977.

105. Mukherjee, S.K.; Pringle, R.M.; Baxter, A.D. Fracture of the lateral process of the talus. A report of thirteen cases. J Bone Joint Surg Br 56:263–273, 1974.

106. Mulfinger, G.L.; Trueta, J. The blood supply of the talus. J Bone Joint Surg Br 52:160–167, 1970.

107. Myerson, M.S. Management of compartment syndromes of the foot. Clin Orthop 271:239–248, 1991.

108. Myerson, M.S.; Mann, R.A.; Coughlin, M.J. Soft tissue trauma: Acute and chronic management. In: Mann, R.A.; Coughlin, M.J., eds. Surgery of the Foot and Ankle, 6th ed. Philadelphia, C.V. Mosby, 1993, pp. 1367–1410.

109. Nevelos, A.B.; Colton, C.L. Rotational displacement of the lower tibial epiphysis due to trauma. J Bone Joint Surg Br 59:331–332, 1977.

110. Nusem, I.; Ezra, E.; Wientroub, S. Closed posterior dislocation of the ankle without associated fracture in a child. J Trauma 46:350–351, 1999.

111. Ogden, J.A. Skeletal Injury in the Child. Philadelphia, Lea & Febiger, 1982, pp. 621–641.

112. Ogden, J.A.; Lee, J. Accessory ossification patterns and injuries of the malleoli. J Pediatr Orthop 10:306–316, 1990.

113. Ogilvie-Harris, D.J.; Sarrosa, E.A. Arthroscopic treatment of osteochondritis dissecans of the talus. Arthroscopy 15:805–808, 1999.

114. Parmar, P.; Letts, M.; Jarvis, J. Injuries caused by water tubing. J Pediatr Orthop 18:49–53, 1998.

115. Peterson, C.A.; Peterson, H.A. Analysis of the incidence of injuries to the epiphyseal growth plate. J Trauma 12:275–281, 1972.

116. Peterson, H.A. Growth plate injuries. In: Morrissy, R.T., ed. Lovell and Winter's Pediatric Orthopaedics, 3rd ed., Vol. 2. Philadelphia, J.B. Lippincott, 1990.

117. Peterson, H.A. Partial growth plate arrest. In: Morrissy, R.T., ed. Lovell and Winter's Pediatric Orthopaedics, 3rd ed., Vol. 1. Philadelphia, J.B. Lippincott, 1990.

118. Peterson, H.A.; Burkhart, S.S. Compression injury of the epiphyseal growth plate: Fact or fiction? J Pediatr Orthop 1:377–384, 1981.

119. Petty, W. The effect of methyl methacrylate on bacterial phagocytosis and killing by human polymorphonuclear leukocytes. J Bone Joint Surg Am 60:752–757, 1978.

120. Petty, W. The effect of methyl methacrylate on chemotaxis of polymorphonuclear leukocytes. J Bone Joint Surg Am 60:492–498, 1978.

121. Pick, M.P. Familial osteochondritis dissecans. J Bone Joint Surg Br 37:142–145, 1955.

122. Poland, J. Traumatic Separation of the Epiphysis. London, Smith, Elder, 1898.

123. Powell, J.H.; Whipple, T.L. Osteochondritis of the talus. Foot Ankle 6:309–310, 1986.

124. Preidler, K.W.; Brossmann, J.; Daenen, B.; et al. MR imaging of the tarsometatarsal joint: Analysis of injuries in 11 patients. AJR Am J Roentgenol 167:1217–1222, 1996.

125. Ralph, B.G.; Barrett, J.; Kenyhercz, C.; DiDomenico, L.A. Iselin's disease: A case presentation of nonunion and review of the differential diagnosis. J Foot Ankle Surg 38:409–416, 1999.

126. Rang, M. Children's Fractures. Philadelphia, J.B. Lippincott, 1974.

127. Rapariz, J.M.; Ocete, G.; Gonzalez-Herranz, P.; et al. Distal tibial triplane fractures: Long-term follow-up. J Pediatr Orthop 16:113–118, 1996.

128. Rendu, A. Fracture intra-articulaire parcellaire de la poulie astragalienne. Lyon Med 150:220–222, 1932.

129. Renner, R.R.; Mauler, G.G.; Ambrose, J.L. The radiologist, the orthopedist, the lawyer, and the fracture. Semin Roentgenol 13:7–18, 1978.

130. Renzi-Brivio, L.; Lavini, F.; de Bastiani, G. Lengthening in the congenital short femur. Clin Orthop 250:112–116, 1990.

131. Salter, R.B.; Harris, W.R. Injuries involving the epiphyseal plate. J Bone Joint Surg Am 45:587–622, 1963.

132. Schindler, A.; Mason, D.E.; Allington, N.J. Occult fracture of the calcaneus in toddlers. J Pediatr Orthop 16:201–205, 1996.

133. Schmidt, T.L.; Weiner, D.S. Calcaneal fractures in children: An evaluation of the nature of the injury in 56 children. Clin Orthop 171:150–155, 1982.

134. Schofield, R.O. Fractures of os calcis. J Bone Joint Surg Br 18:566–580, 1936.

135. Segers, M.J.M.; Wink, D.; Clevers, G.J. Bicycle-spoke injuries: A prospective study. Injury 28:267–269, 1997.

136. Sherry, D.D.; Wallace, C.A.; Kelley, C.; et al. Short and long-term outcomes of children with complex regional pain syndrome type I treated with exercise therapy. Clin J Pain 15:218–223, 1999.

137. Shin, A.Y.; Moran, M.E.; Wenger, D.R. Intramalleolar triplane fractures of the distal tibial epiphysis. J Pediatr Orthop 17:352–355, 1997.

138. Siffert, R.S.; Arkin, A.M. Post-traumatic aseptic necrosis of the distal tibial epiphysis. J Bone Joint Surg Am 32:691–694, 1950.

139. Silas, S.I.; Herzenberg, J.E.; Myerson, M.S.; Sponseller, P.D. Compartment syndrome of the foot in children. J Bone Joint Surg Am 77:356–361, 1995.

140. Simonian, P.T.; Vahey, J.W.; Rosenbaum, D.M.; et al. Fracture of the cuboid in children. A source of leg symptoms. J Bone Joint Surg Br 77:104–106, 1995.

141. Spiegel, P.G.; Cooperman, D.R.; Laros, G.S. Epiphyseal fractures of the distal ends of the tibia and fibula. A retrospective study of 237 cases in children. J Bone Joint Surg Am 60:1046–1050, 1978.

142. Stone, J.W. Osteochondral lesions of the talar dome. J Am Acad Orthop Surg 4:63–73, 1996.

143. Stucky, W.; Loder, R.T. Extremity gunshot wounds in children. J Pediatr Orthop 11:67–71, 1991.

144. Tachdjian, M.O. Pediatric Orthopedics, 2nd ed. Philadelphia, W.B. Saunders, 1990.

145. Takakura, Y.; Takaoka, T.; Tanaka, Y.; et al. Results of opening-wedge osteotomy for the treatment of a post-traumatic varus deformity of the ankle. J Bone Joint Surg Am 80:213–218, 1998.

146. Talkhani, I.S.; Reidy, D.; Fogarty, E.E.; et al. Avascular necrosis of the talus after a minimally displaced neck of talus fracture in a 6 year old child. Injury 31:63–65, 2000.

147. Taranow, W.S.; Bisignani, G.A.; Towers, J.D.; Conti, S.F. Retrograde drilling of osteochondral lesions of the medial talar dome. Foot Ankle 20:474–480, 1999.

148. Thermann, H.; Schratt, H.E.; Hufner, T.; Tscherne, H. Fractures of the pediatric foot. Unfallchirurg 101:2–11, 1998.

149. Thomas, H.M. Calcaneal fracture in childhood. Br J Surg 56:664–666, 1969.

150. Tol, J.L.; Struijs, P.A.; Bossuyt, P.M.; et al. Treatment strategies in osteochondral defects of the talar dome: A systematic review. Foot Ankle 21:119–126, 2000.

151. Tomaschewski, H.K. Ergebnisse der Behandlung des post-traumatischen Fehlwuchses des Fusses bei Kindern und Jugendlichen. Beitr Orthop Traumatol 22:90, 1975.

152. Torg, J.S.; Ruggiero, R.A. Comminuted epiphyseal fracture of the distal tibia. A case report and review of the literature. Clin Orthop 110:215–217, 1975.

153. Trias, A.; Ray, R.D. Juvenile osteochondritis of the radial head. Report of a bilateral case. J Bone Joint Surg Am 45:576–582, 1963.

154. Trillat, A.; Lerat, J.L.; LeClerc, P.; Schuster, P. Tarsometatarsal fracture-dislocations. Rev Chir Orthop 62:685–702, 1976.

155. Vahvanen, V.; Alto, K. Classification of ankle fractures in children. Arch Orthop Trauma Surg 97:1–5, 1980.

156. Vosburgh, C.L.; Gruel, C.R.; Herndon, W.A.; Sullivan, J.A. Lawn mower injuries in the pediatric foot and ankle: Observations on prevention and management. J Pediatr Orthop 15:504–509, 1995.

157. Wagner, H. Operative lengthening of the femur. Clin Orthop 136:125–142, 1978.

158. Walter, E.; Feine, U.; Anger, K.; et al. Szintigraphische diagnostik und verlaufskontrolle bei epiphysenfugen verletzunger. Fortschr Geb Rontgenstr Nuklearmed Erganzungsband 132:309–315, 1980.

159. Waugh, W. The ossification and vascularisation of the tarsal navicular and their relation to Köhler's disease. J Bone Joint Surg Br 40:765–777, 1958.

160. White, J. Osteochondritis dissecans in association with dwarfism. J Bone Joint Surg Br 39:261–267, 1957.

161. Wiley, J.J. Tarsometatarsal joint injuries in children. J Pediatr Orthop 1:255–260, 1981.

162. Xenos, J.S.; Mulligan, M.E.; Olson, E.J.; et al. Tibiofibular syndesmosis: Evaluation of the ligamentous structures methods of fixation and radiographic assessment. J Bone Joint Surg Am 77:847–856, 1995.

163. Zellweger, V.H.; Ebnother, M. Uber eine familiare Skelettstorung mit multilocularen, aseptischem Knochennekrosen, insbesondere mit Osteochondritis dissecans. Helv Paediatr Acta 6:95–111, 1951.

# CHAPTER 17

# Child Abuse

Kathryn E. Cramer, M.D.
Neil E. Green, M.D.

Child abuse has become a social and medical problem of epidemic proportions. The number of abused and neglected children in the United States rose from 1.4 million in 1986 to 2.9 million in 1993.[7] The actual incidence is unknown, and although legal mandates for reporting child abuse have increased awareness and documentation of the problem, many cases are unreported. It is estimated that approximately 2000 children die annually in the United States as a result of child abuse and neglect,[68] and according to the Third National Incidence Study of Child Abuse and Neglect, 1.5 million children were intentionally injured in 1993.[90] Unfortunately, child abuse is still frequently identified in retrospect after a history of repetitive trauma has been established.[42, 49] Even though most orthopaedists are aware of the "classic" skeletal signs of abuse in children, more recent data suggest that other injury patterns are much more prevalent.[51, 64, 69, 74, 111] Whether these findings reflect a true evolution of the syndrome, however, is not known; it is therefore important that physicians treating children be aware of these injuries in order to diagnose and intervene appropriately.

## LEGAL ASPECTS

In 1961, the Children's Bureau of the U.S. Department of Health, Education, and Welfare published a model law that required mandatory reporting by physicians and other medical professionals. Although the exact reading of the law in various communities may differ, all statutes require prompt identification of any child suspected of having been abused. Physicians are granted immunity from civil and criminal liability if a report is made in good faith. Maliciously reporting abuse when it is not the cause of injury, however, may expose an individual to the risk of litigation. In addition, civil suits have been filed against physicians for failure to report acts of child abuse, and most laws impose a criminal penalty for failure to report suspected child abuse. Suspected child abuse must be reported and the examining physician must be aware of the syndrome to recognize it.

## HISTORICAL PERSPECTIVE

Although the radiographic findings of child abuse have been known for more than a century, it was not until 1946 that Caffey studied six children with chronic subdural hematomas and fractures of long bones with no history of injury.[12] He stated that they did not have a systemic disease that could explain the radiographic findings and believed that injury to the children was responsible for the findings. He further suggested that children with unexplained long bone fractures should be investigated for chronic subdural hematomas and vice versa.

In 1953, Silverman described periosteal new bone formation associated with irregular fragmentation of the metaphyses in children and believed that this injury was part of the syndrome that Caffey originally described.[96] In 1960, Altman and Smith reported cases of unrecognized trauma in children, and in 1972, Kempe and Helfer coined the term "battered child syndrome."[5, 50] Since that time, the definition has been expanded to include forms of abuse other than physical.

## FORMS OF ABUSE AND NEGLECT

Although this chapter will deal only with physical abuse, the treating surgeon must be familiar with other forms of child abuse. Recognition of signs of neglect, sexual abuse, or emotional maltreatment may lead the treating physician to consider nonaccidental injury as a possibility.

Child neglect may be defined as the failure of a parent or other legal guardian to provide for the child's basic needs and provide an adequate level of care.[23] Physical neglect is pervasive and may be more common than physical abuse. Neglect tends to be chronic and leads to an inadequate level of love, food, clothing, shelter, medical care, safety, and education. Physical signs of neglect include malnutrition, pica, constant fatigue and listlessness, poor hygiene, and inadequate clothing for the circumstances.[23] Behavioral signs of physical neglect include lack of appropriate adult supervision and even "role reversal," in which the child becomes the parental caretaker. Other signs include drug or alcohol abuse, poor school attendance, and exploitation by the parents, such as being forced to beg or steal.[23]

Child sexual abuse is the sexual exploitation of a child for the gratification or profit of an adult. Sexual exploitation is usually perpetrated by someone known to the child and frequently continues over a prolonged period. It is very prevalent, but this type of abuse is difficult to detect and confirm.[23] A description of the physical signs of sexual abuse is beyond the scope of this text; however, the behavioral signs should be recognized because their presence may alert the physician that the child is a victim of sexual abuse. A child who is a victim of sexual abuse may become withdrawn and have poor peer relationships. These children may demonstrate low self-esteem and seem frightened, especially of adults. They may have feelings of shame or guilt, and their academic performance may deteriorate. They may also show pseudomature personality development. Regressive behavior and even attempted suicide may be the result of child sexual abuse. These children may also become sexually promiscuous and may sexually abuse a sibling.

## PHYSICAL ABUSE

Although soft tissue injuries are the most common finding in child abuse,[69] 10% to 70% of physically abused children manifest some form of skeletal trauma.[2, 37, 43, 45, 63, 69] It is estimated that 30% to 50% of physically abused children are seen by orthopaedists for fractures or other orthopaedic problems.[3, 91] An orthopaedist caring for injured children must be familiar with abuse-related injuries and the clinical manifestations of such injuries to appropriately diagnose and intervene in suspicious cases.

Recognition of physical abuse is extremely important to protect the involved child, as well as any siblings. Of children returned to an abusive home without intervention, 35% to 50% will be abused again, and the second incident may be fatal in 5% to 10%.[41, 88] Early identification and intervention in cases of child abuse cannot be overemphasized, and the results are encouraging. Recurrence rates of less than 10% have been reported after early, appropriate intervention.[37]

### Identifying the Problem

Physicians caring for children must always consider the possibility of nonaccidental trauma when evaluating injuries, particularly in very young children. Almost a third of cases of physical abuse occur in children younger than 1 year, and nearly 50% occur in children younger than 2 years.[64] It has been stated that 10% of the trauma to children younger than 3 years seen in the emergency department is nonaccidental, as are 30% of head and limb injuries in this age group.[47] Although nearly 80% of the deaths from abuse occur in children younger than 5 years, over half of these children are younger than 1 year.[25] Bone tends to be more delicate in very young children, and as a result, more than 50% of the abuse-related skeletal injuries occur in children younger than 1 year.[64] Children older than 5 years account for less than 10% of the fractures related to abuse.[74, 111] Even though only 58% of the children in Herndon's study were younger than 3 years, they accounted for 94% of the fractures.[45] In another study, 65% of the abused children were younger than 18 months.[28] Whereas the incidence of nonaccidental fractures decreases with increasing age, the incidence of accidental fractures increases with increasing age up to 12 years.[110]

### History of Injury

The parent or caregiver's account of the injury is often vague and incomplete. When questioned, they may be evasive or contradictory and fail to volunteer details regarding the incident. The degree of physical injury may be inconsistent with the history given,[20, 31, 44] and often the reported time of injury does not correlate with the obvious age of the injury. A delay in seeking treatment is often noted. A history of repeated trauma with the child treated in several different facilities should arouse suspicion.

The parents' response to the situation may be inappropriate. They may be critical of or angry with the child for being injured, or they may ignore the child completely. Other parents may become overly involved.[40]

The social history will provide additional information in identifying children at risk. Although child abuse is pervasive and occurs in all socioeconomic strata, reporting appears to be higher in lower socioeconomic groups.[23] Socially isolated families with no external support system tend to be more abusive. Abuse is also more common in families in which the parents are involved in a violent interpersonal relationship. Adults who were childhood victims of abuse are more likely to become abusive parents, as are those with unrealistic expectations (i.e., expectations inconsistent with the child's developmental or intellectual abilities) for their children. Families with increased stress are vulnerable. An illegitimate or unplanned pregnancy, a teenage pregnancy, and parental divorce are all factors associated with an increased incidence of child abuse. Unemployment, drug or alcohol abuse, and physical or mental illness enhances the likelihood of child abuse.[23, 47]

Any condition that interferes with normal parent-child bonding and results in lack of normal parental contact increases the risk of child abuse. Irritable or hyperactive children or children with physical or developmental disabilities are more likely to suffer abuse from their parents or caretakers. Premature infants, who may require more care and attention, are abused three times as often as term infants.[4] In a recent report reviewing infant homicide, a mother younger than 17 years, a second or subsequent birth in a mother 19 years or younger, no prenatal care, and a low level of education were cited as the strongest risk factors. Because infanticide occurs most often in the first few months of life, intervention during pregnancy and the postpartum period is recommended.[81]

## Physical Examination

An orthopaedist caring for children's fractures will probably be confronted with children who have sustained musculoskeletal injuries as a result of abuse. The possibility of nonaccidental trauma must always be considered, and a complete and systematic examination of the child must be performed. Careful documentation of skin and soft tissue injuries is required, including the size, shape, location, and estimated stage of healing of any lesions.[23] The entire axial and appendicular skeleton is then examined. The injured area is examined last to lessen the child's anxiety. Whereas tenderness, crepitus, or instability may be present in acute fractures, palpable callus without associated tenderness may be noted in healing fractures. Any of the aforementioned findings warrants radiographic examination.

Soft tissue injuries may include bruises or welts over any part of the body. Areas particularly subject to trauma are the face, head, and neck, including the lips, mouth, ears, and eyes.[69] Bruises about the trunk, back, buttocks, and thighs are also common. Bruises may form regular patterns resembling the shape of the object that was used to inflict the injury, such as a hand, fist, belt or belt buckle, or electrical cord. Multiple body surface involvement or multiple injuries in various stages of resolution suggest abuse and warrant further investigation.[16, 23]

Burns are also commonly seen and may be noted in conjunction with other injuries. Cigarette burns may be present, especially on the palms, soles, back, or buttocks. Immersion burns form a regular pattern. If the child is pushed into a tub or sink of very hot water, the burns will occur around the buttocks and genitalia. However, if one of the extremities is dipped in hot water, a stocking-glove distribution of the burn will be seen. Pattern burns may result if the child is burned with an instrument such as an iron, grill, or some other hot object with a recognizable shape.

Lacerations may occur anywhere on the body, but some common types are rope burns on the wrists, ankles, neck, or torso. Lacerations about the head and face are frequently noted and may even be seen inside the mouth or ears. One must also look for injuries to the genitalia and other body surfaces.

Injuries to the abdomen and to the components of the abdominal cavity may result from child abuse. Bruises of the abdominal wall and bleeding within the wall of the small intestine may be seen. Rupture of an abdominal viscus has been reported, including the intestine, spleen, liver, pancreas, and blood vessels. The kidneys and bladder may also be injured.

Trauma to the central nervous system is common and may be severe. Subdural hematoma may result from either blunt trauma or violent shaking of the infant. More commonly, subarachnoid hemorrhage is a result of the so-called shaken baby syndrome. Ophthalmologic examination will demonstrate the presence of retinal hemorrhage.[109]

An abused child is likely to have behavioral characteristics that may be the result of physical or emotional abuse.[23] Abused children may be less compliant, more negative, and more unhappy than the average child. Abused children may be hypervigilant and wary of any contact with adults.[40] They tend to be angry, feel isolated, and show destructive behavior. They may be abusive toward others and have difficulty developing normal relationships.[87] Parental separation is frequently difficult, but occasionally an abused child will be indifferent to separation from the parents. These children may constantly seek attention and may show developmental delays as well.[23]

## Radiographic Evaluation

Initially, the clinical examination determines the areas to be evaluated with biplanar radiographs.[34, 71] Oblique views may be helpful if a fracture is suspected but not seen on biplanar radiographs. Additional imaging studies, such as ultrasound or arthrography, may be necessary to evaluate cartilaginous areas.[71, 72] In areas where ossification is normally delayed, such as the capital femoral epiphysis and the proximal and distal ends of the humerus, ultrasound has been shown to be particularly helpful.[71] Ultrasound may also demonstrate subperiosteal hemorrhage, occult long bone fractures, and costochondral injuries acutely before these injuries are visible on conventional radiographs.[17]

In cases of suspected physical abuse, conventional skeletal radiography is the primary screening examination. Twenty-two percent of abused children younger than 1 year will have unsuspected fractures detected by the skeletal survey.[74] A complete skeletal survey consists of anteroposterior projections of the extremities (including the hands and feet), frontal and lateral views of the thoracolumbar spine with adequate penetration to visualize the ribs, and an anteroposterior and lateral skull series.[71] A "baby-gram" with the entire child on one radiograph is unacceptable.[71, 83, 84] All physically abused children younger than 2 years and infants younger than 1 year with evidence of significant neglect should be evaluated with a complete skeletal survey.[71] A recent report recommends extending this recommendation to 3 years of age.[69] A more selective approach is used in older children because only 9% of children older than 1 year will have radiographic evidence of fractures not suspected clinically.[74] Routine, complete skeletal surveys are rarely indicated in children older than 5 years.[71, 74]

Follow-up skeletal surveys (approximately 2 weeks after the initial evaluation) have been shown to be helpful in identifying and dating skeletal injuries in cases of suspected child abuse. In one study, additional information regarding skeletal injury was obtained in 14 of 23 cases, and fracture detection increased 27%. The follow-up skeletal survey also assisted in dating injuries in 20%.[61] Digital transmission and display of radiographic images are becoming more common,[39] and a recent study compared the use of digitized images and screen-film radiographs in skeletal surveys performed for the evaluation of child abuse.[112] This study found that digital imaging failed to detect metaphyseal and rib fractures, was of lower quality, and required longer interpretation time. The authors raised concern regarding the adequacy of digital imaging for interpretation of suspected child abuse and recommended further study before accepting digitized images as sufficient evaluation.[112]

Some authors have advocated radionuclide skeletal scintigraphy for initial screening because of its increased sensitivity and decreased radiation dose.[98, 102] Others have argued that the growth plate, as a target organ, actually receives increased radiation exposure during scintigraphy.[104] Epiphyseal-metaphyseal fractures may not be detected on bone scans because of the normally increased radionuclide uptake in this area,[71, 72, 74] and symmetric fractures may also be missed.[71, 74] Most importantly, an abnormal bone scan is not specific for trauma and may be seen in a variety of other conditions.[102] In addition, interpretation of bone scans in children is often difficult, and even minor errors in positioning may simulate focal abnormality.[102] Scintigraphy is, however, quite sensitive for rib, some spine, and subtle diaphyseal trauma, especially in acute situations.[70, 71, 102] Therefore, radionuclide skeletal scintigraphy is recommended as a supplemental examination when the skeletal survey is negative but a strong clinical suspicion of injury exists.[64]

## RADIOGRAPHIC DATING OF INJURIES

A basic knowledge of the stages of fracture healing that can be detected radiographically is imperative for orthopaedists caring for injured children. A fracture in a radiographic stage of healing that does not correspond to the stated date of injury should arouse suspicion. Table 17–1 gives a general timetable for the various stages of fracture healing, and a brief outline is presented here. Very young infants may exhibit an accelerated rate of response, so the timetable should be considered only an estimate.

### Resolution of Soft Tissues

Obliteration of the normal fat planes and muscle boundaries occurs as a result of hemorrhage and inflammation. These changes are the first and sometimes the only evidence of fracture immediately after injury. Depending on the magnitude of injury, these changes may persist for several days.[18, 78]

### Periosteal New Bone

Radiographically, periosteal new bone formation is not evident until it calcifies, usually between 7 and 14 days in an infant; however, it may occur in as few as 4 days.

| **TABLE 17–1** | | | |
|---|---|---|---|
| Timetable of Radiographic Changes in Children's Fractures | | | |

| Category | Early | Peak | Late |
|---|---|---|---|
| Resolution of soft tissues | 2–5 days | 4–10 days | 10–21 days |
| Periosteal new bone | 4–10 days | 10–14 days | 14–21 days |
| Loss of fracture line definition | 10–14 days | 14–21 days | — |
| Soft callus | 10–14 days | 14–21 days | — |
| Hard callus | 14–21 days | 21–42 days | 42–90 days |
| Remodeling | 3 months | 1 year | 2 years to epiphyseal closure |

Adapted from O'Connor, J.F.; Cohen, J. Dating fractures. In: Kleinman, P., ed. Diagnostic Imaging of Child Abuse. Baltimore, Williams & Wilkins, 1987, pp. 103–113.

Continued subperiosteal hemorrhage caused by repetitive trauma to a nonimmobilized fracture may result in extensive or "exuberant" fracture callus.[18, 78]

### Loss of Fracture Line Definition

As necrotic bone is resorbed, the sharply defined margins of fresh fractures become blurred. The fracture gap appears to widen and becomes indistinct. It reaches a peak between 2 and 3 weeks but is not generally apparent before 1 week.[18, 78] Bucket-handle metaphyseal fractures or corner fractures can frequently be dated only by this method because periosteal new bone formation does not occur.[78]

### Soft Callus

The production plus calcification of osteoid results in a subtle increase in density that is visible radiographically and begins soon after the appearance of periosteal new bone.[18, 78]

### Hard Callus

A week or so after soft callus is visible, the fracture site will be bridged by lamellar bone. This phase of healing is complete between 3 and 6 weeks.[18, 78]

### Remodeling

Patient age, the degree of displacement, and the amount of callus formation are all variables involved in bone remodeling. A young child with a nondisplaced fracture may complete remodeling in a few months; however, an older child with a displaced or angulated fracture may continue remodeling for over a year.[18, 78]

## Fracture Patterns

Fractures of almost any bone may occur; the extremities, skull, and rib cage are the most common sites of injury.[28, 45, 51, 63, 66, 74, 79, 111] In one series, fractures of the long bones accounted for 68% of all fractures in patients who were the victims of child abuse.[14] Although no fracture pattern is absolutely pathognomonic of physical abuse, certain fracture patterns have been found to be more specific than others.[3, 8, 28, 37, 63, 71, 74, 79, 84] These patterns include metaphyseal or epiphyseal fractures (corner fractures, bucket-handle fractures, chip fractures), posterior rib fractures, multiple or wide complex skull fractures, scapular and sternal fractures, multiple fractures, and unreported fractures. Single fractures, linear narrow parietal skull fractures, long bone shaft fractures, and clavicular fractures are all associated with child abuse but have low specificity.[52, 63, 66, 105, 111] Whereas spiral fractures were the most common long bone fracture pattern reported by earlier authors,[45, 79] more recent data suggest that single, transverse long bone fractures are the most common fractures in child abuse.[37, 51, 66] Because these fractures are also seen in accidental trauma, they are not specific for abuse.[105]

## DIAPHYSEAL FRACTURES

Spiral, oblique, and transverse fractures of the long bone shafts may result from accidental or nonaccidental trauma (Figs. 17–1 and 17–2). Transverse fractures are the result of direct injury, whereas spiral fractures result from rotational or torsional forces (Fig. 17–3). An abusive parent may use either mechanism, so both fracture patterns may be seen in abuse. An isolated diaphyseal fracture is the most common fracture pattern identified in child abuse,[28, 51, 66] and diaphyseal fractures occur four times as often as "classic" metaphyseal fractures.[74] The humerus, femur, and tibia are the most

frequently injured long bones in cases of child abuse.[3, 37, 45, 51, 66, 79] Fracture of the diaphysis of a long bone in a nonambulatory child suggests child abuse until proved otherwise. Abuse should be suspected if either an unreasonable history of the cause of the fracture is described, such as a fracture occurring during a diaper change, or no true history of trauma is reported. Abuse should also be suspected if the delay in seeking medical care is inappropriate or if physical evidence of other trauma is observed. The diagnosis of abuse should be made if the child has, in addition to a diaphyseal fracture, radiologic evidence of fractures in varying stages of healing or multiple acute fractures without evidence of accidental trauma or bone disease.

Femoral shaft fractures are seen in both accidental and nonaccidental trauma; however, in children younger than 12 months, abuse accounts for 60% to 80% of these fractures.[6, 8, 42, 67, 105] A femur fracture in a nonambulatory child without a significant history of trauma requires investigation. Schwend and colleagues found that the strongest predictor of abuse was a femoral fracture in a child who had not yet achieved walking age and believed that unless other evidence of abuse existed, abuse was unlikely in a walking-age child.[89] Long, spiral fractures of the femur are common in toddlers as a result of accidental trauma and should not be considered solely the result of abuse, and several authors have recently shown that femoral shaft fracture patterns are unreliable in differentiating accidental from nonaccidental in-

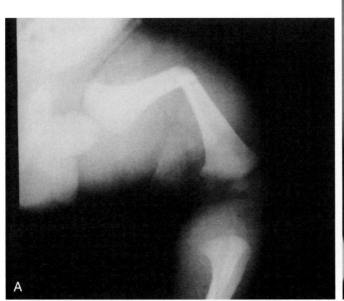
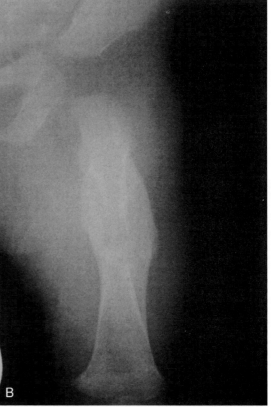

**FIGURE 17–1.** Fracture of the midshaft of the femur in an infant that was caused by nonaccidental trauma. *A,* A radiograph of the femur demonstrates a midshaft fracture of the femur with marked angulation. Fractured femurs in infants that result from child abuse may be spiral fractures but may also be simple transverse diaphyseal fractures such as seen here. This fracture was undoubtedly the result of significant force. *B,* Healing of the fracture is demonstrated after the fracture had been reduced and the limb immobilized in a hip spica cast.

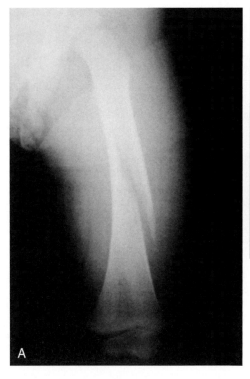
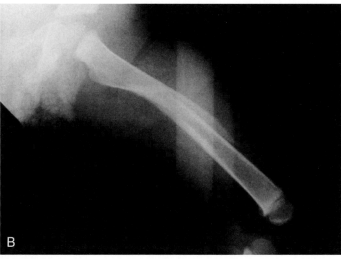

**Figure 17–2.** Fracture of the femur in a toddler that occurred as a result of accidental trauma. *A,* Anteroposterior radiograph of the femur of a 2-year-old child who tripped while running. This fracture pattern is quite typical of fractures in the toddler age group. Investigation of the family showed no evidence for suspicion, and the child had no other injuries or warning signs of abuse. *B,* Lateral radiograph demonstrating the long spiral fracture of the femur.

jury.[9, 85] Humeral shaft fractures in young children have historically had a high association with child abuse and were not generally reported as a result of accidental trauma.[51, 79, 105, 111] Worlock and colleagues found no cases of accidental humeral shaft fracture in children younger than 5 years; all the cases documented were the result of abuse. In contrast, all the supracondylar and condylar fractures of the distal end of the humerus in

their series were the result of accidental trauma.[111] However, more recent reports dispute these findings. In evaluating humeral fractures in children younger than 3 years, Strait and co-workers documented abuse in only 58% of humeral shaft fractures but found that 20% of the supracondylar fractures evaluated were associated with abuse.[101] Abuse-related injuries in this study were significantly associated with an age younger than 15

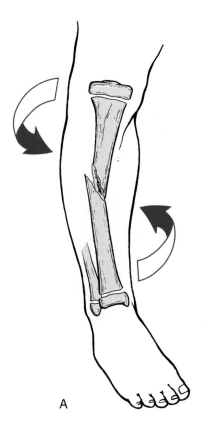
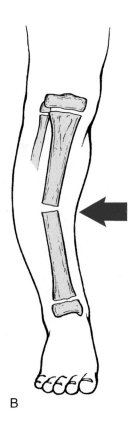

**Figure 17–3.** The mechanism of injury that will produce either a spiral fracture, which is the result of a twisting injury (*A*), or a transverse fracture, which is the result of a direct blow to a long bone (*B*).

A

B

months. Given these data, abuse should be considered an etiology in all humeral fractures (including supracondylar fractures) in children younger than 15 months.[101] Fractures of the radius and ulna, commonly seen in accidental trauma, are the least fractured long bones in child abuse.[3, 37, 45, 51, 66, 79]

One must be careful when assessing the etiology of tibial shaft fractures in children of walking age. A nondisplaced spiral tibial shaft fracture ("toddler's fracture") is very common and is a result of accidental trauma. A "toddler's fracture" typically occurs in the second and third years of life, and frequently the history of trauma is not always clear on initial examination. The parents may be unaware of the trauma because it occurred out of their sight. We are often confronted with a child who has been picked up from daycare and carried to the car and then into the house. The child may eat and go to bed without walking. In the morning, the parents are aware that the child will not walk and at that time they seek medical attention. Normally, the delayed diagnosis and lack of a clear history of trauma alert the physician to possible child abuse; however, such is not usually the case in this injury. The fracture may be difficult to identify on plain radiographs, and oblique radiographs may demonstrate the fracture in the mid- and distal portions of the tibia. In some instances, even these views fail to show the fracture, and empirical treatment is necessary. Repeat radiographs 2 to 3 weeks later will show periosteal healing about the fracture (Fig. 17–4).

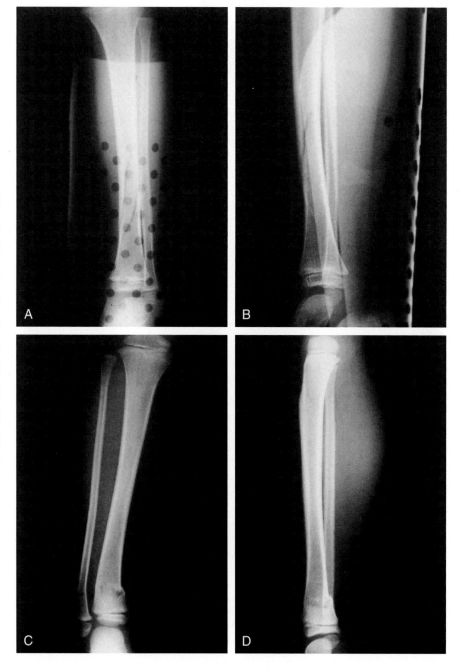

FIGURE 17–4. Fractures of the tibia are commonly seen as a result of accidental trauma in young children. *A* and *B*, Anteroposterior and lateral radiographs of the tibia of a 2-year-old child who sustained this spiral fracture of the tibia when she fell while running. This typical so-called toddler's fracture is well seen on these radiographs, but the fracture may be much more subtle and very difficult to see except on oblique radiographs. Sometimes, the fracture may not be seen on any initial radiograph, but in follow-up, periosteal healing of the fracture may be demonstrated. *C* and *D*, Anteroposterior and lateral radiographs of the tibia of a child who sustained a fracture of the distal end of the tibia in a fall. This fracture, though less common than a spiral fracture, is also the result of accidental trauma. The child and family were investigated, and no suspicion of child abuse was found. The fracture was treated with simple immobilization.

*Treatment*

Diaphyseal fractures of the long bones are optimally treated with immobilization. Fractures of the shaft of the femur are best treated with the application of an immediate spica cast. Some fractures of the shaft of the femur may be very unstable if the trauma has been significant enough to disrupt the periosteum. Therefore, close observation with repeat radiographs is necessary until union of the fracture is complete, usually within 6 weeks. Hospitalization is frequently necessary for completion of a social services investigation of the family and the circumstances of the injury.

Humeral shaft fractures should also be treated with immobilization, which is best accomplished with the application of a Velpeau bandage. This fracture will heal very quickly in an infant (Fig. 17–5).

## PERIOSTEAL NEW BONE FORMATION

Periosteum is firmly attached at the metaphysis; however, it is loosely attached along the shaft and is easily stripped. Separation of periosteum from the bone results in periosteal new bone formation and may be quite subtle.

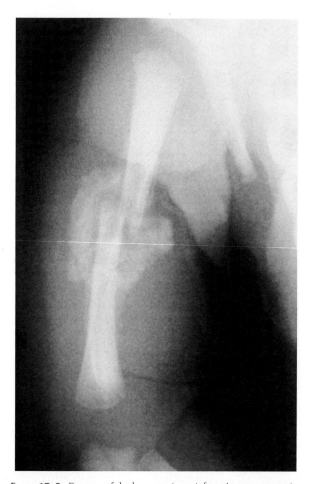

FIGURE 17–5. Fracture of the humerus in an infant. An anteroposterior radiograph of the humerus demonstrates a transverse, mid-diaphyseal fracture of the humerus that was the result of nonaccidental trauma. When the child was seen, the fracture was already healing, as demonstrated by the radiograph. The child was found to have other skeletal and soft tissue injuries.

It may be unnoticeable clinically. Scintigraphy may detect the process before radiographs confirm the injury.[22] Even though periosteal new bone formation is one of the most frequent findings in cases of abuse,[28] it is not specific for trauma and may be present in a variety of disorders.[71]

## EPIPHYSEAL-METAPHYSEAL FRACTURES

Although epiphyseal-metaphyseal fractures are much less common than diaphyseal fractures, they are much more specific for child abuse. The forces necessary to produce such fractures (traction and torsion) are unlikely to be generated from falls or other accidents[14] (Figs. 17–6 and 17–7). It was once believed that these fractures represented focal avulsion of the metaphysis, but recent pathologic radiographic studies have shown that "corner fractures" and "bucket-handle fractures" are probably the same lesion viewed in different projections[57, 59] (Fig. 17–8). The shearing forces associated with rapid acceleration-deceleration in violent shaking cause fracture through the primary spongiosa, with a disc of bone and calcified cartilage left attached to the epiphysis. Subsequent subperiosteal new bone formation does not occur because the periosteum in this area is tightly adherent and is not disrupted.[17] If present at all, periosteal reaction is often subtle. Massive periosteal reaction occurs only with displacement of the metaphyseal fragment or shearing of the periosteum itself[17, 52, 71] (see Figs. 17–7 and 17–9). The fracture margins will become indistinct with further healing.[71] These fractures may be easily overlooked acutely, and high-quality radiographs are necessary to make the diagnosis.[52–56] In addition, the absence of periosteal elevation in the healing phase makes detection of these fractures difficult. As a result, the true incidence of these fractures may be underestimated.[71]

The presence of radiolucent epiphyseal extensions of hypertrophied cartilage into the metaphysis has also been documented during the healing phase. The depth of penetration into the metaphysis is related to the age of the injury, and the configuration of the extensions is related to the degree of injury. These radiolucent epiphyseal extensions are single and focal in minor injuries and multiple and broad in extensive injuries.[80]

True physeal fractures with separation of the epiphysis frequently result from violent traction or rotation rather than shaking and may be complicated by growth disturbance and deformity.[71, 106] These fractures are uncommon in an abused child except in the distal end of the humerus and proximal ends of the humerus and femur.

## TYPE I DISTAL HUMERAL FRACTURES

The exact incidence of this type of fracture is not known because it is underdiagnosed.[26] At one time this injury was thought to be very rare, but it is now recognized more frequently. Two clear associations are seen with this fracture: birth trauma and abuse. Child abuse is the probable cause after the neonatal period. Holda and colleagues reported that a fall from a height was the cause of the fracture in their series.[46] However, three of their

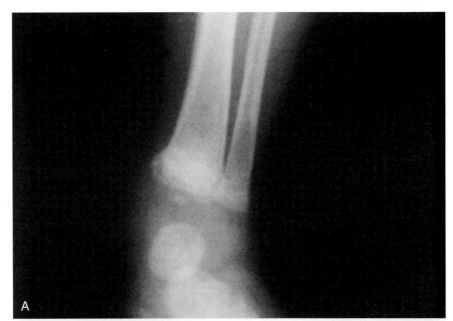

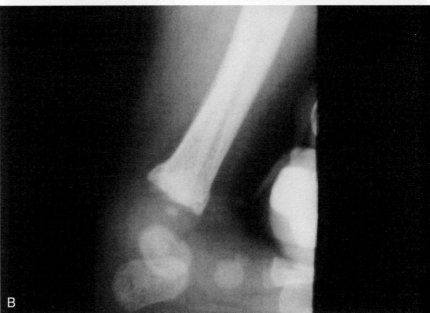

**Figure 17–6.** Corner fractures of the distal end of the tibia in an infant who was abused. *A,* Anteroposterior radiographs showing the corner fractures of both sides of the metaphysis at the level of the physis. Evidence of new bone formation is present and indicates that the fracture is more than a week old. *B,* A lateral radiograph of the same ankle also shows the corner fractures.

seven patients were younger than 18 months, thus making child abuse more likely. DeLee and co-workers reported that child abuse was proved or suspected in 6 of their 16 patients.[26] One must therefore strongly suspect the possibility of child abuse when one sees this fracture in a young child.[75]

These children present with marked swelling about the elbow, and the physical appearance of the elbow resembles a dislocation. Gentle manipulation of the elbow will reveal a muffled crepitus, which is the result of two cartilaginous surfaces rubbing against each another. It must be distinguished from bony crepitus. On an anteroposterior radiograph the radius and ulna are displaced in relation to the humerus. However, the radius and ulna are in their normal relationship to each other (Fig. 17–10). This injury must be distinguished radiographically from an elbow dislocation, a displaced

fracture of the lateral condyle of the distal end of the humerus, and a distal humeral supracondylar fracture.

Unlike a supracondylar fracture, this fracture is usually stable because it occurs through the thicker distal end of the humerus below the thin supracondylar region. Therefore, cubitus varus deformity is less likely to result than after a supracondylar fracture.[26] Holda and co-workers, however, found cubitus varus deformity in five of their seven patients.[46]

DeLee and associates recommend closed reduction if the fracture is fresh, but if the fracture is old, they recommend splinting the arm until the fracture is solid, without any attempt at reduction.[26] The results presented by Holda and colleagues tend to corroborate such management because their results with more aggressive treatment were poor.[46] Mizuno and co-workers obtained

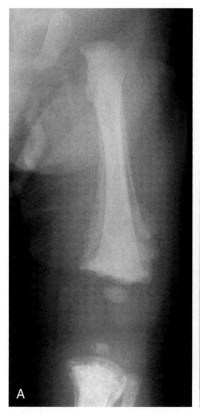
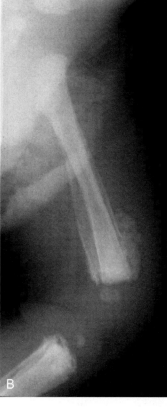

FIGURE 17–7. Infant with multiple injuries sustained as a result of child abuse. *A,* An anteroposterior radiograph of the leg in this child shows significant periosteal reaction about the distal end of the femur and proximal portion of the tibia. The child sustained both distal femoral and proximal tibial physeal fractures. The proximal tibial fracture was a so-called corner fracture. *B,* Lateral radiograph of the same extremity again showing the remarkable periosteal reaction in the femur. The periosteum was significantly stripped well beyond the midpoint of the femur, which indicates the enormous amount of trauma that the infant sustained.

good results with open reduction through a posterior approach.[75]

Our preference is to investigate the possibility of child abuse first. The child may be admitted to the hospital to facilitate this investigation, if necessary. Admission may

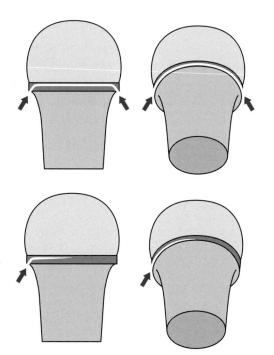

FIGURE 17–8. Corner fractures and bucket-handle fractures have been shown to be the same lesion viewed from different projections.

also be warranted to observe for circulatory change. If reduction is required, closed reduction is performed by placing gentle traction on the forearm. The medial displacement of the distal fragment is then corrected. Any malrotation is corrected, and the elbow is flexed to 90° with the forearm pronated because the medial displacement recurs with the forearm in supination.[26] The arm is splinted for 3 weeks, after which unrestricted motion is allowed.

## TYPE I PROXIMAL FEMORAL FRACTURES

Type I fractures of the proximal end of the femur are very rare and are usually the result of significant trauma, such as a motor vehicle accident or a fall from a great height. Displaced type I fractures may be associated with dislocation of the femoral head. The prognosis, particularly in the case of dislocation, is generally poor because of the extremely high incidence of avascular necrosis.

If a type I fracture of the proximal part of the femur is seen and the history of the injury does not include violent trauma, the orthopaedic surgeon should be suspicious of child abuse, especially in a child younger than 5 years. A 60% prevalence of child abuse has been documented in type I fractures of the proximal end of the femur in young children.[33]

Although the prognosis for a markedly displaced type I fracture is poor, that for a minimally displaced fracture of the proximal femoral physis has been good in our experience. Forlin and colleagues have shown that avascular necrosis of the femoral head is not as common as once feared if the femoral head is not dislocated. They

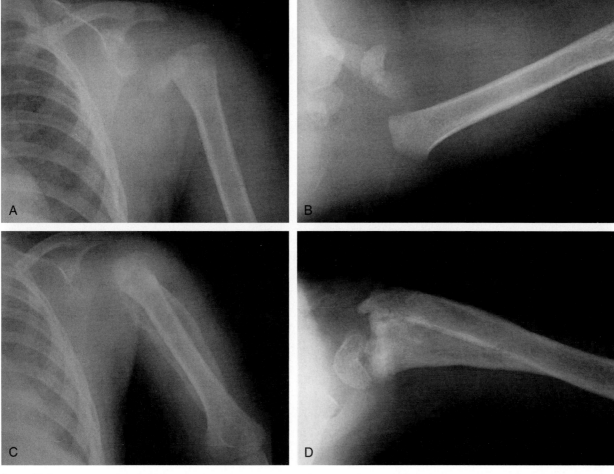

**FIGURE 17–9.** This 20-month-old child sustained a violent injury to her shoulder. When seen, she had an enormously swollen shoulder and would not move her arm. The family gave no history of trauma, but it was subsequently proved that the child had been abused. *A,* This anteroposterior radiograph demonstrates a totally displaced fracture of the proximal humeral physis. The epiphysis sits inferior to the metaphysis and the inferior portion of the glenoid. *B,* A lateral radiograph of the same shoulder and proximal part of the humerus again demonstrates the remarkable displacement of the fracture that occurred through the proximal humeral physis. *C,* This anteroposterior radiograph taken 1 month postinjury demonstrates the enormous amount of periosteal new bone formation that is occupying the entire shaft of the humerus. This finding demonstrates that this fracture was the result of violent trauma with a significant amount of periosteal stripping all the way to the distal humeral metaphysis. *D,* A lateral radiograph of the humerus 5 months after injury demonstrates that the fracture is healed with all the early remodeling. One can expect complete subsequent remodeling. At this juncture, the child had complete full range of motion of the shoulder with no pain and normal use of the arm.

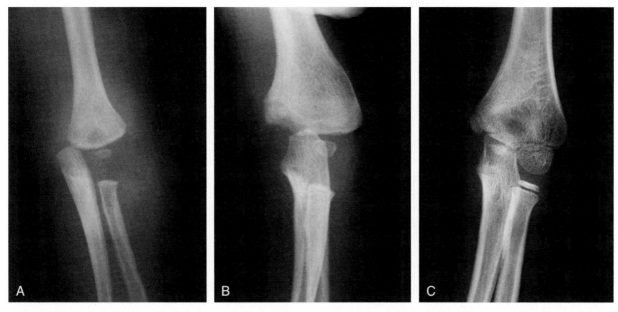

**FIGURE 17–10.** Displaced fracture of the distal humeral physis. *A,* Anteroposterior radiograph of the distal end of the humerus at the time of injury demonstrating medial displacement of the capitellum. Note that the longitudinal axis of the radius intersects the capitellum. *B,* Anteroposterior radiograph of the elbow 3 months after injury. The displacement was not corrected at the time of immobilization. *C,* Follow-up radiograph 5 years postinjury demonstrating remodeling of the distal portion of the humerus. Clinically, the patient had full mobility in the elbow.

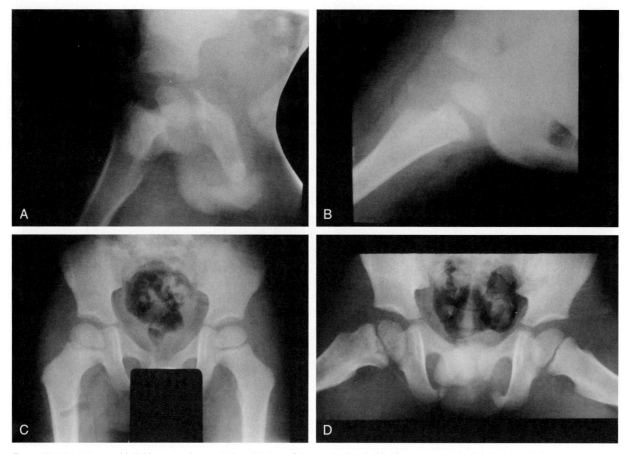

**FIGURE 17–11.** A 3-year-old child sustained a type I physeal injury of the proximal end of the femur as a result of child abuse. *A,* An anteroposterior radiograph demonstrates the angulation of the fracture but without complete displacement. *B,* A lateral radiograph of the hip and proximal end of the femur also shows the displacement of the fracture. *C,* An anteroposterior radiograph of both hips shows nearly complete remodeling of the fracture 1½ years after the injury. The fracture was not reduced, but the child was placed in a hip spica cast for 6 weeks. No evidence of avascular necrosis of the femoral head can be found. *D,* A lateral radiograph of both hips demonstrates nearly complete remodeling of the fracture.

are in accord with treatment of these fractures in a spica cast until union is complete.[33] Remodeling of the fracture is usually extensive because of the wide range of motion of the hip (Fig. 17–11).

Other Salter-Harris injuries of the physis are commonly seen in children as a result of accidental trauma but are only rarely seen in victims of child abuse.

## RIB FRACTURES

The ribs are the third most common site of skeletal injury in children who are abused,[72, 74] and 90% of abuse-related rib fractures are seen in children younger than 2 years.[74] The relatively pliant rib cage of infants and toddlers affords protection against fracture of the ribs from falls, and accidental fracture is rare.[14] Investigators have shown that even cardiopulmonary resuscitation does not cause rib fractures in children.[32] In Worlock and colleagues' series, none of the rib fractures in the infants and toddlers in their series were the result of accidental trauma.[111] Moreover, all the children and infants with rib fractures had an additional skeletal injury. Most of the rib fractures were identified incidentally on skeletal surveys.[111]

Though often clinically unsuspected, rib fractures are usually multiple and symmetric and most occur posteriorly.[64, 74] These posterior fractures result from maximal mechanical stress at the costovertebral junction as the child is grasped and shaken.[17] Lateral rib fractures are much less commonly seen in child abuse and are thought to be caused by anterior compression of the chest (Fig. 17–12). Anterior rib fractures involving the costochondral junctions have also been reported in association with major abdominal visceral injuries.[77] Rib fractures in abused children may be very difficult to diagnose radiographically in the acute setting. In a postmortem study of infants who died with inflicted injuries, only 36% of the rib fractures identified were detected by the skeletal survey.[60] These fractures are best visualized radiographically after fracture callus is evident (Fig. 17–13). Posterior rib fractures and costovertebral junction fractures are best detected acutely with bone scanning.[58]

## FRACTURES OF THE SHOULDER GIRDLE

Most accidental and abuse-related clavicular fractures involve the midshaft of the clavicle, and the diagnosis of

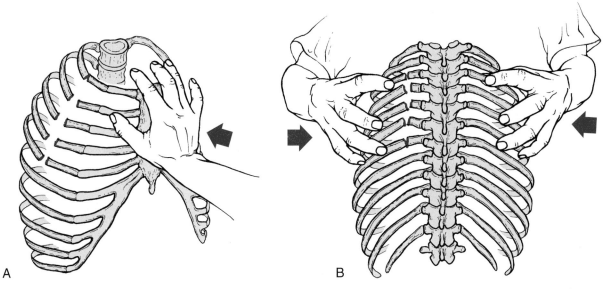

**FIGURE 17–12.** Mechanism of injury that produces rib fractures. Anteroposterior compression of the chest will most commonly result in fractures of the ribs laterally (*A*). Compression of the ribs from the side, however, will produce posterior rib fractures (*B*). This mechanism of injury is most commonly seen in children who have been abused from side-to-side compression of the infant by an adult's hands.

abuse must be made on clinical grounds.[63] Avulsion fractures of either end of the clavicle or an acromion process fracture can result from traction or the violent acceleration-deceleration in shaking.[74] Distal clavicular fractures in an infant are particularly suspicious and may be associated with proximal humeral fractures.[63]

## SPINE FRACTURES

Vertebral fractures are unusual in child abuse,[63, 103] and most involve the vertebral body. They are often found incidentally on a skeletal survey without obvious clinical findings.[45, 72] Anterior compression fractures of the lower thoracic and upper lumbar spine are thought to

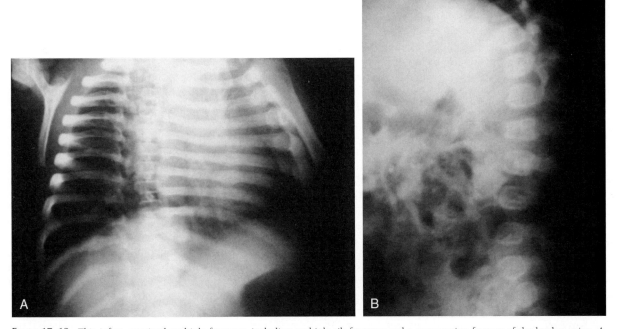

**FIGURE 17–13.** This infant sustained multiple fractures, including multiple rib fractures and a compression fracture of the lumbar spine. *A*, Multiple posterior fractures of the ribs on both sides of the chest in this infant were seen on a radiograph of the ribs taken on the day of admission to the hospital. These fractures were all healed, evidence that these injuries had occurred before admission. *B*, A lateral radiograph of the spine demonstrates a compression fracture of the second lumbar vertebra. Both these injuries were thought to be the result of intentional trauma.

result from hyperflexion of the trunk.[103] Radiographic detection of these fractures may be difficult, and bone scanning is relatively insensitive for body fractures.[62, 74] However, bone scans may demonstrate occult injuries to the transverse and spinous processes.[62, 74] Injury to the spinal cord itself is rare but may be seen in association with particularly violent trauma.[15, 35, 86, 103]

## SKULL FRACTURES

Skull fractures are common in children who have been physically abused. These fractures are second in frequency only to fractures of the long bones.[40, 42] Skull fractures occur far more often as a result of abuse than from accidental trauma.[64] Eighty percent occur in the first year of life, and they are rare after 2 years of age.[51, 74] Most abuse-related skull fractures are linear fractures, similar to those seen in accidental trauma, with the more specific depressed, wide, and complex lesions found less frequently.[73] Planar radiography is the most sensitive imaging study for skull lesions, and bone scanning is unreliable.[84, 102] Computed tomography and magnetic resonance imaging provide further information regarding intracranial injury.[84] Cerebral damage associated with the skull injury is of greatest concern. One most commonly associates cerebral injury with trauma to the skull, but brain injury can occur without external signs of head trauma.[76]

In 1974, Caffey coined the term "whiplash shaken infant syndrome,"[13] today known as the "shaken baby syndrome." This condition refers to cerebral and retinal bleeding in an infant after vigorous shaking.[13] Crying is the most commonly cited provocation for the injury.[30] The infant is held by the thorax and shaken, an action that results in cerebral and retinal bleeding in addition to fractures of the posterior aspect of the ribs.[30] Sustained subarachnoid and subdural hematomas, especially in the posterior hemispheric fissure, are visible with computed tomography.[29] If the child is held by the extremities and shaken, metaphyseal fractures and subperiosteal hemorrhage will result from the traction and shearing forces.[30] Spine and spinal cord injuries are possible with violent shaking.[30]

## Differential Diagnosis

Other conditions may be confused with child abuse. Although a thorough history and physical examination usually provide the diagnosis, additional tests may occasionally be necessary for confirmation.

## NORMAL VARIANTS

Healthy infants may exhibit periosteal new bone formation along the shafts of the long bones during the first few months of life.[38] Spurring and cupping of the metaphysis are also frequently observed.[38] These findings are initially seen between 2 and 3 months and resolve by 8 months.[11, 97] The periosteal new bone formation is identical to that seen in trauma, and the clinical findings must be taken into account.

## BIRTH TRAUMA

Birth trauma should be considered a possible etiology when a child with a fracture is seen during the first few weeks of life. Clavicular fractures are the most common fractures related to birth trauma. Fractures missed in the delivery room or nursery are frequently found incidentally on chest radiographs or when palpable callus is noted by the parents.[11] The humerus is the most commonly fractured long bone in birth trauma,[24] and these fractures usually involve the midshaft.[11] Long bone fractures of the lower extremities occurring during birth are often seen in association with neuromuscular disease or bone abnormality,[11, 24] whereas epiphyseal fractures are most commonly associated with breech delivery.[11] Rib fractures from birth trauma are rare,[11] and rib fractures found incidentally, without a history of severe trauma, are usually due to abuse. Callus will develop in birth fractures within 2 weeks,[11, 24] and lack of callus formation after this time interval strongly suggests that the injury did not occur during delivery.

## OSTEOGENESIS IMPERFECTA

Osteogenesis imperfecta (OI) is the entity that may most closely mimic child abuse. It is divided into four main types that can be further subclassified.[92–95] Type I is most common and accounts for 80% of all cases. It is inherited as an autosomal dominant disorder. The scleras are blue in this type, and it is a milder form of the disease, with fewer fractures and less bone deformity than seen in the other types.[92–95, 99]

Type II is also inherited as an autosomal dominant disorder. It is a very severe form of the disease that leads to intrauterine or early infant death. Type III is similar to type II, but milder; however, both types are characterized by extreme bone fragility, with fractures at birth and obvious bony deformity. Therefore, neither of these two types is likely to be mistaken for child abuse.

Type IV is more like type I in that it is associated with less bone fragility than in types II and III. The scleras are normal or faintly blue in infancy, although they become blue in adulthood. Types I and IV are most likely to be mistaken for child abuse.[92–95, 99] One should look for telltale signs of OI, such as wormian bones and osteopenia. Occasionally, both are absent, thereby making the diagnosis difficult. Although fractures in OI usually involve the shafts of the long bones,[11, 27] Gahagan and Rimsza have reported metaphyseal corner-type fractures also.[36] In one study of children with OI, metaphyseal fractures were seen in 15% of patients.[27] If, in addition, the child is a member of an at-risk family, one may be quick to diagnose child abuse.

A history that is incompatible with the injury is one of the hallmarks of child abuse; however, such is also the case in patients with OI. Fractures in these children may be sustained with minimal, even trivial trauma. A careful family history is important. Because of the occurrence of new mutations, a negative history does not exclude the diagnosis of OI. Currently, no single biochemical or genetic test is completely sensitive in identifying children with OI.[100] Biochemical analysis of skin fibroblast collagen to identify the abnormalities of type I collagen seen in children with OI is available, but 10% to 15% of individuals with nonlethal forms of OI will not be identified with the correct screening test.[108] The determination of OI or abuse can usually be made by careful clinical evaluation by physicians familiar with the variability of OI, and although biochemical studies may provide additional information, routine biopsy of suspected abused patients is unwarranted.[100]

## TEMPORARY BRITTLE BONE DISEASE

"Temporary brittle bone disease" (TBBD) was initially hypothesized by Paterson and colleagues as a temporary deficiency of an enzyme involved in the post-translational processing of collagen. They reported 39 patients who sustained fractures only in the first year of life and had findings similar to those seen in infantile copper deficiency[82]; however, in addition, several features of so-called TBBD (fractures in the first year of life, preponderance of rib and metaphyseal fractures, and lack of an external mechanism of trauma) are also factors proved to be associated with child abuse.[19] This theory has been refuted by others as lacking any scientific data and is not widely accepted.[1, 10, 19] Until scientifically proven, it is the responsibility of the clinician to protect any child suspected of being abused while other diagnoses are being excluded.[1]

## OSTEOMYELITIS

Multifocal metaphyseal lesions with periosteal reaction may be seen in osteomyelitis in young infants. The classic systemic signs and symptoms of infection may not be present in a neonate, thus making the diagnosis difficult. However, true corner fractures are not present, and the metaphyseal radiolucencies are less well defined in osteomyelitis. Over time, the bone destruction seen in osteomyelitis is easily differentiated from the bone formation seen in healing fractures.[11]

## RICKETS

Although metaphyseal abnormalities, fractures, and periosteal reaction may be seen in both rickets and child abuse, the additional radiographic characteristics seen in rickets allow proper diagnosis. Fraying of the metaphysis, widening of the physis, and "Looser's zones" (sharply defined, symmetric, transverse stress fractures in the shafts of long bones) are all seen in rickets but not in child abuse.[11] Multiple long bone and rib fractures are more prominent in premature infants in whom rickets develops in association with total parenteral nutrition.[11] Laboratory tests confirm the diagnosis.

## COPPER DEFICIENCY

Kinky hair disease, or Menkes' syndrome, is associated with inadequate copper absorption. The metaphyseal fractures and periosteal reaction observed in this disorder are similar to those seen with abuse. Long bone metaphyseal spurring and wormian bones in the skull

help differentiate this condition from nonaccidental trauma. Serum levels of copper and ceruloplasmin are reduced and confirm the diagnosis.[11]

## CONGENITAL SYPHILIS

The prevalence of congenital syphilis is increasing in the United States and, if unrecognized, may lead to a delay in treatment, progression of the disease, or a misdiagnosis of child abuse.[21, 48, 65] Congenital syphilis may be mistaken for child abuse because of the periosteal new bone formation and the corner metaphyseal erosions that may be mistaken for corner fractures. The Wimberger sign is a classic finding in congenital syphilis and refers to a medial tibial metaphyseal defect. Congenital syphilis is frequently diffuse and can involve not only the long bones but also the skull and the small bones of the hands and feet.[11] The epiphyses and spine are spared. The bone lesions of congenital syphilis are usually symmetric, and serologic testing confirms the diagnosis (Fig. 17–14).

## CONGENITAL INSENSITIVITY TO PAIN

Inherited as an autosomal recessive trait, this rare syndrome is difficult to differentiate from abuse. Afflicted children are normal in every aspect except for indifference to painful stimuli and occasionally temperature.[11] Multiple fractures and epiphyseal separations may be seen in various stages of healing. A detailed clinical history and careful neurologic sensory examination are required to make the diagnosis.

## CAFFEY'S DISEASE

Infantile cortical hyperostosis is a painful periosteal reaction that results in cortical thickening. It occurs in infants younger than 6 months, and its cause is unknown.[11] Although any bone may be involved, the mandible, clavicle, and ulna are the most common sites.[11] The mandible is involved in 95% of cases. Metaphyseal lesions and fractures are not seen in Caffey's disease,[11] and it is more commonly confused with osteomyelitis because of the associated inflammation (Fig. 17–15).

## VITAMIN A INTOXICATION

Fractures are rare with hypervitaminosis A. However, widening of the cranial sutures and a thick, undulating periosteal reaction of the tubular bones is frequently seen, particularly in the ulna and metatarsals.[11] Acutely, the epiphyseal and metaphyseal areas are radiographically normal, but late deformities secondary to premature epiphyseal fusion have been reported.[11] The diagnosis is confirmed by the history and vitamin A levels.[84]

## LEUKEMIA

Diffuse demineralization and periosteal reaction are both features of leukemia. Multiple localized osteolytic lesions are characteristic of leukemia, whereas sclerotic lesions are unusual. Narrow, radiolucent metaphyseal bands, or

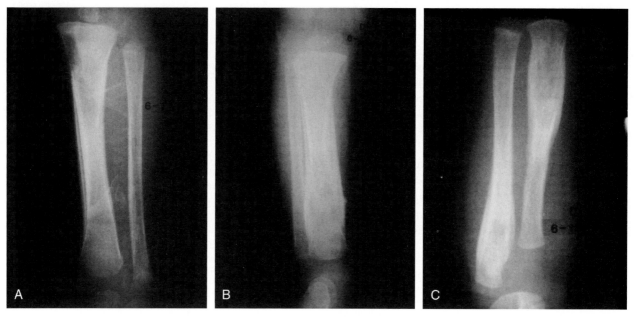

FIGURE 17–14. Radiographs of multiple bones of an infant with congenital syphilis. *A* and *B,* The radiographs show periosteal new bone in both tibias. *C,* Periosteal new bone formation in the radius and ulna.

"leukemic lines," may be seen, but the associated osteopenia and lack of bony fragments easily distinguish them from the metaphyseal lesions in child abuse.[11]

## SCURVY

Scurvy is much less common than rickets and is unusual before the age of 6 months. It is caused by inadequate vitamin C intake. Some of the radiographic changes seen in scurvy, such as subperiosteal hemorrhage and metaphyseal fractures, may also be seen in child abuse. However, bone mineralization in scurvy is impaired, and thin cortices and osteopenia allow differentiation from child abuse.[11]

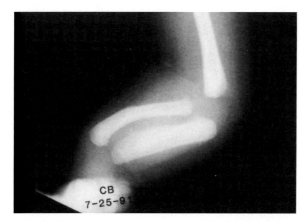

FIGURE 17–15. Caffey's disease is a rare cause of periosteal new bone formation. A radiograph of the forearm in this infant shows periosteal new bone formation in both the radius and, especially, the ulna. Frequently, such children may have fever and evidence of local inflammation, which makes the differential diagnosis of osteomyelitis more common than child abuse.

## DRUG-INDUCED BONE CHANGES

Periosteal reaction of the ribs and long bones may be seen in association with the use of prostaglandin $E_1$. The diagnosis is determined by the history because the radiologic findings are identical to those of traumatic periostitis.[11] Previously, fractures and osteopenia were reported in children treated with methotrexate, but current treatment protocols using lower doses of the drug make such fractures rare today.

A careful history and physical examination combined with thoughtful interpretation of the radiographs and confirmatory laboratory testing will generally allow a correct diagnosis even in obscure etiologies.

## Management

Evaluation of suspected child abuse is best handled by a multidisciplinary team of health care professionals. The team may include a pediatrician, a social worker, a psychiatrist, a nurse, an attorney, and a pediatric orthopaedic surgeon. Consultants may include a pediatric radiologist and a gynecologist. One individual, such as the social worker, should be designated as the contact person for the child abuse team. Such an arrangement will facilitate reporting of suspected abuse in that all contacts are made through the same person or office.

The physician should remain nonjudgmental and, if possible, attempt to establish a normal relationship with the family. If a child presents with a suspicious fracture, the physician should explain to the family that this type of fracture is one that may be seen in children who have been abused. One should never accuse the family, but rather explain in a matter-of-fact way the legal need for investigation of the injury. Most of the time, if the injury is truly accidental, the family will be understanding. If the family becomes argumentative, one's suspicions of abuse increases.

The child should be hospitalized if the suspicion of abuse is strong, even though the injury may not require it. If necessary, the child may be placed in emergency foster care. Abuse of siblings must also be considered, and care must be provided for them. Although orthopaedic surgeons will not usually assume the primary responsibility for complete evaluation and reporting of suspected child abuse, they should be aware of the process so that appropriate steps will be taken to ensure the future safety of the child.

The vast majority of orthopaedic injuries associated with child abuse occur in very young children. Healing is therefore rapid, and treatment primarily consists of simple immobilization of the injured area until the fracture has healed. Frequently, many of these children are seen some time after the original injury, and some degree of healing may already be present. Rarely will the orthopaedic injuries associated with child abuse require operative treatment acutely. Particularly in this young age group, significant remodeling is advantageous and will most often result in complete correction of the deformity over time. Injuries to the physis itself are fortunately rare because these lesions pose the highest risk of permanent deformity.

It is imperative that physicians treating fractures in children have adequate knowledge of the spectrum of injury in child abuse. Although actual treatment of the injury itself may be quite simple, identification of the problem and proper intervention in suspected child abuse are frequently much more difficult and have a much greater impact in the long term.

## REFERENCES

1. Ablin, D.S.; Sane, S.M. Non-accidental injury: Confusion with temporary brittle bone disease and mild osteogenesis imperfecta. Pediatr Radiol 27:111–113, 1997.
2. Akbarnia, B.A.; Akbarnia, N. The role of the orthopedist in child abuse and neglect. Orthop Clin North Am 7:733–742, 1976.
3. Akbarnia, B.; Torg, J.S.; Kirkpatrick, J.; Sussman, S. Manifestations of the battered-child syndrome. J Bone Joint Surg Am 56:1159–1166, 1984.
4. Albert, M.J.; Dvaric, D.M. Injuries resulting from pathologic forces: Child abuse. In: MacEwen, G.; Kasser, J.R.; Heinrick, S.D., eds. Pediatric Fractures: A Practical Approach to Assessment and Treatment. Baltimore, Williams & Wilkins, 1993, pp. 388–400.
5. Altman, D.H.; Smith, R.L. Unrecognized trauma in infants and children. J Bone Joint Surg Am 42:407–413, 1960.
6. Anderson, W.A. The significance of femoral fractures in children. Ann Emerg Med 11:174–177, 1982.
7. Anonymous: Child Maltreatment 1994: Reports from State to the National Center on Child Abuse and Neglect. Washington, DC, National Center on Child Abuse Neglect, U.S. Government Printing Office, 1996.
8. Beals, R.K.; Tufts, E. Fractured femur in infancy: The role of child abuse. J Pediatr Orthop 3:583–586, 1983.
9. Blakemore, L.C.; Loder, R.T.; Hensinger, R.N. Role of intentional abuse in children 1 to 5 years old with isolated femoral shaft fractures. J Pediatr Orthop 16:585–588, 1996.
10. Block, R.W. Child abuse—controversies and imposters. Curr Probl Pediatr 29:253–272, 1999.
11. Brill, P.W.; Winchester, P. Differential diagnosis of child abuse. In: Kleinman, P.K., ed. Diagnostic Imaging of Child Abuse. Baltimore, Williams & Wilkins, 1987, pp. 221–241.
12. Caffey, J. Multiple fractures in the long bones of infants suffering from chronic subdural hematoma. AJR Am J Roentgenol 56:163–173, 1946.
13. Caffey, J. The whiplash shaken infant syndrome: Manual shaking by the extremities with whiplash-induced intracranial and intraocular bleedings, linked with residual permanent brain damage and mental retardation. Pediatrics 54:396–403, 1974.
14. Cameron, J.M.; Rae, L.J. Atlas of the Battered Child Syndrome. Edinburgh, Churchill Livingstone, 1975.
15. Carrion, W.V.; Dorman, J.P.; Drummond, D.S.; Christofersen, M.R. Circumferential growth plate fracture of the thoracolumbar spine from child abuse. J Pediatr Orthop 16:210–214, 1996.
16. Chadwick, D.L. The diagnosis of inflicted injury in infants and young children. Pediatr Ann 21:472–483, 1992.
17. Chapman, S. Radiological aspects of non-accidental injury. J R Soc Med 83:67–71, 1990.
18. Chapman, S. The radiologic dating of injuries. Arch Dis Child 67:1063–1065, 1992.
19. Chapman, S.; Hall, C.M. Non-accidental injury or brittle bones. Pediatr Radiol 27:106–110, 1997.
20. Child Abuse. Guidelines for Intervention by Physicians and Other Health Care Providers. Seattle, Washington State Medical Association, 1990.
21. Connors, J.M.; Schumert, C.; Shapiro, R. Syphilis or abuse: Making the diagnosis and understanding the implications. Pediatr Emerg Care 14:139–142, 1998.
22. Conway, J.J.; Colins, M.; Tanz, R.R.; et al. The role of bone scintigraphy in detecting child abuse. Semin Nucl Med 23:321–333, 1993.
23. Council on Scientific Affairs. AMA diagnostic and treatment guidelines concerning child abuse and neglect. JAMA 254:796–800, 1985.
24. Cumming, W.A. Neonatal skeletal fractures: Birth trauma or child abuse. J Can Assoc Radiol 30:30–33, 1979.
25. Current Trends in Child Abuse Reporting and Fatalities: The Results of the 1991 Annual Fifty State Survey. A Program of the National Committee for Prevention of Child Abuse. Washington, DC, The National Center on Child Abuse Prevention Research. Working Paper No. 808, 1997, pp. 1–24.
26. DeLee, J.C.; Wilkins, K.E.; Rogers, L.F.; Rockwood, C.A. Fracture-separation of the distal humerus epiphysis. J Bone Joint Surg Am 62:46–51, 1980.
27. Dent, J.A.; Paterson, C.R. Fractures in early childhood: Osteogenesis imperfecta or child abuse? J Pediatr Orthop 11:184–186, 1991.
28. Drvaric, D.M.; Morrell, S.M.; Wyly, J.B.; et al. Fracture patterns in the battered child syndrome. J South Orthop Assoc 1:20–25, 1992.
29. Duhaime, A.C.; Gennarelli, T.A.; Thibault, L.E.; et al. The shaken baby syndrome: A clinical, pathological, and biomechanical study. J Neurosurg 66:409–415, 1987.
30. Dykes, L.J. The whiplash shaken infant syndrome. What has been learned? Child Abuse Negl 10:211–221, 1986.
31. Everything You Always Wanted To Know about Child Abuse and Neglect. Washington, D.C., National Center on Child Abuse and Neglect, 1991.
32. Feldman, K.W.; Brewer, D.K. Child abuse, cardiopulmonary resuscitation and rib fractures. Pediatrics 73:339–342, 1984.
33. Forlin, E.; Guille, J.; Kumar, S.; Rhee, K. Transepiphyseal fractures on the neck of the femur in very young children. J Pediatr Orthop 12:164–168, 1992.
34. Franken, E.A.; Smith, J.A. Roentgenographic evaluation of infant and childhood trauma. Pediatr Clin North Am 22:301–315, 1975.
35. Gabos, P.G.; Tuten, H.R.; Leet, A.; Stanton, R.P. Fracture-dislocation of the lumbar spine in an abused child. Pediatrics 101:473–477, 1998.
36. Gahagan, S.; Rimsza, M.E. Child abuse or osteogenesis imperfecta: How can we tell? Pediatrics 88:987–992, 1991.
37. Galleno, H.; Oppenheim, W.L. The battered child syndrome revisited. Clin Orthop 162:11–19, 1982.
38. Glaser, K. Double contour, cupping and spurring in roentgenograms of long bones in infants. AJR Am J Roentgenol 61:482–492, 1949.

39. Goldberg, M.A. Teleradiology and telemedicine. Radiol Clin North Am 34:647–665, 1996.

40. Green, F.C. Child abuse and neglect, a priority problem for the private physician. Pediatr Clin North Am 22:329–339, 1975.

41. Green, M.; Haggerty, R.J. Ambulatory Pediatrics. Philadelphia, W.B. Saunders, 1968, pp. 285–289.

42. Gross, R.H.; Stranger, M. Causative factors responsible for femoral fractures in infants and young children. J Pediatr Orthop 3:341–343, 1983.

43. Habibian, A.; Sartoris, D.J.; Resnick, D. The radiologic findings in battered child syndrome. J Musculoskel Med 4:16–33, 1988.

44. Helfer, R.E.; Slovis, T.L.; Black, M. Injuries resulting when small children fall out of bed. Pediatrics 60:535–553, 1977.

45. Herndon, W.A. Child abuse in a military population. J Pediatr Orthop 3:73–76, 1983.

46. Holda, M.E.; Manolia, A.; LaMont, R.L. Epiphyseal separation of the distal end of the humerus with medial displacement. J Bone Joint Surg Am 62:52–57, 1980.

47. Holter, J.C.; Friedman, S.B. Child abuse. Early case finding in the emergency department. Pediatrics 42:128–138, 1968.

48. Ikeda, M.K.; Jenson, H.B. Evaluation and treatment of congenital syphilis. J Pediatr 117:843–852, 1988.

49. Jackson, G. Child abuse syndrome: The cases we miss. BMJ 2:756–757, 1972.

50. Kempe, C.H.; Helfer, R.E. Helping the Battered Child and His Family. Philadelphia, J.B. Lippincott, 1972.

51. King, J.; Diefendorf, D.; Apthorp, J.; et al. Analysis of 429 fractures in 189 battered children. J Pediatr Orthop 8:585–589, 1988.

52. Kleinman, P.K. Skeletal trauma: General considerations. In: Kleinman, P.K., ed. Diagnostic Imaging of Child Abuse. Baltimore, Williams & Wilkins, 1987, pp. 5–28.

53. Kleinman, P.K.; Marks, S.C., Jr. A regional approach to the classic metaphyseal lesion in abused infants: The proximal tibia. AJR Am J Roentgenol 166:421–426, 1996.

54. Kleinman, P.K.; Marks, S.C., Jr. A regional approach to classic metaphyseal lesions in abused infants: The distal tibia. AJR Am J Roentgenol 166:1207–1212, 1996.

55. Kleinman, P.K.; Marks, S.C., Jr. A regional approach to the classic metaphyseal lesion in abused infants: The distal femur. AJR Am J Roentgenol 170:43–47, 1998.

56. Kleinman, P.K.; Marks, S.C., Jr. A regional approach to the classic metaphyseal lesion in abused infants: The proximal humerus. AJR Am J Roentgenol 167:1399–1403, 1996.

57. Kleinman, P.K.; Marks, S.C., Jr. Relationship of the subperiosteal bone collar to metaphyseal lesions in abused infants. J Bone Joint Surg Am 77:1471–1476, 1995.

58. Kleinman, P.K.; Marks, S.C., Jr.; Adams, V.I.; et al. Factors affecting visualization of posterior rib fractures in abused infants. AJR Am J Roentgenol 150:635–638, 1988.

59. Kleinman, P.K.; Marks, S.C., Jr.; Blackbourne, B. The metaphyseal lesion in abused infants: A radiologic-histopathologic study. AJR Am J Roentgenol 146:895–905, 1986.

60. Kleinman, P.K.; Marks, S.C., Jr.; Nimkin, K.; et al. Rib fractures in 31 abused infants: Postmortem radiologic-histopathologic study. Pediatr Radiol 200:807–810, 1996.

61. Kleinman, P.K.; Nimkin, K.; Spevak, M.R.; et al. Follow-up skeletal surveys in suspected child abuse. AJR Am J Roentgenol 167:893–896, 1996.

62. Kleinman, P.K.; Zito, J.L. Avulsion of spinous processes caused by infant abuse. Radiology 151:389–391, 1984.

63. Kogutt, M.S.; Swischuk, L.E.; Fagan, C.J. Patterns of injury and significance of uncommon fractures in the battered child syndrome. AJR Am J Roentgenol 121:143–149, 1974.

64. Leonidas, J. Skeletal trauma in the child abuse syndrome. Pediatr Ann 12:875–881, 1983.

65. Lim, H.K.; Smith, W.L.; Sato, Y.; Choi, J. Congenital syphilis mimicking child abuse. Pediatr Radiol 25:560–561, 1995.

66. Loder, R.T.; Bookout, C. Fracture patterns in battered children. J Orthop Trauma 5:428–433, 1991.

67. McClellan, C.Q.; Kingsbury, G.H. Fractures in the first year of life: A diagnostic dilemma? Am J Dis Child 136:26–29, 1982.

68. McClain, P.W.; Sacks, J.J.; Froehlke, R.G.; Ewigman, B.G. Estimates of fatal child abuse and neglect, United States, 1979 through 1988. Pediatrics 91:338–343, 1993.

69. McMahon, P.; Grossman, W.; Gaffney, M.; Stanitski, C. Soft-tissue injury as an indication of child abuse. J Bone Joint Surg Am 77:1179–1183, 1995.

70. McNeese, M.C.; Hebeler, J.R. The abused child: A clinical approach to identification and management. Clin Symp 29:1–36, 1977.

71. Merten, D.F.; Carpenter, B.L. Radiologic imaging of inflicted injury in the child abuse syndrome. Pediatr Clin North Am 37:815–837, 1990.

72. Merten, D.F.; Kirks, D.R.; Ruderman, R.J. Occult humeral epiphyseal fracture in battered infants. Pediatr Radiol 10:151–154, 1981.

73. Merten, D.F.; Osborne, R.S.; Radkowski, M.A.; et al. Craniocerebral trauma in the child abuse syndrome. Radiological observations. Pediatr Radiol 14:272–278, 1984.

74. Merten, D.F.; Radkowski, M.A.; Leonidas, J.C. The abused child: A radiological appraisal. Radiology 146:377–381, 1983.

75. Mizuno, K.; Hirohata, K.; Kashiwagi, D. Fracture-separation of the distal humeral epiphysis in young children. J Bone Joint Surg Am 61:570–573, 1979.

76. Morris, M.W.; Smith, S.; Cressman, J.; Ancheta, J. Evaluation of infants with subdural hematoma who lack external evidence of abuse. Pediatrics 105:549–553, 2000.

77. Ng, C.S.; Hall, C.M. Costochondral junction fractures and intra-abdominal trauma in non-accidental injury (child abuse). Pediatr Radiol 28:671–676, 1998.

78. O'Connor, J.F.; Cohen, J. Dating fractures. In: Kleinman, P.K., ed. Diagnostic Imaging of Child Abuse. Baltimore, Williams & Wilkins, 1987, pp. 103–113.

79. O'Neill, J.A., Jr.; Meacham, W.F.; Griffin, J.P.; et al. Patterns of injury in the battered child syndrome. J Trauma 13:332–339, 1973.

80. Osier, L.K.; Marks, S.C.; Kleinman, P.K. Metaphyseal extension of hypertrophied chondrocytes in abused infants indicate healing fractures. J Pediatr Orthop 13:249–254, 1993.

81. Overpeck, M.D.; Brenner, R.A.; Trumble, A.C.; et al. Risk factors for infant homicide in the United States. N Engl J Med 339:1211–1216, 1998.

82. Paterson, C.R.; Burns, J.; McAlion, S.J. Osteogenesis imperfecta: The distinction from child abuse and the recognition of a variant form. Am J Med Genet 45:187–192, 1993.

83. Radkowski, M.A. The battered child syndrome: Pitfalls in radiological diagnosis. Pediatr Ann 12:894–899, 1983.

84. Radkowski, M.A.; Merten, D.F.; Leonidas, J.C. Abused child: Criteria for the radiologic diagnosis. Radiographics 3:262–297, 1983.

85. Rex, C.; Kay, D.R. Features of femoral fractures in nonaccidental injury. J Pediatr Orthop 20:411–413, 2000.

86. Rooks, V.J.; Sisler, C; Burton, B. Cervical spine injury in child abuse: Report of two cases. Pediatr Radiol 28:193–195, 1998.

87. Salzinger, S.; Feldman, R.S.; Hammer, M.; Rosario, M. The effects of physical abuse on children's social relationships. Child Dev 64:169–187, 1993.

88. Schmitt, B.; Clemmens, M. Battered child syndrome. In: Touloukin, R., ed. Pediatric Trauma. St. Louis, Mosby–Year Book, 1990, pp. 161–187.

89. Schwend, R.M.; Werth, C.; Johnston, A. Femur shaft fractures in toddlers and young children: Rarely from child abuse. J Pediatr Orthop 20:475–481, 2000.

90. Sedlak, A.J.; Broadhurst, D.D. Executive Summary of the Third National Incidence Study of Child Abuse and Neglect. Washington, DC, Department of Health and Human Services, National Clearinghouse on Child Abuse and Neglect Information, 1996.

91. Sheinkop, M.B.; Gardner, H.R. Child abuse as seen by the orthopaedic surgeon. Paper Presented at the 41st Annual Meeting of the American Academy of Orthopaedic Surgeons, 1974, Dallas.

92. Sillence, D.O. Abnormalities of density of modeling in the skeleton. In: Behrman, R.E.; Vaughan, V.C., eds. Nelson's Textbook of Pediatrics. Philadelphia, W.B. Saunders, 1983, pp. 1645–1647.

93. Sillence, D.O. Osteogenesis imperfecta: An expanding panorama of variants. Clin Orthop 159:11–25, 1983.

94. Sillence, D.O.; Barlow, K.K.; Cole, W.G.; et al. Osteogenesis imperfecta type III. Delineation of the phenotype with reference to genetic heterogeneity. Am J Med Genet 23:821–832, 1986.

95. Sillence, D.O.; Senn, A.S.; Danks, D.M. Genetic heterogeneity in osteogenesis imperfecta. J Med Genet 16:101–116, 1979.

96. Silverman, F.N. The roentgen manifestations of unrecognized skeletal trauma in infants. AJR Am J Roentgenol 69:413–427, 1953.

97. Silverman, F.N. Radiologic and special diagnostic procedures. In: Kempe, C.H.; Helfer, R.E., eds. The Battered Child, 3rd ed. Chicago, University of Chicago Press, 1980, pp. 215–240.

98. Smith, F.W.; Gilday, D.L.; Ash, J.M.; et al. Unsuspected costo-vertebral fractures demonstrated by bone scanning in the child abuse syndrome. Pediatr Radiol 10:103–106, 1980.

99. Smith, R. Osteogenesis imperfecta. BMJ 289:394–395, 1984.

100. Steiner, R.D.; Pepin, M.; Byers, P.H. Studies of collagen synthesis and structure in the differentiation of child abuse from osteogenesis imperfecta. J Pediatr 128:542–547, 1996.

101. Strait, R.T.; Siegel, R.M.; Shapiro, R.A. Humeral fractures without obvious etiologies in children less than 3 years of age: When is it abuse? Pediatrics 96:667–671, 1995.

102. Sty, J.R.; Strashak, F.J. The role of scintigraphy in the evaluation of the suspected abused child. Radiology 146:369–375, 1963.

103. Swischuk, L.E. Spine and spinal cord trauma in the battered child syndrome. Radiology 92:733–738, 1969.

104. Thomas, S.R.; Gelfand, M.J.; Kerelakes, J.G.; et al. Dose to the metaphyseal growth complexes in children undergoing 99mTc-EHCP bone scans. Radiology 126:193–195, 1978.

105. Thomas, S.A.; Rosenfield, N.S.; Leventhal, J.M.; Markowitz, R.I. Long-bone fractures in young children: Distinguishing accidental injuries from child abuse. Pediatrics 88:471–476, 1991.

106. Thompson, G.H.; Gesler, J.W. Proximal tibial epiphyseal fracture in an infant. J Pediatr Orthop 4:114–117, 1984.

107. Walker, A.; Chernoff, R.; Joffe, A.; Wilson, M.E.H. Office pediatrics. Child abuse, sudden infant death syndrome, infectious disease, and vaccinations. Curr Opin Pediatr 6:225–231, 1994.

108. Wenstrup, R.J.; Willing, M.C.; Starman, B.J.; Byers, P.H. Distinct biochemical phenotypes predict clinical severity in nonlethal variants of osteogenesis imperfecta. Am J Hum Genet 46:975–982, 1990.

109. Wilkinson, W.S.; Han, D.P.; Rappley, M.D.; Owings, C.L. Retinal hemorrhage predicts neurologic injury in the shaken baby syndrome. Arch Ophthalmol 107:1472–1474, 1989.

110. Worlock, P.; Stower, M. Fracture patterns in Nottingham children. J Pediatr Orthop 6:656–660, 1986.

111. Worlock, P.; Stower, M.; Barbor, P. Patterns of fractures in accidental and nonaccidental injury in children: A comparative study. BMJ 293:100–102, 1986.

112. Youmans, D.C.; Don, S.; Hildebolt, C.; et al. Skeletal surveys for child abuse: Comparison of interpretation using digitized images and screen-film radiographs. AJR Am J Roentgenol 171:1415–1419, 1998.

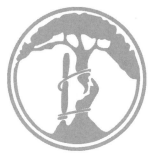

# CHAPTER 18

# Anesthesia and Analgesia for the Ambulatory Management of Children's Fractures

Eric C. McCarty, M.D.
Gregory A. Mencio, M.D.

The goal of anesthesia in the management of fractures in children is to provide analgesia and relieve anxiety to facilitate successful closed treatment of the skeletal injury. Optimal pain management in the emergency department or other ambulatory setting is delivered by the combined efforts of the orthopaedic surgeon and anesthesiologist or emergency medicine specialist. Numerous techniques are available to control pain associated with fractures in children, including *blocks* (local, regional, and intravenous [IV]), *sedation* (conscious, deep), and *general anesthesia*. Important factors in choosing a particular technique include efficacy, safety, ease of administration, cost, and patient/parent acceptance.

Local and regional techniques such as hematoma, brachial plexus, and IV regional blocks are particularly effective for upper extremity fractures. Sedation with inhalational agents such as nitrous oxide, parenteral narcotic-benzodiazepine combinations, and ketamine is not region specific and is suitable for patients over a wide range of ages. With any of these techniques, proper monitoring and adherence to safety guidelines are essential. The purpose of this chapter is to describe current methods of analgesia and sedation for fracture management in children.

## BACKGROUND

Fractures in children are common. The majority (approximately 65%) involve the upper extremity, and most are closed and best treated by closed reduction. Time, logistics, and cost favor treatment in the emergency department or other ambulatory setting, as opposed to the operating room, when possible. In a study of axillary block anesthesia for the treatment of pediatric forearm fractures in the emergency department, Cramer and colleagues estimated a cost reduction of almost 70% when compared with similar treatment in the operating room.[18]

To be able to perform satisfactory closed treatment of musculoskeletal injuries in an ambulatory setting, effective and safe levels of sedation and analgesia are essential to minimize pain and allay apprehensions in the child.[43, 61] A variety of anesthetic techniques are available to an orthopaedic surgeon faced with the challenge of treating a child with a closed fracture.

## PRINCIPLES OF PAIN MANAGEMENT IN CHILDREN

Children with fractures typically have a great deal of pain and apprehension. Psychologically, their perceptions of the emergency department and the impending treatment of their injury often exacerbate their level of discomfort and anxiety.[51] Children with painful injuries who are about to undergo additionally painful treatment are entitled to adequate analgesia and sedation. Despite the rationale of this concept, the problem of undertreatment of pain in children in the emergency department has been documented and is still an all-too-common occurrence.[6, 30, 34, 46, 52–55, 66] Ignorance of the problem of pain in children, lack of familiarity with the methods of anesthesia and sedation in children, and apprehension of complications such as respiratory depression and hypotension are reasons for the often inadequate management of pain in the pediatric population.[30, 34, 46, 48, 50–54, 57, 66]

In recognition of the increase in the number of minor procedures performed on children in a variety of ambulatory settings, the American Academy of Pediatrics (AAP) has developed goals for sedation and analgesia in children: ensure the child's safety and welfare while minimizing the physical discomfort and negative psychologic impact frequently associated with treatment of painful injuries, control the child's behavior, and return the child to a state in which safe discharge is possible.[3]

From a practical perspective, the method of analgesia/sedation must also allow for satisfactory treatment of the primary problem. Thus, efficacy, safety, ease of administration, patient/parent acceptance, and cost are all important factors to be considered when selecting a technique.[61]

From an orthopaedic perspective, the ultimate goal of anesthesia for a child with a closed fracture requiring manipulation is to facilitate satisfactory reduction of the injury and obviate the need for a trip to the operating room. The *ideal* method would be efficacious and safe in eliminating pain, promoting patient compliance, and producing amnesia of the procedure. It would be easy to administer, predictable in its action, and reliable for a wide range of ages. It would have a rapid onset and short duration of action, result in no complications or side effects, and be reversible. Finally, the ideal method would be relatively inexpensive to administer and completely satisfactory to the child and parents.*

## ANESTHETIC TECHNIQUES

A variety of techniques short of general anesthesia have been espoused to achieve analgesia and sedation in children with closed fractures requiring treatment in the ambulatory setting. The techniques can be grouped into two broad categories: *blocks* (local, regional, and IV) and conscious or deep *sedation* (anxiolytics, narcotic analgesics, or dissociative agents alone or in combination). Each technique incorporates various aspects of the "ideal" method just described. It is incumbent on orthopaedic surgeons treating children's fractures to be aware of the various techniques and the potential benefits, side effects, and complications of each to be able to make an educated decision about which to use in a particular situation.

### Techniques to Be Avoided

Vocal or "OK" anesthesia is a technique that entails verbal assurance to the child that manipulation of the fracture will be only briefly painful. The concept that children are somehow more resilient to pain has been disproved as knowledge of the developmental and psychologic makeup of children and their perception of pain has become better understood.[30, 34, 41] The notion that children need to endure pain during the performance of therapeutic or diagnostic procedures has become dated with the evolution of techniques in pediatric pain management.[47, 50, 53] Given the availability of many safe and effective options for pain management during the reduction of children's fractures, the technique of "verbal reassurance" should be avoided if possible.

Chloral hydrate and the so-called lytic cocktail, a combination of Demerol (meperidine), Phenergan (promethazine), and Thorazine (chlorpromazine) (DPT), are two techniques of sedation that have been popular

historically but have fallen out of favor more recently.[4, 8] Chloral hydrate was introduced in 1832 and continues to be the most common sedative for children undergoing *painless* diagnostic procedures.[8] Although it has been demonstrated to be effective for the sedation of young children (younger than 6 years) undergoing therapeutic procedures, it has several disadvantages for the management of fractures in children.[50] The onset of sedation is slow (40 to 60 minutes), and recovery can be prolonged and take up to several hours, with residual effects lasting as long as 24 hours. Moreover, chloral hydrate has no analgesic properties, and children can become disinhibited and agitated in response to painful stimuli. For these reasons, chloral hydrate is, at best, an antiquated technique for sedation in the management of fractures in children.[8, 38, 47, 48, 50, 51, 54]

The DPT combination, also known as the "lytic cocktail," is the second most commonly used method of sedation for children undergoing *painless* diagnostic tests and the one most widely used in children undergoing therapeutic procedures for the last 30 years.[4] This drug "cocktail" is typically administered by a single intramuscular (IM) injection, although it can be given IV and provides sedation with some analgesia.

Despite widespread use, the lytic cocktail has many undesirable characteristics. The combination is poorly titrated with a delayed onset of action (20 to 30 minutes). The duration of sedation can last up to 20 hours, whereas the duration of analgesia is shorter, only 1 to 3 hours. The mixture does not have any anxiolytic or amnestic properties.[4] Recently, it has been argued that the DPT/lytic cocktail is an empirical mixture of drugs not based on sound pharmacologic data that has a relatively frequent occurrence of therapeutic failure (29%) and a relatively high rate (approximately 4%) of serious adverse effects such as seizures, respiratory depression, and death.[4, 50, 56, 60] For these reasons, the use of DPT is discouraged by both the U.S. Agency for Health Care Policy and Research and the AAP.[4, 60]

### Local/Regional Anesthesia

Local anesthetics work by blocking the conduction of nerve impulses. At the cellular level, they depress sodium ion flux across the nerve cell membrane and, in this way, inhibit the initiation and propagation of action potentials.[64] After injection, local anesthetics diffuse toward their intended site of action and also toward the nearby vasculature, where uptake is determined by the number of capillaries, local blood flow, and the affinity of the drug for the tissues. After vascular uptake, elimination occurs by metabolism in the plasma or liver. Vasoconstrictors such as epinephrine are mixed with local anesthetics to decrease vascular uptake and prolong the anesthetic effect.

Local anesthetics are classified chemically as either amines or esters (Table 18–1). After absorption in the blood, esters are broken down by plasma cholinesterase whereas amines are bound by plasma proteins and then metabolized in the liver. Local adverse effects include erythema, swelling, and rarely, ischemia when injected

---

*See references 5, 9, 14, 16–18, 21, 25–27, 31, 32, 36, 47, 48, 50, 51, 56, and 61.

**TABLE 18–1** •••••••••••••••••••••••••••••••••••••••••••••••••••••••••••••••••••••••••••••••••••••••••••••••••••

Local Anesthetics

| Generic Name | Brand Name | Onset | Duration | Maximal Dose |
|---|---|---|---|---|
| **AMINES** | | | | |
| Lidocaine | Xylocaine | Fast | 1.0–2.0 hr | 5 mg/kg, 7 mg/kg (epinephrine) |
| Mepivacaine | Carbocaine | Fast (infiltration) | 1.5–3.0 hr | 5 mg/kg |
| Bupivacaine | Marcaine | Slow | 4.0–12.0 hr | 3 mg/kg |
| **ESTERS** | | | | |
| Chlorprocaine | Nesacain | Fast | 30–60 min | 15 mg/kg |
| Procaine | Novocain | Fast (infiltration) | 30–60 min | 7 mg/kg |
| | | Slow (block) | | |
| Tetracaine | Pontocaine | Slow (topical) | 30–60 min | 2 mg/kg |

into tissues supplied by terminal arteries. Adverse systemic effects are caused by high blood levels of local anesthetics and include tinnitus, drowsiness, visual disturbances, muscle twitching, seizures, respiratory depression, and cardiac arrest. Bupivacaine is particularly dangerous because it binds with high affinity to myocardial contractile proteins and can cause cardiac arrest.

A number of local and regional techniques, including hematoma, IV regional, and regional nerve blocks have been reported to be variably effective in providing anesthesia for fracture treatment in children. These methods require the surgeon to be familiar with regional anatomy, have working knowledge of the pharmacokinetics and dosing of local anesthetic drugs, and be proficient in the techniques of administering them. When compared with adults, these techniques are often technically easier to perform in children because anatomic landmarks are more readily identifiable.[28] Physiologically, the relatively smaller calibers of the peripheral nerves in children are more susceptible to the pharmacologic actions of anesthetic agents.[63]

## Hematoma Block

The hematoma block has been a popular method of anesthesia for the reduction of fractures, particularly in the distal end of the radius, but also about the ankle.[1, 2, 13, 20, 35] This technique entails the injection of a local anesthetic agent directly into the hematoma surrounding the fracture. The anesthetic inhibits the generation and conduction of painful impulses primarily in small nonmyelinated nerve fibers in the periosteum and local tissues.[47] This block is quick and relatively simple to administer. The skin is prepared with a bactericidal agent and draped at the site of infiltration. The fracture hematoma is aspirated with a 20- or 22-gauge needle and then injected with plain lidocaine. The typical dose of lidocaine is 3 to 5 mg/kg, which should be concentrated so that the total amount of fluid injected is limited to less than 10 mL to avoid elevating soft tissue compartment pressure and minimize the risk of creating a compartment syndrome or other neurovascular problem.[65] Although direct injection of the hema-

toma theoretically converts a closed fracture into an open one, infection has not been reported with this technique.[13]

Children as young as 2 years have been included in reports of this technique. However, no studies have involved the exclusive administration of hematoma block anesthesia to a pediatric population. In three separate studies authored by Dinley and Michelinakis (1973), Case (1985), and Johnson and Noffsinger (1991) with a combined total of 491 adult *and* pediatric patients, hematoma block was shown to be effective for the reduction of a variety of fractures of the distal end of the upper extremity in patients of *all* ages.[13, 20, 35] Despite this generally favorable experience with hematoma block anesthesia, other methods of regional anesthesia have been shown to be more effective for the management of upper extremity fractures. A study by Abbaszadegan and Jonsson (1990) found that analgesia during fracture reduction was superior with IV regional (Bier block) anesthesia than with a hematoma block and that fracture alignment after reduction was better as well. The authors concluded that the more favorable outcomes achieved with Bier block were related to better analgesia and muscle relaxation.[1]

## Intravenous Regional Anesthesia

IV regional anesthesia was originally described in 1908 by August Bier, who used IV cocaine to obtain analgesia.[9, 36] Subsequently, a number of studies have described the effective use of this technique of anesthesia for the treatment of upper extremity fractures in children in an ambulatory setting.* The block has also been described with lower extremity fractures but is less commonly used.[37]

The technique for administering a Bier block in the upper extremity involves placement of a deflated pneumatic cuff above the elbow of the injured extremity. Holmes introduced the concept of two cuffs in an effort to minimize tourniquet discomfort with prolonged inflation, but the practice has not proved to be necessary

*See references 5, 7, 9, 12, 15, 16, 22–24, 33, 36, 37, 44, and 58.

for the limited amount of time that it takes for fracture reduction in a child.[5, 9, 16] The tourniquet should be secured with tape to prevent Velcro failure.[44] IV access is established in a vein on the dorsum of the hand of the injured extremity with a 22- or 23-gauge butterfly needle. The arm is exsanguinated by elevating it for 1 to 2 minutes. Although exsanguination with a circumferential elastic bandage is described classically, this method can be more painful and difficult to perform in an injured extremity and is no more efficacious than the gravity method.[9, 16, 27, 36] The blood pressure cuff is then rapidly inflated to either 100 mm Hg above systolic blood pressure or between 200 and 250 mm Hg.[5, 9, 16, 27, 36, 44] The arm is lowered after cuff inflation. Lidocaine is administered, the IV catheter removed, and reduction of the fracture performed. In the traditional technique, the lidocaine dose is 3 to 5 mg/kg,[5, 16, 44] and in the "minidose" technique, it is 1 to 1.5 mg/kg.[9, 22, 27, 36]

The tourniquet is kept inflated until the fracture is immobilized and radiographs are obtained in case repeat manipulation is necessary. In any event, the tourniquet should remain inflated for at least 20 minutes to permit the lidocaine to diffuse and become adequately fixed to the tissues, thus minimizing the risk of systemic toxicity.[44, 59] The blood pressure cuff may be deflated in either a single stage or graduated fashion, although single-stage release has proved to be clinically safe and technically simpler.[22, 36, 44]

During the entire procedure, basic monitoring is required, and cardiac monitoring is suggested in case toxicity occurs. Routine IV access in the noninjured extremity may be beneficial but is not required.[5, 27] Patients should be observed for at least 30 minutes after cuff deflation for any adverse systemic reactions. Motor and sensory function typically returns during this period and allows assessment of the neurovascular status of the injured extremity before discharge.[59]

The literature within the past decade certainly speaks to the effectiveness of the traditional Bier block, with a lidocaine dose of 3 to 5 mg/kg, in managing forearm fractures in children. Four large series with a total of 895 patients undergoing this technique[5, 16, 44, 58] demonstrated satisfactory anesthesia and successful fracture reduction in over 90% of cases (Table 18–2). The most common adverse effect of the procedure in these studies was tourniquet pain in about 6% of patients.[16, 58] One

patient experienced transient dizziness and circumoral paresthesia.[58] Persistent myoclonic twitching developed in one patient after tourniquet deflation, and the patient was admitted for observation.[44]

Despite the efficacy and relatively low number of complications with the "traditional" Bier block (lidocaine, 3 to 5 mg/kg), concern and anecdotal reports of systemic lidocaine toxicity (i.e., seizures, hypotension, tachycardia, arrhythmias) have prompted the development of a "minidose" (lidocaine, 1 to 1.5 mg/kg) technique of IV regional anesthesia.[9, 22, 36] Reports by Farrell and associates and Bolte and co-workers of anesthesia with a lidocaine dose of 1.5 mg/kg and by Juliano and colleagues with a dose of 1.0 mg/kg on a total of 218 patients have shown the minidose Bier block to be effective in achieving adequate anesthesia in 94% of the children studied (Table 18–3).[9, 22, 36]

The primary site of action of the IV regional block is thought to be the small peripheral nerve branches. At this anatomic level, blockade is better achieved with a larger volume of anesthetic that can be distributed more completely to the peripheral nerve receptors. It appears to be the quantity (i.e., volume) and not the dose of anesthetic that predicates success of the block. For any given dose of lidocaine, diluting the concentration permits the administration of a larger volume of fluid (Table 18–4). This mechanism explains the success with the minidose technique. In the series by Juliano and co-workers, forearm fracture reduction was pain free in 43 of 44 patients (98%) after an IV regional block achieved with a very dilute lidocaine solution (0.125%) and a relatively small total dose (1 mg/kg).[36]

IV regional anesthesia using either the traditional or the minidose technique has several advantages. The technique is fairly easy to administer. The onset of action of the block is relatively fast (<10 minutes), but also of relatively short duration, which allows for assessment of neurovascular function in the extremity after fracture reduction and immobilization. An empty stomach is not required. Tourniquet discomfort is the most common adverse side effect. Inadvertent cuff deflation with loss of analgesia or the onset of systemic toxicity is a potentially significant problem. Compartment syndrome has also been reported. Technically, placing the tourniquet and obtaining IV access in the injured extremity can be a challenge in an uncooperative child, and application of

---

**TABLE 18–2**

Results with "Traditional"* IV Regional Anesthesia (Bier Block) for Forearm Fracture Reduction in Children

| Author | Lidocaine Dose | Good/Excellent Anesthesia | Successful Fracture Reduction | Adverse Effects |
|---|---|---|---|---|
| Turner et al. (1986) | 0.5%, 3 mg/kg | 177/205 (86%) | 98% | Tourniquet pain (12), dizziness (1), circumoral paresthesia (1) |
| Olney et al. (1988) | 0.5%, 3 mg/kg | 361/401 (90%) | 98% | Myoclonus (1) |
| Barnes et al. (1991) | 0.5%, 3–5 mg/kg | 100/100 (100%) | 100% | None |
| Colizza and Said (1993) | 0.5%, 3 mg/kg | 139/139 (100%) | 96% | Tourniquet pain (10) |

*The traditional technique uses 3 to 5 mg/kg of 0.5% lidocaine.
Adapted from McCarty, E.M., et al. J Am Acad Orthop Surg 7:84, 1999.

**TABLE 18–3**

Results with the "Minidose"* Bier Block for Forearm Fracture Reduction in Children

| Author | Lidocaine Dose | Good/Excellent Anesthesia | Successful Fracture Reduction | Adverse Effects |
|---|---|---|---|---|
| Farrell et al. (1985) | 0.5%, 1.5 mg/kg | 29/29 (100%) | 100% | None |
| Juliano et al. (1992) | 0.125%, 1.0 mg/kg | 43/44 (98%) | 100% | Tourniquet pain (1) |
| Bolte et al. (1994) | 0.5%, 1.5 mg/kg | 61/66 (92%) | 100% | Tourniquet pain (2), local reaction (3) |

*The "minidose" technique uses 1.0 to 1.5 mg/kg lidocaine.
Adapted from McCarty, E.M., et al. J Am Acad Orthop Surg 7:84, 1999.

the splint or cast can be cumbersome with the tourniquet in place.

## Axillary Block

The brachial plexus supplies all the motor function to the upper extremity and sensation to the lower two thirds of the limb. It is formed from the fifth through eighth cervical and first thoracic nerve roots with occasional contributions from the fourth cervical and second thoracic nerves. A continuous fascial sheath that extends from the cervical transverse processes to the axilla encases it. Regional blockade of the brachial plexus within this sheath may be performed at the interscalene, supraclavicular, infraclavicular, or axillary level (Fig. 18–1).

An axillary block provides excellent anesthesia for the forearm and hand. Initial use of the technique is attributed to Halsted and Hall, who first used an axillary block for outpatient procedures in 1884. The technique has since proved to be a safe and reliable method of anesthesia for a variety of outpatient surgical procedures in the upper extremity in both adults and children.[63] It is an excellent choice of anesthesia for the treatment of fractures below the elbow because it provides muscle relaxation in addition to analgesia. Cramer and coauthors

**TABLE 18–4**

Effect of Lidocaine Dose and Concentration on Infusion Volume

Lidocaine dose (mg/mL) = Lidocaine concentration (mg/dl) × 10
  *Examples:* 1.0% lidocaine = 10 mg/mL; 0.125% lidocaine = 1.25 mg/mL
Calculations of infusion volumes for a 20-kg child with the traditional and minidose techniques
  Dose (mg/kg) × body wt (kg) ÷ lidocaine concentration (mg/mL) = IV infusion volume (mL)
  3 mg/kg × 20 kg ÷ 5 mg/mL (0.5% lidocaine) = 12 mL of 0.5% lidocaine
  1 mg/kg × 20 kg ÷ 1.25 mg/mL (0.125% lidocaine) = 16 mL of 0.125% lidocaine

Decreasing the concentration of lidocaine with the minidose technique permits the infusion of a larger volume (milliliters) of anesthetic with a lower risk of systemic toxicity because the total amount (milligrams) of lidocaine is much lower than with the traditional technique.

reported on the successful use of axillary anesthesia by orthopaedic surgeons in the emergency department for the reduction of forearm fractures in children.[18] In this study, effective anesthesia was achieved in 105 of 111 (95%) children with no complications.

Axillary block anesthesia is administered by placing the child in a supine position with the injured arm abducted and externally rotated 90°. IV access is usually established in the uninjured extremity. Mild sedation may be helpful before the procedure. The axilla is prepared with a bactericidal solution and draped with sterile towels. The block is performed with a 1.0% lidocaine solution at a dose of 5 mg/kg. As with the Bier block, a larger volume of local anesthetic is preferable and can be achieved by using a more dilute concentration of drug. The target for delivery of the anesthetic agent is the axillary sheath, which contains the axillary artery and vein surrounded by the radial nerve (behind), median nerve (above), and ulnar nerve (below). The musculocutaneous nerve courses outside this sheath through the coracobrachialis muscle and, for this reason, may escape blockade, thus explaining the unreliability of this technique for anesthesia above the elbow.

Several techniques have been described to ensure accurate delivery of anesthetic into the axillary sheath, including blind injection into the neurovascular sheath, patient-reported paresthesia, use of a nerve stimulator, and transarterial puncture. Elicitation of paresthesias provides reliable evidence of position within the neurovascular sheath, but it may be uncomfortable and requires a conscious and cooperative patient. For these reasons, it cannot be used in most children. The use of a nerve stimulator and insulated needle to elicit a motor response is another effective method to determine accurate location within the sheath. However, this technique requires special equipment (nerve stimulator and insulated needles) that may not be readily available in an ambulatory setting, and threshold stimulation of the nerves may be distressing in a conscious patient.

The transarterial method is the most popular technique of axillary block and, as described in the study by Cramer and colleagues, has been shown to be an effective way to administer this block in children (Fig. 18–2A and B). With this method, the axillary artery is palpated, and a 23-gauge butterfly needle, connected via extension tubing to a syringe containing lidocaine, is inserted perpendicular to the artery. The needle is advanced while

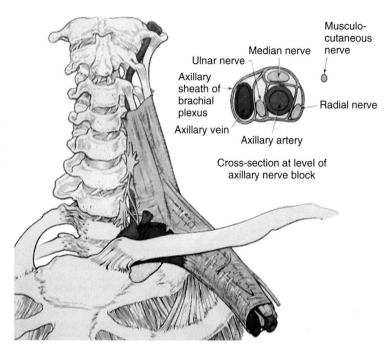

FIGURE 18–1. Brachial plexus sheath. A continuous fascial sheath extending from the cervical transverse processes to just beyond the axillary region completely surrounds the brachial plexus. Common sites for blockade of the brachial plexus within this sheath include the interscalene, infraclavicular, and axillary regions. (Adapted from Bridenbaugh, L.D. In: Cousins, M.J.; Bridenbaugh, P.O., eds. Neural Blockade in Clinical Anesthesia and Management of Pain, 2nd ed. Philadelphia, J.B. Lippincott, 1988, p. 392.)

being continuously aspirated until a flash of arterial blood is seen, and it is then advanced through the artery. Approximately two thirds of the lidocaine is injected into the sheath deep to the artery, with aspiration after every 5 mL to ensure extravascular positioning. The needle is withdrawn to the superficial side of the artery, and the remaining lidocaine is injected. Pressure is held over the puncture site for 5 minutes, and fracture manipulation can usually begin shortly thereafter.

In most children, the axillary sheath is superficial because of the dearth of subcutaneous fat, thus making for a technically easier procedure in a child than an adult. Of course, this advantage can be offset if the child is

obese or uncooperative. From a pharmacokinetic standpoint, the local anesthetic diffuses more rapidly and with enhanced blockade of the nerves, which are smaller in diameter in children than adults.[63] The duration of the block is usually prolonged enough to allow repeat manipulation of the fracture in the event of an unsatisfactory reduction.

Potential complications of axillary block anesthesia include systemic lidocaine toxicity, hematoma formation, and persistent neurologic symptoms. Horner's syndrome has also been reported. In actuality, complications of axillary block anesthesia are rare.[63] None were encountered in the series reported by Cramer and associates of

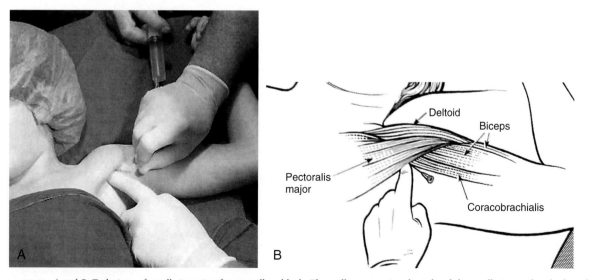

FIGURE 18–2. *A* and *B,* Technique of needle insertion for an axillary block. The axillary artery is palpated and the needle inserted at the lateral edge of the pectoralis major and parallel to the coracobrachialis. (*A,* Courtesy of Stephen Hays, M.D., F.A.A.P., Assistant Professor, Departments of Anesthesiology and Pediatrics, Vanderbilt University Medical Center, Nashville, TN. *B,* Adapted from Bridenbaugh, L.D. In: Cousins, M.J.; Bridenbaugh, P.O., eds. Neural Blockade in Clinical Anesthesia and Management of Pain, 2nd ed. Philadelphia, J.B. Lippincott, 1988, p. 401.)

111 children with displaced forearm fractures treated in an emergency department setting.[18] Contraindications to axillary block anesthesia are the presence of a coagulopathy of any type, a preexisting neurologic or vascular abnormality of the extremity, axillary lymphadenitis, and an uncooperative or combative patient.

## Wrist and Digital Blocks

The efficacy of brachial plexus anesthesia has all but eliminated the need for more distal upper extremity blocks. However, a wrist or digital block may be useful for the treatment of fractures or minor surgical procedures in the hand. Anesthesia to the digits can be achieved by a block of the common digital nerves near their bifurcation between the metacarpal heads or by a block of the radial and ulnar, volar and dorsal digital nerves at the base of each finger. This technique is most useful for the treatment of phalangeal fractures of a single digit. For injuries involving multiple digits or the metacarpals, anesthesia of the hand can be achieved by blocking the three major nerves of the upper extremity at the wrist (wrist block). The median nerve is located on the radial side of the palmaris longus tendon approxi-

mately 2 cm proximal to the wrist crease and is blocked with 3 to 5 mL of local anesthetic (Fig. 18–3A and B). The ulnar nerve is blocked on the radial side of the flexor carpi radialis, about 2 cm proximal to the volar wrist crease, with 3 to 5 mL of local anesthetic, and the dorsal and volar cutaneous branches of the nerve are blocked by subcutaneous injection of an additional 2 to 3 mL of anesthetic (Fig. 18–3A and B). Alternatively, the ulnar nerve may be approached from the ulnar side of the wrist, just dorsal to the flexor carpi ulnaris tendon (Fig. 18–3C). The terminal branches of the radial nerve are blocked by the injection of 1 to 2 mL of anesthetic along the extensor pollicis longus tendon as it crosses the base of the first metacarpal and across the "snuffbox" to the radial side of the extensor pollicis brevis tendon (Fig. 18–3D).

## Femoral Nerve Block

Femoral nerve blockade is another type of regional anesthesia that has been used in the treatment of femoral fractures.[19, 29, 49] Although most children with femoral fractures are not managed on an outpatient basis, femoral nerve blockade can provide excellent

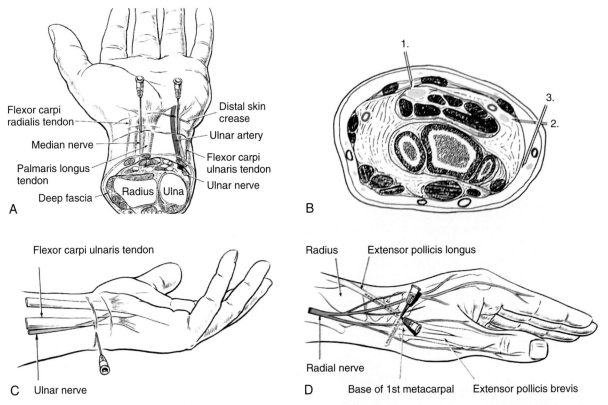

**FIGURE 18–3.** *A* and *B,* Technique for performing a median and ulnar nerve block at the wrist. The median nerve is approached from the palmar side of the wrist between the palmaris longus and flexor carpi radialis. The ulnar nerve can be approached between the flexor carpi ulnaris tendon and the ulnar artery. *C,* Alternative method for ulnar nerve blockade. The ulnar nerve can also be approached from the ulnar side of the wrist just dorsal to the flexor carpi ulnaris tendon. *D,* Technique for performing a radial nerve block at the wrist. The needle is inserted at the point where the extensor pollicis longus tendon crosses the base of the first metacarpal, and approximately 2 to 3 mL of local anesthetic is injected as the needle is advanced along the tendon to the radial tubercle. The needle is then redirected at a right angle across the anatomic "snuffbox" and an additional 1 to 2 mL injected to the radial border of the extensor pollicis longus tendon. (Adapted from Bridenbaugh, L.D. In: Cousins, M.J.; Bridenbaugh, P.O., eds. Neural Blockade in Clinical Anesthesia and Management of Pain, 2nd ed. Philadelphia, J.B. Lippincott, 1988, p. 392.)

anesthesia and analgesia for the initial management of this injury, including manipulation of the fracture, application of an immediate spica cast, or placement of a traction pin. It is a good option for children unable to undergo general anesthesia or be sedated for any reason. This technique is most effective for fractures of the middle third of the femur and less so for fractures of the proximal and distal thirds of the bone, which also receive sensory innervation from branches of the obturator and sciatic nerves, respectively.

Technically, the inguinal area is prepared and draped and the femoral artery palpated. A 22- or 23-gauge needle on a syringe containing a local anesthetic agent (typically 0.5% bupivacaine at 1 to 1.5 mg/kg) is inserted 1 fingerbreadth lateral to the artery and 1 to 2 cm below the inguinal ligament. The needle is advanced at a 30° to 45° angle to the skin and the syringe aspirated as the needle passes through the deep fascia into the femoral triangle. If no blood is aspirated, the anesthetic agent is injected around the femoral nerve. The onset of analgesia occurs within 10 minutes and, with the use of long-acting agents such as bupivacaine, may last up to 8 hours.[19]

With this technique, few inadvertent arterial punctures, no long-term sequelae, and no neurologic complications have been reported.[19, 29, 49] Other potential complications include systemic toxicity from intravascular injection, infection, and injury to the nerve. As with the axillary block, this method may be difficult in obese children, as well as young or uncooperative children. Contraindications include any preexisting neurologic abnormality of the injured lower extremity and the inability to manage systemic toxicity.

## SEDATION

Sedation is a continuum of various states of consciousness. For purposes of classification, two levels are recognized: *conscious* and *deep*. *Conscious sedation* is a state of depressed consciousness in which protective reflexes and a patent airway are maintained and from which the individual can be aroused by physical stimulation or verbal command. *Deep sedation* is a more profound state of unconsciousness with loss of protective airway reflexes. Sedation can be achieved with inhalational agents such as nitrous oxide or with parenteral techniques, including opiate analgesics, benzodiazepines, and neuroleptics (ketamine), alone or in combination. The AAP has established guidelines for equipment and monitoring for all levels and methods of sedation in an attempt to guard patient welfare during sedation and emergence and allow safe discharge home afterward (Table 18–5).[3, 39]

## Nitrous Oxide

Dentists have used nitrous oxide extensively since the 1950s to provide anesthesia for patients undergoing dental procedures in the office setting. Its use in the

**TABLE 18–5**

**American Academy of Pediatrics Guidelines for Conscious Sedation**

**MONITORING**

Preprocedure vital signs
Continuous monitoring of $O_2$ saturation/heart rate
Intermittent monitoring of respiratory rate and blood pressure every 5 min
Personnel responsible *only* for administering drugs/monitoring patients
Individual skilled in airway management

**EQUIPMENT**

Pulse oximeter
Positive-pressure oxygen delivery system and suctioning equipment *in the room*
Emergency cart with appropriate medications, electrocardiographic monitor with defibrillator, equipment for airway management *immediately available*

**RECOMMENDED DISCHARGE CRITERIA**

Cardiovascular function and airway patency are satisfactory and stable
The patient is easily arousable, and protective reflexes are intact
The patient can talk (if age appropriate)
The patient can sit up unaided (if age appropriate)
For a very young or handicapped child incapable of the usually expected responses, the presedation level of responsiveness or a level as close as possible to the normal level has been achieved
The state of hydration is adequate

Adapted from the American Academy of Pediatrics Committee on Drugs. Pediatrics 89:1110–1115, 1992.

ambulatory setting for fracture management is more recent.[21, 31, 32, 62] Nitrous oxide is a relatively weak inhalational anesthetic with low solubility. It acts quickly on the central nervous system and has a fairly short duration of action, which makes it a good anesthetic option for fracture treatment. Other desirable effects of nitrous oxide include a variable degree of analgesia, sedation, anxiolysis, and amnesia.[21, 32, 51]

Nitrous oxide has been shown to be most effective when it is administered as a 50% mixture of nitrous oxide and oxygen.[50, 62] This mixture of gases is most commonly delivered through a machine (Nitronox) that controls the rate of flow of the gases, regulates the mix, and scavenges stray nitrous oxide from the surrounding environment. The gas is self-administered through inspiratory effort with the child holding the facemask. Once adequate sedation occurs, the child relaxes and drops the mask. When the mask seal is broken, the flow of nitrous oxide is stopped. As a safeguard against overdosing, it is important that the mask not be held by anyone but the patient. Fracture reduction can begin within a few minutes of administration of the nitrous oxide.[51] After the fracture has been immobilized, 100% oxygen is administered to the child for approximately 5 minutes to wash out the nitrous oxide and prevent diffusion hypoxia.[21, 32, 51, 62] Guidelines for conscious sedation need to be followed.

This technique of sedation is relatively easy to administer, works quickly, and does appear to be safe.

Nitrous oxide is quickly eliminated and does not seem to suppress laryngeal reflexes. The child does not have to have an empty stomach, and IV access is not required.[32, 62] This method is obviously not region specific and can be used for fractures in all extremities. On the negative side, administration of nitrous oxide can be a problem in a child who is uncooperative or anxious with the facemask and in those who have difficulty obtaining a tight seal with the mask.[31, 62] Other potential problems are nausea, vomiting, diffusion hypoxia, and respiratory depression. Contraindications to the use of nitrous oxide include the presence of significant cardiac or pulmonary disease, previous administration of narcotics or sedatives, the presence of a pneumothorax or abdominal distention, middle ear infection, or altered mental status.

Studies suggest that nitrous oxide does provide effective sedation for the management of fractures but that its analgesic effects are variable.[21, 27, 32, 62] Evans and colleagues found nitrous oxide to provide similar analgesia but also to have a faster onset of action, a shorter recovery time, and better patient satisfaction than IM meperidine.[21] Gregory and Sullivan compared nitrous oxide with IV regional anesthesia (Bier block) in a prospective study of 28 children with upper extremity fractures and found that fracture reduction was completed in less time with nitrous oxide, although the pain response, as measured by a visual analog scale, was worse.[27] In two separate studies by Hennrikus and Wattenmaker and their co-workers with a combined total of 76 children in whom nitrous oxide was used as the sole anesthetic agent, fracture reduction was successful in 95%, and no complications were encountered.[32, 62] However, "moderate" or "significant" pain was observed in 41% percent of the patients during fracture reduction, and in the study by Wattenmaker and colleagues, analgesia was completely ineffective in 9%.

## Nitrous Oxide and Hematoma Block Combination

Because of the unpredictable nature of analgesia with nitrous oxide alone, some have suggested that it be combined with a regional technique. Hennrikus and coauthors reported on the use of nitrous oxide and hematoma block in 100 children 4 to 17 years old with various closed fractures treated in the emergency department.[31] In the combined technique, preliminary administration of nitrous oxide provides sedation and anxiolysis, which facilitates placement of the block, as well as an amnestic response to fracture reduction. The hematoma block provides additional analgesia both during and after the reduction. The study found a significant decrease in behavior suggestive of pain with this technique when compared with an earlier study using nitrous oxide alone.[32, 62]

## Intravenous Sedation

A variety of medications is used for sedation of pediatric patients (Table 18–6). Narcotics and benzodiazepines have been safely administered to children with painful injuries to provide analgesia or to supplement other methods of anesthesia in the emergency department setting for many years.[47, 51] Narcotics produce analgesia by reversibly binding to opioid receptors. In higher doses, they also have some sedative properties. Benzodiazepines are primarily sedatives. They produce hypnosis, anxiolysis, muscle relaxation, and some antegrade amnesia but have no analgesic properties. When given in combination, these two classes of drugs act synergistically to induce a deep level of sedation and analgesia.[47] The IV route of administration is preferred over others (IM, nasal, oral, rectal) because it is the most reliable and manageable.[51] The effect after IV administration is rapid in onset, can be readily titrated, and is reversible if necessary. IV access should be obtained in a noninjured extremity, and the guidelines for conscious sedation should be followed. The benzodiazepine is ideally administered before the narcotic to provide a sedative effect. Low doses of medications should be given initially and titrated for effect within recommended dosage levels (see Table 18–5).[39] Supplemental oxygen should be administered if oxygen saturation falls below 90%. Reversal agents such as naloxone (Narcan) for the

---

**TABLE 18–6** ● ● ● ● ● ● ● ● ● ● ● ● ● ● ● ● ● ● ● ● ● ● ● ● ● ● ● ● ● ● ● ● ● ● ● ● ● ●

Common Medications Used for Sedation in the Reduction of Children's Fractures

| Medications | Dosages | Comments |
|---|---|---|
| Midazolam (Versed) | 0.05–0.2 mg/kg IV | Rapid onset, brief duration of action |
| Diazepam (Valium) | 0.04–0.3 mg/kg IV | Good muscle relaxant |
| Morphine | 0.1–0.2 mg/kg IV | Long duration of action |
| Meperidine (Demerol) | 1–2 mg/kg IV | Long duration of action |
| Fentanyl (Sublimaze) | 1.0–5.0 μg/kg IV | Potent, rapid onset of action; titrate slowly |
| Ketamine | 1–2 mg/kg IV<br>3–4 mg/kg IM | Manage emergency reactions with small doses of midazolam |
| Naloxone (Narcan) | 1.0–2.0 μg/kg IV | Narcotic reversal agent |
| Flumazenil (Romazicon) | 0.003–0.006 mg/kg IV | Benzodiazepine reversal agent |
| Atropine | 0.01 mg/kg IV or IM (maximum, 0.5 mg) | Antisialogogue |
| Glycopyrrolate (Robinul) | 0.05 mg/kg IV or IM (maximum, 0.25 mg) | Antisialogogue |

Adapted from McCarty, E.M., et al. J Am Acad Orthop Surg 7:88, 1999.

narcotic and flumazenil (Romazicon) for the benzodiazepine should be readily available. Fracture reduction can typically begin when the patient becomes drowsy.[61]

The more common benzodiazepines used for IV sedation are midazolam (Versed) and diazepam (Valium). Midazolam is a rapidly acting benzodiazepine that has three to four times the potency of diazepam. Its onset of action is usually within 2 to 3 minutes.[47] It is also eliminated rapidly and thus has the shortest duration of action of any of the benzodiazepines. Because of these characteristics, it has supplanted diazepam as the benzodiazepine of choice for sedation before noxious procedures in most emergency departments. Diazepam has a slightly longer onset and a more protracted duration of action, thus making it less desirable than midazolam from a pharmacokinetic standpoint. However, it is an excellent muscle relaxant and continues to be a good choice for fracture or joint reduction (or both).[50, 51]

Morphine, meperidine (Demerol), and fentanyl (Sublimaze) are the most common narcotics used for the IV management of acute pain and painful procedures in the emergency department.[50] Morphine is the standard by which other narcotics are compared. However, it tends to be more effective for continuous dull pain than the sharp pain typically associated with fractures.[47] It is the least lipid soluble of the narcotics listed and, as a consequence, has a slower onset and longer duration of action (3 to 4 hours). As a result, it is difficult to titrate.[47] Meperidine is the most commonly used narcotic in the emergency department. It is one tenth as potent as morphine but has better euphoric properties. It has a slightly faster onset and shorter duration of action (2 to 3 hours) than morphine. Like morphine, meperidine is also difficult to titrate. Fentanyl (Sublimaze) is a narcotic analgesic that is 100 times more potent than morphine. It is highly lipid soluble and has a rapid onset of action with peak analgesia in 2 to 3 minutes.[47] Its duration of action is shorter than that of either meperidine or morphine (20 to 30 minutes). Infants younger than 6 months metabolize fentanyl more slowly than older children and should receive more conservative doses (one third normal).[51]

When administering IV sedation with both a narcotic and a benzodiazepine, dosing should begin low and be titrated slowly while being mindful of the synergistic effect of these drugs. If respiratory depression occurs, reversal agents should be administered. Typically, the narcotic is reversed first with naloxone. If respiratory depression persists after 1 to 2 minutes, the benzodiazepine should be reversed with flumazenil.[61] Both reversal agents have shorter half-lives than the drugs that they are reversing. Therefore, monitoring must continue until all respiratory effects have dissipated. IV sedation should never be used in children with a history of apnea or airway disease, altered mental status, or hemodynamic instability, or in infants younger than 2 months.

IV sedation has proved to be safe and effective for the management of fractures in children of various ages. In a study by Varela and colleagues, 104 children (age 2 months to 15 years) received IV meperidine (2 mg/kg) and midazolam (0.1 mg/kg) before fracture manipulation in an ambulatory setting.[61] Physician satisfaction with the sedation was good or excellent for 94% of the reductions. Eighty-two of 86 parents (95%) contacted

were satisfied with the sedation as well. Most of the children did display some signs of pain as the fracture was manipulated; however, 93% percent had amnesia for the event. Minor side effects, including oversedation, hallucinations, pruritus, and emesis, occurred in 14% of the patients. No cardiorespiratory complications occurred.

## Ketamine

Ketamine is a pharmacologic analogue of phencyclidine that causes dissociation between the thalamoneocortical and limbic areas of the brain, and it induces a cataleptic, trancelike state. Ketamine interferes with the perception of visual, auditory, and noxious stimuli.[26, 47] Children under ketamine sedation appear to be awake, with eyes open and nystagmus, but are unresponsive to stimuli. Ketamine provides a combination of sedation, analgesia, and amnesia without cardiovascular depression. With ketamine sedation, normal function of the orotracheal airway, including protective reflexes, is preserved.[26] Respiratory depression is rare and dose related. The onset of sedation with ketamine is rapid, the effect is short lived, and recovery is rapid.[25, 26, 51] It can be used for injuries in all extremities.

Ketamine can be administered by either the IV or IM routes.[25, 26] The IV route is attractive because dosing can be titrated and a smaller cumulative dose given to achieve the desired effect. The onset of action is also quicker, and recovery is more rapid.[25] The IV dose of ketamine is 1 to 2 mg/kg and should be administered slowly to avoid respiratory depression. The IM route can be used when IV access is unobtainable. The IM dose is 4 mg/kg. Typically, fracture manipulation may begin within 1 to 2 minutes after IV administration and 5 minutes after IM administration. A repeat IM dose can be given after 10 to 15 minutes if the initial effect is inadequate.[25, 26] The AAP guidelines for equipment and monitoring of patients undergoing deep sedation must be followed.

Ketamine does increase upper airway secretions, and an antisialogogue such as atropine or glycopyrrolate can be effective in minimizing this effect.[26, 47, 51] Ketamine may cause hallucinations during emergence from sedation, although this problem rarely occurs in children younger than 10 years.[25, 26] In older children, prophylactic administration of a low-dose benzodiazepine (midazolam, 0.05 mg/kg) can effectively prevent this side effect from occurring.[47, 51] However, the benzodiazepine may prolong recovery by delaying the metabolism of ketamine.[25]

Other potential problems associated with ketamine include nausea, emesis, rash, elevated intracranial pressure, tachycardia and hypertension, rigidity or hypertonicity, and random movements. Contraindications to the use of ketamine are pulmonary disease or upper respiratory infections, the presence of an intracranial mass, closed head injury, a history of psychiatric problems, age older than 10 years (because of emergence phenomena), hypertension, heart disease, porphyria, glaucoma, penetrating eye injury, and hyperthyroidism.[25, 26]

Ketamine has been in clinical use for more than 30

years. During that time, the safety and efficacy of ketamine sedation in children undergoing painful procedures in an emergency department setting have been established.[25, 26, 47, 50, 51] In 1990, Green and Johnson performed a meta-analysis of 97 studies of ketamine sedation that included administration to 11,589 children.[25] Only two children (0.017%) required intubation for laryngospasm. The incidence of emesis was 8.5%, but no cases of aspiration occurred. Because of its unique properties and safe track record, Sacchetti has described ketamine as having "clearly come to the forefront as the ideal drug for emergency department use in children."[50]

Ketamine has had relatively limited experience in the sedation of children during fracture treatment or management of other musculoskeletal problems. Of the studies reviewed by Green and Johnson in their extensive analysis of the literature on ketamine use in the emergency department, only one mentioned fracture treatment as one of the indications for sedation by this method.[10] A subsequent investigation by Green and colleagues on the use of IM ketamine in the emergency department reported successful sedation in 7 children (out of 108 children) with fractures.[26] Physician satisfaction with the sedation was excellent. Most of the patients (82.9%) were able to undergo fracture reduction within 5 minutes of ketamine injection. Several minor complications did occur, including hypersalivation, hypertonicity, rash, and vomiting, but no major problems were reported. Overall parental satisfaction was high in this study.

In the early 1970s, several reports appeared in the European literature regarding the use of ketamine in children with fractures.[11, 42, 45] More recently, McCarty and associates reported excellent results with ketamine sedation for the treatment of fractures in 114 children in the emergency department.[40] The time from administration of the ketamine to manipulation of the fracture averaged less than 2 minutes after IV dosing and under 5 minutes after IM administration. Pain scale scores reflected minimal or no pain during fracture reduction. Parental satisfaction was high, and 99% of parents responded that they would allow it to be used again in a similar situation. Airway patency and independent respiration were maintained. Minor adverse effects occurred, including nausea (13 patients) and vomiting (8 patients), but only well into the emergence phase of the sedation. No major problems were encountered.

## SUMMARY

Numerous techniques of analgesia and sedation can be used for the outpatient management of fractures in children. The method chosen should be safe, reliable, and efficacious to keep the child free of pain and minimize anxiety, satisfy the parents, and ultimately permit satisfactory treatment of the fracture and thereby obviate a trip to the operating room.

DPT and chloral hydrate are outmoded methods and should *not* be used. Local and regional techniques such as the hematoma block, axillary block, and IV regional anesthesia (Bier block) can be effective for upper extremity fractures. Sedation with nitrous oxide or a parenterally administered narcotic-benzodiazepine combination is not region specific and is suitable for a wide range of ages. Ketamine sedation is an excellent alternative for fractures in any anatomic location in children younger than 10 years. With any method of conscious sedation, institutional guidelines for monitoring should be followed, and equipment/expertise for advanced airway management should be available.

## REFERENCES

1. Abbaszadegan, H.; Jonsson, U. Regional anesthesia preferable for Colles' fracture: Controlled comparison with local anesthesia. Acta Orthop Scand 61:348–349, 1990.
2. Alioto, R.; Furia, J.; Marquardt, J. Hematoma block for ankle fractures: A safe and efficacious technique for manipulations. J Orthop Trauma 9:113–116, 1995.
3. American Academy of Pediatrics Committee on Drugs. Guidelines for monitoring and management of pediatric patients during and after sedation for diagnostic and therapeutic procedures. Pediatrics 6:1110–1115, 1992.
4. American Academy of Pediatrics Committee on Drugs. Reappraisal of lytic cocktail/Demerol, Phenergan, and Thorazine (DPT) for the sedation of children. Pediatrics 95:598–602, 1995.
5. Barnes, C.; Blasier, R.; Dodge, B. Intravenous regional anesthesia: A safe and cost-effective outpatient anaesthetic for upper extremity fracture treatment in children. J Pediatr Orthop 11:717–720, 1991.
6. Beales, J.G.; Kean, J.H.; Holt, P.J. The child's perception of the disease and experience of pain in juvenile chronic arthritis. J Rheumatol 10:61–65, 1983.
7. Bell, H.; Slater, E.; Harris, W. Regional anesthesia with intravenous lidocaine. JAMA 186:544–549, 1963.
8. Binder, L.; Leake, L. Chloral hydrate for emergent pediatric procedural sedation: A new look at an old drug. Am J Emerg Med 9:530–534, 1991.
9. Bolte, R.; Stevens, P.; Scott, S.; Schunk, J. Mini-dose Bier block intravenous regional anesthesia in the emergency department treatment of pediatric upper-extremity injuries. J Pediatr Orthop 14:534–537, 1994.
10. Caro, D. Trial of ketamine in an accident and emergency department. Anaesthesia 29:227–229, 1974.
11. Caroli, G.; Lari, S.; Serra, G. La ketamina in ortopedia e traumatologia: Indicazioni e limiti. Chir Organi Mov 61:99–104, 1972.
12. Carrel, E.; Eyring, E. Intravenous regional anesthesia for childhood fractures. J Trauma 11:301–305, 1971.
13. Case, R. Haematoma block—a safe method of reducing Colles' fractures. Injury 16:469–470, 1985.
14. Chudnofsky, C.R.; Wright, S.W.; Dronen, S.C.; et al. The safety of fentanyl use in the emergency department. Ann Emerg Med 18:635–639, 1989.
15. Colbern, E. The Bier block for intravenous regional anesthesia: Technic and literature review. Anesth Analg 49:935–940, 1970.
16. Colizza, W.; Said, E. Intravenous regional anesthesia in the treatment of forearm and wrist fractures and dislocations in children. Can J Surg 36:225–228, 1993.
17. Cook, B.; Bass, J.; Nomizu, S.; et al. Sedation of children for technical procedures. Clin Pediatr (Phila) 31:137–142, 1992.
18. Cramer, K.E.; Glasson, S.; Mencio, G.; Green, N.E. Reduction of forearm fractures in children using axillary block anesthesia. J Orthop Trauma 9:407–410, 1995.
19. Denton, J.S; Manning, M.P. Femoral nerve block for femoral shaft fractures in children: Brief report. J Bone Joint Surg Br 70:84, 1988.
20. Dinley, R.; Michelinakis, E. Local anesthesia in the reduction of Colles fractures. Injury 4:345–346, 1973.
21. Evans, J.; Buckley, S.; Alexander, A.; Gilpin, A. Analgesia for the reduction of fractures in children: A comparison of nitrous oxide with intramuscular sedation. J Pediatr Orthop 15:73–77, 1995.
22. Farrell, R.; Swanson, S.; Walter, J. Safe and effective IV regional anesthesia for use in the emergency department. Ann Emerg Med 14:239–241, 1985.

23. Fitzgerald, B. Intravenous regional anaesthesia in children. Br J Anaesth 48:485–486, 1976.
24. Gingrich, T. Intravenous regional anaesthesia of the upper extremity in children. JAMA 200:235, 1967.
25. Green, S.; Johnson, N. Ketamine sedation for pediatric procedures: Part 2, review and implications. Ann Emerg Med 19:1033–1046, 1990.
26. Green, S.; Nakamura, R.; Johnson, N. Ketamine sedation for pediatric procedures: Part 1, a prospective series. Ann Emerg Med 19:1024–1032, 1990.
27. Gregory, P.; Sullivan, J. Nitrous oxide compared with intravenous regional anesthesia in pediatric forearm fracture management. J Pediar Orthop 16:187–191, 1996.
28. Grey, W. Regional blocks and their difficulties. Aust Fam Physician 6:900–906, 1977.
29. Grossbard, G.; Love, B. Femoral nerve block: A simple and safe method of instant analgesia for femoral shaft fractures in children. Aust N Z J Surg 49:592–594, 1979.
30. Haslam, D. Age and the perception of pain. Psychonomic Sci 15:86, 1969.
31. Hennrikus, W.; Shin, A.; Klingelberger, C. Self-administered nitrous oxide and a hematoma block for analgesia in the outpatient reduction of fractures in children. J Bone Joint Surg Am 77:335–339, 1995.
32. Hennrikus, W.L.; Simpson, R.B.; Klingelberger, C.E; Reis, M.T. Self-administered nitrous oxide analgesia for pediatric reductions. J Pediatr Orthop 14:538–542g, 1994.
33. Holmes, C. Intravenous regional analgesia: A useful method of producing analgesia of the limbs. Lancet 1:245–247, 1963.
34. Jay, S.; Ozolins, M.; Elliott, C.; et al. Assessment of children's distress during painful medical procedures. Health Psychol 2:133–147, 1983.
35. Johnson, P.; Noffsinger, M. Hematoma block of distal forearm fractures: Is it safe? Orthop Rev 20:977–979, 1991.
36. Juliano, P.; Mazur, J.; Cummings, R.; McCluskey, W. Low-dose lidocaine intravenous regional anesthesia for forearm fractures in children. J Pediatr Orthop 12:633–635, 1992.
37. Lehman, W.L.; Jones, W.W. Intravenous lidocaine for anesthesia in the lower extremity. A prospective study. J Bone Joint Surg Am 66:1056–1060, 1984.
38. Lowe, S.; Hershey, S. Sedation for imaging and invasive procedures. In: Deshpande, J.; Tobias, J., eds. The Pediatric Pain Handbook. St. Louis, Mosby, 1996, pp. 263–317.
39. McCarty, E.C.;, Mencio, G.A.; Green, N.E. Anesthesia and analgesia for the ambulatory management of fractures in children. J Am Acad Orthop Surg 7:81–91, 1999.
40. McCarty, E.C.; Mencio, G.A.; Walker, L.A.; Green, N.E. Ketamine sedation for the reduction of children's fractures in the emergency department. J Bone Joint Surg Am 82:912–918, 2000.
41. McGrath, P.; Craig, K. Developmental and psychological factors in children's pain. Pediatr Clin North Am 36:823–836, 1989.
42. Muncibi, S.; Santoni, R. Utilizzazione della Ketamina in ortopedia e traumatologia. Minerva Anestesiol 39:370–376, 1973.
43. Ogden, J. Skeletal Injury in the Child. Philadelphia, W.B. Saunders, 1990, p. 15.
44. Olney, B.; Lugg, P.; Turner, P.; et al. Outpatient treatment of upper extremity injuries in childhood using intravenous regional anaesthesia. J Pediatr Orthop 8:576–579, 1988.
45. Pagnani, I.; Ramaioli, F.; Mapelli, A.: Prospettive sull'impiego clinico della Ketamina cloridrato in ortopedia e traumatologia pediatrica. Minerva Anestesiol 40:159–162, 1974.
46. Paris, P. Pain management in children. Emerg Med Clin North Am 5:699–707, 1987.
47. Proudfoot, J. Analgesia, anesthesia, and conscious sedation. Emerg Med Clin North Am 13:357–378, 1995.
48. Proudfoot, J.; Roberts, M. Providing safe and effective sedation and analgesia for pediatric patients. Emerg Med Rep 14:207–217, 1993.
49. Ronchi, L.; Rosenbaum, D.; Athouel, A.; et al. Femoral nerve blockade in children using bupivacaine. Anesthesiology 70:622–624, 1989.
50. Sacchetti, A.D. Pediatric sedation and analgesia. Emerg Med Nov:67–87, 1995.
51. Sacchetti, A.; Schafermeyer, R.; Gerardi, M.; et al. Pediatric analgesia and sedation. Ann Emerg Med 23:237–250, 1994.
52. Schecter, N. Pain and pain control in children. Curr Probl Pediatr 15:1–67, 1985.
53. Schecter, N. The undertreatment of pain in children: An overview. Pediatr Clin North Am 36:781–794, 1989.
54. Selbst, S. Managing pain in the pediatric emergency department. Pediatr Emerg Care 5:56–63, 1989.
55. Selbst, S.; Henretig, F. The treatment of pain in the emergency department. Pediatr Clin North Am 36:965–977, 1989.
56. Snodgrass, W.; Dodge, W. Lytic/"DPT" cocktail: Time for rational and safe alternatives. Pediatr Clin North Am 36:1285–1291, 1989.
57. Stehling, L. Anesthesia update #11—unique considerations in pediatric orthopaedics. Orthop Rev 10:95–99, 1981.
58. Turner, P.; Batten, J.; Hjorth, D.; et al. Intravenous regional anaesthesia for the treatment of upper limb injuries in childhood. Aust N Z J Surg 56:153–155, 1986.
59. Urban, B.; McKain, C. Onset and progression of intravenous regional anesthesia with dilute lidocaine. Anesth Analg 61:834–838, 1982.
60. U.S. Department of Health and Human Services, Public Health Service, Agency for Health Care Policy and Research, Acute Pain Management Guideline Panel. Clinical Practice Guideline—Acute Pain Management: Operative or Medical Procedures and Trauma. February 1992.
61. Varela, C.D.; Lorfing, K.C.; Schmidt, T.L. Intravenous sedation for the closed reduction of fractures in children. J Bone Joint Surg Am 77:340–345, 1995.
62. Wattenmaker, I.; Kasser, J.; McGravey, A. Self-administered nitrous oxide for fracture reduction in children in an emergency room setting. J Orthop Trauma 4:35–38, 1990.
63. Wedel, D.; Krohn, J.; Hall, J. Brachial plexus anesthesia in pediatric patients. Mayo Clin Proc 66:583–588, 1991.
64. Winnie, A. Regional anesthesia. Surg Clin North Am 54:861–892, 1975.
65. Younge, D. Haematoma block for fractures of the wrist: A cause of compartment syndrome. J Hand Surg [Br] 14:194–195, 1989.
66. Zeltzer, L.; Jay, S.; Fisher, D. The management of pain associated with pediatric procedures. Pediatr Clin North Am 36:941–963, 1989.

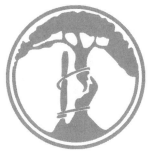

# CHAPTER 19

# Rehabilitation of the Child with Multiple Injuries

Louise Z. Spierre, M.D.
Linda J. Michaud, M.D.

Fractures are the most common type of pediatric trauma.[4] Although uncomplicated fractures seldom result in disability warranting provision of pediatric rehabilitation services, children with multiple injuries can frequently benefit from efforts to minimize disability.

The focus of rehabilitative effort is on maximizing function. In most uncomplicated fractures in children and adolescents, return of function after a period of immobility is merely a matter of regaining range of motion (ROM) and restoring lost strength.[29] With the active nature of a typical child, formal rehabilitation programs are seldom needed to accomplish these goals. However, a child with multiple injuries may have injury-related complications that require prompt recognition and management if maximal functional recovery is to be achieved. Complications may also arise from prolonged immobility, such as contracture and weakness. The longest-lasting functional limitations result from concurrent damage to the central and peripheral nervous system. Children with concurrent brain, spinal cord, plexus, or other peripheral nerve injuries may be left with long-term functional limitations and a need for rehabilitative intervention long after their skeletal injuries have healed. Recently developed outcome measures that take into consideration the functional abilities of children at different ages and developmental stages should prove helpful in future quantification of the short- and long-term impact on levels of activity and participation in children with complicated and multiple injuries (see Chapter 7).[36]

## REHABILITATION OF FRACTURES

### Therapeutic Exercise

Once the period of immobilization is over, the work of regaining ROM and strength and returning to full activity and participation begins. Table 19–1 lists the full ROM and the functional ROM of mature joints.[17] They are listed with measurements standardized by the Committee for the Study of Joint Motion of the American Academy of Orthopaedic Surgeons.[3] ROM is measured as degrees of deviation from the anatomic position. The ranges given in Table 19–1 are for mature limbs. Very young children should be evaluated by someone familiar with pediatric norms. For example, infants have physiologic hip flexion contracture, with normal hip extension that averages −30°, as well as increased external rotation at the hip. These "contractures" resolve slowly as the infant matures.

Exercises to increase ROM may be active (movement generated by the patient) or passive if the child is too young, too weak, or unable to cooperate. Active-assistive ROM exercise consists of having the child actively move through as much of the range as possible and then passively completing as much movement as possible through the normal range. Active ROM exercises are generally preferred if possible. The use of body weight can sometimes increase the effectiveness of ROM exercises, for example, with stretching of the gastrocnemius muscles. These powerful muscles are capable of lifting the entire body weight and are commonly shortened after multiple injury. Unless the child is small, passively ranging these muscles is difficult, and the best stretch is obtained when standing. Every effort should be made to encourage children to participate in their own ROM exercise program. Older children can often complete their exercise programs quite independently. Even young children may be able to perform simple stretches if properly supervised.

In children with spasticity or poor mobility, fracture healing may be complicated by contractures. The best management related to contractures is prevention with proper positioning of joints, early ROM, and splinting.[47] Once a contracture has occurred, a range of management options are available. Flexible contractures may be managed with ROM exercises, dynamic splinting, or serial casting. If associated spasticity is a factor, reducing muscle pull may improve patient tolerance, the effective-

**TABLE 19–1** ....................................................

Normal and Functional Joint Range of Motion

| Joint | Degrees Normal ROM (Functional ROM) |
|---|---|
| **Shoulder** | |
| Abduction | 180 (120) |
| Adduction | 45 (30) |
| Flexion | 180 (120) |
| Extension | 60 (40) |
| Internal rotation (arm in abduction) | 80 (45) |
| External rotation (arm in abduction) | 90 (45) |
| **Elbow** | |
| Flexion | 140–160 (130) |
| Extension | 0--5 (-30) |
| Supination | 80–90 (50) |
| Pronation | 70–80 (50) |
| **Wrist** | |
| Flexion | 75 (15) |
| Extension | 70 (30) |
| Radial deviation | 20 (10) |
| Ulnar deviation | 35 (15) |
| **Hip** | |
| Flexion | 125–128 (90–110) |
| Extension | 0–20 (0–5) |
| Abduction | 45–48 (0–20) |
| Adduction | 40–45 (0–20) |
| Internal rotation | 40–45 (0–20) |
| External rotation | 45 (0–15) |
| **Knee** | |
| Flexion | 130–140 (110) |
| Extension | 0 (0) |
| **Ankle** | |
| Plantar flexion | 45 (20) |
| Dorsiflexion | 20 (10) |
| Inversion | 35 (10) |
| Eversion | 25 (10) |

...................................................................

Compiled from Hoppenfeld, S.; Murthy, V.L. Treatment & Rehabilitation of Fractures. Philadelphia, Lippincott, Williams & Wilkins, 2000.

ness of casting/splinting, and the ease of ROM. Management of spasticity may be accomplished in several ways. Systemic medications such as baclofen and dantrolene are frequently used to decrease generalized spasticity in children. However, in the case of contractures, more localized treatment of spasticity is frequently used. Options include temporary inhibition of function of the neuromuscular junction by the injection of botulinum toxin or neurolysis with phenol. If the contracture is severe and fixed, the only effective option may be surgical.

Evaluation of strength is by manual muscle testing, with muscle strength graded on a 0 to 5 scale[5]:

0 = No contraction
1 = Palpable or visible contraction
2 = Full range of motion with gravity eliminated
3 = Full range or motion against gravity
4 = Full range of motion against moderate resistance
5 = Full range of motion against full resistance

Strengthening exercises may be indicated when bone healing is well established. These exercises usually involve extremely simple equipment such as a ball or putty. More formal strengthening programs may include isometric exercises, which maintain muscle length with increasing tension during contraction, or isotonic exercises, with muscle shortening and steady tension. Isotonic exercises are further subdivided into open kinetic chain exercises, such as with free weights, or closed kinetic chain exercises, such as with pulley systems. Closed kinetic chain exercises are often favored in the early postinjury period because they provide a more predictable path of movement for the exercising limb. For athletes, evaluation by a therapist familiar with the specific motions involved in the sport (cutting, jumping, etc.) will help identify areas of weakness that may lead to re-injury. Return to play should not be allowed until full pain-free strength and ROM have been restored.

## Interventions with Physical Agents

Heat and cold may be used in the rehabilitation of fractures. Generally, cold is used acutely to reduce swelling and inflammation. It is rarely indicated in a patient with severe trauma and is most appropriate for isolated, minor low-energy fractures. In the rehabilitation phase, direct heat from a warm water bath or hot packs warms the skin and may improve comfort. Other measures such as ultrasound, short-wave diathermy, and microwave diathermy are seldom used in children.

## Orthoses and Adaptive Equipment

Plaster or fiberglass splints and casts are often used for acute fracture management, and resting splints may be applied to provide additional support after fracture healing has occurred. A dynamic orthosis may be indicated if the child has a concurrent peripheral nerve injury.[46] Cervical orthoses are used for suspected or actual spinal cord injury (SCI). Halo vests provide the best stabilization of an unstable spine. Rigid cervical collars decrease rotation but still allow movement in the sagittal plane. Soft cervical orthoses do not provide spine stabilization.[38] For thoracic and lumbar spine injuries, a thoracolumbosacral orthosis may be useful.

For extremity fractures, adaptive devices can be helpful to extend reach, provide grasp, reduce force, and improve safety.[46] Such devices can provide increased independence in basic activities of daily living, including feeding, dressing, bathing, grooming, and toileting. Examples include reachers and sock aids (Fig. 19–1), a long-handled sponge or shoe horn, grooming aids, built-up feeding utensils, a rocker knife, a raised toilet seat, tub chair, and built-up door handles.[46] Velcro or elastic shoe closures may be helpful. Evaluation by an occupational therapist for problem-solving and individualized recommendations may prove invaluable in increasing independence and improving the quality of life during recovery for both injured children or adolescents and their parents and other caregivers.

Gait aids such as walkers or crutches may be useful for a child with weight-bearing restrictions on the lower extremity. When used with a "swing-through" gait pattern, crutches can completely eliminate weight bearing on the affected limb. Some initial instruction with crutches is needed to prevent axillary trauma and to ensure that these children are able to understand their limitations. A child who requires additional support because of instability or reduced lower extremity strength may require a walker. Either a walker or crutches can be modified with an upper extremity platform support to distribute the weight through the elbow and along part of the forearm, and such support should be considered in children with concurrent wrist or hand injuries. This modification is also preferred in rheumatologic conditions in which the use of axillary crutches may cause undue stress to the involved wrist and hand. Wheelchair use should be encouraged if both lower extremities are involved.

In the case of multiple fractures, a short stay in a rehabilitation unit may be helpful for provision of adaptive equipment to increase independence in activities of daily living and instruction of the patient and family in safe transfer techniques and wheelchair safety skills. Devices such as a sliding board may be helpful in increasing a child's independence in transfers. At least two limbs must be able to bear weight for patients to participate in their own transfer. If a patient is not weight bearing on three or four limbs, caregivers should be instructed on safe transfers and the use of a lift if needed.

## Pain Control

Adequate pain control in children after traumatic injury is an issue that is gaining increasing attention. The subject of most investigations is acute pain control during procedures such as fracture reduction in the emergency department. However, for a multiply injured child, pain may be an ongoing problem even during the rehabilitation phase. Patients who are uncommunicative because of age or neurologic insult and in whom unexplained agitation or vital sign changes such as tachycardia or hypertension develop should be carefully evaluated for evidence of additional painful injury before ascribing the changes to other factors, including the natural history of concurrent brain injury recovery or autonomic instability.

Observational scales such as the Children's Hospital of Eastern Ontario Pain Scale and the Objective Pain Scale are primarily used in infants and very young children.[44] For children aged 3 to 6 years, visual progression of happy to sad faces is frequently used.

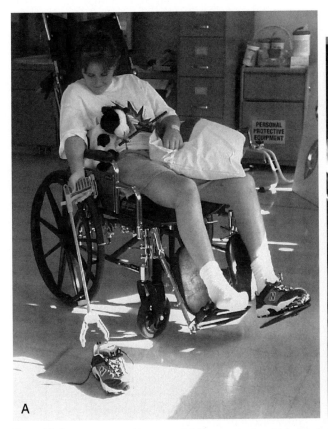

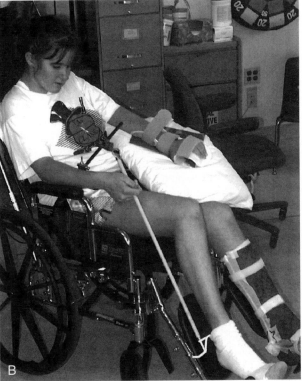

**FIGURE 19–1.** This 17-year-old restrained driver sustained multiple injuries in a motor vehicle crash, including pelvic and sacral fractures, managed with internal and external fixation, and traumatic brain injury resulting in left hemiparesis. She remained non–weight-bearing in bilateral lower extremities until the time of discharge from acute rehabilitation, with significant motor impairment in her left upper extremity due to her neurologic injury. Provision of adaptive equipment, including a reacher *(A)* and sock aid *(B)*, reduced caregiver assistance required in self care from total to moderate (approximately 50%).

Examples include the McGrath Facial Affective Scale and Beyer's Oucher Scale. Providing a description of their pain is difficult for preschool-aged children who do not possess the language ability or the understanding to correctly identify the location and characteristics of the pain.[20] Older children have improved abstract and numeric reasoning and may be able to use more adult measures such as the visual analog scale.[44]

In the rehabilitation setting, the goal is to slowly wean the child from opioid analgesics while managing side effects such as constipation and urinary retention. When a patient has been taking opioid analgesics for a long period, weaning is often better tolerated when the medication is first changed to a longer-acting agent, which is then slowly tapered.

## PERIPHERAL NERVE INJURY AND ELECTRODIAGNOSIS

Screening for evidence of peripheral nerve injury is part of routine care after skeletal injury in children. Nerve injury can occur both as a consequence of the initial injury and as a complication of fracture stabilization.[35]

Clavicle fractures may be associated with brachial plexus injuries. Brachial plexus injuries are subdivided into upper plexus injuries (C5–C6), or those above the clavicle, and lower plexus injuries (C8, T1), or those below the clavicle. The mechanism of injury may give a clue to the location of the lesion even before the physical examination is performed. For instance, the upper plexus is vulnerable to neck traction injuries. The classic example is a newborn with shoulder dystocia in whom Erb's palsy develops because of traction on the neck.[6, 15] The lower plexus may be injured by extreme abduction of the arm that produces a classic Klumpke's palsy. Sports injuries may include both mechanisms, with weakness produced at multiple root levels. Generally, recovery from traction injury is good, but the presence of cervical nerve root avulsion leads to a much poorer prognosis.

Lumbosacral plexopathy is a concern after pelvic fractures.[51] The lumbosacral plexus is usually well protected from trauma because of its posterior location and proximity to the pelvic bones. However, trauma severe enough to produce an unstable pelvic fracture, retroperitoneal hematoma, or fracture-dislocation of the hip joint may also affect the plexus. The injury may be subtle, so a high index of suspicion for peripheral nerve damage needs to be maintained in pelvic trauma.

Supracondylar fracture of the humerus, particularly if displaced, can lead to injury to the anterior interosseus, radial, median, or ulnar nerves alone or in combination. The estimated incidence of nerve injury after a supracondylar fracture varies from 6% to 16%. Because of its lack of sensory distribution, injuries to the interosseus nerve may be overlooked.[6, 12, 13, 15, 40] Median nerve injury is a rare complication of a distal radial fracture.[8] An estimated 5% of children with traumatic fracture or dislocation of the hip suffer nerve injury, usually to the peroneal branch of the sciatic nerve.[11]

Peripheral nerve injury does not always occur acutely. Damage to the growth plate or angulation in a joint may lead to later nerve injury. An example is an angulation deformity at the elbow leading to later ulnar nerve injury.

Greater long-term disability may result from the complicating nerve injury during skeletal trauma than from the skeletal injury itself. Peripheral nerve injuries are divided according to Seddon's classic work into neurapraxia, axonotmesis, and neurotmesis.[23] Neurapraxia is nerve compression or ischemia with subsequent segmental demyelination. No disruption of the axon occurs, and the prognosis for complete return of function is excellent. Recovery usually occurs rapidly within weeks, except in the case of chronic entrapment, which leads to permanent damage. Axonotmesis involves disruption of the axon with maintenance of intact supporting structures. Wallerian degeneration of the distal segment ensues. Resolution of the injury is variable and slow and is dependent on nerve sprouting and regeneration. Neurotmesis is the most severe injury, with disruption of both the axon and supporting structures. Without intact supporting structures, nerve sprouting and regeneration are inefficient and often misdirected, sometimes leading to inappropriate innervation. The prognosis for recovery is poor, and surgical intervention may be indicated.[9, 23]

Recovery after peripheral nerve injury in children is faster and more complete than in adults.[6, 15, 23] In adults after complete resection and anastomosis, peripheral nerves regenerate at a rate of 1.5 to 2.0 mm/day. Maximal recovery can take up to 40 months. Perhaps because of a combination of the shorter length of children's limbs and faster healing, pediatric recovery is maximal in 13 to 19 months.[23] Nerve injuries that fail to demonstrate healing after 5 months may require surgical intervention.[6, 13] In cases in which the location or severity of injury is uncertain, electrodiagnostic studies may provide valuable diagnostic and prognostic information.

Most electrodiagnostic studies include nerve conduction studies and electromyography. In nerve conduction studies, an electrical impulse is transmitted across a sensory or motor nerve and the resulting response is picked up by recording electrodes. In motor studies, the response is called the compound motor action potential (CMAP), whereas in sensory nerve conduction studies, the sensory nerve action potential (SNAP) is recorded. Timing is important. In the first week after a nerve injury, wallerian degeneration has not occurred. If a nerve is stimulated proximal to the lesion and the recording electrode is placed distal to it, the CMAP or SNAP will be significantly decreased. However, if the nerve is stimulated distal to the lesion, the CMAP and SNAP will be within normal limits. This phenomenon is referred to as conduction block. It can be very useful for localization of a nerve injury. However, distinguishing the type of nerve injury electrodiagnostically is difficult in the first week after injury.

Wallerian degeneration occurs within 7 to 11 days. Determination of the location of the lesion becomes more difficult, but estimation of the severity of the nerve injury becomes easier. Neurapraxic lesions (without any wallerian degeneration) may demonstrate conduction block if segmental demyelination is significant, or nerve conduction studies may be normal. In axonotmesis and neurotmesis, the distal nerve segment, which has been severed from the axon, degenerates. CMAP and SNAP are uniformly low in affected nerves, regardless of the location of stimulation.

By 2 to 3 weeks after injury, electromyography will show evidence of denervation in affected muscles, along with muscle membrane instability in the form of positive waves and fibrillations. The distribution of denervation may be useful for localization of the lesion. For instance, footdrop after hip surgery may be due to damage to the peroneal branch of the sciatic nerve at the hip or compression palsy of the common peroneal nerve at the fibular head. Differentiation between the two sites on clinical grounds may be difficult in a postsurgical patient. The short head of the biceps femoris is innervated by the peroneal nerve before it crosses the fibular head. Involvement of this muscle is more consistent with sciatic nerve injury.

Electrodiagnostic studies can be difficult in young and uncooperative children. Children younger than 2 years have different normal values for nerve conduction studies because of the immaturity of the myelin sheath. For these reasons, young children should be evaluated by an electromyographer familiar with the special issues related to electrodiagnosis in children.

## SPINAL CORD INJURY

Spinal cord injury (SCI) is an uncommon complication of pediatric skeletal trauma and occurs in only 2% of reported cases of pediatric trauma.[4] Although the complication is rare, it can be devastating. It is also easily overlooked because of a phenomenon that occurs primarily in children—spinal cord injury without radiographic abnormality (SCIWORA). This phenomenon is possible because of the flexibility of the pediatric spinal canal, which can stretch up to 2 inches in infants. However, the spinal cord will tear after being stretched just 0.25 inches.[2] Children with this condition will have no abnormalities on plain radiographs, but their injuries may be detectable on magnetic resonance imaging. An estimated 16% to 19% of SCIs in children are SCIWORA.[2]

Because almost one in five children with SCI will have no abnormalities on plain radiographs, careful clinical examination in any child with a suspected neck injury is indicated.[2] The American Spinal Injury Association (ASIA) has published a guide to the examination of persons with SCI.[5] Grading involves strength testing in key muscle groups and evaluation of sensation to pinprick and light touch in a dermatomal distribution, including the sacral segments in particular. If any abnormalities are found, they are used to determine the sensory and motor levels of the SCI. The lowest intact motor level is the level at which the strength grade on manual muscle testing is at least a 3 (antigravity) and the level above has a strength of 5 (normal). Any sensation felt on the rectal examination indicates that the patient is sensory incomplete. The ASIA grading scale (which is modified from the original Frankel scale) is as follows:

A = Complete. No sensory or motor function is preserved in the sacral segments S4–S5.

B = Incomplete. Sensory but not motor function is preserved below the neurologic level and includes the sacral segments S4–S5.

C = Incomplete. Motor function is preserved below the neurologic level, and more than half the key muscles below the neurologic level have a muscle grade less than 3.

D = Incomplete. Motor function is preserved below the neurologic level, and at least half the key muscles below the neurologic level have a muscle grade greater than or equal to 3.

E = Normal. Sensory and motor function are normal.

This grading should be determined once the patient is out of spinal shock, which is defined by return of the bulbocavernosus reflex. The level and completeness of SCI have prognostic value for both eventual neurologic recovery and functional independence.

The long-term complications of SCI in children are myriad. They can prolong the rehabilitation process and persist long after discharge from inpatient rehabilitation. Children with lesions at the thoracic and cervical levels need aggressive pulmonary management ranging from assisted ventilation (invasive or noninvasive) to instruction in quad cough techniques. Insensate skin is vulnerable to pressure ulceration. In lesions above T7, the sympathetic nervous system is often affected. Early low sympathetic tone with orthostatic hypotension, which warrants management with abdominal binders and elastic stockings, may give way to later life-threatening autonomic dysreflexia. At the time of discharge, patients at risk should be given a card outlining the symptoms and treatment of autonomic dysreflexia to take with them to a clinic or emergency department that may be unfamiliar with the special health care problems of individuals with SCI. Neurogenic bladder must also be evaluated in a child with SCI. Some of the highest pressures in the bladder can be generated by bladder-sphincter dyssynergia after SCI. This problem must be addressed with a regular catheterization program to keep volumes at or below the maximal bladder volume for age. This volume can be roughly calculated as (age + 2) years = bladder volume in ounces. Neurogenic bowel involvement should not be overlooked. Bowel programs often include timing, stimulation, dietary recommendations, and medications, with the goal of age-appropriate continence. Children should be involved in their own bladder and bowel management as soon as age appropriate. No consensus has been reached on indications for deep venous thrombosis prophylaxis for pediatric SCI. The problem is thought to be less common in preadolescent children. The recommendation for adults is to begin prophylaxis within 72 hours unless contraindicated and continue for 8 to 12 weeks, depending on completeness of the injury and the presence of other risk factors.

Fractures in children with SCI can occur either acutely as a result of the same trauma that caused the SCI or later as chronic immobility leads to osteopenia. A recent review of the National Spinal Cord Injury Database revealed that 28% of individuals at the time of admission for acute SCI also had extraspinal fractures. The most common locations of these fractures were, in decreasing order, the chest, lower extremity, upper extremity, head, other, and pelvis.[48] Children with new SCI should have a thorough evaluation for evidence of swelling, pain, and unusual mobility, with particular attention paid to insensate areas.[16, 31, 50]

Individuals who sustain an SCI in childhood are at risk for long-term musculoskeletal complications.[32] Long-term immobility may lead to osteoporosis in adulthood, particularly in individuals with higher-level lesions.[7, 22, 24, 27, 39, 45] In a recent study of adults who had suffered SCI as children, young adults (median age of 31 years) were showing decreased bone mineral density in the femoral region an average of 19 years after their injuries.[22] Risk factors associated with osteoporosis after SCI include immobilization for surgical treatment and complete injury.[39] Osteoporosis may lead to low-velocity fractures, particularly of the supracondylar distal end of the femur (paraplegic fracture).[39] Traditional approaches to fractures below the level of the SCI in paraplegic and tetraplegic individuals have included closed reduction with traction or a well-padded cast or splint that can be removed to inspect insensate skin.[10, 37] Evaluation of interventions aimed at reducing the loss of bone mineral density, including exercise, supported standing, and functional electrical stimulation, has revealed mixed results.[14, 43] There is no clear indication at this time that these efforts reduce osteoporosis in the long term, although they may have other benefits, such as improved strength, reduced hypercalcemia, and better cardiovascular fitness.[48]

## TRAUMATIC BRAIN INJURY

Traumatic brain injury (TBI) is a major cause of acquired disability in children with an annual incidence of 200 per 100,000.[33] The Glasgow Coma Scale (GCS) is widely used in the classification of TBI severity. After resuscitation, a GCS score of 8 or less indicates severe brain injury, 9 to 12 represents moderate injury, and 13 to 15 indicates mild injury.[19] These criteria must be used with some caution, however, because non-neurologic factors may influence the GCS score. Other indicators of brain injury include loss of consciousness, post-traumatic amnesia, and changes on imaging studies of the brain. Some neurologic deficits may be detected on physical examination; other deficits are subtle and can be more fully evaluated with formal neuropsychologic testing. Prompt recognition is essential for proper monitoring and follow-up. Children with moderate and severe TBI

continue to show deficits in multiple areas of functioning even 3 years after injury.[19] Other delayed complications after brain injury include infection, seizures, pulmonary complications, hypercalcemia, deep venous thrombosis, endocrinologic changes, heterotopic ossification, and hydrocephalus.[33]

Skeletal injury at the time of TBI presents challenges in evaluation and management of both types of injury. Children may not be able to cooperate with the examination to indicate an area of skeletal injury concurrent with the head injury because of either unresponsiveness or agitation. In a recent series of children with TBI and SCI, 49 previously undetected injuries in 60 children were found with bone scanning.[40] The high rate of clinically unsuspected fractures has led to the recommendation that patients with TBI have screening radiographs of the cervical, thoracic, and lumbar spine, as well as the pelvis and possibly the knees.[26] Bone scans may be advisable in young children because of an inability to visualize growth plates on plain films.[26, 40] As discussed earlier, peripheral nerve injury may also occur, so a high index of suspicion should be maintained, especially in children with concurrent TBI whose examinations may be confounded by motor changes resulting from both brain injury and peripheral nerve injury, particularly around fracture sites. If possible, electrodiagnostic studies may be helpful, especially in children whose clinical recovery of motor function is not typical of those recovering from central nervous system injury.[26]

When fractures have been detected in a child with concurrent brain injury, management is somewhat controversial. Newer anesthetic agents and improved intracranial pressure monitoring make early fracture fixation more feasible. In patients with severe cerebral edema, it may be advisable to wait 7 to 10 days for the cerebral edema to decrease.[26] Close attention must also be paid to fluid resuscitation during fixation to prevent secondary brain injury.[21] When possible, the early mobilization afforded by internal fixation is preferred, given the agitation and motor restlessness often encountered in patients after TBI.[26] If closed reduction is chosen, it is important to allow monitoring of the skin in a patient who may not be able to express the pain that may result from excessive skin pressure. Bivalving the cast when possible makes frequent removal and skin examination possible. Given the risk for the development of spasticity and contractures after brain injury, casting in the neutral position is preferred.[26] Fracture evaluation should be undertaken with the assumption that the patient will regain full mobility.

Heterotopic ossification is another adverse skeletal event related to TBI or SCI in children. The incidence is lower than in adults, with rates estimated to be between 3% and 20%. It is more frequent in children with TBI who are 12 years of age or older and who have longer durations of coma.[18] Etidronate disodium prophylaxis is less commonly used in children because of its association with rickets and gastrointestinal upset. Treatments used include observation only, etidronate disodium, nonsteroidal anti-inflammatory drugs, and surgical resection.[18] Currently, no consensus has been reached regarding the most effective management of heterotopic ossification in children. The goal of treatment is to maintain joint mobility and decrease pain.

## PREVENTION OF RE-INJURY

Children with fractures may have higher rates of conduct disorder, psychosomatic complaints, and impulsive/hyperactive behavior.[30] Effort to prevent re-injury is an integral part of the rehabilitation process and includes a discussion of safety equipment such as seat belts, helmets, and proper sports equipment. For certain casts such as a hip spica, commercially available car seats may not be adequate, and specialized car restraint devices should be used for safe transportation. Injury prevention may also include behavioral interventions in an attempt to decrease or at least better manage the impulsive behavior that may have contributed to the child's injury in the first place. Prevention may be a sensitive subject, particularly if the injury was potentially avoidable with improved parental supervision or appropriate use of safety devices. However, if this discussion is avoided, the child and family may incur worse trauma if recurrent injuries are sustained.

## PSYCHOSOCIAL FACTORS

The osteogenic activity of pediatric bone leads to a generally good outcome after skeletal trauma.[28, 34] However, awareness is growing that fractures in children cause limitation in activity at discharge, as well as family stress.[1, 41, 42, 48, 49]

Rehabilitation of children cannot be accomplished without involving the family. The coping ability and stress faced by the family members of children with orthopaedic injuries have only recently been investigated. Family coping strategies such as denial or the use of humor may affect the overall distress levels.[49] Although the negative impact of serious neurologic injuries on family adjustment and functioning is well described, even without neurologic injuries some families of children with fractures may experience family stress up to 6 months after the injury. This scenario is most likely if the child suffered a lower extremity fracture.[41] Activity restriction is more severe and more prolonged with lower extremity fractures.[25] Family stress is worse in families with difficulties in family functioning before the injury.[42] For these reasons, social work and psychology should play an active role in the rehabilitation team to provide family guidance and reassurance. Referrals for short-term assistance with community resources may be helpful in reducing the economic burden on a family with a multiply injured child. Assistance from the rehabilitation team may be helpful in the school reentry process as a child with multiple injuries is reintegrated into the usual roles in the home and community.

## REFERENCES

1. Aitken, M.E.; Jaffe, K.M.; DiScala, C.; et al. Functional outcome in children with multiple trauma without significant head injury. Arch Phys Med Rehabil 80:889–895, 1999.
2. Akbarnia, B.A. Pediatric spine fractures. Orthop Clin North Am 30:521–536, 1999.
3. American Academy of Orthopedic Surgeons, Committee for the Study of Joint Motion: Method of Measuring and Recording Joint Motion. Chicago, American Academy of Orthopedic Surgeons, 1965.
4. American Pediatric Surgical Association. National Pediatric Trauma Registry, 2001.
5. American Spinal Injury Association. International Standards for Neurological Classification of Spinal Cord Injury, 2000.
6. Barrios, C.; de Pablos J. Surgical management of nerve injuries of the upper extremity in children: A 15-year survey. J Pediatr Orthop 11:641–645, 1991.
7. Bauman, W.A.; Spungen, A.M. Metabolic changes in persons after spinal cord injury. Phys Med Rehabil Clin North Am 11:109–140, 2000.
8. Binfield, P.M.; Sott-Miknas, A.; Good, C.J. Median nerve compression associated with displaced Salter-Harris type II distal radial epiphyseal fracture. Injury 29:93–94, 1998.
9. Buchthal, F.; Kuhl, V. Nerve conduction, tactile sensibility, and the electromyogram after suture or compression of peripheral nerve: A longitudinal study in man. J Neurol Neurosurg Psychiatry 42:436–451, 1979.
10. Cochran, T.P.; Bayley, J.C.; Smith, M. Lower extremity fractures in paraplegics: Pattern, treatment, and functional results. J Spinal Disord 1:219–223, 1988.
11. Cornwall, R.; Radomisli, T.E. Nerve injury in traumatic dislocation of the hip. Clin Orthop 377:84–91, 2000.
12. Cramer, K.E.; Green, N.E.; Devito, D.P. Incidence of anterior interosseous nerve palsy in supracondylar humerus fractures in children. J Pediatr Orthop 13:502–505, 1993.
13. Culp, R.W.; Osterman, A.L.; Davidson, R.S.; et al. Neural injuries associated with supracondylar fractures of the humerus in children. J Bone Joint Surg Am 72:1211–1215, 1990.
14. de Bruin, E.D.; Frey-Rindova, P.; Herzog, R.E. Changes of tibia bone properties after spinal cord injury: Effects of early intervention. Arch Phys Med Rehabil 80:214–220, 1999.
15. Frykman, G.K. Peripheral nerve injuries in children. Orthop Clin North Am 7:701–716, 1976.
16. Garland, D.E.; Jones, R.C.; Kunkle, R.W. Upper extremity fractures in the acute spinal cord injured patient. Clin Orthop 233:110–115, 1988.
17. Hoppenfeld, S.; Murthy, V.L., eds. Treatment & Rehabilitation of Fractures. Philadelphia, Lippincott, Williams & Wilkins, 2000.
18. Hurvitz, E.A.; Mandac, B.R.; Davidoff, G.; et al. Risk factors for heterotopic ossification in children and adolescents with severe traumatic brain injury. Arch Phys Med Rehabil 73:459–462, 1992.
19. Jaffe, K.M.; Polissar, N.L.; Fay, G.C.; et al. Recovery trends over three years following pediatric traumatic brain injury. Arch Phys Med Rehabil 76:17–26, 1995.
20. Joseph, M.H.; Brill, J.; Zeltzer, L.K. Pediatric pain relief in trauma. Pediatr Rev 20:75–84, 1999.
21. Kalb, D.C.; Ney, A.L.; Rodriguez, J.L.; et al. Assessment of the relationship between timing of fixation of the fracture and secondary brain injury in patients with multiple trauma. Surgery 124:739–745, 1998.
22. Kannisto, M.; Alaranta, H.; Merikanto, J.; et al. Bone mineral status after pediatric spinal cord injury. Spinal Cord 36:641–646, 1998.
23. Kimura, J. Anatomy and physiology of the peripheral nerve. In: Electrodiagnosis in Diseases of Nerve and Muscle: Principles and Practice. New York, Oxford University Press, 2001, pp. 73–79.
24. Kiratli, B.J.; Smith, A.E.; Nauenberg, T.; et al. Bone mineral and geometric changes through the femur with immobilization due to spinal cord injury. J Rehabil Res Dev 37:225–233, 2000.
25. Kopjar, B.; Wickizer, T.M. Fractures among children: Incidence and impact on daily activities. Inj Prev 4:194–197, 1998.
26. Kushwaha, V.P.; Garland, D.G. Extremity fractures in the patient with a traumatic brain injury. J Am Acad Orthop Surg 6:298–307, 1998.

27. Lazo, M.G.; Shirazi, P.; Sam, M.; et al. Osteoporosis and risk of fracture in men with spinal cord injury. Spinal Cord 39:208–214, 2001.

28. Leach, J. Orthopaedic conditions. In: Campbell, S.K., ed. Physical Therapy in Children. Philadelphia, W.B. Saunders, 2000, pp. 353–382.

29. Lindaman, L.M. Bone healing in children. Clin Podiatr Med Surg 18:97–108, 2001.

30. Loder, R.T.; Warschausky, S.; Schwartz, E.M.; et al. The psychosocial characteristics of children with fractures. J Pediatr Orthop 15:41–46, 1995.

31. Massagli, T.L. Medical and rehabilitation issues in the care of children with spinal cord injury. Phys Med Rehabil Clin North Am 11:169–182, 2000.

32. McKinley, W.O.; Jackson, A.B.; Cardenas, D.D.; et al. Long-term medical complications after traumatic spinal cord injury: A regional model systems analysis. Arch Phys Med Rehabil 80:1402–1410, 1999.

33. McLean, D.E.; Kaitz, E.S.; Keenan, C.J.; et al. Medical and surgical complications of pediatric brain injury. J Head Trauma Rehabil 10(5):1–12, 1995.

34. Moulton, S.L. Early management of the child with multiple injuries. Clin Orthop 376:6–14, 2000.

35. Neiman, R.; Maiocco, B.; Deeney, V.F. Ulnar nerve injury after closed forearm fractures in children. J Pediatr Orthop 18:683–685, 1998.

36. Pencharz, J.; Young, N.L.; Owen, J.L.; et al. Comparison of three outcome instruments in children. J Pediatr Orthop 21:425–432, 2001.

37. Ragnarsson, K.T.; Sell, G.H. Lower extremity fractures after spinal cord injury: A retrospective study. Arch Phys Med Rehabil 62:418–423, 1981.

38. Richter, D.; Latta, L.L.; Milne, E.L.; et al. The stabilizing effects of different orthoses in the intact and unstable upper cervical spine: A cadaver study. J Trauma 50:848–854, 2001.

39. Sabo, D.; Blaich, S.; Wenz, W.; et al. Osteoporosis in patients with paralysis after spinal cord injury: A cross sectional study in 46 male patients with dual-energy X-ray absorptiometry. Arch Orthop Trauma Surg 121:75–78, 2001.

40. Sobus, K.M.L.; Alexander, M.A. Undetected musculoskeletal trauma in children with traumatic brain injury or spinal cord injury. Arch Phys Med Rehabil 74:902–904, 1993.

41. Stancin, T.; Kaugars, A.S.; Thompson, G.H.; et al. Child and family functioning 6 and 12 months after a serious pediatric fracture. J Trauma 51:69–76, 2001.

42. Stancin, T.; Taylor, H.G.; Thompson, G.H.; et al. Acute psychosocial impact of pediatric orthopedic trauma with and without accompanying brain injuries. J Trauma 45:1031–1038, 1998.

43. Stein, R.B. Functional electrical stimulation after spinal cord injury. J Neurotrauma 16:713–717, 1999.

44. Steward, S.; O'Connor, J. Pediatric pain, trauma, and memory. Curr Opin Pediatr 6:411–417, 1994.

45. Sugawara, H.; Linsenmeyer, T.A.; Beam, H.; et al. Mechanical properties of bone in a paraplegic rat model. J Spinal Cord Med 21:302–308, 1998.

46. Thomas, M.A. Assistive devices and adaptive equipment for activities of daily living (ADL). In: Hoppenfeld, S.; Murthy, V.L., eds. Treatment & Rehabilitation of Fractures. Philadelphia, Lippincott, Williams & Wilkins, 2000, pp. 49–56.

47. Thomas, M.A. Therapeutic exercise and range of motion. In: Hoppenfeld, S.; Murthy, V.L., eds. Treatment & Rehabilitation of Fractures. Philadelphia, Lippincott, Williams & Wilkins, 2000, pp. 19–25.

48. Upperman, J.S.; Gardner, M.; Gaines, B.; et al. Early functional outcome in children with pelvic fractures. J Pediatr Surg 35:1002–1005, 2000.

49. Wade, S.L.; Borawski, E.A.; Taylor, H.G.; et al. The relationship of caregiver coping to family outcomes during the initial year following pediatric traumatic injury. J Consult Clin Psychol 69:406–419, 2001.

50. Wang, C.M.; Chen, Y.; DeVivo, M.J.; et al. Epidemiology of extraspinal fractures associated with acute spinal cord injury. Spinal Cord 39:589–594, 2001.

51. Weis, E.B. Subtle neurological injuries in pelvic fractures. J Trauma 24:983–985, 1984.

# INDEX

............................................................................................

Note: Page numbers followed by the letter f refer to figures;
those followed by the letter t refer to tables.

## A

AARF. *See* Atlantoaxial rotary fixation (AARF).
Abdomen, in Modified Injury Severity Scale, 79t
Abdominal injury
  in child abuse, 589
  secondary survey of, 88–89, 88t, 89t
Abduction, traction in, 392t, 393
Absent pulse
  in arterial injuries, 124–126, 125f
  in supracondylar humeral fractures, 275–277, 276f
Abuse, child, 587–605. *See also* Child abuse.
Accessory ossicles, navicular, 540, 541f
  of foot, 537–538, 539f
  of malleoli, 517
Acetabular fracture
  complications of, 389
  management of, 380, 382t, 387
  physical examination of, 374
  prevalence of, 371
  radiographic evaluation of, 378
Achondroplasia, 62t
Acid-base balance, in primary survey, 85
Acromioclavicular joint
  in distal clavicular fracture, 326
  injury to, 326–328, 328f
Acromion fracture, 330
ACS. *See* American College of Surgeons (ACS).
Activity-based physical functional disability scales, 154–155
Activity Scale for Kids (ASK), 153, 160t, 162
Adaptive equipment, for fracture rehabilitation, 620–622, 621f
Adduction injury, varus deformity from, 577
Adolescent Tillaux injury, of ankle, 521t
Age, in physical function scales, 162–163
Air bag deployment, spinal injury from, 353–354, 354f
Airway assessment, in multiple injuries, 82–84, 83t
Alignment. *See* Reduction.
Allman's classification, of acromioclavicular joint injury, 326–327, 328f
Allograft, for pathologic fracture, 65–66
American Academy of Pediatrics (AAP), on conscious sedation, 613, 613t
American College of Surgeons (ACS), on pediatric trauma centers, 81–82, 82t
  on primary survey and resuscitation, 82
American Spinal Injury Association (ASIA) grading scale, 623–624
Amines, 607–608, 608t
Amputation
  for foot injuries, 571–572
  for soft tissue injuries, 110–113, 115f
  traumatic, 121
Analgesia. *See* Pain management.
Anatomic reduction
  of ankle fracture, 523
  of distal tibial fracture, 526–527
  of tarsometatarsal fracture, 557
Anesthetic techniques, 607–613
  for axillary block, 610–612, 611f
  for femoral nerve block, 612–613
  for hand injuries, 242
  for hematoma block, 608
  for intravenous regional anesthesia, 608–610, 610t
  for local/regional anesthesia, 607–608, 608t
  for wrist and digital blocks, 612, 612f
  to avoid, 607

Angular deformity
  after distal femoral physeal fracture, 447–448
  after forearm fracture, 199, 200f
  after proximal tibial physeal fracture, 463, 506
  after tibial and fibular fracture, 505
  of distal fibular growth plate, 579, 582f
  of distal tibial growth plate, 577–579, 578f–581f
  secondary to malunion, 580
Angulation
  late, 134, 136f, 137f
  malunion and, 133
Ankle, range of motion of, 620t
Ankle injuries, 516–537
  anatomy of, 516–517, 517f–519f
  aphorisms for, 583–584
  classification of, 520–523, 521t, 522f–524f
  consequences of, 518
  distal fibular fractures in, 534–536, 536f
  distal tibial fractures in, 524–529.
    *See also* Distal tibial fracture.
  incidence and mechanism of, 517–518
  radiologic evaluation of, 519–520, 519f, 520f
  surgical treatment of, 523–524
  transition fractures in, 529–534
    juvenile fracture of Tillaux and, 529–531, 530f–532f
    triplane fracture in, 531–534, 533f, 534f
Annular ligament, 167, 168f
Anterior approach, to radius, in forearm fracture, 183, 184f
Anterior humeral line, 258–259, 261f
Anterior interosseous nerve
  in forearm fractures, 190
  palsy of, 144, 145f
Anterior talofibular ligament, 516, 518f
Anterior tibiofibular ligament, 516, 518f
Antibiotic therapy, 107–108
Antimicrobials, 107–108
Apophyseal injuries, 48–52, 49f–52f
Apophysiolysis, 51
Apophysitis
  calcaneal, 50
  iliac, 50
  medial epicondylar, 51, 52f
  traction, 49
    of fifth metatarsal, 562–563, 563f
  vertebral, 51, 51f
Appendicular skeleton, 57
Arterial injuries, 124–126, 125f
  of extremities, 90
Arteriography. *See* Radiographic evaluation.
Arthritis, degenerative, after acetabular fracture, 389
Arthrodesis, of cervical spine, 362–364, 363f
Aseptic necrosis, after femoral shaft fracture, 435, 436f
Ashhurst-Bromer classification, of ankle injuries, 520
ASIA grading scale. *See* American Spinal Injury Association (ASIA) grading scale.
ASK. *See* Activity Scale for Kids (ASK).
Asymmetric arrest, of distal tibial growth plate, 577–579, 578f–581f
Atlantoaxial rotary fixation (AARF), 354f, 358–359
Atlas, fractures of, 359, 360f
Atropine, for sedation, 614t
Atypical Scheuermann's disease, 51, 51f
Autogenous bone graft, for pathologic fracture, 65–66
Autonomic dysreflexia, in spinal cord injury, 624
Avascular necrosis
  after acetabular fracture, 389
  after hip dislocation, 403

Avascular necrosis (*Continued*)
  after proximal femoral fracture, 398, 399
  after talar fracture, 546
  of distal tibial physis, 582
Avulsion fracture
  of calcaneus, 552–553
  of fifth metatarsal, 562–563
  of medial epicondyle, 51–52, 52f
  of tibial tubercle, 457, 458f
Axial compression
  atlas fracture from, 359, 360f
  in distal tibial fractures, 528–529, 530f
Axial skeleton, 57
Axillary block, 610–612, 611f
Axis deviation, in forearm fractures, 181–182, 182f
Axonotmesis, 622–623

## B

Backboard, for primary survey and resuscitation, 83, 83f
Bandage, for distal fibular fracture, 536
Barthel Index, 157t
Battered child syndrome. *See* Child abuse.
Baumann's angle, 258, 259f
Bayonet apposition, of radius and ulna, 173, 176f
Bedrest/non–weight-bearing
  for acetabular fracture, 387
  for pelvic fracture, 383–384, 384f
Behavior, of abused child, 589
Bell-Tawse annular ligament reconstruction, with Lloyd-Roberts modification, 229
Bend deformation. *See* Plastic deformation.
Benign bone tumors, 64, 66f
Benzodiazepines, for sedation, 614–615, 614t
Bicipital tuberosity, in forearm fracture, 169, 170f
Bicycle spoke injuries, tibial shaft fracture in, 489–490, 489f
  to foot, 575
Bier block, 608–610, 609t, 610t
Biology, bone, in pathologic fractures, 59–61, 59f–61f
Biopsy, of bone tumor, 58
Birth, fractured clavicular shaft at, 324–325, 325f
Birth trauma, child abuse differentiated from, 600
Bladder, neurogenic, in spinal cord injury, 624
Blood pressure, in primary survey, 84, 84t
Blood volume, 75
  in primary survey, 84, 84t
BMP. *See* Bone morphogenetic protein (BMP).
Bohler traction bow, for pelvic fractures, 384
Bone biology, in pathologic fractures, 59–61, 59f–61f
Bone cysts
  of foot, 540, 541f
  unicameral, 57, 64, 65f
Bone disease, temporary brittle, 600–601
Bone formation, 3, 4f
  ectopic, 129, 129f
    after femoral shaft fractures, 435
  periosteal new, in child abuse, 594
    in radiographic dating of injuries, 590, 590t
Bone graft
  for bone union, 116, 116f
  for nonunion, 141–142, 142f, 143f
    of humeral fracture, 293, 294f
  for pathologic fracture, 65–66
Bone growth and development. *See* Skeletal growth and development.

Bone length inequality
    after distal femoral physeal fracture, 447
    after pelvic fracture, 389
Bone morphogenetic protein (BMP), in fracture
    healing, 4
Bone physiology, in pathologic fractures, 57–59
Bone remodeling. See Remodeling.
Bone resorption, 57–58
Bone scans, of tibial and fibular fractures, 474, 490
Bone strength, in pathologic fractures, 58
Bone union, of fractures, with soft tissue injuries,
    116, 116f–120f
Bowel, neurogenic, in spinal cord injury, 624
Bowing, of radius and forearm, 177, 180f
Boyd approach, to open reduction, of Monteggia
    fracture, 220–221, 222f
Boyd-Syme amputation, 571–572
Brace, for distal femoral fracture, 442
Brachial artery, 257, 258f
    in elbow dislocation, 309
Brachial plexus
    in axillary block, 610, 611f
    injuries to, 622
Brachioradialis muscle, in distal radius fracture,
    202, 204f
Brain injury, in multiple trauma, 624–625
Breathing assessment, in multiple trauma,
    82–84, 83t
Brittle bone disease, child abuse differentiated from,
    600–601
Bucket-handle fracture, in child abuse, 594, 596f
Buckle base injury, 558, 559f
Buckle fracture, 11, 11f
    of distal radius and ulna, 200
    of forearm, 173, 177f
Bupivacaine (Marcaine), 608, 608t
    for femoral nerve block, 613
Burns, in child abuse, 589

C

Caffey's disease, child abuse differentiated from,
    601, 602f
Calcaneal apophysitis, 50
Calcaneal injuries, 549–554
    classification of, 549, 551f, 551t
    complications of, 554
    consequences of, 549–554, 552f–555f
    physeal, 37, 38f
Calcaneofibular ligament, 516, 518f
Calcaneus, 538, 539f
Callus, in radiographic dating of injuries, 590, 590t
Canadian Occupational Performance Measure
    (COMP), 158t
Capability measures, of physical function, 155
Capitellotrochlear sulcus, in humeral fracture,
    287, 287f
Capitellum
    fracture of, 293, 295f
    in fracture-separation of distal humeral
        physis, 281
    in humeral lateral condyle fracture, 287–288,
        287f–289f
    of distal humerus, 258–259, 261f
    ossification of, 257
Carbocaine. See Mepivacaine (Carbocaine).
Cardiac tamponade, in primary survey, 84
Caregiver, in child abuse, 588
C-arm, in closed reduction, of extension-type
    supracondylar fracture, 269–270, 270f
Carpal fracture-dislocation, 239, 239f, 240f
Carpal fractures, 240
Carpometacarpal (CMC) dislocations, 241–242
Carrying angle, of elbow, 259–260
Cast brace treatment, of distal femoral physeal
    fractures, 442
Cast syndrome, 130, 130f
Casting
    in rehabilitation, 620
    of distal femoral fracture, 440–442, 440f, 441f
    of distal fibular fracture, 536
    of distal radius fracture, 202, 203f

Casting (Continued)
    of distal tibial fracture, type I, 525
        type II, 526
        type IV, 527
    of extension-type supracondylar fracture,
        267–268
    of femoral fracture, 411, 411t, 412t
    of femoral physeal fracture, 136
    of forearm fracture, 175, 179f, 180, 181f, 182f
    of isolated tibial shaft fracture, 486–487
    of juvenile fracture of Tillaux, 530
    of navicular fracture, 555
    of open tibial and fibular fractures, 497, 503
    of pelvic fractures, 378
    of proximal tibial fracture, 477–478
    of talar neck fracture, 543
    of tarsometatarsal fracture, 557
    of tibial and fibular shaft fractures, 481, 484–485
    of tibial spine fracture, 454
    of toddler's fracture, 487, 488f
    of triplane fracture, 534
    of triquetrum fracture, 240
    spica. See Spica cast.
Cefamandole, for infection, 107
Cefazolin, for infection, 107
Central nervous system trauma, in child abuse, 589
Cephalosporin, for infection, 107
Cervical seat belt syndrome, 353
Cervical spine
    anatomy of, 345–347, 346f
    anomalies of, 347
Cervical spine injuries, 356–364
    atlantoaxial rotary fixation in, 354f, 358–359
    fractures and dislocations of C3-C7 in,
        362–364, 363f
    fractures of atlas in, 359, 360f
    fractures of axis in, 359–362, 360f, 361f
    occiput-C1 in, 356–357, 356f
    subluxation of C1 on C2 in, 357–358
Cervical vertebrae, anatomy of, 344
Cervicobasilar relationship, radiology of, 347
Chance's fracture, 78
CHAQ. See Childhood Health Assessment
    Questionnaire (CHAQ).
Chemotherapy, pathologic fracture healing and, 61
Chest, in Modified Injury Severity Scale, 79t
Chest injuries, secondary survey of, 87–88
Child abuse, 587–605
    differential diagnosis of, 600–602, 602f
    examination of, 589
    femoral fractures in, 408
    forms of, 587–588
    fracture patterns in, 590–600
        diaphyseal, 591–594, 591f–594f
        epiphyseal-metaphyseal, 594, 595f–597f
        periosteal new bone formation and, 594
        rib, 598, 599f
        shoulder girdle, 598–599
        skull, 599
        spine, 599–600
        type I distal humeral, 594–596, 597f
        type I proximal femoral, 596–598, 598f
    historical perspective of, 587
    history of injury in, 588–589
    identification of, 588
    in fracture-separation of distal humeral physis, 281
    legal aspects of, 587
    management of, 602–603
    radiographic evaluation of, 589–590, 590t
    rib fractures in, 77
    thoracolumbar spine fractures in, 364, 364f
    tibial shaft fractures in, 487–489
Child Health Questionnaire (CHQ), 161t
Childhood Health Assessment Questionnaire
    (CHAQ), 160t, 162
Chip fracture, of navicular bone, 555–556, 556f
Chloral hydrate, 607
Chloroprocaine (Nesacain), 608t
Chlorpromazine (Thorazine), in lytic cocktail, 607
Chondrodiastasis, for complete growth arrest, 42
Chondroepiphysis, of second metatarsal, 561
Chopart-level amputation, 571, 572
CHQ. See Child Health Questionnaire (CHQ).
Ciprofloxacin, for infection, 107
Circulation, assessment of, 84–85, 84t

Clavicle, 322–326
    anatomy of, 322
    fractures and dislocations of, 322–326
        at birth, 324–325, 325f
        diagnosis of, 322–323, 323f, 324f
        distal, 326, 327f
        in childhood, 325–326, 326f
        incidence of, 322
        mechanism of injury in, 322
        peripheral nerve injury and, 622
        treatment of, 323–324
Clindamycin (Cleocin Phosphate),
    for gas gangrene, 107
Closed fractures
    of tibial and fibular shafts, 480
    with soft tissue injuries, 105, 106t
Closed reduction
    of carpometacarpal dislocation, 242
    of distal femoral fracture, 443, 444f
    of distal femoral physeal fracture, 445
    of distal tibial fracture, 525–527, 528f, 529f
    of elbow dislocation, 307
    of extension-type supracondylar fracture, 265
        casting and, 267–268
        percutaneous pinning and, 268–272, 270f,
            271f, 273f
    of forearm fracture, 166, 175–177, 180–183,
        180f–182f, 212
    of fracture-separation of distal humeral physis,
        284–285
    of glenohumeral dislocation, 333, 333f
    of greenstick forearm fracture, 178
    of hand fracture and dislocation, 242
    of hip dislocation, 401, 402
    of humeral shaft fracture, 339
    of juvenile fracture of Tillaux, 530, 532f
    of lateral humeral condyle fracture, 290
    of medial clavicular fracture, 324
    of Monteggia fracture, 223–225
    of multiple injuries, 94–95
    of patellar dislocation, 467
    of patellar fracture, 452
    of pelvic fracture, 378–380, 380f, 382t, 386
    of physeal injury, 32
    of proximal femoral fracture, 391–392
        internal fixation and, 393
        percutaneous pinning and, 396
        pin fixation and, 392t, 393
        screw fixation and, 394
        spica casting and, 392–394, 392t, 396
    of proximal humeral fracture, 335, 336f
    of proximal radial fracture, 303
    of proximal tibial fracture, 477–478
    of proximal tibial physeal fracture, 461
    of radial head subluxation, 317
    of tarsometatarsal fracture, 557
    of tibial and fibular shaft fractures, 481, 483–485
    of tibial spine fracture, 454
    of triplane fracture, 533, 534f
Closing wedge osteotomy, for cubitus varus,
    278–280, 279f, 280f
Clostridial infection, in soft tissue injuries, 106–107
CMAP. See Compound motor action potential
    (CMAP).
CMC dislocations. See Carpometacarpal (CMC)
    dislocations.
Cold, in rehabilitation, 620
Collar bone. See Clavicle.
Collateral ulnar ligament, in medial epicondylar
    fracture, 297–298, 299f
Comminuted fracture
    of distal tibia, 521t
    of patella, 451
    of supracondylar humerus, 272, 274f
    of tibial and fibular shafts, 480
COMP. See Canadian Occupational Performance
    Measure (COMP).
Compartment syndrome, 126–128, 127f
    after femoral shaft fracture, 433
    after foot injuries, 565–566
    after forearm fracture, 175, 190–194, 193f, 194f
    after soft tissue injuries, 109–110
    after tibial and fibular fractures, 508–510
    of extremities, 90–91, 91f, 92f
Complete displacement, of forearm fracture, 179–180

Complete fracture, 12, 12f
  of distal radius and ulna, 200–201, 202f
  of forearm, 173, 179f
  of proximal tibial metaphysis, 474
  of radial shaft, 205
  of tibial diaphysis, 485
Complete growth arrest, after physeal injury, 21,
  42–44, 44f
Complex regional pain syndrome (CRPS), in foot
  injuries, 575–577
Compound motor action potential (CMAP), 623
Compression
  in distal tibial fractures, 528–529, 530f
  in extension-type supracondylar fracture,
    264–265, 264f
  in humeral fracture, 286
  in multiple trauma, 74
  in physeal injuries, 19
  in thoracolumbar spine fractures, 364
Compression dressing
  for distal fibular fracture, 536
  for free tissue transfer, 569
  for tarsometatarsal fracture, 557
Compression fracture
  of distal tibia, 528–529, 530f
  of proximal tibial metaphysis, 474
  of talar dome, 544
Computed tomography (CT). See Radiographic
  evaluation.
Congenital dislocation, of radius, 314
Congenital insensitivity to pain
  child abuse differentiated from, 601
  foot fractures and, 575, 575f
Congenital syphilis, child abuse differentiated from,
  601, 602f
Conscious sedation, 613, 613t
Contamination, wound, 106
Contracture
  therapeutic exercise for, 619–620
  Volkmann's ischemic, 126–127, 127f
Copper deficiency, child abuse differentiated
  from, 601
Coracoid fracture, 330–331, 331f
Corner fracture, in child abuse, 594, 595f, 596f
Coronoid process, of elbow, 257–258
Cost-benefit analysis, 154
Cost-effectiveness analysis, 154
Cost-utility analysis, 154
Coxa vara, after proximal femoral fracture,
  398, 399, 400f
Cross union, 134, 135f
  of forearm fracture, 212
CRPS. See Complex regional pain syndrome
  (CRPS).
CT (computed tomography). See Radiographic
  evaluation.
Cubitus valgus, after humerus fracture,
  293, 294f
Cubitus varus deformity, after supracondylar
  fracture, extension-type, 278–280,
  279f–281f
  management of, 264–265, 264f
  of humerus, 130, 131f
Cuboid bone, 538
Cuboid fracture, 556
Cuneiform bone, 538
Cysts
  of foot, 540, 541f
  unicameral bone, 57, 64, 65f

**D**

Dameron and Rockwood classification, of distal
  clavicular fractures, 326, 327f
Darrach procedure, for distal radioulnar joint
  dislocation, 239
Débridement
  for clavicular shaft fracture, 325
  for free tissue transfer, 569
  for gas gangrene, 107
  for humeral shaft fracture, 341
  for lawn mower injuries, 568–569

Débridement (Continued)
  for open fractures
    of forearm, 215
    of knee, 465
    tibia and fibula, 504
  for soft tissue injuries, 108–109, 108f–114f
Decompression, 91–92, 91f
  of compartment syndromes, 127–128
  of forearm, 193–194, 194f
  of nerve injuries, 144
Deep sedation, 613
Deep vein thrombosis, spontaneous, 130
Degenerative arthritis, after acetabular fracture, 389
Delayed open reduction, of lateral condyle of
  humerus fracture, 292–293, 292f
Delayed union
  of closed tibial fracture, 474
  of open tibial and fibular fractures, 502–503
  of tibial and fibular fractures, 504–505
  of tibial and fibular growth plate injuries, 582
Deltoid ligament, 516, 518f
Demerol. See Meperidine (Demerol).
Development, in physical function scales, 162–163
Diaphyseal fractures, from child abuse, 591–594,
  591f–594f
  isolated fibular, 494, 495f
  isolated tibial, 485–487, 486f
  with soft tissue injuries, 121
Diaphysis, 10
Diazepam (Valium), for sedation, 614t, 615
Digital block, 612, 612f
Dilantin. See Phenytoin (Dilantin).
DIP joint. See Distal interphalangeal (DIP) joint.
Direct measures, of physical function, 155
Disability
  in hip dislocations, 403
  in pelvic fractures and dislocations, 388
  in proximal femoral fractures, 398
Dislocation(s)
  of ankle joint, 536–537, 537f
  of C3-C7, 362–364, 363f
  of carpal bones, 239, 239f, 240f
  of carpometacarpal joint, 241–242
  of clavicle, 322–326
  of distal radioulnar joint, 235–239, 237f, 238f
  of elbow, 307–314. See also Elbow.
  of foot joints, 565, 565f, 566f
  of glenohumeral joint, 331–334, 332f, 333f
  of hand, 248–250, 249f, 250f
  of hip, 399–404. See also Hip dislocations.
  of interphalangeal joint, 248, 249f, 565, 565f
  of knee, 469
  of metacarpophalangeal joint, 248, 249f
  of metatarsophalangeal joint, 565, 566f
  of patella, 466–468, 466f–468f
  of pelvis, 371–389. See Pelvic fractures and
    dislocations.
  of radial head, 314, 317f
  of thumb, 250, 250f
Displaced fractures, comminuted, 274f
  of forearm, growth plate injuries and, 196–198,
    197f, 198f
    management of, 180–181
  of metatarsals, 558
  of navicular bone, 556
  of proximal tibial epiphysis, 460, 461f
  of proximal tibial metaphysis, 465
  of supracondylar humerus, 272, 273f, 275f
  of tibial and fibular shafts, 480
    management of, 481, 485
Distal clavicular fracture, 326, 327f
Distal femoral fracture, 439–449
  anatomy of, 439–440
  of metaphysis, 440–443, 440f, 441f, 444f
  of physis, 443–449
    classification of, 444–445
    complications of, 447–449, 449f
    diagnosis of, 445
    management of, 445–447, 446f–448f
    mechanism of injury in, 443–444
Distal femur, physeal injuries of, characteristics of, 35
  growth arrest and, 48
Distal fibular fracture, 534–536, 536f
Distal fibular growth plate, growth arrest of,
  579, 582f

Distal humeral fracture, 257–260, 258f–261f
  from child abuse, 594–596, 597f
Distal humeral physeal fracture-separation, 280–285
  classification of, 281
  diagnosis of, 281–283, 283f–285f
  incidence of, 280
  mechanism of injury in, 286
  treatment of, 283–285, 285f
Distal humerus
  ossification of, 257, 258f
  physeal injuries of, 40, 40f, 41f, 43f
  supracondylar fracture of, 260–263, 261f
Distal interphalangeal (DIP) joint
  dislocation of, 248, 249f
  in forearm fractures, 174
Distal phalangeal epiphyseal fracture, 564, 565f
Distal phalangeal fracture, 244
Distal radioulnar dislocation, 235–239, 237f, 238f
Distal radius
  fractures of, 199–201, 201f, 202f
  growth plate injuries to, 195–199, 195f, 197f–200f
  physeal injuries of, characteristics of, 40
    growth arrest and, 48
Distal third of radius, fractures of, 201–204, 203f,
  204f
Distal tibia, physeal injuries of
  characteristics of, 35–37, 37f, 38f
  growth arrest and, 48
Distal tibial fracture, Salter-Harris, 524–529
  type I, 524–525, 525f
  type II, 525–526, 526f
  type III, 526–527, 526f
  type IV, 527–528, 527f–529f
  type V, 528–529, 530f
  type VI, 529
Distal tibial growth plate, asymmetric arrest of,
  577–579, 578f–581f
Distal tibial metaphyseal fracture, 494–495, 496f
Distal tibial physis, 517, 519f
  avascular necrosis of, 582
Distal ulna, physeal injuries of, 40–41, 44f
Distraction injury, in thoracolumbar spine fractures,
  365, 366f
Divergent dislocation, of elbow joint, 314, 316f
Double-pin traction, for distal femoral metaphyseal
  and physeal fractures, 441
Down syndrome, cervical instability in, 357–358
Drug-induced bone changes, child abuse differenti-
  ated from, 602
Dunlop's traction, for extension-type supracondylar
  fracture, 265–266
Dysreflexia, autonomic, in spinal cord injury, 624

**E**

Ectopic bone formation
  after femoral shaft fractures, 435
  in fracture complications, 129, 129f
Education, multiple injuries and, 97
Elbow, 257–321
  carrying angle of, 259–260
  dislocation of, 307–314
    classification of, 307
    complications of, 309–312, 316f
    divergent, 314, 316f
    incidence of, 307
    mechanism of injury of, 307, 313f, 314f
    median and ulnar nerve entrapment after, 145
    posterior, 227–228
    radial head, 314, 317f
    recurrent, 312–314
    treatment of, 307–309, 315f
  distal humeral fracture of, 257–260, 258f–261f
  distal humeral physeal fracture-separation of,
    280–285. See also Distal humeral physeal
    fracture-separation.
  floating, 299, 305f, 306f
  lateral condyle of humerus fracture of, 286–293.
    See also Lateral condyle of humerus fracture.
  lateral epicondyle fracture of, 299
  medial condyle of humerus fracture of, 293–297,
    296f

Elbow (*Continued*)
  medial epicondyle fracture of, 297–299, 297t,
    298f–303f
  olecranon fracture of, 305–307, 312f, 313f
  proximal radial fracture of, 299–305.
    *See also* Proximal radial fracture.
  radial head subluxation of, 314–317
  range of motion of, 620t
  supracondylar fracture of, 260–263, 261f
    extension-type, 263–280. *See also*
      Extension-type supracondylar fracture.
    flexion-type, 280, 282f
    T-condylar fracture of, 299, 304f–306f
Electrodiagnosis, of peripheral nerve injury, 623
Electromyography, in peripheral nerve injury, 623
Embolism, fat, 128
Embryonic bone formation, 3
Enchondroma, 57, 67, 67f
Encroachment, malunion and, 133
Endochondral bone formation, in fracture healing, 5
Endochondral ossification, 3
Endotracheal tube, for resuscitation, 82–83
End-stage renal osteodystrophy, foot fractures
  and, 575
Epicondyle
  lateral, fracture of, 299
  medial, fracture of, 297–299, 297t, 298f–303f
Epiphyseal fracture, 12–14, 13f
  management of, 93
Epiphyseal-metaphyseal fracture, from child abuse,
  594, 595f–597f
Epiphysis, 9
Essex-Lopresti fracture, 230, 234f
Esters, 607–608, 608t
Ewing's sarcoma, 62t
Exercise, for fracture rehabilitation, 619–620, 620t
Extension-type supracondylar fracture, 263–280
  complications of, 275–280
    cubitus varus in, 278–280, 279f–281f
    neurologic injury in, 277–278
    vascular compromise in, 275–277, 276f
  history of, 263
  management of, 264–265, 264f, 266f
  physical examination of, 263–264
  treatment of, 265–274
    closed reduction and casting in, 267–268
    closed reduction and percutaneous pinning in,
      268–272, 270f, 271f, 273f
    open reduction and internal fixation in, 272,
      274f, 275f
    skeletal traction in, 266–267, 267f
    skin traction in, 265–266
External fixation, for free tissue transfer, 569
  of distal femoral fracture, 442–443
  of distal tibial fracture, 527, 528f, 529f
  of femoral fracture, 412t
  of femoral shaft fracture, 416–419, 417f–419f
    complications from, 432–433, 434f, 435, 435f
  of fractures, with soft tissue injuries, 119–121
  of multiple injuries, 95
  of open tibial and fibular fractures, 497–500,
    503, 504
  of pelvic fracture, 378–380, 380f, 385–386
  of tibial and fibular shaft fractures, 481, 482–483,
    482f
External rotation, traction in abduction and,
  392t, 393
Extra-articular fracture, of calcaneus, 549, 551f
Extremities
  in Modified Injury Severity Scale, 79t
  injuries to, secondary survey of, 89–91, 89t, 90t,
    91f, 92f
  mangled, 105, 105t


F

Face, in Modified Injury Severity Scale, 79t
Facet dislocation
  cervical, 363, 363f
  thoracolumbar, 365, 367f
Facet joint, 344
Facial injuries, spinal injury and, 76–77

Falls
  in calcaneal fractures, 551, 552f
  in distal radioulnar joint dislocation, 237
  in forearm fractures, 172
  in tibial and fibular fractures, 473
  mechanism of injury in, 76
Familial dysautonomia
  child abuse differentiated from, 601
  foot fractures and, 575, 575f
Family
  in child abuse, 588
  in rehabilitation, 625
Fasciotomy
  for compartment syndrome, 91–92, 92f
  of forearm, 193
Fat embolism, in fracture complications, 128
Fat pads, of elbow, 257–258, 259f
Femoral fracture, distal. *See* Distal femoral fracture.
  in battered child syndrome, 487–489
  ipsilateral, 491, 492f–493f
  nerve block for, 612–613
  proximal, 389–399. *See also* Proximal femoral
    fracture.
  recurvatum deformity of tibia after, 22
  supracondylar, arterial injuries in, 124, 125f
Femoral nerve block, 612–613
Femoral physeal fracture, growth disturbances in, 136
Femoral shaft fracture, 407–438
  anatomy and development in, 407–408
  classification of, 410
  decision making for, 410–411, 411t
  diagnosis of, 408–410
  in child abuse, 591, 591f, 592f
  management of, 411–436, 412t
    complications of, 432–435, 433f–436f
    external fixation in, 416–419, 417f–419f
    immediate spica casting in, 412–414, 413f
    in multiply injured child, 429–432
    medullary nailing in, 419–424
    pins and plaster in, 416
    plate fixation in, 424–429, 428f–432f
    preferred treatment for, 435–436
    skeletal traction in, 414–416, 415f
    skin traction in, 412
  mechanism of injury in, 408
Femur, physeal injuries of
  characteristics of, 35, 36f
  growth arrest and, 48
Fentanyl (Sublimaze), for sedation, 614t, 615
FGF. *See* Fibroblast growth factor (FGF).
Fiberglass splints and casts, in rehabilitation, 620
Fibroblast growth factor (FGF), in fracture
  healing, 4
Fibroma, nonossifying, 67–68
Fibrous cortical defect, 64, 66f
Fibrous dysplasia, 62t, 67, 67f
Fibula
  anatomy of, 516, 517f
  growth disturbances and, 137, 137f, 138f
Fibular fracture, 472–515
  angular deformity from, 505
  compartment syndrome in, 508–510
  delayed union of, 504–505
  diagnosis of, 472–473, 473t
  distal, 534–536, 536f
  from bicycle spokes, 489, 489f
  lower extremity length inequality from, 506–507
  malrotation of, 505–506
  neurologic injury in, 508
  nonunion of, 505
  of diaphysis, 494, 495f
  of shaft, 480–485
    authors' preferred treatment for, 484–485
    follow-up and rehabilitation of, 484
    in multiple trauma, 481
    treatment for, 480–484, 480t, 482f, 483f
  open, 495–504. *See also* Open fractures, of tibia
    and fibula.
  pathology of, 472–473, 473t
  proximal, 465
  vascular injury in, 507–508
Fibular growth plate injuries, 577–582
  angular deformity from, 577–580, 578f–582f
  avascular necrosis of, 582
  leg length discrepancy from, 580–582

Fibular growth plate injuries (*Continued*)
  nonunion or delayed union of, 582
  osteoarthritis from, 582
  rotational deformities from, 582
Field management, before transport, for multiple
  injuries, 81
Fifth metatarsal, 561–564, 563f
Finger
  anesthesia to, 612, 612f
  dislocation of, 248–250, 249f
Finger traps, in traction, 180, 181f
First metatarsal, 558–559, 559f
Fixation
  atlantoaxial rotary, 354f, 358–359
  external. *See* External fixation.
  for cubitus varus, after supracondylar fracture,
    278–279
  internal. *See* Internal fixation.
  of fractures, with soft tissue injuries, 116–121
  pin. *See* Pin fixation.
  plate. *See* Plate fixation.
  rod, of ipsilateral tibia and femur fractures, 491
    of tibial and fibular shaft fractures, 483–484
  screw. *See* Screw fixation.
Fixed forefoot, in tarsometatarsal injury, 556, 557f
Flagyl. *See* Metronidazole (Flagyl).
Flexion
  in cervical fractures and dislocations, 362
  in closed reduction, of extension-type supracondy-
    lar fracture, 268
  in forearm fractures, 172, 172f
  in olecranon fracture, 305–307, 312f, 313f
  in supracondylar fracture, 261, 280, 282f
  in thoracolumbar spine fractures, 364
Flexion distraction fracture, lumbar, 365
Floating elbow, 299, 305f, 306f
Floating knee, 133
Fluids, for circulation and resuscitation, 84, 84t
Flumazenil (Romazicon), for sedation, 614t, 615
Foot injuries, 537–577
  amputation for, 571–572
  anatomy of, 537–538, 539f
  aphorisms for, 583–584
  calcaneus in, 549–554. *See also* Calcaneal injuries.
  compartment syndrome in, 565–566
  cuboid fractures in, 556
  dislocations in, 565, 565f, 566f
  foot pain in, 574–577, 575f, 576f
  foreign bodies in, 572–574, 574f
  free tissue transfer for, 569–571, 570f–571f
  from lawn mowers, 566–569, 567f, 568f
  laceration, 572
  metatarsal fractures in, 557–564. *See also* Metatar-
    sal fractures.
  navicular bone in, 555–556, 555f
  osteochondroses and variants in, 539–540,
    540f–542f
  phalangeal fractures in, 564–565, 564f, 565f
  puncture, 572, 573f, 574f
  talus in, 542–549. *See also* Talar injuries.
  tarsometatarsal fractures in, 556–557, 557f
  to growth plates, 577–582. *See also* Growth plate
    injuries, of tibia and fibula.
  types of, 541, 542f
Foot pain, miscellaneous causes of, 574–577,
  575f, 576f
Forearm, in extension-type supracondylar
  fracture, 263
Forearm fractures, 166–234
  anatomy of, 167–171, 167f–171f
  Bier block for, 609, 609t, 610t
  classification of, 173, 177f–179f
  complications of, 184–195
    compartment syndrome in, 190–194, 193f, 194f
    infection in, 194
    malunion in, 185–190, 187f–189f
    nerve and vessel injuries in, 190
    nonunion in, 190
    overgrowth in, 195
    reflex sympathetic dystrophy in, 195
    refracture in, 190, 191f
    tendon entrapment in, 190, 192f
  deforming muscular forces in, 171–172, 172f
  diagnosis of, 173–175
  Galeazzi, 229–234. *See also* Galeazzi fracture(s).

Forearm fractures (*Continued*)
  growth plate injuries in, 195–199, 195f, 197f–200f
  ipsilateral, 214–215, 214f
  management of, 175–184, 179f
    closed reduction in, 180–183, 180f–182f
    surgical approaches to, 183–184, 184f–186f
    with complete displacement, 179–180
    with greenstick fractures, 178–179
    with plastic deformation, 177–178, 179f, 180f
    with undisplaced fractures, 177
  mechanism of injury in, 172–173, 172f
  Monteggia, 216–229. *See also* Monteggia fractures.
  of distal radius and ulna, 199–201, 201f, 202f
  of distal third of radius, 201–204, 203f, 204f
  of shafts of radius and ulna, 204–214
    classification of, 205
    complications of, 212, 213f
    diagnosis of, 205
    follow-up care and rehabilitation of, 212
    management of, 205–206, 206f, 207f
    surgical management of, 206–212, 208f–211f
  open, 215–216
  remodeling potential in, 173, 174f–176f
Forefoot, 538
Foreign body, in foot, 572–574, 574f
Fourth metatarsal, 561, 561f, 562f
Fracture(s)
  avulsion. *See* Avulsion fracture.
  bucket-handle, in child abuse, 594, 596f
  buckle, 11, 11f
    of distal radius and ulna, 200
    of forearm, 173, 177f
  chance's, 78
  chip, of navicular bone, 555–556, 556f
  classification of, 11–14, 11f–13f
  closed, of tibial and fibular shafts, 480
    with soft tissue injuries, 105, 106t
  comminuted. *See* Comminuted fracture.
  complete. *See* Complete fracture.
  complications of, 124–151
    compartment syndromes in, 126–128, 127f
    ectopic bone formation in, 129, 129f
    fat embolism in, 128
    growth disturbances in, 136–141
      partial growth arrest and, 138–141, 138f–141f
      physeal fractures and, 136–137, 137f, 138f
    hypercalcemia of immobilization in, 128–129
    injury to triradiate cartilage in, 134–135
    late angulation in, 134, 136f, 137f
    ligamentous instability in, 143–144, 144f
    malunion in, 130–133, 131f–134f
    nerve injuries in, 144–145, 145f
    nonunion in, 141–142, 142f, 143f
    overgrowth phenomenon in, 136
    reflex sympathetic dystrophy in, 145–146, 146t
    refracture in, 143
    spontaneous deep vein thrombosis in, 130
    superior mesenteric artery syndrome in, 130, 130f
    synostosis in, 134, 135f
    traction-induced hypertension in, 130
    vascular injuries in, 124–126, 125f
  compression. *See* Compression fracture.
  corner, in child abuse, 594, 595f, 596f
  from child abuse, 590–600. *See also* Child abuse, fracture patterns in.
  greenstick. *See* Greenstick fractures.
  hangman's, 359–362, 360f, 361f
  in child abuse, 589
  in multiple trauma, rehabilitation of, 619–622, 620t, 621f
  ipsilateral, of tibia and femur, 491, 492f–493f
    of upper extremity, 214–215, 214f
  isolated. *See* Isolated fractures.
  Jefferson, 359, 360f
  Jones, 562
  Monteggia, 216–229. *See also* Monteggia fractures.
  nondisplaced, of medial condyle of humerus, 294
    of third and fourth metatarsals, 561, 561f
  oblique, 12
    in child abuse, 591, 592f
    of tibial and fibular shafts, 480
  of acetabulum. *See* Acetabular fracture.
  of acromion, 330
  of atlas, 359, 360f

Fracture(s) (*Continued*)
  of axis, 359–362, 360f, 361f
  of C3-C7, 362–364, 363f
  of calcaneus, 549, 551–553, 551f, 555f
  of capitellum, 293, 295f
  of carpal bones, 240
  of clavicle, 322–326. *See also* Clavicle.
  of coracoid, 330–331, 331f
  of cuboid, 556
  of diaphysis. *See* Diaphyseal fractures.
  of distal femur, 439–449. *See also* Distal femoral fracture.
  of distal fibula, 534–536, 536f
  of distal humerus, 257–260, 258f–261f
    from child abuse, 594–596, 597f
  of distal phalanx, 244
    epiphyseal, 564, 565f
  of distal radius, 199–201, 201f, 202f
  of distal third of radius, 201–204, 203f, 204f
  of distal tibia. *See* Distal tibial fracture.
  of elbow, 257–321. *See also* Elbow.
  of epiphysis, 12–14, 13f
    management of, 93
  of epiphysis-metaphysis, from child abuse, 594, 595f–597f
  of femur. *See* Femoral fracture.
  of fibula, 472–515. *See also* Fibular fracture.
  of forearm, 166–234. *See also* Forearm fractures.
  of glenoid, 329–330, 330f
  of hand, 243–248, 243f. *See also* Hand injuries.
  of humerus. *See* Humeral fracture.
  of ischial tuberosity, 23, 27f
  of lateral epicondyle, 299
  of medial clavicle. *See* Medial clavicular fracture.
  of medial epicondyle, 297–299, 297t, 298f–303f
  of medial malleoli, 577, 578f
  of metaphysis, distal femoral, 439–449, 440–443, 440f, 441f, 444f. *See also* Distal femoral fracture.
    distal tibial, 494–495, 496f
    proximal tibial, 463–465, 464f
  of metatarsals, 557–564. *See also* Metatarsal fractures.
  of middle phalanx, 244, 245f
  of olecranon, 227, 305–307, 312f, 313f
  of patella, 451–452, 451f–453f
    osteochondral, 23, 28f
  of pelvis, 371–389. *See also* Pelvic fractures and dislocations.
  of phalanx. *See* Phalangeal fracture.
  of ribs, from child abuse, 598, 599f
    in multiple injured child, 77
  of scapula, 328–329, 329f
  of tarsometatarsals, 556–557, 557f
  of thoracolumbar spine, 364–368, 364f–367f
  of thumb, 247–248, 248f
  of tibia, 472–515. *See* Tibial fracture.
  of tibial spine, 452–455, 453f–456f
  of tibial tubercle, 455–459, 458f, 459f
  of Tillaux, 529–531, 530f–532f
  of triquetrum, 240–241, 241f, 242f
  of ulna. *See* Ulnar fracture.
  open. *See* Open fractures.
  osteochondral, of foot, 546–549, 547f, 548f, 550f
    of knee, 449–451, 450f
    of patella, 23, 28f
  outcomes assessment in, 153–165.
    *See also* Outcomes assessment.
  pathologic, 57–71. *See also* Pathologic fractures.
  spiral, 12
    in child abuse, 591, 592f
  stress. *See* Stress fractures.
  subtrochanteric, in osteopetrosis, 59, 59f, 60
  supracondylar, 260–263, 261f
    extension-type, 263–280. *See also* Extension-type supracondylar fracture.
    flexion-type, 280, 282f
  T-condylar, 299, 304f–306f
  transverse, 12, 12f
    in child abuse, 591, 592f
    of patella, 451
  unstable. *See* Unstable fractures.
  with soft tissue injuries, 104–123. *See also* Soft tissue injuries.
Fracture-dislocation, carpal, 239, 239f, 240f

Fracture healing. *See* Healing.
Fracture management, 91–96
  epiphyseal, 93
  open, 95–96
  surgical, 91, 93t
    principles of, 93–94
    techniques of, 94–95
  timing of, 92–93
Fracture-separation, of distal humeral physis, 280–285. *See also* Distal humeral physeal fracture-separation.
Free tissue transfer, for foot injuries, 569–571, 570f–571f
Freiberg's disease, 560, 560f
Functional Independence Measure for Children (WeeFIM), 156t
Fusion
  in distal tibial physis, 517, 519f
  of cervical fractures and dislocations, 363, 363f


                                    **G**

Gait aids, in rehabilitation, 620–622
Galeazzi fracture(s), 229–234
  classification of, 229–230, 232f–234f, 232t
  complications of, 233–234, 235f–236f
  diagnosis of, 233
  management of, 233
  mechanism of injury in, 230–232
Galeazzi fracture dislocation, 232
Gas gangrene, 107
Gastric distention, ventilation abnormalities in, 84
GCS. *See* Glasgow Coma Scale (GCS).
Genu recurvatum deformity, after proximal tibial physeal fracture, 506
Giant cell tumors, 57
Glasgow Coma Scale (GCS), 78, 80t
  in traumatic brain injury, 624
Glenohumeral joint dislocation, 331–334, 332f, 333f
Glenoid fracture, 329–330, 330f
Glycopyrrolate (Robinul), for sedation, 614t
Graft
  bone
    for bone union, 116, 116f
    for humeral fracture, 293, 294f
    for nonunion, 141–142, 142f, 143f
    for pathologic fracture, 65–66
  skin, for wound coverage, 113–115
Greenstick fractures, 11–12
  in multiple trauma, 74
  of distal radius and ulna, 200, 201f
  of forearm, 173, 178–179, 178f, 179f
  of proximal tibial metaphysis, 474
  of radial shaft, 205
  of tibial diaphysis, 485
  valgus, 463–465, 464f
Growth, in physical function scales, 162–163
Growth acceleration, after physeal injuries, 41–42
Growth and development. *See* Skeletal growth and development.
Growth arrest, 138–141, 138f–141f
  after physeal injury, 42–48
    complete, 21, 42–44, 44f
    partial, 21–22, 44–48, 45f–47f
Growth disturbance, 136–141
  after distal femoral physeal fracture, 447
  after epiphyseal injury, 14
  after femoral shaft fracture, 432
  after forearm fracture, 199, 200f
  after pelvic fracture, 373, 373f
  after physeal fracture, 136–137, 137f, 138f
  after triradiate cartilage injury, 134–135
  partial growth arrest and, 138–141, 138f–141f
Growth plate injuries
  of distal radius and ulna, 195–199, 195f, 197f–200f
  of metatarsals, 558
  of proximal phalanx, 564, 564f
  of tibia and fibula, 577–582
    angular deformity from, 577–580, 578f–582f
    avascular necrosis of, 582
    leg length discrepancy from, 580–582

Growth plate injuries (Continued)
  nonunion or delayed union of, 582
  osteoarthritis from, 582
  rotational deformities from, 582
Gunshot wounds
  of foot, 572–574, 574f
  to knee, 466
Gunstock deformity
  after supracondylar fracture, extension-type,
    278–280, 279f–281f
    management of, 264–265, 264f
  of humerus, 130, 131f


H


Halo application, for subluxation, of C1 on C2, 357
Hand injuries, 242–250
  dislocations in, 248–250, 249f, 250f
  fractures in, 243–248, 243f
    of distal phalanx, 244
    of metacarpals, 246–247
    of middle phalanx, 244, 245f
    of proximal phalanx, 244–246, 245f–247f
  incidence of, 242
  of thumb, 247–248, 248f
  treatment of, 242–243
Hangman's fracture, 359–362, 360f, 361f
Hard callus, in radiographic dating of injuries,
    590, 590t
Harris lines, 44
Head injuries
  secondary survey of, 86–87
  spinal injury and, 76–77
Healing, fracture, 4–11
  biology of, 4–6
  growth and, 3
  inflammatory phase of, 4–5
  pathologic, 58
  pediatric versus adult, 6–11, 7f
    anatomy in, 7, 8f, 9–10, 10f
    biomechanics in, 10–11, 11f
    remodeling in, 7–9, 8f, 9f
  remodeling phase of, 6
  reparative phase of, 5
Heat, in rehabilitation, 620
Heel pain, 550
Heel-to-toe compression, in tarsometatarsal injury,
    556, 557f
Hemarthrosis, in patellar dislocation, 467
Hematoma block, 608
  nitrous oxide and, 614
Hemorrhage, in primary survey, 84–85
  pelvic fractures with, 381
Henry approach, to decompression, of forearm,
    91, 91f
Hepatic injuries, 89
Heterotopic ossification, in traumatic brain
    injury, 625
Hindfoot, 538
Hip, range of motion of, 620t
Hip dislocations, 399–404
  complications of, 403–404
  diagnosis of, 401
  management of, 401–403
    results of, assessment of, 403
      expected, 403
  pathology of, 399–401
Hippocratic method, of reduction, of glenohumeral
    dislocation, 333, 333f
HIS. See Rand Health Insurance Study Scale (HIS).
Humeral fracture
  distal, 257–260, 258f–261f
    from child abuse, 594–596, 597f
  in battered child syndrome, 487–489
  of lateral condyle, 286–293. See also Lateral
    condyle of humerus fracture.
  of medial condyle, 293–297, 296f
  of shaft, 337–341, 338f–340f
    in child abuse, 592, 594, 594f
  proximal, 334–337, 334f, 335t, 336f, 337f–338f
  supracondylar
    arterial injuries in, 124, 125f

Humeral fracture (Continued)
  cubitus varus deformity after, 130, 131f
  peripheral nerve injury and, 622
  vascular injuries with, 126
Humeral physis
  distal, fracture-separation of, 280–285.
    See also Distal humeral physeal
    fracture-separation.
    injuries to, 40, 40f, 41f, 43f
  proximal, injuries to, 37–40, 39f
Humerus, anatomy of, 257–258
Humerus-elbow-wrist (HEW) angle, 280f–281f
Hypercalcemia, of immobilization, 128–129
Hyperextension injury, in supracondylar humeral
    fracture, 261, 262
Hyperparathyroidism, rickets of, 62t, 63–64, 63f
Hypertension, traction-induced, 130
Hypotension, orthostatic, in spinal cord injury, 624
Hypothermia, 75
  in primary survey, 85
Hypovolemia, 75


I


Iliac apophysitis, 50
Ilium, 371, 372f
ILs. See Interleukins (ILs).
Immediate spica casting, of femoral shaft fracture,
    412–414, 413f
Immobilization
  hypercalcemia of, 128–129
  of coracoid fracture, 330–331
  of distal clavicular fracture, 326
  of distal femoral fracture, 442
  of distal radius fracture, 202, 203f
  of elbow dislocation, 308
  of extension-type supracondylar fracture, 264
  of femoral physeal fracture, 136
  of forearm fracture, 166, 175, 179f, 180,
    181f, 182f
  of fracture-separation of distal humeral physis,
    285, 285f
  of glenoid fracture, 329
  of hand injuries, 242–243
  of hip dislocation, 403
  of humeral fracture, 288
  of isolated tibial shaft fracture, 486–487
  of juvenile fracture of Tillaux, 530
  of medial epicondylar fracture, 297
  of osteochondral fracture, 450
  of pelvic fractures and dislocations, 387–388
  of proximal femoral fractures, 397–398
  of proximal humeral fractures, 335–336
  of proximal radial fracture, 304–305
  of proximal tibial fracture, 477–478
  of proximal tibial physeal fracture, 462–463
  of scapulothoracic dissociation, 330
  of tibial and fibular shaft fractures, 481, 483,
    484–485
  of tibial spine fracture, 454
  of tibial tubercle fracture, 458
  of toddler's fracture, 487, 488f
Immunization, tetanus, 89, 89t, 106–107
Impact injury, to tarsometatarsals, 556, 557f
Implant removal
  in distal tibial fractures, 527
  in hip dislocations, 403
  in pelvic fractures and dislocations, 388
  in proximal femoral fractures, 398
Incomplete tension-compression fracture.
    See Greenstick fractures.
Index finger, dislocation of, 248–250, 249f
Indirect measures, of physical function, 155
Infection
  after distal femoral fracture fixation, 443
  after femoral shaft fracture, 432–433, 434f,
    435f
  after forearm fracture, 194
  after lawn mower injury, 566
  after open tibial and fibular fractures, 502
  after puncture trauma, 572
  clostridial, 106–107

Inflammatory phase, of fracture healing, 4–5
Insensitivity, to pain, congenital, 601
Interfragmentary screw fixation
  of distal tibial fractures, 527, 527f
  of juvenile fracture of Tillaux, 530, 532f
Interleukins (ILs), in fracture healing, 4
Internal fixation
  of capitellum fracture, 293, 295f
  of clavicular shaft fracture, 325
  of distal tibial fracture, 528
  of humeral lateral condyle fracture, 293
  of humeral shaft fracture, 341
  of ipsilateral tibia and femur fractures, 491
  of multiple injuries, 94–95
  of open forearm fracture, 215–216
  of open tibial and fibular fractures, 500
  of patellar fracture, 452, 453f
  of pelvic fracture, 386–387
  of proximal femoral fracture, 391–392, 393
  of proximal radial fracture, 303–304, 308f
  of tibial and fibular shaft fractures, 481,
    483–484, 483f
  of tibial spine fracture, 454, 456f
  open reduction and. See Open reduction and
    internal fixation (ORIF).
Interosseous membrane, of forearm, 169, 169f
Interosseous nerve, in forearm fractures,
    174–175, 190
Interphalangeal (IP) joint, in forearm fractures, 174
Interphalangeal (IP) joint dislocation, 248, 249f,
    565, 565f
Intervertebral disc calcification, in thoracolumbar
    trauma, 365
Intoxication, vitamin A, 601
Intra-abdominal injury
  in thoracolumbar spine fractures, 365
  pelvic fractures with, 381
Intra-articular fractures
  of calcaneus, 549, 551–553, 551f, 555f
  with soft tissue injuries, 121
Intramedullary fixation
  for tibial and fibular shaft fractures, 483–484
  of femoral fracture, 411, 411t, 412t
  of forearm fracture, 206–209, 208f, 209f
  of fractures, with soft tissue injuries, 117–118
  of ipsilateral tibial and femoral fractures, 491
Intravenous regional anesthesia, 608–610, 610t
Intravenous sedation, 614–615, 614t
Intubation, for resuscitation, 82–83
IP joint. See Interphalangeal (IP) joint.
Ipsilateral fractures
  of tibia and femur, 491, 492f–493f
  of upper extremity, 214–215, 214f
Irradiation, pathologic fracture healing and, 61
Irrigation, for fractures, with soft tissue injuries,
    108–109, 108f–114f
Ischial tuberosity fracture, 23, 27f
Ischium, 371, 372f
Iselin's disease, 562–563, 563f
Isolated fractures
  of diaphysis, in child abuse, 591
  of femur, 408–409
  of fibular diaphysis, 494, 495f
  of metatarsals, 558
  of second metatarsal, 559
  of tibial diaphysis, 485–487, 486f


J


Jefferson fracture, 359, 360f
Joint space, loss of, after acetabular fractures, 389
Jones fracture, 562
Juvenile fracture of Tillaux, 529–531, 530f–532f


K


Karnofsky Scale, 157t
Ketamine, for sedation, 614t, 615–616
Klein-Bell ADL Scale, 157t

Knee, 439–471
  dislocation of, 469
  distal femoral fractures of, 439–449. See also Distal
      femoral fracture.
  ligamentous instability of, 143, 144f
  open fractures of, 465–466
  osteochondral fractures of, 449–451, 450f
  patellar dislocation of, 466–468, 466f–468f
  patellar fractures of, 451–452, 451f–453f
  proximal fibular fractures of, 465
  proximal tibial fractures of, 459–465.
      See also Proximal tibial fracture.
  range of motion of, 620t
  tibial spine fracture of, 452–455, 453f–456f
  tibial tubercle fracture of, 455–459, 458f, 459f
Kocher approach, for humeral fracture, 291
Kocher-Langenbeck approach, for acetabular
    fractures, 387
Köhler's disease, navicular fracture versus, 555, 555f
K-wires, for ankle fractures, 523

L

Lacerations
  in child abuse, 589
  of foot, 572
Lap belt injuries
  cervical, 353
  in multiple injured child, 78
  thoracolumbar, 365
Late angulation, in fracture complications, 134,
    136f, 137f
Lateral condyle of humerus fracture, 286–293
  capitellum fractures and, 293, 295f
  classification of, 286–288, 287f–291f
  complications of, 293, 294f
  diagnosis of, 288
  incidence of, 286
  mechanism of injury in, 286, 286f
  treatment of, 288–293
      delayed open reduction in, 292–293, 292f
Lateral epicondyle fracture, 299
Lauge-Hansen classification, of ankle injuries, 520
Lawn mower injuries
  amputation and, 110, 115f
  calcaneal fractures from, 551, 553f
  open fractures in, 104–105
  to foot, 566–569, 567f, 568f
Leg length discrepancy
  after pelvic fractures, 389
  after tibial and fibular growth plate injuries,
      506–507, 580–582
Length discrepancy, malunion and, 133
Lesions, Monteggia, 216–217
Letournel and Judet classification, of pelvic fractures,
    374, 376f
Leukemia
  child abuse differentiated from, 601–602
  thoracolumbar spine fractures and, 364
Lidocaine (Xylocaine), 608t
  for axillary block, 610–612
  for Bier block, 609, 609t, 610t
  for hematoma block, 608
Ligamentous instability
  in cervical fractures, 363, 363f
  in fracture complications, 143–144, 144f
Ligaments, of ankle, 516, 518f
Limb salvage, in arterial injuries, 126
Liver, in abdominal trauma, 89
Lloyd-Roberts modification, Bell-Tawse annular
    ligament reconstruction with, 229
Local anesthesia, 607–608, 608t
  in axillary block, 610–612
  in wrist and digital blocks, 612
Long bone, growth of, 3
Lower extremity trauma, Mangled Extremity Severity
    Score for, 105, 105t
Lumbar flexion distraction fracture, 365
Lumbar spine
  anatomy of, 344
  anomalies of, 347
  fractures of, 364–368, 364f–367f

Lumbosacral plexopathy, pelvic fractures and, 622
Lytic cocktail, 607

M

Magnetic resonance imaging (MRI). See Radiographic
    evaluation.
Malalignment, of hand fractures, 243
Malleolar fracture, medial, 577, 578f
Malleoli, accessory ossicles of, 517
Malrotation, of tibial and fibular fractures, 505–506
Malunion, 130–133, 131f–134f
  of forearm fractures, 185–190, 187f–189f,
      198–199, 212
  of Galeazzi fracture, 233–234
  of Monteggia fracture, 229
Mangled Extremity Severity Score (MESS), 105, 105t
  amputation and, 111
Manipulation, for hand injuries, 242
Marble bone disease, 59, 59f, 60, 62t
Marcaine. See Bupivacaine (Marcaine).
MCA. See Motor Control Assessment (MCA).
Medial clavicular fracture, 322–326
  at birth, 324–325, 325f
  diagnosis of, 322–323, 323f, 324f
  in childhood, 325–326, 326f
  incidence of, 322
  mechanism of injury in, 322
  treatment of, 323–324
Medial condyle of humerus fracture, 293–297, 296f
Medial epicondylar apophysitis, 51, 52f
Medial epicondylar epiphyseal angle, 258, 260f
Medial epicondyle fracture, 297–299, 297t,
    298f–303f
Medial malleolar fracture, angular deformity from,
    577, 578f
Median nerve block, 612, 612f
Median nerve entrapment, after elbow disloca-
    tion, 145
Median nerve injury, in elbow dislocation, 309
Medullary nailing, for femoral shaft fractures,
    419–424, 422f–427f
  flexible technique of, 421–424, 425f–427f
  reamed, locked, antegrade technique of, 420–421,
      422f–424f
Membranous bone formation, 3, 4f
Meperidine (Demerol)
  for sedation, 614t, 615
  in lytic cocktail, 607
Mepivacaine (Carbocaine), 608t
MESS. See Mangled Extremity Severity Score (MESS).
Metabolic disease, foot fractures and, 575
Metabolic rate, 75
Metacarpals
  anesthesia to, 612, 612f
  fractures of, 246–247
Metacarpophalangeal (MP) joint dislocation,
    248, 249f
Metaphyseal fractures, distal femoral, 439–449.
    See also Distal femoral fracture.
  distal tibial, 494–495, 496f
  proximal tibial, 463–465, 464f
Metaphysis, 10
Metatarsal fractures, 557–564
  fifth, 561–564, 563f
  first, 558–559, 559f
  second, 559–561, 559f–561f
  third and fourth, 561, 561f, 562f
  treatment for, 558, 558f
Metatarsals, 537–538, 539f
Metatarsophalangeal dislocation, 565, 566f
Metronidazole (Flagyl), for gas gangrene, 107
Microtrauma, repetitive, apophyseal injury and, 49
Midazolam (Versed), for sedation, 614t, 615
Middle phalangeal fracture, 244, 245f
Midfoot, 538
Milch classification, of humeral fracture, 287, 287f,
    289f, 293f
Minerva jacket, for atlantoaxial rotary fixation, 359
Minidose technique, of intravenous regional
    anesthesia, 609–610, 610t
MISS. See Modified Injury Severity Scale (MISS).

Mobilization
  for hip dislocations, 403
  for pelvic fractures and dislocations, 388
  for proximal femoral fractures, 398
Modified Injury Severity Scale (MISS), for multiple
    injuries, 78–80, 79t, 80t
Monteggia fractures, 216–229
  classification of, 216–218, 216f–218f
  complications of, 228–229, 228f, 230f–231f
  diagnosis of, 219, 219f, 220f
  follow-up and rehabilitation of, 228
  management of, 219–228
      of Monteggia-equivalents, 225–228, 226f, 227f
      of type I, 219–223, 221f–224f
      of type II, 223
      of type III, 223–224
      of type IV, 224–225
  mechanism of injury in, 218–219
Monteggia lesions, 216–217
  malunion and, 131, 131f
Morphine, for sedation, 65, 614t
Motor Control Assessment (MCA), 156t
Motor vehicle accidents, mechanism of injury in,
    76, 76t
MP joint dislocation. See Metacarpophalangeal (MP)
    joint dislocation.
MRI (magnetic resonance imaging). See Radiographic
    evaluation.
Multiple injuries, 73–103
  anatomic differences in, 73–74, 74f
  biomechanical differences in, 74–75
  consequences of, 80–81
  femoral shaft fractures in, 429–432
  field management of, before transport, 81
  fracture management for, 91–96
      epiphyseal, 93
      open, 95–96
      surgical, 91, 93t
          principles of, 93–94
          techniques of, 94–95
      timing of, 92–93
  hip dislocations in, 402
  incidence of, 75
  injuries associated with, 76–78, 77f
  mechanism of, 75–76, 76t
  pathology of, 73
  pelvic fractures and dislocations in, 381–383,
      383f
  physiologic differences in, 75
  primary survey and resuscitation of, 82–85,
      83t, 84t
  proximal femoral fractures in, 392
  proximal tibial metaphysis fracture in, 477
  rehabilitation of, 96–97, 97t, 619–626
      brain injury in, 624–625
      fractures in, 619–622, 620t, 621f
      peripheral nerve injury in, 622–623
      psychosocial factors in, 625
      re-injury prevention in, 625
      spinal cord injury in, 623–624
  secondary survey of, 85–91
      abdominal injuries in, 88–89, 88t, 89t
      chest injuries in, 87–88
      extremity injuries in, 89–91, 89t, 90t, 91f, 92f
      head injuries in, 86–87
      spine and spinal cord injuries in, 87
      trauma radiographic series in, 85–86
  tibial and fibular shaft fractures in, 480–485, 480t,
      482f, 483f
  trauma centers for, 81–82, 82t
  trauma scoring systems for, 78–80, 79t, 80t
  trauma team for, 82
Musculoskeletal-related disorders, 61, 62t

N

Nail fixation
  of femoral fracture, 411, 411t, 412t
  of femoral shaft fracture, 419–424, 422f–427f
      flexible technique of, 421–424, 425f–427f
      reamed, locked, antegrade technique of,
          420–421, 422f–424f

Nail fixation (*Continued*)
    of forearm fracture, 206–208, 208f, 209f
    of fractures, with soft tissue injuries, 117–118
Naloxone (Narcan), for sedation, 614–615, 614t
Narcan. *See* Naloxone (Narcan).
Navicular bone injuries, 555–556, 555f
Neck, in Modified Injury Severity Scale, 79t
Necrosis
    aseptic, after femoral shaft fracture, 435, 436f
    avascular. *See* Avascular necrosis.
Neer-Horwitz classification, of proximal humeral
    fractures, 335, 335t
Neglect, child, 587–588
Neonates, spinal injury in, 351, 352f
Nerve conduction studies, in peripheral nerve
    injury, 623
Nerve entrapment, after elbow dislocation, 145
Nerve injuries
    from forearm fracture, 190
    from Monteggia fracture, 229, 230f–231f
    from supracondylar fracture, 262
    in fracture complications, 144–145, 145f
    in multiple trauma, 622–623
Nervous system trauma, in child abuse, 589
Nesacain. *See* Chloroprocaine (Nesacain).
Neurapraxia, 622
Neurofibromatosis, 60, 60f, 62t
Neurogenic bladder, in spinal cord injury, 624
Neurogenic bowel, in spinal cord injury, 624
Neurologic injury
    after dislocation of elbow joint, 309–312, 316f
    after extension-type supracondylar fracture,
        277–278
    from tibial and fibular fractures, 508
Neuromuscular disorders, tibial fractures in, 473–494
Neurotmesis, 622, 623
Nitrous oxide, for sedation, 613–614
Nondisplaced fractures
    of medial condyle of humerus, 294
    of third and fourth metatarsals, 561, 561f
Nonossifying fibroma, 67–68
Nonunion, 141–142, 142f, 143f
    of forearm fracture, 190, 212, 213f
    of lateral condyle of humerus fracture, 293, 294f
    of open tibial and fibular fractures, 503
    of proximal femoral fracture, 398, 399
    of tibial and fibular fractures, 505
    of tibial and fibular growth plate injuries, 582
Novocain. *See* Procaine (Novocain).
Nursemaid's elbow, 314
Nutritional rickets, 62t, 63–64, 63f


O

Objective outcome measures, 154
Oblique fractures, 12
    in child abuse, 591, 592f
    of tibial and fibular shafts, 480
Occiput-C1 injuries, 356–357, 356f
Occult fracture, of calcaneus, 549–550
Odontoid, 346
    fractures of, 360–361
    radiology of, 347, 348f
Ogden classification, of ankle injuries, 521
    of physeal injury, 23, 24f, 27f, 28f
OI. *See* Osteogenesis imperfecta (OI).
Olecranon
    anatomy of, 257–258
    fracture of, 227, 305–307, 312f, 313f
Olecranon apophysitis, 51
Open fractures
    infection of, 107–108
    management of, 95–96
    of clavicular shaft, 325
    of femur, 410
    of forearm, 215–216
    of humeral shaft, 341
    of knee, 465–466
    of phalanges, 564–565
    of tibia and fibula, 495–504
        assessment and classification of, 497
        follow-up care and rehabilitation of, 500

Open fractures (*Continued*)
        free tissue transfer for, 570
        treatment for, 497–500, 498f–499f
            authors' preferred method of, 504
            results of, 500–504, 501f, 502f
    with soft tissue injuries, 104–105, 105t
Open reduction
    of acetabular fracture, 387
    of ankle fracture, 524
    of capitellum fracture, 293, 295f
    of clavicular shaft fracture, 325
    of distal femoral physeal fracture, 445
    of distal tibial fracture, 527, 527f, 528f
    of forearm fracture, 183–184, 184f–186f
        rotation and, 170
    of fractures, in multiple trauma, 91, 93t
    of glenoid fracture, 329
    of hip dislocation, 402–403
    of lateral condyle of humerus fracture, delayed,
        292–293, 292f
    of medial clavicular fracture, 324
    of Monteggia fracture, 220–221, 222f
    of osteochondral knee fracture, 450
    of proximal femoral fracture, screw fixation and,
        394–395, 395f
        smooth pin fixation and, 392t, 393
    of proximal humeral fracture, 336
    of proximal radial fracture, 303–304, 308f
    of proximal tibial fracture, 478
    of proximal tibial physeal fracture, 461
    of talar neck fracture, 543
    of tibial and fibular shaft fractures, 481
    of tibial spine fracture, 454, 455f
    of triplane fracture, 533
    of valgus greenstick fracture, 463
Open reduction and internal fixation (ORIF)
    of acetabular fracture, 387
    of compartment syndrome, 566
    of distal femoral fracture, 443
    of distal femoral physeal fracture, 445–446
    of extension-type supracondylar fracture, 272,
        274f, 275f
    of forearm fracture, 206–212, 208f–211f
    of ipsilateral tibia and femur fractures, 491, 492f
    of multiple injuries, 94
    of pelvic fracture, 378, 382t
    of physeal injury, 32–33
    of proximal femoral fracture, 394, 394f, 396–397,
        397f
    of tibial and fibular shaft fractures, 483
    of tibial tubercle fracture, 458
OPG. *See* Osteoprotegerin (OPG).
ORIF. *See* Open reduction and internal
    fixation (ORIF).
Orthoses, for fracture rehabilitation, 620–622, 621f
Orthostatic hypotension, in spinal cord injury, 624
Os acromiale, 328, 328f
Os odontoideum, 361–362, 361f
Os peroneum, 540, 540f
Os trigonum, 540, 541f, 546
Os vesalianum, 540, 540f
    fracture of, 561, 563f
Osgood-Schlatter disease, 49
Ossification
    endochondral, 3
    heterotopic, in traumatic brain injury, 625
    in distal humeral fracture, 257, 258f
    of femur, 407, 439
    of forearm, 167, 167f
    of patella, 451
    of spine, 344, 345f, 346f
Osteoarthritis
    after hip dislocation, 403
    from tibial and fibular growth plate injuries, 582
Osteoblast, 57
Osteochondral fracture
    of foot, 546–549, 547f, 548f, 550f
    of knee, 449–451, 450f
    of patella, 23, 28f
Osteochondritis, of first metatarsal, 558–559
Osteochondritis dissecans, 546
Osteochondromatosis, 62t
Osteochondrosis
    in foot injuries, 539–540, 540f–542f
    of second metatarsal, 560, 560f

Osteoclasis, for malunion, of forearm fractures,
    186, 187f
Osteoclast, 57
Osteogenesis imperfecta (OI), 62–63, 62t, 63f
    child abuse differentiated from, 600–601
Osteology, of forearm, 167
Osteomyelitis
    after open tibial and fibular fractures, 503
    child abuse differentiated from, 601
Osteopenia
    in neuromuscular disorders, 492
    in spinal cord injury, 624
Osteopetrosis, 59, 59f, 60, 62t
Osteoporosis, in spinal cord injury, 624
Osteoprotegerin (OPG), 59–60
Osteosarcoma, 57, 58t, 62t
    surgical resection for, 68–69, 68f
Osteosynthesis, plate, for femoral fracture, 412t
Osteotomy
    after distal femoral physeal fracture, 448–449
    after proximal tibial physeal fracture, 463
    for cubitus varus, 131
        after supracondylar fracture, 278–280,
            279f, 280f
    for late angulation, 134
    for malunion, of forearm fractures, 186, 188f
    for valgus deformity, 475, 479
Outcomes assessment, 153–165
    approaches to, 153–155
    measures of, 155–162, 156t–161t
        methodologic difficulties of, 162–164
Overgrowth
    after femoral shaft fracture, 136, 432
    after forearm fracture, 195
Overhead skeletal traction, for extension-type
    supracondylar fracture, 267


P

Pain
    congenital insensitivity to, 601
    foot, miscellaneous causes of, 574–577, 575f,
        576f
    in extension-type supracondylar fracture, 263
Pain management, 606–617
    anesthetic techniques in, 607–613.
        *See also* Anesthetic techniques.
    background of, 606
    for fracture rehabilitation, 622
    for reflex sympathetic dystrophy, 576–577
    principles of, 606–607
    sedation in, 613–616, 613t, 614t
Parents, in child abuse, 588
Partial growth arrest, after physeal injury, 21–22,
    44–48, 45f–47f
    in fracture complications, 138–141, 138f–141f
Patella
    dislocation of, 466–468, 466f–468f
    fracture of, 451–452, 451f–453f
        osteochondral, 23, 28f
Pathologic fractures, 57–71
    bone tumors in, 57, 58t
    of foot, 575, 575f, 576f
    of thoracolumbar spine, 364, 365f
    of tibia, 494
    outcome triangle for, 58f, 59–70
        bone biology in, 59–61, 59f–61f
        function in, 69–70
        pathology in, 61–69, 62t, 63f, 65f–68f
        physiology of, 57–59
Paucilaceration injury, from lawn mower, 566,
    568f
PDGF. *See* Platelet-derived growth factor (PDGF).
Pearson attachment, for pelvic fractures, 385
PEDI. *See* Pediatric Evaluation of Disability
    Inventory (PEDI).
Pediatric Evaluation of Disability Inventory
    (PEDI), 159t
Pediatric Musculoskeletal Functional Health
    Questionnaire, 160t
Pediatric trauma centers, 81–82, 82t
Pediatric Trauma Score (PTS), 80, 80t

Pelvic fractures and dislocations, 371–389
  avulsion, 50–51, 50f
  complications of, 389
  diagnosis of, 374–378, 377f, 379f
  in multiple injured child, 77–78, 77f
  management of, 378–388
    bedrest/non–weight-bearing in, 383–384, 384f
    closed reduction in, 386
    evolution of, 378–381, 380f, 381f, 382t
    external fixation in, 385–386
    follow-up care in, 387–388
    for acetabular fractures, 387
    for polytrauma patients, 381–383, 383f
    internal fixation in, 386–387
    pelvic sling in, 385
    results of, assessment of, 388
      expected, 388–389
    skeletal traction in, 384–385
    spica cast in, 385
  pathology of, 371–374, 372f, 373f,
    375f–377f, 375t
  peripheral nerve injury and, 622
Pelvic girdle, in Modified Injury Severity Scale, 79t
Pelvic sling, for pelvic fracture, 378, 385
Penetrating trauma, to abdomen, 89
Penicillin, for infection, of open fractures, 107
Pennal-Tile classification, of pelvic fractures,
    374, 375f
Peptide signaling proteins, in inflammatory phase, of
    fracture healing, 4
Percutaneous pins
  for ankle fracture, 523
  for distal femoral fracture, 443, 444f
  for distal tibial fracture, 527
  for extension-type supracondylar fracture,
    268–272, 270f, 271f, 273f
  for proximal femoral fracture, 396
  for proximal humeral fracture, 335, 336f
  for triplane fracture, 533, 534f
Performance measures, of physical function, 155
Periarticular fracture, with soft tissue injuries, 121
Periosteal hinge, in reduction, of forearm fractures,
    171, 171f
Periosteal new bone formation
  in child abuse, 594
  in radiographic dating of injuries, 590, 590t
Periosteum, 9
  in forearm fractures, 171, 171f
Peripheral nerve injury, in multiple trauma, 622–623
Peritoneal lavage, for abdominal injuries, 88–89,
    88t, 89t
Peroneal nerve, 439
Pes anserinus, in proximal tibial osteotomy, 475
Peterson classification, of physeal fractures, 26, 28f
Pfannenstiel approach, to internal fixation, of pelvic
    fracture, 386
Phalangeal fracture, 564–565, 564f, 565f
  digital block for, 612, 612f
  distal, 244
  middle, 244, 245f
  proximal, 244–246, 245f–247f
Phalanx, 537–538, 539f
Phenergan. See Promethazine (Phenergan).
Phenytoin (Dilantin), rickets from, 575, 576f
Physeal fractures
  distal femoral, 443–449
    classification of, 444–445
    complications of, 447–449, 449f
    diagnosis of, 445
    management of, 445–447, 446f–448f
    mechanism of injury in, 443–444
  growth disturbances and, 136–137, 137f, 138f
  proximal tibial, 460–463, 461f, 462f
    closure of, 506
Physeal injuries, 17–56
  characteristics of, 35–41
    calcaneal physis in, 37, 38f
    distal femur in, 35
    distal humerus in, 40, 40f, 41f, 43f
    distal radius in, 40
    distal tibia in, 35–37, 37f, 38f
    distal ulna in, 40–41, 44f
    proximal femur in, 35, 36f
    proximal humerus in, 37–40, 39f
    proximal tibia in, 35, 37f

Physeal injuries *(Continued)*
  complications of, 41–52
    apophyseal injuries in, 48–52, 49f–52f
    growth acceleration in, 41–42
    growth arrest in, 42–48
      complete, 42–44, 44f
      partial, 44–48, 45f–47f
  diagnosis of, 26–31, 30f
    differential, 31, 32f
    radiographic evaluation in, 27–28, 31f
    special studies in, 28–31, 31f
  distal femoral, 439–449. See also Distal femoral
    fracture.
  fracture-separation of distal humerus in.
    See Distal humeral physeal
    fracture-separation.
  management of, 31–35, 34f
  mechanisms of, 19–26
    associated injuries in, 22–23, 22f
    classification in, 23–26, 24f–29f
    consequences in, 19–22, 20f, 21f
    pathology of, 17–19, 18f
Physical function scales, 155–162, 156t–161t
Physical interventions, for fracture rehabilita-
    tion, 620
Physical therapy
  for hip dislocations, 403
  for multiple injuries, 96–97
  for pelvic fractures and dislocations, 388
  for proximal femoral fractures, 398
Physis, 9–10
  distal humeral, fracture-separation of, 280–285.
    See also Distal humeral physeal
    fracture-separation.
  distal tibial, avascular necrosis of, 582
Pin fixation
  of carpometacarpal dislocation, 242
  of cervical fractures and dislocations, 363, 363f
  of cubitus varus, after supracondylar fracture,
    278–279
  of distal femoral fracture, 442–443
  of distal radius fracture, 204, 204f
  of extension-type supracondylar fracture, 265,
    266f
  of femoral fracture, 416–419, 417f–419f
  of femoral shaft fractures, 416
  of forearm fracture, 206–208, 208f, 209f
  of pelvic fracture, 385
  of proximal femoral fracture, 391–392
    closed reduction and, 392t, 393
  of proximal radial fracture, in open reduction,
    303–304, 308f
  percutaneous. See Percutaneous pins.
Pin tract infection
  after femoral shaft fractures, 432–433, 434f, 435f
  after open tibial and fibular fractures, 502
Pin traction
  for femoral fracture, 414–416, 415f
  for pelvic fractures, 384
  for proximal humeral fractures, 335
PIP joint. See Proximal interphalangeal (PIP) joint.
Plaster splints and casts
  for femoral shaft fractures, 416
  in rehabilitation, 620
Plastic deformation, 11
  in anterior dislocation of radial head, 225
  in forearm fractures, 177–178, 179f, 180f
    of radius and ulna, 173, 177f
  in multiple trauma, 74
  in radial shaft fracture, 205
Plate fixation
  of femoral shaft fracture, 424–429, 428f–432f
  of fractures, with soft tissue injuries, 117
  of hand fractures and dislocations, 243
  of Monteggia fracture, 220
Plate osteosynthesis, for femoral fracture, 412t
Platelet-derived growth factor (PDGF), in fracture
    healing, 4
Play Performance Scale, 159t
Pneumatic antishock garments, for pelvic
    fractures, 381
Pneumothorax, tension, ventilation abnormali-
    ties in, 84
Poland classification, of physeal injury, 24f
Polyostotic disease, 57

Polytrauma patients. See also Multiple injuries.
  hip dislocations in, 402
  pelvic fractures and dislocations in, 381–383, 383f
  proximal femoral fractures in, 392
Pontocaine. See Tetracaine (Pontocaine).
Popliteal artery, 439
POSNA Pediatric Musculoskeletal Functional Health
    Questionnaire, 160t
Posterior approach, to radius, in forearm fractures,
    183–184, 185f
Posterior interosseous nerve, in forearm fractures,
    174–175
Posterior talofibular ligament, 516, 518f
Posterior triceps-dividing approach, to open
    reduction, for extension-type supracondylar
    fracture, 272
Premature closure, of proximal femoral fracture,
    398, 399
Prevertebral soft tissue trauma, radiology of, 347–348
Primary hyperparathyroidism, rickets of, 62t,
    63–64, 63f
Primary survey, of multiple injuries, 82–85, 83t, 84t
Procaine (Novocain), 608t
Promethazine (Phenergan), in lytic cocktail, 607
Pronation, in forearm fractures, 172, 172f
Pronation-eversion–lateral rotation injury, of ankle,
    521t, 522f
Proximal femoral fracture, 389–399
  complications of, 399, 400f
  diagnosis of, 390–391
  from child abuse, 596–598, 598f
  management of, 391–398
    evolution of, 391–392
    follow-up care in, 397–398
    for polytrauma patients, 392
    for type I fractures, 392–393
    for type II fractures, 393–394, 394f
    for type III fractures, 394–395, 395f–397f
    for type IV fractures, 395–397, 397f
    results of, assessment of, 398, 398t
      expected, 398
  pathology of, 389–390, 391f
Proximal femoral physeal injuries, 35, 36f
Proximal fibular fracture, 465
Proximal humeral fracture, 334–337, 334f, 335t,
    336f–338f
Proximal humeral physeal injuries, 37–40, 39f
Proximal interphalangeal (PIP) joint, in forearm
    fractures, 174
Proximal phalangeal fracture, 244–246,
    245f–247f, 564
Proximal radial fracture, 299–305
  anatomy of, 301
  classification of, 302, 307t
  diagnosis of, 302–303
  incidence of, 299–301
  management of, 303–305, 308f–311f
  mechanism of injury in, 301–302, 307f
Proximal radioulnar joint complex, 167, 168f
Proximal tibial fracture, 459–465
  anatomy of, 459–460, 460f–462f
  metaphyseal, 463–465, 464f
  physeal, 460–463, 461f, 462f
Proximal tibial metaphyseal fracture, 474–480, 479f
  follow-up care and rehabilitation of, 478
  in multiple trauma, 477
  treatment for, authors' preferred method of,
    479–480, 479f
    current algorithm of, 477
    evolution of, 476–477
    options of, 477–478
    results of, 478
Proximal tibial physeal fracture, 506
Proximal tibial physeal injuries
  characteristics of, 35, 37f
  growth arrest and, 48
Pseudarthrosis, of tibia, from neurofibromatosis,
    60, 60f
Pseudoepiphysis, at distal end of metatarsal,
    540, 540f
Pseudosternoclavicular joint dislocation, 322–326
  at birth, 324–325, 325f
  diagnosis of, 322–323, 323f, 324f
  in childhood, 325–326, 326f
  incidence of, 322

Pseudosternoclavicular joint dislocation (Continued)
    mechanism of injury in, 322
    treatment of, 323–324
Pseudosubluxation, of cervical vertebrae,
    348–349, 348f
Psychologic rehabilitation, in multiple trauma,
    97, 97t
Psychosocial factors, in rehabilitation, of multiply
    injured child, 625
PTS. See Pediatric Trauma Score (PTS).
Pubis, 371, 372f
Pulled elbow, 314
Pulmonary management, for spinal cord injury, 624
Pulse
    in arterial injuries, 124–126, 125f
    in primary survey, 84, 84t
    in supracondylar humeral fractures, 275–277, 276f
Puncture wounds, of foot, 572, 573f, 574f

Q

Q angle, 466, 466f
Quality of Well-being, 158t
Questionnaires, in physical function scales, 163

R

Radial fracture
    distal, 199–201, 201f, 202f
    malunion of, 132, 132f
    of distal third, 201–204, 203f, 204f
    of shaft, 204–214
        classification of, 205
        complications of, 212, 213f
        diagnosis of, 205
        follow-up care and rehabilitation of, 212
        management of, 205–206, 206f, 207f
        surgical management of, 206–212, 208f–211f
    proximal, 299–305. See also Proximal radial
        fracture.
Radial head dislocation, 314, 317f
    anterior, 225–227
Radial head subluxation, 314–317
Radial neck fracture, 225, 226f
Radial pulse, in supracondylar humeral fractures,
    275–277, 276f
Radiation therapy, pathologic fracture healing and, 61
Radiographic evaluation
    of abdominal injuries, 88–89
    of ankle injuries, 519–520, 519f, 520f
    of atlantoaxial rotary fixation, 358, 359f
    of atlas fracture, 359
    of carpal bone fractures, 240
    of chest injuries, 87–88
    of child abuse, 589–590, 590t
    of distal femoral metaphyseal and physeal
        fractures, 440
    of distal femoral physeal fractures, 445
    of distal humeral fracture, 258–259, 259f–261f
    of distal radioulnar joint dislocation, 237
    of femoral shaft fractures, 409–410
    of fracture-separation of distal humeral physis,
        281–283
    of hangman's fracture, 360
    of head injuries, 86–87
    of hip dislocation, 401
    of humeral fracture, of medial condyle,
        296–297, 296f
    of knee dislocation, 469
    of medial clavicular fractures and pseudosterno-
        clavicular dislocations, 323, 323f, 324f
    of medial epicondylar fracture, 297, 298f
    of multiple injuries, 85–86
    of osteochondral fractures, of knee, 449–450
    of patellar dislocation, 467
    of patellar fractures, 452
    of pelvic fractures and dislocations, 376–378,
        377f, 379f
    of physeal injuries, 27–31, 31f

Radiographic evaluation (Continued)
    of proximal femoral fracture, 390
    of proximal radial fracture, 302–303
    of proximal tibial epiphyseal fractures, 460,
        461f, 462f
    of scapular fractures, 329, 329f
    of spinal cord injury, 354–355
    of spine, 347–350, 348f–350f
    of spine and spinal cord injuries, 187
    of stress fractures, of tibia and fibula, 490
    of tarsometatarsal injury, 556–557
    of thoracolumbar spine fractures, 365
    of tibial and fibular fractures, 474
    of tibial spine fractures, 454
    of tibial tubercle fractures, 457–458
    of toddler's fracture, 487
Radiotherapy, physeal damage from, 19
Radioulnar joint
    dislocation of, 235–239, 237f, 238f
    in forearm fractures, 167–169, 168f, 169f
Radius
    growth plate injuries to, 195–199, 195f,
        197f–200f
    in forearm anatomy, 167, 168f
    in forearm fractures, anterior approach to,
        183, 184f
        bayonet apposition of, 173, 176f
        plastic deformation of, 173, 177f
        posterior approach to, 183–184, 185f
    physeal injuries of, characteristics of, 40
        growth arrest and, 48
    rotation of, on ulna, 169–170, 170f
Rand Health Insurance Study Scale (HIS), 159t
Rang classification, of physeal injury, 24, 26f
Range of motion (ROM), in therapeutic exercise,
    619–620, 620t
Ratliff's classification, of treatment of hip fracture
    results, 398, 398f
Recurrent dislocation
    of elbow joint, 312–314
    of hip, 404
    of patella, 468
Recurvatum deformity, of tibia, after femoral
    fractures, 22
Reduction, anatomic
    of ankle fracture, 523
    of distal tibial fracture, 526–527
    of tarsometatarsal fracture, 557
    closed. See Closed reduction.
    loss of, after femoral shaft fracture, 432, 433f
    of ankle fracture, 523
    of distal radius fracture, 202, 203f, 204f
    of distal tibial fracture, 525
    of extension-type supracondylar fracture, 265
        skeletal traction and, 267
    of foot deformities, after fractures, 538
    of forearm fracture, 177
        Bier block for, 609, 609t, 610t
        periosteum and, 171, 171f
    of interosseous space, 170
    open. See Open reduction.
    sedation for, 614–615, 614t
Reflex sympathetic dystrophy (RSD)
    from forearm fracture, 195
    in foot injuries, 575–577
    in fracture complications, 145–146, 146t
Refracture, 143
    after distal femoral metaphyseal and physeal
        fracture, 443
    after femoral shaft fractures, 432–435,
        434f, 435f
    after forearm fracture, 190, 191f
Regional anesthesia, 607–608, 608t
    intravenous, 608–610, 610t
Rehabilitation, for multiple injuries, 96–97, 97t
Re-injury, prevention of, 625
Reliability, of physical function scales, 162
Remodeling, 7–9, 8f, 9f, 57
    in fracture healing, 5
    in radiographic dating of injuries, 590, 590t
    of extension-type supracondylar fracture, 265
    of femoral shaft fractures, 432
    of forearm fractures, 166, 173, 174f–176f
        of rotational malalignment, 171
    of humeral shaft fractures, 339–341

Reparative phase, of fracture healing, 5
Repetitive microtrauma, apophyseal injury and, 49
Resolution of soft tissues, in radiographic dating of
    injuries, 590, 590t
Respiration, in primary survey, 84, 84t
Responsiveness, of physical function scales, 162
Resuscitation, for multiple injuries, 82–85, 83t, 84t
Retropharyngeal spaces, radiology of, 347
Retrotracheal spaces, radiology of, 347
Rib fractures
    from child abuse, 598, 599f
    in multiple injured child, 77
Rib stabilization, in clavicular shaft fractures,
    325–326, 326f
Rickets, 62t, 63–64, 63f
    child abuse differentiated from, 601
Rigid fixation, of tibial and fibular shaft fractures, 481
Robinul. See Glycopyrrolate (Robinul).
Rod fixation
    of ipsilateral tibia and femur fractures, 491
    of tibial and fibular shaft fractures, 483–484
ROM. See Range of motion (ROM).
Romazicon. See Flumazenil (Romazicon).
Rotation
    after forearm fractures, 166
    forearm, 169–171, 170f
    traction in abduction and, 392t, 393
Rotational deformities, from tibial and fibular growth
    plate injuries, 582
RSD. See Reflex sympathetic dystrophy (RSD).

S

Sacrum, 371, 372f
Salter-Harris classification
    of ankle injuries, 521, 523
    of distal femoral physeal fractures, 445–447,
        447f, 448f
    of distal tibial epiphyseal fractures, 522f
    of distal tibial fractures, 524–529
        type I, 524–525, 525f
        type II, 525–526, 526f
        type III, 526–527, 526f
        type IV, 527–528, 527f–529f
        type V, 528–529, 530f
        type VI, 529
    of epiphyseal injuries, 13, 13f
    of forearm fractures, 196–198, 197f–199f
    of hand fractures, 244–246, 245f–247f
    of humeral lateral condyle fractures, 287
    of physeal injuries, 20–21, 21f, 23f–26f
    of proximal tibial physeal fractures, 461–462
    T-condylar fracture, 299, 304f–306f
Sarcoma, 57, 58t
    Ewing's, 62t
    surgical resection for, 68
Satisfaction, in outcome measures, 155
Scapula, 328–331, 328f–331f
Scapulothoracic dissociation, 329, 329f
Scheuermann's disease, atypical, 51, 51f
SCI. See Spinal cord injury (SCI).
Sciatic nerve injury, after hip dislocation, 403
SCIWORA. See Spinal cord injury without
    radiographic abnormality (SCIWORA).
Scoliosis, thoracolumbar spine fractures and,
    364, 365f
Screw fixation
    of acetabular fracture, 387
    of capitellum fracture, 293, 295f
    of cubitus varus, 279, 279f
    of distal tibial fracture, 527, 527f
    of extension-type supracondylar fracture,
        266–267, 267f
    of hand fractures and dislocations, 243
    of juvenile fracture of Tillaux, 530, 532f
    of Monteggia fracture, 220
    of pelvic fracture, 386–387
    of proximal femoral fracture, 394–395, 395f
    of tibial tubercle fracture, 458, 459f
Scuderia and Bronson classification, of triradiate
    cartilage fractures, 26, 29f
Scurvy, child abuse differentiated from, 602

Seat belt injuries
  cervical, 353
  in multiple injuries, 78
  thoracolumbar, 365
Second metatarsal, 559–561, 559f–561f
Secondary survey, of multiple injuries, 85–91,
    88t–90t, 91f, 92f
Sedation, 613–616, 613t, 614t
  principles of, 606–607
Sensory nerve action potential (SNAP), 623
Separation, of distal humeral physis, 280–285.
    See also Distal humeral physeal
    fracture-separation.
Sesamoids, 537–538, 539f
Sever's disease, 50, 539, 540f
Sexual abuse, 588
Shock, in primary survey, 84, 84t
Shoulder, 322–343
  acromioclavicular joint injury and, 326–328, 328f
  clavicle and, 322–326. See also Clavicle.
  girdle fractures of, from child abuse, 598–599
  glenohumeral joint dislocation and, 331–334,
    332f, 333f
  humeral shaft fractures and, 337–341, 338f–340f
  proximal humeral fractures and, 334–337, 334f,
    335t, 336f–338f
  range of motion of, 620t
  scapula and, 328–331, 328f–331f
Shredding injury, from lawn mower, 566, 567f
Sidearm traction, for extension-type supracondylar
    fracture, 266–267
Sinding-Larsen-Johansson syndrome, 49
Skeletal growth and development, 1–15
  bone formation in, 3, 4f
  fractures and, classification of, 11–14, 11f,
    12f, 13f
  healing of, 4–11. See also Healing.
  in history and diagnosis, 1–3, 2f
Skeletal traction
  for acetabular fractures, 387
  for distal femoral metaphyseal and physeal
    fractures, 440
  for extension-type supracondylar fracture,
    266–267, 267f
  for femoral fracture, 412t
  for femoral shaft fractures, 414–416, 415f
  for metatarsal fractures, 558, 558f
  for pelvic fractures, 384–385
  for proximal femoral fractures, 395–396
  for proximal humeral fractures, 336–337
Skin, in spinal cord injury, 624
Skin graft, for wound coverage, 113–115
Skin traction
  for extension-type supracondylar fracture,
    265–266
  for femoral shaft fractures, 412
Skull, spine and, 345
  radiology of, 347
Skull fractures, from child abuse, 600
Sling
  for coracoid fractures, 330–331
  for distal clavicular fractures, 326
  for glenoid fractures, 329
  for pelvic fractures, 378, 385
  for scapulothoracic dissociation, 330
SNAP. See Sensory nerve action potential (SNAP).
Social history, in child abuse, 588
Soft callus, in radiographic dating of injuries,
    590, 590t
Soft tissue injuries
  fractures with, 104–123
    amputation and, 110–113, 115f
    antimicrobials for, 107–108
    bone union of, 116, 116f–120f
    characteristics of, 104
    classifications of, 104–105, 105t, 106t
    clostridial infections in, 106–107
    fixation of, 116–121
    initial care of, 106
    wound care for, 108–110, 108f–114f
    wound contamination in, 106
    wound coverage and, 113–115
  physical examination of, in child abuse, 589
Soft tissue reconstruction, of distal radioulnar joint
    dislocation, 238–239

Soft tissues, resolution of, in radiographic dating of
    injuries, 590, 590t
Somatosensory evoked potential (SSEP), in spinal
    trauma, 354
Spasticity, therapeutic exercise for, 619–620
Spica cast
  for femoral fractures, 411, 411t, 412t
  for femoral physeal fractures, 136
  for femoral shaft fractures, 412–414, 413f
  for pelvic fractures, 378, 385
  for proximal femoral fractures, 391
    type I, 392–393, 392t
    type II, 393
    type III, 394
    type IV, 396
Spinal blockade, for reflex sympathetic dystrophy,
    576–577
Spinal cord injury (SCI), 351–356
  characteristics of, 353–355, 354f
  in multiple trauma, rehabilitation of, 623–624
    secondary survey of, 87
  SCIWORA in, 351–353, 353f
  syndromes of, 355–356
Spinal cord injury without radiographic abnormality
    (SCIWORA), 351–353, 353f
  rehabilitation for, 623–624
Spinal cord syndromes, 355–356
Spine, 344–370
  anatomy of, 344–347, 345f, 346f
  anomalies of, 347
  injury to, in multiple trauma, 76–77
  radiology of, 347–350, 348f–350f
  trauma to, cervical, 356–364. See also Cervical
    spine injuries.
    from child abuse, 599–600
    in neonates, 351, 352f
    incidence of, 350–351
    secondary survey of, 87
    spinal cord injury and, 351–356
      See also Spinal cord injury (SCI).
    thoracolumbar, 364–368, 364f–367f
Spinous process, 346
Spiral fracture, 12
  in child abuse, 591, 592f
Spleen, in abdominal trauma, 89
Splints
  for femoral fracture, 411, 411t
  for forearm fractures, 175, 179f
  for open tibial and fibular fractures, 497
  for pelvic fractures, 385
  for triquetrum fractures, 240
  in rehabilitation, 620
Split-thickness skin graft, for wound coverage,
    113–115
Spontaneous deep vein thrombosis, 130
SSEP. See Somatosensory evoked potential (SSEP).
Stable diaphyseal fractures, 121
Steinmann pins
  for ankle fractures, 523
  for distal tibial fractures, 527
  for extension-type supracondylar fracture, 266
  for open tibial and fibular fractures, 503
  for pelvic fractures, 384
  for proximal femoral fractures, 392, 392t
  for proximal tibial fracture, 479
  for triplane fracture, 533, 534f
Stimson method, of reduction, for glenohumeral
    dislocation, 333, 333f
Strengthening exercise, 620
Stress, physiologic, 75
Stress fractures
  of calcaneus, 549–550
  of femur, 408
  of foot, 575
  of patella, 451
  of second metatarsal, 559, 559f, 560f
  of tibia, 490–491
Subjective outcome measures, 154
Sublimaze. See Fentanyl (Sublimaze).
Subluxation
  of C1 on C2, 357–358
  patellar, 468, 468f
  radial head, 314–317
Subtrochanteric fracture, in osteopetrosis, 59, 59f, 60
Superior mesenteric artery syndrome, 130, 130f

Supination, in forearm fractures, 172, 172f
Supination-inversion injury, of ankle, 521t, 522f
Supination–lateral rotation injury, of ankle, 521t
Supination–plantar flexion injury, of ankle,
    521t, 522f
Supracondylar fracture, 260–263, 261f
  anterior interosseous nerve palsy from, 144, 145f
  extension-type, 263–280. See also Extension-type
    supracondylar fracture.
  flexion-type, 280, 282f
  of femur, 124, 125f
  of humerus, arterial injuries in, 125f, 126
    cubitus varus deformity after, 130, 131f
    peripheral nerve injury and, 622
    vascular injuries with, 126
Synostosis, 134, 135f
  of forearm fractures, 212
Syphilis, congenital, child abuse differentiated from,
    601, 602f
Systemic antibiotics, 107–108
Systolic blood pressure, in primary survey, 84, 84t


                        T

Talar injuries, 542–549, 543f, 544f
  complications of, 546
  os trigonum in, 546
  osteochondral fractures in, 546–549, 547f,
    548f, 550f
  types of, 542–546, 545f
Talofibular ligament, 516, 518f
Talus
  anatomy of, 516, 517f
  osteochondritis dissecans of, 546–549, 547f,
    548f, 550f
TAMP. See Tufts Assessment of Motor Performance
    (TAMP).
Tarsometatarsal fracture, 556–557, 557f
TBBD. See Temporary brittle bone disease (TBBD).
TBI. See Traumatic brain injury (TBI).
Technetium bone scans, of tibial and fibular fractures,
    474, 490
Temporary brittle bone disease (TBBD), 600–601
Tendon entrapment, from forearm fracture, 190, 192f
Tension-compression, in multiple trauma, 74
Tension pneumothorax, ventilation abnormali-
    ties in, 84
Tetanus, 89, 89t, 106–107
Tetracaine (Pontocaine), 608t
TGF-β. See Transforming growth factor β (TGF-β).
Therapeutic exercise, for fracture rehabilitation,
    619–620, 620t
Third metatarsal, 561, 561f, 562f
Thomas splint, for pelvic fractures, 385
Thompson approach, to radius, in forearm fractures,
    183–184, 185f
Thoracic spine, anatomy of, 344
Thoracolumbar spine
  anomalies of, 347
  fractures of, 364–368, 364f–367f
Thoracotomy, for clavicular shaft fractures,
    325–326, 326f
Three-point fixation, of forearm fractures, 171, 171f
Thumb
  dislocation of, 250, 250f
  fractures of, 247–248, 248f
Thurston-Holland sign, in physeal fractures, 23, 27
Tibia
  anatomy of, 516, 517f
  avascular necrosis of, 582
  growth disturbances and, 137, 137f, 138f
  physeal injuries of, characteristics of, 35–37,
    37f, 38f
    growth arrest and, 48
  pseudarthrosis of, from neurofibromatosis,
    60, 60f
  recurvatum deformity of, after femoral fractures, 22
Tibial fracture, 472–515
  angular deformity from, 505
  compartment syndrome in, 508–510
  delayed union of, 504–505
  diagnosis of, 473–474

Tibial fracture (Continued)
  free tissue transfer for, 570
  from bicycle spokes, 489, 489f
  in battered child syndrome, 487–489
  in bicycle spoke injuries, 489–490, 489f
  in neuromuscular disorders, 492–494
  in toddlers, 487, 488f
  ipsilateral, 491, 492f–493f
  lower extremity length inequality from, 506–507
  malrotation of, 505–506
  neurologic injury in, 508
  nonunion of, 505
  of diaphysis, 485–487, 486f
  of distal metaphysis, 494–495, 496f
  of metaphysis and diaphysis, valgus after, 22
  of proximal metaphysis, 474–480, 479f
    follow-up care and rehabilitation of, 478
    in multiple trauma, 477
    treatment for, algorithm for, 477
      authors' preferred, 479–480, 479f
      evolution of, 476–477
      options of, 477–478
      results of, 478
  of proximal physis, closure of, 506
  of shaft, 480–485
    etiology of, 593, 593f
    follow-up and rehabilitation of, 484
    in multiple trauma, 481
    treatment for, authors' preferred, 484–485
      current algorithm of, 480
      evolution of, 480, 480t
      options of, 481–484, 482f, 483f
      results of, 484
  of spine, 452–455, 453f–456f
  of tubercle, 455–459, 458f, 459f
  open, 495–504. See also Open fractures, of tibia
    and fibula.
  pathologic, 494
  pathology of, 472–473, 473t
  stress, 490–491
  vascular injury in, 507–508
Tibial growth plate injuries, 577–582
  angular deformity from, 577–580, 578f–582f
  avascular necrosis of, 582
  leg length discrepancy from, 580–582
  nonunion or delayed union of, 582
  osteoarthritis from, 582
  rotational deformities from, 582
Tibial nerve, 439
Tibial valgus, after tibial fractures, 22
Tibiofibular syndesmosis, 516–517, 518f
Tile's classification, of pelvic fractures, 374, 375t
Tillaux injury, 521t, 529–531, 530f–532f
Toddler's fracture, 487, 488f, 593, 593f
Tornadoes, open fractures from, 104–105
Torsion
  in isolated tibial fractures, 485
  in osteochondral fractures, 546
Torus. See Compression.
Total blood volume, 75
Traction
  for acetabular fractures, 387
  for atlantoaxial rotary fixation, 359
  for distal femoral metaphyseal and physeal
    fractures, 440–442, 440f, 441f
  for distal radial fractures, 202, 203f
  for elbow dislocation, 307–308
  for extension-type supracondylar fracture,
    265–266, 266f–267f, 267f
  for femoral shaft fractures, 412, 414–416, 415f
  for forearm fractures, 180, 181f, 182f
  for pelvic fractures, 384–385
  for proximal femoral fractures, 392t, 393–396
  for proximal humeral fractures, 335
  for supracondylar humeral fractures, 277
Traction apophysitis, 49
  of fifth metatarsal, 562–563, 563f
Traction-induced hypertension, 130
Transarterial method, of axillary block,
  610–611, 611f
Transforming growth factor β (TGF-β), in fracture
  healing, 4
Transition fractures, of ankle, 529–534
  juvenile fracture of Tillaux in, 529–531, 530f–532f
  triplane fracture in, 531–534, 533f, 534f

Transport, field management before, for multiple
  injuries, 81
Transverse fracture, 12, 12f
  in child abuse, 591, 592f
  of patella, 451
Transverse ligament, of spine, 345–346
Trauma, growth and development related to, 1–15.
  See also Skeletal growth and development.
Trauma centers, pediatric, 81–82, 82t
Trauma scoring systems, 78–80, 79t, 80t
Trauma team, 82
Traumatic arterial spasm, after tibial and fibular
  fractures, 508
Traumatic brain injury (TBI), in multiple trauma,
  rehabilitation of, 624–625
Triangular fibrocartilage complex (TFCC), in forearm
  fractures, 167–168, 169f
Triplane injury, of ankle, 521t, 522f, 531–534,
  533f, 534f
Triquetrum, fractures of, 240–241, 241f, 242f
Triradiate cartilage injury
  in fracture complications, 134–135
  Scuderia and Bronson classification of, 26, 29f
Trochlea, ossification of, 257
Trochlear groove, in humeral fracture, 287, 287f, 289f
Tufts Assessment of Motor Performance (TAMP), 156t
Tumors, bone, 57–58, 58t
Two-pin traction, for distal femoral fractures, 441


U

UBCs. See Unicameral bone cysts (UBCs).
Ulna
  anatomy of, 257–258
  bayonet apposition of, in forearm fractures,
    173, 176f
  distal physeal injuries of, 40–41, 44f
  growth plate injuries to, 195–199, 195f, 197f–200f
  in forearm anatomy, 167, 168f
  plastic deformation of, after anterior dislocation
    of radial head, 225
  in forearm fractures, 173, 177f
  rotation of radius on, 169–170, 170f
  surgical approach to, in forearm fractures,
    184, 186f
Ulnar bow line, 219, 219f
Ulnar fracture, 199–201, 201f, 202f
  malunion of, 132, 132f
  Monteggia lesion and, 131, 131f
  of diaphysis, 227
  of metaphysis, 225–227
  of shaft, 204–214, 225, 226f
    classification of, 205
    complications of, 212, 213f
    diagnosis of, 205
    follow-up care and rehabilitation of, 212
    management of, 205–206, 206f, 207f
    surgical management of, 206–212, 208f–211f
Ulnar ligament, in medial epicondylar fracture,
  297–298, 299f
Ulnar nerve, in medial epicondylar fracture, 299
Ulnar nerve block, 612, 612f
Ulnar nerve entrapment, after elbow dislocation, 145
Ulnar nerve injury, in elbow dislocation, 309
  in supracondylar fracture of humerus, 622
Ultrasound. See Radiographic evaluation.
Undisplaced fractures, of forearm, growth plate
  injuries and, 196
  management of, 177
Unicameral bone cysts (UBCs), 57, 64, 65f
Union. See also Malunion; Nonunion.
  cross, 134, 135f
    of forearm fracture, 212
  delayed. See Delayed union.
  of fractures, with soft tissue injuries, 116,
    116f–120f
Unstable fractures
  of diaphysis, 121
  of tibial and fibular shaft, 480
    management of, 481, 485

V

Valgus angulation, 134
Valgus deformity
  after distal femoral fracture, 443
  after proximal tibial fracture, 475, 479
  after tibial metaphyseal and diaphyseal
    fractures, 22
Valgus greenstick fracture, 463–465, 464f
Valgus instability, in medial epicondylar fracture,
  297–298, 299f
Valgus osteotomy, for cubitus varus, 278
Validity, of physical function scales, 162
Valium. See Diazepam (Valium).
Varus deformity, 134
  after distal femoral fracture, 443
  from adduction injury, 577
Varus-valgus angulation, 259–260
Vascular anatomy, in distal humeral fracture,
  257, 258f
Vascular compromise
  after elbow dislocation, 309
  after extension-type supracondylar fracture,
    275–277, 276f
Vascular injuries
  from tibial and fibular fractures, 507–508
  in fracture complications, 124–126, 125f
  to extremities, 90
  with supracondylar fracture, 262
Ventilation abnormalities, life-threatening, 84
Versed. See Midazolam (Versed).
Vertebrae, anatomy of, 344, 345f, 346f
Vertebral apophysitis, 51, 51f
Vessel injuries, from forearm fracture, 190
Vineland Adaptive Behavioral Scales, 158t
Vitamin A intoxication, child abuse differentiated
  from, 601
Volar splint, for triquetrum fractures, 240
Volkmann's ischemia
  from supracondylar humeral fractures, 277
  in compartment syndromes, 126–127, 127f


W

Waddell's triad, 76
Wallerian degeneration, in peripheral nerve
  injury, 623
Watson-Jones classification, of tibial tubercle
  fractures, 457
Watts classification, of pelvic fractures, 374
Wedge osteotomy, for cubitus varus, 278–280,
  279f, 280f
WeeFIM. See Functional Independence Measure
  for Children (WeeFIM).
Wires
  for ankle fractures, 523
  for type II extension-type supracondylar
    fracture, 265
Wound care, for fractures, with soft tissue injuries,
  108–110, 108f–114f
Wound contamination, in fractures, with soft tissue
  injuries, 106
Wound coverage, for fractures, with soft tissue
  injuries, 113–115
Wrist, range of motion of, 620t
Wrist block, 612, 612f
Wrist injuries, 235–242
  carpal bone fractures in, 240
  carpal fracture-dislocations in, 239, 239f, 240f
  carpometacarpal dislocations in, 241–242
  dislocation of distal radioulnar joint in, 235–239,
    237f, 238f
  fractures of triquetrum in, 240–241, 241f, 242f


X

Xylocaine. See Lidocaine (Xylocaine).